Leddy & Pepper's

Professional Nursing

TENTH EDITION

Leddy & Pepper's

Professional Nursing

TENTH EDITION

Lucy Jane Hood, RN, PhD

Professor Emeritus
Saint Luke's College of Health Sciences at Rockhurst
University
Kansas City, Missouri

Wolters Kluwer

Philadelphia • Baltimore • New York • London
Buenos Aires • Hong Kong • Sydney • Tokyo

Not authorised for sale in United States, Canada, Australia, New Zealand, Puerto Rico, and U.S. Virgin Islands.

Director of Nursing Education and Practice Content: Jamie Blum
Acquisitions Editor: Michael Kerns and Susan Hartman
Supervisory Development Editor: Staci Wolfson
Editorial Coordinator: Anju Radhakrishnan
Editorial Assistant: Molly Kennedy
Senior Production Project Manager: Alicia Jackson
Manager, Graphic Arts & Design: Stephen Druding
Art Director: Jennifer Clements
Senior Manufacturing Coordinator: Margie Orzech
Marketing Manager: Brittany Riney
Prepress Vendor: S4Carlisle Publishing Services

10th edition

Library of Congress Cataloging-in-Publication Data

Names: Hood, Lucy Jane, author.
Title: Leddy & Pepper's professional nursing/Lucy Jane Hood.
Other titles: Leddy & Pepper's conceptual bases of professional nursing |
    Leddy and Pepper's professional nursing
Description: Tenth edition. | Philadelphia : Wolters Kluwer Health, 2022. |
    Includes bibliographical references and index.
Identifiers: LCCN 2021026545 | ISBN 9781975172626 (paperback)
Subjects: MESH: Nursing Theory | Nurse's Role | Nursing—trends | BISAC:
    MEDICAL/Nursing/Social, Ethical & Legal Issues
Classification: LCC RT82 | NLM WY 86 | DDC 610.7306/9—dc23
LC record available at https://lccn.loc.gov/2021026545

CCS0821

To all professional nurses and nursing students who have a passion for nursing that enables them to share their values, beliefs, and skills to make differences in the lives of others and to shape the nursing profession. To all professional nurses who risk their own lives to care for persons during the COVID-19 pandemic, you make me proud to be a member of this wonderful profession. To Dr. Susan Leddy and Dr. Mae Pepper, who saw the need for a textbook to meet the needs of registered nurses who returned to school to complete nursing degrees. To all the readers of this text who have the courage to take the risk of returning to school or pursuing a professional nursing career. To the following persons whose actions, values, and beliefs enabled me to live out my dream of being a professional nurse: my parents, Bob and Helen Chamberlin; Mary Belle Hickey, RN, my first nurse manager, who always challenged me to be the best possible nurse and gave me the confidence to pursue higher education; my dear mentor, Dr. Susan Leddy, professor of nursing, who showed me the essence of nursing scholarship; and my loving husband, Michael, who selflessly gives me the time, support, and humor to live out my dreams.

Lucy Jane Hood

In Memory

J. Mae Pepper

January 18, 1936–March 19, 1997

For 20 years, Mae was Susan Leddy's colleague, coauthor, mentor, and friend. In 1977, Mae joined the faculty at Mercy College in Dobbs Ferry, New York. Mae's previous teaching experience at the University of North Carolina-Chapel Hill, New York University, and Bronx Community College, as well as her vision, wisdom, and dedication, was crucial to the development and accreditation of the new baccalaureate program for registered nurses and to the subsequent development of the first master's program at the college.

Mae held the position of chairperson of the nursing program from 1981 until her sudden death in March 1997. She was devoted to the students and faculty, and very conscientious in her service to the College and many civic and professional organizations.

Mae found time to read voraciously, listen to music, care for animals, and enjoy outdoor white water rafting, camping, and bird watching. She loved her garden, was a careful craftsperson in her furniture refinishing, and liked to go to garage sales and flea markets looking for collectibles. Mae had a good sense of humor and loved a good time. Devoted to her friends and family, she willingly gave time and attention to anyone who asked. She was a great listener, and her counsel was always wise and kind. Mae lived her belief in mutuality, genuineness, and respect for others.

Susan Kun Leddy

February 23, 1939–February 23, 2007

For 14 years, Susan was my mentor and friend. We met in 1993 when I became a doctoral student at Widener University. Susan had a long distinguished career in nursing education. She set high academic standards for herself and also expected her students to attain them.

Susan taught in all levels of nursing education. She and three other faculties founded the RN-BSN program at Pace University. Along with Mae Pepper, Susan opened the first RN-BSN program at Mercy College in 1977. The two of them realized the need for a textbook to meet the needs of registered nurses returning to school for BSN education and cowrote *Conceptual Bases for Nursing Practice* that was first published in 1981. Susan served as the first dean of the School of Nursing at the University of Wyoming in 1981 and was later promoted to the dean of the College of Health Sciences. In 1988, she returned to the East Coast where she served as the dean of the School of Nursing at Widener University until 1993 when she gave up her administrative responsibilities to teach in the doctoral program.

Susan was a prolific scholar and has many journal publications. In addition to previous editions of this text, she authored *Integrative Health Promotion: Conceptual Bases for Nursing Practice* and *Health Promotion: Mobilizing Strengths to Enhance Health, Wellness & Well-Being*. Both of these books received Book of the Year Awards from the *American Journal of Nursing*.

Susan made time to travel and visited nearly every place in the world. She found her trips exhilarating and stimulating. She incorporated many of the ideas from her travels into her Human Energy Model. Susan also enjoyed quilting, weaving, and dabbling in watercolors. She was very energetic and always had a project to accomplish.

Susan deeply loved her daughters, Deborah and Erin. She adored her granddaughter, Katie, who always got her to laugh and smile even through some very rough times.

Susan exemplified the life of a true scholar, superb teacher, and devoted mother. It is my hope to live up to the standards of my beloved mentor and friend. I miss her great words of wisdom and support.

Reviewers

Elizabeth W. Black, MSN, RN
Assistant Professor
Gwynedd Mercy University
Gwynedd Valley, Pennsylvania

Billie Blake, RN, MSN, BSN, EdD, CNE
(Retired) Associate Dean of Nursing
St. Johns River State College
Orange Park, Florida

Laura Blank, RN, MSN
Associate Clinical Professor
Northern Arizona University
Flagstaff, Arizona

Annie Boucher, RN, MScN
Professor
Cambrian College
Sudbury, Canada

Mary Boylston, EdD, MSN, BSN, AHN-BC
Assistant Professor
Eastern University
St. Davids, Pennsylvania

Beryl K. Broughton, MSN, CRNP, CS, CNE
Nursing Faculty
ARIA Health School of Nursing
Trevose, Pennsylvania

Jennifer Bryer, PhD
Acting Assistant Dean, Chairperson, Associate Professor
Farmingdale State College
Farmingdale, New York

Kathy Burlingame, EdD, MSN, RN
Dean of Nursing
Galen College of Nursing
Louisville, Kentucky

Paula Byrne, DNP, RN
Assistant Professor and Chair
The College of St. Scholastica
Duluth, Minnesota

Ruth Chaplen, DNP, MSN, BSN
Associate Professor
Rochester College
Rochester Hills, Michigan

Betty Daniels, PhD, RN
Assistant Professor
Brenau University
Gainesville, Georgia

Karen Davis, DNP, RN, CNE
Clinical Assistant Professor
University of Arkansas for Medical Sciences
Little Rock, Arkansas

Lori A. Edwards, DrPH, MPH, RN, PHCNS-BC
Assistant Professor, Associate Director for Global
    Occupational Health
University of Maryland
Baltimore, Maryland

Marcus M. Gaut, DNP, RN
Assistant Professor
The University of Southern Mississippi
Hattiesburg, Mississippi

Evalyn J. Gossett, MSN, RN
Lecturer
Indiana University Northwest
Gary, Indiana

Debra Kantor, PhD, RN
Associate Professor
Molloy College
Rockville Centre, New York

Coleen Kumar, PhD, RN
Dean of Nursing
SUNY Downtown Medical Centre College of
    Nursing
Brooklyn, New York

Kathleen M. Lamaute, EdD, MS, FNP-BC, NEA-BC, CNE
Associate Professor
Molloy College
Rockville Centre, New York

Debra Lee, PhD, BSN, RN
Assistant Professor, Dean of School of Nursing and
    Health Sciences
Malone University
Canton, Ohio

Rosemary Macy, PhD, RN, CNE, CHSE
Associate Professor
Boise State University
Boise, Idaho

Kari Mardian, MEd, BN, RN
Instructor
Medicine Hat College
Medicine Hat, Canada

Tammie McCoy, BA, BSN, MSN, PhD
Professor/Chair
Mississippi University for Women
Columbus, Mississippi

Valerie O'Dell, DNP, RN, CNE
Associate Professor/MSN Program Director
Youngstown University
Youngstown, Ohio

Teresa O'Neill, PhD, APRN, RNC
Distance Education Coordinator, Professor Emerita
University of Holy Cross
New Orleans, Louisiana

Cheryl Passel, PhD
Assistant Professor
Marian University
Fond du Lac, Wisconsin

JoAnne Pearce, MS RNC, APRN-BC
Assistant Professor
Idaho State University
Pocatello, Idaho

Theresa T. Quell, PhD, RN
Assistant Dean for Academic Programs
Fairfield University
Norwalk, Connecticut

Janet Reagor, RN, PhD
Interim Dean, Assistant Professor
Avila University
Kansas City, Missouri

Debra Simons, PhD, RN, CNE, CHSE, CCM
Associate Dean
College of New Rochelle
New Rochelle, New York

Diane Spoljoric, PhD, RNC, FNP
Associate Professor
Purdue Northwest
Westville, Indiana

Nancy Steffen, MSN
Instructor
Century College
White Bear Lake, Minnesota

Alicia Stone, PhD, MS, RN, FNP
Professor
Molloy College
Rockville Centre, New York

Wendy Wheeler, RN, BScN, MN
Continuous Nursing Faculty
Red Deer College
Red Deer, Canada

Sylvia K. Wood, DNP, APRN, ANP-BC
Assistant Professor
St. Joseph's College
Brooklyn, New York

Ronda Yoder, PhD, ARNP
Faculty
Pensacola Christina College
Pensacola, Florida

Karen Zapko, PhD, CNS, MSN, RN
Assistant Professor
Kent State University at Salem
Salem, Ohio

Tamara Zurakowski, PhD
Clinical Associate Professor
Virginia Commonwealth University
Richmond, Virginia

About the Author

Lucy Hood, PhD, RN, is the daughter of an American auto worker. She graduated from St. Luke's Hospital of Kansas City Diploma Nursing School. She returned to school and earned a BSN from Webster College (now Webster University), an MSN from UMKC, and a PhD in nursing from Widener University, Chester, Pennsylvania. With 14 years of experience in the areas of medical-surgical and neuroscience nursing, she embarked on a career in nursing education. Dr. Hood taught undergraduate and graduating nursing at St. Luke's College of Health Sciences for 25 years. She then taught in the RN-to-BSN and MSN nursing programs in the School of Nursing and Health Sciences at MidAmerica Nazarene University in Olathe, Kansas. From 2016 to 2019, Dr. Hood served as the Department Chair of Pre-Licensure Nursing Education, in the School of Nursing at MNU. She has also taught in the Clinical Pastoral Education Program at St. Luke's Hospital of Kansas City. Current professional nursing activities include membership in the ANA, MONA, and Sigma Theta Tau International. She serves on the MONA Advocacy Committee, which involves political activism. She is a volunteer musician for St. Margaret of Scotland Catholic Church. She enjoys swimming, walking, gardening, reading, and finding collectibles at flea markets. She lives with her husband of 35 plus years, and they enjoy caring for their rescue, dachshund, Yoda.

Preface

In the early 1980s, Susan Leddy and Mae Pepper realized the need for a professional development textbook for registered nurses who were returning to school to earn baccalaureate degrees in nursing. This edition builds on the previous contributions that Leddy and Pepper made in earlier editions of *Professional Nursing*. So that the memory of Susan Leddy and May Pepper will continue, their names have appeared as part of the book title since 2003.

I express my sincere appreciation to the following persons for their creativity and attention to detail during the revision process: Staci Wolfson, supervisory development editor; Michael Kerns and Susan Hartman, acquisitions editors; Molly Kennedy, editorial assistant; Anju Radhakrishnan, editorial coordinator; Jennifer Clements, art director; Stephen Druding, design coordinator; Jennifer Clements, art director; Kalpagam Rao and Jeethu Abraham and the production team staff at S4Carlisle. Without the members of this talented team, the book would have never been published.

Organization

The tenth edition is organized into the following sections:

- Section 1, Exploring Professional Nursing
- Section 2, Professional Practice in an Ever-Changing Health Care Context
- Section 3, Professional Nursing Roles
- Section 4, Envisioning and Creating the Future of Professional Nursing

Content revisions to the tenth edition include the following.

Chapter 1: The Professional Nurse

Presentation of information found in *The Essentials: Core Competencies of Professional Nursing Education* that were revised and released in April 2021.

Chapter 2: The History Behind Today's Professional Nursing

New content addressing discrimination in health care delivery, the contributions to professional nursing made by Black women, and updated information on racial segregation in nursing education. In addition, lessons learned from the influenza pandemic of 1918 to 1919 were highlighted in relation to the COVID-19 pandemic.

Chapter 3: Contextual, Philosophical, and Ethical Elements of Professional Nursing

New content presenting Eastern and African philosophical and ethical approaches to life.

Chapter 4: Establishing Helping and Healing Relationships

The Core Competencies for Interprofessional Practice were added.

Chapter 5: The Health Process and Self-Care of the Nurse

This chapter is presented earlier in the book because nursing students may find some of the presented strategies for self-care as they take courses early in the curriculum and semester. Content from *Healthy People 2030* is provided as well as a brief introduction to mindfulness. New content regarding professional well-being from the National Academy of Medicine and National Academies of Science, Engineering, and Medicine has been added.

Chapter 11: Multicultural Issues in Professional Practice

New content for this chapter includes the social determinant of health outlined in *Healthy People 2030* that explains some of the causes of health disparities, content related to White privilege, cultural humility, information for gender-sensitive care, and information on human trafficking. Information on human trafficking was included because according to the Polaris Project, 40% of the homeless population are youth who are struggling with gender-affirming issues and homeless youths are the highest-risk group for human trafficking.

Chapter 13: Environmental and Global Health

Updated information regarding the global environment and new content related to mass shootings, electromagnetic sensitivity, and the impact of incivility and racism on the work environment has been added.

Chapter 14: Informatics and Technology in Nursing Practice

Expanded content on how nurses can use social media in professional development, clinical practice, and showcasing the profession of nursing to the public. Addition of content related to the potential insecurity of protected health information due to cyber-attacks.

Chapter 15: Nursing Approaches to Client Systems

Updated content on person- and family-centered care, and how this is incorporated into clinical practice. Expanded content on the concept of community as clients appears in this chapter along with career opportunities for nurses in community health settings.

Chapter 16: The Professional Nurse's Role in Teaching and Learning

Updated content to include the 2020 U.S. Department of Health and Human Services definitions of personal and organizational health literacy and the inclusion of the newest vital sign, a 3-minute assessment for personal health literacy.

Chapter 17: Leadership and Management in Professional Nursing

New content added on planning and leading meetings and expanded information on dysfunctional leadership and the change process to promote divergent thinking, agility, and flexibility to cultivate an environment that supports change and innovation.

Chapter 18: Continuous Quality Improvement: Enhancing Client Safety and Health Care Quality

Expanded information on benchmarking, balanced score card, updated Baldrige Award criteria, and additional art illustrating the Pareto chart and fishbone diagram. The Leapfrog Group was added as a collaborative effort to promote continuous quality improvement in health care.

Chapter 19: The Professional Nurse's Role in Public Policy

Updated information to address the current American Nurses Association legislative priorities and highlights about nurses currently representing the profession in the public policy arena along with new information on how to create a legislative fact sheet and new tips for preparing and providing testimony.

Chapter 20: Career Options for Professional Nurses

Updated information on legal nurse consulting, revised content on nurse entrepreneurs and private consulting, expanded information on occupational health nursing, and presentation of new nursing specialty area, travel health nursing.

Chapter 21: Development of a Professional Nursing Career

New information on Shirey's nursing career phases and how they can be used to set the stage for a desired professional career and expanded content to include presentation of mentoring models.

Chapter 22: Shaping the Future of Nursing

Revised information on the future of nursing practice based on predictions from the U.S. Health Resources and Services Administration, the messages from *The Future of Nursing 2020-2030: Charting a Path to Create Health Equity* (2021), and from current futurists who analyze current trends to predict the future along with potential future health issues arising from the COVID-19 pandemic, vaping, and legalized cannabis.

Learning Tools

Continued efforts have been made to make this book more "user-friendly" and to engage students in the learning process and in the application of this material to practice. In addition to such textbook standards as **Key Terms and Concepts, Learning Outcomes,** and **References,** each chapter also includes:

- **Real-Life Reflections:** Case studies are presented at the beginning of each chapter and revisited at chapter's end, highlighting for students the application of the chapter's content to practice and providing questions for thought as they read the chapter.
- **Questions for Reflection:** Questions posed throughout the text help students think about their own life experiences in the context of their learning.
- **Focus on Research:** Current journal articles are synopsized to relate research to learning and practice.
- **Concepts in Practice:** Hypothetical clinical situations teach professional nurses how they can best incorporate text concepts into real-life practice.
- **From Theory to Practice:** End-of-chapter questions ask students to think about each chapter's content in the context of their own lives.
- **Nurse as Author:** Short writing exercises designed to strengthen critical thinking and writing skills. The nature of the written exercise in each chapter relates to and depends upon the nature of chapter content.
- **Your Digital Classroom:** At the end of each chapter, online resources are brought together to provide students with opportunities for further study and reflection. These include *Online Exploration* (compilation of websites appropriate to each chapter's content); *Expanding Your Understanding* (Internet-based exercises); and *Beyond the Book* (a link to and instructions for accessing the numerous online resources now available with this text).

Text boxes have been categorized to help students identify the purpose of their content.

- **Professional Building Blocks:** Highlight clinical and professional implications.
- **Learning, Knowing, and Growing:** Provides students with information to help them grow both personally and professionally.
- **Professional Prototypes:** Provide examples of documents, concepts, philosophies, and more with suggestions for personal and professional growth.

Students who follow the Beyond the Book link to thePoint® can access

- Fully searchable eBook
- Learning Objectives
- Spanish–English Audio Glossary
- Weblink Exercises
- Journal Articles
- Critical Thinking Activities

To facilitate reading, this edition is being printed in full color and photographs have been added to break up large chunks of printed material.

As Mae Pepper and Susan Leddy noted in the preface to the third edition,

> During these changing times, we have been pleased with the utilization of our book in many educational settings, particularly in baccalaureate and graduate programs. Although the first edition of the book was targeted for upper division RN baccalaureate programs, we have become aware of its utilization in generic baccalaureate programs, masters programs, and practice settings.

It is my hope that this 10th edition of *Professional Nursing* will carry on the tradition of previous editions and continue to make a meaningful contribution to the profession.

Lucy Jane Hood

Contents

1

EXPLORING PROFESSIONAL NURSING

To people outside the nursing profession, being a nurse means taking care of those who are ill or injured in a variety of complex and sometimes chaotic situations. Nurses make key contributions in the delivery of health care services by providing safe, high-quality care to individuals, families, and groups. The profession is continuously evolving in order to attain all criteria for attaining true professional status. The therapeutic relationships nurses establish with clients play a significant role in making differences in the lives of the people they serve. In an ideal world, nurses should be role models of physical, mental, and spiritual health for their clients. Learning the art and science of nursing requires time and perseverance. When nurses provide solid evidence of their impact on client outcomes, the unique contributions they make become apparent to the other members of the health care team and to the public. Professional nurses engage in lifelong learning to remain competent in the areas of clinical practice.

The Professional Nurse

KEY TERMS AND CONCEPTS

Professional nurses
Professional nurse con-
  tributions model
Core competency
Nurse of the Future Nurs-
  ing Core Competencies
Caregiver
Client advocate
Teacher
Change agent
Coordinator
Counselor
Colleague
Peer-reviewed
Socialization
Resocialization
Role theory

Role
Role conflict
Returning-to-school
  syndrome
Transitions
Professional self-concept
Novice-to-expert model
Characteristics of a
  profession
Associate degree in nurs-
  ing (ADN)
Diploma nursing program
Bachelor of science in
  nursing (BSN)
Differentiated competencies
Graduate nursing
  education

Postgraduate nursing
  education
Critical thinking
Creative thinking
Reflective thinking
Reflection in action
Reflection on action
Nursing process
Licensure
Autonomy
State boards of nursing
Professional
  organizations
General-purpose nursing
  organizations
Specialized nursing
  organizations

National League for Nurs-
  ing (NLN)
American Association
  of Colleges of Nursing
  (AACN)
National Council of State
  Boards of Nursing
  (NCSBN)
American Nurses Associa-
  tion (ANA)
International Council of
  Nurses (ICN)
Sigma Theta Tau Interna-
  tional (STTI)
National Student Nurses'
  Association (NSNA)
Ethical codes

LEARNING OUTCOMES

By the end of this chapter, the learner will be able to:

1. Outline key elements for professional nursing contributions to health care.
2. Explain the significance of core competencies to professional nursing practice.
3. Describe the multiple roles assumed by professional nurses.
4. Identify strategies for thriving in the nursing education environment.
5. Specify a process for socialization into the profession.
6. Discuss methods to facilitate socialization and resocialization into the nursing profession.
7. Outline a process for developing a professional self-concept.
8. Identify the characteristics of a profession.
9. Explain how nursing meets the characteristics of a profession.
10. Discuss additional work that needs to be done to fulfill all characteristics of a profession and attain professional status on a par with that of other professions.

REAL-LIFE REFLECTIONS

Sue graduated from an associate degree in nursing (ADN) program and has been work-
ing as a night charge nurse on a medical-surgical unit. She likes working with Martin, a
nursing student enrolled in a local bachelor of science in nursing (BSN) degree program.
Her nurse manager is interested in hiring Martin when he graduates from college. When

(continued on page 4)

speaking with a nurse friend, Sue says, "I am a good nurse even though I do not have a BSN. I really do not see how going back to school to earn one will improve the patient care I give. However, I see how it would make my charge nurse position secure." What assumptions has Sue made relative to the importance of education in nursing practice?

- *How would you respond to her?*
- *If you are a registered nurse (RN) student, what are your thoughts about the BSN degree and higher education for nurses?*
- *If you are not an RN student, why did you decide to go to a BSN program before starting your nursing career?*

Professional nurses comprise the largest group of health care workers in the United States. The National Council of State Boards of Nursing (NCSBN) (2020b) reported that 4,195,750 individuals hold active RN licenses. This figure includes nurses who are actively working or who have left the profession but maintain their licenses. The U.S. Bureau of Labor Statistics (USBLS) (2021b) reported that close to 3.1 million of these nurses are actively employed RNs (including retirees) who volunteer their professional services; in order to do so, they must possess an active RN license. **Professional nurses** are RNs with a broad scope of practice that is determined by each state.

Some people consider all caregivers to be "nurses." This logical confusion stems from the fact that people who tend to the sick, injured, disabled, or older adults commonly have the word "nurse" in their job titles, such as nursing assistants or licensed practical/vocational nurses (LPN/LVNs). However, professional nurses offer a specialized service to society. In return, nurses expect certain things from society to promote their work. They assume ultimate accountability for client outcomes, and they supervise and educate LPN/LVNs and unlicensed assistive personnel (UAP) as they assist in nursing care delivery. Although they frequently perform tasks that could be done by other health care team members, professional nurses bring an ability to improvise while individualizing client care in a variety of settings. Professional nurses use science and theories as a basis for professional practice along with the art of modifying care approaches. Thus, nursing is often considered both an art and a science (see Box 1.1, Professional Prototypes, "Essential Features of Professional Nursing").

 1.1 Professional Prototypes

Essential Features of Professional Nursing

Professional nurses assume responsibility to the public for using the best evidence to provide safe, high-quality health-related services for all those they serve. In return, nurses expect certain things from society. In *Nursing's Social Policy Statement*, the American Nurses Association (Fowler, 2015b) identified the following "key essential features of professional nursing" (p. 20).

What Society Expects From Nurses

1. Provide nursing care with compassion without prejudice to protect, promote, and optimize health of care recipients, to prevent illnesses and injuries, alleviate suffering through the diagnostic and treatment processes of the human response, and to advocate for individuals, families, communities, and populations (p. 20).
2. Place the needs of the client first and above all needs of others, including those of the nurse and the institution where care is delivered.

3. Maintain current knowledge, skills, and competence by following standards of care; oversee education through accreditation; and develop methods to deal with incompetent, unprofessional, impaired, or unethical practice.
4. Provide hazardous service under conditions that are not required by individuals outside of the profession, including infectious pathogens, weather emergencies, power failures, man-made disasters, and tending to combative or violent clients.
5. Bear responsibility and accountability for practice such as engagement in self-regulation, being transparent when care lapses occur, participating in peer review, and establishing and overseeing nursing professional policies.
6. Progress and develop by incorporating new findings in science and humanities into professional practice, expanding the knowledge of the profession through

nursing theory development, research, and best clinical evidence.

7. Assure ethical practice by developing, affirming, and upholding a code of ethics to which each nurse should adhere.

8. Collaborate with other health care professionals and other disciplines to promote the health of society.

9. Promote the health of the public, addressing each client's problems, confronting issues of health disparities, developing health policies at all governmental levels, and engaging in whistle-blowing when needed to protect clients and the public.

What to Expect in Return From Society

1. Support autonomy by trusting nurses to practice within their designated scope of practice.

2. Support self-governance by allowing the nursing profession to regulate itself via state boards of nursing, professional associations, and accrediting its own educational programs.

3. Facilitate title and practice protection by enabling the nursing profession to develop and administer nursing licensing exams, require mandatory licensure, provide legal protection for using the term "registered nurse (RN)" as a title, and prevent others from encroaching on nursing practice.

4. Maintain respectful and just renumeration through societal accord of professional respect, support nursing education and research efforts, payment of a just wage, provision of humane working conditions, and facilitation of nursing influence regarding any health policies that affect professional nursing practice.

5. Allow freedom to practice by providing nurses with the authority and liberty to practice the profession to the full extent of their education and preparation, including that of specialized and advanced practice roles.

6. Facilitate workforce sustainability by societal development of a strategic plan for addressing shortages, replacement of workers as nurses retire and leave, and increased access to nursing education and developing structures for upward mobility.

7. Provide protection from hazardous service by requiring health care organizations to provide nurses with equipment to limit the risks of hazardous service, such as personal protection equipment, to limit chance of contracting an infection, and lifting devices to prevent back injuries.

CHARACTERISTICS OF PROFESSIONAL NURSING PRACTICE: THE HOOD PROFESSIONAL NURSE CONTRIBUTIONS MODEL

As interdisciplinary health care team members, nurses make many unique contributions to health care delivery in clinical settings. The **professional nurse contributions model** (Fig. 1.1) synthesizes the affective, cognitive, behavioral, and psychomotor domains of professional practice. The model's circular form illustrates how the interprofessional health care team surrounds health care consumers. A solid outer circle emphasizes the importance of all team members working cohesively for the benefit of care recipients. Each of the concepts in this model is integrally connected to the others to result in a unified whole.

In an ideal world, all health care team members would share an altruistic attitude toward the individuals they serve. Many people enter the nursing profession because they genuinely care (caring) about other people and have a desire to help others in times of need (compassion). *Caring, compassion,* and *commitment* are the key affective domains for optimal professional nursing that are intricately linked and comprise the outer circle of the model. The concepts of caring, compassion, and commitment are key for nurses to view nursing as a profession rather than just a job. Two additional attributes of nurses that are closely linked are competence and confidence. Clients expect *competence* from health care providers. Likewise, health care providers expect competence from each other. To provide safe, effective client care, nurses must have competence with clinical skills and decision making. Many nursing education programs use simulations with high- or low-fidelity manikins to provide students with the opportunities to learn essential clinical skills and clinical decision making in a safe learning environment (Bradshaw et al., 2020). Current literature emphasizes that students gain and retain knowledge, learn clinical skills, and develop confidence in nursing abilities from simulated learning experiences (Alexander et al., 2015; Bortolato et al., 2018).

Before competence can be achieved, however, professional nurses must have *confidence* in their ability to execute the clinical, communication, and cognitive skills needed for effective practice. Simulated clinical experiences in nursing education also build confidence in nursing students (Bradshaw et al., 2020). As the nurse's confidence improves, they

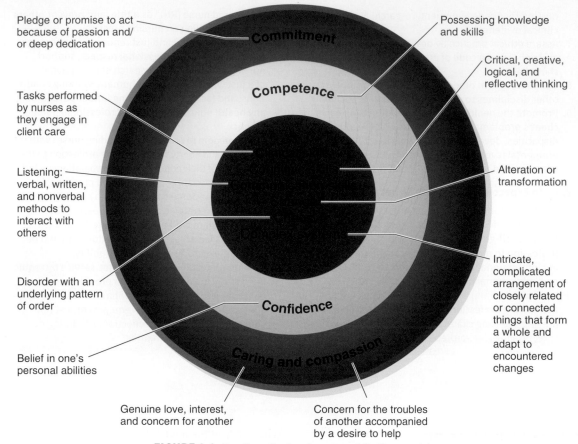

Pledge or promise to act because of passion and/or deep dedication

Possessing knowledge and skills

Critical, creative, logical, and reflective thinking

Tasks performed by nurses as they engage in client care

Listening: verbal, written, and nonverbal methods to interact with others

Alteration or transformation

Disorder with an underlying pattern of order

Intricate, complicated arrangement of closely related or connected things that form a whole and adapt to encountered changes

Belief in one's personal abilities

Genuine love, interest, and concern for another

Concern for the troubles of another accompanied by a desire to help

Commitment

Competence

Confidence

Caring and compassion

FIGURE 1.1 Hood's professional nurse contributions model.

become willing to question orders and actions by others that may not appear to be logical or safe. Clients and families feel more at ease when receiving care from a confident nurse. For example, the nurse who knows how to start an intravenous (IV) line and has confidence in their ability will attempt to start IVs. As the nurse gains experience in starting IVs, they refine their technique and eventually possess the ability to start IVs in any client. The nurse's colleagues identify them as the IV starting expert on the unit (confidence booster). The nurse gains more experience starting IVs even when colleagues cannot (increasing competence). Thus, there appears to be a symbiotic relationship between confidence and competence in nursing practice.

The innermost circle in the model depicts the overlapping skills and circumstances with which nurses must work and cope. The roles assumed by nurses require that they have a repertoire of *clinical*, *cognitive*, and *communication skills*. The nurse must always have sound reasons behind clinical decisions and actions

and be able to communicate the reasons well. A broad knowledge base related to all information and strategies available enable the nurse to decide the best course of action to take in any given clinical situation. Highly refined clinical, cognitive, and communication skills delineate professional nurses from all other members of the health care team.

Nurses deliver health care in *complex systems*, so it is important that they understand the nature of these systems and are able to manipulate them. Wiggins (2008) describes health care systems as complex adaptive systems in which interdependency exists among individuals and groups. Each individual's actions within complex adaptive systems are based on current knowledge and past experiences. Just like the human body is composed of interacting systems, the client is part of a community; communities form states, states form nations, and nations are part of the global community. The earth is part of a solar system, which is part of a galaxy, which is part of the universe.

Nurses frequently encounter complicated client situations and must adapt to *change* as new scientific evidence emerges, reforms occur in legal aspects of health care delivery, and, most importantly, client conditions fluctuate. Finally, professional nursing practice has an element of unpredictability and disorder that is conceptualized as *chaos*. Nurses must continuously make complex and multiple decisions to help bring order to today's clinical environments. Once order is achieved, something may occur that results in disorder. The pattern of ever-emerging chaos creates constant challenges for nurses. Upon acknowledgment of the deeper underlying, uniform pattern of chaos, nurses understand that they cannot control all clinical practice events. Even though a clinical setting may have a well-defined organization, nurses must adapt to and work in an ever-changing, highly complex, and chaotic environment.

CORE COMPETENCIES FOR PROFESSIONAL NURSES

The concept of core competency arose in the 1990s. A **core competency** can be defined as "a skill that is needed to be successful at a job or other activity" (Dictionary.com, 2020). In professional nursing, core competencies comprise the fundamental knowledge, abilities, and skills that enable nurses to provide safe, effective care to clients in health care settings. In many health care settings, professional nurses are expected to display competence in a particular area of practice on an annual basis. Frequently, nursing staff development departments design and deploy activities to verify that nurses possess a certain level of competence with the knowledge and skills appropriate to their specific clinical practice areas.

In 1973, the American Nurses Association (ANA) published the first *Standards of Nursing Practice*. The goal was to develop a generic list of standards for professional nurses that would apply across practice settings. The standards primarily focused on nursing process (assessment, diagnosis, planning, implementation, and evaluation), which at the time articulated a thinking model for all nurses to use in clinical practice. As time passed, the original standards of nursing practice have evolved into the *Scope and Standards of Nursing* that outline all key elements of professional nursing practice, including nursing process and key competencies (knowledge and skills) for meeting each standard of professional practice. Although the competencies are distinguished from one another, the execution of each

competency may be context dependent. For example, Standard 3, "Outcome Identification," and Standard 4, "Planning," specify that the client, significant others, and other health team members should be involved in determining the desired outcomes and how to achieve them (ANA, 2021). If the client is unconscious or has been legally declared mentally incompetent, then the client is unable to be an active participant in the determination of care goals and planned actions to attain them.

By the 1990s, the ANA recognized the need to develop standards of practice for nursing specialty areas and collaborated with nursing specialty organizations to develop context-based scope and standards of practice, including those for psychiatric mental health; faith community; holistic, pediatric, school, forensic, hospital, and palliative care nursing; and nursing administration. The ANA's (2021) fourth edition of the *Nursing: Scope and Standards of Practice* contains 6 standards addressing nursing process (assessment, diagnosis, outcome identification, planning, implementation, and evaluation) and 12 standards related to professional performance (ethics, advocacy, respectful and equitable practice, communication, collaboration, leadership, education, scholarly inquiry, quality of practice, professional practice evaluation, resource stewardship, and environmental health) (ANA, 2021). Disposing used needles and sharp implements (e.g., needles, disposable scissors) into hard, impermeable boxes labeled "biohazard" is an example of a competency related to environmental health and worker safety.

In the 1990s, the Institute of Medicine (IOM) published a series of reports outlining safety and quality concerns within the American health care system. The Robert Wood Johnson Foundation provided funding to Linda Cronenwett, PhD, as principal investigator and the American Association of Colleges of Nursing (AACN) for the Quality Safety Education for Nursing (QSEN) initiative to develop strategies for nursing practice and education for continuously improving and enhancing safety in health care delivery. During the first phase of the project, the following six core competencies were identified for professional nursing: client-centered care, teamwork and collaboration, evidence-based practice, quality improvement, informatics, and safety (QSEN Institute, 2014). Along with identifying the competencies, the initiative developed sets of knowledge, skills, and attitudes for each of them. The project initially addressed prelicensure nursing education but was eventually expanded to address graduate nursing education (QSEN Institute, 2014). Over the years, the core competencies have remained the same, but the developed sets of knowledge, skills, and attitudes demonstrating attainment have been revised. The QSEN Institute serves as a repository for all information regarding the competencies. Its mission is to be "a collaborative of healthcare professionals focused on education, practice, and scholarship to improve the quality and safety of healthcare systems" (QSEN Institute, 2020).

In March 2006, the Massachusetts Department of Higher Education and the Massachusetts Organization of Nurse Executives held a workshop called "Creativity and Connections: Building the Framework for the Future of Nursing Education and Practice" that was attended by 32 key stakeholders in nursing education and practice. An outcome of the workshop was the formation of a subcommittee to develop a set of core professional nursing competencies to facilitate a seamless continuum for progression in nursing education and a statewide program for transitioning for new graduate nurses into the world of professional practice. Between 2006 and 2009, the committee reviewed the best practices, standards, and initiatives of education progression to create a list of nursing

competencies for each level of nursing education. Results of the review were compiled into a set of 10 core competencies that were then compared to outcomes required for associate degree and baccalaureate degree program accrediting agencies. Funded by the Massachusetts Department of Higher Education and the Johnson and Johnson Promise of Nursing for the Massachusetts Nursing School Grant Program, the Nurse of the Future Competency Committee identified 10 core competencies that are essential for professional nursing practice known as the **Nurse of the Future Nursing Core Competencies** (Fig. 1.2). The identified competencies are client-centered care, professionalism, leadership, systems-based practice, information and technology, communication, teamwork and collaboration, safety, quality improvement, and evidence-based practice. Each competency in the model has specific knowledge, attitudes/behaviors, and skills associated with it for planning, implementing, and evaluating education of its mastery (Massachusetts Department of Higher Education, 2016).

In 2021, the AACN (2021) revised the essential elements for baccalaureate nursing education. The changes appear in *The Essentials: Core Competencies*

MASSACHUSETTS DEPARTMENT OF HIGHER EDUCATION
Nurse of the Future Nursing Core Competencies
The Art and Science of Nursing

K – Knowledge
A – Attitudes
S – Skills

FIGURE 1.2 Massachusetts Nurse of the Future Nursing Core Competencies.

for Professional Nursing Education. Revisions focus on competencies for providing the highest quality and value of health care. They identified the following 10 key areas encountered in the domain of professional nursing: knowledge for nursing practice; person-centered care; population health; scholarship for nursing practice; quality and safety; interprofessional partnerships; systems-based practice; information and health care technologies; professionalism; and personal, professional and leadership development. AACN also identified the following four key concepts for professional nursing, which are applicable for all areas of nursing practice: (a) clinical judgment, (b) communication, (c) compassionate care, and (d) diversity, equity, and inclusion (AACN, 2021). AACN outlined that the following four spheres of care has to be included in the education of the nurse generalist: wellness and disease prevention, regenerative/restorative care (care for acutely ill clients and including rehabilitation to an optimal level of wellness), chronic disease management, and hospice/palliative care. The competencies for each domain describe what professional nurses are capable of doing over time and across settings, incorporating certain knowledge, attitudes, and skills.

Caring, compassion, commitment, and confidence are the key attitudes that make up the affective domain of professional nursing practice. Caring and compassion involve the nurse's genuine concern for others and a desire to help them. When a nurse displays confidence in what is being done as a professional, recipients of nursing care, other health care team members, and the public perceive that the nurse possesses the knowledge, skills, and attitude for effective role performance. Competence means that nurses are capable of performing skills (cognitive, clinical, and communication) effectively to provide safe, optimal care. Complex systems, chaos, and change describe the clinical practice environments of professional nurses.

THE MULTIPLE ROLES OF THE PROFESSIONAL NURSE

Nurses assume multiple roles while meeting the health care needs of clients. They serve as **caregivers** when providing direct client care. Their **client advocate** role emerges when they intervene on behalf of clients to ensure that adequate information and decision-making resources are provided and that client wishes are respected at all times. They assume the role of **teacher** when providing education to UAP, clients, family members, students, each other, and interprofessional

colleagues. When working to reform public policy, modify work processes, or transform workplace environments, nurses become **change agents**. They accept the role of **coordinator** when assuming supervisory and managerial responsibilities. Nurses also act as **counselors**, providing emotional and spiritual support to clients. Finally, they assume the role of **colleague** to all health team members. To execute these multiple roles effectively and with genuine compassion, nurses must commit themselves to lifelong learning.

Take Note!
Nurses must commit themselves to lifelong learning if they are to effectively and compassionately execute their multiple professional roles.

CHALLENGES FOR THE PROFESSIONAL NURSING STUDENT

Anyone who assumes the role of professional nursing student will need to make lifestyle changes to be successful. The added responsibilities of nursing school mean that life as previously known will be greatly altered. Previous routines will be disrupted and personal sacrifices will be needed. Money once used for recreation may be spent on tuition, student fees, books, and other school supplies. Less time is available to spend with family and friends. Families and friends have different reactions as the nursing student role is assumed. The reactions vary from feeling neglected (which may result in actions to derail the educational process) to intense pride (as they watch the nursing student grow). Ongoing communication between the new student, family, and friends enables all involved parties to understand how roles will be altered and what lifestyle changes will need to occur (Dunham, 2008; Quan, 2006).

Meeting job and school responsibilities may be challenging for employed students. Employers may not support educational endeavors. Some coworkers may add to the difficulties by complaining about or refusing work schedule changes; others may express pride in their colleague and help accommodate the student's schedule.

Part of the toll of returning to school is entering into unfamiliar learning situations. The once-confident honor student or professional nurse may question their ability to survive in an intense academic program. The educational process is designed to change people. During times of change, people frequently encounter feelings of discomfort.

SKILLS FOR EDUCATIONAL SUCCESS

In ideal educational situations, students and faculty interact with each other as colleagues. Faculty design educational experiences and students bear the responsibility for active engagement in learning activities. In traditional education, faculty members serve as authoritarian experts who impart knowledge to students and may create oppressive climates. In educative-caring education, students and faculty members hold equal status, and faculty members strive to create effective learning climates based on active and participative learning (Bevis & Watson, 2000; Billings & Halstead, 2020). Such egalitarian interactions with faculty members provide students with experience in collegiality.

When students assume responsibility for learning, they reap maximum benefits from the educational process. To make professional transitions, nurses focus their educational efforts on refining previously learned skills while establishing theoretical foundations for professional practice. Theory-based practice enables professional nurses to understand complex situations and anticipate potential complications in clinical settings. Learners need a variety of skills to be successful in the educational process.

Take Note!
To make the most of the educational process, students must assume responsibility for learning and utilize a variety of skills.

Reading, Listening, and Speaking

Reading constitutes a major component of a successful education experience, but finding time to read remains a challenge for today's busy students—especially as they juggle multiple roles. Effective reading skills streamline the study process. Trying to read and digest each word printed on a page or screen is inefficient. When students master the skill of reading for major ideas within a passage, reading becomes more efficient

(Dunham, 2008; Osuna, 2014). Strategies to develop reading effectiveness and efficiency include reading for general understanding of ideas, using learning outcomes to identify key concepts, taking notes while reading, highlighting key points, and taking brief reading breaks between major headings within a chapter. During reading breaks, some students find it beneficial to paraphrase what has been read.

In educational settings, effective speaking and listening skills are essential to success. Students listen to faculty members as they share their nursing expertise. Taking time to think before responding to faculty-posed questions enables better organization of thoughts and selection of the best words to convey an answer. Most nursing programs require that students give oral classroom presentations to facilitate refinement of public speaking skills.

Asking questions is essential to avoid making errors in both education and health care settings. Most people (especially clinical nursing faculty and nurses) welcome questions from students. However, fear prevents some students from asking questions. Sometimes, the most difficult task to master is learning what questions need to be asked and having the courage to ask them.

Because nursing relies on teamwork, faculty frequently assign group projects. Some students dread group projects because of the difficulty finding time to connect with group members. Osuna (2014) offers the following suggestions to thrive when working on group projects:

1. Provide all members of the group with contact information to facilitate the sharing of project information.
2. Appoint a group leader who organizes the project timeline, requests member project sections, pulls the entire project together for a finished product (edits writing for consistent style and finalizes required formatting), serves as a resource person, and tackles issues when they arise.
3. Develop a project timeline with the equal input of all group members.
4. Define specific tasks (including the format for each member to submit the section to the leader) required for the project and make group assignments.
5. Hold all members accountable for their sections of the project.
6. Communicate openly, in a timely fashion, and respectfully.

Hopefully, by following these suggestions, the project gets completed in accordance with the course syllabus. When problems arise, the group should be able to manage them. However, sometimes faculty involvement may be needed should an irreconcilable issue arise.

Writing

Writing is another critical skill for educational and career success. Professional nurses use writing skills to document client care, develop clinical practice policies, compose email messages and letters, publish articles, develop budgets, and submit change proposals (Fig. 1.3). Writing requires nurses to use critical and reflective thinking (Broussard & Oberleitner, 1997).

Written course assignments provide opportunities to polish writing and thinking skills. Success requires understanding the purpose of the writing assignment, setting a timeline for completion by the designated deadline, allowing time for multiple drafts, and having a trusted friend or family member proofread the work before submission.

Perhaps the most difficult aspect of preparing an assignment is narrowing the topic appropriately to fit assignment criteria and enabling a realistic approach for gathering relevant and reputable resources among the vast sources of information. Librarians and faculty welcome the opportunity to help students secure reliable resources such as books, peer-reviewed journal articles (online, in print, or on microfilm), nursing experts, government documents, and online information from academic, nonprofit organizational nurse specialty groups and government websites (Dunham, 2008; Stebbins, 2006).

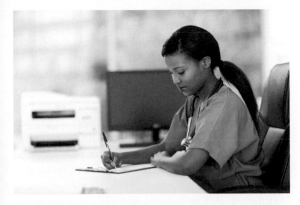

FIGURE 1.3 Writing by hand in the clinical setting enables the professional nurse to have key information readily available for change of shift reports, report key client information to physicians, and record client assessments in the event of computer failure.

When students use a database from a library, there is an option to perform an advanced search to limit the findings to peer-reviewed sources and the dates of publication. **Peer-reviewed** materials have been reviewed by a panel of experts in a given field for accuracy, relevance, and novel ideas that contribute to the knowledge within their areas of expertise. Online journal articles gathered from such a database typically have undergone this process. Articles found in some online open-access resources may not have this rigorous scholarly quality, especially if they are generated by companies that charge authors or special interest organizations that have an agenda to communicate. In addition, the peer-review process for some open-access journals may lack the academic rigor compared to established publications (Adams, 2019). Frequently, faculty may require references for an assignment to be no more than 5 years old unless they are considered to be seminal references (e.g., Hans Selye's work on general adaptation syndrome).

Students should be cautious when considering information from for-profit sources, some special interest organizations, and the news media. For-profit sources want to sell a product. Some special interest groups and news media outlets may be biased to retain reader interest, rather than just presenting facts. Social media, blogs, online videos, and podcasts may offer some valuable information if they are connected to large, fact-based organizations such as TED conferences, for example (Adams, 2019; Purdue University Online Writing Lab, n.d. b). However, some websites serve as a "virtual soapbox" for any person, organization, or company. The Purdue University Online Writing Lab (n.d. a) suggests that if these sources are used, students should cross-check the information, investigate the qualifications and affiliations of the author(s), check for biased language, and look for the presence and quality of a reference list. Health professionals and students must carefully evaluate the validity and appropriateness of information from websites used for personal, professional, and client education (Table 1.1).

Hyperlinks that appear within a website may send viewers to websites of lesser quality. Some website information can disappear without warning, and unless the website has security mechanisms, the information may be susceptible to unauthorized and accidental changes (Adams, 2019; Hasan & Abuelrub, 2009). For example, any person who accesses the online encyclopedia, Wikipedia, has the capability to change posted information. Therefore, this particular site should not be considered a reliable resource.

TABLE 1.1	Guidelines for Evaluating Online Information
Criteria	**Questions to Ask Yourself**
Content accuracy	■ Is the material written at a level of reading appropriate to health care consumers (for client use) or health professionals (for professional use)? ■ Is the information error free? ■ Does the information conflict with known scientific information? ■ Does the site contain any unvalidated scientific information? ■ Does the information cover the entire scope of what is known about the health issue or topic of concern?
Authority	■ What are the qualifications of the expert(s) or organization providing the information? ■ Are there any references cited or sources stated? ■ Is there a way to contact author(s) or organization?
Objectivity	■ Does the information seem biased or attempt to sway the reader, such as by selling a product or advocating a specific viewpoint? ■ Is there any emotionally charged language used?
Currency	■ Are the initial posting dates and update dates presented? ■ When was the site last updated?
Site format and design	■ Is there an index or map for the site? ■ Do the tabs for the content on the site work? ■ How many clicks does it take to reach the desired information? ■ Is the site visually appealing? ■ Is the font on the site easily read? ■ Are there headings to guide the reader? ■ Are there space breaks between narrative sections? ■ How well does scrolling work? ■ Do video and sound inputs download and play effectively? ■ Are there menu tabs that are easily found, and do they work? ■ Do hyperlinks to related sites work?
User considerations	■ Is the site available to everyone, or do you need to register by providing a username and password? ■ Is there a fee for using part of or the entire site? ■ Is there specific content available for members only? ■ Does the site require the use of cookies? ■ Is the site secure for paying when purchasing content or products? ■ Is the site free of any racial or ethnic biases? ■ For users not fluent in English, does the site offer multilingual versions of content?

Adapted from Hasan, L., & Abuelrub, E. (2009). *Assessing the quality of websites.* https://www.researchgate.net/publication/228686530_Assessing_the_Quality_of_Web_Sites/fulltext/00006b4f0cf275ecfef0faf9/Assessing-the-Quality-of-Web-Sites.pdf; Adams, P C. (2019). Geographies of media and communication III: Academic communication and the digital communication environment. *Progress in Human Geography, 43*(4), 739–748 https://doi.org/10.1177/0309132518763849

Writing style for student work varies according to assignment criteria. Nonfiction prose can be developed using description, narration, exposition, and argumentation. Description is used to create a dominant impression. When storytelling is the goal, narration serves as an effective tool. Exposition, which is used to show the "how" and "why" of something, can employ one or more of the following tools: (1) exemplification (providing illustrations or examples for a concept); (2) process analysis (giving step-by-step instructions for how to do something); (3) compare and contrast (outlining similarities and differences); (4) analogy (comparing something unknown to something familiar); (5) classification (placing into groups based on common features); (6) definition (explaining the meaning of something);

and (7) causal analysis (outlining cause-and-effect relationships). Finally, argumentation can be used to present an objective rationale to support a position. A casual or informal debate among friends or colleagues involves a presentation of diverse viewpoints based on personal opinions. However, a scholarly debate consists of having some form of evidence (scientific, statistical, research, or ideally information from a peer-reviewed reference) to substantiate the various views being discussed (Hacker & Sommers, 2019).

Effective writing requires that authors select words to convey messages clearly. Reading serves as a vehicle to expand vocabulary that can be used in writing. Dictionaries and thesauri provide rich source of words for use in writing. Many dictionaries also provide grammatical rules for written language, and word-processing programs offer spelling and grammar check features. Some writers feel it is useful to read aloud passages they have written to hear how they sound (Hacker & Sommers).

Most educational programs have standard formats for written assignments. Students enrolled in these programs should purchase the publication manual for the selected format. Students also may find internet sites that provide assistance with questions about frequently encountered formats such as the American Psychological Association guidelines for manuscript preparation. However, nothing supersedes proofreading by another person to verify that what is written clearly communicates the intended ideas and follows the proper writing guidelines.

In recent years, much attention has been paid to plagiarism. Use of computers and the internet can entice students to cut and paste large pieces of text into assignments and then pass it off as their own work. Plagiarism is best avoided by citing all sources used, avoiding the use of too many citations, paraphrasing and summarizing information carefully, limiting the use of direct quotations, and never purchasing a paper from a friend or paper mill (Stebbins, 2006). Many colleges subscribe to plagiarism detection programs for faculty use. The nursing profession requires that its practitioners be honest and forthright. Most nursing programs have penalties for plagiarized assignments that vary from a warning to removal from the program.

Organizational Skills

Scholastic success requires good organizational skills. Previously learned organizational skills transfer readily in helping to balance personal and professional responsibilities. Work–life–school balance means having a feeling of control, achievement, and enjoyment in daily life (Young & Koopsen, 2011). Key organizational skills for success include managing information, refining test-taking skills, and managing personal time.

Managing Information

The enormous amount of information that one must review, evaluate, and study to remain current in today's professional practice environment challenges all nurses, not just students. Scientific discoveries and changes in health care delivery systems surface quickly. Students and professional nurses spend much time sorting through large volumes of correspondence, publications, advertisements, and professional information. Going through information immediately as it arrives eliminates clutter. Setting priorities for action facilitates meeting professional, personal, and school deadlines. Organizing personal libraries and files saves time by making available resources easier to find (Dunham, 2008; Osuna, 2014; Quan, 2006). To stay abreast of the latest information, some nurses subscribe to online newsletters and service lists (LISTSERV) that offer summaries of new developments in the health care arena.

Refining Test-Taking Skills

Testing serves as a means for assessing learning, yet many students find test taking stressful. Optimal test preparation, which increases the chance of a favorable performance, includes reading all required class assignments, attending class, asking questions during class, taking notes, reviewing learning objectives for each class, reviewing class materials frequently, attending test reviews (if available), and talking with faculty members to clarify content when needed. Some students find they are better prepared if they participate in a peer study group, establish a study schedule, make audiotapes of class sessions (if permitted), outline readings, recopy notes, or create study cards (Dunham, 2008; Osuna, 2014).

Some students become overly anxious during examinations, which may result in poor performance. For some students, a bit of stress may be helpful. Each student perceives stress in a different manner. However, when stress produces anxiety, the following tips might be helpful: arriving 15 minutes early to the test site; practicing relaxation techniques (deep breathing exercises, visualizing success, and guided imagery); skimming notes and textbooks; and talking with classmates. Quan (2006) and Osuna (2014) suggest that study groups offer the opportunity to talk with others about the content covered in courses while also helping to establish new friendships. Complementary health practices such as aromatherapy (e.g., smelling mandarin essential oil, which evokes feelings of calmness, thereby allaying anxiety) may also be useful (Leddy, 2003).

Managing Personal Time

Time takes on paramount importance for all students enrolled in a nursing program because of role conflicts. Balancing work, professional, student, and family responsibilities is an art. Family members may feel neglected. Scheduling time to tend to the needs of family and friends may provide a welcome study break and facilitate the maintenance of optimal mental and spiritual health (Dunham, 2008; Osuna, 2014).

Success in education requires a team effort. Learning to say no and asking for help without feeling guilty are essential time management techniques. Delegation of household tasks (such as cooking, cleaning, and laundry) to other family members frees time for study while providing other family members with an opportunity to learn or refine their own life survival skills (Dunham, 2008; Quan, 2006). Finally, networking with one's colleagues can result in time-saving ideas, such as sharing quick, easy recipes.

IMAGE AND PHYSICAL APPEARANCE

Physical appearance plays a role in projecting a professional image. Nursing caps became obsolete in the 1970s, and nurses quickly abandoned their white uniforms for colorful scrub suits and dresses. Clean, pressed scrubs and dresses present a professional appearance. However, when nurses wear printed scrubs with cartoon characters, they may fail to project the desired professional image unless they are working with children.

Cleanliness and safety should be priorities when preparing for professional practice. Clean clothing, well-manicured natural nails, and clean shoes decrease the spread of infection. Dangling earrings and necklaces can create hazards for nurses if they encounter confused or combative clients. Tongue piercings may impair the clarity of a nurse's speech. When engaging in clinical learning experiences, nursing students must abide by the clinical facility's dress code for staff. Additionally, students must also have clear identification of their student status. Clients must know the name and status of all care providers. Other health care team members need to know when a student is providing care so that they do not have unrealistic expectations. Overall, clients have more confidence in nurses who display a professional appearance.

SOCIALIZATION AND RESOCIALIZATION INTO THE NURSING PROFESSION

Nurses who assume different roles undergo the processes of socialization and resocialization. In simple terms, **socialization** is the process of preparing someone for a particular societal role. The definition of professional socialization is expanded to include the

"formation and internalization of a professional identity congruent with the professional role" (Lynn et al., 1989, p. 232). **Resocialization** occurs when someone adapts their role to a new setting. As they pursue new jobs or educational endeavors throughout their careers, professional nurses have many socialization and resocialization experiences.

Traditionally, the study of socialization emphasizes how external factors, such as family, peers, school, and other institutions, affect a person's development. Professional socialization addresses the processes by which a person develops a professional identity along with how a profession accepts an individual into its ranks.

Significant environmental changes (e.g., changing a job, moving to a different practice setting, returning to school) stimulate the resocialization process. Thus, resocialization is also a lifelong occurrence. Nurses can reduce the discomfort of resocialization by understanding all aspects of the change processes required for successful professional transitions.

For example, some nursing students select a path of educational mobility as their route to entering the nursing profession. These students start health careers as UAP, then become LPN/LVNs or associate degree nurses before pursuing a baccalaureate or higher nursing degree. Resocialization is needed at each level of education to help the nurse synthesize a changed theoretical foundation for practice, adapt to new professional role expectations, and form a new professional identity.

Nurses returning to school provide a rich source of information to educational programs. Because of previous client care experiences, they already possess a sense of self as a nurse; know how to use current health care technologies; understand governmental and accrediting agency regulations; know how to interact with other health care team members; have encountered human suffering and death; have coped with personal fears, anxiety, concerns, and shortcomings; have worked within complex organizations; have seen others who model lifelong learning; and acknowledge the inevitability of change (Diekelmann & Rather, 1993).

Despite their knowledge and expertise, nurses returning to school still face the process of resocialization. Nurses typically undergo a transformation in the way they practice after earning a new degree. In some cases, however, resocialization may be ineffective and students may finish programs with more knowledge but without changes in their internalized professional self-image.

Take Note!
Throughout their education and careers, nurses will face numerous circumstances in which adaptability—their ability to socialize and resocialize—will be key to their success.

REAL-LIFE REFLECTIONS

- *Describe the resocialization process that Sue might experience if she decides to return to school.*
- *How might she make the process easier?*
- *What advice would you give to a student just beginning their nursing education to help them navigate the socialization process?*

Role Theory

Role theory serves as the basis for socialization. As a concept, roles link persons and society. Linton (1945) proposed that a **role** contains three key pieces: values, attitudes, and behaviors. Professional socialization focuses on preparation for a particular role that offers service to society rather than life in general. Because roles are viewed as separate and discontinuous, it is assumed that stress occurs when a person takes on a new role or new expectations within an existing role (Bradby, 1990). When getting married, for example, a person adopts the new role of spouse, and new expectations might be assumed as part of that role (e.g., homemaker, financial supporter, and child caregiver). Adult nursing students often hold multiple roles that sometimes compete for attention, such as employee, relationship partner, and parent. When a new role is assumed (becoming a "student" again), students must adjust how they meet all current life roles. **Role conflict** arises when roles assumed by a person compete with each other for time and attention (Bradby, 1990). The newly acquired student role competes with other roles because of school demands.

Most students enter nursing because they want to help others. In contrast, the professional educational image of the nurse differs somewhat from societal views. These differences include "an increased emphasis on health maintenance and promotion, establishment of analytic and therapeutic nurse–client relationships, strong technical skills along with a broad scientific knowledge base to guide professional interventions, use of critical inquiry processes to creatively individualize nursing care to address client concerns and needs, and the assumption of responsibility and accountability for

patient care decisions" (Hinshaw, 1976, p. 5). Clearly, the socialization process involves changes in knowledge, skills, attitudes, and values that may trigger strong negative emotional reactions.

Take Note!
The changes in knowledge, skills, attitudes, and values required by the socialization process may trigger strong negative emotional reactions.

▐ QUESTIONS FOR REFLECTION

1. What potentially competing roles may surface in your life as you begin your nursing education or return to school?
2. Why is it important to identify potentially competing roles?
3. List your roles in order of priority. Why did you list them in this order?

Shane's Returning-to-School Syndrome

Shane (1980) described a **returning-to-school syndrome** encountered by RNs seeking to earn higher nursing degrees. Although the syndrome was described decades ago, it remains relevant today.

The first phase, the honeymoon phase, is positive. Nurses identify similarities between their previous educational experiences and their present experiences that reinforce their original role identity as a nurse. The nurse feels energetic about learning new things.

The next stage, conflict, is characterized by turbulent negative emotions. Conflict arises during the first nursing theory or clinical nursing course when faculty challenge nurses to change their ways of thinking and/or practicing. Feelings of professional inadequacy may emerge during this stage and may be expressed by angry outbursts, feelings of helplessness, or depression.

Successful resolution of conflict results in the next stage, the beginning of reintegration. Here, nurses struggle to hold on to cherished beliefs about practice and frequently wonder why they decided to pursue a higher degree. Hostile feelings toward the nursing program and faculty are common during this phase.

Once the nurse works through the first three stages, the final stage of integration emerges. This stage is characterized by the ability to blend the original culture of work with the new culture of school. The integration of the old with the new results in a positive resolution of the returning-to-school syndrome. Nurses recognize that a transformation has occurred. They notice that their clinical practice has forever changed, and they incorporate their newly acquired theoretical knowledge into practice. Using in practice what they have learned in school stimulates these nurses and fosters a new curiosity to learn more.

Moving into a new practice arena or position may mean that despite years of clinical experience and specialized education, an expert nurse becomes a novice again. By recognizing the various stages of socialization and resocialization processes, nurses can identify sources of actual and potential feelings of discomfort and work effectively by steering rather than reacting to the processes of change.

REAL-LIFE REFLECTIONS

- *Thinking back to Sue, what assumptions can you identify that she has made about the benefit of seeking a baccalaureate degree in nursing?*
- *What personal transitions will be required of Sue to successfully work through resocialization using Shane's returning-to-school syndrome?*
- *Why are these transitions important?*

Bridges's Managing Transitions

The work of William Bridges offers an explanation of the personal changes that occur when someone returns to school. In his original work (2003), he proposed that individuals undergo **transitions** (psychological adaptations to changes) whenever they are exposed to changes. Bridges developed a three-step process to facilitate transitions that "starts with an ending and finishes with a beginning" (p. 5). According to Bridges, people do not move sequentially through the phases; instead, they experience the phases, sometimes simultaneously. Bridges and Bridges (2019) updated the model specifying that change begins with an ending and ends with a new beginning. Between the ending and the new beginning, there is a neutral zone that must be effectively managed to make the new beginning possible.

The first phase is "ending" previous behaviors and identities and envisioning a new reality (Bridges & Bridges, 2019). Professional nursing students frequently experience stress as they embark on a new educational program because they realize that what they have done in past practice may not have always been the best practice. Beginning nursing students encounter stress because they are uncertain if they can do what is needed to become a professional nurse.

Bridges's second phase is called "the neutral zone," which is when the old identity has vanished but the new one is not fully developed. People going through this phase experience an unsettled feeling because they may not know how to act or what questions to ask. They try new ways of looking at and doing things without discarding the old ways. They are uncertain about the new expectations to attain the new way of being. When starting a new course or educational program, students sometimes do not know how to begin. In a beginning nursing program (ADN or BSN), students assume a new role of nurse. Nurses returning to college for a bachelor's or advanced nursing degree must assume the role of a student and reconcile with the new role of a professional or advanced practice nurse (APRN). Feelings of fearful uneasiness surface as the person tries to reconcile the new with the old. If a person leaves the neutral zone before repatterning is solidified, the change will most likely not be successful. Bridges and Bridges (2019) describe the neutral zone as being a lonely place; interpersonal communication is therefore essential. When in the neutral zone, individuals experience distress and need the support of others. Creative use of the neutral zone involves setting short-term goals, spending time in personal reflection to examine the meaning of change, discovering new ways of doing things, experimenting with the new role, taking time to embrace setbacks and losses, and networking with others in similar transitions. Students enrolled in the same program frequently and effectively support each other while experiencing the neutral zone. After working through the uncertainty and obscurity of the neutral zone, they make an emotional commitment to start anew.

Bridges (2003) called the final phase the new beginning, which is a mental image or experience hallmarked by "a release of new energy in a new direction" (p. 57). A new beginning means a new commitment and identity. Bridges specified that new beginnings require four Ps: "the purpose, a picture, the plan, and a part to play" (p. 60). Quick successes such as the accomplishment of small goals facilitate the process of internalizing a new identity. For example, professional nursing students who actually use theories derived from best evidence to guide clinical practice may see the positive effects of a theoretically based practice. Take the situation of a nurse caring for a client who is having difficulty sleeping. A theoretical approach to the problem analyzes and addresses the environmental, psychological, and spiritual factors that may be interfering with the client's ability to sleep. Instead of immediately administering a sedative, the nurse rubs the client's back and spends time talking with the client who expresses concern about the impact of the current illness on their family. After sharing the concerns with the nurse and with the muscle relaxation that occurs from the massage, the client is able to sleep without a sedative.

DEVELOPING A PROFESSIONAL SELF-CONCEPT

As a person develops patterns of behavior, the self-system becomes organized and strives to actualize itself, though it is continually being repatterned. The self-system interacts symbiotically with the environment, providing the conditions from which a personal view of the self emerges—the self-concept. The self-concept encompasses all beliefs about oneself and personal interpretations about the past, present, and future (Jones, 2004). Because humans develop personal selves first, those personally organized sets of behaviors form the basis of the selves brought into the profession. Thus, the personal self strongly influences the emerging professional self.

The development of the **professional self-concept** (how a person perceives oneself as a nurse) follows the same path as that of development of the personal self. In every profession, the professional has significant others. During various stages of professional growth and development, nurses have different significant others who help them during times of transitions. For example, beginning nursing students may view faculty members as significant others, whereas novice nurses may identify experienced nursing colleagues and/or nurse managers as significant others.

Significant others in professional self-development serve as role models or mentors as nurses adjust to changing situations and try to be the kind of person capable of meeting situational demands. Role models provide nurses with examples of how to be, and mentors provide guidance and emotional support. Professional self-concept development also requires that individual nurses engage in episodic self-appraisal along with a willingness to accept the challenges and criticisms of mentors and role models. The personal self-concept cannot be separated from the professional self-concept, though professional significant others are different from personal significant others.

Successful implementation of professional nursing roles and tasks reinforces one's perception of the professional self. Repeated successes in practice solidify the concept of being a competent professional nurse, resulting in increased self-confidence. Because the development of a professional self requires interactions with others in the profession, separating the developmental from the socialization processes may be impossible.

Benner's Novice-to-Expert Model

Benner (1984) devised a model of stages from novice to expert that has relevance for experienced nurses. Benner's **novice-to-expert model** describes stages in the progression of client care expertise that can result from practicing nursing experience (Table 1.2). This model, based on the work by Dreyfus and Dreyfus (1980), suggests the following three general aspects of skilled performance:

1. Movement from reliance on abstract principles to the use of past concrete experience as paradigms
2. Change in perception of what is needed in a particular situation from a compilation of equally important bits of information to a more or less complete whole in which only certain parts are relevant
3. Passage from detached observer to involved performer who is engaged in the situation

Stage I, the novice stage, corresponds to the student experience in nursing school. Because no background understanding exists, the novice depends on context-free rules to guide actions. Although this approach enhances safety, "rule-governed behavior is extremely limited and inflexible" (Benner, 1984, p. 21). When nursing students encounter situations that do not conform to the rules learned, they become highly critical of what happened and cling steadfastly to what they learned in class.

TABLE 1.2	**Benner's Stages From Novice to Expert**				
	Stage I	**Stage II**	**Stage III**	**Stage IV**	**Stage V**
Title	Novice	Advanced beginner	Competent	Proficient	Expert
Experience level	Student	New graduate	2–3 years in same setting	3–5 years in same setting	Extensive time in one or many settings
Characteristics of performance	Is inflexible Exhibits rule-governed behavior	Formulates principles Needs help with priority setting	Plans Has feelings of mastery	Perceives "wholes" Interprets nuances	Has an intuitive grasp

Data from Benner, P. (1984). *From novice to expert: Excellence and power in clinical nursing practice* (pp. 21–34). Addison-Wesley.

The new nursing graduate demonstrates marginally acceptable performance as an advanced beginner in stage II. The advanced beginner relies on basic theory and principles and believes that "clinical situations have a discernible order" (Benner et al., 1996, p. 54). The advanced beginner can formulate principles for actions, but because all actions are viewed as equally important, help is needed for priority setting. Advanced beginners typically become uncomfortable when they encounter chaotic clinical situations.

The competent practitioner, who has reached stage III, has typically worked in the same setting for 2 to 3 years. This person has conscious awareness of long-range goals and can engage in deliberate planning based on abstract and analytical contemplation. As a result of this planning activity, the practitioner has a feeling of mastery and the ability to cope with contingencies and feels efficient and organized. Competent practitioners must typically think about what can be done before acting in novel or chaotic situations.

By stage IV, which requires 3 to 5 years of experience, the nurse is a proficient practitioner. The proficient nurse perceives situations as "wholes" rather than as accumulations of aspects, and performance is guided by maxims. Actions do not need to be thought out, and meanings are perceived in relation to long-term goals. In addition, the proficient practitioner can interpret nuances in situations and recognize which aspects of a situation are most significant. Proficient practitioners automatically use creative adaptive strategies when they encounter complex, unfamiliar, or chaotic clinical situations.

The fifth and final stage—expert practitioner—is achieved only after extensive experience. The expert has an intuitive grasp of situations and thus does not have to think through actions analytically. In fact, experts are so skilled at grasping the situation as a whole that they are often unable to think in terms of steps. Expert nurses instinctively act effectively for the client's welfare in any clinical situation.

Professional Nursing Roles

Benner (1984, p. 6) recognized that nurses use many competencies as they engage in clinical practice. She organized them into the following seven categories according to the roles and key functions that fall within the domain of professional nursing.

1. "The helping role" provides the foundation for the roles of caregiver (provider of direct client care), colleague (helpful team member), and client advocate (person looking out for the client's best interests).

2. "The teaching–coaching function" provides the foundation for the roles of teacher (provider of education and information) and counselor (one who provides emotional support and encouragement).

3. "The diagnostic and patient-monitoring function" provides the foundation for the caregiver and critical thinker (someone who uses complex thought processes) roles.

4. "Effective management of rapidly changing situations" provides the foundation for the caregiver, change agent (person who initiates and guides the change process), and coordinator (person who manages, leads, and verifies that things get done) roles.

5. "Administration and monitoring of therapeutic interventions and regimens" provide the foundation for the caregiver and change agent roles.

6. "Monitoring of and ensuring the quality of health care practices" provide the foundation for the roles of coordinator, client advocate, and change agent.

7. "Organizational and work-role competencies" provide the foundation for the client advocate, change agent, and coordinator roles.

According to Benner, experience is absolutely necessary for the development of professional expertise.

CHARACTERISTICS OF A PROFESSION

The **characteristics of a profession** (what differentiates a professional from a technician) have been debated for many years. The Flexner Report issued by the Carnegie Foundation in 1910 served as the criteria for determining medicine as a profession. Since the 1950s, the nursing profession has been analyzed using sociologic theories that define a "profession."

Although considered a profession for many years, an assessment of the characteristics of a profession reveals that nursing fails to meet all required criteria and is more accurately classified as an "emerging profession" (Table 1.3). Although nursing does use a specialized knowledge base, has autonomy and control over its work, requires specialized competence, regulates itself, possesses a collegial subculture, and has public acceptance (Freidson, 1994; Miller et al., 1993), nursing fails to have standardized education criteria for entry into the profession.

 Take Note!
Although considered a profession for many years, an assessment of the characteristics of a profession reveals that nursing fails to meet all required criteria and is more accurately classified as an "emerging profession."

TABLE 1.3 Professional Status Progress: How Nursing Meets Characteristics of a Profession

Professional Characteristics	How Nursing Meets the Criteria or Characteristic
Authority to control its own work	■ Nurses work for physicians or health care agencies unless engaged in private advanced nursing practice. ■ State boards of nursing set rules and regulations for practice in nurse practice acts.
Specialized body of knowledge	■ Nurses pull from a variety of fields to provide holistic nursing care. ■ Nursing research generates new scientific knowledge for practice.
Specialized plan of formal education	Currently, there are three levels of education for entry into professional nursing practice: associate degree, diploma, and baccalaureate nursing programs.
Specialized competence	■ Nurses demonstrate assessment skills; possess an understanding of pharmacology, various branches of physical sciences, pathophysiology, diagnostic tests, and surgical procedures; and have skills to manage the technical equipment used in client care. ■ Many nurses hold certifications in specialized areas of nursing practice.
Control over work performance	■ Nurses make independent judgments based on client situations and area of practice. ■ Some nurses work in organizations that use shared governance and quality management frameworks.
Service to society	■ Nursing care focuses on the client system. ■ Caring for others serves as a major theme in most nursing theories. ■ Nurses receive middle-income pay for taking care of others.
Self-regulation	■ Nurses abide by the nurse practice act of the state in which they practice. ■ Individual state boards of nursing regulate nursing practice.
Credentialing systems to certify competence	■ Nurses take the National Certification Licensing Examination (NCLEX) developed by nurses, which measures minimum competence for safe nursing practice. ■ Nurses obtain certification in specialized areas of nursing practice from nurse specialty organizations. ■ Some states require continuing education for continued licensure.
Legal reinforcement of professional standards	■ All nurses are held liable for their actions based on what a reasonable and prudent nurse would do in a given client care situation. ■ Individual state boards of nursing have the power to restrict the practice of nursing within a state.
Ethical practice	The ANA and ICN have both published codes of ethics for nurses.
A collegial subculture	Professional nursing organizations offer networking opportunities, shared governance, and clinical practice partnership models, and they enhance collegiality among staff nurses and nursing administration.
Intrinsic rewards	■ Many nurses derive deep personal satisfaction from making a difference in the lives of clients and families. ■ Some nurses view the profession as an opportunity to practice religious beliefs on a daily basis.
Societal acceptance	Nursing has been ranked as the most honest and ethical of all the professions for 18 years according to polling done by Gallup in 2019 (Reinhart, 2020).

Currently, three levels of education qualify individuals to take the licensing examination for professional nurse registration. The **associate degree in nursing (ADN)** consists of 2 years of concentrated study focused on clinical skills in the community college setting. The **diploma nursing program** offers 3 years of nursing education focused on learning nursing skills in a hospital-based setting. In diploma nursing programs, students typically receive the most clock hours of clinical instruction. The **bachelor of science in nursing (BSN),** or baccalaureate, degrees consist of 4 years of nursing education in institutions of higher learning (4-year colleges and universities). Along with education focused on the art and science of nursing, BSN programs also emphasize the importance of a liberal education, nursing research, and community health nursing. The U.S. Health Resources and Service Administration's Health Workforce Bureau (2020) reported that 63.3% of all practicing nurses held a BSN or higher degree in nursing.

Trends in the initial preparation of professional nurses have changed over time. Table 1.4 summarizes key changes. Diploma nursing programs prepared the majority of new nurses until 1971. Associate degree

TABLE 1.4   Percentage of Graduates From Baccalaureate, Associate Degree, and Diploma Nursing Programs, 1960–2015

Year	Baccalaureate (%)	Associate Degree (%)	Diploma (%)
1960–1961	13	3	84
1970–1971	21	31	48
1980–1981	33	50	17
1990–1991	27	65	8
2001	36	60	4
2010	39.3	58	2.7
2015	44.9	53.4	1.7
2019*	492	49.5	1.3

Note: The National Council of State Boards of Nursing reporting years changed from July 1 to June 30 to a traditional calendar year in 1997.
*2020 NCLEX-RN statistics will not be available until summer 2021.
From Hood, L. J., & Leddy, S. K. (2006). *Leddy & Pepper's conceptual base of professional nursing* (6th ed.). Lippincott Williams & Wilkins; National Council of State Boards of Nursing. (2012). *Revised 2010 nurse licensee volume and NCLEX® examination statistics.* http://www.ncsbn.org/12_REVISED_2010NCLEX-ExamStats_Vol52.pdf; National Council of State Boards of Nursing . (2016a). *2015 Number of candidates taking NCLEX examination and percent passing by type of candidate*. https://www.ncsbn.org/Table_of_Pass_Rates_2015_(3).pdf; National Council of State Boards of Nursing. (2000). *NCSBN research brief: 2019 NCLEX® exam statistics*. https://www.ncsbn.org/2019_NCLEXExamStats.pdf

nursing programs prepared most of the new nurses by the mid-1970s and continue to be the dominant form of educational preparation for newly licensed professional nurses. However, the number of baccalaureate-prepared nurses appears to be continually rising. In 2019, the number of newly educated graduate nurses from associate degree programs was 84,798; 84,282 graduate nurses completed BSN degrees (NCSBN, 2020c).

Intellectual Characteristics

Because nurses make decisions that affect clients' lives, they need the intellectual capability to master scientific concepts, understand the impact of themselves on others, use this information in clinical practice, and understand potential consequences of alternative actions (AACN, 2008). Professional nurses possess the following three intellectual characteristics:

1. A body of knowledge on which professional practice is based
2. A specialized education to transmit this body of knowledge to others
3. The ability to use their knowledge in critical and creative thinking

Because of the global nature of professional nursing to meet client care needs, nurses frequently use knowledge that originated in other professional disciplines. However, they use the cognitive skills of critical and creative thinking to adapt this knowledge to the realm of professional nursing practice.

Specialized Body of Knowledge

Professional practice is based on a body of knowledge derived from experience (leading to expertise) and research (leading to theoretical foundations for knowledge and practice). Most state boards of nursing (SBNs) specify that an ADN serves as the minimum educational qualification for practice as an RN. However, according to the IOM's extensive 2011 literature review, clients who receive care from baccalaureate-prepared nurses had better outcomes than those who received care from associate degree–prepared nurses. Areas of improved outcomes included reduced incidences of hospital-acquired pneumonia, urinary catheter–associated infections, and failure to rescue (recognition of early signs of life-threatening complications and taking action before clients experienced a respiratory or cardiac arrest).

Most states require advanced education and professional certification for nurses who assume advanced practice roles. Professional nurses make clinical judgments based on solid, scientific rationales. They modify plans and actions to meet the demands of specific client situations. ADN programs tend to emphasize technical skills over theoretical concepts. New nurses and nurses who have been educated with a skills focus seek out a single "right" answer when delivering client care. However, seasoned nurses use theory in practice, anticipate complications before they occur, analyze all aspects that affect health care delivery, and adapt institutional policies and procedures when needed to address complex client care situations.

Liberal arts education serves as a hallmark of professional education. A liberal arts education provides a knowledge base that enhances a person's ability to practice citizenship, communicate effectively, appreciate advantages of diverse viewpoints, and understand more deeply what it means to be human. Liberal arts courses foster the development of thinking and communication skills, cognizance of historical contributions, understanding of science, exploration of personal values, appreciation of the fine arts, and sensitivity of human diversity (AACN, 2008, 2021). ADN educational programs require nearly 2 years of liberal education, especially in science and mathematics, and baccalaureate degree programs include courses in fine arts, statistics, and social sciences that provide baccalaureate degree nurses with a broader perspective of what it means to be human. Knowledge and skills derived from a liberal arts education enhance the nurse's ability to adapt knowledge and skills to novel situations through the use of global rather than narrow thinking.

Whether nursing has a unique body of knowledge or applies knowledge borrowed from the fields of medical, behavioral, or physical science has long been a matter of debate. In the early days of nursing, nurses derived knowledge through intuition, tradition, and experience or by borrowing it from other disciplines (Kalisch & Kalisch, 2004). Today, the nursing profession uses nursing models and frameworks as a foundation for practice. These models and frameworks provide guidance for nurse researchers to scientifically substantiate the unique contributions that nurses make in health care delivery.

Specialized Plan of Formal Education

The NCSBN coordinates efforts to license registered and practical nurses. The NCSBN Nursing Licensure Examination for Registered Nurses (NCLEX-RN) provides computer-adaptive testing that measures minimal competence for safe professional nursing practice. Examination content includes health promotion, pharmacotherapeutics, nursing assessment, clinical decision making, nursing interventions, and client care outcome evaluation.

Education for other health care professions (pharmacists, social workers, physical therapists, occupational therapists, chaplains, and physicians) requires postbaccalaureate education. Some nursing leaders have proposed requiring a master's degree (or even a doctorate) as the educational entry level for professional nursing. The IOM (2011) recommends that by 2020, 80% of all RNs hold bachelor degrees in nursing. The IOM report also recommends interdisciplinary education of all future health team members, including professional nurses. Some collegiate health science programs offer interdisciplinary learning experiences that provide nursing students an opportunity to collaborate with other future interprofessional health team members.

In 1965, the ANA issued a white paper (a detailed proposal) that specified that the entry level into professional nursing should be the BSN degree. The AACN concurs with this position. Efforts during the mid-1980s resulted in **differentiated competencies** for ADN- and BSN-prepared nurses. Professional nursing has two accrediting agencies for nursing education programs—the National League for Nursing (NLN) (all levels of nursing education from practical/vocational nursing through doctoral programs) and the AACN for baccalaureate and higher-degree programs (Kumm et al., 2014). Distinguishing program outcomes and competencies for each level of nursing education has been difficult. According to a study by Kumm and colleagues (2014), the following six outcomes and competencies are present exclusively in BSN nursing programs: liberal education; organizational and system leadership for client safety and quality care; evidence-based practice and nursing scholarship; health care policy, financing, and regulatory systems; interprofessional communication and collaboration to improve client outcomes and clinical prevention; and population health.

In 2010, the NLN developed a list of differentiated competencies for professional nurses based upon earned degrees. The NLN differentiated competencies fall under the domains of human flourishing, nursing judgment, professional identity, and spirit of inquiry (NLN, 2010). Table 1.5 outlines the different expectations of ADN- and BSN-prepared nurses. All nurses advocate for their clients and act as interprofessional colleagues. ADN competencies tend to center around caregiver, counselor, and educator roles with clients and families, whereas BSN competencies include working with communities. However, in recent years, ADN nurses are educated to provide nursing care following established evidence-based policies and procedures while using critical thinking skills to make decisions when deviations to policies and procedures are needed.

TABLE 1.5   Differentiated Core Competencies for ADN- and BSN-Prepared Nurses

ADN-Prepared Nurses	BSN-Prepared Nurses
Advocate for clients and families when needs arise during the provision of nursing care services	Advocate for clients, families, and communities during the provision of nursing care services and in the political process to affect health care policy development
Make evidence-based practice judgments to provide safe, high-quality care to promote client health, recognizing the effects of the client's family and community	Make evidence-based and theoretical-based nursing judgments using nursing and borrowed theories to provide safe, quality care to promote the health of clients, families, and communities
Practice professional nursing with diverse clients and families in a responsible, ethical manner with utmost integrity and develop an ever-changing professional self-identity with a commitment to caring for others using evidence to guide practice and serving in an advocacy role when needed	Practice professional nursing with diverse clients, families, and communities in a responsible, ethical manner with utmost integrity and develop an ever-changing professional self-identity with a commitment to caring for others, using evidence to guide practice, serving in an advocacy role when needed, providing leadership to others, and assuming leadership in the change process to improve care services
Challenge the status quo of clinical practices, examine evidence underlying assumptions for current practice, and offer suggestions to improve the quality of care for clients and families	Challenge the status quo of clinical practices, identify questions to ask to guide accessing evidence to answer clinical questions, seek out high-quality evidence, critique the available evidence to either substantiate current practice or identify key areas for practice changes, propose nursing innovations when needed, and follow established processes for making changes within the context of care delivery to improve the quality of care for clients, families, and communities Use concepts and theories from liberal arts studies to guide professional practice and engage with clients, families, health care team members, and communities while understanding, appreciating, and respecting care variation, increased complexity, and increased use of all available resources (organizational, private, and public) required for attaining, maintaining, and retaining optimal health for all Develop, design, manage, and coordinate care for clients, families, and communities
Use computer technology effectively for direct client care to access reliable evidence for practice and obtain relevant and accurate client and family education materials	Use computer technology effectively for direct client care to access reliable evidence for practice and obtain relevant and accurate client, family, and community education materials Effectively conduct computerized database searches for relevant and valid evidence for critique
Use critical thinking and nursing process effectively	Use critical and *creative* thinking and nursing process effectively and incorporate reflection in action and reflection on action into daily clinical practice
Follow rules, laws, and regulations when engaging in professional practice	Engage in legal professional practice and participate in political and legislative processes to improve health care policies, regulations, and laws
Conduct physical, psychological, and spiritual client assessments	Conduct holistic client, family, and community assessments by paying close attention to environmental factors that affect the quality of human life
Use material, financial, and human resources effectively to implement health care services to clients and families	Use and coordinate material, financial, and human resources to maximize access to and implementation of health care services to clients, families, and communities
Identify issues and trends that affect the nursing profession, clinical practice, and health care delivery	Identify and analyze technology to understand and generate possible solutions for issues and trends affecting the nursing profession, clinical practice, health, quality of life, and health care delivery for clients, families, communities, and society
Apply basic principles of disaster preparedness and contagious disease control and prevention for clients and families	Use principles and theoretical models of epidemiology for contagious disease and control, evidence-based risk reduction, and theoretical models for disaster preparedness and response and recovery when providing services to clients, families, and communities

Form National League for Nursing. (2010). *Outcomes and competencies for graduates of practical/vocational, diploma, baccalaureate and masters nursing programs.* New York: National League for Nursing; American Association of Colleges of Nursing. (2021). *The essentials: Core competencies for professional nursing education.* https://www.aacnnursing.org/Portals/42/AcademicNursing/ pdf/Essentials-Final-Draft-2-18-21.pdf. Texas Board of Nursing. (2011). *Differentiated essential competences (DECs) of graduates of Texas nursing programs evidenced by knowledge, clinical judgment and behaviors.* Texas Board of Nursing.

BSN-prepared nurses are educated to engage in independent thinking, analyze current evidence-based practices, critique new research findings, and spearhead efforts to change practice standards for improved nursing care. ADN and BSN nurses practice in a variety of settings. Because of the independence required and the complexity of community health nursing, BSN preparation has become the minimal education preparation for this specialized area of professional nursing practice.

However, implementation of the different levels of practice has been difficult because after gaining years of valuable clinical experience, ADN-prepared nurses have effectively assumed leadership and supervisory roles in many health care organizations. Still, many health care organizations require at least BSN and sometimes graduate nursing degrees for nursing management positions. Some health care organizations use clinical ladders for promoting staff nurses, and many of these require a BSN degree to reach higher levels. Along with organizational requirements, multiple research studies have demonstrated that clients have improved outcomes when receiving care from BSN-prepared nurses and nurses who hold certifications in specialized areas of clinical practice.

▌ QUESTIONS FOR REFLECTION

1. Which of the BSN outcomes/competencies listed in Table 1.5 do you think will be of utmost interest to you as you pursue your degree? Why do these interest you the most?

2. Which of the BSN outcomes/competencies listed in Table 1.5 do you not find particularly interesting to you? Why do you find these less interesting?

3. Do you agree with the list of differentiated competencies for ADN- and BSN-prepared nurses found in Table 1.5? Why or why not?

Currently, LPNs provide direct resident care in extended facilities, and RNs provide supervision. Many times, the RN supervisor in an extended care facility has been prepared at the associate degree level. The Pew Health Professions Commission (1998) emphasized the importance of strengthening career mobility paths within the nursing profession and proposed a seamless educational path from nursing assistant to RN and RN to nursing doctorate. Aiken et al. (2003) published a landmark study that found that surgical client outcomes differed based on the educational level of RNs

caring for them. The study findings suggest that when clients receive care in an acute care unit staffed with 50% BSN-prepared nurses, mortality is reduced by 5% and substantial reductions are found in incidences of failure to rescue, nosocomial pneumonia, and pulmonary failure. In 2007, the Agency for Healthcare Research and Quality examined the findings of 94 studies using meta-analysis techniques and found that lower client mortality rates were apt to occur when nurses had BSN preparation and had more than 7 years of nursing experience. The study also showed that statistically significant reductions occurred in failure to rescue, client falls, urinary tract infections, nosocomial pneumonia, and pulmonary failure when nurse-to-client ratios fell from 1:5 to 1:4. This and other studies also found that the likelihood of a nurse making a medication or treatment error increased threefold when shift lengths exceeded 12.5 hours. Harrison and colleagues (2019) found that clients who suffered cardiac arrest who were cared for by BSN-prepared nurses had a 24% greater chance of having better cerebral function outcomes. These and other studies consistently support BSN preparation for all nurses as a means to improve the quality of health care in hospitals.

Graduate nursing education programs offer advanced education for nurses interested in pursuing careers in advanced practice nursing (certified nurse midwifery, nurse practitioners, or clinical nurse specialists) or in nursing education, nursing administration, or nursing informatics. Most graduate nursing education programs offer master's degrees, which can usually be completed within 3 years if a student assumes a full-time plan of study. The majority of programs give students up to 7 years to complete graduate work.

In 2004, the AACN noted several issues with the educational preparation of APRNs at the master's degree level. First, the amount of time spent by nurses engaged in nursing graduate study surpassed the amount of time spent by members of other health care disciplines earning master's degrees (60 vs. 45 credit hours, respectively). Second, some APRNs specified a need for more education to meet the demands of advanced practice. The AACN set a goal that all APRNs would hold a doctor of nursing practice (DNP) degree by 2015. However, this goal was not achieved even though many other members of the interprofessional health care team (e.g., physical therapists, pharmacists, physicians) do. The AACN proposed that graduate nursing programs prepare the clinical nurse leader, who would provide "care in all health settings at the point of care, and assumes accountability for client care outcomes by coordinating, delegating, and supervising the care provided by the health care team" (AACN, 2004, p. 10). Currently, there is much debate over the implementation of the DNP requirement for APRN certification and practice.

Postgraduate nursing education leads to a doctorate in nursing. Traditional doctoral nursing programs offer a philosophy degree (PhD) to prepare nurse researchers and collegiate faculty. Nurses engaged in PhD programs have the expectation to generate new nursing knowledge through a rigorous, scientific research study. The DNP is a clinically focused degree targeted toward an advanced area of nursing practice. Nurses engaged in DNP programs conduct a final, extensive, evidence-based project that is practice- and application oriented. Instead of generating new nursing knowledge, DNP students are expected to translate new scientific advancement to practice situation. Nurses with DNP preparation have the credentials to be clinical faculty in nursing education programs (AACN, 2015). Although less common, some institutions of higher learning still offer clinical doctorates such as doctor of nursing (DN) or the doctor of nursing science (DNS or DNSc). Grants and scholarships are available for nurses interested in doctoral work.

Using Knowledge by Thinking Critically

Critical thinking has cognitive and affective characteristics. **Critical thinking** imposes standards (Paul, 1992) and prevents illogical thinking. Rubenfeld and Scheffer (2015) identify the following habits of the mind associated with critical thinking: "confidence, contextual perspective, creativity, flexibility, inquisitiveness, intellectual integrity, intuition, open-mindedness, perseverance, and reflection" (p. 7). They also identify the cognitive skills of critical thinking as "analyzing, applying standards, discriminating, information seeking, logical reasoning, predicting, and transforming knowledge" (p. 7).

Creative Thinking

As a key component of critical thinking (Rubenfeld & Scheffer, 2015), **creative thinking** generates alternative approaches to clinical situations. Creative thinking requires an ability to think outside of what usually is done and results in novel approaches to client care. If not tempered with critical thinking, however, solutions generated with creative thinking may be hazardous.

For example, when using therapeutic touch to relieve a client's pain, the nurse notes that the client experiences a substantial fall in blood pressure resulting in hypotension. If the hypotension results in the client fainting when getting out of bed after the therapeutic touch session and sustaining an injury, the nurse is accountable for the adverse outcome. Nurses engage in creative thinking when confronted with clients who have complex integrative health problems that require individually designed plans to attain desired outcomes.

Reflective Thinking

Reflective thinking is engaging in purposeful analysis about what one is currently doing and about what one has done (Schon, 1987). Reflection plays a key role in professional nursing practice (Fig. 1.4). Consider the following clinical situation:

> *Ms. S has advanced cancer and lives in constant pain. Because the pain is unbearable, Ms. S's physician orders patient-controlled analgesia (PCA) with morphine. Ms. S is fearful that the morphine will not ease her pain, will result in addiction, and will produce a loss of consciousness. Her fear and anxiety cause increased muscle tension. As the nurse initiates the morphine drip, she remembers the pharmacologic action and potential adverse effects of the morphine. She educates Ms. S about morphine and how best to use the PCA device for optimal pain control. As the nurse talks with Ms. S, she performs a back massage, knowing the evidence-based benefits of human touch and the physiologic response to muscle massage.*

When nurses think about theoretical and scientific principles while delivering client care, they engage in **reflection in action** (Clarke et al., 1996; Kim, 1999; Powell, 1989; Schon, 1983).

FIGURE 1.4 Reflective thinking enables nurses to analyze and improve their professional performance.

Schon (1983, 1987) advocated for reflection on action, another form of professional reflection. **Reflection on action** occurs when the professional practitioner conducts a retrospective analysis of the action taken (Clarke et al., 1996; Schon, 1987). Returning to the previous example, the nurse analyzes care given to Ms. S considering what interventions were implemented and whether they were successful. Reflection on action enables the practitioner to develop a deeper understanding of practice and provides a vehicle to learn from experience (Clarke et al., 1996; Schon, 1987). Journal writing also provides practice with reflection on action.

Take Note!
Cognitive skills such as critical, creative, and reflective thinking help nurses make sound clinical decisions when providing client care.

Independent Clinical Decision Making

Professional nurses make independent decisions to solve problems in clinical practice. Sometimes, nurses act prematurely because of inadequate information and insufficient time to generate alternative approaches.

When nurses critical thinking and logical reasoning to support the actions taken, they make effective clinical decisions.

Concepts in Practice

Visiting Hours

Which of the following actions would you take with a client whose visitors insist on staying beyond the visiting hours established by hospital policy?

1. *Possible action 1:* Tell the client and the visitors that the visitors must leave.
2. *Possible action 2:* Allow the visitors to stay for an additional hour.
3. *Possible action 3:* Explore the reasons why the visitors want to stay and the significance of having the visitors spend time with the client. Base your decision on the result of information generated.

As a nurse, you would use critical thinking to realize that collecting more information surrounding the situation will result in an optimal decision. Perhaps the visitors have arrived from out of town and have no place to stay. Maybe the client has not seen them in a long time or the client may be afraid to be left alone in the hospital the night before a potentially life-threatening procedure.

Nursing Process

Nurses use the **nursing process**, a systematic thinking method, to process information about specific client care situations. This problem-solving process consists of five interacting steps: assessment, diagnosis, planning, implementation, and evaluation (Fig. 1.5). Assessment consists of collecting subjective (what clients say) and objective (measured or verifiable by the care provider) information about clients. Nurses then categorize data into clusters to determine nursing diagnoses (an actual or potential client response) upon which a care plan is developed. After the care plan is implemented (executed), nurses evaluate the effectiveness of the plan and start the process again with assessment. Effective use of the nursing process requires critical, creative, and reflective thinking.

Service to Society

Ever since nursing began, it has been associated with serving others. However, the intrinsic motivation "to care" is only one way to look at caring. Morse et al. (1991, p. 122) identified the following five conceptualizations of caring: (1) caring as a human trait; (2) caring as a moral imperative; (3) caring as an affect; (4) caring as an interpersonal interaction; and (5) caring as a therapeutic intervention. Obviously, caring encompasses more than just intuitive concern for others. Several nursing theories use caring as a major concept or central theme.

Professional service to society requires impeccable integrity, individual responsibility for ethical practice, and lifelong commitment. However, some nurses view nursing as a job rather than a profession.

Many nurses leave the profession (permanently or temporarily) to pursue personal interests or to care for families. Some nurses work to supplement family incomes, and others work because they are the sole or primary income providers for their family. Nurses who need job security avoid confronting less-than-ideal nursing practice situations. Employing agencies sometimes exploit these nurses. Regardless of high client-to-nurse ratios, rotating shifts, and floating, some nurses maintain the status quo. However, other nurses confront poor working conditions and always do what is best for clients.

Service to others involves ethical and legal responsibilities. Nurses must have the integrity to do what is right, especially in situations that may cause moral dilemmas. The International Council of Nurses (ICN) has published a code of ethics (2012) and the ANA

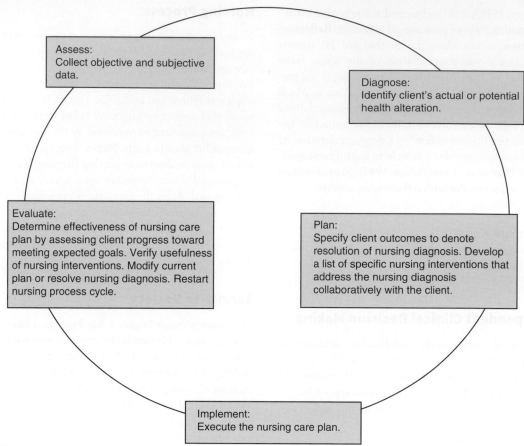

Assess:
Collect objective and subjective data.

Diagnose:
Identify client's actual or potential health alteration.

Evaluate:
Determine effectiveness of nursing care plan by assessing client progress toward meeting expected goals. Verify usefulness of nursing interventions. Modify current plan or resolve nursing diagnosis. Restart nursing process cycle.

Plan:
Specify client outcomes to denote resolution of nursing diagnosis. Develop a list of specific nursing interventions that address the nursing diagnosis collaboratively with the client.

Implement:
Execute the nursing care plan.

FIGURE 1.5 Nursing process as a continuous cycle.

(2015) also has published a code of ethics and social policy statements for nurses to follow. Fowler (2015b) articulates that the *ANA's Nursing's Social Policy Statement* serves as a reciprocal contract between nurses and society. Society expects nurses to offer caring services with the client as the primary concern of the nurse when services are offered. Nurses are expected to have the necessary knowledge, skill, and competence to execute their professional duties. Nurses also acknowledge that there are hazards associated with client care (violent clients, exposure to contagious diseases, and placing oneself in peril to negotiate hazardous weather conditions to report for duty). Nurses as individuals and as members of the profession are accountable and responsible for professional practice endeavors. Professional nurses are expected to develop and stay abreast of new scientific knowledge to improve the health of all people. They also must engage in ethical practice as specified by professional nursing codes of ethics. As members of an interprofessional health care team, they are expected to collaborate with other team members and recipients of care to identify care needs, set care

outcomes, and plan care. Nurses are also expected to promote the health of the public by addressing health disparities and intervening to protect the public via whistle-blowing and advocacy efforts. In return, nurses expect society to authorize practice autonomy, extend self-governance, protect the title of RN and scope of practice, receive respect and fair remuneration for services, be free to practice nursing to the full extent of educational preparation, receive support to sustain the nursing profession, and be protected from hazardous service activities.

Service to society requires legal assurances that practitioners are competent. Credentialing systems, such as licensure, provide a means to certify minimal competence for safe practice by a person legally permitted to use the title "registered nurse." State nurse practice acts also provide legal reinforcement against incompetence. Upon initial state licensure, the nurse receives a copy of their state's nurse practice act. Printed copies of specific nurse practice acts can be obtained from individual SBNs (a fee usually is charged), or copies may be downloaded from SBN websites. When litigation occurs, courts hold nurses accountable for what a typical and prudent nurse would do in a particular client care situation.

Autonomy and Self-Regulation

Autonomy means professionals have control over their practice and are not controlled by others. In the early days of nursing, nurses followed physician orders while tending to the basic needs of clients. As practice evolved, nurses could be held accountable for executing physician orders that resulted in harm to clients under their care. Levels of autonomy vary according to professional nursing practice roles and regulations. The following Focus on Research box outlines how perceptions of autonomy vary among professional nurses.

Autonomy involves independence, a willingness to take risks, and accountability for one's actions, as well as self-determination and self-regulation. In the United States, each state has a nursing board that governs practice that occurs within its borders. **State boards of nursing** regulate professional nursing practice by issuing professional licenses to qualified individuals. Through licensure and the legal system, society protects consumers from unsafe nursing practice by holding nurses responsible for their professional actions. SBNs have legal authority to ensure that all nurses follow the state's nurse practice act. Thus, the nursing profession regulates itself.

FOCUS ON RESEARCH

Registered Nurses' Perceptions of and Experiences with Autonomy

Because of differences in nurse perceptions of autonomy worldwide (especially in England and the United States), the investigators conducted a descriptive phenomenology analysis of 48 interviews with nurses from two different hospitals in Britain's National Health Service. The aim of the study was to see how British nurses conceptualized and experienced autonomy in everyday nursing practice.

The primary investigator of the study interviewed all participants and asked the nurses four questions while the nurses were on break; each interview lasted between 6 and 18 minutes. The questions asked about each nurse's understanding and meaning of autonomy to provide an experience of autonomous practice and to comment about what they thought was missing in autonomous practice. The primary investigator interviewed nurses from 28 units that were located in two large general hospitals (one with 500 beds and the other with 600 beds). Interviews were conducted with 26 nurses at one hospital and 22 nurses at the other hospital. Of the participants, 45 were female; all had varying years of practice; 22 practiced at the bedside; 2 were charge nurses; 11 were ward sisters (i.e., head nurses or nurse managers); 22 were ward managers. No new themes or patterns emerged after 48 interviews were completed.

The interview transcripts were transcribed verbatim. The primary investigator read and sorted interviewee quotes into meaningful units that were then condensed and consolidated into subthemes, which were later merged into general themes. The other members of the interview team independently read and confirmed the identified meaningful units, subthemes, and themes.

Six main themes emerged from the interviews, starting with *working independently.* According to the interviews, this meant working independently and on their own without direct supervision to plan their day without the input of others. The nurse linked working independently with being accountable for their actions. They also acknowledged that working independently requires a certain level of self-assurance and confidence in one's abilities. Finally, they noted that the work of nursing can be unpredictable and that sometimes nurses had to take risks.to make the right choices for their clients.

The second theme was *working in a team.* The nurses identified that health care delivery was a team activity. Each member of the team has a certain set of skills and complementary knowledge bases to be considered when providing health care services. The nurses emphasized that they bring unique knowledge to be considered when making decisions about clients. They articulated that sometimes team members other than nurses can be a valued source of support.

The third theme identified was *having professional skills and knowledge.* The nurses believed having and using unique knowledge and skills was a key element in autonomy. They used their knowledge and skills to make clinical decisions when caring for clients, considering interpreting client information an independent function of the nurse. Nurses with more experience were viewed as having better ability to make independent decisions, whereas less experienced nurses might need to consult a colleague with more experience. The participants linked knowledge and skills with a certain level of professional competence. Using clinical judgment for making decisions also contributed to autonomy, and these decisions surrounding client care are to be made on information and evidence.

The fourth theme that emerged was *involvement in autonomy*. The nurses expressed having autonomy in daily practice and when providing basic client care. They also equated autonomy when making decisions related to basic procedural tasks such as discontinuing IV fluids from a client who had an adequate oral intake of fluids. This concept of involvement meant practicing autonomously in exceptional circumstances. The nurses reported anticipating what the physician would need when a client's condition would deteriorate. They would order anticipated tests and, if needed, administer oxygen. They also reported making spur-of-the-moment independent decisions to save the life of a client in any emergency situation. In the absence of ward or unit sisters, the bedside nurses reported making more independent decisions about ward activities.

The fifth theme was *boundaries around autonomy*. Nurses identified that the profession sets boundaries on their practice by establishing standards of practice and codes of conduct. Other boundaries surrounding autonomy included organizational structure and hierarchy, managerial attitudes, following governmental rules and regulations, and acknowledging their own professional limitations. They reported practicing outside the established boundaries when acting in the best interest of the client.

The final theme was that *developing autonomy requires support*. The nurses identified the importance of supporting junior members of the nursing staff as they make decisions. Supporting them enhances the development of self-confidence. This is most effectively accomplished when junior nurses are assigned to senior nurses to care for the same client group, but the junior nurse is the one expected to make the decisions surrounding care delivery. When the decisions are confirmed prior to implementation or affirmed afterward, the junior nurse gains confidence. However, if things go awry and the junior nurse is blamed, the junior nurse loses self-confidence in the ability to be a professional nurse. Support from nurse managers is also needed for senior nurses. And new managers need support from senior managers to develop the confidence to engage in autonomous practice.

This study has significance for the nursing profession and clinical practice in several ways. First, RN perceptions and experiences with autonomy vary between the United States and Great Britain. The British nurses tend to view autonomy to occur at the level of care delivery. They do not perceive themselves as having the autonomy to determine organizational clinical practice policies and protocols. In contrast, U.S. nurses report being involved and able to initiate updates and revisions to clinical practice policies and protocols for their employing institutions. Secondly, there is a certain level of professional self-confidence required for autonomous clinical practice. This is gained by having the knowledge and skills to make effective clinical judgments and perform nursing tasks successfully and independently while receiving support from nursing colleagues and other health care team members. Finally, nurses everywhere are willing to engage in autonomous practice when acting in the best interest of clients under their care.

Oshodi1, T. O., Bruneau, B., Crockett, R., Kinchington, F., Nayar, S., & Wests, E. (2019). Registered nurse's perceptions and experiences of autonomy: A descriptive phenomenological study. *BMC Nursing, 18*, 51. https://doi.org/10.1186/s12912-019-0378-3.

Nurse practice acts define various levels of nursing practice, determine rules that guide each level of nursing practice, and provide specific guidelines for continued licensure. The SBN has legal authority and accountability to implement the nurse practice act. Most SBNs are composed of a group of individuals typically appointed by the state's governor, with nurses holding most of the positions. Requirements for RN licensure appear in each state's practice act. Most nurse practice acts contain information related to reasons for licensure, nursing definitions, minimum standards for nursing education programs, licensure requirements, licensure exemptions, reasons for license revocation, endorsement provisions for nurses licensed in other states, development of a state board of examiners, nursing board responsibilities, and penalties for practicing

1.2 Professional Building Blocks

Licensure Versus Registration

Licensure refers to "a form of credentialing whereby permission is granted by a legal authority to do an act; without such permission, action would be illegal, trespass a tort, or otherwise not allowable" (Loquist, 1999, p. 105). A professional nursing license is a legal document that certifies that an individual has met minimum standards for qualified practice. As a state function, licensure protects citizens from unsafe or incompetent health care providers. Upon licensure, nurses become registered in a particular state to practice professional nursing according to the state's nurse practice act.

Registration denotes "enrolling or recording the name of a qualified individual on an official roster by an agency of government" (Loquist, 1999, p. 15). Although licensure is permanent (unless it is revoked for illegal or immoral behavior), registration must be renewed periodically (usually every 1 to 2 years) by paying a fee to each state in which current registration is desired.

nursing without a license or not in accordance with the state nurse practice act (see Box 1.2, Professional Building Blocks, "Licensure Versus Registration"). Each SBN has the responsibility for carrying out activities covered in its nurse practice act.

Recognizing the need for a united approach to nursing licensure and education, the 50 SBNs formed the NCSBN in 1978. This national board has developed licensure examinations for professional and practical nursing, a mutual compact for interstate nursing licensure, and educational materials for new and experienced nurses.

As in the United States, Canadian legislation to regulate nursing practice is passed by the provincial and territorial governments. In all provinces (except Ontario, where the College of Nurses of Ontario assumes responsibility), regulation of professional nurse registration lies with the provincial or territorial professional nursing associations. Canadian nursing regulatory bodies determine educational and practice standards and define the scope of nursing practice. They also specify who may use the title RN and outline mechanisms for professional discipline. Finally, the regulatory bodies also approve educational programs to prepare individuals for entry into practice and to establish continuing educational and competency requirements for members of the nursing profession (McDonald & McIntyre, 2019).

Because the profession of nursing defines nursing practice, sets practice standards, and has established mechanisms to discipline members failing to meet practice standards, nursing fulfills the element of autonomy and self-regulation. In some cases, the regulatory bodies also provide a means for professional nurses to engage in the activities, resulting in the creation of a collegial subculture, another hallmark of a profession.

A Collegial Subculture (Accrediting, Professional, and Student Nursing Organizations)

Professions also have a collegial subculture that helps their members support one another and ensure continuance. Like other professions, nursing has many national and international **professional organizations** that set practice standards, advocate, and provide networking opportunities for members. More than 200 professional specialty nursing associations have been formed to date in the United States (Nurse.org, 2020), each of which creates its own collegial subculture. Some of the specialty groups for nurses are linked to disease-specific organizations.

Professional nursing organizations can be divided into two categories: **general-purpose nursing organizations** (which address the issues and concerns of all nurses) and **specialized nursing organizations** (which address specific issues and concerns of nurses practicing within a specific specialized practice arena). Specialized nursing organizations link nurses who practice in a particular area and create subcultures of nurses with common interests within the profession. Each organization specifies its mission, goals, and constituency.

In 2018, 55,000 nurses were ANA members, representing less than 2% of all RNs in the United States (ANA, 2019). Some nurses believe that membership in specialty organizations (e.g., Oncology Nursing Society, American Assembly for Men in Nursing) better fits their professional needs than membership in a general nursing organization. Others (Milstead, 2008; Shinn, 2012) have argued that if all professional nurses would join a single, general-purpose organization, nurses would become more influential in health care delivery and policy formation. In 2001, the Nursing Organization Alliance was formed to bring all nursing organizations together so that a strong, cohesive voice and action plan could address common issues of concern to all professional nurses (Shinn, 2012). The following sections introduce some of the major broad-purpose organizations.

National League for Nursing

The **National League for Nursing (NLN)**, which may be the oldest nursing organization in the United States, was formed in 1893 (Dock & Stewart, 1920; NLN, 2020a). The NLN is committed to advancing the quality of all levels of nursing education, from LPNs to nursing doctorates. Membership is open to nursing education institutions, nurses and other health care professionals, health care agencies, and anyone interested in improving the quality of nursing education. The NLN has over 40,000 individual members and 1,200 institutional memberships (NLN, 2020b); core values are caring, integrity, diversity, and excellence, guiding its work and services. Its mission is to promote "excellence in nursing education to build a strong and diverse nursing workforce to advance the health of our nation and the global community" (NLN, 2020b, para 1). The NLN has the four following key goals: (a) serve as "the leader in nursing education by enhancing its impact as a well-respected and recognized leader in nursing education, (b) display commitment to members by being engaging empowering, and responsive to all nurse educators at any time in their academic careers; (c) serve as the champion for nurse educators by being their voice and forwarding their interests in the academic, political, and professional domains; and (d) advance the science of nursing education" by promoting the scholarship of teaching and evidence-based nursing education practice (NLN, 2020c). The NLN Commission for Nursing Accreditation accredits vocational, associate degree, diploma, baccalaureate, and upper-degree nursing programs to foster high-quality nursing education (NLN, CNEA, 2020).

Along with its accreditation activities, the NLN provides consultation services, continuing education programs, analysis of statistical data related to nursing education and nursing workforce resources, various examination and testing services, information about legislative affairs affecting nursing, journals, continuing education seminars, grants for nurse educators conducting research, nurse educator certification, and a variety of information packages to promote recruitment and the image of professional nursing.

American Association of Colleges of Nursing

The **American Association of Colleges of Nursing (AACN)** acts to guide and increase the quality of baccalaureate and higher-degree programs in nursing. Its mission reads, "To serve as the collective voice for academic nursing, AACN serves as the catalyst for excellence and innovation in nursing education" (AACN, 2020a). AACN envisions "nurses transforming health care and improving health" and its core values are "leadership, innovation, diversity and inclusion, and integrity" (AACN, 2020a). Membership consists of 840 nursing programs in private and public institutions of higher learning. The association offers seven leadership networks for faculty and staff who engage in instruction, research, leadership, faculty practice, business operations, research, graduate student recruitment, and communications and development. To standardize program curricula, AACN publishes essential documents for baccalaureate, graduate, and postgraduate nursing programs that outline competency expectations for program graduates (AACN, 2020b).

Along with developing standards for nursing programs, the AACN provides government advocacy, research and data services, conferences and webinars, and special projects such as integrating and certifying clinical nurse leaders, determining best practices for end-of-life nursing care, establishing cultural competency, developing and implementing quality and safety in nursing education competencies, and facilitating the requirement of the DNP as the minimal education level for advanced nursing practice (AACN, 2020b).

The AACN has an autonomous entity, the Commission on Collegiate Nursing Education (CCNE), that accredits baccalaureate and graduate nursing programs. The CCNE specifies the criteria that outline the hallmarks of nursing education programs to prepare effective professional nurses. Through program identification and assessment, the CCNE serves the public by publishing a list of accredited programs. CCNE accreditation means that a program offers effective educational practices (AACN, 2020c).

National Council of State Boards of Nursing

The **National Council of State Boards of Nursing (NCSBN)** and individual SBNs work together on common issues and concerns that might affect public health, safety, and welfare, including setting standards for minimal competence for safe nursing practice (measured by the NCLEX). The NCSBN assumes the responsibility for development and administration of the NCLEX for professional and practical/vocational nurses. Along with licensure examination, the NCSBN keeps records on nursing license suspensions, tracks professional nursing demographics, spearheads the effort toward interstate licensure, and conducts research to develop evidence-based regulation for nursing practice. In collaboration with the ANA and other advanced nursing practice groups, the NCSBN and SBNs set guidelines for licensure of APRN at state levels (NCSBN, 2020a). Membership is limited to the boards of nursing from the 50 U.S. states. Associate membership includes five colleges and seven associations of nursing from Canadian provinces, the Bermuda and New Zealand Nursing Councils, Nursing and Midwifery Boards of Ireland and Australia, and the Singapore Nursing Board. Over 48 million nurses are regulated through the NCSBN (2020a).

American Nurses Association

In 1896, 10 representatives from 10 different alumni association of nursing programs met at the Manhattan Beach Hotel with the aim of starting a national professional nursing organization and named it the Nurses' Associated Alumnae of the United States and Canada. The name was changed to the **American Nurses Association (ANA)** in 1911 and officially established the current organization (Flanagan, 1976). The ANA has over 55,000 members, representing only about 10% of the licensed RNs in the United States (ANA, 2019). The ANA is part of the ANA Enterprise, which also includes the American Nurses Foundation and the American Nurses Credentialing Center (ANCC). The three organizations share the same mission to "lead the profession to shape the future of nursing and health care," envisioning "a healing world through the power of nursing." The values of the three organizations are that nurses are trusted, innovative, inclusive, and empowered (ANA Enterprise, 2020). Membership criteria require professional nursing licensure. When professional nurses join the national organization, they obtain membership at the state and local district levels. The ANA represents nurses in all 50 states, the District of Columbia, Guam, and the U.S. Virgin Islands. The ANA offers a wide variety of services to members, including promoting healthy workplaces for nurses through continuing education programs; certification programs for specialized and advanced practice; maintaining nurse workforce data; participating in political activism and public policy analysis; providing programs to promote the economic and general welfare of nurses; and the

development and publication of nursing practice standards, handbooks, journals, newsletters, social policy statements, and an ethical code. Members receive discounts on nurse liability insurance, publications, journal subscriptions, conferences, and online educational programs (ANA, 2020a). The ANA addresses national nursing issues through membership in various national nursing councils that meet regularly to discuss the issues and concerns about nursing practice.

The ANA also sponsors activities of the American Academy of Nursing, a group of distinguished nurses who have made major contributions to the nursing profession, and the American Nurses Foundation, a program that provides funding for nursing research and other projects to advance the profession (ANA, 2019). The ANCC provides certification examinations for nurse practitioners and clinical specialists and recognizes organizations that provide empowering and safe nurse working environments so nurses can thrive (Pathway to Excellence) as well as organizations that value professional nurse contributions to care delivery, have data substantiating excellence in nursing care, shared governance structures, established nursing research programs, and an emphasis on keeping nurses content (Magnet Recognition) (ANA, 2020b). The ANA is also a member organization of the ICN (ANA, 2019).

The International Council of Nurses

Founded by nurses in Great Britain, Canada, Germany, Scandinavia, and the United States, and located in Geneva, Switzerland, the **International Council of Nurses (ICN)** unites national nursing organizations from 130 nations in a single confederation. Since 1899, the ICN has worked to preserve the professional welfare of nurses, address interests of women, and improve global health (ICN, 2020b). The mission of the ICN is "to represent nurses worldwide, advance the nursing profession, promote the well-being of nurses, and advocate for health in all policies" (ICN, 2020a). The ICN vision statement specifies a desired state in which "the global community recognises, supports, and invests in nurses and nursing to deliver health for all" (ICN, 2019). The ICN espouses the following core values—accountability, inclusiveness, innovativeness, and social justice (2019). It addresses a wide array of nursing concerns, including nursing regulatory issues, the global standardization and credentialing of nurses, human rights, ethics, socioeconomic welfare of nurses, occupational safety, health policy formation, career development, and position statements on health issues.

The ICN serves as an advocate for more than 20 million nurses and for all the people of the world (ICN, 2020a). Current efforts by the ICN focus on fighting the problems of substandard and fake health products, promoting community health, securing access to health care for people in areas of armed conflicts, protecting human rights, safeguarding health workers and clients, investing in women and girls, promoting early childhood development and effective parenting, and combating heart disease and stroke (ICN, 2020a). The organization has advised the United Nations on global health issues. In addition to its *Code of Ethics for Nurses* (2012), the ICN has published position statements that have been presented for consideration to governments when making health care policy decisions (ICN, 2020a).

Sigma Theta Tau International

Four nursing students at the University of Indiana formed Sigma Theta Tau in 1922. In 1985, **Sigma Theta Tau International (STTI)** became an international honor society for nurses. The organization has more than 135,300 active members from 100 countries. The society has more than 540 chapters in close to 700 institutions of higher education throughout the world. Chapters are located on every continent except Antarctica. STTI holds membership in the Association of College Honor Societies. The mission of STTI is "developing nurse leaders anywhere to improve health care everywhere" (STTI, 2020a). The vision for STTI is "connected, empowered nurse leaders transforming global health care" (STTI, 2020a).

To become a member of STTI, a nurse must demonstrate superior scholastic achievement, professional leadership potential, and/or marked achievement in the nursing field. STTI contributes to the advancement of nursing via research grants, scholarships, monetary awards to nursing, online continuing education programs, conferences, and publications. The organization publishes *The Journal of Nursing Scholarship*, *Worldview on Evidence-Based Nursing*, scholarly books, *Chapter Leader Emphasis*, and *Sigma Update* (a monthly electronic member newsletter). *Nursing Centered* is a resource of articles, stories from members, Sigma-Cast (podcast) episodes, webinars, and videos. STTI also sponsors writers' seminars, offers a media development program, and bestows awards for outstanding contributions to the nursing profession. Local chapters present educational programs, awards, and scholarships (STTI, 2020a). STTI manages the Sigma e-repository that houses thousands of full-text academic articles and a clinical repository. All nurses are invited to submit scholarly papers to the repository. Before they are posted, each paper undergoes a peer-review process (STTI, 2020b).

National Student Nurses' Association

The **National Student Nurses' Association (NSNA)** is an inclusive association for students from all types of nursing educational programs. Sixty thousand student members finance and run the autonomous organization. Members live in all 50 states, the District of Columbia, Puerto Rico, and the U.S. Virgin Islands. NSNA goals, according to the group's mission statement, are "to mentor the nursing students preparing for initial licensure as RNs and to convey the standards, ethics, and skills that students will need as responsible and accountable leaders and members of the profession" (NSNA, 2020).

NSNA offers a variety of activities and services to implement its mission. The association participates on NLN, ANA, and ICN committees. The NSNA Foundation administers a scholarship program and publishes the journal *Imprint*, the newsletter *NSNA News*, and a variety of reports and handbooks. The organization hosts an annual convention and a mid-year meeting. As members of NSNA, students enjoy discounts on health insurance, publications, conference attendance fees, mobile device applications, cell phones, and state board review courses (NSNA, 2020).

▮ QUESTIONS FOR REFLECTION

1. Are you currently a member of a professional nursing organization? Why or why not?

2. If you are a member of an organization, how would you go about recruiting another nurse to join your organization?

3. If you are not a member of an organization, what factors prevent you from joining one?

4. Is a nurse more professional if they hold membership in a professional organization? Why or why not?

Ethical Practice

Ethical professional practice has been defined by several broad-purpose nursing organizations through published **ethical codes** (statements defining honest, honorable, humane, and fair practice). Ethics permeates all areas of professional practice. Nurses with solid professional identities possess strong individual and professional values that provide the foundation for ethical dimensions of professional practice. Caring emerges as a shared value within the nursing profession. Clients trust nurses with their lives, and professional nurses must never violate this sacred trust.

Sometimes, a nurse's professional duties will be in conflict. Nurses have individual, professional, and societal duties (Bandman & Bandman, 1995; Fowler, 2015a). As science and technology advance and resources dwindle, nurses confront increasingly difficult, complex, and conflicting issues in daily practice. Ethical systems provide nurses with a set of values and behaviors to use when situations without clearly right or wrong answers arise. By studying ethics, nurses identify and examine personal biases and values. A code of ethics assists nurses to make decisions when confronted with ethical dilemmas.

Bandman and Bandman (1995) stated, "Effective nurses function as moral agents" (p. 46). When acting as moral agents, nurses assume responsibility and accountability to do no harm. Nurses assume responsibility for action when they assume blame or credit for their own actions. Accountability encompasses the ability to provide sound reasons, explanations, and defenses for the actions taken (Sullivan & Christopher, 1999). When nurses encounter practice situations with multiple correct actions and answers, they often agonize about which of the imperfect and alternative choices would serve the best interests of the client. Table 1.6 identifies some common ethical dilemmas encountered by nurses in clinical practice.

Nurses use multiple ethical codes depending upon the context in which they practice. Common principles appear in original versions of the *ICN Code of Ethics for Nurses* (ICN, 2012) and the ANA *Code of Ethics for Nurses with Interpretive Statements* (Fowler, 2015a). Nurses can read specific ethical codes online. Although ethical codes are often updated, all ethical codes contain the following common principles:

- Respect for human dignity and uniqueness
- Protection of confidential information
- Actions to safeguard persons receiving nursing care
- Responsibility and accountability for nursing actions
- Maintenance of nursing competence
- Use of informed judgment
- Participation in research and other activities to generate new nursing knowledge
- Participation in activities to improve and implement nursing standards
- Integrity of the nursing profession
- Collaboration with coworkers, other health care professionals and consumers

Ethical codes are morally, not legally, binding.

Societal Acceptance: Legal Reinforcement of Professional Standards

Nurses must know and function within the legal parameters of nursing practice in the state where nursing services are offered. People know what services professional services nurses provide and hold them accountable for providing high-quality, safe, and effective nursing care. If nurses have ethical or legal concerns about medical treatment or client situations, they must share their concerns with medical and institutional authorities. Because nurses are responsible for client well-being, they may refuse to execute a treatment, but they must not attempt to circumvent the physician by interfering with treatment without the physician's knowledge. Nurses and physicians must collaborate, not compete, with each other. Members of society trust nurses. For the past 18 years, Gallup poll findings reveal that Americans have consistently rated nursing as the most honest and ethical of all professions (Reinhart, 2020).

Future Work for the Nursing Profession to Attain Full Professional Status

In nursing, several barriers to fulfilling all criteria for professional stature exist. First, while most professions have a single, specialized plan of study before individuals can enter them, professional nursing has multiple levels of education for entry. Many recipients of nursing services do not know the differences in educational preparation. To them, a nurse is a nurse.

Along with an inconsistent educational entry level, many nurses have become specialists in a particular area of practice (e.g., oncology, cardiology, critical care). Frequently, some of these nurses find themselves having to choose between joining a specialty or general-purpose nursing organization because of limited time and monetary resources. Other nurses may not even join a professional organization (Shinn, 2012). By failing to unite, nurses reduce their political effectiveness and collective identity, which may create opportunity for others to exploit them.

In addition, society tends to devalue nurses more than other health care team members. Although nurses hold the lives of their clients in their hands when they practice, some clients view nurses simply as "hired help." In a capitalistic society, the amount of money received for a service is based on the perceived value of the service. Professional nurses tend to receive comparatively less compensation than other interprofessional health team members. According to the USBLS

TABLE 1.6   Ethical Issues Encountered by Professional Nurses in Practice

Ethical Principle	Definition	Practice Dilemmas
Sanctity of human life	Human life is sacred and must be preserved at all costs	▪ Quality vs. quantity of life ▪ Pro-choice vs. pro-life ▪ Capital punishment ▪ Withholding life-saving treatments ▪ Euthanasia and assisted suicide
Autonomy	Individual freedom to make rational and unconstrained decisions	▪ Lack of client knowledge about available treatments ▪ Coercive power ▪ Paternalism ▪ Individuals with cognitive impairment ▪ Individual decisions that interfere with another person's rights
Veracity	Truth telling	▪ Whistle-blowing ▪ Concealing a chemical or physical abuse pattern ▪ Falsification of legal documents to cover errors ▪ Covering up reasons for care errors or poor performance ▪ Informed consent
Distributive justice	Allocation of limited resources	▪ Managed care ▪ Reduced access to care based on inability to pay for services ▪ Judicious use of high-tech equipment for prolonging life ▪ Deciding who gets resources based on fitness, cost–benefit analysis, equal chance, equal share, or equal consideration
Respect for personal beliefs	Accepting individual beliefs as a basis for decision making	▪ Religious preferences not to subject self or family to "impure" acts ▪ Conflicts of research evidence on personal health habits
Nonmaleficence	Do no harm	▪ Securing court orders for life-saving therapies ▪ Withholding therapy ▪ Assisted suicide ▪ Right to leave clients alone
Beneficence	Do only good	Balancing what is morally right with what is legal and practical; highly individualized for each situation and shares actions with many of the principles presented earlier
Confidentiality	Keeping privileged information private	▪ Reporting health problems that interfere with safe driving to state officials ▪ Telling families about poor prognoses before informing clients ▪ Disclosing alternative lifestyles
Fidelity	Keeping promises	▪ Not keeping one's word ▪ Failing to follow up with what one says one will do
Justice	Treating people fairly	▪ Treating clients differently based on their ability to pay or other sociocultural characteristics ▪ Singling out special clients for extra nursing care ▪ Denying health care access to anyone

(2020a), the average salary for full-time employed RNs in 2014 was $77,460 and certified RN anesthetists, nurse midwives, and nurse practitioners earned an average annual salary of $115,800 (USBLS, 2020c). In comparison, the 2020 Medscape Physician Compensation Report states the mean salary for a physician was $243,000. The lowest paid specialty was pediatrics with a mean income of $232,000 and the highest paid was orthopedic surgeons with a mean income of $511,000 (Tank, 2020) and is consistent with salaries reported by the USBLS (2020b). Pharmacists earned a median income of $128,710 (USBLS, 2021a), and physical therapists earned $89,440 (USBLS, 2020d). The disparities in salary could be related to the fact that all the aforementioned health team members typically hold at least a master's degree in their practice area and some require doctorates for entry into practice.

Professional nurses must work together to showcase the contributions they make to society while developing ways to overcome the barriers to attaining full status as a profession. There are more professional nurses than any of the other members of the interdisciplinary health team. If efforts by the profession were channeled toward cooperation rather than competition, nurses could make substantial contributions toward the betterment of health for all.

REAL-LIFE REFLECTIONS

Recall the situation of Sue, who is considering returning to school. What advice would you give to Sue as she enters a baccalaureate nursing program? Why do you think each piece of advice you will give her is important?

Summary and Significance to Practice

Because nursing fails to meet all criteria for a profession, it is sometimes referred to as an emerging profession. The process of becoming a professional nurse involves change and growth throughout various stages of a career. Over time, being a professional nurse may become embedded into one's personal identity and being. The profession calls on nurses to engage in moral and ethical practice to provide what is best for clients. Through educational and occupational experiences, the nurse develops attitudes, beliefs, and skills as knowledge expands and deepens. A professional nurse should expect to commit to a life of continuous learning, growth, and development. Any change in clinical specialty practice area and formal education results in resocialization. The professional nurse assumes many roles when engaged in clinical practice. Effective implementation of these roles requires deep commitment; authentic caring; genuine compassion; technical competence; self-confidence; cognitive, clinical, and communication skills; and the ability to work in and cope with nonstop change, highly complex systems, and chaos.

From Theory to Practice

1. Has your perception of professional nursing changed since reading this chapter? Why or why not?
2. What do you think is a major barrier to nursing achieving status as a profession? Why do you think

this is a major barrier? What steps could the nursing profession take to eliminate this barrier to attaining full status as a profession?

Nurse as Author

Write a 400- to 500-word essay about why you have decided to pursue a BSN in nursing and how this will affect your future nursing career. Remember that an essay has an introductory paragraph, several supporting paragraphs, and a concluding paragraph. If you need a refresher in how to write an essay, visit the Writing Center at the University of Minnesota:

http://writing.umn.edu/sws/assets/pdf/quicktips/academicessaystructures.pdf

Be certain to follow instructions found in your course syllabus for this and any other written course assignment.

Your Digital Classroom

Online Exploration

American Association of Colleges of Nursing: **https://www.aacnnursing.org/**

American Nurses Association: **www.nursingworld.org**

International Council of Nurses: **www.icn.ch**

National Council of State Boards of Nursing: **www.ncsbn.org**

National League for Nursing: **www.nln.org**

Sigma Theta Tau International: **www.nursingsociety.org**

Expanding Your Understanding

1. Visit www.nursingworld.org, the official website of the ANA Enterprise/ANA to analyze the benefits and costs of membership. Click on the "ANA" tab at the top left of the page, then click on "Membership" at the top center of the next page. Would you join the ANA? Why or why not?
2. Search the internet for any specialized area of nursing practice and see if you can find a professional nursing organization to support nurses practicing in that field of nursing. Analyze the benefits and costs of membership. Compare and contrast two professional nursing organizations.
3. Visit www.ncsbn.org, the website for the NCSBN. Identify key issues surrounding safe nursing practice. What states have enacted the multistate compact for professional nursing practice? Visit your

SBN website by clicking on "Contact Details" in the "Contact a Member" section on the home page of the NCSBN website. Then click on the state desired on the provided map to learn about and identify key information surrounding initial licensure, license renewal, announcements, and news.

Beyond the Book

Visit thePoint® at **www.thePoint.lww.com** for activities and information to reinforce the concepts and content covered in this chapter.

REFERENCES

Adams, P. C. (2019). Geographies of media and communication III: Academic communication and the digital communication environment. *Progress in Human Geography, 43*(4), 739–748. https://doi.org/10.1177/0309132518763849

Aiken, L. H., Clarke, S. P., Cheung, R. B., Sloane, D. M., & Silber, J. H. (2003). Educational levels of hospital nurses and surgical patient mortality. *Journal of the American Medical Association, 290*, 1617–1623. https://doi.org/10.1001/jama.290.12.1617

Alexander, M., Durham, C. F., Hooper, J. I., Jeffries, P. R., Goldman, N., Kardong-Edgren, S. S., Kesten, K. S., Spector, N., Tagliareni, E., Radtke, B., & Tillman, C. (2015). NCSBN simulation guidelines for prelicensure nursing programs. *Journal of Nursing Regulation, 6*(3), 39–42. https://doi.org/10.1016/S2155-8256(15)30783-3

American Association of Colleges of Nursing. (2004). *AACN position statement on the practice doctorate in nursing.* https://www.aacnnursing.org/Portals/42/News/Position-Statements/DNP.pdf

American Association of Colleges of Nursing. (2008). *The essentials of baccalaureate education for professional nursing practice.* Author.

American Association of Colleges of Nursing. (2015). *The doctor of nursing practice: Current issues and clarifying recommendations.* Report from the task force on the implementation of the DNP. https://www.aacnnursing.org/Portals/42/DNP/DNP-Implementation.pdf

American Association of Colleges of Nursing. (2020a). *Vision and mission.* https://www.aacnnursing.org/About-AACN/AACN-Governance/Vision-and-Mission

American Association of Colleges of Nursing. (2020b). *Who we are.* https://www.aacnnursing.org/About-AACN

American Association of Colleges of Nursing. (2020c). *CCNE accreditation.* https://www.aacnnursing.org/CCNE

American Association of Colleges of Nursing. (2021). *The essentials: Core competencies for professional nursing education.* Retrieved May 11, 2021, from https://www.aacnnursing.org/Portals/42/AcademicNursing/pdf/Essentials-2021.pdf

American Nurses Association. (2015). *Code of ethics for nurses with interpretive statements.* Author.

American Nurses Association. (2019). *2018 annual report.* https://www.nursingworld.org/~49d621/globalassets/docs/ana/ana-annual-report-for-2018.pdf

American Nurses Association. (2020a). *Member benefits.* Retrieved August 30, 2020, from https://www.nursingworld.org/membership/member-benefits/

American Nurses Association. (2020b). *Organizational programs.* Retrieved August 30, 2020, from https://www.nursingworld.org/organizational-programs/

American Nurses Association. (2021). *Nursing Scope and standards of practice* (4th ed.). Author.

ANA Enterprise. (2020). *2020–2023 strategic plan.* Retrieved August 30, 2020, from https://www.nursingworld.org/ana/about-ana/anae-strategic-plan-2020---2023/

Bandman, E. L., & Bandman, B. (1995). *Nursing ethics through the life span* (3rd ed.). Appleton & Lange.

Benner, P. (1984). *From novice to expert: Excellence and power in clinical nursing practice.* Addison-Wesley.

Benner, P., Tanner, C. A., & Chesla, C. A. (Eds.). (1996). *Expertise in nursing practice: Caring, clinical judgment and ethics.* Springer.

Bevis, E. O., & Watson, J. (2000). *Toward a caring curriculum: A new pedagogy for nursing.* Jones & Bartlett Learning.

Billings, D., & Halstead, J. (2020). *Teaching in nursing: A guide for faculty* (6th ed.). Elsevier Saunders.

Bohm, D. (1980). *Wholeness and the implicate order.* Routledge.

Bortolato, C., Perez, J., Mattei da Silva, A. Mantovani, M., Felix, J., & Boostel, R. (2018). Contributions of the simulation for undergraduate nursing students. *Journal of Nursing UFPE/Revista de Enfermagem UFPE, 12*(6), 1751–1762. https://doi.org/10.5205/1981-8963-v12i6a230633p1751-1762-2018

Bradby, M. (1990). Status passage into nursing: Another view of the process of socialization. *Journal of Advanced Nursing, 15*, 1220–1225. https://doi.org/10.1111/j.1365-2648.1990.tb01715.x

Bradshaw, M. J.; Hutlquist, B. L., & Hagler, D. (2020). *Innovative teaching strategies in nursing and related health professions* (8th ed.). Jones & Bartlett Learning.

Bridges, W. (2003). *Managing transitions, making the most of change.* Perseus.

Bridges, S., & Bridges, W. (2019). *Transitions: Making the most of change.* Lifelong Books.

Broussard, P. C., & Oberleitner, M. G. (1997). Writing and thinking: A process to critical understanding. *Journal of Nursing Education, 36*(7), 334–336.

Clarke, B., James, C., & Kelly, J. (1996). Reflective practice: Reviewing the issues and refocusing the debate. *International Journal of Nursing Studies, 33*, 171–180. https://doi.org/10.1016/0020-7489(95)00045-3

Dictionary.com. (2020). *Core competency.* https://www.dictionary.com/browse/core-competency

Diekelmann, N. L., & Rather, M. L. (Eds.). (1993). *Transforming RN education: Dialogue and debate.* National League for Nursing.

Dock, L., & Stewart, I. (1920). *A short history of nursing.* Putnam.

Dreyfus, S., & Dreyfus, H. (1980). *A five-stage model of the mental activities involved in directed skill acquisition.* Storming Media. www.dtic.mil/cgi-bin/GetTRDoc?AD=ADA084551&Location=U2&doc=GetTRDoc

Dunham, K. S. (2008). *How to survive and maybe even love nursing school!* (3rd ed.). F. A. Davis.

Flanagan, L. (1976). *One strong voice.* Lowell Press.

Fowler, M. D. M. (2015a). *Guide to the code of ethics for nurses with interpretive statements, development, interpretation and application* (2nd ed.). American Nurses Association.

Fowler, M. D. M. (2015b). *Guide to Nursing's social policy statement: Understanding the profession from social contract to social covenant.* American Nurses Association.

Freidson, E. (1994). *Professionalism reborn: Theory, prophecy and policy.* University of Chicago Press.

Hacker, D., & Sommers, N. (2019). *The Bradford handbook* (11th ed.). Bedford/St. Martins MacMillan Learning.

Harrison, J. M., Aiken, L. H., Sloane, D. M., Brooks-Carthon, J. M., Merchant, R. M., Berg, R. A., & McHugh, M. D. (2019). In hospitals with more nurses who have baccalaureate degrees, better outcomes for patients after cardiac arrest. *Health Affairs, 38,* 1087–1094. https://doi.org/10.1377/hlthaff.2018.05064

Hasan, L., & Abuelrub, E. (2009). *Assessing the quality of websites.* https://www.researchgate.net/publication/228686530_Assessing_the_Quality_of_Web_Sites/fulltext/00006b4f0cf275ecfef0faf9/Assessing-the-Quality-of-Web-Sites.pdf

Hinshaw, A. S. (1976). *Socialization and resocialization of nurses for professional nursing practice (National League for Nursing Publication No. 15–1659).* National League for Nursing.

Institute of Medicine. (2011). *The future of nursing: Leading change, advancing health.* National Academies Press.

International Council of Nurses. (2012). *The ICN code of ethics for nurses.* Revised 2012. https://www.icn.ch/sites/default/files/inline-files/2012_ICN_Codeofethicsfornurses_%20eng.pdf

International Council of Nurses. (2019). *Strategic Plan 2019–2023: ICN mission, vision and strategic plan.* https://www.icn.ch/who-we-are/icn-mission-vision-constitution-and-strategic-plan

International Council of Nurses. (2020a). *What we do: Campaigns.* https://www.icn.ch/what-we-do/campaigns

International Council of Nurses. (2020b). *Who we are.* Retrieved August 31, 2020, from https://www.icn.ch/who-we-are

Jones, R. (2004). The science and meaning of the self. *Journal of Analytical Psychology, 49,* 217–233. https://doi.org/10.1111/j.1465-5922.2004.00454.x

Kalisch, P., & Kalisch, B. (2004). *The advance of American nursing: A history* (4th ed.). Lippincott Williams & Wilkins.

Kim, H. S. (1999). Critical reflective inquiry for knowledge development in nursing practice. *Journal of Advanced Nursing, 29*(5), 1205–1212. https://doi.org/10.1046/j.1365-2648.1999.01005.x

Kumm, S., Godfrey, N., Martin, D., Tucci, M., Muenks, M., & Spaeth, T. (2014). Baccalaureate Outcomes Met by Associate Degree Nursing Programs. *Nurse Educator, 39*(5), 216–220. https://doi.org/10.1097/nne.0000000000000060

Leddy, S. K. (2003). *Integrative health promotion.* Slack.

Linton, R. (1945). *The cultural background of personality.* Appleton.

Loquist, R. S. (1999). Regulation: Parallel and powerful. In J. A. Milstead (Ed.), *Health policy and politics: A nurse's guide.* Aspen.

Lynn, M. R., McCain, N. L., & Boss, B. J. (1989). Socialization of RN to BSN. *The Journal of Nursing Scholarship, 21,* 232–237. https://doi.org/10.1111/j.1547-5069.1989.tb00149.x

Massachusetts Department of Higher Education. (2016). *Nurse of the Future Core Competencies© Registered Nurse.* https://www.mass.edu/nahi/documents/NOFRNCompetencies_updated_March2016.pdf

McDonald, C., & McIntyre, M. (2019). *Realities of Canadian Nursing: Professional, practice and power issues* (5th ed.). Wolters Kluwer

Miller, B. K., Adams, D., & Beck, L. (1993). A behavioral inventory for professionalism in nursing. *Journal of Professional Nursing, 9*(5), 290–295. https://doi.org/10.1016/8755-7223(93)90055-H

Milstead, J. A. (2008). *Health policy and politics: A nurse's guide* (3rd ed.). Jones & Bartlett Learning.

Mish, F. C. (Ed.) (2020). *Meriam-Webster's Collegiate Dictionary* (11th ed.). Merriam-Webster, Inc.

Morse, J. M., Bottorff, J., Neander, W., & Solberg, S. (1991). Comparative analysis of conceptualizations and theories of caring. *The Journal of Nursing Scholarship, 23*(2), 119–126. https://doi.org/10.1111/j.1547-5069.1991.tb00655.x

National Council of State Boards of Nursing. (2020a). *About NCSBN: History.* https://www.ncsbn.org/history.htm

National Council of State Boards of Nursing. (2020b). *Active RN licenses.* https://www.ncsbn.org/6161.htm

National Council of State Boards of Nursing. (2020c). *NCSBN research brief: 2019 NCLEX® examination statistics.* https://www.ncsbn.org/2019_NCLEXExamStats.pdf

National League for Nursing. (2010). *Outcomes and competencies for graduates of practical/vocational, diploma, associate degree, baccalaureate, master's, practice doctorate and research doctorate programs in nursing.* National League for Nursing.

National League for Nursing. (2020a). *Overview.* http://www.nln.org/about/overview

National League for Nursing. (2020b). *Core values.* http://www.nln.org/about/core-values

National League for Nursing. (2020c). *Mission and strategic plan.* http://www.nln.org/about/mission-goals

NLN Nursing Commission for Nursing Education Accreditation. (2020). *Who we are.* https://cnea.nln.org/about

National Student Nurses Association. (2020). *About NSNA.* https://www.nsna.org/about-nsna.html

Nurse.org. (2020). *List of nursing organizations.* https://nurse.org/orgs.shtml

Osuna, M. (2014). *Nursing school thrive guide.* Author.

Paul, R. (1992). *Critical thinking: What every person needs to survive in a rapidly changing world* (2nd rev. ed.). Foundation for Critical Thinking.

PEW Health Professions Commission. (1998). *Recreating health professional practice for a new century.* University of California, San Francisco Center for the Health Professions.

Powell, J. H. (1989). The reflective practitioner in nursing. *Journal of Advanced Nursing, 14*(10), 824–832. https://doi.org/10.1111/j.1365-2648.1989.tb01467.x

Purdue University Online Writing Lab. (n.d.a). *Evaluating Sources: General guidelines.* https://owl.purdue.edu/owl/research_and_citation/conducting_research/evaluating_sources_of_information/general_guidelines.html

Purdue University Online Writing Lab. (n.d. b). *Evaluating digital sources.* https://owl.purdue.edu/owl/research_and_citation/conducting_research/evaluating_sources_of_information/evaluating_digital_sources.html

QSEN Institute. (2014). *Project overview.* http://qsen.org/about-qsen/project-overview/

QSEN Institute. (2020). *About QSEN.* https://qsen.org/about-qsen/

Quan, K. (2006). *The everything new nurse book.* Adams Media.

Ray, M. (1998). Complexity and nursing science. *Nursing Science Quarterly, 11*(3), 91–93. https://doi.org/10.1177/089431849801100302

Reinhart, R. J. (2020). *Nurses continue to rate highest in honesty, ethics.* https://news.gallup.com/poll/274673/nurses-continue-rate-highest-honesty-ethics.aspx

Rubenfeld, M. G., & Scheffer, B. K. (2015). *Critical thinking tactics for nurses* (3rd ed.). Jones & Bartlett Learning.

Schon, D. A. (1983). *The reflective practitioner.* Temple Smith.

Schon, D. A. (1987). *Educating the reflective practitioner: Toward a new design for teaching and learning in the professions.* Jossey-Bass.

Shane, D. L. (1980). The returning-to-school syndrome. In S. Mirin (Ed.), *Teaching tomorrow's nurse.* Nursing Resources.

Shinn, L. (2012). Current issues in nursing associations. In D. Mason, J. Leavitt, & M. Chaffee (Eds.), *Policy & politics in nursing and health care* (6th ed.). Elsevier Saunders.

Sigma Theta Tau International. (2020a). *From library to repository.* https://www.sigmarepository.org/history/

Sigma Theta Tau International. (2020b) *Sigma organizational fact sheet.* https://www.sigmanursing.org/why-sigma/about-sigma/sigma-organizational-fact-sheet

Stebbins, L. F. (2006). *Student guide to research in the digital age.* Libraries Unlimited.

Sullivan, M. C., & Christopher, M. M. (1999). Ethical issues. In E. J. Sullivan (Ed.), *Creating nursing's future.* Mosby. https://www.bon.texas.gov/pdfs/publication_pdfs/delc-2010.pdf

Tank, A. (2020). *Physician salary report 2020: Salaries rising prior to COVID-19 impacts.* https://weatherbyhealthcare.com/blog/annual-physician-salary-report

United States Bureau of Labor Statistics. (2020a). *Occupational Employment Statistics: Registered nurses.* https://www.bls.gov/oes/current/oes291141.htm

United States Bureau of Labor Statistics. (2020b). *Occupational Outlook Handbook: Physicians and surgeons.* https://www.bls.gov/ooh/healthcare/physicians-and-surgeons.htm

United States Bureau of Labor Statistics. (2020c). *Occupational Outlook Handbook: Nurse anesthetists, nurse midwives and nurse practitioners.* https://www.bls.gov/ooh/healthcare/nurse-anesthetists-nurse-midwives-and-nurse-practitioners.htm

United States Bureau of Labor Statistics. (2020d). *Occupational Outlook Handbook: Physical therapists.* https://www.bls.gov/ooh/healthcare/physical-therapists.htm

United States Bureau of Labor Statistics. (2021a.) *Occupational Outlook Handbook: Pharmacists.* Retrieved June 10, 2021 from https://www.bls.gov/oes/current/oes291051.htm

United States Bureau of Labor Statistics. U.S. Department of Labor (2021b). *Occupational Outlook Handbook. Registered nurses.* Retrieved May 11, 2021, from https://www.bls.gov/ooh/healthcare/registered-nurses.htm#tab-3

US Department of Health & Human Services, Bureau of Health Workforce. (2020). *National Sample of Registered Nurses: 2018 key findings.* https://bhw.hrsa.gov/health-workforce-analysis/data/national-sample-survey-registered-nurses

Wiggins, M. (2008). The challenge of change. In C. Lindberg, S. Nash, & C. Lindberg (Eds.), *On the edge: Nursing in the age of complexity.* Plexus Press.

Young, C., & Koopsen, C. (2011). *Spirituality, health and healing: An integrative approach.* Jones & Bartlett Learning.

The History Behind Today's Professional Nursing

KEY TERMS AND CONCEPTS

Ancient nursing practice
Roots of holistic nursing
  practice
White magic
Roman matrons
Early Christian nurses
Nurses from religious
  orders
Kaiserworth
Careful nursing

Florence Nightingale
Mary Seacole
Public health nurse
Civil War nursing
State registration
Work redesign
Clinical pathways
Case management
Consilience

LEARNING OUTCOMES

By the end of this chapter, the learner will be able to:

1. Trace the history of nursing from ancient to current times.
2. Outline the key societal trends that affected recruitment and retention of nurses in the workforce.
3. Explain the parallels between past nursing history and current nursing practice.
4. Discuss various ways nurses have been portrayed in the media.
5. Describe how history could be used to address current and future nursing issues.

REAL-LIFE REFLECTIONS

Marita, Carol, and Joe received an assignment to give a class presentation on nursing history that could be used to prepare the nursing profession for a future challenge. At first, they view this assignment as busywork. However, as they explore the history of nursing, they come to appreciate significant events and persons. They acknowledge that the profession may need to look at history to solve current and future problems.

- *How much do you know about the history of nursing?*
- *Do you think knowing the history of the profession might be helpful as you embark on this phase of your education? Why or why not?*

With advances in technology, the field of health care is increasingly initiating targeted efforts to explain the interrelationships of health, longevity, multiculturalism, socioeconomics, and spirituality. In many ways, nursing has helped forge the path to this holistic view of health care. An examination of nursing history provides professional nurses with an understanding of the profession's unique place within the health care arena and may offer answers for current and future challenges.

Take Note!
An examination of nursing history provides professional nurses with an understanding of the profession's unique place within the health care arena and may offer answers for current and future challenges.

NURSING IN ANCIENT CIVILIZATIONS (BEFORE 1 CE)

Humans learned how to care for one another by observing how animals relied on each other in times of need (Nutting & Dock, 1935a), such as uninjured animals bringing food to injured companions and helpless offspring. By watching animals, humans learned therapies such as licking wounds as a form of an antiseptic cleaning (from canines and felines), applying pressure to control bleeding (from apes), amputating extremities when ensnared in traps (from rats), ingesting salt (from deer, cows, and antelope), wrapping wounds in a spiral fashion (from birds), applying splints (from snipe), traveling great distances to soak in healing water (from deer), and entombing the dead (from bees).

Early cultures believed that a person's soul (or life-giving spirit forces) existed independently of the body. Human tragedy, including illness, was blamed on the spirit world. Early therapies for illnesses and injuries focused on the religious domain, and ancient societies believed that some of their members possessed special powers that could ease suffering, enhance healing, and cure diseases by appeasing the spirits. Techniques used by early healers included pummeling (a form of massage), administering herbs, exposing persons to smoke, squeezing, starving, purging, applying roots or balms to the skin, or twisting the body into various positions. Along with touch, ancient healers frequently applied warm poultices and held healing ceremonies using drumming, smoking, and chanting to drive out evil spirits (Nutting & Dock, 1935a).

Egypt

The oldest written recordings about medicine and nursing come from Egypt and date to 3000 BCE. The Ebers Papyrus outlines over 700 therapies derived from minerals, plants, and animals. Compounded prescriptions were made up in the forms of decoctions, pills, tablets, injections, infusions, lozenges, powders, potions, inhalations, lotions, ointments, and plasters (Kalisch & Kalisch, 2004; Nutting & Dock, 1935a). The art of medicine in ancient Egypt consisted of two branches. The theurgic class devoted themselves to magical cures, while the practitioners used natural cures. Along with disease treatment, the Egyptians practiced public hygiene and sanitation. Although there is no evidence of hospitals or nursing in ancient Egypt, there is mention of temple priestesses without reference to their duties (Nutting & Dock, 1935a).

India

Details of nursing are also recorded in Lesson IX of the *Charaka Samhita*. This ancient Indian record describes the following four qualifications for a nurse: (1) knowledge of drug preparation, (2) cleverness, (3) devotion to clients, and (4) purity of body and mind (Nutting & Dock, 1935a). The ancient Indians were the first to link hygiene to health (Jamieson & Sewall, 1954; Kalisch & Kalisch, 2004; Nutting & Dock, 1935a).

In the 3rd century BCE, King Ashoka of India developed community institutes to care for sick travelers. These precursors of hospitals were described as spacious and roomy mansions protected from strong winds, breezes, smoke, sun, dust, and rain. In **ancient nursing practice**, the sick were cared for by male attendants noted for their purity and cleanliness of habits; they were characterized as kind, clever, and skillful in providing service to others. Along with providing good nutrition, ventilation, and a clean environment, the attendants read stories, chanted hymns, played musical instruments, and conversed with the infirm while attending to all their needs. In many ways, these earliest known nursing interventions were the **roots of holistic nursing practice**. At the same time, records from Ceylon wrote about women who provided care for the sick as part of the Buddhist tradition of mercy, compassion, justice, and humane treatment for all living things. Caring for the infirm in ancient Eastern cultures was done by both men and women (Nutting & Dock, 1935a).

Babylonia

The Babylonians shared some ideas with the Egyptians, but they also believed that numbers possessed magical powers, and they displayed a great interest in astrology (Jamieson & Sewall, 1954). Like the Egyptians, the Babylonians viewed illness as punishment for displeasing or sinning against the gods and they used methods to banish demons and avoid evil spirits. However, the Babylonians also left records outlining surgical procedures, and in 1900 BCE, King Hammurabi developed a code that provided the first sliding scale of fees for goods and services. Hammurabi's code of laws also specified that citizens had to compensate each other equally for transgressions. Therefore, a surgeon could have his hands amputated if he performed an unsuccessful surgery (Jamieson & Sewall, 1954; Nutting & Dock, 1935a).

China

The ancient Chinese developed the concept of yin (the passive, negative, feminine energy force) and yang (the active, positive, masculine energy force) and defined health as a balance of these two forces. By 2000 BCE, the Chinese were practicing dissection, performing acupuncture, and prescribing herbal therapies to enhance health and cure illness. They used baths to reduce fever and bloodletting to remove evil spirits from the body. The Chinese were the first to outline detailed principles of physical examination (look, listen, ask, and feel) (Jamieson & Sewall, 1954).

Take Note!
Practices for taking care of the ill date back to the beginning of civilization.

Persia

A Persian epic dated back to 642 BCE mentions three kinds of physicians: one who healed by the knife, another by exorcism and incantations, and a third by using plants. The Persians excelled at chemistry; they tested bodily fluids, studied drugs, and were the first to introduce medications derived from plants. They built beautiful hospitals and cared for clients in specialized wards. Clients were treated with skill and kindness. Although Persian records make no mention of nurses, they describe numerous procedures, many of which fall within the domain of current nursing practice, such as detailed ways to care for wounds, provide hydration, and control discomfort (Nutting & Dock, 1935a).

Palestine

The Hebrew culture adopted sanitary measures from Egypt during the period of enslavement around 1200 BCE. The ancient Hebrews adopted natural cures but rejected magical therapies. The Old Testament outlines food inspection, vital statistics records, and infectious disease quarantine followed by fumigation. Hebrew law also placed an obligation on people to show sympathy, cheer, and aid to the sick. One of the seven acts of charity mentioned in rabbinical literature is visiting the sick. The Hebrews developed sick houses that were connected to rest houses for travelers and the destitute (Nutting & Dock, 1935a).

Greece

Like Egypt, Greece traced medical arts to divine myths. The Greeks also divided the healing arts into two branches, with one retaining priestly powers and the other having medical functions.

In *The Iliad*, Homer identifies Asklepios, the father of Machaon and Podalirius, as the "blameless physician." Temples of Asklepios were reported to exist as early as 1134 BCE.

Hospitality was a sacred obligation in Greek culture. In large Greek cities, the "xenodochium" served as a municipal inn for strangers, the poor, and the sick (Nutting & Dock, 1935a). In addition to the public xenodochium, the Greeks established "iotrions" (temples for healing services) where surgery was performed and dispensaries were located. Only individuals who could be cured were admitted to the iotrions. Temples had a place devoted to the sick called the "abaton." Ruins reveal that the abaton contained a large room with an altar surrounded by smaller rooms that could accommodate a single person. The abaton was staffed with priests and a variety of others, including physicians, bath attendants, slaves, and priestesses. The Greeks believed that birth and death caused permanent pollution where they occurred. Therefore, the terminally ill were left on the street to die (Nutting & Dock, 1935a).

The great physician Hippocrates outlined the role of physicians as assisting nature to bring about a cure. Hippocrates set standards for bathing, bandaging, and other cures. Although he provided no treatise on nursing, his work specified that he used assistants (Kalisch & Kalisch, 2004; Nutting & Dock, 1935a).

Rome

The Greeks introduced the Romans to medicine sometime in the 3rd century BCE. Before then, Romans believed that lost health could only be restored by the gods. The Romans constructed drains, aqueducts, good roads, sewage systems, and proper cemeteries, as well as an organized system of medicine that enhanced public health. Nero organized a Roman medical service and appointed a superintendent of court physicians. Slaves of rich families cultivated knowledge of practical medicine. Many slaves earned freedom by curing owners with their skills. The Romans reserved the best medical and nursing care for their soldiers (Kalisch & Kalisch, 2004; Nutting & Dock, 1935a).

Northern Europe

Civilization in northern Europe at the time of the Roman Empire was less organized. The ancient Teutons, Norsemen, and Druids revered their wise women. These women, usually elders, gathered herbs that they knew had medicinal and remedial qualities.

As time progressed, various superstitions followed both wise women and medicine men. According to Finnish mythology, the ancient healers practiced **white magic** or healing magic, which was primarily medicinal in nature. However, society grew to believe that these persons with special healing powers also had connections to evil spirits and could use "black magic," which caused natural catastrophes or human illness and injury (Nutting & Dock, 1935a). The healing women may have been seen as early prototypes of witches.

Germany

Like the northern Europeans in the last millennium before the Christian era, the Gauls and Germans held certain women in high regard. They believed that these women could communicate readily with the gods. Many women also possessed great knowledge and skill in medicine and surgery. German women established expertise in treating wounds from war, providing obstetric care, and treating animals (Nutting & Dock, 1935a).

▌ QUESTIONS FOR REFLECTION

1. Are any ancient nursing interventions used today to tend to the ill and infirm?
2. Why do you think that some ancient nursing interventions and medical therapies had to be "rediscovered?"

NURSING IN THE EARLY CHRISTIAN ERA (1–500 CE)

Roman Matrons

As early as the 2nd century CE, Roman converts to Christianity transformed their homes into places to care for the sick and poor. Women from well-established Roman families enjoyed dignified and respected positions in the society. Wives in such families were considered equal to their husbands. These **Roman matrons** organized and delivered care to people in need.

The earliest female workers in the Catholic Church who were concerned with nursing were the deaconesses and widows. Early converts to Christianity, especially affluent women, viewed comforting the afflicted as a sacred duty. Deaconesses were married women who were commissioned to serve in a church-related agency such as a hospital or social outreach program, though men also performed nursing duties. In 60 CE, Phoebe became the first parish worker, friendly visitor, and district nurse and is credited as the mother of visiting nursing (Nutting & Dock, 1935a).

Early church deacons and deaconesses sought out those in need, established a system of visiting nurses, and

sometimes brought the ill into their homes. As home hospitals were organized, the deaconate became associated with the work of nursing. Eventually, the bishops followed the deaconate example and opened their homes to tend to the sick. As congregations grew and more poor people joined them, the church established the Christian xenodochium, or home for strangers. The xenodochium contained one section for ordinary travelers and another section for the poor and infirm. Nursing the sick was seen as proper penance for past sins and solace for unhappy lives (Nutting & Dock, 1935a).

Between 249 CE and 263 CE, an extensive epidemic hit Rome, resulting in many deaths among the deaconate. In 350 CE, another epidemic hit the city of Edessa, where desperate wealthy inhabitants freely gave money to Ephrem to provide care for the ill. Ephrem, who was later canonized as a saint, used the donations to build the first hospital. Along with the matrons, widows, old men, and the disenfranchised provided nursing care in the hospital established by Ephrem.

In the 5th century CE, Emperor Justinian granted the bishops authority over hospitals. With great zeal, the bishops built shelters, hospices, foundling asylums, and nosocomials (nursing hospitals) within the confines of monasteries. Nursing religious orders were formed and flourished. Men and women joined the religious orders. Because arranged marriages were common in this era, women could join a religious order and embark on a life of caring for the ill within these establishments resulting in living a life that was intellectually stimulating and personally satisfying (Jamieson & Sewall, 1954; Nutting & Dock, 1935a).

Advances in Greece

Although **early Christian nurses** were instrumental in the development of modern nursing, other groups played key roles in the advancement of nursing practice. In 100 CE, Aretaeus emphasized the necessity for strict cleanliness of bed clothes, the use of powders on moist skin, and mouthwashes for clients who were not allowed to drink. He directed that for fevers, rooms should be light and airy and clients should be lightly covered and receive only liquids for nourishment. Excitable clients should be kept in small, undecorated rooms kept at a constant temperature. Aretaeus outlined strategies for pain control that included hot baths, fomentations, hot water bladders, light massage, plasters, and salves. Music was also used to soothe and lull persons in distress.

In 138 CE, the Greeks established a maternity hospital and a home for the dying (Nutting & Dock, 1935a).

NURSING IN THE MIDDLE AGES (500–1500)

The first mention of a nursing uniform surfaced in 1190, when a Bavarian monk insisted that religious women wear distinctive dress to be recognized when out in public performing charitable acts. As monasteries flourished as centers of learning, nuns became distinguished for work in academia and service. By the 13th century CE, monks and nuns were said to have more medical knowledge than the rest of the society (Nutting & Dock, 1935a).

Because of the societal power monks and nuns possessed from their medical knowledge, the Lateran Council in 1123 forbade monks and priests from the practice of medicine. The Benedictine sisters, however, covertly and actively continued to expand the knowledge of medicine and practiced medicine and nursing without the support of the church. Monks secretly joined the nuns and they conjointly cared for the sick; the monks cared for men and the nuns cared for women. The nuns took charge of the hospital while the monks served as priests (Nutting & Dock, 1935a).

Hildegarde, a nun, perhaps heralded the beginning of female dominance in nursing. She possessed extraordinary intellectual powers and amassed great knowledge of medicine through her nursing experiences. Between 1151 and 1159, she wrote volumes devoted to medical works that include accurate physiology related to reproduction, circulation, and the nervous system (Nutting & Dock, 1935a).

The Crusades and Nursing Knights

During the Crusades, hospitals were built on the routes to and in Jerusalem where men delivered care to travelers and battle-scarred warriors. The Knights Hospitallers of St. John of Jerusalem started as an exclusive nursing order. The Teutonic Knights had both nursing and military duties. The Knights of St. Lazarus was a nursing order from the great hospital in Jerusalem built by Basil in 329 AD. Along with the Knights of St. Lazarus, the Sisters of St. Lazarus, an order of nuns, provided care.

In England, the Order of St. John consisted of men devoted to charitable work, including the formation of cottage hospitals, convalescent homes, and nurse training for the poor (Kalisch & Kalisch, 2004; Nutting & Dock, 1935a).

In the 11th century, two hospitals were built in England—one to care for those afflicted with leprosy and another to care for others. Religious brothers attended to the sick men, and nuns attended to the sick women. The hospital for leprosy (St. Giles) was run by an order of nuns known as the Poor Clares. Ladies of noble birth added attending to the sick as a social duty (Nutting & Dock, 1935a).

Religious Orders of Nursing for Women

In 12th century France, nursing became part of the manual labor performed by several orders of Roman Catholic sisters. Secular orders of nuns also engaged in nursing. One French hospital staffed itself with laywomen who were either widowed or repenting from sins of impurity (Nutting & Dock, 1935a). **Nurses from religious orders** provided a structured approach to the care of the ill and infirm, while other women haphazardly cared for them. In Paris, the Augustinian order of nuns provided nursing care in hospitals. Those in the Augustinian order shared with one another information on how to care for the sick. In 1212, the Catholic Church passed statutes to regulate the nursing orders to exercise control over them. To join, both men and women took permanent vows of poverty, chastity, and obedience. Within 150 years, the various orders became corrupt and many leaders skimmed off donated resources for personal gain. The men and women actually caring for the sick became demoralized because they had no respite from the unrelenting toil. Religious orders, especially the nuns, accumulated much money and many possessions and focused their efforts to manage them. When an epidemic of syphilis spread, hospitals became centers of infection. During this time, many individuals left monasteries and convents taking whatever they could carry, further depleting resources for the care of the infirm (Nutting & Dock, 1935a).

THE ESTABLISHMENT OF NURSING IN EUROPE, ENGLAND, AND THE NEW WORLD (1500–1819)

France

In 1505, France's King Louis XII decreed that jurisdiction of the hospitals be temporarily removed from the Catholic Church and governed by secular directors. In 1526, the rectors of a hospital located in Lyons directed staff members to wear white uniforms to denote purity of character. In 1562, the dress changed from white to black, with a white linen apron and an unstarched white cap. The apron was worn when directly caring for the sick. By the middle of the

16th century, the secular rectors introduced stringent regulations and required nursing service members to become part of a religious order. Male nurses were required to wear blue robes and silver crosses. Female nurses could only leave nursing to marry or to care for aging parents. Nursing service members worked in hospitals, visited the sick at home, and distributed herbal medications (Nutting & Dock, 1935a).

England

In England, control of hospitals moved from the church to become the responsibility of the cities. Philanthropy and state aid became the major funding sources. Members of religious orders were replaced by ordinary lay servants and attendants hired by civic authorities who had little knowledge about caring for the infirm. The matron, who had the status of an untrained housekeeper, usually had some knowledge of how to run a hospital, supervised all attendants, and was responsible for finding staff. Frequently, the matron found care attendants from jails and debtor prisons. The title "sister" was bestowed on the head nurse of a ward. A "sister" had no formal nursing education but assumed responsibility for the staff that cared for clients and the work performed on a ward. An ordinance passed in 1699 decreed that only wives of free men could hold the position of sister because of their social status. Clients received care from heartless attendants and nurses (female servants who were hired by the matron, but learned how to care for clients from a sister), who were required to work 12 to 48 hours without breaks. In some cases, clients nursed each other as the servant nurses slept (Nutting & Dock, 1935a).

The late 1700s marked the earliest beginning of the worldwide hospital reform movement. John Howard's work on reforming hospitals evolved from his crusade to reform prisons (Jamieson & Sewall, 1954). In his 1789 notes on the state of hospitals throughout Europe and England, Howard wrote that hospitals staffed by members from religious orders tended to be quiet, neat, and clean, with careful attention to client hygiene and infection prevention. When describing secular hospitals, he wrote that clients were dirty, pest infested, and without bed linens (Nutting & Dock, 1935b).

Nursing in the New World

As the New World was settled, French and Spanish religious orders opened hospitals. In what is now Canada, the Jesuits opened a hospital for settlers and native people. The native people shared remedies for scurvy with the French. Likewise, the Jesuits shared their knowledge of medicine with the native populations. The nuns assumed most of the client care in hospitals. As the load of hospital labor for nuns grew heavier, native women also quickly began providing client care (Nutting & Dock, 1935b).

Sometime before 1524, Cortez built the Hospital of the Immaculate Conception in what is now Mexico City. Nursing staff consisted primarily of a religious order of men. In 1531, the second oldest hospital of the New World was founded in what is now Santa Fe, New Mexico, where a community of over 30,000 members of the Pueblo tribe practiced hospitality and charitable works (Nutting & Dock, 1935b).

In the English colonies, the growth of hospitals was slow. Often, a ship's captain assumed the role of religious deacon, and frequently his wife assumed midwife responsibilities. Early treatment for illness in the English colonies consisted of prayer and superstitious practices. Early American hospitals admitted the poor and destitute along with the sick. Care was provided by uneducated persons from public work houses and houses of correction. When hospitals opened in New York in 1751 and Philadelphia in 1771, they admitted only ill individuals. Although the New York and Philadelphia hospitals relied solely on private donations for support, administrators exercised care in selecting the person who provides client care services. The hospitals offered basic training in client care. Dr. Valentine Seaman of the New York Hospital was the first physician known to have lectured American nurses in the areas of anatomy, physiology, maternal nursing, and care of children (Jamieson & Sewall, 1954; Kalisch & Kalisch, 2004).

Take Note!
As the New World was colonized, members of religious orders established the earliest health care systems.

During the American Revolutionary War, Catholic nuns were the only organized group of nurses. Women followed husbands to the battlegrounds and provided nursing care to the wounded and infirm soldiers. Many homes and barns became hospitals. In 1786, the Quakers established the Philadelphia Dispensary, where physicians practiced disease prevention. In New York, a residential insane asylum was founded in 1798. In Canada, the Augustinian nuns from France established hospitals, visiting nurse programs, schools, and orphanages (Jamieson & Sewall, 1954; Nutting & Dock, 1935b).

THE MOVEMENT OF NURSING TO A RESPECTABLE PROFESSION (1820–1917)

Although efforts to educate nurses did not become formalized until the early 19th century, at the end of the 18th century, nursing manuals began to appear. Some contained commonsense information, while others were scientifically based. Dr. J.D. Phahler's manual gave specific instructions on how to arrange and maintain a sick room, procedures for various treatments, instructions for use of equipment, and maintenance of written records. Along with procedures, Phahler's manual emphasized the importance of attending to clients' psychological needs. Dr. Franz May's nursing manual provided more general approaches to client care and also emphasized the importance of maintaining the health of caregivers. In 1836, Pastor Gossner, who assumed responsibility for a German evangelical hospital, favored the word "Pflegerin" (nurse) to title care attendants in Prussia (Nutting & Dock, 1935b).

In 1821, Pastor Theodor Fliedner arrived in Kaiserworth, Germany, to find himself the pastor of a financially depressed congregation. Fliedner founded a hospital there for two purposes: to care for the sick and to provide a field for deaconess instruction. In 1836, Gertrud Reichardt, a physician's daughter who helped with her father's practice, became the first probationer of the hospital. A probationer was a young woman who expressed an interest in becoming a nurse but was uncertain if she had the stamina, fortitude, and determination to learn how and to provide client care services. Under the leadership of Pastor Fliedner's wife Fredrike, the hospital tended to the sick and probationers received clinical and theoretical instruction on the art of nursing. Upon completion of their education, the newly ordained deaconesses provided services to the poor, imprisoned, and infirm (Jamieson & Sewall, 1954; Nutting & Dock, 1935b). The deaconesses from Kaiserworth established an honorable reputation of nursing that spread worldwide. In 1850, Fliedner took several deaconesses to Pittsburgh, Pennsylvania, where they staffed a hospital. The movement progressed to Milwaukee, Wisconsin, where the Deaconess Home and Hospital was founded (Jamieson & Sewall, 1954; Nutting & Dock, 1935b).

In 1811, Stephen Grellet, a French American, became appalled at the living conditions of the children who had been born in prison. He consulted Elizabeth Fry, an English friend, to help. Fry had developed a program for the female prisoners to make and sell goods. Revenue generated from the sale of the goods provided funds to feed, clothe, and care for the children. As she traveled throughout Europe setting up similar programs, Fry became acquainted with **Kaiserworth**, a German training program for nurses. Fry referred Florence Nightingale to Kaiserworth upon learning of Nightingale's interest in nursing (Jamieson & Sewall, 1954; Nutting & Dock, 1935b).

In 1831, a group of Irish women under the leadership of Catherine McAuley formed the Religious Sisters of Mercy and provided nursing services throughout Ireland and the world. The Irish sisters devised a system of **careful nursing** that comprised "physical care and emotional consolation provided from a spiritual perspective" (Meehan, 2003, p. 99). In the realm of careful nursing, each client was cared for with great tenderness, gentleness, kindness, and patience. Clients received highly skilled care from nurses who practiced with spiritual love, sought to create an environment of calmness, created restorative environments, strove for perfection in keeping clients safe and comfortable, provided health education, collaborated with physicians and other health care providers, and took care of themselves. During the Asian cholera epidemic of 1832, there was a substantially lower mortality rate among recipients of nursing services from McAuley and her colleagues (Meehan, 2003).

The Nursing Society of Philadelphia was founded in 1836 and primarily provided home maternity services. This group selected its nurses from the applicants who displayed stable character. In 1850, the Nursing Society opened a home and school where systematic instruction was given on cooking and obstetrics. Students received clinical instruction in client homes (Jamieson & Sewall, 1954).

In the antebellum south, some Black slaves were recognized for their healing gifts and skills in nursing and midwifery. Most of the slave nurses and midwives used their nursing skills to tend to the ill and injured on the plantations where they resided. However, there were some Black slave nurses who provided care to the sick and delivered babies out in the wider community. The slave owners would charge for the nursing and midwifery services. Sometimes, they would share the fee with the Black midwives. Jensey Snow is one such midwife who received praise for the extraordinary care she provided for the ill while risking her own health and safety. In 1825, her owner, Benjamin Harrison, granted her freedom. She continued working as a nurse and opened a hospital in Petersburg, Virginia (Kirchgessner, 2018).

FIGURE 2.1 Florence Nightingale (1820–1910) photograph, circa 1880.

Florence Nightingale and the Birth of Nursing as a Profession

The beginnings of nursing reform evolved from efforts to reform prisons and hospitals. **Florence Nightingale** (Fig. 2.1) led the efforts to reform client care and establish nursing as a profession.

Nightingale was born into an affluent English family. Her father delighted in teaching her Latin, Greek, and other languages, as well as mathematics, science, and reading. According to her diary entries, Nightingale identified nursing as her life passion from her experiences accompanying her mother on hospital visits. Although the elder Nightingale expressed concern about her daughter keeping company with drunken, immoral nurses and tending to the needs of people with unhealthy bodies in prisonlike, dirty, smelly hospitals, when Nightingale turned 25, her parents allowed her to attend a British hospital–based nurse's training program. Nightingale did not practice nursing fulltime after her training, but continued to travel with her parents.

After visiting with nuns in Rome, Nightingale explored the option of starting a community of trained nurses. A friend of the Nightingale family informed Nightingale about Kaiserworth. Nightingale attended Kaiserworth in 1850 and 1851, where she was instructed in the art of nursing (Jamieson & Sewall, 1954; Kalisch & Kalisch, 2004; Nutting & Dock, 1935b). At age 34, Nightingale became the superintendent of a small London institution that provided shelter to homeless women and nursing services to sick governesses.

When the British became involved with the Crimean War, they discovered that they had no sisters to assist with injured and infirm troops. In 1854, the British government appointed Nightingale as the superintendent of the nursing staff because of her demonstrated ability to obtain and organize resources for the homeless and to provide effective nursing services care. She and 38 other women (including Joanna Bridgeman, a colleague of Catherine McAuley) went to Scutari, Turkey, where they found two hospitals in deplorable condition. Nightingale obtained funding and supplies from friends and transformed the hospitals into clean, well-ventilated buildings that provided nutritious meals for the clients. The hospitals' mortality rate of 40% declined to 2% after the implementation of Nightingale's reforms (Jamieson & Sewall, 1954; Kalisch & Kalisch, 2004; Meehan, 2003). Nightingale also considered the physical and psychosocial needs of the ill and injured. She wrote letters for soldiers, employed wives who had accompanied spouses to the battlefield, and made night rounds in the wards with a lamp. Power, admiration, and fame came to Nightingale. Before long, army nursing under Nightingale evolved into a health service valued by the British government.

During the Crimean War, Nightingale met **Mary Seacole** (Fig. 2.2), a Jamaican nurse volunteer who also nursed the soldiers. Seacole saw the need for holistic outreach nursing services for civilians who had been injured or displaced. She set up a hotel where she provided shelter, relaxation, and excellent food. When guests became ill, she prescribed medicines. After the war, Seacole dedicated her life to elevating nursing to a respectable profession (Wheeler, 1999).

In 1855, prominent British citizens established the "Nightingale fund" to enable Nightingale to establish a school to train women in the art of nursing. Nightingale expected graduates of her school to teach nursing to the entire world. Besides establishing a formalized program of nursing education, Nightingale continued her efforts at reforming hospitals, public health, and nursing (Jamieson & Sewall, 1954; Nutting & Dock, 1935b).

Along with Nightingale, several American women influenced the reform of health care and nursing. In

FIGURE 2.2 A postage stamp printed in the United Kingdom circa 2006, bearing the portrait of Mary Seacole (1805–1881), highlights how the profession of nursing has been shaped by nurses from diverse cultural backgrounds.

1893, Lillian Wald and Mary Brewster opened a Nurses' Settlement House in New York City. They used the term **"public health nurse"** to describe the trained nurses who responded to nursing needs outside the hospital. These nurses responded to calls from individuals as well as physicians to provide home nursing services. The program provided services regardless of the ability of recipients to pay. In 1895, Wald and Brewster moved to larger accommodations that became known as the Henry Street Settlement House. By 1900, 20 district nursing organizations employed 200 trained nurses across the United States (Roberts, 1954).

▌ QUESTIONS FOR REFLECTION

1. Did you know about the contributions of people other than Florence Nightingale to professional nursing in the 19th century?

2. Why do you suppose these contributions may have been overlooked?

THE BIRTH OF FORMAL NURSING EDUCATION

In the Victorian era (1837–1901), upper- and middle-class women led circumscribed lives: They were deemed the property of their fathers or husbands, had no independent rights, and were considered incapable of intellectual development. Some in Victorian society even thought that education would damage women's reproductive organs. Women from lower classes, for whom work was a necessity, found socially acceptable employment as retail clerks, factory workers, governesses, or domestic servants. Nursing, however, was considered an unacceptable profession and reserved for female paupers from work houses or those who served prison time for drunkenness, vagrancy, or prostitution.

Nightingale's service in the Crimean War elevated the nursing profession. Society began thinking of nursing as an art that "must be raised to the status of a trained profession" (Kjervik & Martinson, 1979, p. 22), and efforts to standardize training were made. Although Nightingale established a theoretical model for nursing practice, she proposed that nurses should follow protocol rather than use independent thinking. She emphasized that nurses should be taught how to carry out physicians' orders. To maintain discipline, Nightingale delineated a strict nursing service hierarchy. Good character superseded intellectual ability when the Nightingale nursing school selected students. Education in Nightingale's school focused on teaching nurses what to do and how to do it, following physicians' orders, knowing why, training the senses, and linking these things with reflection to decide what should be done (Kalisch & Kalisch, 2004).

Civil War Nursing

As nursing became more acceptable, women volunteered during the Civil War to be nurses. American women transformed the ballrooms of their homes into wards for injured and infirm soldiers, resulting in the birth of **Civil War nursing**. Dorothea Dix, who was appointed as the superintendent of female nurses in the Union Army, founded the first American Army Nursing Corps and was given full power to organize human and material resources to care for sick and injured soldiers.

Along with the Army Nursing Corps, female volunteers and family members also provided nursing services to Civil War casualties. Author Louisa May Alcott served as a nurse during the war and wrote about her tragic experiences caring for soldiers. Mary Ann "Mother" Bickerdyke diligently searched to find living soldiers who had been wounded in battle but had been mistakenly placed among the dead. Clara Barton, a former schoolteacher from New England, independently organized a large relief effort to provide supplies to care for those injured or displaced on both sides of the battle and occasionally provided nursing care. In 1881, Barton persuaded the U.S. government to ratify the Geneva treaty of the Red Cross and is credited with starting the American Red Cross.

Jane Stuart Woolsey, a Union hospital nurse, kept detailed records of her observations. She and her sister served as supervisors of the nursing and cooking department for a Union hospital located on a Virginian hillside. Woolsey had the opportunity to visit various types of hospitals during the Civil War and noted that the hospitals run by nuns seemed to have a system for client care along with discipline and order in contrast to the haphazard care provided by most military and public hospitals (Kalisch & Kalisch, 2004). Along with female volunteers, Young Men's Christian Association (YMCA) members volunteered to serve as nurses (Jamieson & Sewall, 1954).

In Confederate states, most of the nursing care was delivered by Southern "matrons" who volunteered their services. Efforts made by these women focused on cooking, making bandages, and sewing. Slaves and plantation mistresses and daughters worked together at times to provide care for wounded and sick soldiers (Kalisch & Kalisch, 2004).

American Hospital Training Programs and Diploma Schools

In the United States, nursing training programs started simultaneously when society accepted and provided opportunities for college education for upper-class women. As medical education moved into the postgraduate university, nursing education became established as apprenticeship training under the control of physicians and hospitals. The first nursing training programs were established in 1872 and 1873 in Boston, New Haven, and New York City. In 1879, Mary E.P. Mahoney earned a diploma in nursing "from the School of Nursing of the New England Hospital for Women and Children in Boston" (Kalisch & Kalisch, 2004). Nursing programs were opened for Black nursing students in the 1880s (Kalisch & Kalisch, 2004). By 1880, 15 programs existed. Within a decade, the number of programs had grown to 432, and 3,465 nurses had graduated (Burgess, 1928).

The early hospital training schools had some autonomy in determining the nursing program of study but rapidly became dependent on hospitals for financial support, eventually becoming nursing service departments within the affiliated hospitals. Students worked

7 days a week, 50 weeks per year for 1 to 2 years in exchange for on-the-job training, a few lectures, and a small allowance. Only unmarried women (single or widowed) were accepted as students. Students followed strict rules and schools tolerated no misconduct. Staffing the hospitals with students and faculty proved financially advantageous, and hospitals without training programs quickly established them. Hospitals quickly discovered that they could care for more clients and reap large profits when they provided nursing education. Between 1880 and 1926, the number of hospital-based nursing programs increased from 15 to 2,155 (Burgess, 1928).

The United States was not the only nation to provide formal nursing education in hospitals; Australia and Great Britain also educated nurses within the confines of hospitals. Hospital training programs became the dominant form of nursing education in the early part of the 20th century. However, untrained nurses continued to practice nursing, especially in rural areas where they filled a need and held the respect of their communities (Kalisch & Kalisch, 2004; Madsen, 2005). Unlike their trained counterparts, untrained nurses willingly provided housekeeping services along with client care. They also filled the need for caregivers in long-term care institutions (Madsen, 2005).

Nursing program graduates found themselves in hospital supervisory positions or in homes as private duty nurses. Hospitals with nursing students used the students as staff or contracted their services with families and pocketed the money for the services rendered. Typical private duty nursing cases required the nurse to live with families and be available 24 hours a day. The average wage earned was $120 per month. The nurse remained idle if not on a private case. As nurses aged, they lacked the stamina required for all-night vigils and the hard work required for safe, effective client care (Goldmark, 1923).

Not all nursing program graduates became licensed when the process of registration and licensure was initiated because they could provide nursing services without one. The first state to require registration of nurses was North Carolina in 1903. To qualify for registration, the program graduate had to complete the curriculum of a recognized hospital training program or diploma school. The state provided an exam to ensure that the nurse was competent. The exam consisted of two parts, a written knowledge exam regarding safe client care and the actual demonstration of a skilled nursing procedure. Meeting these requirements provided the nurse with a permissive license to use the title "registered nurse" (RN). Hospitals would employ one RN to supervise nursing program graduates and nursing students (Benefiel, 2011).

Early efforts to establish autonomy and a collegial subculture started during this era. To maintain records of RNs, North Carolina formed the first state board of nursing. The National League for Nursing (NLN) Education was established by the American Society of Superintendents of Training Schools in Nursing in 1893 and started drafting a standardized curriculum for nurse training programs, which was published in 1917 (NLN, 2020). Ten nurses who had graduated from nursing programs organized the Nurses' Associated Alumnae of the United States and Canada in a Manhattan Beach hotel in 1896, and 2 years later, nearly 10,000 nurses attended the organization's convention. The association recognized the need to publish information exclusively for nursing and published *The American Journal of Nursing* starting in 1900. The association changed its name to the American Nurses Association (ANA) in 1911 (Benefiel, 2011). Because Black nurses were barred from ANA membership, Martha Minerva Franklin founded the National Association of Colored Nursing Graduates (NACNG) in 1908. The association kept a registry of professional nurses, promoted the welfare of Black nurses, and addressed issues related to racial discrimination in the profession (African American Registry, 2020).

In the late 1890s and early 20th century, medical and public health journals published articles that asserted that diseases were carried by African Americans and that they posed a direct threat to White Americans. Due to discrimination in health care, African American churches, physicians, and institutions established their own hospitals; some were segregated while others provided care exclusively to African Americans. Some of the hospitals established nurse training programs to ensure a constant supply of nurses would meet future staffing needs. Like their White counterparts, Black nurses were subjected to hospital exploitation and experienced low social status. However, they were also subject to discrimination and inequality when working in segregated health care organizations (Hehman, 2018). For these reasons, Black women avoided joining the nursing profession. There were more untrained Black midwives than there were professional nurses at this time (Hehman, 2018).

■ QUESTIONS FOR REFLECTION

1. Do you think today's nursing students and professional nurses are exploited by their employers? Why or why not?
2. How do you think today's employers exploit professional nurses if you believe they do?
3. What safeguards are in place to prevent exploitation of nurses by employers? Why are these important?

Proliferation of Nursing Education Programs

The proliferation of nursing programs between 1880 and 1900 resulted in widespread variance in nursing education quality. Linda Richards, a graduate of a Canadian nursing program and the first trained American nurse, led reforms in major American nursing programs (Jamieson & Sewall, 1954). Isabel Hampton Robb questioned the qualifications of nursing faculty and spearheaded the first educational program for nursing faculty at Teacher's College in New York in 1901 (Dock, 1912).

Widespread public concern arose regarding the safety of nursing and medical care. Reforms in nursing education followed reforms in medical education. In 1910, the Flexner Report broadcasted problems with the quality of medical education, resulting in drastic reforms (Flexner, 1910). Nursing leaders of the time hoped the Flexner Report would also result in nursing education reform. The Goldmark Report (1923) and other studies and surveys conducted at the time indicated that the root of most of the difficulties related to nursing training stemmed from the nursing schools' dual purpose of providing both education and nursing service. Unfortunately, these studies resulted in limited reform. Table 2.1 highlights the development of modern nursing education programs.

Baccalaureate Programs

In 1893, the School of Medicine at Howard University (Washington, D.C.) established the first nursing diploma program within a university setting. The program, designed for African American students, lasted only 1 year before being assumed by Freedmen's Hospital. The University of Texas recognized nursing in the early 1890s and gave an endowed professorial chair to Hanna Kindborn, who lectured to both nursing and

TABLE 2.1   The Development of Modern Nursing Education Programs

Year	Event
1897	First school for training practical nurses opens.
1898	Daughters of the American Revolution serve as the examining board for military nurses.
1903	North Carolina becomes the first state to require registration of nurses.
1909	University of Minnesota starts a baccalaureate degree nursing program.
1911	1006 hospital-based nursing training programs and 90 mental health institution–based nursing programs exist.
1920s	Apprenticeship approach dominates nursing educations.
1923	The Goldmark Report proposes that additional education beyond the basic diploma is needed for practice in public health, nursing education, and supervision.
1926	25 nursing programs grant Bachelor of Arts (BA) or a Bachelor of Science degree in Nursing (BSN), with Yale opening the first separate university nursing department in 1924.
1930	11 practical nursing programs operate in the United States.
1936	1,472 hospital-based education programs, 70 collegiate nursing education programs, and 36 practical nursing programs exist.
1941	Crash programs are developed to train nursing aides to alleviate the nursing shortage of World War II.
1948	The Brown Report ranks nurses as important to society as teachers and ranks collegiate nursing education as equal to other professional education programs.
1952	Accreditation programs are created for practical and professional nursing schools.
1954	296 practical nursing programs are in existence.
1958	Birth of ADN programs in community colleges.
1963	*Toward Quality in Nursing Needs and Goals. A Report of the Surgeon General's Consultant Group in Nursing* is released by the U.S. Public Health Service.
1964	The Nursing Training Act is enacted.
1965	The ANA releases its *Position Paper on Education for Nursing*.
1966	797 hospital-based, 218 ADN, and 210 BSN programs exist.
1982	288 hospital-based, 742 ADN, and 402 BSN programs exist.
2003	60 hospital-based, 890 ADN, and 661 BSN programs exist.

From Kalisch, P. A., & Kalisch, B. J. (2004). *American Nursing: A History* (4th ed.). Lippincott Williams & Wilkins.

medical students (Dock, 1912). In 1909, the University of Minnesota established a 3-year diploma nursing program within its College of Medicine. In subsequent years, colleges adopted the pattern of combining academic and professional courses that led to both a diploma and a Bachelor of Science in Nursing (BSN) degree. Students attended academic courses at the university and received professional nursing courses using the apprenticeship model at the hospital (Dock, 1912; Jamieson & Sewall, 1954). In 1909, Dr. Richard Olding Beard instituted a plan to make nursing a college major at the University of Minnesota (Jamieson & Sewall, 1954).

In 1923, Yale University established a nursing program that had its own dean and endowed funds. Other universities that established baccalaureate nursing programs included Case Western Reserve University

in 1923, the University of Chicago in 1925, and Vanderbilt University in 1930. As nursing education moved to the collegiate setting, physicians voiced opposition because they thought higher education and theoretical knowledge might lead nurses to question their authority (Kalisch & Kalisch, 2004).

Associate Degree Programs

The Brown Report (Brown, 1948) and the Ginzberg Report (Ginzberg, 1949), two privately commissioned reports, specified that professional nursing education should be removed from hospitals and transferred to the collegiate setting. In her 1951 doctoral dissertation, Mildred Montag suggested that education for the technical nurse should occur in community college settings. She proposed that technical nurse education would result in a terminal degree and that technical nursing would attain a unique and semiprofessional identity (Montag, 1951). Upon graduation, the technical nurse would be completely prepared for hospital or nursing home employment. Community college nursing programs flourished. Graduates of Associate Degree in Nursing (ADN) programs were given the same professional nursing licensure examination as graduates from diploma and baccalaureate nursing programs.

▣ QUESTIONS FOR REFLECTION

1. How did the associate degree nursing program affect the nursing profession?
2. What differences do you see between nurses educated at the associate degree, diploma, and baccalaureate degree levels?

THE AMERICAN PUBLIC HEALTH MOVEMENT

As the field of public health nursing grew, basic principles specific to the specialty emerged. Reform efforts indicated a need to provide nursing services to all who were sick without considering the ability to pay, religious affiliation, or ethnic background. District nurses identified the need to keep formal client records to facilitate consistency in service. To avoid duplication of services and prevent gaps in fulfilling client needs, nurses learned the importance of cooperation with other groups providing community care. During the rise of the public health movement, the family became the basic care unit (Spradley, 1990). Some public health nurses acknowledged the limitations of their hospital-based educations and sought additional education in institutions of higher learning to develop a global approach for community nursing.

Public health nursing prospered from 1900 until the outbreak of World War I. The client home served as the major location for nursing practice as hospitals had become places to receive charity, contract infection, and die.

Other Social Reform Movements

Other social reform movements in the early 1900s impacted the nursing profession. William Booth founded the Salvation Army to protect the poor, the ex-prisoners, the old, the young, and any who were miserable and had been perceived by the society as having fallen from the grace of God. Jane Addams established Hull House in Chicago, which provided day care, kindergarten, and library services to immigrant women and children. Christian associations of young men and women were formed to build character and provide community services. These associations were the forerunners of today's YMCA and Young Women's Christian Associations (YWCA). Medicine experienced reforms that emphasized science and invention over superstitious practices. The spread of the telegraph and telephone also helped spread the word of these movements across the United States and throughout the world (Jamieson & Sewall, 1954; Kalisch & Kalisch, 2004).

NURSING DURING THE EARLY 20TH CENTURY, THE WORLD WARS, AND THE POST-WORLD WAR II ERA (1890–1960)

North Carolina led the efforts in **state registration** of nurses in 1903 by establishing guidelines for professional registration. Requirements included graduation from an established diploma nursing school. New Jersey and New York quickly followed. By 1912, 29 states and the District of Columbia had registration requirements for nurses. To renew initial registration, nurses were given a 3-year grace period to practice, then were required to take a licensing examination that emphasized dietetics, client comfort, skilled handling of clients, and general management (Dock, 1912).

Registration as a professional nurse was not limited to women. But the few male nurses suffered discrimination in professional practice. According to Kalisch and Kalisch (2004), male nurses were described in a 1914 hospital administration manual as being a composite of genius and drunkenness but seemed more easygoing than their female colleagues. They were accused of taking sips of whiskey while on duty to cope with the daily stresses of clinical practice. During World War I, trained male nurses were assigned to National Guard units and gained expertise in psychiatric mental health nursing (Kalisch & Kalisch, 2004).

As the United States entered World War I in 1917, unmarried trained nurses entered the Army and Navy Nurse Corps. Volunteers from well-to-do families served as nurses' aides at their own expense. The government launched a publicity campaign to recruit women into nursing. Advertisements glamorizing nursing appeared in newspapers and magazines. However, on the battlefields, the nurses encountered the horrors of battlefield injuries. At times, the nurse-to-client ratio rose to as high as 1:60. Nurses were required to perform surgery to save lives. The flu epidemic of 1918 to 1919 only compounded the need for more nurses (Kalisch & Kalisch, 2004).

Nursing sustained an image problem in the 1920s. Movies portrayed nursing in unrealistic and unflattering ways. Reduced prestige for the profession resulted from several factors: (1) 95% of nurses were women, (2) most nursing leaders were unmarried, (3) societal expectations were that the woman's place was in the home as a devoted wife and mother, and (4) nursing was portrayed as an altruistic, self-sacrificing profession in a time that valued frivolity and self-indulgence.

By the 1920s, most trained nurses were employed as private duty nurses. However, technologic advances in client care and improvements in hospital facilities led to more clients being hospitalized for treatment and surgery. Public acceptance of going to the hospital for acute and serious illnesses reduced the demand for private duty nurses working in home settings (Kalisch & Kalisch, 2004). Hospitals relied on student nurses for client care, leaving program graduates unemployed. In 1939, the NLN reported that the typical hospital connected with a school of nursing. By the 1920s, most trained nurses were employed as private duty nurses. However, technologic advances in client care and improvements in hospital facilities led to more clients being hospitalized for treatment and surgery. Public acceptance of going to the hospital for acute and serious illnesses reduced the demand for private duty nurses working in home settings (Kalisch & Kalisch, 2004). Hospitals relied on student nurses for client care, leaving program graduates unemployed. In 1939, the NLN reported that the typical hospital connected with a school of nursing during 1938 employed only an average of 10 graduate nurses for general duty (NLN, 1939, 2020).

During the Great Depression, trained nursing graduates willingly worked for room and board. As the economic state improved, hospitals kept these trained nurses on staff while paying them an hourly wage. Medical advances increased the demand for educated RNs. A few nurses found employment with the new aviation industry as nurse-stewardesses. Other nurses participated in the Civil Works Administration (CWA) and Works Progress Administration (WPA) programs and became employed in public hospitals, clinics, and public health agencies.

Efforts to find best practices for nursing procedures started during this era. Even though nursing research was not a formalized process, nursing all over the world disseminated information through publications such as *The American Journal of Nursing, The Canadian Nurse,*

and *Kai Tiaki* in New Zealand. A description of nurses during this era is explained in the following Focus on Research box that examines artifacts from these times to specify the process for determining best practices for nursing procedures.

Although most nurses were women in 1940, there were five nursing schools that exclusively educated male nurses. Of these, four were accredited by the NLN and enrolled 212 men. There were also 63 coeducational programs with a combined enrollment of 710 men and 3,798 women. When more men were available to provide direct bedside care, hospital administrators noted improvements in the care of male clients, especially in the areas of psychiatric and genitourinary nursing (Kalisch & Kalisch, 2004).

In 1941, President Franklin Roosevelt issued an executive order that declared that all Americans were encouraged to fully participate in national defense programs. He proclaimed that the nation could only be defended with success if all Americans could work together. In addition, Roosevelt extended steps toward equality in America by appointing the Fair Employment Practices Committee. The efforts of the committee opened up new employment opportunities for all Americans because of the need for increased production of war-related products. Between 1940 and 1944, Black employment in manufacturing rose by close to 700,000 persons and the number of Black people employed in governmental service more than tripled (Kalisch & Kalisch, 2004).

By World War II, graduate nurses and RNs had become accepted members of hospital staffs. When hospitals discovered that hiring RNs could cut costs, many nursing schools closed. However, as news of war loomed in Europe, the government took steps to promote the entry of young women into nursing. Recruitment methods included advertisements in printed media and the Cadet Nurse Corps. The Cadet Nurse Corps was designed to provide nurses for essential and military nursing for the duration of World War II. The program was open to all young women who wanted to become nurses. Two thousand young Black women entered the program with 20 all-Black nursing schools enrolling 1,600 of them (Kalisch & Kalisch, 2004). As RNs joined the military, a civilian nurse shortage resulted. Hospitals employed civilian workers who held certificates from the Red Cross and hired the volunteers who had been helping nurses with nonprofessional duties.

In addition, Black nurses were permitted to join the ANA but only if they secured membership in a state nurse association that specified no restrictions for race

FOCUS ON RESEARCH

Standardized Nursing Practice: Striving for Best Practice

In the 1930s, nurses identified the need to standardize nursing procedures to improve client care and to strengthen nursing education. In New Zealand, the head of the National Nursing Association, Mary Lambie, held responsibility for all nursing matters in the country. She formed a Nursing Education Committee (NEC) with members of nurses from a variety of practice areas. The NEC goal was to develop best practices for nursing procedures. The committee sent surveys about two to three nursing procedures to nurse administrators of all training hospitals. They combined the survey responses and constructed a model method for each nursing procedure. These results were published in *Kai Tiaki*. The journal was then circulated to all nurse training schools by the Department of Health.

Starting in the 1940s, the model procedures consisted of a series of recommended steps but also contained rationales for underlying key principles for nurse consideration. Nurses then could vary the procedure steps and supplies according to local conditions but would pay close attention as to not violate the key principles. The model procedures were reviewed by a medical committee of physicians, and many times, they specified that more study was required.

Some of the standardized procedures developed by the NEC included the following: hand hygiene, cleanliness of nursing uniforms, isolation procedures, sterile dressings, bedsore prevention, bedpan use, oral care, temperature taking, urine testing, and all routes of medication administration. Before finalizing each procedure, the NEC submitted them to a medical advisory committee who agreed with them but did not approve them. The goal was to have the training hospitals develop film strips and guidelines for test questions, but World War II derailed the project.

Formalized nursing research studies can be traced back to the early 1930s when research studies were performed in the United States and Canada for establishing the effectiveness of intramuscular injections of camphor oil to ease postpartum breast engorgement, comparing ways to optimally disinfect thermometers and to determine the effectiveness of cod liver oil use to treat wounds and burns. In New Zealand, a nurse compared two treatments of scales, two treatments for impetigo, and four treatments for pediculosis and compared costs, number of required treatments, and days of treatment needed to obtain a cure.

At the 1927 International Council of Nurses (ICN) conference, the organization cautioned against the use of standardized practice because it might interfere with the best interest of the client or the well-being of the nurse. However, the group also concluded that identification of standardized practices could be applied to develop scientific nursing practice. The search for the "one" way to perform nursing procedures became the search for the best way.

Results of this reveal the importance of having key underlying scientific principles to guide professional nursing practice in order to provide optimal nursing care. The perception of standardized practice as becoming monotonous routine practice without being able to individualize client care to best meet client needs persists today. Like the search for standardized procedures, evidence-based practice protocols will continually be challenged as ways of health care delivery change.

Wood, P., & Nelson, K. (2013). Striving for best practice: Standardizing New Zealand nursing procedures, 1930–1960. *Journal of Clinical Nursing, 22*, 3217–3224. https://doi.org/10.1111/jocn.12456

---

as a condition for membership (Kalisch & Kalisch, 2004). Previously, these nurses could join the National Association of Colored Graduate Nurses (NACGN) that was founded by Martha Minerva Franklin. Like the ANA, the NACGN worked toward advancing the welfare of its members. In addition, the NACGN fought to win integration of African American RNs into all nursing employment opportunities,

nursing education programs, and nursing organizations (African American Registry, 2020). By 1951, the NACGN merged with the ANA.

After World War II, the United States experienced a time of great economic growth. Companies offered health insurance as a fringe benefit for workers and a concession for not increasing wages. Workplace reforms led to an 8-hour workday and a 40-hour workweek.

Scientific advancements transformed health care delivery and everyday life. Nurses embraced the scientific method and established a four-step process (assessment, planning, implementation, and evaluation) to deliver client care starting in the 1950s. This process, called the nursing process, guided education and became the basis for professional nursing licensing exams. The NLN Committee on Testing managed the nursing license examination process, including test construction and administration, starting in 1944. In 1955, the ANA assumed control over nursing licensure test administration (Benefiel, 2011; NLN 2020). See Chapter 8, "Professional Nursing Processes" for more about nursing process.

Insurance reimbursement of hospital care resulted in an increase in the number of hospital beds. Hospitals also became profitable and provided a central location for advancements in medical technology. However, the nursing shortage worsened as more hospital beds became available. Many nurses left practice to pursue marriage, better-paying jobs outside the profession, and more autonomous positions in industry or public health.

Segregation became outlawed in the United States in 1954 with the Supreme Court ruling in the *Brown v. Board of Education in Topeka* case. This decision overturned the long-held doctrine of "separate but equal" and espoused that all students, regardless of race, are offered "equal protection of the law." This landmark case created opportunities for all Americans to pursue educational endeavors that had previously been unavailable to them. Before the ruling, the NLN had issued a position that nursing education should be open to all individuals. Prior to World War II, only 42 American nursing schools would admit Black students. This number rose to 710 programs following the NLN's 1953 position statement on the need to open nursing program enrollment to all students (Kalisch & Kalisch, 2004).

NURSING IN THE MODERN ERA (1960–1999)

The 1960s

The 1960s ushered in a time of great change in American culture. The civil rights movement to end racial segregation, begun more than a decade earlier, accelerated, and marches and acts of civil disobedience increased awareness among all Americans about the inequalities that were present in everyday life. In 1965, Congress enacted President Lyndon B. Johnson's

"Great Society" legislation to create a society in which all citizens would have equal access to employment, education, and health care. Many of today's current social programs, such as Medicare and government grants for education, grew out of the civil rights movement and this legislation. Equal rights meant equal rights for all, including all women. In the early 1960s, the health care system consisted primarily of independent, not-for-profit hospitals; small, independent physician offices; and neighborhood pharmacies and medical supply stores. Individuals unable to afford care sought health care services in local government-managed hospitals and clinics. By working independently or in small practices, physicians enjoyed autonomy and control over client care. Hospitals recruited physicians to join medical staffs. Private insurance companies or clients reimbursed physicians based on fee-for-service payment systems. In the health care system of the 1960s, nurses were viewed as subservient to physicians.

Although the NLN denied accreditation to hospital diploma schools that used students to staff hospitals in the 1960s, hospital-based diploma schools remained the dominant educational pattern for registered nursing until the early 1970s. Educational reforms instituted in the 1960s resulted in increased expenditures for hospitals that sponsored diploma programs. Some hospitals offered solid nursing education but at a marked financial deficit. The federal government offered hospitals with diploma programs direct reimbursement for the number of student practice days to defray education-induced costs. In response to a predicted need for 680,000 additional professional nurses by 1970, the federal government increased funding for nursing education through a series of initiatives, including professional nurse traineeships, the Nurse Training Act of 1964, and the Health Professions Educational Act of 1963 (Kalisch & Kalisch, 2004).

In 1965, ANA published the *ANA Position Paper on Education for Nursing*, which specified that the minimum educational level for beginning professional nursing practice should be the BSN, the minimum educational preparation for technical nursing practice should be the ADN, and all unlicensed care assistants should receive education in vocational education centers instead of just on-the-job training. The proposal assumed that hospital diploma nursing schools would collaborate with either baccalaureate degree-granting institutions or community colleges to develop either professional or technical nursing programs. However, instead of collegial collaboration among hospitals and other educational institutions, the result was a deep division among members within the nursing profession (Flanagan, 1976; Kalisch & Kalisch, 2004).

Growth of the Professional Nurse Workforce

In addition to societal upheavals, the 1960s was also a time of biomedical advancements leading to expensive, life-saving technologies. Complex surgical procedures, new pharmaceuticals, the establishment of intensive care units (ICUs), and new technologies increased not only the cost of health care delivery but also the need for highly skilled and educated nurses. By this time, employers offered health care insurance as a standard benefit to workers. Health care expenditures accounted for 5% of the gross domestic product (GDP) in 1960 (Kornfeld et al., 2020). In 1965, the federal government introduced Medicare and Medicaid to provide health care coverage to the older population and the poor. Improved insurance coverage meant improved access to health care services for the employed and the older citizens. Demand for hospital care and physician services increased. Hospital admissions rose, and along with that came the need for highly educated, clinically competent professional nurses for client care.

ADN programs were viewed as a means to provide a quick way to increase the number of nurses capable of hospital practice. Many hospitals that provided nursing diploma programs found themselves struggling to maintain their nursing programs because of the financial costs. The U.S. Public Health Service (1963) issued a report, *Toward Quality in Nursing: Needs and Goals*, that outlined the following concerns: severe deficiencies in the current nursing education, not enough young people entering the nursing profession, high turnover within the nursing profession, the need for collegiate and university-based nursing programs, the persistent low socioeconomic status of nurses, the ineffective use of available nursing personnel, and not enough research being conducted to advance the practice of professional nursing. The report served as evidence for the Nurse Training Act of 1964, which provided federal funding for diploma nursing schools to defray nursing education costs. The act also provided federal monetary support for ADN programs in community colleges and BSN programs in 4-year colleges and universities (Kalisch & Kalisch, 2004).

During the days of the early Vietnam conflict, the Army Student Nurse Program (instituted in 1956) enabled diploma nursing students to receive a free nursing education in return for 2 years of service in the Army Nurse Corps. However, because of the unpopularity of the Vietnam War (1955–1975), the number of nurses willing to serve in the military declined. In 1966, a bill was passed authorizing male nurses to serve as regular forces in the Air Force, Army, and Navy Nurse Corps. By 1967, 22% of the Army Nurse Corps consisted of male professional nurses (Kalisch & Kalisch, 2004). Some military reservists and soldiers who had served in the military opted to use military education benefits toward acquisition of a professional nursing education.

The 1970s

The 1970s saw an increase in inflation and unemployment. Consumers revolted against tax increases. To decrease the economic burden of supplying health care, the government employed mechanisms to monitor health care delivery to Medicare and Medicaid recipients. Although ineffective, these mechanisms, such as utilization review to reduce lengths of hospital stays and physician peer review programs, have become common practice. Hospitals and physicians are still required to participate in these programs or lose Medicare and Medicaid reimbursement.

Insurance providers also carried increased risks as consumers and employers exerted pressure on them to keep premiums from rising. In 1974, the Employment Retirement Security Act added incentives to businesses to self-insure their employees. A few for-profit investor hospitals were established, but medical and hospital care proceeded as usual. Self-insurance enabled employers to negotiate with health care organizations to become preferred providers for an employer-based health insurance program in attempts to curb health care costs. Some professional nurses found differences in working conditions between for-profit and not-for-profit hospitals with higher workloads in the for-profit hospitals.

Health care providers began identifying some disadvantages to using complex and expensive life-saving measures for all clients. Quality of life emerged as more important than the sanctity of life. Most hospitals established "do not resuscitate" protocols because of the futile efforts of attaching the terminally ill or individuals with no brain function to life-supporting machines. Keeping such clients alive began to be considered dehumanizing and a wasteful use of resources (Kongsuwan et al., 2016).

During this era, community colleges prospered as society placed emphasis on equal opportunity for all

American citizens to education. ADN-prepared nurses successfully passed the professional nursing licensure examination and soon filled vacant nursing positions, where they provided effective nursing care services. Costs for hospital-based nursing education programs continued to rise.

Graduate nursing education programs proliferated in the 1970s, offering advanced study in clinical specialty areas, nursing education, and nursing administration. Nurse practitioner programs were started to improve health care delivery while reducing costs. Nursing research became a hallmark of advanced nursing education and practice.

In 1971, the National Institutes of Health (NIH) noted the importance of nursing research and established the National Center for Nursing Research. Compared to medical research, nursing research has been hampered by inadequate financial support. Between 1971 and 1981, the government awarded $40 million to the National Center for Nursing Research. During the same period, the NIH received $1.7 billion for general biomedical research.

The 1970s also ushered in the women's rights movement, sometimes called women's liberation, the modern feminist movement, or second-wave feminism (Malka, 2007). Equality for all oppressed persons became a dominant societal theme during this decade. The perception of nursing as a vocation became outdated. For many individuals, the selection of a professional career focused upon high salary and status rather than pursuing a career as a religious calling (Bradshaw, 2010). Women strove to discover their authentic selves, find personal meaning in their existence, and enjoy social equality. Women found they could pursue other careers besides nursing and teaching, and the nursing profession no longer attracted the best and brightest young women. The ability of women to select other careers seems to have contributed to the current nursing shortage (Gore et al., 2017).

A shift also occurred in the societally accepted goal of women's behavior and attitude toward pleasing men to an opportunity for self-expression and fulfillment. Medicine, a male-dominated profession, dictated how health care was delivered, resulting in further oppression of some nurses. However, other nurses saw the feminist movement as a means to assert themselves and use female empowerment to transform the role of nurses from dutiful servants to competent professionals with an obligation to question physician orders when needed to protect clients. Many nurses asserted their rights as individuals and professionals. Changes proliferated in

practice settings; nurses no longer stood when physicians entered nursing units, gathered charts for rounds, or got coffee for them. However, other nurses found second-wave feminism antithetical to their profession of service. Early years of the feminist movement resulted in further divisions within the nursing profession (Malka, 2007). Nurses began to assert themselves with physicians, administrators, and each other.

Health care teams began to identify client problems that could be managed exclusively by nurses or collaboratively with physicians. These client problems evolved into "nursing diagnoses," and the step "nursing diagnosis" was added as the second step of the established nursing process. Many physicians argued with using the term "diagnosis," as they believed that diagnosing was a process exclusive to medical practice.

In 1975, nursing licensing exams were administered twice annually across multiple testing sites necessitating test delivery by trucks. Disruptions to test security and developing multiple versions of valid and reliable tests were cumbersome. In 1978, the National Council of State Boards of Nursing (NCSBN) was established to give state boards of nursing increased autonomy over nursing licensure, including administration of the licensing exam. Each board of nursing had a representative on the council. Along with enhanced state regulation of nursing licensure, the NCSBN was formed to ensure the public safety and quality of care delivered by nurses (Benefiel, 2011; NCSBN, 2020).

Also during the 1970s, many military-trained paramedics (predominately male) entered the nursing profession. Some nursing programs offered academic credit for previous military training in order to meet admission criteria.

The 1980s

Health care costs continued to skyrocket during the 1980s, despite a weak economy. More expensive and sophisticated diagnostic equipment and treatments became common as new advances in health care were discovered and consumers demanded them. In 1983, Medicare introduced a prospective payment system known as "diagnosis-related groups." The goal of the program was to reduce cost rate increases for hospital care by reducing the length of hospitalization. Employers selected health insurance programs offering preferred provider organizations that negotiated discounted services from participating health care organizations. By the end of the decade, hospitals experienced decreased profits as beds remained empty.

Hospitals consolidated, resulting in a decreased demand for hospital nurses.

In attempts to alleviate the high costs of health care, the nursing profession embarked on expanding the roles of professional nursing. Collegiate nursing programs offered education for nurse practitioners, clinical nurse specialists, and certified nurse midwives along with established advanced education to prepare nursing faculty.

As the number of hospital beds decreased, inpatient acuity increased substantially, thereby requiring highly skilled nurses to care for clients. Primary nursing became the dominant nursing care delivery system and brought the professional nurse back to the bedside. In primary nursing, the RN planned individualized care, implemented the plan, and also provided health education for hospitalized clients and families. Clients were sent home to recover from surgery and illnesses once their conditions stabilized. In response, the demand for nurses working in home health care and ambulatory health care increased.

Feminism further flourished in the 1980s. Carol Gilligan (1982) published *In a Different Voice*, which highlighted key differences between the communication styles of men and women and in the socialization of boys and girls. Gilligan emphasized that women preferred to be connected to each other. Various approaches to feminism arose. Although devised in the 19th century, the liberal feminist view promoted by Gilligan grew in popularity because of its continued commitment toward achieving equality between men and women. Nursing education embraced feminist traditions. Educators and students alike strove to become their authentic selves, use intuition as one means of clinical decision making, and embark on teaching–learning partnerships (Chinn, 2013).

However, some professional nurses would not accept the feminist movement because some in the movement made derogatory comments about the nature of the work of nursing. Many nursing contributions to client care remained invisible (Malka, 2007). People did not see nursing assessments and surveillance activities that save lives, but omissions and adverse effects, such as the failure to reposition bedridden clients leading to pressure ulcer development, were readily apparent. The feminist movement also devalued nursing as a profession because of nursing's subservient status to the medical profession (Malka, 2007).

The 1990s

The 1990s heralded the movement toward cost containment in health care. By 1990, "95% of insured employees were enrolled in some form of managed care, including fee-for-service plans with utilization management, preferred provider organizations, or [health maintenance organizations (HMOs)]" (Bodenheimer & Grumbach, 1995, p. 87). Hospitals, physicians, and insurance companies joined forces and created integrated health care networks. Large surpluses of specialist physicians and a shortage of generalists occurred. Nurse practitioners offered primary care services to fill the void. Physicians increasingly formed large practices, while large commercial companies dominated the insurance market. For-profit companies took control of many nursing homes, home health care companies, and multihospital system networks. Physicians lost control of their medical practices. Third-party payers dictated reimbursement rates to hospitals. Eighty-five million Americans were uninsured, underinsured, or enrolled in Medicaid (Ginzberg, 1995). Insurance providers employed tactics to avoid enrolling potentially high users of health care services, expanded managed care, and emphasized case management.

As hospital and home health care agencies' profits declined, efforts to control costs of services led to reductions in professional nursing staff even as the acuity level of inpatients continued to rise. Use of unlicensed assistive personnel (UAP) became popular despite the evidence that RNs improved client care quality (Brooten & Naylor, 1995). The change in skill mix reduced professional nurse positions, added more delegation responsibilities, and further devalued the contributions of RNs to client care (Buerhaus, 1995).

Client-focused care and work redesign efforts were developed to increase client and staff satisfaction. Key elements of client-focused care included the formation of specialty care units for clients with similar diagnoses, unit-based support services, and cross-training client care teams (Greenberg, 1994). Critical and acute care staff who were cross-trained would develop an appreciation for all things that occurred across the continuum of care within the hospital.

Work redesign efforts expanded the responsibility and job scope for nonprofessional staff. UAP replaced RNs and licensed vocational (practical) nurses. With minimal on-the-job training, UAP perform the basic tasks of client hygiene, ambulation, vital signs, and intake–output determination while assuming phlebotomy, electrocardiography, bladder catheterization, and simple dressing changes in some institutions. In addition, some institutions assigned social workers, housekeeping personnel, dietary workers, respiratory therapists, and clinical laboratory staff to a nursing department under the supervision of a nurse manager.

To improve quality of care by minimizing variance in care-providing procedures, hospitals instituted clinical pathways. **Clinical pathways** outlined standardized plans of care (nursing diagnoses, outcomes, interventions, and projected length of hospital stay) for clients with specific health conditions that required hospitalization. With clinical pathway implementation, individualization of nursing care declined. However, standardized work processes resulted in superior client outcomes. Work redesign resulted in a change of the RN role from direct care provider to one that required more delegation and supervision. Nurses focused work efforts at verifying that client care processes were followed, evaluating client outcomes, and looking for ways to improve care.

■ QUESTIONS FOR REFLECTION

1. How do you think the expanded use of unlicensed personnel in health care settings has affected professional nursing practice?

2. What are the consequences for the nursing profession of increased use of unlicensed care providers?

3. What are the consequences for clients of increased use of unlicensed care providers?

To ensure efficient and effective use of health care resources without sacrificing client satisfaction and care quality, health care providers and insurers developed **case management** systems in order to streamline health care delivery and to ensure continuity of care across care settings. Case management systems varied in setting and implementation. Table 2.2 outlines seven components common to all case management models.

Although social workers served as the first case managers, when it became evident that they were unable to see the entire client situation, health care institutional administration and social workers turned to nurses for assistance. Case management required thought processes frequently used by nurses in clinical practice. Early efforts using nurses as case managers improved client outcomes, increased consumer satisfaction with care, and decreased health care costs (Cohen & Cesta, 2001).

Research in nursing continued to be hampered by inadequate financial support. In 1993, the National Institute for Nursing Research (NINR) was established within the NIH by an act of Congress with the purpose of identifying nursing research priorities,

distributing grants to nurse researchers, and disseminating findings of nursing research to the public and other health professions. In 2000, NINR received $90 billion in federal support to achieve its mission.

By the 1990s, the nursing profession continued to have difficulty in attracting the best and brightest women because other professions were now welcoming them. Ironically, successful and highly educated nurses moved away from bedside care. Advanced practice nurses worked in collaborative partnerships with physicians, although some physicians began to see nurse practitioners and certified nurse midwives as competitors rather than partners (Malka, 2007). Nurses attended to all ranges of human responses to health and illness while providing a caring relationship to facilitate health and healing, according to the 1995 ANA *Social Policy Statement* (ANA, 1995).

NURSING IN THE EARLY POSTMODERN ERA

Scholars debate when the postmodern era actually began. Some feel it began in the 1960s; others claim it started with the introduction of the computer and the internet. Another group of scholars considers the beginning of the postmodern age when questioning with the scientific method was established as the best approach for discoveries to answer the questions surrounding humanity, the environment, and health-related issues (Watson, 1999). Wilson (1998) introduced the term *consilience* to describe unity of knowledge, thereby emphasizing the effects of the past on the present and future. **Consilience** represents the point at which scientific, artistic, ethical, spiritual, social, environmental, and personal knowledge intersect. Some research has discovered that spirituality plays a key role in health and healing, and qualitative research methods hold the same promise as quantitative research in generating health care knowledge. Consilience explains the intertwining of all aspects of human experience and being one with the world, a key characteristic of the postmodern era.

The First Decade of the Postmodern Era (2000–2010)

During the first decade of the 21st century, professional nurses continued to adapt to changes in practice and the society. Scientific advances increased the complexity and costs of health care. Mandatory use of electronic health records for all health care providers became

TABLE 2.2 Common Components of Case Management Systems

Component	Case Manager Duties
Client identification and outreach	Receive clients through referrals, interviews, and networking
Client assessment and diagnosis	Perform comprehensive holistic client assessments to identify physical, psychological, sociocultural, and spiritual problems
Planning of services and resource identification	Determine what services will be used in collaboration with the client, then assume the responsibility for planning and coordinating the services
Linking clients to required services	Serve as brokers to expedite and follow through with the coordination and planning of services for clients
Coordination and implementation of services	Verify that the identified needs are met and abide by formal agreements made with the service-providing agencies by keeping extensive documentation and records focused on the efficiency, effectiveness, and quality of case-managed care services
Service delivery monitoring	Collaborate with interdisciplinary team members who are providing client services and verify that clients are receiving appropriate, quality services from the agencies
Client advocacy	Work on behalf of clients to ensure clients are receiving services contracted for, making progress in the designated program, and receiving satisfactory services
Evaluation of services and outcomes	Bear responsibility for specific and general client outcomes; continually monitor and reassess services in order to promptly identify the need for change or problems to ensure timely intervention and replanning

the norm. According to the Centers for Medicare & Medicaid Services (CMS, 2010), health care accounted for 17.6% of the GDP in 2010. The population of individuals over age 65 increased 15.1% from 2000 to 2010 (U.S. Census Bureau, 2011). The CMS estimated that close to 80% of health care resources are used by the people in this age group. Efforts to contain health care costs resulted in further reduction in inpatient stays, leading to the transfer of health care services from acute care to either the home or rehabilitation settings.

The gap between the rich and the poor continued to widen, resulting in an increase in governmental funding for health care services. Sources of health care insurance include employers, private purchase, or the government. In 2010, nearly 50 million Americans joined the ranks of the uninsured, and 39 million persons participated in Medicaid programs (Holahan & Chen, 2011).

By virtue of education and practice, nurses demonstrated that they had the best knowledge and skill base to assume the gatekeeper and advocacy roles required of case managers. Nurse practitioners also demonstrated the ability to deliver high-quality health care economically without compromising care quality. Hospitals employed 62.2% of working RNs; many other RNs worked in extended-care facilities, homes, clinics, and community health settings (U.S. Department of Health and Human Services, Health

Resources and Services Administration, & Bureau of Health Professions, 2010).

The Great Recession that began in 2007 resulted in rises in unemployment (with resultant loss of employer-sponsored health insurance coverage), reduced income for the average American, increased home foreclosures, and less money to spend on health care (The Kaiser Family Foundation, 2012). Many RNs (especially those over 50 years of age) returned to the active workforce because spouses had lost their jobs (Buerhaus & Auerbach, 2011).

The confluence of economic factors and reduced access to health care for increased numbers of Americans resulted in the 2010 enactment by Congress of the Patient Protection and Affordable Care Act (ACA). This law mandated incremental reforms in the way health care is delivered and financed, and required all individuals to have health insurance by 2014.

According to the ACA, employers with more than 50 workers must offer health care insurance. The ACA specifies the following services must be covered by the policy: hospitalization, prescription medications, emergency care, comprehensive pediatric health services (including dental and vision coverage), ambulatory (or outpatient) services; pregnancy, maternity, and newborn care; laboratory tests; mental health and substance disorder services; rehabilitative and habilitative (assist the disabled or injured to regain skills for independent living) services and devices; and services for disease prevention, wellness promotion, and chronic disease management (Healthcare.gov, n.d.). Heath insurance exchanges became available to consumers to compare and purchase the best care based on health needs and affordability, and government-financed public health insurance programs were expanded. Programs emphasizing wellness, early detection of illnesses, and disease prevention were established. In addition, programs offering strategies to keep elders at home and out of long-term care institutions were implemented. Health care providers were and continue to be held accountable for outcomes based on comparative effectiveness research. Health care providers including nurses were and are expected to follow evidence-based or best practice guidelines for disease management and prevention.

Reform initiatives, the ever-increasing use by consumers of the internet for health information, and increased use of alternative health care practices created new demands on professional nurses. In some cases, health care consumers (especially those with rare medical conditions) sometimes knew more about their disorders than nurses. Nurses acknowledged that sometimes consumers used sources of unreliable health information and found themselves coaching consumers in strategies to find scientific-based health information.

Because of increasing use of complementary and alternative health care practices, the NIH received funding in 1999 to form the National Center for Complementary and Alternative Medicine (NCCAM) and published its first strategic plan in 2000 (NIH, 2016). In 2008, the NCCAM reported that 38% of Americans used some form of complementary or alternative practices to manage their health (U.S. Department of Health and Human Services, NIH, & NCCAM, 2008). Natural products were the most frequently used form to treat conditions or maintain health (e.g., glucosamine for arthritis, ginseng for mental health and memory). Because of widespread use, many health care organizations added use of complementary and alternative approaches to health history forms as some of these practices could result in serious adverse effects when combined with drugs and surgeries. Nurses also became responsible for knowing more about these health care practices.

Additionally, the federal government published best practice protocols for various disease processes. Watson (2012) warned of the possibility of depersonalization of care when nurses may be pressured to abide strictly by rigid policies and protocols required for institutional reimbursement. Nurses had to spend increasing amounts of time documenting client care to comply with government-approved protocols (e.g., standardized documentation for influenza vaccines for Medicare recipients). Electronic health records began to trigger messages to health care providers to alert them to guidelines that needed to be followed to comply with government recommendations in order to maximize reimbursement for rendered services.

The Second Decade of the Postmodern Era and Beyond (2010–Present)

Along with different settings for professional nurse employment, many nurses have found that the complexity of information in any given practice area requires ongoing education. Continuing education and nurse specialty certification persists today. More than 130 professional nursing organizations provide opportunities for further education in such specialized practice fields as critical care, oncology, neuroscience, faith community, maternal–child, psychiatric, public health, and administration. Nurse specialty organizations provide certification programs that attest to the nurse member's knowledge and skill in the specialized area of practice. Some professional nursing positions require certification, yet many organizations fail to provide financial rewards for professional certification. Many individuals consider certification prestigious, but in a 2011 study, researchers found that nursing specialty certification had no effect on client outcome unless the nurse also held a BSN (Kendall-Gallagher et al., 2011).

Along with specialty certification, nurses in a variety of practice settings participate in health care quality improvement programs. The use of evidence-based standards for client nursing care assessments and interventions reduces client injuries and complications. Regulatory and accrediting agencies such as The Joint Commission (TJC, formerly the Joint Commission on Accreditation of Healthcare Organizations [JCAHO]) require that certain national and international standards for client care be met before being designated as accredited centers. All TJC-accredited organizations must have quality improvement programs in place (see Chapter 18, "Quality Improvement: Enhancing Patient Safety and Health Care Quality") and meet all requirements to receive reimbursement for rendered services. If an organization fails to meet accreditation criteria, it loses the ability to receive federal funds for delivered health care services. In addition, the CMS has identified hospital-associated conditions for which Medicare and Medicaid may deny reimbursement (see Box 2.1,

2.1 Professional Building Blocks

Hospital-Associated Conditions Resulting in Denial of Reimbursement

- Foreign object remaining in a client following surgery
- Infection at surgical site
- Air embolism
- Stage III and IV pressure injuries
- Transfusion of incompatible blood or blood products
- Falls and trauma that occur as inpatients
- Manifestations of poor blood sugar control
- Urinary catheter–associated infections
- Intravascular catheter–associated infections
- Deep venous thrombosis or pulmonary embolism

Professional Building Blocks, "Hospital-Associated Conditions Resulting in Denial of Reimbursement"). The CMS plans to add more conditions to the list in the future.

Since the enactment of the ACA, more Americans have secured health insurance. The U.S. Census Bureau reported that 89.6% of Americans had health care insurance. The sources of health care insurance policies are private 66%, employer-based 55.4%, and government sponsored 36.5%. Many people, especially those over age 65, have private Medicare tie-in plans. Only 80.7% of individuals living below the poverty level had secured health insurance coverage (Smith & Medalia, 2015). The percentage of GDP consumed by health care was 17.7% in 2018 and is expected to rise to 19.7% by 2028 (Kornfeld et al., 2020). The increase reflects increased use of prescription medications and hospitalizations as well as increased costs related to sophisticated technologic advances now used in health care delivery.

The gap between the wealthy and poor further expanded. According to Eggleston and Hays (2019), home equity and retirement accounts were the two major contributing factors to the wealth of Americans. Eggleston and Hays also reported that 37% of Americans did not own a home in 2015, and 47.1% did not have retirement accounts. Characteristics of individuals with more wealth included those with fulltime employment, those who had completed undergraduate college degrees, and those identifying as Asian American and non-Hispanic White American.

Besides being knowledgeable in a specific practice area, informatics, and quality improvement, today's nurses realize the importance of being well versed in current consumer health care practices. Some complementary therapies, such as aromatherapy, guided imagery, therapeutic touch, and massage, may ease some adverse effects of conventional medical and surgical therapies. The NIH has added research on complementary and alternative health care practices to its list of research priorities. The National Center for Complementary and Integrative Health serves as the key American governmental agency that provides scientific information about unconventional medical practices to consumers and health care providers as well as provides grant funding to substantiate their effectiveness and safe use (NIH, 2021). Thus, the knowledge required for effective nursing practice continues to expand, evolve, and increase in complexity. In the second decade of the 21st century, nurses were depicted as leaders with advanced skills. In the series *Chicago Med* (2015–2017), a nurse named Maggie performed direct client care skills, solved complex problems, arranged for spiritual care from a shaman for a dying client, and advocated for clients. She also warned the nursing staff of the need to protect the clients from new residents whose lack of knowledge and experience could kill people (Summers & Summers, 2017).

However, in these same years, nurses were not always depicted positively. For example, in *Carol's Second Act* (CBS 2019–2020), a male nurse named Dennis serves as a cruel gatekeeper of a nursing unit as its charge nurse. He bullies medical students and takes bribes for providing them with information that they need for success. However, when he interacts with staff physicians and clients, he acts professionally and compassionately. *Grey's Anatomy*, which began in 2005 and is still on air, generally ignores nurses even though many scenes in the series occur in the hospital setting.

The mainstream media highlighted the contributions made and risks taken by nurses, other health care team members, and first responders in providing care during the COVID-19 pandemic in 2020. They praised nurses as heroic when they left home during times of lockdown to provide nursing services in areas hit hard by the virus. Unfortunately, as of March 2021, over 3,000 nurses have died from COVID-19 according to 60 nations that track this information (France-Presse, 2021) and 3 million health care workers had contracted the disease (ICN, 2020). By risking their lives, health, and well-being, nurses have earned the respect of the communities and individuals they serve.

USING HISTORY TO GUIDE CURRENT AND FUTURE PROFESSIONAL PRACTICE—AN EXAMPLE

Regardless of media portrayal, nursing has been a respectable profession for more than 200 years. This has been achieved by the efforts of many people over the years.

Additional current and future influences on nursing include an increasing older population, ever-expanding reliance on technology for health care delivery and general living, political instability, the widening gap between the affluent and poor, natural and man-made ecologic disasters, climate change, and the emergence of new and once eliminated contagious diseases (both with and without cures). Nurses will be there to help clients and families adapt and adjust to whatever the future may bring. In order to accomplish the task, professional nurses will need to be able to work within complex systems with confidence, competence, and compassion.

Because history has a tendency to repeat itself, there are lessons from the past that can apply to present and future professional nursing practice. Historical accounts from the 1918 to 1919 influenza pandemic provide people (including health care professionals) information and interventions that can influence the trajectory of the COVID-19 pandemic. The first lesson is that the earlier pandemic swept across the globe in two waves; the second wave was worse than the first (Esparza, 2020; Mozes, 2020). Most flu epidemics last 2 to 4 years (Esparza, 2020). Even though little was known about viruses at the time, scientists understood that the 1918 virus was transported by respiratory droplets expelled during coughing and sneezing (Mozes, 2020). There was no vaccine for that flu virus, and it targeted younger people, coming on suddenly (Esparza, 2020; Mozes, 2020). Cases markedly declined once 30% of the population contracted the disease (Esparza, 2020).

Controlling the 1918 pandemic required crowd control, mask wearing, and trying to prevent public panic (Esparza, 2020; Mozes, 2020). Communities that immediately closed venues where large numbers of people gathered (e.g., theaters, churches, schools) when a case of the virus was identified had a lower incidence of the disease and fewer deaths. Community members soon recognized the value of staying away and distancing themselves from others (Esparza, 2020; Mozes, 2020). Some locales instituted mandatory mask wearing outside of the home. However, this was not as effective as controlling crowds (Esparza, 2020).

During this pandemic, government officials stifled the severity of the pandemic to avoid public panic and did not truly make the severity well known until 1925 (Mozes, 2020). They also expressed concern that the health care system would crumble under the pressure of caring for all those stricken with the flu.

The COVID-19 pandemic has many similarities to the 1918 pandemic. Many of the strategies for containment are similar (social distancing, effective hand washing, donning masks, and limiting the number of persons attending events). However, many people, especially in the United States, avoided abiding by these containment interventions. Former President Donald Trump attempted to hide the severity of COVID-19 from Americans, saying he did not want them to panic. The health care system periodically became overwhelmed in different locations, and there was a severe shortage of personal protective equipment for first responders and health care professionals. Pressure was applied to state governors to close everything except essential businesses in the first few months of the pandemic, resulting in economic insecurity and uncertainty. In professional practice, an old nursing intervention common for clients with pneumonia, having clients assume a prone position, was found to be effective in preventing posterior lung atelectasis. By doing what was done in the past, the world will survive the COVID-19 pandemic and will be better prepared for the next one.

REAL-LIFE REFLECTIONS

Remember Marita, Carol, and Joe from the beginning of the chapter. What topic area should they use for their class presentation? Why do you think this might be a useful topic to be presented? Why is it important for them to have knowledge about nursing history? How might they use history to guide their current and future nursing practice?

Summary and Significance to Practice

Recognition of nursing as a respected profession continues in the ever-changing, complex, and chaotic world. The existence of three entry levels of education remains a barrier to nursing attainment of full professional status. Scientific advances are providing an opportunity for the profession to establish its own body of knowledge as well as increasing the need for highly educated nurses. Hard science continues to be intertwined with ethics, spirituality, and philosophy and points to the validity of individualized holistic nursing care. Professional nurses must focus efforts toward looking at all aspects that affect human health and healing. For many generations, nurses have made remarkable, but sometimes invisible contributions to the delivery of health care. Hopefully, as a result of nurses exhibiting compassion, confidence, and competence, current and future societies will more highly value the contributions of nurses in health care. By showcasing their clinical, cognitive, and communication skills with confidence, today's nurses can shape the image of the nursing profession.

From Theory to Practice

1. What are some current issues in health care that might be solved by looking at nursing history?
2. What are the similarities among ancient and current nursing practices?
3. How does current professional practice compare with nursing in various stages of human history?
4. How did the feminist movement affect the nursing profession?

Nurse as Author

This chapter has provided a broad overview of the history of nursing. Visit www.internurse.com to view pictures and read more about the nurses who have shaped our profession. Listen to the voice of Florence Nightingale at the following website: http://publicdomainreview.org/collections/the-voice-of-florence-nightingale/. Take time to reflect on what you just heard. Then write a paragraph or two describing your thoughts, feelings, and perceptions about nursing history.

Your Digital Classroom

Online Exploration

The American Association for the History of Nursing: **www.aahn.org**

The Barbara Bates Center for the Study of the History of Nursing: **www.nursing.upenn.edu/history**

History of the American Association of Men in Nursing: **https://www.aamn.org/history**

Brief biography of Mary Seacole, Nurse and War Hero: **https://www.thoughtco.com/women-and-war-4133255**

History of the American Nurses Association (ANA): **https://www.nursingworld.org/ana/about-ana/history/**

History of Sigma Theta Tau International (STTI): **https://www.sigmanursing.org/why-sigma/about-sigma/sigma-organizational-fact-sheet**

STTI founders: **https://www.sigmanursing.org/why-sigma/about-sigma/sigma-organizational-fact-sheet/stti-founders**

National League for Nursing (NLN): **http://www.nln.org/about/history-of-nln**

Current and past media portrayals of nurses: **https://blog.truthaboutnursing.org/category/media/**

Expanding Your Understanding

Select a historical era that interests you. Explore nursing and health-related issues encountered during this time in history. Identify at least one issue confronted during this historical time and relate it to current professional nursing practice. What did nurses do during this time to address the identified issue? Is it possible that the same issue might appear again in the future? Do you think that a similar solution that was used during the historical area might be useful? Why or why not?

Beyond the Book

Visit the Point® at **www.thePoint.lww.com** for activities and information to reinforce the concepts and content covered in this chapter.

REFERENCES

African American Registry. (2020). *National Association of Colored Graduate Nurses founded*. https://aaregistry.org/story/national-association-of-colored-graduate-nurses-founded/

American Nurses Association. (1965). *ANA position paper on education for nursing*. Author.

American Nurses Association. (1995). *Social policy statement*. Author.

Benefiel, D. (2011). The story of nurse licensure. *Nurse Educator, 36*(1), 16–20. https://doi.org/10.1097/NNE.0b013e3182001e82

Bodenheimer, T., & Grumbach, K. (1995). The reconfiguration of U.S. medicine. *Journal of the American Medical Association, 274*, 85–90. https://doi.org/10.1001/jama.1995.03530010099050

Bradshaw, A. (2010). An historical perspective on the treatment of vocation in the Briggs Report (1972). *Journal of Clinical Nursing, 19*, 3459–3467. https://doi.org/10.1111/j.1365–2702.2010.03359.x

Brooten, D., & Naylor, M. D. (1995). Nurses' effect on changing patient outcomes. *Image, 27*, 95–99. https://doi.org/10.1111/j.1547-5069.1995.tb00829.x

Brown, E. L. (1948). *Nursing for the future (Brown Report)*. Russell Sage Foundation.

Buerhaus, P. I. (1995). Economic pressures building in the hospital employed RN labor market. *Nursing Economics, 13*, 137–141. https://pubmed.ncbi.nlm.nih.gov/7783787/

Buerhaus, P. I., & Auerbach, D. (2011). The recession's effect on hospital registered nurse employment growth. *Nursing Economics, 29*(4), 163–167. https://pubmed.ncbi.nlm.nih.gov/21919412/

Burgess, M. A. (1928). *Committee on the grading of nursing schools: Nurses, patients and pocketbooks*. Commonwealth Fund.

Centers for Medicare & Medicaid Services. (2010). *National health expenditure projections 2010–2020*. https://www.cms.gov/Research-Statistics-Data-and-Systems/Statistics-Trends-and-Reports/NationalHealthExpendData/NationalHealthAccountsHistorical

Chinn, P. L. (2013). *Peace and power, new directions for building community* (8th ed.). Jones & Bartlett Learning.

Cohen, E. L., & Cesta, T. G. (2001). *Nursing case management from essentials to advanced practice applications* (3rd ed.). Mosby.

Dock, L. L. (1912). *A history of nursing* (Vol. 3). Putnam.

Eggleston, J., & Hays, D. (2019). *Many U.S. households do not have biggest contributors to wealth: Home equity and retirement accounts*. https://www.census.gov/library/stories/2019/08/gaps-in-wealth-americans-by-household-type.html

Esparza, J. (2020). Lessons from history: What can we learn from 300 years of pandemic flu that could inform the response to COVID-19? *American Journal of Public Health, 110*(8), 1160–1161. https://doi.org/10.2105/AJPH.2020.305761

Flanagan, L. (1976). *One strong voice: The story of the American Nurses Association*. American Nurses Association.

Flexner, A. (1910). *Medical education in the United States and Canada: A report to the Carnegie Foundation for the Advancement of Teaching*. Merrymount Press.

France-Presse, A. (2021). *3000 nurses dead, COVID exodus looming: global federation*. Retrieved March 16, 2021, from https://mb.com.ph/2021/03/11/3000-nurses-dead-covid-exodus-looming-global-federation/

Gilligan, C. (1982). *In a different voice*. Harvard University Press.

Ginzberg, E. (1949). *A pattern for hospital care*. Columbia University Press.

Ginzberg, E. (1995). A cautionary note on market reforms in health care. *Journal of the American Medical Association, 274*, 1633–1634. https://doi.org/10.1001/jama.1995.03530200069041

Goldmark, J. (1923). *Nursing and nursing education in the United States*. Macmillan.

Gore, J., Rickards, B., Fray, L., Holmes, K., & Smith, M. (2017). Profiling Australian school students' interest in a nursing career: insights for ensuring the future workforce. *Australian Journal of Advanced Nursing, 35*(2), 12–22. https://www.researchgate.net/publication/321499814_Profiling_Australian_school_students'_interest_in_a_nursing_career_Insights_for_ensuring_the_future_workforce

Greenberg, L. (1994). Work redesign: An overview. *Journal of Emergency Nursing, 20*, 28A–32A. https://pubmed.ncbi.nlm.nih.gov/8007512/

Healthcare.gov. (n.d.) *What Marketplace health insurance plans cover*. https://www.healthcare.gov/coverage/what-marketplace-plans-cover/

Hehman, M. C. (2018). The rise of a profession: "An art and a science" 1873-1901 (Chapter 3). In A. W. Keeling, M. C. Hehman, & J. C. Kirchgessner (Eds.), *History of professional nursing in the United States, toward a culture of health* (pp. 44-71). Springer Publishing Co.

Holahan, J., & Chen, V. (2011). *Changes in health insurance coverage in the great recession, 2007–2010*. https://www.kff.org/medicaid/issue-brief/changes-in-health-insurance-coverage-in-the/

International Council of Nurses. (2020). *New ICN report show governments are failing to prioritize nurses as number of confirmed COVID-19 nurse deaths passes 1000*. https://www.icn.ch/news/new-icn-report-shows-governments-are-failing-prioritize-nurses-number-confirmed-covid-19-nurse

Jamieson, E. M., & Sewall, M. F. (1954). *Trends in nursing history* (4th ed.). WB Saunders.

Kaiser Family Foundation. (2012). *Making sense of the census uninsured numbers*. http://kff.org/health-reform/event/making-sense-of-the-census-uninsured-numbers/

Kalisch, P. A., & Kalisch, B. J. (2004). *The advance of American nursing* (4th ed.). Lippincott Williams & Wilkins.

Kendall-Gallagher, D., Aiken, L., Sloane, D., & Cimiotti, J. (2011). Nurse specialty certification, inpatient mortality and failure to rescue. *Journal of Nursing Scholarship, 43*(2), 188–194. https://doi.org/10.1111/j.1547-5069.2011.01391.x

Kirchgessner, J. C. (2018). Nursing in the colonial era and early days of the United States. (pp. 1–21). In Keeling, A. W., Hehman, M. C., & Kirchgessner, J. C. (Eds.), *A history of professional nursing in the United States, toward a culture of health*. Springer.

Kjervik, D. K., & Martinson, I. J. M. (1979). *Women in stress: A nursing perspective*. Appleton-Century-Crofts.

Kornfeld, R. J.; Hartman, M.B.; Espinoza, N. A., Butler, R. L., & Catlin, A. C. (2020). *A reconciliation of health care expenditures in the national health expenditures accounts and in gross domestic product*. Retrieved August 23, 2020, from https://www.bea.gov/system/files/papers/BEA-WP2020-8.pdf

Kongsuwan, W; Keller, K. B., & Chase, S.K. (2016). Evolution of caring for dying patients in intensive care units in the United States from 1960–1980. *International Journal of Human Caring, 20*(1), 2–7. https://doi.org/10.20467/1091-5710.20.1.2

Madsen, W. (2005). Early 20th century untrained nursing staff in the Rockhampton district: A necessary evil? *Journal of Advanced Nursing, 51*(3), 307–313. https://doi.org/10.1111/j.1365-2648.2005.03492.x

Malka, S. G. (2007). *Daring to care*. University of Illinois Press.

Meehan, T. C. (2003). Careful nursing: A model for contemporary nursing practice. *Journal of Advanced Nursing, 44*, 99–107. https://doi.org/10.1046/j.1365-2648.2003.02772.x

Montag, M. (1951). *The education of nursing technicians*. Putman.

Mozes, A. (2020). *Four lessons from the 1918 Spanish flu pandemic*. https://www.webmd.com/lung/news/20200420/four-lessons-from-the-1918-spanish-flu-pandemic#1

National Council of State Boards of Nursing. (2020). *Explore NCSBN through the years*. Retrieved August 21, 2020, from https://timeline.ncsbn.org/index.htm

National Institutes of Health. (2016). *The NIH Almanac: National Center for Complementary & Integrative Health*. http://www.nih.gov/about-nih/what-we-do/nih-almanac/national-center-complementary-integrative-health-nccih

National Institutes of Health (2021). *NIH National Center for Complementary and Integrative Health*. About NCCIH. Retrieved March 16, 2021, from https://www.nccih.nih.gov/about

National League for Nursing. (1939). More graduate duty nurses. *American Journal of Nursing, 39*, 898.

National League for Nursing. (2020). *History of the national league for nursing: 1893–2018.* http://www.nln.org/docs/default-source/default-document-library/nln-timeline-june-2020.pdf?sfvrsn=2

Nutting, M. A., & Dock, L. L. (1935a). *A history of nursing: The evolution of nursing systems from the earliest times to the foundation of the first English and American training schools* (Vol. 2). Putman.

Nutting, M. A., & Dock, L. L. (1935b). *A history of nursing: The evolution of nursing systems from the earliest times to the foundation of the first English and American training schools* (Vol. 3). Putman.

Roberts, M. M. (1954). *American nursing: History and interpretation.* Macmillan.

Smith, J., & Medalia, C. (2015). *Health insurance coverage in the United States: 2014.* Current population. Reports Number: P60–253. http://www.census.gov/content/dam/Census/library/publications/2015/demo/p60–253.pdf

Spradley, B. W. (1990). *Community health nursing: Concepts and practice.* Scott Foresman/Little Brown.

Summers, S., & Summers, H. (2017). *Gotta keep em from killing people.* https://blog.truthaboutnursing.org/2020/04/chicago-med-s1-s2/

U.S. Census Bureau. (2011). *Age and sex composition: 2010 Census briefs.* http://www.census.gov/prod/cen2010/briefs/c2010br-03.pdf

U.S. Department of Health and Human Services, Health Resources and Services Administration, & Bureau of Health Professions. (2010). *The registered nurse population: Findings from the 2008 National Sample Survey of Registered Nurses.* Retrieved June 10, 2021, from https://data.hrsa.gov/DataDownload/NSSRN/GeneralPUF08/rnsurveyfinal.pdf

U.S. Department of Health & Human Services, National Institutes of Health, & National Center for Complementary and Alternative Medicine. (2008). *The use of complementary and alternative medicine in the United States.* https://nccih.nih.gov/sites/nccam.nih.gov/files/camuse.pdf

U.S. Public Health Service. (1963). *Toward quality in nursing: Needs and goals. A report of the surgeon general's consultant group in nursing.* Author.

Watson, J. (1999). *Postmodern nursing and beyond.* Churchill Livingstone.

Watson, J. (2012). *Human caring science a theory of nursing* (2nd ed.). Jones & Bartlett Learning.

Wheeler, W. (1999). Florence: Death of an icon? *Nursing Times, 95,* 24–26. https://pubmed.ncbi.nlm.nih.gov/10437484/

Wilson, E. O. (1998). *Consilience: The unity of knowledge.* Alfred A. Knopf.

Contextual, Philosophical, and Ethical Elements of Professional Nursing

LEARNING OUTCOMES

By the end of this chapter, the learner will be able to:

1. Identify environmental factors that constitute the context for nursing practice.
2. Outline the essential elements of a nursing philosophy.
3. Develop a personal nursing philosophy.
4. Outline key steps for effective analysis of ethical dilemmas.
5. Use a structured method for making ethical decisions.
6. Specify fallacies that might occur when making ethical decisions.
7. Explain how demographic, cultural, economic, environmental, and ethical factors influence professional practice.

REAL-LIFE REFLECTIONS

Jane has been working as a hospital nurse for 15 years. Because of her high level of nursing expertise, local nursing programs assign students to work with her during their clinical experiences. Lately, Jane often feels detached from her clients and perceives herself as a "client care machine." She is fearful that she might impart her feelings of frustration to nursing students and discourage them from pursuing nursing. Jane is thinking about leaving the profession and pursuing another career. As you work with Jane, you notice that she does not seem happy and fulfilled. You want to ask her about your observations, but you are not certain how to proceed. Jane yearns for the "good old days" when client care was focused on people rather than on business. However, she knows in her heart that she does make a difference in her clients' lives, and she derives profound satisfaction from helping others.

- *What do you think would be an effective way to confront Jane about her unhappiness at work? Why do you think this would be a good approach?*
- *For RN students, in what ways do you think nursing has become less focused on person-centered care?*
- *For BSN students, how would you respond to Jane if she expresses a desire to leave the profession?*
- *List three possible options to keep Jane engaged in the profession of nursing.*
- *In what ways do you think nursing has become less focused on client care?*
- *What advice would you give to Jane?*

As a science, nursing focuses on humanity in a highly objective manner, using interventions based on scientific evidence. As technologic advances create a more complex world, making sense of the world becomes more important. A well-defined set of **values** (principles, or what things are important) and **beliefs** (ideas regarded as truths) provides a firm foundation for nursing practice. If nurses relied exclusively on thinking and approached nursing using only hard science, they would appear cold and distant to their clients. However, professional nurses connect emotionally and spiritually with clients, thereby allowing genuine warmth and authentic compassion to guide clinical practice. Values and beliefs influence perceptions, thoughts, and feelings.

> **Take Note!**
> Because values and beliefs strongly influence our perceptions, thoughts, and feelings, a well-defined set of values and beliefs provides the best foundation for nursing practice.

Context can be defined as "the interrelated conditions in which something exists or occurs: the whole situation, background, or environment relevant to a particular event" (Mish, 2020, p. 270). Environmental and situational conditions create the context of nursing practice. This also includes the people involved in the nursing situation. Each nurse brings to the context their personal set of beliefs about people, the world, health, and nursing. This set of beliefs constitutes a **philosophy** of nursing. When providing care, nurses interact with the environment, which is composed of contextual factors in which the nurse's philosophy plays a key role:

- The pragmatic professional self seeks cause-and-effect relationships and looks for the practical nature of nursing and how it can be used to solve issues that arise in daily clinical practice.
- The idealistic professional self pays serious attention to the ideal conceptualizations of nursing practice and views nursing as a means for forming authentic and caring relationships with others to help them achieve their maximum health potential.
- The realistic professional self emphasizes facts and scientific principles during nursing practice.
- The existentialist professional self displays great regard for individuals and respects their choices with an acceptance of responsibility for those choices made as nursing care is delivered.

Some degree of congruence with the vastly different worldviews is desirable for authentic, humane, scientific-based, nonpaternalistic nursing practice.

Development of an individual nursing philosophy helps nurses come to terms with diverse worldviews. However, to begin developing a personal nursing philosophy, nurses need to be cognizant of the **contextual elements of nursing practice**. These elements comprise the demographic, economic, environmental, and ethical factors that surround a client care situation. Contextual elements surrounding a clinical situation affect a nurse's professional roles and the clinical decisions they make. Along with a personal nursing philosophy, contextual elements help nurses develop a meaningful and thoughtful practice.

CONTEXTUAL BASIS OF NURSING PRACTICE

What is the world of nursing like today? Before that question can be answered, we must look at the world environment—the place where nursing occurs. Professional nursing practice does not occur in isolation; rather, nursing is embedded in and integral to the complex health care delivery system. When one area of health care experiences a change, all areas of health care delivery experience change. Dramatic changes in health care over the past two decades have profoundly affected professional nursing practice. Future changes may occur so quickly that nurses and other health care workers may have difficulty fully comprehending the effects of change and coping with its implications (Porter-O'Grady & Malloch, 2015).

Professional nursing practice is a complex concept affected by many contextual elements; it is impossible to present all of these elements in a single chapter. To capture an accurate picture of current professional practice, the following discussion focuses on quantum science, which requires relational and whole-systems thinking; technology, communication, safety, and consumerism; the global community; and the desire for equality while maintaining personal identity.

Quantum Science: Relational and Whole-Systems Thinking in Health Care

Change is constant; no one can avoid it (Hawking, 2002). To survive change, humans must learn new ways of thinking. The world is a complex place full of chaos where everything is interconnected. Structure becomes defined by wholes rather than individual parts (Hawking, 2002; Porter-O'Grady & Malloch, 2015).

When looking into a hologram, the entire picture can be seen on any-sized fraction of the image. Such is the nature of the overall structure.

The smallest structural unit of a system mirrors its entire system in terms of organization pattern and behavior. Systems work continuously to renew and reinvent themselves while maintaining their basic integrity. Systems are composed of multiple interacting feedback loops. Structure has disorder, and disorder has structure. Quantum science eliminates dualistic or "either/or" thinking and envisions new possibilities of combining ideas through the use of synthesis.

Synthesis involves putting ideas or things together in a new way. For example, the human body synthesizes food eaten into muscle, fat, energy, and waste products. It takes chemicals from the consumed food and transforms them into a new state. In Hegelian philosophy, it means to reconcile two opposites and make a new whole, which is a form of dialectical thinking. For the author of this book, work and play are two opposing concepts. Therefore, all work and all play would be polar opposites. However, a synthesis of work and play within one's personal life would result in a balance between them. However, if a person immensely enjoys an activity (such as writing) and has a contract to produce a book (work), a synthesis of the two concepts could result in playing while working. The coined terms "playwork" and "workplay" could be used to describe this synthesis.

Relational thinking involves recognition of the interconnectedness of all things. All things become interdependent. A complex algorithm (series of steps or events) is required for things to occur or exist (Porter-O'Grady & Malloch, 2015). For example, human health is a complex process that involves a safe environment, intact physical and mental capabilities, meaningful interpersonal relationships, and spiritual dimensions. The link between mental and physical health has been studied extensively in the field of psychoneuroimmunology. Studies have established relationships among health status, mental outlook, and finding meaning in life (Antonovsky, 1987; Ferreira & Sherman, 2007; Hatala, 2008; Iwarrsson et al., 2007; Lewis, 2008a, 2008b). As client advocates, caregivers, coordinators, teachers, and counselors, nurses look at the client holistically to determine what resources are required to promote health.

The holistic approach also requires **whole-systems thinking**, in which many smaller interacting systems aggregate to create the larger (whole) system (Porter-O'Grady & Malloch, 2015). For example, a hospital consists of many departments (e.g., surgery,

radiology, laboratory, pharmacy, nursing, dietary), each of which assumes responsibility for an integral part of client care. In the case of nursing departments, client care is delivered 24 hours a day, 7 days a week. Thus, different nursing care teams staff the hospital during the different shifts. Each nursing unit represents an additional system. The nursing team on a unit may be broken down even further to represent the professional nurse, a vocational (or practical) nurse, and unlicensed care providers. Each individual providing client care is also a complex system with many personal needs.

When engaging in whole-systems thinking, one must look at the complex nature of all the interacting systems. Consider the hospital as only one system in the larger health care delivery system. Waste byproducts of health care therapies must be either discarded or recycled. The impact of waste affects the global environment.

When nurses use whole-systems thinking in daily clinical practice, they assume the role of care coordinator. They look for ways to use human and material resources optimally to meet client care needs (e.g., staffing nursing units and judicious use of medical supplies). When assuming the role of client advocate, nurses frequently refer clients to community agencies for assistance if needs remain unmet and resources are unavailable in the practice setting.

Take Note!

Whole-systems thinking requires an awareness of the numerous smaller systems that make up the larger system and note the interrelationships among them.

Because of the complex nature of clinical practice and health care delivery, nurses consider many factors when providing client care. Quantum science and relational and systems thinking provide nurses with the ability to consider the impact of clinical decisions not only on clients but also on the institutional, national, and global communities. Because change remains constant, nurses must stay abreast of factors that influence professional practice. The ability to use relational and systems thinking enables the nurse to appraise the entire client care situation before making decisions focused on the client's best interest. The following discussion provides a broad overview of factors that affect professional nursing practice.

Technology, Communication, Safety, and Consumerism in Health Care

Technology has transformed human lives. Increased use of technology in health care has resulted in people surviving illnesses once thought to be untreatable, enabled instant access to information, increased the costs of health care, and created increasingly savvy health care consumers. In the United States, consumers drive the delivery of health care and frequently rely on information obtained from the internet. Pharmaceutical companies post new information about medications on the internet and target consumers with advertising. When assessing client knowledge of health-related information, nurses must find out what clients know and the sources of their information. As educators, nurses should assist clients in determining the quality of information accessed from the internet (see Chapter 14, "Informatics and Technology in Nursing Practice"). Clients sometimes demand the newest (but not always the best) health care treatments from providers (Herzlinger, 2004).

Take Note!

Because of the array of health information found online, nurses must stay abreast of developments in health promotion and disease management to remain effective caregivers and educators.

In some cases, clients may know more about their health problems than health care providers (Herzlinger, 2004). For example, a young woman, newly diagnosed with myasthenia gravis, finds detailed information about her disease from visiting the National Myasthenia Gravis Foundation website. She learns what medications may result in increased muscle weakness. When she needs surgery that requires hospitalization, she brings the long list of medications known to increase muscle weakness in individuals with myasthenia gravis to the hospital so that she will not receive them. Although her actions may have been unnecessary because nurses and physicians providing her care have access to the same information, they can still save the health care providers' time.

Many health care organizations provide nurses with pagers or cell phones so they can receive instant messages in case of client emergency or other client needs. These devices may distract and interrupt nurses from paying full attention to clients when providing care. This can disrupt the development and maintenance of therapeutic client relationships, a critical element of professional practice. Clients expect nurses to care for them by ensuring their safety, being competent in nursing, taking action that is in their best interests, and listening to them. In addition, some clients become distracted by their cell phones while receiving health care and may miss critical information on how to best manage their health (Herzlinger, 2004). Most health care provider offices post signs requesting clients not to use their cell phones during office visits. Box 3.1, Professional Building Blocks, "Technologic Devices: Patient Care Enhancement or Distraction?" highlights how technologic devices have the potential to both enhance and distract nurses and clients during the delivery of care.

Along with the latest developments in traditional medical care, many clients have knowledge of complementary and alternative health care therapies. Some consumers expect health care professionals, including nurses, to have knowledge of, provide them with, and offer advice about these therapies (Blasko-Helming et al., 2022; Herzlinger, 2004). Nurses must inquire as to all health care practices used by clients to ensure the safety of prescribed, traditional medical therapies and to determine if any complementary and alternative therapies may pose potential health hazards.

Today, clients and health care providers work as partners toward common goals. Looking out for one's own safety or the safety of a loved one has become a factor in care delivery and health maintenance. With the COVID-19 pandemic of 2020, much attention has been placed upon ways to avoid getting the disease. Public health departments, governmental agencies, health care facilities, accrediting agents, the media, and health care professionals provide clients and families with information about how to remain safe during such times. When hospitalized, inpatient facilities provide clients and families with educational materials about health promotion techniques like infection control, fall prevention, and the importance of hand hygiene. Professional nurses and all health care team members strive to keep clients safe. Technologic devices such as barcode machines reduce the incidence of errors in medication dosing, and bedside acquisition of blood and body fluid specimens for laboratory testing makes the delivery of care quicker, more convenient, and more accurate.

Because of the complex nature of health care delivery, various members of the health care team assume different aspects of care. Breakdowns in communication frequently result in client care errors,

3.1 Professional Building Blocks

Technologic Devices: Client Care Enhancement or Distraction?

Device	Enhancement	Distraction
Pager	Increased and immediate awareness of a significant client care need or another staff member's need for help	Interruption while working with a client or client's family
Cell phone	■ Quicker notification of a significant client care need, another staff member's need for help, or to speak directly to another health care provider or client's family ■ Access to a variety of clinical resources ■ Increased availability of health education applications that could be shared with clients and families	■ Client distraction while receiving health care services ■ Nurse interruption during care delivery ■ Potential for photographing or videotaping care delivery
Personal digital device	Access to a variety of clinical resources	Perceptions of being used for personal rather than professional reasons
Bedside computers	■ Immediate access to key client information ■ Elimination of the need for multiple care providers to ask clients the same questions ■ Increased safety of care delivery ■ Instantaneous documentation of nursing assessments, interventions, and evaluations	Focus on getting documentation completed with the potential of ignoring concerns of client and significant others

and when errors occur, the system involving the entire team bears the blame rather than a single person (Institute of Medicine, 2000, 2010; Porter-O'Grady & Malloch, 2015).

Take Note!
Effective communication is crucial in ensuring that all health care team members involved in the client's care are aware of specific needs and anything that might adversely affect the client.

The Global Community and Health Care

The emergence of a single world economy and the acknowledgment of earth's finite resources have resulted in a changed context for professional practice. Today, the nations of the world are connected as a global economic community. Political and social unrest and economic instability in one nation have the potential to disrupt the economies of many.

Various nations have different forms of health care delivery systems. How health care is delivered has an impact on whether people use organized health systems or rely on alternative modes. Developed nations

have well-refined health care delivery systems along with access to sophisticated treatments, whereas underdeveloped nations (especially those in political turmoil) may have no organized systems to meet the health care needs of their residents (UNDP, 2021; World Health Organization [WHO], 2019). Other disparities in quality of life and health care are becoming more evident than ever before. Whereas underdeveloped and overpopulated nations are looking for ways to combat malnutrition and infectious diseases, citizens of highly developed nations suffer from health problems related to a life of excess, such as obesity, diabetes mellitus, and cardiovascular disease (WHO, 2020).

In 2015, the United Nations (UN) identified 17 "sustainable development goals" (SDGs) that all 191 UN member states agreed to attain by 2020. Because the goals were not met, the UN extended the deadlines for attainment to 2030 (UN, 2020a). The UN efforts focus on the goals that are related to human health and well-being:

1. No poverty: Eliminate all forms of poverty everywhere (UN, 2020b).
2. Zero hunger: Eliminate hunger, attain food security, and improve nutrition while promoting sustainable agriculture (UN, 2020c).

3. Good health and well-being: Ensure healthy lives and promote well-being in all persons (UN, 2020d).
4. Quality education: Provide equitable, high-quality education and provide lifelong learning opportunities for all (UN, 2020e).
5. Gender equality: Attain gender equality and empowerment for women and girls (UN, 2020f).
6. Clean water and sanitation: Ensure access to clean water and effective sanitation for all (UN, 2020g).
7. Affordable and clean energy: Ensure access to affordable, reliable, and sustainable modern energy for all (UN, 2020h).
8. Decent work and economic growth: Provide inclusive economic growth, employment, and decent work for everyone (UN, 2020i).
9. Industry, innovation, and infrastructure: Construct resilient infrastructure, ensure sustainable industrialization, and promote innovation (UN, 2020j).
10. Reduced inequalities: Reduce economic and power inequalities within and among all nations (UN, 2020k).
11. Sustainable cities and communities: Transform and create cities and communities that are resilient, safe, and sustainable (UN, 2020l).
12. Responsible consumption and production: Promote sustainable patterns of production and consumption (UN, 2020m).
13. Climate actions: Take urgent steps to combat climate change and its impact on the planet and people (UN, 2020n).
14. Life below water: Conserve and wisely use the oceans, seas, and marine resources (UN, 2020o).
15. Life on land: Manage forests sustainably, reduce desertification, stop and reverse land degradation, and stop loss of biodiverse plants, animals, and organisms (UN, 2020p).
16. Peace, justice, and strong institutions: Facilitate the development and maintenance of inclusive, just, and peaceful societies (UN, 2020q).
17. Partnerships for the goals: Develop and renew global partnerships for the achievement of the SDGs (UN, 2020r).

All the SDGs influence health, and health in turn influences the goals. Other factors that threaten health around the world include war, accidents, community and domestic violence, natural and man-made disasters, human trafficking, health care provider errors, the emergence of drug-resistant infections, pandemics, obesity, and chemical abuse (see Concepts in Practice, "The Need for Global Cooperation").

Concepts in Practice

The Need for Global Cooperation

One of the worst potential threats to global health is the emergence of a new, highly contagious, and lethal virus, which came to pass when the novel coronavirus, severe acute respiratory syndrome (SARS)-CoV-2 or COVID-19, became a pandemic in 2020. Because of worldwide air travel, such a virus could and did spread throughout the world in as few as 100 days. Clusters of cases popped up simultaneously around the world, and thousands died, in this case as a result of respiratory failure. Global cooperation among public health officials in the past has been instrumental in preventing such a disaster, including a pandemic of SARS in 2003 (Enserink, 2004); a potential tuberculosis epidemic in 2007; a polio epidemic in the Middle East in 2014; Ebola in 2015; and Zika virus in 2016.

When the WHO declares a health emergency, member nations are expected to share data on the incidence of the disease and its health risks and complications; control the vector (if insect-borne or animal-borne illness); issue health risk warnings, travel recommendations, and safety measures; and share research findings about the disease and any new products developed to contain, control, or treat it (WHO, 2019). However, world cooperation faltered in 2020, and COVID-19 ravaged the world.

Desire for Equality While Maintaining a Personal Cultural Identity

Despite globalization and access to information from around the world, people strive to maintain ties to their own cultures. Many people immigrate to developed nations to escape political persecution or less-than-ideal economic situations. Others may come to developed nations to secure treatment for health problems. Although they have left their nations of birth, many of these individuals maintain cultural ties and traditions with their homelands. In addition, many of those born in developed nations whose parents or other ancestors came from other countries also value their cultural heritage.

Culturally sensitive care enables the health care system to accommodate client needs to abide by specific cultural practices. Some health care facilities use computers that permit printing of discharge instructions in more than one language and have interpreters for staff to use when working with clients from different cultures. In some cases, folk healers are permitted to practice in inpatient settings (Blasko-Helming et al., 2022). As client advocates, nurses sometimes have to work with specific cultural practices that might be detrimental to client health. (More detailed information on multicultural issues in professional practice is presented in Chapter 11, "Multicultural Issues in Professional Practice.")

The ability to determine if and when a client's health practices are potentially unsafe depends in part on the individual nurse's knowledge, values, and beliefs. Part of the education involves discovery of things unknown about oneself. The section that follows offers a discussion about philosophy and its significance to professional nursing practice.

FIGURE 3.1 *The School of Athens.* This 16th century fresco by Raphael symbolizes the spirit of philosophical inquiry. "Philosophy" derives from Greek and means "love of wisdom."

Take Note!
Nurses who deliver culturally sensitive nursing care acknowledge the cultural needs of clients.

NURSING PHILOSOPHY

Philosophy is a conceptual discipline involving things that cannot be directly touched or observed. The word "philosophy" is derived from the Greek *philia* (love or friendship) and *sophia* (wisdom). Philosophy provides a foundation for understanding the world, examining what it means to be human and determining moral values. When people engage in philosophical thought, they are reflecting upon their lives and attempting to find meaning in human existence (Rosen et al., 2018). People have been searching for meaning and happiness in their lives for centuries (Fig. 3.1). Development of a personal philosophy requires examination of beliefs and values about life and requires a little time. However, development of a collective (group) philosophy requires much time and consolidation of individual beliefs and values. Philosophies may change as people gain new knowledge and skills through life journeys.

Anyone can be a philosopher. Tools used by philosophers include analyzing concepts, doubting everything, and determining what it truly means to be human. Philosophers think carefully, analytically, deeply, logically, critically, and ambitiously. When they disagree with each other, philosophers present solid reasoning for their contrary thoughts (Rosen et al., 2018). A process known as concept analysis is used to arrive at a clear, concise definition of a concept. During concept analysis, philosophers identify the antecedents (things that must occur prior to something existing or occurring) and consequences (what happens as the result of something existing or occurring). The process then involves the development of a model case of the concept to provide a clear example of the concept. To further clarify the concept, the person conducting the concept analysis designs related and contrary cases (Fitzpatrick & McCarthy, 2016). When philosophers engage in the process of doubting everything, the mere existence of all ideas, events, and tangible objects is questioned (Rosen et al., 2018). The process of doubting everything enables individuals to generate personal or scientific evidence for the existence of things and events. What is deemed to be true for one person may not be true for another (e.g., religious beliefs, historical events, and even personal strategies that promote health). The variance in beliefs about what is true can be considered a key way of how individuals are unique. People possess common functional and structural elements. However, each person also possesses differences in genetic composition, cultural background, and belief systems. A person's belief system provides a perceptual foundation of what it means to be human. Rosen and colleagues (2018) articulate that learning about what it means to be human requires detailed descriptions of human lived experiences and making meaning of one's existence. Finding meaning in one's life enables people to survive harsh conditions (Frankl, 1963) and promotes health (Antonovsky, 1987; Lewis, 2008b; Malloy et al., 2015). The following Focus on Research box, "Finding Meaning in the Work of Nursing: An International Study," discusses how nurses find meaning in their work.

FOCUS ON RESEARCH

Finding Meaning in the Work of Nursing: An International Study

After receiving approval from ethical research boards, 60 nurses with diverse backgrounds from Canada, India, Ireland, Japan, and Korea participated in 11 focus groups and responded to questions to explore how they perceive and find meaning in their professional nursing practice. Group sizes ranged from nine to 14 participants. The nurses worked in various areas of nursing practice including long-term care, geriatric care, oncology, diabetes, intensive care, and care in the home setting. Each group was asked the same question—"Do you consider your work meaningful?" (para. 12).

The primary investigator conducted the interviews in Canada and Ireland and was present at the interviews led by members of the research team who lived in the other countries. Interviews were recorded, and the investigative team analyzed the content to discover commonalities and themes.

The transcript analysis revealed four themes emerging from all focus group discussions. These themes were relationships, compassionate caring, identity, and a mentorship culture. The relationships with clients and each other enabled the nurses to create a special community (especially for the nurses working in long-term care facilities with older clients).

The commitment to compassionate caring was the impetus for many of the nurses to enter the profession, and they expressed deriving satisfaction from helping others. The nurses articulated that being a nurse was a part of their personal identity and that nursing was more than just the work they performed. Finally, creating a culture of mentorship by mentoring new nurses gave them deep satisfaction because sharing their knowledge and skills enabled them to help new nurses, recruit new staff, and develop meaningful long-term professional relationships.

Limitations to this study include the inability to generalize the findings beyond the study participants, the potential for some participants to not want to share their true feelings in front of others, and potential errors in translating some of the interview transcripts.

Although the study findings cannot be generalized to the entire nursing profession, the study supports that nurses find meaning in their careers. This is important in preventing professional exhaustion and burnout when encountering the stressors associated with clinical practice.

Malloy, D. C., Fahey-McCarthy, E., Murakami, M., Lee, Y., Choi, E., Hirose, E., & Hadjistavropoulos, T. (2015). Finding meaning in the work of nursing: An international study. *Online Journal of Issues in Nursing, 20*(3), 1. https://doi.org/10.3912/OJIN.Vol20No03PPT02

Building the Foundation

Box 3.2, Professional Building Blocks, "Major Disciplines of Philosophy," outlines the nine major disciplines of philosophy and the questions each seeks to answer. This can serve as a general guide to understanding and developing a philosophy.

Philosophy focuses on conceptual clarity and requires an individual journey while providing a foundation for human action (Rosen et al., 2018). For clarity, **nursing philosophy** is defined as the intellectual and affective outcomes of the professional nurses' efforts to

1. understand the ultimate relationships between humans, environment, and health;
2. approach nursing as a scientific discipline;
3. integrate a sense of value into practice;
4. appreciate aesthetic elements that contribute to health and well-being;
5. define the mission of nursing;
6. articulate a personal belief system about human beings, the environment, health, and nursing.

Significance of Philosophy for Nursing

Over time, the study of philosophy has accrued great benefits for individuals, societies, and, particularly, specific sciences. Essentially, science benefits from philosophy because philosophy governs scientific methods through logic and ethics.

Pursuing the objectives of philosophy provides individuals with opportunities to develop an understanding of the world around them and to exercise value judgments. Development of a personal system of values requires making ethical and aesthetic decisions. The quest for reason develops understanding. Achievement of intellectual enlightenment is considered better protection than ignorance against potentially calamitous mistakes.

3.2 Professional Building Blocks

Major Disciplines of Philosophy

1. **Logic:** Systematic study of arguments for logical or illogical reasoning
   - *Does this make sense?*

2. **Epistemology:** Study of knowledge
   - *What is knowledge? How do people acquire it?*

3. **Philosophy of science:** Explanation of the successes of science
   - *How is science used? What are the benefits of hard sciences to humans?*

4. **Metaphysics (ontology):** Analysis of issues surrounding the ultimate nature of existence, reality, and experience; also addresses the reality of abstractions (from mathematical constructs such as numbers to religious concepts such as God, angels, and the human soul) and the existence of abstractions in the absence of human thought
   - *What is there?*

5. **Philosophy of mind:** Study of the nature of the mental dimension of people
   - *What is the mind? How should we understand intentions, desires, beliefs, emotions, pleasure, and pain? How do mental processes explain human behavior?*

6. **Ethics (moral philosophy):** Study of the appropriateness of possible courses of action based on a system of moral principles and values
   - *What is morality? What actions are obligatory, morally permissible, or impermissible?*

7. **Sociopolitical philosophy:** Study of the control and regulation of people living in a society and the means to improve their lives
   - *Where do states come from? What does it mean to be a citizen of a state? Must we obey laws, and why? When should laws be changed?*

8. **Philosophy of religion:** Study of the meaning of human life
   - *Is religious language meaningful? Does God exist? Is there good and evil? What other basis can give meaning to life if the religious assumptions were to be proven false?*

9. **Aesthetics:** Study of what constitutes beauty
   - *What is beauty? What makes something a work of art? Why are art and other forms of artistic expression important?*

The nursing profession needs philosophers who articulate visions for nursing as a scientific discipline, emphasize concern for the ultimate good of humankind, develop belief systems reflecting sound ethics, reflect on the meaning of nursing, and conduct periodic reviews of nursing philosophies.

Nurses need personal philosophies that reflect a belief in recasting the health system to benefit all humankind rather than ensuring institutional survival. Nursing philosophers analyze current health care systems and conceptualize the bases for nursing practice, research, and education. These nursing philosophers also concern themselves with moral issues surrounding nursing and health care while promoting behavior based on a professional code of ethics.

Rafael (1996) coined the term "empowered caring" to denote leadership as a unity of power and caring that values the characteristics and experiences of individuals and a system of ethics that "stems from a heightened awareness of interrelatedness and emerges as a sense of responsibility toward others" (p. 15). Rafael's writing demonstrates the work of a nursing philosopher who provides novel thinking and uses this to shift from a hierarchical approach to nursing to one in which nurses and nurse leaders share knowledge and expertise with clients and each other.

Nurse leaders have identified a system of values to guide the nursing profession. According to the American Association of College of Nursing (2021), a professional nurse's behavior is driven by ethics. "Ethics is closely tied to moral philosophy involving the study of or examination of morality through a variety of different approaches" (p. 13). Many nurses enter the profession for altruistic reasons. When these are accompanied by a deep respect for the dignity and worth of all persons, their right to autonomy, and social justice, nurses have a solid foundation for acting with personal and professional integrity. Ethical and honest behavior by professional nurses promotes social respect for nurses and enhances client safety. A strong professional value set facilitates decision making in ethically charged clinical situations.

Developing a Personal Nursing Philosophy

A personal nursing philosophy provides an individualized perspective for nursing practice, research, and scholarship (Salsberry, 1994). Articulation of a personal nursing philosophy enables nurses to make and find meaning about being a professional nurse. Rew (1994) explains that a well-articulated philosophy combines ways of doing with ways of being. Determining ways of being involves an examination of one's personal beliefs and values. For example, how nurses view their professional activities, such as doing a job, engaging in a professional career, and/or living out one's calling to help others, affects how they practice nursing and what it means to be a professional nurse. Marchuk (2014) suggests that a personal nursing philosophy promotes the integration of nursing knowledge into compassionate clinical care. Additionally, Hountras (2015) asserts that having a personal nursing philosophy facilitates personal motivation and provides reasons behind the work of professional nursing for each nurse. A personal nursing philosophy is never complete; rather, it evolves as knowledge and experience expand. Because the nursing profession concerns itself with people, health, nursing, and the environment, most personal nursing philosophies address these key concepts.

Take Note!
Never carved in stone, nursing philosophy remains a constant work in progress.

Carper (1978) identified four patterns of knowing in nursing: personal knowledge, empirics, aesthetics, and ethics (presented in more detail in Chapter 6, "Patterns of Knowing and Nursing Science"). A well-developed nursing philosophy represents personal knowledge related to professional nursing.

To construct a personal philosophy of nursing, one must engage in reflective thinking about one's relationship to the universe. Discovery of a personal **mission** or goal within the realm of nursing solidifies the decision to practice professional nursing. Because nursing focuses on individuals and the environment, a beginning nursing philosophy should minimally address these concepts (Box 3.3, Learning, Knowing, and Growing, "Developing a Nursing Philosophy").

The greatest opportunity to begin developing answers to the questions asked in Box 3.3, Learning, Knowing, and Growing, "Developing a Nursing Philosophy," begins with the first nursing course. Likewise, as nurses attain higher levels of education, beginning a new course becomes an opportune time to continue to evaluate and modify one's professional nursing philosophy. A nurse's professional self-concept is built on the foundation of their personal life and educational and

---

 ### 3.3 Learning, Knowing, and Growing

Developing a Nursing Philosophy

To develop a nursing philosophy, nurses must examine and answer questions that address the key concepts of professional nursing, the elements of nursing as a scientific discipline, and the valuation elements of nursing.

Key Concepts of Professional Nursing

- What is the environment, and what is the nature of the relationship between humans and the environment?
- What is your central belief about the individual person and that person's potential?
- What is your central belief about the family and its potential?
- What is your central belief about the community and its potential?
- What are your central beliefs about the relationship between society and health?
- What is your view on health? Is it a continuum? A state? A process?
- How do illness and wellness relate to health?
- What is the central reason for the existence of nursing?
- Who is the recipient of nursing care?

Nursing as a Scientific Discipline

- Is nursing a science, an art, or both?
- From what cognitive base does the professional nurse operate?
- What is the nursing process? How is it implemented?
- What is necessary to apply nursing knowledge?
- How is the theory base for nursing derived?
- What is the theoretical framework for the profession? Is there more than one theoretical framework?
- What are the purposes and processes of nursing research?

Valuation Elements of Nursing

- What are the essential rights and responsibilities of the professional nurse?
- What are the essential rights and responsibilities of recipients of nursing care?
- What are the governing ethical principles in the delivery of nursing care and the conduct of nursing research?
- What are your beliefs about the educational requirements for the practice of the profession?
- What are your beliefs about the teaching–learning process?
- What is the ultimate goal of professional nursing care?

clinical practice experiences. As a nurse progresses on their life journey, finding meaning in one's personal and professional existence remains a constant challenge.

Take Note!
Articulation of a personal nursing philosophy helps the nurse find purpose, create meaning, and increase commitment to the profession of nursing.

Box 3.4, Professional Prototypes, "Sample Professional Nursing Philosophy," presents a brief sample nursing philosophy that employs analogy to present philosophical views about nursing. Analogies can be useful when presenting deeply held beliefs. However, a nursing philosophy does not require using an analogy; statements about personal beliefs serve just as well. As you develop your philosophy, realize that there is no one "right" nursing philosophy. You may also find over time that your nursing philosophy may change.

3.4 Professional Prototypes

Sample Professional Nursing Philosophy

Nursing is like a diamond. Special conditions must exist for a diamond to be created, and special care must be taken to maximize its luster.

Nurses hold a sacred trust with their clients when clients put their lives in the nurse's hands. The nurse's mission is to focus on what is best for the client when making decisions concerning care. When possible, the nurse and clients work as partners to promote health. Together they carve out a multifaceted plan of care that integrates the needs of body, mind, and spirit. The nurse always considers client choices for care. However, when the client is no longer able to choose, the nurse abides by the information left previously by the client or by the family's wishes. Along with caring for individuals, the nurse cares for families and communities.

A diamond never shows its luster if left in a box. Likewise, a nurse fails to shine when they are unable to care for others.

Once you have an established nursing philosophy, you can use it in many ways. When seeking employment, ask to see the potential employer's organizational philosophy and see how closely it matches your own. A recent trend in health care is the development of a unit-based philosophy. To engage in the process, all unit staff meet and draft a philosophy. This process is time consuming and creates interesting debates among staff members. When organizational and personal philosophies match, people have a stronger commitment to work processes and increased job satisfaction.

MORALITY AND ETHICS IN NURSING PRACTICE

Within any practice context, nurses feel compelled to do what is "right" for their clients. **Morality**, as defined by O'Neill (1995, p. 224), encompasses "the oughts of a given society." **Ethics** is "the philosophical study of morality" (Noddings, 1984, p. 1). Nurses confront many situations in which they rely on their conscience for decision making. When working with coherent clients, nurses provide information and share the process of decision making with them.

Many nurses acknowledge that a desire to care for others was the impetus for them to enter the nursing profession (Malloy et al., 2015; Streubert, 1994). The science and art of nursing center around the concept of caring. Experts in caring theory emphasize that before one can effectively care for others over a lifetime, one must be able to care for oneself (Benner, 2000; Benner & Wrubel, 1989; Watson, 1988, 2012). Watson (1988, 2012) called caring a moral imperative. Nurses enter the profession with the intent to care, and society expects them to care.

Changes in health care delivery often prevent nurses from having the time to express caring in practice. Some institutions treat nurses as replaceable technicians who have sophisticated skills. Clients have become consumers. Instead of individualized care, health care consumers receive treatment from standardized plans. Nurses feel pressure to streamline care to maximize the use of health care resources.

The shift of nursing care to a "trade service" is most apparent with the advent of managed care. Managed care looks for cost-cutting measures such as increased use of unlicensed care providers. Health insurers limit covered health care services and an individual's right to choose health care providers. Access to and justification for care supersede the more important, close interpersonal relationships that nurses build with clients. Therefore, the main stimulus for entering nursing—caring—becomes less valued by health care providers, especially administrators whose main concern is financial viability.

Moral Development

Gilligan (1982, p. 19) identified two ways of thinking about moral development. She associated these concepts of morality with what she called "male" and "female" modes of describing relationships between others and oneself:

1. Fairness: Connecting moral development to the understanding of rights and rules (male mode)
2. Concern with the activity of care: Connecting moral development to the understanding of responsibilities and relationships (female mode)

Traditional views of moral development emphasize "rights" over relationships and responsibilities. In the traditional view of moral development, a person progresses through a series of stages. The first is a preconventional level, which encompasses the first two stages with obedience to avoid punishment (stage 1) followed by a self-interest orientation (stage 2). The next level is conventional, when people are concerned with interpersonal accord and conforming to expectations (stage 3) and following authority and social orders such as obeying the law (stage 4). The third and final level is the postconventional level in which individuals assume a social contract orientation by displaying mutual respect and acknowledging pluralism (stage 5) and then applying universal ethical principles based on conscience and reasoning (stage 6) (Kohlberg, 1981).

Noddings (1984) proposed that morality and ethics should be "rooted in receptivity, relatedness, and responsiveness" (p. 2). Haegert (2004) adapted Noddings's work on the ethics of caring to professional nursing practice. For Noddings, caring involves two aspects of human nature in the embodied self and ethical self. The embodied self describes an idealized self that is "synonymous with caring" and the "vision that implied a picture of goodness toward the one caring (the nurse) and the one cared for (the patient)" (Haegert, 2004, p. 434). Nurses devote energy to the development of authentic, therapeutic, and caring relationships with clients. The ethical self involves nurses considering the legal and institutional standards of care along with client rights for self-determination and equal access to care. Therefore, nursing presents a unique opportunity for blending different approaches to morality and ethics. However, as long as society values fairness and responsibility over receptivity, relatedness, and responsiveness, contributions made by professional nurses may not be as valued as those made by members of other health professions.

Morality supersedes status when people entrust their lives to others. Therefore, moral principles guide health care providers in practice. Some of the moral principles central to nursing include beneficence, fidelity, and veracity. According to Flynn (1987), the principle of beneficence is to do only good. This principle also requires that individuals act to prevent harm. Aroskar (1987) viewed fidelity as undisputed and primary loyalty and faithfulness to the client. Finally, veracity requires absolute truth telling.

In 1948, the *United Nations Declaration of Human Rights* mentioned human dignity but failed to define its meaning. One definition of dignity is a state of being worthy, having esteem, and possessing honor (Mish, 2020). Depending upon one's secular or religious views, human dignity may mean different things. The Judeo-Christian perspective espouses that humans are made in the image of God. Sulmasy (2008) identified three different ways to conceptualize dignity from a moralistic perspective: attributed (worthiness based on social status, reputation, or merit based upon societal contributions); intrinsic (people have value and worth just because they are human); and inflorescent (the flourishing of the human as they act in manners expressing the intrinsic value of humanity).

Fowler (2015) specifies that it is inflorescent dignity that is observed in nurses as they deliver skilled nursing care to others with genuine caring and compassion while displaying the utmost regard for the care recipient's humanity. In the nursing ethical literature, human dignity is inherent (permanently fixed); intrinsic (within and part of the natural innerness and belonging); and inviolable (it must not be violated, broken, or disturbed). By embracing human dignity as a moral concept, human dignity becomes the foundation for respect, protection, caring, and preservation of the human rights of clients.

However, because nurses are also humans, attention needs to be made to the human dignity of the nurse (Fowler, 2015). The recognition of the dignity of the nursing profession is an emerging concept for the profession and is being recognized by society, especially with legal efforts to protect nurses from physical and verbal assaults from health care consumers, exploitation from employers, sexual harassment, and lateral violence.

Take Note!

Professional nurses use the principles of beneficence, fidelity, and veracity daily when providing care to clients.

Moral and Ethical Dilemmas

Moral and ethical principles create dilemmas for nurses. Disagreements surface regarding what is good for a client depending on the situation (Flynn, 1987). Individual health care team members may disagree on what is best for a terminally ill person. Fidelity specifies that nurses should always remain loyal and faithful to the client and abide by the client's wishes. Sometimes, nurses encounter situations that require them to deceive clients or withhold information from them to protect the institutions for which the nurses work or the physicians whom they serve. Although most institutions require nurses to report errors using some form of incident reporting, many institutional policies specify that the nurse should not document completion of an incident report.

When nurses encounter situations in which there is no good outcome, the principle of double effect (known as choosing the "lesser evil") guides practice. Burkhardt (2016, p. 122) outlined four conditions that should be met to justify double-effect actions:

1. The act itself must be morally good or at least indifferent.
2. The good effect must not be achieved by means of the bad effect.
3. Only the good effect must be intended, though the bad effect is foreseen and known.
4. The good effect intended must be equal to or greater than the bad effect.

As client advocates, nurses must act on behalf of clients. To assess a particular clinical situation, nurses use critical thinking skills to collect and analyze information and to formulate possible courses of action. As critical thinkers, nurses also anticipate consequences of actions before choosing the best course to take. Professional nurses use values and philosophical beliefs to set priorities and establish action plans in ethically and morally charged situations (see Concepts in Practice, "An Ethical Dilemma: The Case of Mrs. G").

Concepts in Practice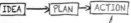

An Ethical Dilemma: The Case of Mrs. G

Mrs. G, a 96-year-old woman, is comatose due to a head injury from an automobile accident in which she was the driver. Before the accident, she lived independently and volunteered at the library teaching adults to read. Mrs. G has been unresponsive and ventilator-dependent for 3 days. She has shown no improvement, but her son is insisting on a tracheotomy so that his mother can be maintained on the ventilator until she regains consciousness.

QUESTIONS FOR REFLECTION

1. How should the nurse respond to the ethical dilemma presented in the case of Mrs. G?
2. What ethical principles should be applied in this case?
3. What roadblocks might the nurse encounter in providing the best care for Mrs. G?

ETHICAL DECISION MAKING

According to Bandman and Bandman (1995), nursing ethics focuses on doing good and avoiding harm. The nurse bears responsibility for valuing choices that clients make. For example, choices may be clearly articulated when people complete living wills before becoming incapacitated. However, when people fail to make their desires known before they are unable to do so, health care professionals rely on families for treatment-related decisions. In the absence of family, moral and ethical tenets guide actions.

Nurses, like scientists and philosophers, base their decisions on outcomes of inquiry. Munhall linked nursing inquiry to ethical reflection, with the ultimate ethical question being "toward what goal and what end?" (Munhall, 1988, p. 151). Munhall added that "many of our research endeavors focus on facilitating health. The search for a means to produce a desired health outcome requires critical ethical reflection" (p. 152).

> **Take Note!**
> Ethical dilemmas are messy, heart-wrenching situations with no clear-cut answers.

Principlism, Care, and Contextualism

Traditionally, three perspectives provide a foundation for and influence ethical thinking: principlism, care, and contextualism.

- Of the three, the most prevalent framework is **principlism**, which can be defined as using a set of principles or general guidelines for analyzing a situation considering general norms that have been derived from common morality. It involves incorporating professional duties, rights, and principles (Beauchamp & Childress, 2013; Fowler, 2015). Beauchamp and Childress (2013) identify four key ethical principles (Table 3.1) to guide ethical

TABLE 3.1   Key Ethical Principles

Principle	Definition	Examples
Nonmaleficence	To do no harm to others	*Due diligence*: Exercise care in a situation so that one does not harm another (e.g., carefully checking medications before administering them). *Double effect*: The outcomes outweigh the potential harm (e.g., administration of chemotherapy [adverse effects] to kill cancer cells).
Beneficence	To do only good for others	*Compassion*: Caring with a desire to help others (e.g., attending to the psychological needs of a person who has a new colostomy). *Veracity*: Being honest and telling the truth (e.g., informing clients about all options for the treatment of a health condition). *Fidelity:* Being faithful in relationships and in matters of trust (e.g., maintaining the confidentiality of personal health information and disclosing information when obtaining informed consent). *Proportionality*: Choosing the option that produces more good than harm (e.g., determining the best treatment options for clients).
Autonomy	The right of people to make free and informed choices	*Privacy*: Respecting another's personal space and business (e.g., asking for permission prior to touching a client). *Confidentiality*: Keeping personal information about clients secret (e.g., not holding an end-of-shift report where visitors and other clients may be able to hear). *Advocacy*: Hearing and respecting client wishes, needs, and values (e.g., abiding by a terminally ill client's desires to not be connected to life support). *Informed consent*: Ensuring that clients receive all pertinent information surrounding a prescribed treatment so they can make the best possible decision (e.g., explaining all potential hazards of a surgical procedure).
Justice	Fairness and impartiality to provide equality of service according to individual needs and contributions	*Respect*: Preserving or maintaining personal dignity and rights (e.g., providing equal services for all clients despite their ethnicity or culture). *Allocation of resources*: Fairly distributing limited services based on need rather than ability to pay (e.g., using complex life-saving technology on individuals with the potential for survival).

Adapted from Mish, F. C. (Ed.). (2020). *Merriam-Webster's Collegiate Dictionary* (11th ed.). Merriam-Webster, Inc.; Bosek, M., & Savage, T. (2007). *The ethical component of nursing education, integrating ethics into clinical experience*. Lippincott Williams & Wilkins; Beauchamp, T., & Childress, J. (2013). *Principles of biomedical ethics* (7th ed.). Oxford University Press; Fowler, M. D. M. (2015). *Guide to the code of ethics for nurses with interpretive statements* (2nd ed.). American Nurses Association.

decision making—respect for autonomy (an individual's right to self-determination and making their own decisions); nonmaleficence (to do no harm); beneficence (to do good); and justice (fairness, impartiality, and what is right). This perspective values rationalism. However, a health care professional must analyze individual situations, sensitivity to the needs of others, and relationship dynamics when using principlism to guide ethical decision making.

■ The care perspective can be used only when the caregiver and care receiver have a reciprocal relationship. Fowler (2015) identifies **four phases of caring**: caring about, taking care of, care giving, and care receiving. The four moral elements of an ethic of care are attentiveness, responsibility, competence, and responsiveness. When using the ethic of care, the nurse communicates with everyone involved in the decision-making process to identify and consider individual needs and preferences. Nursing based on the care perspective recognizes that time must be spent to discover what is meaningful to clients.

■ Finally, in **contextualism**, individual situations become the paradigm cases that provide "rules of thumb" to follow. In the contextualist perspective, practical experience in client care is highly valued (O'Neill, 1995). Nursing based on contextualism supports detailed analysis of individual nursing situations and determines the best approaches to fit each situation.

In a postmodern world, people tend to discount the simpler, monolithic approach to life and prefer pluralism. McCarthy (2006) proposed a pluralistic view of nursing ethics that blends the traditional and theory views of nursing ethics.

The traditional view asserts that nursing ethics is a subcategory of health care ethics. Nurses engage in identifying, analyzing, and making decisions using the concepts of deontology (acting on the basis of moral duty and obligations), utilitarianism (acting to bring about the greatest good), or principlism (using duties, rights, and rules based on truth, laws, or doctrine) to navigate ethical challenges encountered in daily practice.

In contrast, the pluralistic theory view of ethics espouses a nursing-focused, ethical approach based on philosophical approaches derived from "virtue ethics, care ethics, or feminist ethics" (McCarthy, 2006, p. 160). This approach also uses ethical standards developed by international, national, and specialty nursing organizations. The theory view of ethics is contextual and emphasizes the power relationships among individuals, societies, and organizations. An understanding of many views of ethics is important when considering using a pluralistic approach when encountering ethically charged situations. In a pluralistic view of nursing ethics, nurses use a combination of approaches to reflect on and make decisions about ethical dilemmas.

The nursing literature also presents additional ethical theories and approaches. Consequentialism requires a person to use the outcomes of one's action as the most important thing to consider prior to taking action. *Prima facie* ("on the face," or first impression) rights declare that something is correct unless it is shown to be wrong. Preventing distress, keeping promises, repaying kindness, and helping others are classified as *prima facie* good actions until classified otherwise. For example, a nurse who promises her family that she will be home in time to leave for a family outing is late because she had to stay at work to attend to a client who had a medical emergency during the change of shift. Casuistry is an inductive approach to making decisions based upon individual cases. Narrative ethics are based on storytelling, considering clients as moral agents who make choices. When using a narrative approach, nurses consider human relationships and how individuals evolved to be who they currently are and how they became involved in the current situation. Critical theory arises from the worldview that powerful groups dominate others, and this theory focuses on freeing the oppressed from their oppression. Feminist ethics addresses how ethical approaches differ between men and women. This approach possesses political connotation and looks at the oppression of women by dominating social groups, especially men. The feminist approach to ethics is a form of critical theory that espouses the differences between how men and women approach moral reasoning. Instead of focusing on duty, fairness,

impartiality, and objectivity, the ethics of care focuses on women's concern for others and emphasizes love, compassion, and sympathy. The emotional component is viewed as complementary to the rational element of decision making (Rich, 2020).

Eastern Philosophical and Ethical Approaches

Eastern philosophical and ethical approaches concentrate on understanding the interconnectedness of the self with the universe. In this approach, people do not exist as individual selves but are integrated within the universe. The actions taken by a person result in fair consequences. Hinduism emphasizes cosmic unity. People live in an illusory, temporary, everyday experience. Karma (fate) is a series of reincarnations that are based on previous actions. Eventually, the soul of each individual becomes one with the cosmic self and the absolute reality of Brahman (Rich, 2020, p. 22).

In contrast, Buddhism developed when Siddhartha Gautama, a Hindu prince, became a spiritual teacher as he left the confinement of his father's palace and saw human suffering. He spent his life trying to understand and end suffering. The Buddhist Four Noble Truths act as a framework for understanding existence. Human suffering or lack of satisfaction is an inherent part of all forms of existence. Suffering arises when individuals become egocentric and cling to temporary things. This attachment must be let go of to alleviate suffering. The Fourth Noble Truth is renouncing attachment to relieve suffering, called the Eightfold Path. It consists of eight right practices—"right view, right thinking, right mindfulness, right speech, right action, right diligence, right concentration, and right livelihood" (Rich, 2020, p. 23).

Taoism extends from the work of Lao-tzu (571 BCE) who authored the Taoist guide to life. When translated into English, the Chinese word *tao* means "way" or "path," but its essence is the natural harmony or order of all things. Nature and humans cannot be separated. Taoist philosophy espouses the balance of nature's dark (*yin*) and light (*yang*) elements. An ethical life requires authenticity, simplicity, unselfishness, and being in harmony with nature and oneself (Rich, 2020, p. 23).

Confucianism arose out of K'ung Fu-tzu's set of fundamental truths, principles, rules, and sayings to guide how people should live. Early Christians visiting China called him Confucius. Two key concepts *li* and *yi* are part of the system of Confucian ethics. *Li* guides social order and interpersonal relations (social etiquette and rituals). *Yi* focuses on righteousness and morality through sincerity, teamwork, and balance. *Ren* (human goodness or benevolence) is the primary virtue of this belief system. Confucianism espouses a more communitarian approach that places importance of human relationships, social goals, and what is good for society over the individual (Rich, 2020, pp. 23–24). The communal approach to ethics emphasizes what is best for others rather than focusing on the rights of individuals and what is best for each. Individuals believe it is their duty to make sacrifices for the benefit of others. This is often a common theme of conversations surrounding community and public health.

African Philosophical and Ethical Approaches

African philosophy, morals, and ethical principles diverge somewhat from Western thought, being more collective than individualistic. Many principles have been passed down through generations via storytelling (Wareham, 2017). There are numerous varying philosophies and ethical approaches among different tribes and geographical populations. Moral beliefs are influenced by culture and environment. Decisions are made by *indaba* (group discussion or conference), *baraza* (public meeting), or storytelling (Mish, 2020; Wareham, 2017). Ibanga (2016) explains that "either/or" thinking is not always prevalent in African cultures; "both/and" thinking is more commonplace.

Some of the moral and philosophical tenets of sub-Saharan Africa are based on highly prized communal relationships (Wareham, 2017). Box 3.5 presents some of the beliefs, values, and morals among these cultures. The African approach to ethics is holistic and promotes a dialectic approach to addressing ethical issues when they arise. The need to "be right" is eliminated because when polarity occurs in a given situation, either way of managing the situation can be the best course of action.

Take Note!
Eastern and African philosophies espouse a view of individuals being one with the universe and the importance of community over individuals.

Box 3.5 Beliefs, Morals, and Philosophical Tenets Common in Africa

1. The good of those with whom one shares a communal relationship is most important (Ibanga, 2016; Wareham, 2017).
2. "A person is a person through other persons" (Wareham, 2017, p. 682).
3. Moral people are created via initiation rites (Manomi, 2019).
4. What a person does defines who they are (Manomi, 2019).
5. Who we are is more important than who I am (Manomi, 2019).
6. All people have full humanity and are equal (Manomi, 2019).
7. Steadiness of body and mind (self-control) is desired and regarded as a key aspect of social order, not a means of self-aggrandizement (Manomi, 2019).
8. Man shares the environment with nonhumans, including spirits (Ibanga, 2016).
9. Self-preservation is a law of nature (Ibanga, 2016).
10. Pastors and spiritual men speak the truth of God or the Great Being, and their words cannot be faulted (Ibanga, 2016).
11. Man has a relational order with the environment (Ibanga, 2016).
12. Humans should peacefully "coexist with the universe and treat it with some concern for its worth survival and sustainability" (Ibanga, 2016, p. 10).
13. "Live and let live" (Ibanga, 2016, p. 11).
14. Man and nature are intricately intertwined so the well-being of each is tied to the other (Ibanga, 2016).
15. We share our food with the land because we are an extension of the land.
16. Humans and animals share the same food chain.
17. Humans share the same being with animals.
18. Animals should be treated using the same cordial manner as one would use to treat a person.
19. Each should work for the good of all and for the entire community as a whole.
20. "I am because you are" (Ibanga, 2016, p. 14).
21. Humans and nonhumans can only attain bliss and harmony if they are in a complementary relationship with each other (Ibanga, 2016).
22. Man is a being of others in the universe of being (Ibanga, 2016).

Sources: Ibanga, F. D. A. (2016). Logical and theoretical foundations of African environmental ethics. *Africology: The Journal of Pan African Studies, 9*(9), 3–24; Manomi, D. J. (2019). Towards an African-Biblical virtue ethics: Reflection on the letter to Titus through a progressive-negotiated-ethics. *Acta Theologica, 39*(2), 114–129. https://doi.org/10.18820/23099089/actat.v39i2.7; Wareham, C. S. (2017). A duty to explore African ethics? *Ethical Theory Moral Practice, 20,* 857–872. https://doi.org/10.1007/s10677-017-9826-x

Polarized Thinking

In practice, nurses (and other health care professionals) must make decisions with which they can live and perhaps use to make better decisions in the future. Some individuals make decisions by deferring to rules, principles, and strong philosophical views. When they hold steadfast to a certain view (e.g., liberalism, conservativism), they engage in **polarized thinking**. However, this can lead to confusion and discomfort in how to figure out life and find meaning in it when rules are abandoned. Individuals often desire finding the "right" answer, even when there are no clear-cut answers, and develop radical, steadfast approaches that fuel political debates and conflict.

Consider the debate about whether nursing is an art or a science. Emphasis on technology, scientific evidence, and quality improvement suggests that nursing is a science. However, considering the beauty of the deep, meaningful, interpersonal relationships between nurses and clients and capturing how it unfolds suggests that nursing may be an art. Conventional thinking would require the person to decide whether nursing is an art *or* science. Both/and thinking is a pluralistic view that considers all arguments and blends the two into a combined view. In this instance, it can be argued nursing is simultaneously an art and a science.

▌ QUESTIONS FOR REFLECTION

1. What are your beliefs and values about human life?
2. How strong are these beliefs and values?
3. What would you do if you encountered a client care situation in which decisions were made that were against your values and beliefs? Why would you act this way?

REAL-LIFE REFLECTIONS

Jane is the charge nurse, and Sheila and Ben are working with her today. A 50-year-old client just received a diagnosis of advanced cancer, and the physician told him that he has less than 6 months to live. The client has three children: 17-year-old John, 15-year-old Ruth, and 12-year-old Daniel. The client and the family have opted for hospice care, and all cancer treatments are being stopped. While the family is at lunch, Ben spends time talking with the client and learns about his concerns. Because his

wife never understood the financial side of running a household, the client decided that John should assume this responsibility for the family in anticipation of his death. The client asks Ben for ideas of how to tell his son about this wish. What would you do if you were in Ben's situation? Why do you think that you would act this way? Is there a correct decision to be made in this situation? Why or why not?

An Ethical Decision-Making Process

Nurses frequently encounter moral and ethical problems in practice, thereby creating a need for a workable method with which to analyze and resolve ethical dilemmas (see Concepts in Practice, "Ethical Decision Making in Action"). Fowler and Levine-Ariff (1987) proposed a systematic **ethical decision-making process** that incorporates principlism, care, and contextualism to help nurses thoughtfully address moral problems in practice (Table 3.2). Consistent use of a sequential process for ethical decision making enables nurses to consider all aspects surrounding a situation before taking action. Once the situation has resolved, engagement in evaluation allows the nurse to reflect on actions taken and to generate ideas for managing a similar situation in the future.

▌ QUESTIONS FOR REFLECTION

1. Can you identify the steps Mary and her colleagues took in their ethical decision-making process?
2. What else could Mary and her colleagues have done to remedy this situation?

Bandman and Bandman (1995, p. 110) discussed the pitfalls—or "fallacies"—that nurses may encounter when using an ethical decision-making process. These errors in reasoning include:

1. Arguing that because something (X) is the case, something else (Y) ought to be the case
2. Making someone accept the conclusion of another based on force alone (appealing to force)
3. Abusing the person rather than addressing the person's reasons for making a particular decision
4. Arguing that because everybody does something, it must be good
5. Appealing to inappropriate authority to justify a decision

TABLE 3.2　Process for Ethical Decision Making

Steps	Thoughts and Actions
Identify the problem.	■ Analyze the situation to clearly identify the problem. ■ Determine the presence of more than one ethical concern. ■ Look for any conflict of duties with personal or professional values. ■ Determine whether the ethical conflict rightly belongs to you.
Identify the morally relevant facts.	■ Examine the complete context of the dilemma (how it occurred, likelihood of arising again). ■ Identify the key players and their views and vested interest(s). ■ Identify administrative, political, economic, legal, medical, and aesthetic concerns.
Evaluate the ethical problem.	■ Examine the ethical norms by reviewing the literature, code of ethics for nursing, and moral traditions in the profession. ■ Based on this information, identify guides for moral actions that are appropriate for the situation. ■ Consider broader ethical principles, such as justice and autonomy, to provide directions for action. ■ Consider aspects that are unique to the dilemma. ■ Examine the dilemma using each ethical principle. ■ Assign priorities to each of the ethical principles according to professional and personal values.
Identify and analyze action alternatives.	■ Determine all possible options for action. ■ Create new options not found elsewhere. ■ Analyze each alternative action for potential harms and benefits. ■ Speculate on the possible outcomes of each action for the key players. ■ Identify which actions will produce subsequent dilemmas. ■ Analyze each alternative according to institutional procedures.
Choose and act.	■ Choose a course of action (preferably in consultation with others). ■ Modify the plan in accordance with legal, institutional, or other values while remaining true to your moral values and norms. ■ Implement the action selected.
Evaluate and modify the plan.	■ Identify the result of action taken. ■ Clarify your moral feelings about your actions. ■ Generate modifications to the plan used if you encounter similar situations in the future. ■ Modify the current plan if the ethical dilemma persists.

Adapted from Fowler, M. D. M., & Levine-Ariff, J. (Eds.). (1987). *Ethics at the bedside: A source-book for the critical care nurse.* Lippincott Williams & Wilkins.

6. Assuming that if one exception is made to a rule, then uncontrolled events with unwanted circumstances will occur (called the "slippery slope fallacy")

7. Refusing to allow evidence to be shared if it contradicts one's personal position

Concepts in Practice　IDEA ⟶ PLAN ⟶ ACTION

Ethical Decision Making in Action

Mary is a nurse who works the night shift on an acute general surgical unit. Because of budget cuts, the hospital has eliminated two night shift professional nursing positions, resulting in a consistent staffing pattern of one nurse for 15 clients. Mary has always valued her ability to provide individualized nursing care to postoperative clients. However, under the new staffing pattern, Mary believes clients are receiving substandard care. She realizes that the hospital has been losing revenue, but she also thinks this staffing pattern is unsafe. Her recent complaints to her nurse manager have been futile. Because of unsafe care situations, Mary knows that she will have to inform her nurse manager's supervisor and possibly the director of nursing and hospital administration to analyze the entire situation. Mary reads current literature, identifies serious gaps in the accepted standards of practice, and examines the effects of the new staffing practice on each ethical principle. After sharing her concerns with her coworkers and manager, Mary and her colleagues work as a team to develop three action plans. They discuss the pros and cons of each plan and then meet with the director of nursing to share their concerns. The director of nursing thanks the nurses for informing her of the situation and promises action to increase the number of professional nurses for the night shift on the unit. Two months pass with no change in staffing. The nurses decide to meet with hospital administration to voice their concerns.

Bandman and Bandman (1995) suggested ways to avoid these fallacies by using the following principles for ethical decision making:

1. Valuing and respecting the client's self-determination
2. Serving the client's well-being in practice in a manner that prevents harm and does good
3. Treating clients fairly and equally by respecting their rights and treatment options and by making them equal partners in shared health care decisions

Nursing practice, education, and research provide many opportunities for the professional nurse to make ethical decisions and to experience the satisfaction of resolving ethical dilemmas. Situations that generate ethical dilemmas arise from the nurse's efforts to determine what is right. In dealing with each of these ethical issues, the primary responsibility of the nurse in caring for the client is always to respect the person as a unified being. Despite variations in the definition of responsibility in nursing, most nurses would probably agree that the goal for resolving ethical issues is to achieve what is best for clients while attending to the responsibility to self, colleagues, and the profession.

Examples of ethical concerns of nurses include the quality of client care, unfair organizational practices, poor quality work environments, disagreements about end-of-life issues, and conflicts with physicians. When ethical issues arise, nurses may act with power or be powerless. Displays of passivity include silence, "submission, obedience, and powerlessness" (Peter et al., p. 403). Empowered nurses confront ethical issues directly through the exercise of resistance (e.g., whistle-blowing, refusal to follow physician orders, acts of disobedience, and direct confrontation). Failure to abide by one's moral principles has been identified as a reason why nurses leave a job and, in some cases, the profession. Nurses who use resistance to solve ethical dilemmas display great courage because of possible retaliation against them from the people (or the organization) with whom they disagree (Peter et al., 2004).

Achieving Ethical Competence

Achieving ethical competence takes time and practice. **Ethical competence** means nurses have the knowledge, confidence, and courage to take action to do what is right in an ethically charged situation. In nursing education programs, time is allotted for presentation and discussion of ethical concepts and dilemmas. Read the Concepts in Practice box, "When an Endangered Adult Patient Refuses Help." Consider this situation commonly

encountered in practice in emergency departments and how the nurse in this scenario possesses a strong knowledge base about escalation of intimate partner abuse and uses it to provide ethically competent care.

Concepts in Practice

When an Endangered Adult Client Refuses Help

A young married woman with injuries consistent with intimate partner abuse is seen in the emergency department. When the nurse informs the client that by law, the nurses need to contact the local law enforcement agency, the client pleads with the nurse to keep the suspicious nature of her injuries secret. However, the nurse reports the injuries to the legal authorities who confirm that the injuries are the result of being abused. The woman refuses to file charges, speaks with a social worker who arranges legal aid for divorce assistance, and insists upon returning home with her husband. Knowing that the incidence of intimate partner homicide greatly increases when the abused partner plans to dissolve a marriage, the nurse provides the woman with this information and urges her to go to a shelter instead of home. What factors should be considered prior to releasing this client from the hospital?

Key concepts related to nursing ethics include understanding basic theoretical approaches to ethics such as principlism, utilitarianism, and deontology. In addition, nurses need to understand the key ethical principles outlined in Table 3.1. Without basic knowledge of ethical principles, nurses may be unaware of ethical dilemmas and how to handle them when they occur.

Before nurses can address ethical dilemmas, they need to have confidence in their nursing knowledge and clinical decision-making skills. They also need to have refined communication skills to collect information about the relevant events and share professional nursing ideas to manage the ethically charged situation. As nurses gain experience in handling ethical issues, their confidence in their ability to manage them increases. Confident nurses have the courage to tackle ethical issues as they arise in clinical practice.

Take Note!
Knowledge, confidence, and courage are the foundations of ethical competence.

MAJOR CONTEXTUAL ELEMENTS AFFECTING NURSING PRACTICE

To understand the moral and ethical dimension of nursing more fully, the nurse needs to understand the contextual elements of nursing practice that either reinforce or challenge belief and value systems. As noted at the outset of this chapter, contextualism refers to the constellation of all factors that impact any given situation. In contextualism, the nurse analyzes a whole situation, including its background, environmental and personality factors, and relationships. Box 3.6, Professional Building Blocks, "Five Major Contextual Elements Affecting Professional Nursing Practice," presents select demographic, economic, cultural, environmental, and ethical factors that characterize the contexts of nursing practice. Public policy, another significant contextual element, is discussed in Chapter 19, "The Professional Nurse's Role in Public Policy."

The following discussion offers a general overview of the factors most influential to professional nursing practice.

Demographics

Americans are growing older and living longer. By 2040, approximately 80.1 million Americans will be 65 years of age or older, an increase of approximately 24 million persons since 2010 (U.S. Census Bureau, 2020). In 2030, the life expectancy for American men and women will be 79.5 and 83.3 years, respectively (Imperial College London, 2017). By 2030, the percentage of older adults will also increase in Europe, Asia, and Latin America (He et al., 2016). Older adults use more health care resources and have different care needs than younger people. Nurses need to consider the specific needs of older clients when providing care to them.

The increased older population may strain current health care resources because this age group is at increased risk for chronic illness. Individuals older than 65 have higher rates of hospital admittance and may have greater need for assistance with activities of daily living. Many people over age 65 have chronic illnesses, more than half of which involve some mobility limitations; 32% experience problems performing complex activities (National Center for Health Statistics, 2019). Many of these individuals rely on family or friends so they can remain in their own homes.

However, not all older individuals can safely remain at home and need to live in residential facilities. Throughout much of the COVID-19 pandemic, clusters of cases occurred in long-term care facilities. Because of age-related reductions in immune function, the rate of hospitalization for individuals aged 65 to 74 was five times higher, 75 to 84 eight times higher, 85 years and older 13 times higher, putting a strain on the U.S. health care system (Centers for Disease Control and Prevention, 2020). Some older adult clients were able to recover from the virus without hospitalization.

3.6 Professional Building Blocks

Five Major Contextual Elements Affecting Professional Nursing Practice

- **Demographic elements** reflect social and economic conditions. The demographics of a population influence the opportunities an individual has to form or maintain cooperative and interdependent relationships with fellow humans.

- **Cultural elements** provide organization and structure for groups of people. Within a culture, people share common values, beliefs, norms, and practices (Giger & Davidhizar, 1999). Culture plays a key role in the development of human behavior patterns. Sometimes cultural beliefs clash with science-based health care practices.

- **Economic elements** focus primarily on the considerations of costs and return for provided services. In cultures in which health services are viewed as commodities, providers must be reimbursed for their services. However, when societies view health care as a basic right, governments usually provide a national health insurance plan for all citizens.

- **Environmental elements** consist of global health influences. Along with safe food sources, humans require clean air and water for survival. Kleffel (1996) presents an ecocentric view of the world by describing that "the environment is considered to be whole, living, and interconnected" (p. 1).

- **Ethical elements** encompass the moral obligations and duties that emerge from an individual's struggle with good and bad, right and wrong. Ethical nurses act in accordance with approved standards or codes for professional behavior. Nurses confront ethical issues in daily practice. Ethical dilemmas occur when nurses confront situations in which alternatives for action produce unsatisfactory results. Sometimes, what is ethically right can be legally or morally wrong.

However, many died from the virus. In the United States, 80% of the COVID-19 deaths were among individuals 65 years and older (Freed et al., 2020).

The nursing shortage in the United States is a reflection of the worldwide professional nursing shortage. According to the *Occupational Outlook Handbook* published by the U.S. Bureau of Labor Statistics (USBLS, 2020), an additional 221,900 nurses will be needed to meet the health care needs of the aging U.S. population. Increased numbers of older clients, higher prevalence of chronic diseases, and more retiring nurses are fueling the shortage (USBLS, 2020). Overworked nurses and a lack of proper personal protective equipment during the COVID-19 pandemic may also result in nurses who once worked in acute care settings to seek employment outside of hospitals or to leave the profession entirely.

Perhaps the most important health care need for the American population is health promotion and disease prevention services. *Healthy People 2030* is the fifth version of the framework of health promotion goals for Americans established by the U.S. Department of Health and Human Services (USDHHS), and it is based upon all evidence and information gathered over the past 40 years (USDHHS, 2020). The vision of Healthy People is to create "a society in which all people can achieve their full potential for health and well-being across the lifespan" (USDHHS, 2020, para. 3). The program's mission is "To promote, strengthen, and evaluate the nation's efforts to improve the health and well-being of all people" (USDHHS, 2020, para. 4). In it, 355 measurable objectives are identified to attain progress to improved health and well-being of Americans. It includes five overarching goals:

1. Attainment of "healthy, thriving lives and well-being free of preventable disease, disability, injuries, and premature death"
2. Elimination of health disparities to "achieve health equity and attain health literacy to improve the health and well-being of all"
3. Creation of "social, physical, and economic environments that promote" the attainment of the "full potential for health and well-being for all"
4. Promotion of "healthy development, healthy behaviors, and well-being across all life stages"
5. Engagement of "leadership, key constituents, and the public across multiple sectors to take action to design policies that improve the health and well-being of all" (USDHHS, 2020, para. 6)

Keeping people healthy reduces long-term health expenditures and increases the quality of life for people of all ages. Nurses play a key role in imparting health information to clients when they assume client education responsibilities. As the population ages, many middle-aged adults find themselves torn between meeting career obligations, raising teenagers, and caring for aging parents. In the role of counselor, professional nurses can support clients (and their families) by inquiring about the stresses associated with fulfilling multiple role responsibilities, thus strengthening client mental health.

Culture

The U.S. population is diverse and will continue to become more so (Fig. 3.2). The 2019 population estimates revealed 57 possible racial combinations of American citizens; approximately 77% of Americans reported that they were of one race. Individuals completing census forms sometimes responded positively to more than one category, making data analysis difficult. The increasing diversity among Americans increases the complexity of providing effective nursing care. Although the heritage profile among nurses is also diverse, it does not mirror that of the overall population (see Fig. 3.2).

Many immigrant groups tend to settle within specific communities. In such locations, nurses may need to communicate with clients who are not fluent in English. Nurses need to be aware of culturally diverse population clusters and the usual health practices of these groups to provide effective nursing care. Meeting the health care demands of a culturally diverse population means that nurses need to understand the biophysiologic variations related to the risk for specific health problems, development, and medication metabolism, along with specific cultural values, beliefs, and health practices (see Chapter 11, "Multicultural Issues in Professional Practice").

Economics

The economic gap between the wealthy and the poor in the United States continues to expand. Factors associated with increased poverty levels include age, ethnicity, and education. In 2018, the USDHHS reported that 63.17 million Americans, or 11.88% of the population, lived in poverty (20.82% Black/African Americans, 17% Hispanic Americans, 10.10% Asian Americans, and 81% White/non-Hispanic Americans; no data were reported for Hawaiian/Pacific Islanders or Native Americans). The poverty guidelines determined by the Office of Management and Budget set the following poverty guidelines: an annual income

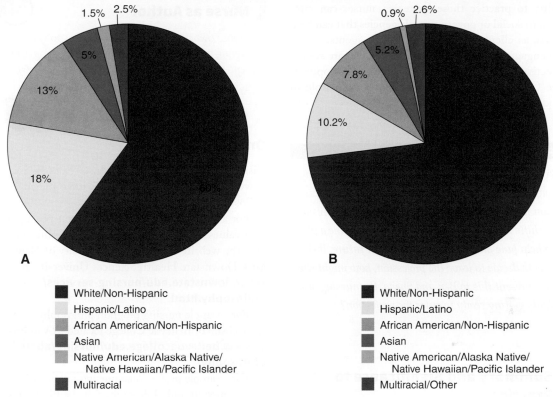

FIGURE 3.2 **A.** Heritage profile of the U.S. population in 2019. **B.** Heritage profile of U.S. nurses in 2018. (*Sources:* U.S. Census Bureau. (2019). *Quick Facts: Population estimates July 1, 2019*. https://www.census.gov/quickfacts/fact/table/US/PST045219; U.S. Department of Health and Human Services, Health Resources and Services Administration, & National Center for Health Workforce Analysis. (2019). *Brief summary results from the 2018 National Sample Survey of Registered Nurses*. HRSA Health Workforce.)

of $56,613 for a family of nine; $46,231 for a family of eight; $41,336 for a family of seven; $35,925 for a family of six; $31,234 for a family of five; $25,000 for a family of four; $19,642 for a family of three; $16,815 for two people under age 65; $15,178 for two people aged 65 years or older; $13,064 for a single person under age 65; and $12,043 for a single person aged 65 or older (Semega et al., 2020). Individuals living in poverty had a 16.9% rate of not carrying health insurance. In 2018, the uninsured rate for Americans was 8.5%, a 0.6% increase from 2017 (Berchick et al., 2019). Individuals with health care insurance have improved access to health care services compared with those without it.

Health care spending is expected to increase. In 2017, health care expenditures accounted for 17.9% of the gross domestic product (National Center for Health Statistics, 2018). Employers providing health care insurance to employees have seen 22% increases in premiums over the past 5 years. Employer costs for individual health insurance depend upon the type of plan and the number of individuals covered. In 2018, the cost of an average family plan was $20,576, and the cost for a single-person plan was $7,188 (Kaiser Family Foundation, 2019). Employers have in turn passed the increases on to the employees. When health care insurance premiums become too expensive, employees may opt out of employer-provided insurance plans and instead choose high-deductible, less expensive plans. This results in a state of being underinsured, placing these individuals at risk for bankruptcy because of debt incurred for health-related reasons despite being insured.

Uninsured Americans have limited access to health care. Personal health-promoting habits require that individuals know what lifestyle behaviors promote health and that they have the resources to obtain them. People without health insurance may use free clinics and public health departments for primary health care services. In these settings, advanced practice nurses frequently assume the role of primary health provider. Other clients may prefer a more holistic approach to health care, seeking out nurses rather than physicians for primary care services. As educators, professional nurses can teach clients health promotion strategies. For clients who do not have the ability to practice these strategies, nurses can refer them to social or governmental agencies that can help (nurse as client advocate). As change agents, nurses can engage in efforts to change the health care system by actively participating in public policy development (see Chapter 19, "The Professional Nurse's Role in Public Policy").

REAL-LIFE REFLECTIONS

After reading this chapter, you find yourself talking with Jane. How would you help Jane with her decision making about leaving the profession as a result of shifts in the focus of nursing care? Outline a plan to help Jane make a decision about her future. If she was to decide to leave the profession, how might she best present this to Ben and Sheila, the nursing students getting ready to enter the profession?

Summary and Significance to Practice

Professional nursing centers on caring for others. When delivering care to individuals, groups, and communities, nurses use individual value systems as a basis for some clinical decisions. Many contextual elements affect health care delivery and clinical practice. Sometimes the contextual elements create ethical dilemmas that need to be resolved. Nurses who have examined their beliefs and have developed a personal nursing philosophy have a basis for finding meaning in professional practice. By becoming cognizant of ethical principles and the multiple factors contributing to ethical dilemmas in clinical practice, nurses can readily identify them as they arise. Nurses who have a strong value system and philosophical stance are armed with effective tools to confront ethically charged situations with confidence.

From Theory to Practice

1. What does it mean to be a professional nurse?
2. How do nurses make a difference in the lives of others?
3. Look at your nursing program's philosophy and/or the developmental and organizational philosophies at your place of employment. Compare these with your own personal philosophy and outline key similarities and differences.

Nurse as Author

Write your own professional nursing philosophy by answering the questions found in Box 3.3, Learning, Knowing, and Growing, "Developing a Nursing Philosophy."

Your Digital Classroom

Online Exploration

Visit the International Philosophy of Nursing Society at www.ipons.online to learn more about nursing philosophy and philosophical inquiry.

For a sample nursing department purpose, policy, core values, theoretical framework, and philosophy, visit the website of the State University of New York Downstate Health Sciences University at **www.downstate.edu/nursing-services/ philosophy.html**

For a sample nursing program philosophy, visit the website of Bellevue College located in Virginia at **www.bellevuecollege.edu/nursing/about/ philosophy/**

For a sample professional nursing organization vision, mission, and philosophy, visit the Philippine Nurses Association of San Diego County, California, at **https://pnasandiego.wildapricot.org/About-Us**

Expanding Your Understanding

1. Search the internet for any college- or university-based nursing program and see if it has the philosophy of its school of nursing posted on the home page.
2. Select a nursing organization that interests you and visit its website to see whether you can find the organization's values, mission, and philosophy. Based on a review of available information, outline reasons why you might or might not join the organization.

Beyond the Book

Visit thePoint® at **www.thePoint.lww.com** for activities and information to reinforce the concepts and content covered in this chapter.

REFERENCES

American Association of Colleges of Nursing (2021). The essentials: Core competencies for professional nursing education. February 18, 2021. Retrieved March 21, 2021 from https://www.aacnnursing.org/Portals/42/AcademicNursing /pdf/Essentials-Final-Draft-2-18-21.pdf?ver=hNeCl7O jgamIA9sHgDi_Yw%3D%3D&timestamp=1613742420447

Antonovsky, A. (1987). *Unraveling the mystery of health.* Jossey-Bass.

Aroskar, M. A. (1987). Fidelity and veracity: Questions of promise keeping, truth telling, and loyalty. In M. D. M. Fowler & J. Levine-Ariff (Eds.), *Ethics at the bedside: A source-book for the critical care nurse*. Lippincott Williams & Wilkins.

Bandman, E. L., & Bandman, B. (1995). *Nursing ethics through the lifespan* (3rd ed.). Appleton & Lange.

Beauchamp, T., & Childress, J. (2013). *Principles of biomedical ethics* (7th ed.). Oxford University Press.

Benner, P. (2000). *From novice to expert: Excellence and power in clinical nursing practice* (Commemorative ed.). Addison-Wesley.

Benner, P., & Wrubel, J. (1989). *The primacy of caring: Stress and coping in health and illness*. Addison-Wesley.

Berchick, E. R., Barnett, J. C., & Upton, R. D. (2019). *Health insurance coverage in the United States: 2018*. U.S. Census Bureau, Current Population Reports, P60-267(RV). U.S. Government Printing Office. https://www.census.gov/library/publications/2019/demo/p60-267.html

Blaszko-Helming, M., Shields, D., Avino, K., & Rosa, W. (2022). *Dossey and Keegan's holistic nursing: A handbok for practice*. Jones & Bartlett Learning.

Burkhardt, M. L. (2016). Holistic ethics. In B. M. Dossey, L. Keegan, C. C. Barrere, M. B. Helming, D. A. Shields, & K. Avino (Eds.), *Holistic nursing: A handbook for practice* (7th ed., pp. 121–134). Jones & Bartlett Learning.

Carper, B. A. (1978). Fundamental patterns of knowing in nursing. *Advances in Nursing Science, 1*, 13–23. https://doi.org/10.1097/00012272-197810000-00004

Centers for Disease Control and Prevention. (2020). *COVID-19 hospitalization and death by age*. https://www.cdc.gov/coronavirus/2019-ncov/covid-data/investigations-discovery/hospitalization-death-by-age.html

Enserink, P. M. (2004). Influenza: Girding for disaster. Looking the pandemic in the eye. *Science, 306*, 392–394. https://doi.org/10.1126/science.306.5695.392

Ferreira, V., & Sherman, A. (2007). The relationship of optimism, pain and social support to well-being in older adults with osteoarthritis. *Aging and Mental Health, 11*(1), 89–98. https://doi.org/10.1080/13607860600736166

Fitzpatrick, J., & McCarthy, G. (2016). *Nursing concept analysis: Application to research and practice*. Springer Publishing Co. LLC.

Flynn, P. A. R. (1987). Questions of risk, duty, and paternalism: Problems in beneficence. In M. D. M. Fowler & J. Levine-Ariff (Eds.), *Ethics at the bedside: A source-book for the critical care nurse*. Lippincott Williams & Wilkins.

Fowler, M. D. M. (2015). *Guide to the code of ethics for nurses with interpretive statements* (2nd ed.). American Nurses Association.

Fowler, M. D. M., & Levine-Ariff, J. (Eds.). (1987). *Ethics at the bedside: A source-book for the critical care nurse*. Lippincott Williams & Wilkins.

Frankl, V. (1963). *Man's search for meaning*. Washington Square Press.

Freed, M., Cubanski, J., Neuman, T., Kates, J., & Michaud, J. (2020). *What share of people who have died of COVID-19 are 65 and older and how does it vary from state to state?* https://www.kff.org/coronavirus-covid-19/issue-brief/what-share-of-people-who-have-died-of-covid-19-are-65-and-older-and-how-does-it-vary-by-state/

Giger, J. N., & Davidhizar, R. E. (1999). *Transcultural nursing assessment and intervention* (3rd ed.). Mosby.

Gilligan, C. (1982). *In a different voice: Psychological theory and women's development*. Harvard University Press.

Haegert, S. (2004). The ethics of self. *Nursing Ethics, 11*, 434–443. https://doi.org/10.1191/0969733004ne722oa

Hatala, A. R. (2008). Spirituality and aboriginal mental health: An examination of the relationship between aboriginal spirituality and mental health. *Advances in Mind-Body Medicine, 23*(1), 6–12. https://www.researchgate.net/publication/45389091_Spirituality_and_Aboriginal_Mental_Health

Hawking, S. (2002). *The theory of everything*. New Millennium Press.

He, W., Goodkind, D., & Kowal P. (2016). *An aging world: 2015*. U.S. Census Bureau, International Population Reports, P95/16-1. U.S. Government Publishing Office. https://www.census.gov/library/publications/2016/demo/P95-16-1.html

Herzlinger, R. (2004). *Consumer-driven health care*. Jossey-Bass.

Hountras, S. (2015). What guides your nursing practice? *Journal of Christian Nursing, 32*(3), 179–181. https://doi.org/10.1097/CNJ00000000000181

Ibanga, F. D. A. (2016). Logical and theoretical foundations of African environmental ethics. *Africology: The Journal of Pan African Studies, 9*(9), 3–24. https://www.researchgate.net/publication/311228436_Logical_and_Theoretical_Foundations_of_African_Environmental_Ethics

Imperial College London. (2017). *Average life expectancy set to increase by 2030*. ScienceDaily. Retrieved March 20, 2021, from www.sciencedaily.com/releases/2017/02/170221222528.htm

Institute of Medicine. (2000). *To err is human: Building a safer health care system*. National Academies Press.

Institute of Medicine. (2010). *The future of nursing: Leading change, advancing health*. National Academies Press.

Iwarrsson, S., Horstmann, V., & Slaug, B. (2007). Housing matters in very old age—Yet differently due to ADL dependence level differences. *Scandinavian Journal of Occupational Therapy, 14*, 3–15. https://doi.org/10.1080/11038120601094732

Kaiser Family Foundation. (2019). *2019 Employer health benefits survey*. https://www.kff.org/report-section/ehbs-2019-section-1-cost-of-health-insurance/

Kleffel, D. (1996). Environmental paradigms: Moving toward an ecocentric approach. *Advances in Nursing Science, 18*, 1–10. https://doi.org/10.1097/00012272-199606000-00004

Kohlberg, L. (1981). *The philosophy of moral development: Moral stages and the idea of justice*. Harper & Row.

Lewis, S. (2008a). Helping people live between office visits: An interview with Bernie Siegel, MD. *Advances in Mind-Body Medicine, 23*, 24–27. https://pubmed.ncbi.nlm.nih.gov/20664138/

Lewis, S. (2008b). The emerging field of spiritual neuroscience: An interview with Mario Beauregard, PhD. *Advances in Mind-Body Medicine, 23*, 20–23. https://pubmed.ncbi.nlm.nih.gov/20664137/

Malloy, D. C., Fahey-McCarthy, E., Murakami, M., Lee, Y., Choi, E., Hirose, E., & Hadjistavropoulos, T. (2015). Finding meaning in the work of nursing: An international study. *Online Journal of Issues in Nursing, 20*(3), 1. https://doi.org/10.3912/OJIN.Vol20No03PPT02

Manomi, D. J. (2019). Towards an African-Biblical virtue ethics: Reflection on the letter to Titus through a progressive-negotiated-ethics. *Acta Theologica, 39*(2), 114–129 https://doi.org/10.18820/23099089/actat.v39i2.7

Marchuk, A. (2014). A personal nursing philosophy in practice. *Journal of Neonatal Nursing, 20*, 266–273. https://doi.org/10.1061/jnn.2014.06.004

McCarthy, J. (2006). A pluralist view of nursing ethics. *Nursing Philosophy, 7*, 157–164. https://doi.org/10.1111/j.1466-769X.2006.00272.x

Mish, F. C. (Ed.). (2020). *Merriam-Webster's Collegiate Dictionary* (11th ed.). Merriam-Webster, Inc.

Munhall, P. (1988). Ethical considerations in qualitative research. *Western Journal of Nursing Research, 10*, 150–162. https://doi.org/10.1177/019394598801000204

National Center for Health Statistics. (2018). *Fast Stats: Health expenditure.* https://www.cdc.gov/nchs/fastats/health-expenditures.htm

National Center for Health Statistics. (2019). *Data table for Figure 12. Functional limitation among adults aged 18 and over, by age and level of difficulty: United States, 2010–2017.* https://www.cdc.gov/nchs/data/hus/2018/fig12.pdf

Noddings, N. (1984). *Caring: A feminine approach to ethics and moral education.* University of California Press.

O'Neill, J. (1995). Ethical decision making and the role of nursing. In G. L. Deloughery (Ed.), *Issues and trends in nursing* (2nd ed.). Mosby-Year Book.

Peter, E., Lunardi, V., & McFarlane, A. (2004). Nursing resistance as ethical action: Literature review. *Journal of Advanced Nursing, 46*, 403–416. https://doi.org/10.1111/j.1365-2648.2004.03008.x

Porter-O'Grady, T., & Malloch, K. (2015). *Quantum leadership: Building better partnerships for sustainable health* (2nd ed.). Jones & Bartlett Learning.

Rafael, A. R. (1996). Power and caring: A dialectic in nursing. *Advances in Nursing Science, 19*, 3–17. https://doi.org/10.1097/00012272-199609000-00003

Rew, L. (1994). Commentary. In J. F. Kikuchi & H. Simmons (Eds.), *Developing a philosophy of nursing.* Sage.

Rich, K. L. (2020). Introduction to ethics. In J. B. Buts & K. L. Rich (Eds.), *Nursing ethics across the curriculum and into practice* (5th ed.). Jones & Bartlett Learning.

Rosen, G., Byrne, A., Cohen, J., Harman, E., & Shiffrin, S. (2018). *The Norton introduction to philosophy* (2nd ed.). W. W. Norton & Co.

Salsberry, P. J. (1994). A philosophy of nursing: What is it? What is it not? In J. F. Kikuchi & H. Simmons (Eds.), *Developing a philosophy of nursing.* Sage.

Semega, J., Kollar, M., Creamer, J., & Mohanty, A. (2020). *Income and poverty in the United States: 2018.* U.S. Census Bureau, Current Population Reports, P60-266(RV). U.S. Government Printing Office. https://www.census.gov/library/publications/2019/demo/p60-266.html

Streubert, H. (1994). Male nursing students' perceptions of clinical experience. *Nurse Educator, 19*, 28–32. https://doi.org/10.1097/00006223-199409000-00018

Sulmasy, D. (2008). Dignity and bioethics: History, theory and selected applications. In *Human dignity and bioethics: Essays commissioned by the President's Council on Bioethics* (pp. 469–504). U.S. Government Printing Office. https://repository.library.georgetown.edu/bitstream/handle/10822/559351/human_dignity_and_bioethics.pdf?sequence=1&isAllowed=y

United Nations. (2020a). *Sustainable development goals: About the sustainable development goals.* https://www.un.org/sustainabledevelopment/sustainable-development-goals/

United Nations. (2020b). *Goal 1: No poverty.* http://www.undp.org/content/undp/en/home/sustainable-development-goals/goal-1-no-poverty.html

United Nations. (2020c). *Goal 2: Zero hunger.* https://www.un.org/sustainabledevelopment/hunger/

United Nations. (2020d). *Goal 3: Good health and well-being.* https://www.un.org/sustainabledevelopment/health/

United Nations. (2020e). *Goal 4: Quality education.* https://www.un.org/sustainabledevelopment/education/

United Nations. (2020f). *Goal 5: Gender equality.* https://www.un.org/sustainabledevelopment/gender-equality/

United Nations. (2020g). *Goal 6: Clean water and sanitation.* https://www.un.org/sustainabledevelopment/water-and-sanitation/

United Nations. (2020h). *Goal 7: Affordable and clean energy.* https://www.un.org/sustainabledevelopment/energy/

United Nations. (2020i). *Goal 8: Decent work and economic growth.* https://www.un.org/sustainabledevelopment/economic-growth/

United Nations. (2020j). *Goal 9: Industry, innovation and infrastructure.* https://www.un.org/sustainabledevelopment/infrastructure-industrialization/

United Nations. (2020k). *Goal 10: Reduced inequalities.* https://www.un.org/sustainabledevelopment/inequality/

United Nations. (2020l). *Goal 11: Sustainable cities and communities.* https://www.un.org/sustainabledevelopment/cities/

United Nations. (2020m). *Goal 12: Responsible consumption and production.* https://www.un.org/sustainabledevelopment/sustainable-consumption-production/

United Nations. (2020n). *Goal 13: Climate action.* https://www.un.org/sustainabledevelopment/climate-change/

United Nations. (2020o). *Goal 14: Life below water.* https://www.un.org/sustainabledevelopment/oceans/

United Nations. (2020p). *Goal 15: Life on land.* https://www.un.org/sustainabledevelopment/biodiversity/

United Nations. (2020q). *Goal 16: Peace and justice, strong institutions.* https://www.un.org/sustainabledevelopment/peace-justice/

United Nations. (2020r). *Goal 17: Partnerships for the goals.* https://www.un.org/sustainabledevelopment/globalpartnerships/

United Nations Development Programme. (2021). About us. Overview. Looking to the future. Retrieved March 20, 2021, from https://www.undp.org/content/undp/en/home/about-us.html

United States Bureau of Labor Statistics. (2020). *Occupational outlook handbook.* Health Care, Registered Nurses. https://www.bls.gov/ooh/healthcare/registered-nurses.htm

U.S. Census Bureau. (2019). *Quick Facts: Population estimates July 1, 2019.* https://www.census.gov/quickfacts/fact/table/US/PST045219

U.S. Census Bureau. (2020). *2017 National Populations Projection Tables: Main series.* https://www.census.gov/data/tables/2017/demo/popproj/2017-summary-tables.html

U.S. Department of Health and Human Services. (2020). *Healthy People 2030 framework.* https://health.gov/healthypeople/about/healthy-people-2030-framework

Wareham, C. S. (2017). A duty to explore African ethics? *Ethical Theory Moral Practice, 20*, 857–872. https://doi.org/10.1007/s10677-017-9826-x

Watson, J. (1988). A case study: Curriculum in transition. In National League for Nursing (Ed.), *Curriculum revolution: Mandate for change.* Author.

Watson, J. (2012). *Human caring science, a theory of nursing* (2nd ed.). Jones & Bartlett Learning.

World Health Organization. (2019). *WHO Annual Report 2018. WHO's work in emergencies: prepare, prevent, detect and respond.* Author. https://apps.who.int/iris/handle/10665/312267

World Health Organization. (2020). *Noncommunicable diseases progress monitor 2020.* Author. https://apps.who.int/iris/handle/10665/330805

Establishing Helping and Healing Relationships

LEARNING OUTCOMES

By the end of this chapter, the learner will be able to:

1. Specify the importance of communication in professional nursing.
2. Outline the major purposes of communication.
3. Discuss principles to establish helpfulness in nurse–client communication.
4. Outline the stages of nurse–client relationship development.
5. Identify the mutuality in helping relationships.
6. Differentiate therapeutic from nontherapeutic communication strategies and relationships.
7. Discuss how nurses use relationships to promote client healing.
8. Explain how health care team members can develop meaningful professional partnerships.
9. Describe strategies that health care team members can use to enhance quality and safety when delivering health care.

REAL-LIFE REFLECTIONS

Marcia, an emergency department nurse, has just arrived at work and is assigned to be the triage nurse. A Latino middle-aged man with severe chest pain and dyspnea arrives with his family. Marcia gets immediate help for the man, who is rushed to the cardiac catheterization lab. Marcia notices that the family members seem anxious and distressed. When she asks them if they would like anything, they reply, "No," but the wife tries to hold back tears as she wrings her hands, the daughter's hands shake, and the son paces. Marcia notes that the nonverbal behavior of the family seems to be incongruent with their verbal messages. As she interacts with the family, Marcia wonders what would be the best course of action to help this distressed family.

Most nurses enter the profession with a desire to help others, and they do so in many ways:

- Assisting clients in meeting basic physical, psychological, and spiritual needs
- Alleviating pain and suffering

- Imparting health care information
- Doing things for clients that they are incapable of doing for themselves
- Guiding clients and families through the complex health care delivery system

91

- Advocating for clients
- Helping clients achieve maximal health potentials
- Keeping clients safe
- Using clinical, cognitive, and communication skills to deliver high-quality health care services

Along with helping clients, families, and communities, professional nurses also help each other and other team members. **Communication**—the sharing of information, thoughts, and feelings—is an essential element of helping others. The verbal and nonverbal messages exchanged during human relationships determine the structure and function of interpersonal relationships. This chapter focuses on communication as a key factor for effective nursing practice and an essential element of helping relationships.

COMMUNICATION AS INTERACTION

Nurses establish relationships with clients, each other, and members of the health care team. To participate effectively in all these relationships, nurses must understand the structure and the functions of communication.

The Interpersonal Component of Professional Nursing

In striving to maximize the client's potential for optimal health, nurses must clearly understand the power of communication in shaping professional relationships. Without well-refined communication skills, nurses cannot establish therapeutic relationships with clients. **Helping relationships** are those in which nurses communicate with clients to assist them in attaining optimal health or to support them through difficult situations. The quality of communication between the nurse and the client is an essential determinant of the success of the helping relationship (Fig. 4.1).

Take Note!

Communication is an essential element of helping others. Mutual goals cannot be defined or achieved without effective communication.

People influence each other. This reciprocal process suggests that the most important human attributes are not only openness to interpersonal experiences but also power to influence oneself and others. Nurses may be perceived as having power over the individuals they serve because of their specialized knowledge of and skills in health care. In order to maintain a therapeutic

FIGURE 4.1 Careful use of humor enhances the nurse–client relationship.

relationship, there needs to be professional boundaries. **Professional boundaries** are imaginary lines that separate the nurse from the client to maintain the integrity of the therapeutic relationship. Clients possess vulnerability when receiving professional nursing services. Boundary crossings are brief incursions across the invisible barriers. They occur when the nurses use clients for personal gain or when there is confusion about the nature of the special therapeutic relationship either on the nurse's or the client's part. Some examples of boundary crossing are overinvolvement, excessive personal disclosure on the nurse's part, secretive behavior, providing "special treatment" to a single client, flirtatious actions, and even sexual misconduct. Nurses must be alert to warning signs of potential and actual boundary violations. Careless use of social media increases the likelihood of boundary encroachment. When nurses engage in self-reflection to evaluate client interactions, they might become more self-aware of the effectiveness of their communication to optimize the nurse–client relationship (National Council of State Boards of Nursing, 2018).

Humans influence one another primarily through communication, which can be defined as the "exchange of meanings between and among individuals through a shared system of symbols that have the same meaning for both the sender and the receiver of the message" (Vestal, 1995, p. 51). Through communication during nurse–client interactions, the nurse hopes to enable the client to acknowledge the importance of and live a healthier lifestyle. This goal can be achieved only if the nurse is knowledgeable about the content and process of the nurse–client relationship. To understand content in nursing situations, the nurse must have knowledge of each client as a complex adaptive human system that strives for "a higher degree of harmony that fosters self-knowledge, self-reverence, self-caring, self-control, and self-healing processes" (Watson, 2012, p. 61).

Nursing has not always been successful in establishing its desired image of autonomy, cohesiveness, and professionalism. Disagreement among nursing theorists, practitioners, and educators about the purpose and meaning of nursing and key concepts such as nursing diagnosis has led to multiple, sometimes conflicting images of nursing. Nurses today generally agree that contemporary nursing practice approaches the client holistically to address the full range of human responses and illness. Nurses also agree that assessment of objective and subjective factors related to client health is essential. They concur that scientific, intuitive, experiential, or mystical evidence may be used to guide practice. However, most nurses in practice acknowledge that establishing authentic, caring relationships with clients is essential to promote health and healing.

Nursing's unique service to society consists of dealing with human responses in health and illness. These responses are the substance of communication. Thus, purposeful communication is an essential dimension in the establishment of effective nurse–client relationships, which should be "characterized by compassion, continuity, and respect for the client's choice. The focus is on the process: the process of the client–environment interaction and the process of the nurse–client relationship" (Newman et al., 1991, p. 406).

The Structure of Communication

Not only does human communication convey information and influence others, but "communication is the relationship" (Sundeen et al., 1998, p. 94). It is the dynamic interaction between two or more people in which ideas, goals, beliefs and values, feelings, and feelings about feelings are exchanged. Even brief communication exchanges may change all involved parties.

Communication is defined only in the context of process. Holistic communication is "a free flow of verbal and nonverbal interchange between and among people and significant beings such as pets, nature, and God/Life Force/Absolute/Transcendent, that explores meaning and ideas leading to mutual understanding and growth" (Mariano, 2016, p. 54). Each person is always affected by others and is always affecting others. As one constantly communicates, changes occur in the self, others, and perhaps the environment.

Although communication is a dynamic process, it is possible to identify components and to analyze the interrelationships among the components. Berlo (1960) traced the various models of communication from the time of Aristotle (circa 350 BCE) to the 1960s. Aristotle identified the related components as the speaker, the speech, and the audience. After analyzing behavioral science research and several points of view, Berlo (1960, pp. 30–32) formed a communication model that is generally accepted today:

1. A (interpersonal) source: Some individuals with ideas, needs, intentions, information, and a reason for communicating
2. A message: A coded, systematic set of symbols representing ideas, purposes, intentions, and feelings
3. An encoder: The mechanism for expressing or translating the purpose of the communication into the message (in people, these are the motor mechanisms—the vocal mechanism for oral messages, the muscles of the hands for written messages, and the muscle systems elsewhere in the body for gestures)
4. A channel: The medium for carrying the message
5. A decoder: The mechanism for translating the message into a form that the recipient can use (in people, the sensory receptor mechanisms)
6. A receiver: The target or recipient of the message.

In this model, the transmission of meaning occurs via a dynamic transactional process in which:

1. A person has an intention or purpose (the communication source).
2. The purpose is translated into a communicable form by the person's set of motor mechanisms and skills (encoder).
3. The message is transmitted through a channel.
4. The message is translated into receivable form by the recipient's sensory mechanisms and skills (decoder).
5. The recipient receives the message (the communication receiver).

Since Berlo's model was developed, systems theorists have further explained the reciprocal relationship between participants in the communication process. At any given time, the individual person is both an active initiator and a recipient of meanings in an interpersonal situation. Thus, it is important for nurses to understand that they are simultaneously acting and reacting when working with clients and that clients' meanings have an equal effect on the outcome of purposeful relationships.

The dynamic nature of the communication process requires nurses to evaluate their actions and reactions when working with clients. Without such awareness and evaluation, the professional will be less likely to experience the feeling of satisfaction associated with transmitting clear meanings and the validation that the message intended was the message received.

Take Note!
Validation of meanings is essential to achieving any therapeutic goals in helping relationships.

Functions and Types of Communication

Synthesizing from several communication models, Ceccio and Ceccio (1982) proposed four major purposes of communication: to inquire, to inform, to persuade, and to entertain. The nurses may attempt to achieve any of these purposes with clients, the health care delivery system, peers, other health care team members, and even themselves. In attempts to achieve one or more of these purposes, the nurse transmits messages.

Messages may be transmitted verbally and nonverbally. Implicit in all models of communication is the concept that communication has two interacting components: the content value of the message and the interactional or perceptual value of the message and its participants. The content value of the message, or its informational aspect, is expressed in verbal or nonverbal forms. The interactional or perceptual value of the message (referred to as metacommunication) identifies how participants interpret content and how they perceive the interpersonal relationship. Metacommunication may be expressed in verbal and nonverbal forms.

Verbal Communication

Verbal communication consists of the spoken word and requires functional, physiologic, and cognitive mechanisms that produce, recognize, and receive speech. Although a major influence, specific words are not the *greatest* influences on communication. Language comprises an elaborate system of symbols. Words symbolize actual objects or concepts. Lack of congruence in language between the nurse and the client usually interferes with initiating relationships and creates obstacles to validation of meanings—the essential characteristic of an effective message.

Two primary influences on verbal communications are developmental age and cultural heritage. Developmental age affects verbal ability (the person's physiologic ability to change sounds into words) and cognitive ability (to symbolize through language) (see Box 4.1, Professional Building Blocks, "Potential Problems in Communication"). Through the process of acculturation, an individual develops culture-based variations from others in defining meanings for words. Although denotative (i.e., explicit) definitions of words

4.1 Professional Building Blocks

Potential Problems in Communication

Nurses need to be aware of three possible types of problems associated with words being symbols of communication (Ceccio & Ceccio, 1982):

1. The technical problem: How accurately can one transmit the symbols of communication?
2. The semantic problem: How precise are the symbols in transmitting the intended message?
3. The influential problem: How effectively does the received meaning affect conduct?

are the same among different persons, connotative (i.e., associated) meanings often vary because of cultural difference, acculturation, and past experiences.

The verbal content of communication generates the content theme during the communication process. If one evaluates the seemingly varied topics of discussion, the words that underlie or link together several ideas will reflect the "what" (or content) of the communication.

Nonverbal Communication

Nonverbal communication usually exerts more influence on communication than does verbal communication. Hunsaker and Alessandra (1980) suggest that 90% of meaning comes from nonverbal communication. **Nonverbal communication** consists of all forms of communication that do not involve the spoken or written word. Perception of nonverbal communication involves all the senses, including hearing, that are used for the perception of verbal communication. Kinesics (facial expressions, gaze, gestures, and all body movements that are not specific signs), objects (all intentional and unintentional display of material things), and proxemics (the use of space) are powerful nonverbal messages perceived by the senses (Hosley & Molle, 2006; Northouse & Northouse, 1998).

Take Note!
Nonverbal communication usually exerts more influence on communication than does verbal communication.

Sundeen et al. (1994, p. 99) identified several purposes of nonverbal communication: expressing emotion and interpersonal attitudes; establishing, developing, and maintaining social relationships; presenting oneself; engaging in rituals; and supporting verbal communication.

The tactile senses represent the most primitive sensory process developed by humans. Bonding between the infant and the parent figure (important to infant development) occurs largely through nonverbal tactile communication. As a child develops into an adult, touch as nonverbal communication takes on specific cultural and personal meanings and remains a powerful communication tool throughout life.

Nurses must understand taboos concerning touch and distance to engage in purposeful communication. For example, a touch on the knee might mean concern to one person but seduction to another. Touch can be a powerful nonverbal tool for the nurse but only when it is used at the proper time and within the context of the client's culture (see Box 4.2, Professional Building Blocks, "Culture and Nonverbal Communication").

All the sensory processes become powerful components of communication throughout life. For example, the olfactory (smell) and gustatory (taste) senses make it possible for people to distinguish pleasant from unpleasant odors and tastes, respectively. Therefore, nurses need to control odors in health care environments.

The sense of hearing the spoken word also has a nonverbal component: interpreting the qualities of the voice. Hunsaker and Alessandra (1980) identified the following voice qualities as strong determinants of effective communication: resonance (the intensity with which the voice fills the environmental space); rhythm (the flow, pace, and movement of the voice); speed (how fast the words are spoken); pitch (the highness or lowness of the voice that relates to the tightening of the vocal cords); volume (loudness); inflection (the change in pitch or volume of voice); and clarity (the articulation and enunciation capacity of the voice).

During communication, people perform various movements of which they may be unaware or have little awareness. Body movements are largely determined through socialization. Developed in a particular psychosocial and cultural setting, motor actions vary by gender, socioeconomic status, age, and ethnic background. Misinterpretations of culturally variable kinesthetic behaviors produce barriers to effective communication. For example, eye motions involved with eye contact communicate culturally specific messages. If the nurse and the client assign different meanings to this nonverbal communication, the effectiveness of the nurse–client relationship may be hampered.

4.2 Professional Building Blocks

Culture and Nonverbal Communication

Culture affects all aspects of nonverbal communication (Hosley & Molle, 2006; Leininger & McFarland, 2006). For example:

- Proximity/spacing: People from various cultures define appropriate personal space differently. For example, compared to individuals of Latino heritage, White Americans prefer more personal space (6 in. to 4 ft). Nurses must acknowledge and respect client preferences for personal space to facilitate effective communication.
- Touching: Any physical contact or touching that is part of an individual's communication style can create problems or discomfort for people from many cultures. Nurses need not abandon hands on a shoulder or arm to show support and caring. Rather, clients should be made to feel empowered to tell the nurse if such touching makes them feel uncomfortable.
- Gestures: People from some cultures may be more animated than others, using hand gestures and body language to communicate. Gestures that have a positive meaning in one culture may be considered insulting and rude in another.
- Eye contact: Traditionally, Americans have valued direct eye contact as a sign of confidence and respect, whereas not making eye contact has negative connotations. However, in many cultures, making eye contact with an authority figure is considered an insult.
- Silence: People from some cultures prefer active verbal interactions and are uncomfortable with silence. Other cultures may value periods of contemplative silence. Cultural characterizations of the meaning of silence may lead to potential misunderstandings of communication style and motivation.
- Body language: The body is one of the more subtle ways people communicate meaning and sincerity. For example, a nurse may say all the right things but communicate tension through their body language.

Kinesics, the meaning of motor actions, and **proxemics**, the function of space in nonverbal communication, also play important roles in all aspects of life. Space is a constant that may be perceived either as surrounding people or existing between them. The nurse can use their awareness of what a client perceives as acceptable use of space and how body position and direction affect the meaning of the relationship to create optimal personal and environmental space to enhance nurse–client relationships.

Metacommunication

Occurring on both verbal and nonverbal levels, **metacommunication** defines the "what," the "who," and the relationship between the "what" and the "who" in the communication process. Because metacommunication is influential in determining the effectiveness of relationships, the nurse must evaluate communication in terms of its context and the relationships among its parts. Understanding themes of the relationship helps the nurse evaluate the metacommunication occurring in the nurse–client interaction.

Three interacting themes occur during metacommunication. The content encompasses the central idea or multiple ideas linked together, that is, the main message being conveyed (the "what"). The mood theme includes the emotions being communicated during the interaction (the "who" and "how"). Finally, the interaction theme involves the dynamics between the participants who are communicating with each other. Metacommunication occurs at all levels of the human experience.

Knowing that change occurs more readily and more effectively if congruence exists between the verbal and nonverbal components of communication, the nurse must be alert to indicators of the degree of agreement on the meaning of the content and on the process of the relationship. When a discrepancy arises between the verbal and nonverbal components, the nonverbal component is usually the more accurate indicator. However, nonverbal behavior is more open to subjective meaning and variations; thus, it must be verbally validated. This validation process plays an important part in effectively using metacommunication in nursing practice.

Take Note!
Communication has both verbal and nonverbal components. When these are not in congruence, the nonverbal components typically dominate the communication.

Interpretation and Perception

The capacity for interpretation makes communication between people possible. When engaged in **interpretation**, people assign meaning to the interpersonal interaction. Interpretation involves perception, symbolization, memory, and thinking. Perhaps the most important of these is perception, the basic component from which the others follow. Taylor (1977) described **perception** as the selection and organization of sensations so that they are meaningful. Taylor proposed that humans learn perceptions and that what they learn depends on their socialization experiences. Perceptual expectations are influenced by emotions, language, and attitude and vary widely from one individual to another. Thus, a person's interpretation ability highly depends on their individual perceptual ability.

Several factors affect perception in the nurse–client relationship: the capacity for attention (reception of sensations) by the nurse and the client, the perspective each brings to the relationship, and the physical condition of the receptors. Anxiety (the tension state resulting from the actual or anticipated negative appraisal of the significant other in the communication process) in the nurse or the client limits the ability to be attentive in the communication process, interferes with the validation of individual perspectives, and decreases physical capacities. Therefore, anxiety must be controlled in the nurse–client relationship. Validated perceptions between the nurse and the client are essential to goal setting and achievement. The nurse must constantly be aware of the power and influence of perception on the outcomes of a communication, regardless of its form.

Self-Concept and Interpersonal Relationships

The relationships among participants greatly affect communication. The self-concept of each participant largely determines the nurse–client relationship. When nurses and clients have healthy self-concepts, both parties respect each other. Nurses and clients recognize and value the contributions made by each person in the relationship, thereby setting the stage for true collaboration, mutual goal setting, individualization of nursing interventions, and recognition of the effectiveness of the interpersonal relationship. Clients receiving care from a nurse who has low self-esteem will question the nurse's competence and actions more frequently, while clients receiving care from a confident, self-assured nurse will feel more comfortable.

According to Brill (1990, p. 7), "In dealing with people it is essential that workers possess awareness of themselves, their own needs, the ways in which they satisfy these needs, (and) the ways in which they use themselves in relationship with others." In addition to self-awareness, other factors involved in the self-concept are essential to effective communication, including the ability to:

- Share ideas, thoughts, and feelings with individuals (a function of achievement of interpersonal developmental tasks)
- Establish, maintain, and terminate the kind of relationship in which one is comfortable (a function of the human need to perpetuate a personal self-concept)
- Share power (a reflection of the person's view of self and others)

If the major reason for nurses' communication with clients is to influence clients toward better health, nurses must develop concepts of self that are most effective in facilitating the client's growth potential. These concepts include an awareness of one's perceptions of and feelings about the self, the ability to derive satisfaction by sharing with the client the responsibility for the nurse–client relationship, the ability to view the self as a therapeutic tool, and an appreciation for shared power in activities directed toward change.

▌ QUESTIONS FOR REFLECTION

1. How do you come across as a professional nurse? (You may have to ask a colleague for the answer to this one; it may surprise you.)
2. Why is it important to know how others perceive you as a professional nurse?
3. What happens to informal communication when the nonverbal behavior is incongruent with what is being said?
4. What occurs when nonverbal behavior contradicts what is being said?
5. Think of the last time that you got angry with or lost patience with someone in your life. What happened during the interaction? What verbal and nonverbal behavior cues resulted in anger or lack of patience?

REAL-LIFE REFLECTIONS

Remember Marcia from the beginning of the chapter. What should she do when the nonverbal behavior of her client's family does not match their verbal messages? Why is it important for her to act when she sees this incongruence? How does culture play a role in communication? What aspects of the client's culture might affect the family's reaction to her outreach?

Principles of Communication in Collaborative Relationships

When engaged in communication with clients, nurses empathize with, demonstrate respect for, and respond genuinely to them. When nurses and clients equally share the responsibility and authority for care, they enter into collaborative relationships. During nursing assessments, **collaborative relationships** promote client sharing of all key information and involve nurse verification of interpretations and conclusions based on assessment data. The nurse and the client work together to identify and prioritize nursing diagnoses and determine a plan of care for implementation. They also decide collaboratively how to execute the plan of care. Finally, the client and the nurse evaluate the effectiveness of the care plan and, if it is deemed unsuccessful, they explore and propose alternative courses of action. If the plan is successful, the nurse and the client work together to develop another care plan to address a different health concern. Presence, empathy, respect, and genuineness are the **principles of communication** that facilitate successful collaboration.

Presence

Presence is an important part of several nursing conceptual models, including those of Parse (1996), Paterson and Zderad (1988), and Watson (1996, 2012). "The core element in presence is 'being there …' It is described as a gift of self and is equated with a use of self that is conveyed through open and giving behaviors of the nurse" (Osterman & Schwartz-Barcott, 1996, p. 24). Table 4.1 describes the characteristics of four ways of "being there." These "reflect degrees of intensity in the context of another" (Osterman & Schwartz-Barcott, 1996, p. 29).

By synthesizing these theoretical conceptions of presence, the nurse focuses all of their energy on the client during interactions. The nurse can be present without speaking. Clients and nurses engaged in true presence during an encounter describe an experience that cannot be captured with words and results in a deep personal connection for both participants with possible resultant personal transformations.

Take Note!
Presence is integrally related to genuineness and a necessary antecedent to empathy.

TABLE 4.1   Presence: Characteristics of Four Ways of "Being There"

Characteristics of Presence	Presence	Partial Presence	Full Presence	Transcendent Presence
Being there	Physically present with another	Physically present with another	Physically present (there) (physical attending behavior—eye contact, leaning toward) Psychologically present (with) (attentive listening behavior)	Physically present Psychologically present (metaphysical beliefs) Holistic
Focus of energy	Self-absorbed	Objects or tasks in environment, relevant to the other individual but none of the energy is directed at the other	Self/other (focusing on another influences response)—reciprocal	Centered (drawing from universal energy) Subject/subject—leads to oneness
	Personal, subjective reality	Mechanical/technical reality	Present-oriented (here and now)—anchoring in present reality	Transcending and oriented beyond here and now—sustaining while transforming reality
Nature of interaction	No interaction; self-absorbed, intrapersonal encounter	Interaction with part of other encounter	Interactive; essential communication; boundaries—role constraints; professional relationship; dyad caring	Relationship; high degree of skilled communication; role-free; human intimacy/love; humanistic caring, no boundaries, monad relationship
Positive outcomes	Reduces stress; reassurance that someone is there; may be quieting and restorative; facilitates creative thinking	Reduces stress; solving a mechanical problem; reduces amount of stimuli in an encounter	Solving of a human problem; relief of a here-and-now distress	Transformations decreased loneliness expansion of consciousness; spiritual peace, hope, and meaning in one's existence (love/connectedness); nice feeling generated in the environment; transpersonal (oneness)
Negative outcomes	No interpersonal engagement—missed communication; isolation, withdrawn, increased anxiety	No interpersonal connectedness	May be too much energy for recipient or feel negative to a recipient; energy not always available for full presence; increased anxiety	Fusion and possible loss of objective reality; danger of taking on recipient's problems

Data from Osterman, P., & Schwartz-Barcott, D. (1996). Presence: Four ways of being there. *Nursing Forum, 31*, 23–30. https://doi.org/10.1111/j.1744-6198.1996.tb00490.x

▌ QUESTIONS FOR REFLECTION

1. Why is it important to be truly present with clients?
2. What factors in your clinical practice setting prevent you from being truly present with clients?
3. How could you proceed with changing the clinical practice setting?

Empathy

Empathy, the ability to understand, sense, share, and accept the feelings of another (Keegan, 1994), enables the nurse to develop helping relationships with clients.

Therapeutic, helping relationships focus on change. Understanding the potential impact of change on clients enables the nurse to identify obstacles for clients to change behaviors and attitudes. When using an empathetic approach, the nurse becomes more tolerant of behaviors, attitudes, and values that differ and could impede progress toward goal attainment. Wiseman (1996, p. 1165) identified four defining attributes of empathy: seeing the world as others see it, being nonjudgmental, understanding another's feelings, and communicating the understanding.

Nurses who possess empathy show awareness of the uniqueness and individuality of clients. They listen and respond as clients share feelings and concerns. They care about clients as humans like themselves. If clients perceive that nurses care about them and how they feel, both nurses and clients benefit from (Keegan, 1994):

- More trusting relationships with open communication
- Increased feelings of being connected to another
- Enhanced client and nurse self-esteem
- Genuine acceptance of others just as they are
- Increased self-awareness for both the nurse and the client
- Increased self-caring and less self-criticism on the part of the client

To be truly empathic, nurses as helpers must listen carefully so they can act as intended, perceive and accept the inner feelings and experiences of clients as the clients experience them, and paraphrase feelings, ideas, and intentions accurately. Two essential actions are necessary for a nurse to develop empathy:

1. Awareness and acceptance of self as a feeling person open to one's experiences
2. Ability to listen to each message of the client, to identify the client's feelings associated with it, and to respond to those feelings

Thus, empathy involves far more than the cognitive or thinking part of the self. It involves the acceptance that we are *feeling* beings, commonly experiencing multiple emotions simultaneously. In effective communication, the nurse and the client know that the nurse perceives and accepts the client's feelings.

Respect

Respect is "feeling or showing deferential regard or esteem for another" (Agnes, 2005, p. 1221). It is the nonpossessive caring for and affirmation of another's personhood as a separate individual. Respect builds self-esteem and positive self-image. In the nurse–client relationship, respect is demonstrated by equality, mutuality, and shared thinking.

Certain behaviors convey respect toward others. Nurses act respectfully toward clients when they look directly at them when providing care; give them full, undivided attention; maintain eye contact if culturally appropriate; smile appropriately; determine how each client wants to be addressed and call clients by their preferred means of address; introduce themselves to clients; and make physical contact such as a handshake or gentle touch. Clients who are members of a cultural group unlike that of the nurse may have special needs

for respect, and sometimes the aforementioned actions should be avoided because they conflict with cultural norms and values (Leininger & McFarland, 2006).

According to Bradley and Edinberg (1990, p. 226), clients may view nurses "as being powerful, one-up, and, if from a different racial group, nonempathic. In addition, nurses might view the clients as powerless, one-down, and different." Respecting the client's dignity is critical to therapeutic communication, "even when the client is in dire social, economic, or health circumstances" (Bradley & Edinberg, 1990, p. 226). Respect toward the client facilitates the development of effective helping relationships.

Genuineness

Genuineness is the state of being real, honest, and sincere. Clients readily detect dishonesty and insincerity when interacting with health care providers. Frequently, genuineness is used synonymously with authenticity.

When defining authenticity, phrases such as "being actually and precisely what is claimed," "genuine," "good faith," and "sincere" are used. Nurses who are genuine display their real selves to clients and do not let themselves become distorted or different because of thoughts or emotions. They act from their hearts and do not need to rehearse or contrive actions. In previous times, nurses were expected to be neutral to attain and maintain a helping relationship (Rogers, 1951). However, neutral behavior often seems depersonalized and sends messages of ambiguity. Ambiguous messages may cause client anxiety because clients may not understand their roles or positions within the relationship.

Nurses take risks to be genuine because such behavior frequently involves expressing negative thoughts and confronting others. However, there may be even more risk when incongruence surfaces between nurse intentions and behaviors. When clients detect incongruence in the nurse–client relationship, feelings of distrust, confusion, and suspicion may arise. Clients may begin to question the credibility of the nurse and the value of the health information being shared. They may only believe the nonverbal messages sent and discount the verbal ones. Finally, therapeutic rapport erodes if clients believe that the nurse is attempting to impress them rather than connect with them (Dinc & Gastmans, 2013).

When a nurse is genuine, action occurs spontaneously. "Being real does not mean being overly familiar"; what the client wants "is an emotionally available, calm, caring proficient resource that can protect, care about, and above all, listen to him or her" (Arnold & Boggs, 1989, p. 439).

Internalizing the principles of empathy, respect, and genuineness makes it possible for the nurse to demonstrate these behaviors and experience satisfaction in professional nursing practice. These principles also help nurses establish healthy, helping relationships with clients and their families.

HELPING RELATIONSHIPS: THE NURSE AS HELPER

The nurse–client relationship is a special helping relationship that has the power to transform the lives of both the client and the nurse. Nurses tailor this private, platonic relationship to fit the needs of the individual client. Because the nurse has specialized knowledge and expertise to serve humanity, the nurse assumes the role of helper.

Rogers (1958) set the following essential conditions of a helping relationship, which are applicable to professional nursing:

1. The individual is capable of and expected to be responsible for themselves.
2. Each individual (the nurse and the client) has a strong drive to become mature and to be socially responsible.
3. The climate of the helping relationship is warm and permits the expression of both positive and negative feelings.
4. Mutually agreed upon limits are set on behavior only, not on attitudes.
5. The helper communicates understanding and acceptance.

These characteristics of helping have positively influenced many health care professionals and serve as criteria for nurses as they develop effective helping relationships.

Nurses bear the responsibility to fulfill a helper role, regardless of the specific parameters and purposes of each relationship. The nurse must validate that the client knows why help was sought. The nurse also assumes that both the client and the nurse will share the responsibility for the outcomes of the nursing encounter. The nurse's helping role is viewed as a facilitative one in which the nurse uses self and expertise as therapeutic tools to assist the client in overcoming threats to health and well-being or to obtain optimal health.

The nurse and the client bring unique talents, skills, and characteristics that affect the development of a helping relationship (Table 4.2) (Benner, 1984, 2001; Northouse & Northouse, 1998; Riley, 2017). The nurse uses client strengths to facilitate the helping relationship. When the client is confused or unresponsive, their significant others (e.g., family members, close friends, those having medical power of attorney) bring these attributes into the therapeutic relationship. At times, as the nurse delivers physical care to the client, efforts are made to fulfill the psychosocial and spiritual needs of the client's significant others.

Theories on Therapeutic Relationship Development

Although the nurse always assumes the roles of facilitator, advocate, and coordinator, their specific functions and purposes evolve as the relationship proceeds through predictable sequential stages. **Stages of the nurse–client relationship** vary according to the relationship's helping purpose. For example:

- The facilitator helps the client move toward improved health.
- The advocate protects the client from stress inherent in the petitioner role and acts on behalf of the client in promoting access to and use of health care services.
- The coordinator attempts to organize and articulate all the services related to meeting the client's health care needs.

The knowledge base needed to act as a helper in professional nursing was largely developed by Dr. Hildegard Peplau more than 50 years ago. Her book, *Interpersonal Relations in Nursing* (1952), presented a thorough analysis of Sullivan's (1953) interpersonal theory in psychiatry and gave nursing a sound conceptual model for practice. Although other nurse scholars have developed models and changed forms of the interpersonal model, Peplau's phases of the nurse–client relationship remain applicable today. Box 4.3, Professional Building Blocks, "Peplau's Phases of the Nurse–Client Relationship," provides associated functions of the nurse in each phase.

Travelbee (1964, 1966, 1971) designated five phases of the nurse–client relationship:

1. During the original encounter, the client and the nurse work to view each other as individual human beings rather than as "nurse" and "client."
2. Once the nurse and client transcend their respective roles, they enter the phase of emerging identities, in which each perceives the other's uniqueness, values the other, and decides to make an emotional investment to begin the therapeutic relationship.
3. Once the client and the nurse have established their identities in the relationship, they enter the phase

■ TABLE 4.2 Interchange of Knowledge, Attitudes, and Skills Between the Client and the Nurse in the Helping Relationship

What the Client Brings to the Relationship	What the Nurse Brings to the Relationship
Cognitive	
■ Individual ways of perceiving the world ■ Preferred ways of making judgments ■ Knowledge and beliefs about health and illness in general ■ Specific knowledge related to current personal health status, usual general health status, and meaning of the current particular illness or altered health status ■ Knowledge and beliefs about health promotion and maintenance in general and information about own health care routines and activities ■ Ability to solve problems and knowledge of preferred methods of doing so ■ Ability to learn ■ Preferred ways to learn based on individualized learning style ■ Preferred communication patterns ■ Knowledge of how current health affects role responsibilities ■ Expectations of encounter with this nurse based on previous encounters with nurses	■ Individual ways of perceiving the world ■ Preferred ways of making judgments ■ Knowledge and beliefs about health and illness in general ■ Knowledge about own clinical specialty ■ Knowledge about what should help this particular client ■ Knowledge and beliefs about health behaviors that prevent illness and promote, regain, and maintain health ■ Ability to solve problems and knowledge of preferred methods of doing so while using nursing cognitive and clinical skills ■ Knowledge about factors that increase client compliance with treatment regimens ■ Expectations of client based on previous encounters with other clients ■ Knowledge of available resources to assist client with this particular health problem ■ Ability to perceive if help is needed for effective nursing management of client health problem
Affective	
■ Cultural and spiritual values ■ Self-perceptions ■ Feelings about seeking help from a nurse ■ Attitudes toward nurses in general ■ Attitudes related to previous encounters with nurses ■ Attitudes toward previous and currently prescribed treatment regimens ■ Values regarding illness prevention ■ Attitude of either being willing or fighting actions to take the required measures to improve the health status at this time with this particular nurse ■ Personal meaning of current health status and encounter with this nurse	■ Cultural and spiritual values ■ Professional nursing values ■ Self-perceptions ■ Feelings about being a nurse helper ■ Attitudes toward clients in general ■ Attitudes toward this particular client system ■ Intuitive feelings about the client system ■ Biases about nursing treatment regimens ■ Values placed on being healthy ■ Values placed on people actively preventing illness or enhancing well-being ■ Willingness to help client take positive action to improve their well-being ■ Personal meaning of current client encounter
Psychomotor[a]	
■ Ability to relate to and communicate with others ■ Ability to carry out own health care management ■ Ability to learn new methods of self-care	■ Ability to relate to and communicate with others using therapeutic communication techniques ■ Proficiency in administering general and specialized nursing interventions (in some cases the nurse has developed expertise) ■ Ability to teach nursing interventions to client

[a]Clients may not always be capable of these if health problem has impaired cognitive or motor abilities.
Adapted from Riley, J. B. (2000). *Communications in nursing* (4th ed., p. 28). Mosby; Benner, P. (1984). *From novice to expert: Excellence and power in clinical nursing practice.* Addison-Wesley; Northouse, L. L., & Northouse, P. G. (1998). *Health communication: Strategies for health professionals* (3rd ed.). Appleton & Lange.

of empathy, during which they predict each other's behaviors but fail to genuinely share feelings.

4. After the empathy phase, the nurse and the client enter the phase of sympathy, when the nurse translates sympathy into helpful nursing actions.

5. Following the sympathy phase is the phase of rapport, in which the nurse and the client enter into a personal, meaningful relationship where they genuinely communicate deeply with each other.

Unlike Peplau, Travelbee never addressed the need to end a helping relationship with the client.

Hames and Joseph (1980) outlined the following four stages in the development of a professional helping relationship that is not specific to nursing:

■ Stage 1: Trust formation—The client trusts the nurse because the nurse consistently displays honesty, respect, positive regard, and empathy.

4.3 Professional Building Blocks

Peplau's Phases of the Nurse–Client Relationship

Orientation Phase
- Introduction of nurse and client
- Elaboration of the client's need to recognize and understand their difficulty and the extent of help needed
- Acceptance of the client's need for assistance in recognizing and planning to use services that professional nurses can offer
- Agreement that the client will direct energy toward the mutual responsibility for defining, understanding, and productively meeting the problem at hand
- Clarification of limitations and responsibilities in the delivery system environment

Identification Phase
- Provision of the opportunity for the client to respond to the helper's offer to assist
- Encouragement for the client to express feelings, reorient those feelings, and strengthen positive forces
- Provision of the opportunity for the nurse and the client to clearly understand each other's preconceptions and expectations

Exploitation Phase
- Full utilization of the nurse–client relationship to mutually work on the solution to problems and the changes needed to improve health
- Provision of opportunities for the client to explore earlier experiences and behaviors and to have emerging needs met

Resolution Phase
- Provision of opportunity to formulate new goals
- Encouragement of gradual freeing of the client from identifying with the nurse
- Promotion of the client's ability to act more independently

- Stage 2: Resistance—The client pulls away from the relationship but the nurse continues to show concern.
- Stage 3: Working—The client and the nurse become actively involved in working together to help the client achieve health-related goals.
- Stage 4: Termination—The client and the nurse end the relationship by engaging in closure activities, such as saying goodbye, shaking hands, and extending good wishes for the future.

Northouse and Northouse (1998) designated four phases of the nurse–client relationship that differ slightly from those of Peplau (1952) and Hames and Joseph (1980). They also proposed that each phase may overlap, depending on various contextual factors:

- Phase 1: Preparation—For the nurse, this involves preparing the setting and oneself for client interactions. The client prepares by making plans to actively seek assistance from a health care provider, such as making an appointment or arranging for a hospital stay.
- Phase 2: Initiation—The nurse uses a variety of therapeutic communication techniques and demonstrates genuine concern, compassion, and respect for the client. The nurse and the client also clarify client needs and establish mutual agreement on expected outcomes for the professional encounter.
- Phase 3: Exploration—The client and the nurse examine and work on client needs and concerns. The nurse creates an environment to foster client sharing of needs and concerns. The nurse also helps the client manage anxiety resulting from discussion of sometimes potentially embarrassing personal issues. The nurse and the client work together to outline a plan to help the client. Finally, the nurse helps the client develop new skills to learn how to live with or resolve the concern (or need) for which the client sought assistance.
- Phase 4: Termination—The nurse assesses the client's ability to independently manage and cope with the health-related issues. During this phase, the nurse summarizes client issues and accomplishments. The client and the nurse mutually agree to end the relationship.

Take Note!
Most of the approaches for developing a helping relationship address the need for the nurse to establish trust with clients by demonstrating the utmost respect for them.

Sometimes, the therapeutic relationship has permanent life-changing effects on clients. Occasionally, the nurse may encounter a former client in a social setting or the client may return to the health care setting for a brief visit. When this happens, memories of previous encounters may surface, resulting in an affirmation of the benefits of the helping relationship.

Roles of the Nurse in Therapeutic Relationships

The nurse assumes various roles depending on the stage or phase of therapeutic relationship development

TABLE 4.3 Roles Assumed by the Nurse During the Therapeutic Relationship

Therapeutic Stage or Phase	Professional Nursing Role
Peplau (1952)	
1. Orientation	Stranger (someone who may or may not be trusted)
2. Identification	Unconditional mother surrogate, resource person, teacher, counselor
3. Exploitation	The above roles plus that of support person or coach
4. Resolution	Primarily a support person as client has attained independence in managing own health
Travelbee (1971)	
1. Original encounter	Stranger
2. Emerging identities	Listener, information giver
3. Empathy	Physical caregiver, but client remains uncomfortable sharing deep personal concerns, early counselor
4. Sympathy	Caregiver, counselor, facilitator, coach, support person, client advocate
5. Rapport	Caregiver, counselor, teacher, facilitator, coach, supporter, client advocate, change agent
Hames and Joseph (1980)	
1. Trust formation	Stranger
2. Resistance	Counselor (especially in offering self-continuously despite rejection)
3. Working	Caregiver, counselor, facilitator, leader, resource person, coach, support person, client advocate, change agent
4. Termination	Counselor, support person
Northouse and Northouse (1998)	
1. Preparation	Critical thinker in deciding how to prepare self and setting for client
2. Initiation	Stranger, counselor
3. Exploration	Caregiver, counselor, resource person, coach, client advocate, change agent, support person, teacher
4. Termination	Counselor and support person

(Table 4.3). Success of the therapeutic relationships relies on the nurse's consistency in demonstrating deep respect, listening intently, and affirming client thoughts, concerns, and needs throughout all phases. As the relationship unfolds, the client dependence on the nurse decreases, and the nurse's role changes primarily to one of offering supports. The relationship ends when the client assumes independence, responsibility, and accountability for meeting their own health care needs.

During the various therapeutic relationship phases, the nurse moves back and forth in some of these roles, depending on the client's needs. The nurse uses client responses as a guide to determine which role to assume at a particular time. Role selection requires that the nurse analyze the client response, weigh the pros and cons of the best role to assume, and anticipate consequences of nursing actions. Thus, the nurse constantly assumes the role of a critical thinker. However, as the client's needs are met, the nurse essentially assumes the roles that promote client independence. The helping roles can be characterized as follows:

- Stranger: In the role of stranger, the client perceives the nurse as an unknown individual who may or may not be trustworthy and competent. Peplau (1952) pointed out that it is essential for the nurse in this role to accord the client respect and convey genuine interest to promote open communication.

- Surrogate: A surrogate is a substitute figure who, in the client's mind, reactivates the feeling generated in the earlier relationships. The nurse's responsibility in this role is to help the client become aware of likenesses and differences and to differentiate the nurse as a person. By permitting clients to reexperience old feelings, the nurse who is acting as surrogate sets up the opportunity for growth experiences.

- Resource person: The resource person role involves the nurse providing specific information that has been formulated to address the client's holistic needs. When clients cannot perform activities of daily living or complex care procedures independently, the nurse assumes the role of caregiver.

- Teacher: The teacher role involves the nurse sharing information and promoting the client's learning through experience and requires the development of novel alternatives with open-ended outcomes in the nurse–client relationship.
- Leader: The leader role involves the nurse facilitating the client's work in solving problems and coaching the client to continue when obstacles are encountered. (The nurse also assumes the leader role when working with other members of the nursing and interdisciplinary health care teams.) For clients to become independent in meeting their health care needs, they experience change in knowledge, behavior, or attitude.
- Change agent: When the nurse facilitates change, the professional role of change agent emerges.
- Counselor: The counselor role incorporates all of the activities associated with promoting experiences leading to health. The counselor helps the client become aware of health behaviors, evaluates them, and plans how to improve them. Counseling focuses primarily on how clients feel about themselves and what is happening to them (Peplau, 1952).
- Critical thinker: The critical thinker determines what nursing assessment data to collect based on information shared by the client. The critical thinker also generates multiple approaches to develop and maintain a therapeutic relationship with clients. By using knowledge of and rationale for nursing interventions, the critical thinker anticipates potential complications and then makes clinical decisions based on consequences of possible actions aimed at achieving optimal care outcomes.

Throughout the entire relationship, nurses frequently assume the counselor and critical thinker roles.

Mutuality in Responsibility and Decision Making

Every person involved in a communication process affects and is affected by every other person involved. Rogers (1970, p. 97) called this phenomenon "reciprocity." Reciprocal relationships are the basis of nursing practice. Having the potential to affect and

be affected by the client offers the nurse the potential to assist the client with changing behaviors in the direction of improved health. Reciprocity can be a powerful tool in problem-solving and decision-making situations that determine the nature and direction of change.

The concept of reciprocity is similar to that of mutuality. Reciprocity "is characterized as an interpersonal exchange, customarily expected to be symmetrical or equivalent" (Mendias, 1997, p. 435). By contrast, **mutuality** is characterized by having the same relationship toward another person and sharing things in common (Agnes, 2005). Mutuality appears as a concept in Peplau's (1952), Watson's (1996, 2012), and Leddy's (2004) conceptual models in terms of mutual gain in a nurse–client relationship. Leddy expanded the use of the term "mutual" in terms of shared and connected processes humans have with environments.

Developing these ideas of mutual exchange and gain, Marck (1990, pp. 49, 57) discussed the concept of therapeutic reciprocity as follows:

> one phenomenon of caring, (which) allows both the nurse and the client to benefit from their relationship in a mutually empowering manner… Therapeutic reciprocity is a mutual, collaborative, probabilistic, instructive, and empowering exchange of feelings, thoughts, and behaviors between the nurse and client for the purpose of enhancing the human outcomes of the relationship for all parties concerned.

Akpotor and Johnson (2018) conducted a concept analysis on client empowerment in the context of community health nursing. They proposed that social motivation, availability of information, multiple possible choices, active participation of all involved, and a willingness to share power must be present before client empowerment can occur. The results of client empowerment identified were social justice, independence, and confidence. The researchers defined client empowerment in community health nursing "as a process by which the community health nurse and her client institute therapeutic relationship within a supportive social climate characterized by respect, mutual decision making, and power sharing leading to client independence, increased confidence, self-reliance, and self-management" (p. 748).

All of the previously specified roles represent elements of presence, empathy, respect, and genuineness.

Communication in these role relationships evolves from diagnostic interactions to therapeutic interactions, including education and support, as the client moves toward achievement of optimal health. The absolute element of all these roles is mutuality in responsibility and decision making if both the nurse and the client are expected to grow and experience satisfaction from the caring experience.

Communication and Anxiety

Nurses facilitate client change. The nature of change includes alternatives of cognitive repatterning (using new information to increase understanding), affective adjustment (using the relationship to become aware of, accept, and express feelings), and synthesis of cognition and feelings in interpersonal repatterning (using the relationship to learn to interact with others in the social system). The direction of change can be toward health enhancement or deterioration. Obviously, the nurse and the client want to direct change toward enhanced health or a peaceful death.

Every social system has role behaviors for constituents to follow. The way a person communicates is greatly affected by their perceived role in the system. Roles "are structures that are imposed on behavior" (Berlo, 1960, p. 153). Three aspects of roles must be understood in trying to positively affect the other person in a relationship:

1. Role prescription: The formal, explicit statement of what behaviors should be performed by each individual in a given role.
2. Role description: A report of the behaviors that are performed by each individual in a given role.
3. Role expectations: The images that people have about the behaviors that are performed by each individual in a given role (Berlo, 1960, p. 153).

In the ideal nurse–client relationship, congruence exists among these three aspects. Together, the nurse and the client agree on the structure and dynamics of their purposeful communication. However, when differences arise regarding the prescriptions, descriptions, and expectations of role behavior between the nurse and the client, communication breakdowns can occur, leading to uncertainty. Uncertainty and ambiguity in turn create increased tension and discomfort in the interpersonal system. Such tension in the human interpersonal system leads to dissipation of energy and decreased ability to use the energy for healing and growth. In interpersonal systems, this tension is often called "anxiety."

Anxiety is the tension state resulting from the actual or anticipated negative appraisal regarding uncertainty in any given situation. Prolonged or intense anxiety consumes available energy that could be better used for decision making or problem solving aimed at changing behavior and attitudes toward enhanced health.

Anxiety in one person is readily communicated to others. Sullivan (1953) attributed great power to anxiety and its effect on a person's interpersonal growth, development, and ability in all stages of life. The actual or anticipated negative appraisals by others that lead to anxiety are perceived as threats to one's self-image. If the anxiety is limited in amount and duration, it simply leads to an increased state of alertness, mediated through physiologic reactions and behavior to reduce the tension. However, if the state of anxiety is prolonged or intense, the individual may experience a state of high alert and be unable to engage in successful tension-reducing behaviors.

Sullivan (1953) postulated that learning occurs through an anxiety gradient extending from mild to severe. A client with mild anxiety can focus energy on most of what is actually occurring. A client with moderate anxiety has limited ability to focus on what is actually occurring and tends to distort reality. A client with severe anxiety cannot focus energy on what is actually happening and thus cannot participate effectively in problem solving or decision making. Sometimes nurses encounter anxiety when they feel overwhelmed from heavy workloads, encounter new clinical situations, become uncertain of actions to take in ambiguous situations, or experience communication problems with clients, families, and other health team members. Nurse anxiety hampers effective clinical decision making. Effective health care demands that both the health care provider and the client control anxiety and focus energy upon what is actually happening in a particular situation so that optimal decisions can be made.

Nurses have two primary responsibilities in controlling anxiety: (1) to be aware of their own feelings of anxiety and structure interactions in such a way that limited anxiety is transferred to the client; and (2) to use effective strategies for intervening in the client's anxiety. Therapeutic intervention for anxiety relies on the ability of nurses to recognize client anxiety as well as monitor and relieve their own.

Clinical practice settings are often stressful. Clients find themselves on unfamiliar turf when they enter the health care system. Nurses realize the importance of learning stress reduction strategies for themselves that they can share with clients. Techniques to help clients (and nurses) recognize, gain insight into, and cope with threats of anxiety are discussed in the following section.

Take Note!
Nurses and clients need to control their anxiety so that optimal care decisions can be made.

Caring and Noncaring Nursing Practices: Therapeutic and Nontherapeutic Communication Techniques

Nightingale wrote about the importance of caring in nursing in the same way that many contemporary nursing theorists espouse the critical nature of caring in the development of helping and healing relationships with clients. Wagner and Whaite (2010) analyzed Nightingale's writings and identified the following themes about caring in nursing:

- "Attend to": The behaviors and actions needed to respond effectively to meet client and environmental needs.
- "Attention to": The nurse's ability to maintain focus and identify the needs of clients using thinking and observation skills.
- "Nurture": Nurses conduct themselves in a manner that "cherishes, strengthens, encourages, supports, and promotes growth, and protects [their] patients" (p. 230).
- "Competent": The nurse's ability to provide effective, safe, and excellent care using science and art.
- "Genuine": Truthful, honest, and sincere character and the ability to display real concern for clients.

Today's health care clients expect that nurses genuinely care for them as people and rely on the nurse's ability to remain focused while engaging in nursing assessments, performing complex nursing skills safely, meeting the clients' holistic needs, helping them in times of distress, creating a safe and therapeutic milieu, and providing education about health issues. Nightingale's caring themes address many key elements of the knowledge, skills, and attitudes presented in the Quality and Safety Education for Nurses (QSEN) competencies.

Because of its abstract nature, the concept of caring is difficult to define. Many nurses identify caring as the essence of nursing. The following actions are frequently used by nurses to show that they care: presence (being physically, emotionally, and spiritually with another to enter the world of the other); sharing (giving of one's skills, thoughts, and knowledge to help another); supporting (providing fortifying help, displaying concern, trusting others, and affirming individuals in their actions); and competence (education and clinical skill). A **caring interaction** creates the uplifting effects for the people involved: feelings of being respected, feelings of belonging, personal growth, personal transformation, wanting to learn to care, and desire to care (Beck, 2001). In daily client interactions, nurses primarily use communication to demonstrate caring or noncaring. Caring communication strategies empower clients while being therapeutic. In contrast, **noncaring communication** typically creates a nontherapeutic "power-over" relationship, with the nurse dominating the client. Noncaring communication creates feelings of ill will among clients, nurses, and other members of the health care team. Table 4.4 presents differences between therapeutic and nontherapeutic communication strategies.

Sundeen et al. (1998) stated that it is devastating to the formation of a helpful relationship if the nurse fails to listen. Listening transmits the message "I value and am interested in you." Effective listening requires the use of various techniques (Hosley & Molle, 2006; Schiavo, 2013; Sundeen et al., 1998; Videbeck, 2014), many of which include ignoring internal and external environmental distractions (Box 4.4, Learning, Knowing, and Growing, "Guidelines for Effective Listening").

▌ QUESTIONS FOR REFLECTION

1. As a health care consumer, what caring behaviors have you experienced?
2. What caring behaviors have you experienced as a nursing student from your student colleagues or faculty?
3. What caring behaviors have you seen in a clinical practice setting?
4. What caring behaviors do you display as a nurse?

To listen effectively and to get clients to share thoughts and feelings, the nurse must use verbal communication techniques that facilitate the client's verbal and nonverbal expressiveness. Such techniques, generally referred to as **therapeutic communication**, facilitate the client's efforts at problem solving, self-expression, and health improvement. Nurses spend time early in their nursing careers learning caring

TABLE 4.4 Therapeutic Versus Nontherapeutic Communication Techniques

Therapeutic Communication Techniques	Description and Outcome(s)	Nontherapeutic Communication Techniques	Description and Outcome(s)
Focused listening	Focusing intently on what the client is saying results in reception of the client's message, equal power, and genuine interest in the client.	Inattentive listening	Failure to receive the client's intended message gives the perception of the nurse's disinterest in and power over the client.
Silence	Periods of nonverbal communication signify client acceptance.	Uncomfortable silence (a prolonged period of silence signifying nothing)	Silence becomes awkward resulting in the client feeling ill at ease.
Guideline establishment	Establishing guidelines clarifies roles, responsibilities, purposes, and limitations so the client understands expectations.	Nurse constantly talking	When the nurse does not let the client speak, the nurse is perceived as being superior or perhaps even uninterested in what the client has to say.
Open-ended questions or broad opening	Comments or questions that require more than one- or two-word responses let the client determine what should be shared.	Closed-ended questions or comments	One- or two-word responses facilitate data collection but fail to get at the entire story, resulting in the client's impression that the nurse may be rushed.
Distance reduction	Decreasing the amount of physical space between the provider and the client conveys the desire to become involved.	Inappropriate use of space	Being too close invades a client's personal space; being too far away conveys an unwillingness to touch or be involved with the client.
Acknowledgment or acceptance	Recognition of the client demonstrates the importance of the client in the interaction, thereby equalizing the power balance.	False reassurance	Attempting to solve or soothe the client with words or platitudes negates the client's feelings or fears.
Restating	Repeating one's perception of the client's main point enhances the validity of the nurse's interpretation of what was said.	Parroting	Restating word for word what the client says conveys that the nurse is not listening or may be incompetent with verbal communication skills.
Reflection	Stating back client ideas, thoughts, questions, and perceptions shows clients their ideas are important.	Rejection	Refusal to discuss topics with clients conveys potential rejection or that the nurse is disinterested or uncomfortable with the topic of concern, thereby enhancing the nurse's power.
Clarification	Requesting more information helps the nurse fully understand the client's views.	Giving advice	Telling the client what should be done negates partnership in decision making and emphasizes the nurse's power over the client.
Consensual validation	Attempting to attain a mutual direct and underlying meaning of what was said shows the nurse's desire to understand the client more fully.	Judging	Approval or disapproval of what is said promotes a client's dependent relationship on the nurse and results in the nurse having power over the client.
Focusing	A question or statement that invites the client to expand ideas in more detail conveys true interest.	Failure to probe	Inadequate data collection results in a lack of individualization of client care and increases the chance for errors.
Summarizing	Stating the key points raised in an encounter helps distinguish relevant from irrelevant information, provides a review, validates the accuracy of interpretation, and closes the interaction.	Defensiveness	Protecting someone or something against negative feedback negates the client's right to question, thereby giving the perception that the nurse has power over the client.

(continued)

TABLE 4.4   Therapeutic Versus Nontherapeutic Communication Techniques (*continued*)

Therapeutic Communication Techniques	Description and Outcome(s)	Nontherapeutic Communication Techniques	Description and Outcome(s)
Collaboration	Mutual decision making about future actions fosters equality.	Giving advice	Telling the client what should be done negates client participation in decision making, resulting in shifting the power balance to the nurse.
Stating direct and implied observations	Stating direct observations or verbalizing what the client says may indirectly remove communication barriers for the client when they may be avoiding or fearing expressing thoughts.	Introduction of an unrelated subject or changing topics	When the nurse directs the nature of the interaction, thereby determining what useful information is, it negates the concerns of the client, and the nurse is perceived as having power over the client.
Offering self	By making oneself available, the nurse presents an unconditional offer to be with, understand, and meet the client's perceived needs, letting the client know that the nurse is available.	Patronization, stereotyping comments	Condescending comments by the nurse place the nurse in a superior position. Use of trite, meaningless, perhaps fashionable verbal expressions negates the importance of what the client has said.
General leads	Statements or phrases that invite clients to express ideas or feelings facilitate client sharing of information and ideas.	Relentless probing	Insisting that the client talk about a particular issue or concern sets a tone of nurse power over the client and negates the client's right to privacy.
Concentrating on a single point	Homing in on a single point focuses the interaction to refine information while preventing the overwhelming nature of the multiple factors contributing to a client care situation.	Interpreting	By telling the client the hidden meaning behind the client's thoughts and feelings, the nurse blocks the client's understanding because only the client can identify or confirm their thoughts and feelings.

From Hosley, J., & Molle, E. (2006). *A practical guide to therapeutic communication for health professionals.* Saunders Elsevier; Schiavo, R. (2013). *Health communication: From theory to practice* (2nd ed.). Jossey-Bass; Sundeen, S. J., Stuart, G. W., Rankin, E. A. D., & Cohen, S. A. (1998). *Nurse–client interaction: Implementing the nursing process* (6th ed.). Mosby; Videbeck, S. L. (2014). *Psychiatric-mental health nursing* (6th ed.). Wolters Kluwer Health/Lippincott Williams & Wilkins.

 4.4 Learning, Knowing, and Growing

Guidelines for Effective Listening

- Give the other person your full attention by facing them directly.
- Focus solely on the current interaction by resisting all external distractions that cause your mind to stray.
- Listen for central ideas and validate them with the client.
- Ignore gut-feeling traps that confirm prejudices and/or produce biases.
- Do not become defensive.
- Watch for both nonverbal and verbal messages.
- Do not prejudge worth based on appearance or delivery of the speaker.
- Listen for ideas and underlying feelings.
- Do not interrupt the person as they speak or when brief pauses in the conversation occur.
- Try to see the situation from the other person's point of view.
- Do not try to have the last word.

---

communication techniques. At first, some nursing students will find the techniques artificial and phony because of current culture values on speed and multitasking. However, nurses must take the time to refine the use of each technique so that it becomes natural and genuine.

To be helpful, the caring nurse must show empathy, attempt to understand the meaning of health and illness for clients, and respond with respect and authenticity.

- *The empathetic nurse* attends carefully and intensely, responds reciprocally to verbal and nonverbal messages, uses appropriate language, times responses appropriately, clarifies and confirms ideas, explores the world from the client's viewpoint, and paces verbal and nonverbal behavior to the client's abilities.

■ *The caring nurse* spends time with clients, identifies relationships, makes connections based on knowledge, conceptualizes trends and patterns, summarizes appropriately, explains purposes of activities, and identifies nonverbal meanings while engaging in clinical practice activities. Some nurses, especially in inpatient or residential settings, make unexpected visits to client rooms to offer professional nursing services. Caring nurses make clients feel as though they are the most important people in the world.

■ *The respectful nurse* verbalizes a clear commitment to understand, conveys acceptance, and clearly affirms the client's worth as a unique person while affirming the client's strengths and ability to assume self-responsibility. By offering oneself unconditionally and allowing clients when feasible (in situations in which the client is not at risk for harming self or others) to direct the nurse–client interactions, the nurse shares power with the client and enhances client self-worth and personal identity. The nurse who displays the utmost respect toward clients works actively to maintain client dignity at all times.

■ *The authentic nurse* consistently responds with genuine thoughts and feelings, resists all urges to play-act, assumes ownership of ideas and feelings, and freely shares emotions with clients. Other expressions of authenticity include extending a hand for the client to grasp in times of loneliness or distress, being present with the client in times of need, and connecting with the client on a spiritual level. Authentic nurses do not assume the role of imposter and acknowledge their limitations.

Noncaring or nontherapeutic communication strategies typically make clients feel inferior to the nurse. At times, nurses may demonstrate noncaring behaviors, which communicate the following attitudes: "You have no value," "I am not interested," "I'm bored," or "I have more important things to do than to spend time listening to you." Other unhelpful nurse behaviors include being judgmental (e.g., putting one's personal values, beliefs, or expectations above the client's), making stereotypical responses (e.g., negating the uniqueness of the client by using platitudes or clichés as responses), and changing the subject (e.g., verbally directing the interaction to a new topic of importance to the nurse or by nonverbally signaling that the topic being discussed

is not important). When nurses distinguish the main differences between caring and noncaring communication strategies, they can determine how to avoid the strategies that disvalue clients (see Table 4.4).

Take Note!
Failing to listen to clients is perhaps the most noncaring behavior a nurse can exhibit.

Nurses display noncaring behaviors for several reasons. In today's health care system, which values cost over care, some nurses find themselves overwhelmed by professional care tasks and have little time to spend engaging in caring interactions with clients. In addition, some nurses may enter the profession with a high need for control. This need, accompanied by increasing anxiety, sometimes leads nurses to adopt an attitude of superiority that is expressed in negative actions, such as moralizing, rejecting, or reacting with hostility.

Defensive behavior commonly occurs in regressive states. For example, a person might demonstrate denial, unconsciously evading or negating the real factors in a situation. Regressive states also may be marked by distortions, rote habitual actions, dogmatic responses, loss of control, invalidated assumptions (jumping to conclusions), parroting, inappropriate timing, and poor judgment. These behaviors represent important components of noncaring and nontherapeutic nursing strategies.

Because therapeutic communication is essential for effective professional nursing practice, nurses should periodically evaluate their communication techniques. This includes reflecting on how and what is said during nurse–client interactions or keeping a written journal. If a pattern of nontherapeutic behaviors is identified, the nurse should seek help from a colleague or counselor, or attend classes or workshops to improve communication techniques. Nurses should let their own feelings be a guide to evaluate the effectiveness of communication during nurse–client interactions. A persistent feeling of anxiety or tension is perhaps the best cue that the nurse may be unwittingly communicating in a noncaring, nontherapeutic, and unhelpful way.

Take Note!
Nurses should periodically evaluate the therapeutic communication techniques that they use in practice to verify how well they work with various clients and their significant others.

Although views vary on the advantages and disadvantages of nurses being characterized as caring persons, the fact is that nurses do care about their fellow humans. One dilemma for nurses is that they are not always permitted to care for clients to the best of their knowledge or ability. Many factors in clinical environments (e.g., short staffing, increased focus on cost reduction, increased turnover, frustration with new technology, and ineffective working relationships with other health care team members) impede the ability of nurses to care for clients as desired and result in feelings of frustration. However, when nurses have the opportunity to share their specialized knowledge and compassion, all involved in health care delivery become enriched as desired outcomes are attained.

▌ QUESTIONS FOR REFLECTION

1. As a health care consumer, what noncaring behaviors have you experienced?

2. What noncaring behaviors have you seen in the clinical practice setting?

3. What noncaring behaviors have you displayed as a nurse? What factors contributed to this behavior?

4. How might you change the characteristics of your clinical or practice setting to keep you from displaying noncaring behaviors to clients and families?

Outcomes of Helping Relationships

The nurse–client relationship has three major desired outcomes:

1. Increased client self-awareness and understanding of how to better use personal responsibility to assume accountability for one's own health (learning)
2. Attainment of optimal health
3. Perceived satisfaction in the relationship

Knowing that clients have adequate knowledge and skills to solve problems or take steps to adopt healthy lifestyles is the goal. Clients who are adequately prepared can make educated choices, expend the required energy, and assume greater responsibility for their own health.

In the nurse–client relationship, change occurs as an outcome of learning in terms of either information gained and understood, or finding meaning in the personal experiences with nurses. The quality of communication plays the paramount role in change. When change and its effects are not communicated clearly, the change cannot be understood. Lack of understanding leads to resistance.

Nurses should continually evaluate their own communication behaviors (see Box 4.5, Learning, Knowing, and Growing, "Self-Evaluation of Communication Patterns"). In addition, feedback should be sought from the client about what has been said and about how the client feels the relationship is going. The value of nurse–client interactions should be explored at regular intervals to promote mutual benefits to the nurse and the client. A focus on asking the client, "How are we doing in terms of meeting your needs and expectations?" tells the client that the nurse values them and cares how the communication

---

4.5 Learning, Knowing, and Growing

Self-Evaluation of Communication Patterns

Hunsaker and Alessandra (1980) proposed a schema for self-evaluation of communication patterns of persons in management positions that apply equally well to nurses when working with clients. The questions below can be used as a starting point for reflection and journaling.

- Did I comprehend each point made?
- Did I make judgments of the words before the speaker was finished speaking?
- Did I make decisions in my own mind while the speaker was still speaking?
- Did I search for evidence that would prove the speaker right? Wrong?
- Did I search for evidence that would prove myself right? Wrong?

- Did I become upset while listening?
- Did I generally jump to conclusions while listening?
- Did I let the speaker speak at least 50% of the time?
- Did I understand the words in terms of their intended meanings?
- Did I restate ideas and feelings accurately?
- Did I study voice, posture, actions, and facial expressions as the speaker talked?
- Did I listen between the lines for unspoken meanings behind the words?
- Did I really try to listen to the speaker?
- Did I really want to listen to the speaker?
- Did I really show the speaker I was, in fact, motivated and interested in listening to them?

Adapted from Hunsaker, P. L., & Alessandra, A. J. (1980). *Art of managing people*. Prentice-Hall.

affects them. In addition, effective therapeutic communication enables clients to feel free to speak out when they have questions or concerns about their care and may result in error reduction (Finkelman & Kenner, 2007).

Along with individual evaluations of nurse–client relationships, much work needs to be done to validate the benefits of the helping relationships nurses build. Therapeutic communication is an independent nursing intervention and has positive effects on client self-confidence and well-being. However, nurses frequently fail to make entries in client records such as "therapeutic listening" or "explored feelings about the meaning of (client health concern)" when documenting delivered care. Most nursing research studies addressing caring are qualitative or descriptive in nature and there are few current studies addressing the effects of therapeutic communication. Client satisfaction data offer the potential to identify the benefits of caring communication and helping relationships only from recipients of nursing care. Nursing job satisfaction studies have the potential to explore provider benefits of being a helper. Perhaps a nursing research program exploring the positive outcomes of helping relationships needs to be established.

HEALING RELATIONSHIPS: THE NURSE'S ROLE IN HEALING

A **healing relationship** might be considered a special type of helping relationship. Because "to heal is the activity of becoming whole" (Kritek, 1997, p. 11), healing has been defined as "a lifelong journey into wholeness, seeking harmony and balance in one's own life and in family, community, and global relations" Healing occurs both within the person and by external interventions

FOCUS ON RESEARCH

Effects of Therapeutic Communication on Clients With Tuberculosis

Rustan and Hasriani (2019) wanted to determine the effects of nurses' therapeutic communication on the self-concept and anxiety levels of individuals infected with tuberculosis (TB). The researchers conducted a cross-sectional study using a stratified random sample of 24 people with TB who received care in a community health center. The study was reviewed by a research ethics board, and participants completed informed consent forms. Participants completed questionnaires that addressed the therapeutic communication of nurses, rating it as bad, average, or good; measured participant self-confidence level; and assessed participant anxiety level.

The 10 male and 14 female participants were 15 years or older. Of them, 50% rated the therapeutic communication as good, and 62.5% of participants reported having a positive self-concept.

Using encoded data to maintain participant confidentiality, the investigators used path analysis to determine the effects of nurse therapeutic communication on participant self-confidence and anxiety. The path analysis revealed that nurse therapeutic communication had moderate and positive effects on participant self-confidence ($r^2 = 0.653$, $p < .05$)

and anxiety ($r^2 = 0.537$, $p < .05$). The statistical analysis also revealed a statistically significant strong and positive effect of nurse therapeutic communication through participant self-confidence, resulting in lower anxiety levels ($r^2 = 0.797$, $p < .05$).

The investigators concluded that therapeutic communication has a direct effect on client self-confidence and anxiety; when a person has a positive self-concept the effects are magnified. They also concluded that therapeutic communication fosters trust in the nurse–client relationship. Nurses can use this information to boost motivation and promote a positive self-concept in their clients. Clients with positive self-concepts are more apt to practice adaptive coping that can reduce anxiety.

The clinical significance of this study is that it provides an objective, mathematical model that demonstrates the positive effect of therapeutic communication on client self-concept and can reduce client anxiety levels. More research addressing the positive effects of nurse therapeutic communication needs to be conducted.

Rustan, E., & Hasriani, R. N. (2019). Application of therapeutic nurse communication to self-concept as reviewed from the anxiety level of tuberculosis patients. *International Journal of Caring Sciences, 12*(2), 979–986. Retrieved March 21, 2021, from http://www.internationaljournalofcaringsciences.org/docs/41_rustan_original_12_2_2.pdf

that mobilize the client's inner healing resources (Micozzi, 1996). Healing encompasses the improvement of the whole person (body, mind, and spirit). Healing is not synonymous with curing—persons with terminal illness can become whole in the process of dying (Dossey & Keegan, 2016).

Dossey and Keegan (2016) identified many healing modalities used by nurses in practice, including:

- Body–mind healing: Cognitive therapy, self-reflection, relaxation techniques
- Nutritional healing: Healthy diets, dietary restrictions, herbs, vitamin and mineral supplements
- Exercise and movement therapy: Tai chi, walking, dance, yoga
- Spiritual healing: Faith healing, miracles, play, humor, use of fine arts
- Energetic healing: Meridians, chakras, aura, smells, sounds, colors, magnets, therapeutic touch, healing touch
- Environmental healing: Reducing toxins, recycling, feng shui

Along with these integrative healing modalities, nurses engage in healing activities based on traditional scientific medicine when administering medications to clients and following preprocedure and postprocedure protocols.

Lerner (1994) differentiated among universal, common, and unique conditions of healing. Examples of universal conditions are inner peace and a deep experience of love. Attention and care from friends and family, deeply enjoying work, laughter, moving music, and great art are examples of common conditions. However, Lerner indicated that the unique conditions of healing are some of the most important. Unique conditions are those that apply only to a single individual as a result of life experiences or personal relationships. As a healer, the nurse must assess clients as individuals to identify the particular needs that are most meaningful for each.

Given that healing occurs within the client, the nurse's role as healer is to facilitate another person's growth and life processes toward wholeness or to assist with illness recovery, a healthier lifestyle, or transition to a peaceful death (Dossey & Keegan, 2016). The nurse assists and responds to the client, who is the central force in the healing process. "Nurses assume that their actions, as professionals, aim to facilitate wholeness in others through an interaction based on a mutuality of purpose" (Kritek, 1997, p. 14). Kritek (p. 21) stated that four fundamental elements are always present in the healing encounter:

1. The nurse and client interact within a given context.
2. The encounter is in response to a health experience.
3. The nurse works in a pattern of mutuality with the client.
4. Healing is facilitated in response to a client's eliciting of nursing involvement and expertise.

Healing is facilitated within a helping relationship, which is characterized by principles such as presence (being rather than doing), intention and purpose, empathy, guiding, creativity, imagery, and spirituality (Dossey & Keegan, 2016; Keegan, 1994; Lerner, 1994).

As a healer, the nurse must assess all life dimensions for potential positive and negative forces that might influence the energy available to use when healing another. Effective healers have heightened sensitivity and awareness as they act with conscious intent. Nurses must recognize that not only is healing a unique life gift, but it also must be nurtured. Before healing another, some nurse healers practice preparation rituals. Healing fosters personal growth and the ability to live life to its fullest for both the client and the nurse (Conti-O'Hare, 2002; McKivergin, 2005).

Healing relationships produce interpersonal connections. Nurses often display intensity and unconditional love when acting as instruments of healing. Nurse healers usually perceive "that healing does not come from them, but through them" (McKivergin, 2005, p. 243). The potential healing does not come from the healer, but rather it is a mysterious phenomenon involving a higher power and energy within the environment. McKivergin suggested that the following factors may increase the nurse's capacity as "an instrument of healing" (p. 245):

- Self-care in all of life's dimensions to ensure a personal flow of energy and healing
- Personal interpretations of life's lessons and meanings
- Rootedness and expansiveness—balancing grounded approaches with intuitive inspirations
- Understanding the complex dynamics of holographic nature, the systems metaphor, and the essential nature of life, health, and healing
- Expansion of consciousness—broadening one's thinking, shifting perspectives, and embracing new approaches to life
- Growth in love
- Courage
- Alignment with the divine
- Openness to being an instrument of the creator's healing grace
- Ability to detach self from the outcomes

- Groundedness and reliability
- Patience
- Authenticity
- Mindfulness
- Integrity

The healing process requires exchange of energy and truth during authentic communication to create an environment of support while helping others become attuned to their own healing capabilities. Outcomes of healing include deep relaxation and the profound change of becoming more whole.

■ QUESTIONS FOR REFLECTION

1. What types of Keegan's types of healing have you personally experienced?

2. Which of Keegan's factors that may increase your capacity as "an instrument of healing" do you currently use in your life and which might you want to adopt as a professional nurse?

3. Which of Dossey and Keegan's (2016) types of healing, if any, have you used in clinical practice?

4. What would be the potential consequences if you used a nontraditional healing technique with clients?

HELPING AND HEALING RELATIONSHIPS WITH COLLEAGUES AND OTHER HEALTH CARE TEAM MEMBERS

Nurses and other health care team members must work together to achieve the common goal of providing the best possible care for clients. Each member of the interdisciplinary team brings a unique perspective to and skill set for providing health care to clients.

Conflict among the health care team has been present since the beginning of health care delivery. As health care professionals find fewer resources for client care, they sometimes turn against each other instead of working together effectively. Historically and today, physicians have exerted power over nurses. Nurses must compete with other health care team members, such as pharmacists, laboratory technologists, radiology technicians, and dietitians, for scarce resources. Unlicensed assistive personnel may experience a lack of respect from professional nurses.

To meet the increasingly complex needs of today's clients, patterns of conflict and competition must end, and members of the health care team must establish effective professional partnerships. Currently, many health care organizations do not have healthy working environments. Health care team members tend to blame each other for shortcomings in client care. The needs of the clients, physicians, and organizational administrators frequently supersede the needs of the nursing staff. In today's fast-paced environment, people communicate with each other just to get jobs done. Civility and politeness have gone by the wayside in an age of instant gratification and ever-present electronic devices as the mainstay for communication.

Professional partnerships help dispel competition, exploitation, and frustration in the delivery of health care. Early work in the establishment of professional partnerships that are now critical to client safety was done in the 1990s. A **professional partnership** is a relationship based on mutual respect to achieve a common mission while each participant lives out their life's purpose. "Partnerships join hearts and minds around a common purpose" (Wesorick et al., 1997, p. 3). Among health care team members, the common mission is client care, and each member plays a key role. For a physician, a life purpose may be curing illness in the sick. For a professional nurse, a life purpose may be to care for and help people as they respond to health alterations. For an unlicensed nursing staff member, a life purpose may be helping people who are incapable of caring for themselves.

The theoretical foundations and concepts related to the development of healthy helping relationships with clients also apply to all health care team members. Healthy working relationships among health care providers require meaningful conversations, which result when people use the following communication principles:

- Intention: Creation of a safe place to foster collaborative learning and to share and listen to the thinking of others to connect at a deeply human level (body–mind–spirit)
- Listening: Truly hearing oneself and others, using physical, mental, and spiritual connections to learn
- Advocacy: Willingness to share spontaneous personal thinking along with reasons behind the thinking, with the intention only to disclose thoughts, not to defend them
- Inquiry: Willingness to ask others questions to discover new insights and learn by connecting diverse ideas and feelings
- Silence: Time of quiet reflection to learn lessons from unspoken words; personal awareness of "the quiet of the soul" (Wesorick & Shiparski, 1997, p. 40)

Taking time to abide by these principles could foster the development of more respectful and healthy working relationships among health care team members. Development of professional partnerships might assist team members with helping each other, bolster team member esteem, and heal wounds. Then all team members can appreciate each person's contribution to the common mission—excellent client care and establishing meaningful relationships with each other.

Take Note!
Applying the communication components used for clients to the members of the health care team can lead to respectful, healthy workplace relationships.

■ QUESTIONS FOR REFLECTION

1. How could you develop professional partnerships with your student colleagues and faculty in your nursing program?
2. How can you develop professional partnerships with health care team members in your clinical practice setting?
3. What personal behaviors or attitudes would you have to change to develop these professional partnerships?

Many times, professional nursing students are afraid to speak to physicians in clinical care settings. Ineffective communication among health care team members is associated with client care errors, delays in executing treatments, and increased numbers of inpatient care days. (Agency for Healthcare Research and Quality, 2019; Porter-O'Grady & Malloch, 2018; Zikhani, 2016). The Interprofessional Education Collaborative (IPEC) was formed in 2009 to improve the education of future health care team members related to interprofessional collaboration. Currently, representatives from 60 health-related professions have participated in IPEC's programs (IPEC, 2016). In 2013, IPEC published **four core competencies for interprofessional collaborative practice** for individuals entering the health care industry and updated them in 2016. Each core competency has a list of 8 to 11 subcompetencies describing expected skills, attitudes, and behaviors. The core competencies include:

■ Work with individuals of other professions to maintain a climate of mutual respect and shared values (values/ethics for interprofessional practice).

■ Use the knowledge of one's own role and those of other professions to appropriately assess and address the health care needs of clients and to promote and advance the health of populations (roles/responsibilities).

■ Communicate with clients, families, communities, and professionals in health and other fields in a responsive and responsible manner that supports a team approach to the promotion and maintenance of health and the prevention and treatment of disease (interprofessional communication).

■ Apply relationship-building values and the principles of team dynamics to perform effectively in different team roles to plan, deliver, and evaluate client- and population-centered care and population health programs and policies that are safe, timely, efficient, effective, and equitable (teams and teamwork) (IPEC, 2016, p. 10).

IPEC does not specify any particular methods to use to attain these competencies. Achievement of each competency requires well-refined communication skills.

In 2002, Patterson et al. developed a framework for communication when addressing high-stakes issues. They describe this concept as a **crucial conversation**. Characteristics that distinguish a crucial conversation from other forms of discussion are that the participants perceive that they are addressing a high-stakes situation, there is divergence of opinion on how best to handle the situation or problem, and emotions of those involved are highly charged.

Health care team members participate in crucial conversations on a daily basis. Crucial conversations can be used in highly emotionally charged situations and when disagreements occur related to client care, work processes, and team relationships (Patterson et al., 2002). Figure 4.2 outlines the steps and goals of a crucial conversation using a flow chart format.

Take Note!
Using the crucial conversations framework, health care team members can build more effective helping and healing relationships with each other.

Quality and safety for clients rely on effective communication among all health team members. In all health care settings, an ideal situation would place clients first, team members would have equal contribution to care delivery, and the goal of care would be to provide the highest quality care possible. In 2006, the Agency

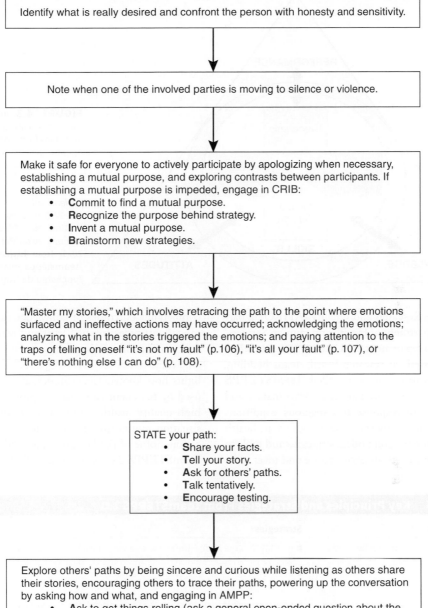

Identify what is really desired and confront the person with honesty and sensitivity.

Note when one of the involved parties is moving to silence or violence.

Make it safe for everyone to actively participate by apologizing when necessary, establishing a mutual purpose, and exploring contrasts between participants. If establishing a mutual purpose is impeded, engage in CRIB:
- **C**ommit to find a mutual purpose.
- **R**ecognize the purpose behind strategy.
- **I**nvent a mutual purpose.
- **B**rainstorm new strategies.

"Master my stories," which involves retracing the path to the point where emotions surfaced and ineffective actions may have occurred; acknowledging the emotions; analyzing what in the stories triggered the emotions; and paying attention to the traps of telling oneself "it's not my fault" (p.106), "it's all your fault" (p. 107), or "there's nothing else I can do" (p. 108).

STATE your path:
- **S**hare your facts.
- **T**ell your story.
- **A**sk for others' paths.
- **T**alk tentatively.
- **E**ncourage testing.

Explore others' paths by being sincere and curious while listening as others share their stories, encouraging others to trace their paths, powering up the conversation by asking how and what, and engaging in AMPP:
- **A**sk to get things rolling (ask a general open-ended question about the conversation content).
- **M**irror to confirm feelings (confront incongruent verbal and nonverbal messages).
- **P**araphrase the other person's story.
- **P**rime when getting nowhere (ask open-ended questions).
  and using ABCs:
  - **A**gree with the perceptions of others.
  - **B**uild a complete story of what led up to the conversation.
  - **C**ompare the paths of all participants.

FIGURE 4.2 Flow chart for a crucial conversation. (Adapted with permission from Patterson, K., Grenny, J., McMillan, R., & Switzler, A. (2002). *Crucial conversations: Tools for talking when stakes are high*. McGraw-Hill.)

FIGURE 4.3 Improving patient safety and care quality—principles and steps from TeamSTEPPS. (From Agency for Healthcare Research and Quality. (2020). *Pocket guide: TeamSTEPPS—Team strategies & tools to enhance performance and patient safety* (AHRQ Publication No. 14-0001-2 Replaces AHRQ Publication No. 06-0020-2). Revised January 2020. Retrieved March 21, 2021, from https://www.ahrq.gov /teamstepps/instructor/essentials /pocketguide.html

for Healthcare Research and Quality (AHRQ), a part of the U.S. Department of Health and Human Services, and the U.S. Department of Defense Patient Safety Program released a research-based, team-building, and communication program called **TeamSTEPPS** (Strategies and Tools to Enhance Performance and Patient Safety) in response to dangerous conditions outlined in various reports on client safety in health care settings. The program offers strategies and tools to enhance health care team performance and meet team competency outcomes of knowledge (a shared mental model), attitudes (mutual trust and team orientation), and performance (adaptability, accuracy, productivity, efficiency, and safety) (AHRQ, 2019). Figure 4.3 highlights how knowledge, attitudes, and performance are used by the client care team to provide safe, effective, high-quality health care services through leadership, situation monitoring, mutual support, and communication. Some of the key principles and strategies from TeamSTEPPS 2.0 are outlined in Table 4.5. A complete

TABLE 4.5   Key Principles and Strategies From TeamSTEPPS 2.0

Key Principles	Strategies
Team structure: Determining the fundamentals of team size, membership, leadership, composition, identification, and distribution	▪ Identify the core team—the client, coordinating team, ancillary and support services, and administration—that collaborates with contingency teams when situation arises. ▪ Clearly delineate all roles and responsibilities of team members.
Leadership: Coordinating team member activities by ensuring that team actions are understood, changes in information are shared, and team members have necessary resources	▪ Effective team leaders organize the team, articulate clear goals, make decisions using the collective input of members, empower members to speak up and challenge (when appropriate), actively promote and facilitate good teamwork, and are skillful in conflict resolution. ▪ Team events include planning (short briefing sessions), problem solving (huddling), and process improvement (debriefing to improve performance and effectiveness after the event and during action review).
Situation monitoring: Actively scanning and assessing situational elements to gain information or understanding or to maintain awareness to support team functioning	▪ Continuous environmental scanning develops situational awareness (knowing what is going on around you). Along with a shared mental model, all team members are "on the same page." ▪ Cross-monitoring is an error-reduction strategy that involves monitoring actions of other team members, providing a safety net within the team, ensuring mistakes or oversights are quickly and easily caught, and "watching each other's back." ▪ STEP (*s*tatus of the client, *t*eam members, *e*nvironment, *p*rogress toward goals) ▪ I'M SAFE checklist (check *i*llness, *m*edication, *s*tress, *a*lcohol and drugs, *f*atigue, and *e*ating and elimination)

Key Principles	Strategies
Mutual support: Anticipating and supporting other team members' needs through accurate knowledge about their responsibilities and workload	■ Task assistance: Team members protect each other from work overload situations, place all offers and requests for assistance in the context of client safety, and foster a climate in which it is expected that assistance will be actively sought and offered. ■ Feedback: Information is provided for the purpose of improving team performance. Feedback should be timely, respectful (focused on behavior, not personal attributes), specific (outline desired behavior changes), directed toward improvement (specific expectations and direction to meet them), and considerate (consider each team member's feelings and deliver negative information with fairness and respect). ■ Advocacy and assertion: Advocate for the client whenever a team member's viewpoint is inconsistent with those of the decision maker and assert corrective action in a firm and respectful manner (make an opening, state the concern, offer a solution, and obtain an agreement). If an initial assertion is ignored, the person with the concern must invoke the two-challenge rule and present the opposing view a second time, while the challenged team member must acknowledge the concern. If the outcome remains unacceptable, the team member who is advocating for the client should take a stronger action or engage a supervisor and follow up with the chain of command. ■ CUS (I am *c*oncerned, I am *u*ncomfortable, and this is a *s*afety issue!) ■ DESC script for conflict resolution (*d*escribe the situation or behavior using concrete data; *e*xpress how the situation makes you feel/what your concerns are; *s*uggest other alternatives and seek agreement; and state *c*onsequences in terms of impact on established team goals); strive for consensus ■ Collaboration: Achieve a mutually satisfying solution resulting in the best outcome by winning for the client care team (including client, team member, and entire team).
Communication: Process by which information is clearly and accurately exchanged among team members	■ Report critical information that requires immediate attention and action regarding a client's condition. ■ SBAR (*s*ituation, *b*ackground, *a*ssessment, *r*ecommendation, and request) ■ Call-out: Communicates critical information to all team members during emergent situation; helps team members anticipate next steps with a designated person holding the direct responsibility for carrying out this important task (e.g., leader of a code blue team). ■ Check-back: Closed-loop communication involving the sender initiating the message, the receiver accepting the message and providing feedback, and the sender verifying the accuracy of the message delivered (e.g., read back verification of verbal or telephone orders). ■ Hand-off: Transfer of information via the I PASS the BATON strategy: *I*ntroduction (introduce self, including role/job and client by name); *p*atient (age, gender, and location); *a*ssessment (summary of chief complaint, vital signs, symptoms, diagnoses, and concerns); *s*ituation (current status/circumstances, including code status, level of uncertainty, recent changes, and response to treatment); *s*afety (critical laboratory values/test reports, socioeconomic factors, allergies, and alerts, such as fall risk, isolation procedures, risk for violence, etc.); *b*ackground (comorbidities, previous episodes, current medication, and family history); *a*ctions (what actions were taken or are required along with a brief rationale for each); *t*iming (level of urgency, explicit timing needed, and prioritization of actions); *o*wnership (who is the responsible team member/team, including client/family); *n*ext (what is scheduled to happen next, including anticipated changes, sharing of plan of care, and contingency plans).

Adapted from Agency for Healthcare Research and Quality. (2020). *Pocket guide: TeamSTEPPS—Team strategies & tools to enhance performance and patient safety* (AHRQ Publication No. 14-0001-2 Replaces AHRQ Publication No. 06-0020-2). Revised January 2020. Retrieved March 21, 2021, from https://www.ahrq.gov/teamstepps/instructor/essentials/pocketguide.html

description and educational materials can be found at the TeamSTEPPS website (AHRQ, 2019).

Standardization of interprofessional health care team communication eliminates oversights related to effective sharing of client information and conflicts that may arise in the course of providing client care. When team members follow specific communication guidelines, they verify what is to be done in a given situation as well as being able to anticipate the next steps required for optimal client outcomes. Any team member is expected to share concerns about a given client care situation especially if the safety of a client is questioned (AHRQ, 2020). Clinical simulations incorporating TeamSTEPPS principles and strategies provide opportunities for health care professionals and students to master essential communication and teamwork skills for optimal client care (Sweigart et al., 2016).

Summary and Significance to Practice

Professional nurses develop helping and healing relationships with clients. All people have visions of what they would like to accomplish and noble intentions about acting on their dreams. Mastery of communication skills is necessary for carrying out the mission of safe, effective, high-quality health and nursing care to clients, families, and communities.

REAL-LIFE REFLECTIONS

Think about Marcia and the situation at the beginning of the chapter. Which of the communication models you have learned might help her as she works with the client and family? What would you do if you were the nurse? What would be the consequences of your proposed actions? Are there other actions that you could take?

From Theory to Practice

1. Think about encounters you have had with health care providers as a consumer. Make a list of positive and negative encounters, and compare the lists. What are the characteristics of caring encounters? What are the characteristics of the noncaring encounters?
2. Has this exercise changed you as a professional nurse? Why or why not?

Nurse as Author

1. Access the National Council of State Boards of Nursing (2018) brochure, *A Nurse's Guide to Professional Boundaries* at https://www.ncsbn.org/ProfessionalBoundaries_Complete.pdf. Identify one of the red flags and one example in which a nurse might violate a professional boundary. For each identified professional boundary, design a strategy to use for yourself or to help a nursing colleague if it is encountered in your future professional practice.
2. Think about the last time you encountered a client care situation that required urgent action. Write about

the situation and how it was managed. Compare and contrast the communication that was used with the strategies outlined by TeamSTEPPS. Write examples of effective and ineffective communication and how a strategy from TeamSTEPPS would have enhanced client safety and teamwork for the identified client care situation.

Your Digital Classroom

Online Exploration

American Holistic Nurses Association: **www.ahna.org**

American Psychiatric Association Help Center: **www.apa.org/helpcenter/index.aspx**

American Psychiatric Nurses Association: **www.apna.org**

TeamSTEPPS Pocket Guide: **http://www.ahrq.gov/sites/default/files/wysiwyg/professionals/education/curriculum-tools/teamstepps/instructor/essentials/pocketguide.pdf**

National Council of State Boards of Nursing Resources on professional nurse–client relationships: Professional Boundaries in Nursing (video): **https://www.ncsbn.org/464.htm**

Social Media Guidelines for Nurses (video): **https://www.ncsbn.org/347.htm**

Expanding Your Understanding

Access the Nurses Association of New Brunswick's (2015) *Standard for the Therapeutic Nurse–Client Relationship* at http://www.nanb.nb.ca/media/resource/NANB-StandardsNurseClientRelation-E-2015-10.pdf. Outline those behaviors that you perceive are unacceptable and list reasons to justify your position. What would you do if you witnessed a nursing colleague engaging in behaviors identified in the document as unacceptable and those that you have identified as unacceptable with a client?

Beyond the Book

Visit thePoint® at **www.thePoint.lww.com** for activities and information to reinforce the concepts and content covered in this chapter.

REFERENCES

Agency for Healthcare Research and Quality. (2019). *About TeamSTEPPS*. Retrieved March 21, 2021, from https://www.ahrq.gov/teamstepps/about-teamstepps/index.html

Agency for Healthcare Research and Quality, (2020). *Pocket Guide: TeamSTEPPS*. Retrieved March 21, 2021, from https://www.ahrq.gov/teamstepps/instructor/essentials/pocketguide.html

Agnes, M. (Ed.). (2005). *Webster's new world college dictionary* (4th ed.). Wiley.

Akpotor, M. E., & Johnson, E. A. (2018). Client empowerment: A concept analysis. *International Journal of Caring Sciences, 11*(2), 743–750. Retrieved March 21, 2021, from http://internationaljournalofcaringsciences.org/docs/14._akpotor_original_10_2.pdf

Arnold, E., & Boggs, K. (1989). *Interpersonal relationships: Professional communication skills for nurses.* W. B. Saunders.

Beck, C. T. (2001). Caring within nursing education: A metasynthesis. *Journal of Nursing Education, 40*(3), 101–109. https://doi.org/10.3928/0148-4834-20010301-04

Benner, P. (1984). *From novice to expert: Excellence and power in clinical nursing practice.* Addison-Wesley.

Benner, P. (2001). *From novice to expert: Excellence for clinical nursing practice, commemorative edition.* Prentice-Hall, Inc.

Berlo, D. K. (1960). *The process of communication.* Holt, Rinehart & Winston.

Bradley, J. C., & Edinberg, M. A. (1990). *Communication in the nursing context* (3rd ed.). Appleton & Lange.

Brill, N. I. (1990). *Working with people: The helping process* (4th ed.). Longman.

Ceccio, J. F., & Ceccio, C. M. (1982). *Effective communication in nursing theory and practice.* Wiley.

Conti-O'Hare, M. (2002). *The nurse as wounded healer: From trauma to transcendence.* Jones & Bartlett.

Dinc, J., & Gastmans, C. (2013). Trust in nurse–patient relationships: A literature review. *Nursing Ethics, 20*(5), 501–516. https://doi.org/10.1177/0969733012468463

Dossey, B., & Keegan, L. (2016). *Holistic nursing: A handbook for practice* (7th ed.). Jones & Bartlett.

Finkelman, A., & Kenner, C. (2007). *Teaching IOM: Implications of the Institute of Medicine reports for nursing education.* American Nurses Association.

Hames, C. C., & Joseph, D. H. (1980). *Basic concepts of helping: A holistic approach.* Appleton-Century-Crofts.

Hosley, J., & Molle, E. (2006). *A practical guide to therapeutic communication for health professionals.* Saunders Elsevier.

Hunsaker, P. L., & Alessandra, A. J. (1980). *Art of managing people.* Prentice-Hall.

Interprofessional Education Collaborative. (2016). *Core competencies for interprofessional collaborative practice: 2016 update.* Author.

Keegan, L. (1994). *The nurse as healer.* Delmar.

Kritek, P. B. (1997). Healing: A central nursing construct—Reflections on meaning. In P. B. Kritek (Ed.), *Reflections on healing: A central nursing construct* (pp. 11–27). National League for Nursing.

Leddy, S. K. (2004). Human energy: A conceptual model of unitary nursing science. *Visions: The Journal of Rogerian Scholarship, 12*, 14–27. Retrieved March 21, 2021, from https://www.thefreelibrary.com/Human+energy%3a+a+conceptual+model+of+of+unitary+nursing+science.-a0161397669

Leininger, M., & McFarland, M. (2006). *Cultural care diversity and universality: A worldwide theory for nursing* (2nd ed.). Jones & Bartlett.

Lerner, M. (1994). *Choices in healing: Integrating the best of conventional and complementary approaches to cancer.* MIT Press.

Marck, P. (1990). Therapeutic reciprocity: A caring phenomenon. *Advances in Nursing Science, 13*(1), 49–59. https://doi.org/10.1097/00012272-199009000-00007

Mariano, C. (2016). Holistic nursing: Scope and standards of practice. In B. M. Dossey & L. Keegan (Eds.), *Holistic nursing: A handbook for practice* (7th ed., pp. 53–76). Jones & Bartlett.

McKivergin, M. (2005). The nurse as an instrument of healing. In B. Dossey, L. Keegan, & C. Guzzetta (Eds.), *Holistic nursing: A handbook for practice* (pp. 233–254). Jones & Bartlett.

Mendias, E. P. (1997). Reciprocity in the healing relationship between nurse and patient. In P. B. Kritek (Ed.), *Reflections on healing: A central nursing construct* (pp. 435–451). National League for Nursing.

Micozzi, M. S. (Ed.). (1996). *Fundamentals of complementary and alternative medicine.* Churchill Livingstone.

National Council of State Boards of Nursing. (2018). *A nurses' guide to professional boundaries.* Retrieved September 7, 2020, from https://www.ncsbn.org/ProfessionalBoundaries_Complete.pdf

Newman, M., Lamb, G. S., & Michaels, C. (1991). Nurse case management: The coming together of theory and practice. *Nursing & Health Care, 12*(8), 404–408. Retrieved March 21, 2021, from https://pubmed.ncbi.nlm.nih.gov/1922978/

Northouse, L. L., & Northouse, P. G. (1998). *Health communication: Strategies for health professionals* (3rd ed.). Appleton & Lange.

Osterman, P., & Schwartz-Barcott, D. (1996). Presence: Four ways of being there. *Nursing Forum, 31*(2), 23–30. https://doi.org/10.1111/j.1744-6198.1996.tb00490.x

Parse, R. R. (1996). The human becoming theory: Challenges in practice and research. *Nursing Science Quarterly, 9*(2), 55–60. https://doi.org/10.1177/089431849600900205

Paterson, J. G., & Zderad, L. T. (1988). *Humanistic nursing.* National League for Nursing.

Patterson, K., Grenny, J., McMillan, R., & Switzler, A. (2002). *Crucial conversations: Tools for talking when stakes are high.* McGraw-Hill.

Peplau, H. (1952). *Interpersonal relations in nursing.* G. P. Putnam and Sons.

Porter-O'Grady, T., & Malloch, K. (2018). *Quantum leadership: Creating sustainable value in health care* (5th ed.). Jones & Bartlett Learning.

Riley, J. B. (2017). *Communication in nursing* (8th ed.). Elsevier.

Rogers, C. R. (1951). *Client-centered therapy: Its current practice, implications, and theory.* Houghton Mifflin.

Rogers, C. R. (1958). Characteristics of a helping relationship. *Personnel and Guidance Journal, 37*(1), 6–16. https://doi.org/10.1002/j.2164-4918.1958.tb01147.x

Rogers, M. E. (1970). *An introduction to the theoretical basis of nursing.* F. A. Davis.

Rustan, E., & Hasriani, R. N. (2019). Application of therapeutic nurse communication to self concept as reviewed from the anxiety level of tuberculosis patients. *International Journal of Caring Sciences, 12*(2), 979–986. Retrieved March 21, 2021, from http://www.internationaljournalofcaringsciences.org/docs/41_rustan_original_12_2_2.pdf

Schiavo, R. (2013). *Health communication: From theory to practice* (2nd ed.). Jossey-Bass.

Sullivan, H. S. (1953). *The interpersonal theory of psychiatry.* W. W. Norton & Co.

Sundeen, S. J., Stuart, G. W., Rankin, E. A. D., & Cohen, S. A. (1994). *Nurse–client interaction* (5th ed.). Mosby.

Sundeen, S. J., Stuart, G. W., Rankin, E. A. D., & Cohen, S. A. (1998). *Nurse–client interaction: Implementing the nursing process* (6th ed.). Mosby.

Sweigart, L. I., Umoren, R. A., Scott, P. J., Carlton, K. H., Jones, J. A., Truman, B., & Gossett, E. J. (2016). Virtual TeamSTEPPS® simulations produce teamwork attitude changes among health professions students. *Journal of Nursing Education, 55*(1), 31–35. https://doi.org/10.3928/01484843-20151212-08

Taylor, A. (1977). *Communicating*. Prentice-Hall.

Travelbee, J. (1964). What's wrong with sympathy? *American Journal of Nursing, 64*, 68–71. https://journals.lww.com/ajnonline/Citation/1964/01000/What_s_Wrong_with_Sympathy_.19.aspx

Travelbee, J. (1966). *Interpersonal aspects of nursing*. F. A. Davis.

Travelbee, J. (1971). *Interpersonal aspects of nursing* (2nd ed.). F. A. Davis.

Vestal, K. W. (1995). *Nursing management: Concepts and issues* (2nd ed.). J. B. Lippincott.

Videbeck, S. L. (2014). *Psychiatric-mental health nursing* (6th ed.). Wolters Kluwer Health/Lippincott Williams & Wilkins.

Wagner, D., & Whaite, B. (2010). An exploration of caring relationships in the writings of Florence Nightingale. *Journal of Holistic Nursing, 28*(4), 225–234. https://doi.org/10.1177/0898010110386609

Watson, J. (1996). Watson's theory of transpersonal caring. In P. H. Walker & B. Neuman (Eds.), *Blueprint for use of nursing models: Education, research, practice and administration* (pp. 141–184). National League for Nursing.

Watson, J. (2012). *Human caring science: A theory of nursing* (2nd ed.). Jones & Bartlett.

Wesorick, B., & Shiparski, L. (1997). *Can the human being thrive in the workplace? Dialogue as a strategy of hope*. Practice Field Publishing.

Wesorick, B., Shiparski, L., Troseth, M., & Wyngarden, K. (1997). *Partnership council field book*. Practice Field Publishing.

Wiseman, T. A. (1996). A concept analysis of empathy. *Journal of Advanced Nursing, 23*(6), 1162–1167. https://doi.org/10.1046/j.1365-2648.1996.12213.x

Zikhani, R. (2016). Seven-step pathway for preventing errors in healthcare. *Journal of Healthcare Management, 61*(4), 271–281. https://doi.org/10.1097/00115514-201607000-00006

The Health Process and Self-Care of the Nurse

LEARNING OUTCOMES

By the end of this chapter, the learner will be able to:

1. Compare and contrast the interaction and integration worldviews of health.
2. Distinguish illness from disease.
3. Differentiate wellness from health.
4. Describe how health/illness can be explained as a unitary concept.
5. Identify factors that contribute to individual variability in wellness.
6. Differentiate health protection from health promotion.
7. Specify factors that promote professional well-being.
8. Outline strategies for changing lifestyle behaviors and health patterning in clients and nurses.
9. Identify signs and symptoms of work-related stress, compassion fatigue, and burnout.
10. Describe strategies for enhancing personal health and personal and professional well-being.
11. Distinguish resilience from mindfulness.

REAL-LIFE REFLECTIONS

After an exhausting shift, two nurses, Michael and Nadine, discuss how ironic it seems that they have worked all day to help others get better at the expense of their own health. Michael says, "The hospital doesn't seem to care about the health and well-being of the staff. We never have time to eat or even take bathroom breaks. Within a few months we'll all be ready to occupy one of the beds." Nadine responds, "You know, I never thought about the toll this job is taking on my health. I wonder what we could do to make this a more healthful place in which to work."

Most nurses enter the nursing profession "to help people." One key way that nurses do this is by supporting and educating clients as they embark on their journeys to enhanced health and well-being. Unfortunately, nurses sometimes neglect their own health because of the perception that professional obligations supersede their personal needs.

Curing disease remains the major focus of medicine despite high costs and sometimes futile efforts. Americans are inundated with public service announcements regarding the importance of good nutrition, regular exercise, and routine disease screenings. Reports on the role of nutrition and exercise in preventing debilitating and fatal illness permeate the airways, internet, and print media. The World Health Organization's (WHO) Sustainable Development Goals and Healthy People 2030 are efforts to improve the health and well-being for all individuals at the global level (see Chapter 3, "Contextual, Philosophical, and Ethical Elements of Professional Nursing"). Professional nurses have the opportunity to influence the health and well-being of clients by sharing their knowledge and expertise. When working with health care consumers, nurses can emphasize the importance of health promotion, enhance general health and well-being, and offer positive reinforcement for healthy behaviors. Health promotion is an essential nursing activity in all nursing care settings, including acute care.

This chapter presents the interaction and the integration worldviews of health, organizing frameworks for alternate views of the concepts of health, well-being, wellness, disease, illness, and sickness. Models and nursing interventions for the protection, promotion, and patterning of health are outlined, and strategies for nurses to attain optimal health are presented.

WORLDVIEWS OF HEALTH

Basic philosophical assumptions about the nature of reality, including humans and the human–environment relationship, are referred to as worldviews. Nursing scholars have described several approaches to worldviews of health, including change/persistence (Hall, 1981), totality/simultaneity (Parse, 1987), particulate–deterministic/interactive–integrative/unitary–transformative (Newman, 1992), and reaction/reciprocal interaction/simultaneous action (Fawcett, 1993). The interaction and integration worldviews of health presented here synthesize elements of these approaches.

The Interaction Worldview of Health

In the **interaction worldview**, as in the totality worldview (Parse, 1987), the individual is conceptualized as a whole comprised of parts, who interacts with a physically separate environment. The environment exerts stressors on people to which they must react. The interaction worldview supports a belief in linear, predictable, and quantifiable cause-and-effect relationships.

In the interaction worldview, people strive to maintain a balance or state of stability. When the environment changes, people must change. Effective reactions to environmental changes result in personal changes without negative effects on well-being, wellness, or health. However, ineffective reactions may negatively affect personal well-being, resulting in disease, illness, or sickness.

Disease

Disease is a medical term consistent with the interaction worldview of health. **Disease** can be defined as a dysfunction of the body with signs and symptoms that impair normal functioning. Medical interventions seek to cure diseases. Many nursing interventions support the medical regimen as nurses administer medications, perform treatments, encourage rest, and evaluate the effects of these interventions.

For infectious diseases, a variety of factors related to the person (host), agent (e.g., virus, bacterium), and environment are considered interrelated in the cause and effective treatment of disease. These interactions must be considered in determining a plan of care.

Illness

Illness is a subjective feeling of being unhealthy that may or may not be related to disease. A person may have a disease without feeling ill and may feel ill in the absence of disease. For example, a person may have hypertension (a disease) controlled with medication, diet, and exercise and be symptom-free (no illness). Another person may have pain and feel ill but may not have an identifiable disease. What is important is how people feel and what they do as a result of those feelings.

Nursing interventions address the human response to illness, the identification of reasons for symptoms, and efforts to decrease symptoms if possible. In contrast, medical interventions focus on efforts to label and treat symptoms and cure disease. When a person's illness is accepted by society and thus given legitimacy, it is considered a "sickness."

Sickness

According to Twaddle and Hessler (1977, p. 97), **sickness** is "a status, a social entity usually associated with disease or illness, although it may occur independently of them." Once a person fulfills criteria for being sick, others condone various dependent behaviors that otherwise might be considered unacceptable. Nurses assist people who are sick until they can reassume responsibility for independent decision making and functioning.

Well-Being

Well-being is a subjective perception of vitality and feeling that is a component of health within the interaction worldview. Although well-being is a variable subjective trait, it can be described objectively, experienced, and measured. Experienced at the lowest degrees, people might feel ill. Experienced at the highest levels, people perceive maximal life satisfaction, feel in perfect harmony with the universe, and believe they have made or are making significant contributions to humanity.

Health as Wellness

Health is difficult to define. Various nurse scholars describe it as a value judgment, a subjective state, a relative concept, a spectrum, a cycle, a process, and an abstraction that cannot be measured objectively (Dossey & Luck, 2016; Leddy, 2006; Mariano, 2013; McElligott, 2013). In many definitions, physiologic and psychological components of health are dichotomized. Other subconcepts that might be included in definitions of health comprise environmental and social influences, freedom from pain or disease, optimal capability, ability to adapt, purposeful direction and meaning in life, and a sense of well-being.

In the interaction worldview of health, **health** indicates the absence of disease and the ability to function independently and perform one's life roles. In this book, health is defined as a state or condition of integrity of functioning (functional capacity and ability) and perceived well-being (feeling well). As a result, a person is able to

- function adequately (can be observed objectively);
- adapt adequately to the environment;
- feel well (as assessed subjectively).

Wellness, as defined in the literature, is similar to the open-ended and eudemonistic models of health described in this chapter, and in this book, it is considered synonymous with health. Dunn (1977, p. 9), in his classic work on high-level wellness, described wellness as "an integrated method of functioning which is oriented toward maximizing the potential of which the individual is capable, within the environment where he is functioning." Jensen and Allen (1994) characterize wellness–illness as "the human experience of actual or perceived function–dysfunction" (p. 349). Indications of wellness (health) might include:

- A person's capacity to perform to the best of their ability
- The ability to adjust and adapt to varying situations
- A reported feeling of well-being
- A feeling that "everything is together"

Smith (1981, p. 47) presented four models of health consistent with the interaction worldview that "can be viewed as forming a scale—a progressive expansion of the idea of health"—the clinical model, the role performance model, the adaptive model, and the eudemonistic model.

The clinical model is the narrowest view. People are seen as physiologic systems with interrelated functions. Health is identified as the absence of signs and symptoms of disease or disability. Thus, health might be defined as being free of disease or illness, not being sick, or being in a "relatively passive state of freedom from illness … a condition of relative homeostasis" (Dunn, 1977, p. 9). The current health care delivery system, which is based on this model of health, expends more resources on dealing with disease and illness after they occur. In the clinical model of health, the opposite end of the continuum from health is disease.

Next on the scale is the idea of health as role performance. This model adds social and psychological dimensions to the concept of health. The critical criterion for health is that the person has the ability to fulfill societal roles effectively. If a person becomes unable to perform expected roles, this inability can mean illness, even if the individual appears clinically healthy. In other words, "Somatic health is … the state of optimum capacity for the elective performance of valued tasks" (Parsons, 1958, p. 168). In the role performance model of health, the opposite end of the continuum from health is sickness.

In the adaptive model, which combines the clinical and role performance models, health is perceived as a condition in which the person can engage in effective interaction with the physical and social environments. This model addresses continuous and simultaneous growth and change in people and the environment. For example, McWilliam et al. (1996, p. 1) defined health as "the individual's ability to realize aspirations, satisfy needs, and respond positively to the challenges of the environment." The adaptive model suggests that health may be a process rather than a state of being. In the adaptive model of health, the opposite end of the continuum from health is illness.

The eudemonistic model provides an even more comprehensive concept of health. In this model, health is "the actualization of inherent and acquired human potential" (Pender et al., 2002, p. 22). Health "transcends biologic fitness. It is primarily a measure of each person's ability to do what he wants to do and become what he wants to become" (Dubos, 1978, p. 74). In the eudemonistic model, health is consistent with high-level wellness and at the opposite end of the continuum is disabling illness.

Examples of nursing conceptual models that are consistent with the interaction worldview are King's systems interaction model, Neuman's health care systems model, Roy's adaptation model, and Orem's self-care deficit model (see Chapter 7, "Nursing Models and Theories").

Take Note!
In the interactive worldview of health, effective reactions to change promote a state of well-being; ineffective reactions lead to a state of disease, illness, and sickness.

The Integration Worldview of Health

In the **integration worldview**, as in the simultaneity worldview (Parse, 1987), individuals are considered to be unitary, indivisible wholes, embedded in and inseparable from their environments. Because the person is in mutual process with the environment, multiple "causes" and "effects" and nonlinear changes make prediction probabilistic and sometimes imprecise.

In the integration worldview, the goal is for people to develop their potential toward increased diversity (becoming the fully unique person that they are meant to be). Change is inevitable and provides an opportunity for growth. Health is viewed as a unitary pattern. A pattern can be described as a "configuration of relationships" (Crawford, 1982, p. 3) or a consistency in all the interconnections among all energy processes that are not detectable through human perception processes (Leddy, 2006). Thus, a person's health (critically ill to optimally well) is a manifestation of the energy patterns that reflect the whole of the person.

Disease and Illness as Manifestations of Health

In the integration worldview, health is viewed as encompassing both disease and "nondisease" (Newman, 1994). Disease can be considered "a manifestation of health . . . a meaningful aspect of health" (Newman, 1994, p. 5) and "a meaningful aspect of the whole" (p. 7). Illness and health are viewed as a single process of ups and downs that are manifestations of varying degrees of organization and disorganization. Disputing that death is the antithesis of health, Newman (1994, p. 11) proposed that disease and nondisease are not opposites but rather are complementary to determine health, a unitary process. Illness, like health, simply represents a pattern of life at a particular moment. The tension characteristic of disease throws one off-balance, which promotes growth toward a new level of evolving capacities, personal uniqueness, and complexity. The person may transform into a new pattern of being.

Therefore, health can be conceptualized as an actively continuing process that involves initiative, ability to assume responsibility for health, value judgments, and integration of the total person. It is a goal, a fluid process, rather than an actual state. Thus, health is difficult to quantify for objective evaluation. In clinical practice, nurses collaborate with clients while trying to help them attain optimal health. Nurses help clients by focusing on client strengths while getting them to acknowledge the factors impeding growth toward maximal health potential. Client goals and feelings direct nursing interventions.

Nursing models and theories that are consistent with the integration worldview include Rogers's science of unitary human beings; Parse's theory of human becoming, Neuman's theory of health as expanding consciousness, and Leddy's human energy model (see Chapter 7, "Nursing Models and Theories"). These models and theories describe health as an evolving or emerging process, a forward movement with mutual person–environment patterns.

Take Note!
In the integration worldview of health, health can be conceptualized as an actively continuing process that involves initiative, ability to assume responsibility for health, value judgments, and integration of the total person.

1. Which of the worldviews on health appeals to you the most? Why?
2. Do you view health as a state or a process?
3. How do your views about health affect your professional practice or your life? Can you provide an example from your professional or personal experiences?

HEALTH PROMOTION AND PROTECTION

Health promotion has been defined as "activities directed toward increasing the level of well-being and actualizing the health potential of people, families, community, and society" (Hravnak, 1998, p. 284). Murdaugh et al. (2019) concur with this approach to health promotion and refer to health promotion as developing and implementing regulations and fiscal controls to prevent exposure to environmental toxins (e.g., contaminated air, water, or soil) or to avert serious injury (e.g., following laws and/or regulations for seat belt use, child car seats, or workplace hazardous materials). They propose that health promotion is "a process to facilitate movement toward accomplishment of health goals" (p. 33). According to Pender et al. (2002), "Health promotion spans from the prevention of disease, to empowering individuals, to promoting environmental and policy change" (p. 23). Individual motivation plays an important role in health promotion.

In contrast, **health protection** focuses on active avoidance of disease and injury. It also includes preventing oneself and others from contracting an infectious disease or sustaining injury. For example, when individuals receive vaccinations against a communicable disease, they are protecting themselves and others from contracting the illness. Regulations requiring vaccines before a child attends school exist in many states. In addition, driving while not under the influence of any substance (e.g., alcohol, opiates, or marijuana) protects the driver and anyone else on the road or in the car.

Early detection of disease and maintaining optimal functioning within the confines of an illness fall within the realm of the health promotion process. Compliance with disease screening protocols and regular exercise are examples of health promotion behaviors that may sometimes cause pain or take motivation and determination. However, health promotion expands the potential for sustainable, optimal health, well-being, and quality of life for all.

Goals for Health Promotion and Protection

The U.S. health care system remains disease oriented despite increased efforts toward health promotion and fitness. With its goal of curing and controlling illness, the United States spends more on health care than all other nations. Health promotion, disease prevention, and health education receive less funding, and health education efforts mainly address illness prevention. For example, children are taught to brush their teeth to avoid cavities (not because the mouth will feel, look, taste, and smell better).

Governmental action aimed at improving the health of Americans started in 1979 under the Carter administration (Office of Disease Prevention and Health Promotion [ODPHP], 2020b). In the 1990s, recognizing the need to promote the health of Americans, the federal government initiated Healthy People 2000. In 2000, the USDHHS (2000) issued its Healthy People 2010 report, which described national objectives for health promotion and disease prevention, including to "increase quality and years of healthy life" (p. 8) and to "eliminate health disparities" (p. 11). The outcomes of Healthy People 2010 were mixed. Between 2000 and 2010, the incidence of Americans dying from heart disease and stroke declined, overall life expectancy rose, and access to and acceptance of mental health services increased. However, health disparities for socially, economically, or environmentally disadvantaged persons rose 13%, millions of Americans lost health insurance coverage, and obesity rates increased dramatically (the percentage of obese individuals increased by 54.5% for children ages 6 to 11 years, 63.6% for adolescents ages 12 to 19 years, and 48% for adults) (USDHHS, 2011).

In 2011, the federal government completed work on the next version, Healthy People 2020, a collaborative process among the ODPHP, a division of the USDHHS, other federal agencies, members of the public, and an advisory committee. No nurse was part of the development of the program. Healthy People 2020 envisioned a society in which all citizens can "live long, healthy lives" (ODPHP, 2017, para. 3). The outcomes for the initiative were yet to be evaluated late in 2020 because the COVID-19 pandemic delayed data analysis and dissemination.

In 2018, the fifth iteration, Healthy People 2030, was initiated (ODPHP, 2020a). Hundreds of experts (including nurses) in various specialties of disease management and public health were involved in setting goals. Healthy People 2030 envisions "A society in which all people can achieve their full potential for health and well-being across the lifespan" (ODPHP,

2020a, para. 2). The mission for Healthy People 2030 is "to promote, strengthen, and evaluate the nation's efforts to improve the health and well-being of all people" (ODPHP, 2020a, para. 3). Healthy People 2030 identifies the following broad domains for social determinants of health—economic stability, education access and quality, health care access and quality, neighborhood and built environment, and social and community context (ODPHP, 2020c). Healthy People 2030 identified 23 leading indicators of health that were determined based on the preventable risk factors and behaviors of disease; how much the indicator would affect the nation; high-priority public health issues with major impacts on public health outcomes; response to evidence-based interventions and strategies to modify the incidence at the national, state, local, and community levels; and addressing the social determinants of health, health disparities, and health equity (ODPHP, 2020b). The leading health indicators in the initiative include increased use of the oral health system, reduced

sugar consumption, prevent drug overdose deaths, improve indoor and outdoor air quality, reduce homicides, eliminate hunger and household food insecurity, improve compliance to annual influenza vaccines, increase the number of persons who are aware of their HIV status, increase the numbers of persons with medical insurance, eliminate suicides, reduce infant deaths, improve reading skills, assure that adolescents receive treatment for major depressive episodes, reduce obesity rates, eliminate use of tobacco products, decrease binge drinking episodes, improving the numbers of persons attaining minimum recommendations for aerobic exercise and muscle strengthening activities, achieving compliance to colorectal cancer screening guidelines, improving control of hypertension, improving employment rates, reducing maternal deaths, and reducing new cases of diabetes (U.S. Department of Health and Human Services, 2020).

Box 5.1, Professional Building Blocks, "Goals, Measurement Categories, and Progress Measures for Healthy

---

 5.1 Professional Building Blocks

Goals, Measurement Categories, and Progress Measures for Healthy People 2030 and Professional Nurse Roles

Health People 2030 Overarching Goal	Measurement Category	Progress Measures	Professional Nurse Roles
Attain high-quality, thriving lives and well-being free of preventable disease, disability, injury, and premature death.	Status of general health and well-being	■ Life and healthy life expectancy ■ Number of physical and mental unhealthy days ■ Self-reported health status ■ Activity limitations ■ Prevalence of chronic diseases ■ International comparisons if available	■ Inquire about client perception of health status. ■ Assess all clients for mobility limitations. ■ Provide education and support on how to enhance health through optimal nutrition, exercise, and ways to avoid chronic illness.
Eliminate health disparities, achieve health equity, eliminate disparities, and attain health literacy to improve the health and well-being of all.	Disparities and inequality	■ Assessment of disparities using the following criteria: race/ethnicity, gender, socioeconomic status, disability statistics, gender preference and transgender status, and geographical location	■ Assess client's socioeconomic status, disabilities, gender identification, and location of primary residence. ■ Advocate for clients when disparities are identified. ■ Create a health delivery environment that provides equal care to all individuals. ■ Use community activism to remove social and economic disparities.

5.1 Professional Building Blocks

Goals, Measurement Categories, and Progress Measures for Healthy People 2030 and Professional Nurse Roles

Health People 2030 Overarching Goal	Measurement Category	Progress Measures	Professional Nurse Roles
Create social and physical environments that promote attaining the full potential for health and well-being for all.	Social determinants of health	■ Social and economic factors ■ Natural and man-made environments ■ Educational status ■ Current policies and programs	■ Develop and implement healthy environmental policies in health care organizations and educational facilities. ■ Perform detailed environmental assessments in homes, workplaces, schools, neighborhoods, and public and private facilities.
Promote healthy development, health behaviors, and well-being across all life stages	Health-related quality of life and well-being	■ Self-reports of well-being and life satisfaction ■ Physical, mental, and social health-related quality of life ■ Participation in common activities	■ Assess client growth and development levels. ■ Educate clients on developmentally appropriate health promotion, disease prevention, and early detection of illness based on age. ■ Perform detailed sociocultural assessments that include participation in some form of community involvement. ■ Perform spiritual client assessments.
Engage leadership, key constituents, and the public across multiple sectors to take action and design policies that improve the health and well-being of all.	Community engagement in policy development New policies related to improvement of economic stability, access and quality of education, access and quality of health care, quality of buildings and neighborhoods, and the social and community context	■ Evidence of citizen and health provider involvement in health care policy development ■ Evidence of citizen engagement in policy development and revisions at the national, state, and local levels	■ Educate the public about the importance of their engagement in the public policy development and revision process. ■ Become involved in the public policy development and revision process at all levels of government. ■ Participate in nursing organizations that have a record of being involved in action regarding public policy.

Adapted from U.S. Department of Health and Human Services. (2020). *Healthy People 2030, framework.* Retrieved September 11, 2020, from https://health.gov/healthypeople/about/healthy-people-2030-framework

People 2030 and Professional Nurse Roles," summarizes the program's highlights and the professional nurse's role in relation to them. The program identifies 62 topics, including such areas as health services access, ag-specific areas (e.g., early and middle childhood through older adult), genomics, immunizations and infectious diseases, injury and violence prevention, food safety, nutrition and weight status, preparedness, sleep health, substance abuse, and social determinants of health. Each topic area has overview information, objectives and data, and evidence-based resources (ODPHP, 2020d). In the future, the federal government may require health care providers to address these determinants of health with each health care consumer encounter.

Take Note!
Concepts of health protection and promotion are consistent with the interaction worldview.

The next section discusses various models and strategies for use in clinical practice to guide nurses in interventions targeted for health promotion and protection.

■ QUESTIONS FOR REFLECTION

1. Think about the last time you engaged in clinical practice as a student or registered nurse. Write down examples of when your practice focused on health promotion and health protection. Why is it important for nurses to engage in client health promotion and protection?

2. Do you have any of the unhealthy conditions or habits outlined in the Healthy People 2030 initiatives? How can you work to become a role model of health for your clients?

3. How do you and your family focus on health protection currently? Where did you get these ideas for health protection?

Models for Changing Lifestyle Behavior

Health Belief Model

Why do people behave in certain ways in certain situations? What kinds of nursing intervention would be most effective in modifying a person's behavior to reduce the risk for disease? Rosenstock's (1966) "health belief" model still has relevance for today's health care situations. Although the model is more than 60 years old, it still serves as a theoretical foundation for research studies in the field of nursing, medicine, psychology, and public health. In a recent literature search using the Cumulative Index for Nursing and Allied Health, the model was cited in more than 45 peer-reviewed, English language published studies within the last year. The model includes the following factors:

1. Perceived susceptibility: The client's perception of the likelihood of experiencing a particular illness

2. Perceived severity: The client's perception of the seriousness of the illness and its potential impact on their life

3. Benefits of action: The client's assessment of the potential of the health action to reduce susceptibility or severity

4. The client's perception of the threat of disease

5. Costs of action: The client's estimate of financial costs, time and effort, inconvenience, and possible side effects, such as pain or discomfort

6. Cues that trigger health-seeking behaviors: For example, information in newspapers or on television; internal signals, such as symptoms; and interpersonal relationships with health care providers and significant others.

The health belief model, called a "rational model," explains how people work toward improving their general well-being and health. The model assumes that all people value well-being and that different actions taken to promote health and well-being vary according to individual perceptions, beliefs, interactions, and motivations. In a review of 10 years of studies related to the model, Janz and Becker (1984) concluded that only two of the model components, perceived barriers (e.g., costs of actions that are too great) and perceived susceptibility, explained or predicted preventive behaviors. Perceived susceptibility has been found to be strongly related to compliance with medical advice (Vincent & Furnham, 1997).

Revised Pender's Health Promotion Model

Nola Pender developed the health promotion model (HPM) in the early 1980s. The model has undergone several revisions based on later research findings (Murdaugh et al., 2019). The HPM provides a framework for combining professional nursing and behavioral science outlooks on various determinants of health behaviors. Pender categorized the determinants of health-promoting behavior into cognitive-perceptual factors (individual perceptions), modifying factors, and variables affecting the likelihood of action. Pender distinguished the HPM from other models explaining health action because it eliminates the "fear" and "threat" perceptions for health action.

Based on extensive research, the HPM was revised in 1996 (Murdaugh et al., 2019; Pender, 1996). The revised model proposes that health-promoting behavior is related to direct and indirect influences among the 10 determinants of individual characteristics and experiences (e.g., previous related behavior and personal factors); behavior-specific cognitions and affect (e.g., perceived benefits of action, perceived barriers to action, perceived self-efficacy, activity-related affect, interpersonal influences, and situational influences); commitment to a plan of action; and immediate competing demands. Pender (1996) considered the behavior-specific cognitions and affect category of variables "to be of major motivational significance … [and to] constitute a critical 'core' for intervention, because they are subject to modification through nursing actions" (p. 68).

A review of studies testing the revised HPM (Murdaugh et al., 2019) reveals that the following factors contribute to health-promoting behaviors:

- Perceived benefits of action
- Perceived barriers to action
- Perceived self-efficacy
- Activity-related deficit
- Interpersonal influences
- Situational influences

Additional research is needed to validate Pender's HPM. Identified areas for future research include how mood and attitude affect success of health-promoting activities, the effects of commitment level to successful health promotion, and the relationship between competing demands and personal preferences when determining specific health promotion actions to take (Murdaugh et al., 2019).

The Transtheoretical Model

The transtheoretical model assumes that change requires movement through discrete motivational stages over time with the active use of different processes of change at different stages. The model has been supported in the studies of a number of lifestyle behaviors, including smoking cessation, weight control, sunscreen use, exercise acquisition, mammography screening, and condom use (Prochaska, Velicer, et al., 1994).

According to Prochaska, Redding, et al. (1994), the stages of change in this model represent a continuum of motivational readiness for behavior change. The stages include:

1. Precontemplation: Not intending to change
2. Contemplation: Intending to change within 6 months
3. Preparation: Actively planning change
4. Action: Overtly making changes
5. Maintenance: Taking steps to sustain change and resisting the temptation to relapse.

Westberg and Jason (1996, p. 147) described steps of successful change that are consistent with the stages of the transtheoretical model. These steps are:

1. Acknowledging that something is not right in one's life
2. Deciding that a change is wanted
3. Setting one or more goals
4. Exploring options for the achievement of goals
5. Deciding on and trying to implement a plan
6. Assessing progress
7. Guarding against backsliding.

Also included in the transtheoretical model is the concept of decisional balance. The model proposes that part of the decision to move toward the action stage of change is based on the relative weight given to the pros and cons of changing behavior to reduce risk. "The pros represent the advantages or positive aspects of changing behavior, and may be thought of as facilitators of change. The cons represent the disadvantages or negative aspects of changing behavior, and may be thought of as barriers to change" (Prochaska, Redding, et al., 1994, pp. 478–479).

This model provides a rationale for individualizing interventions based on a client's readiness for change. It remains to be demonstrated whether stage-appropriate interventions are effective not only in encouraging behavior change progress but also in promoting maintenance of the desired change.

Take Note!
The effectiveness of interventions to modify an individual's lifestyle behavior will depend on the individual's perceptions, values, beliefs, and motivations.

Lifestyle Behavior Change

Lifestyles and Health

Lifestyle can be described as the general way of living based on the interconnectedness of living conditions, socioeconomic factors, and individual behavior patterns. Many health promotion and disease prevention researchers have suggested that lifestyle contributes 33% to a person's health status (Logan, 2007; O'Keefe & O'Keefe, 2006; Rau & Wyler, 2007). The ongoing Nurses' Health Study revealed that close to 80% of coronary heart disease, 81% of sudden cardiac death, and 54% of ischemic strokes could be prevented by adopting healthier lifestyle habits (Yu et al., 2016). Some people elect to incorporate health practices that fall outside traditional scientific-based medicine. When these health practices are used exclusively, they are known as **alternative health practices**. However, when they are used in combination with traditional scientific-based medicine, they become **complementary health practices**. When alternative and conventional therapies are used in a coordinated, complementary manner, integrative health care is being practiced (National Center for Complementary and Integrative Health [NCCIH], 2020a). In the digital age, people can easily access information to learn about complementary health practices. A few examples of complementary health practices include:

- Isopathic remedies (disarming viruses and bacteria by pairing them up with neutralizing agents)
- Chelation therapy (giving intravenous medication that binds body toxins to the blood for renal excretion)
- Chiropractics (spinal manipulation)
- Myoreflex therapy (acupressure points and meridian theory)
- Homeopathy (usually diluted organic substances to stimulate the immune system)
- Cleanses (detoxifying programs with specific diets, juices, and colonic irrigations)
- Hyperthermia or sauna treatment
- Acupuncture
- Nutritional supplements (e.g., vitamins and minerals, protein powder supplements)

Recent evidence shows that modifying simple lifestyle habits can increase the length and quality of life. Lifestyle habits include the following:

- Getting 7 to 8 hours of sleep nightly
- Maintaining a body mass index between 19 and 25 kg/m^2
- Consuming a healthful diet (eating breakfast and at least nine servings of fruits and vegetables)
- Exercising (aerobic, flexibility, and muscle strengthening) on a regular schedule (5-6 days/week)
- Participating in recreational activities
- Drinking at least 64 oz of water daily
- Scheduling quiet time for reflection, mediation, prayer, or other relaxation techniques
- Maintaining an optimistic attitude
- Having and using a social support network
- Securing an integrated approach between allopathic and complementary health practices (Leddy, 2006; Murdaugh et al., 2019; Mariolle, 2020).

Murdaugh and colleagues (2019) suggested that a healthy lifestyle incorporates both health-protecting behaviors and health-promoting behaviors. Health-promoting behaviors include:

- Optimal nutrition
- Perceived self-efficacy
- Supportive relationships
- Regular exercise
- Adequate sleep

People choose their lifestyles. Many assume responsibility for their own lifestyle choices; however, some people may refuse to accept the consequences of personal actions, resulting in an unhealthy lifestyle. Before facilitating lifestyle behavioral changes, the nurse must assess the client's perceived interpretation of what it means to live a healthy lifestyle, perception of health promotion, current health promotion behaviors, level of motivation to change, and expected outcomes of lifestyle changes. The client and the nurse collaborate to determine what changes need to be made and how the nurse can facilitate and support identified changes, thereby shifting thinking from using professional expertise to overcome client weaknesses to empowering clients to help themselves by building on their own strengths.

Health Strengths

A large body of literature associates illness with stress. Stress is assumed to arise when a situation is appraised as threatening or otherwise demanding and an appropriate coping response is not immediately available (Lazarus & Folkman, 1984). When an event is appraised as stressful, emotionally linked responses occur that result in vulnerability to illness.

Certain characteristics, including social support, self-efficacy, and internal locus of control, seem to decrease the relationship between stress and illness. Two models explain the process by which these characteristics might influence well-being. One model suggests that the person is protected, or buffered, from the potentially pathogenic influence of stressful events. In this case, these characteristics would be related to well-being only (or primarily) for individuals under stress (Cohen & Wills, 1985, p. 310). The alternative model suggests that health strengths have a beneficial effect regardless of whether the person is under stress.

Some research suggests that certain personality characteristics reduce the perception of stress or increase resistance to stress and thus may be considered health strengths. In her theory of hardiness, Kobasa (1979) assumed that life is always changing and thus is inevitably stressful. However, people who have a sense of commitment (an overall sense of purpose), control (a belief that one can influence the course of events), and challenge (a view of change as opportunity and incentive for personal growth) are thought to be more resistant to stress. In coherence theory, Antonovsky (1987) proposed that confidence in comprehensibility (a cognitive sense that information is consistent, clear, and ordered), manageability (a belief that resources are adequate to meet demands), and meaningfulness (a motivational commitment and engagement) provides generalized resistance resources and promotes health.

Strategies for Lifestyle Behavior Change

A **lifestyle behavior change** means that people assume different activities in multiple aspects of their lives. The idea of changing a health behavior is uncomfortable for many people. Deeply ingrained habits, even harmful ones, can be difficult to change, and most people have difficulty making even minor changes. According to Westberg and Jason (1996, pp. 147–148), people tend to resist change because change of behavior may:

- require giving up pleasure (e.g., eating high-fat ice cream).
- create an unpleasant feeling (e.g., doing certain exercises).
- cause overt pain (e.g., discontinuing addictive substances).
- produce stress (e.g., facing social situations without alcohol).
- jeopardize social relationships (e.g., engaging in unprotected adolescent sex).
- seem unimportant anymore (e.g., in the case of older individuals).
- require alteration in self-image (e.g., in the case of a hard-working executive learning how to relax).

As a result, giving up long-standing habits and attitudes is not easy for most people.

Given that health behavior change is difficult for most people, Westberg and Jason (1996, pp. 148–150) suggested that to promote "what it takes" to make meaningful, lasting changes in lifestyle, the individual should:

- endorse the need for change.
- have "ownership" of the need for change.
- feel that there is more to gain than to lose.
- develop an enhanced sense of self-worth.
- identify realistic goals and workable plans.
- seek gradual change rather than a "quick fix."
- have patience.
- address starting new behaviors, instead of just focusing on what behaviors should be stopped.
- practice new behaviors.
- seek the support of family, friends, colleagues, and/or health professionals.
- gain positive reinforcement for the desired behavior.
- have a strategy for monitoring progress and making needed changes.
- seek constructive feedback.
- have a mechanism for follow-up to reduce backsliding.

Learning how to help people adopt and sustain healthy attitudes and habits is a challenge for health professionals. "There are no miracle drugs available for helping people change long-standing patterns of living. Simply telling people to stop smoking, eat less fat, have safe sex, exercise more, discontinue their abusive practices, or reduce their life stresses seldom works" (Westberg & Jason, 1996, p. 146). Clients often do not follow the advice of nurses or physicians, particularly when authoritarian "orders" are given. Clients must be actively involved as collaborative partners who assess their current health, develop a health promotion plan, and monitor its effectiveness. Rewards facilitate adherence to health promotion plans. The nurse can best assist in promoting and changing health behaviors by providing education (see Box 5.2, Professional Prototypes, "Teaching the Benefits of Exercise"), facilitating changes (e.g., positive reinforcement for adhering to a plan), and sustaining

 5.2 Professional Prototypes

Teaching the Benefits of Exercise

Disease Prevention/Treatment

Exercise…

- Reduces the lipids and lipoproteins that are associated with atherosclerosis development, helping prevent cardiovascular disease and stroke.
- Has antiinflammatory effects by reducing C-reactive protein and white blood cells associated with cardiovascular disease.
- Reduces fibrinogen levels, thereby reducing thrombus formation.
- Is associated with a reduced incidence of some types of cancer (colon, breast, endometrial, lung) and cancer recurrence (breast).
- Stabilizes the release of insulin and reduces the risk for type 2 diabetes mellitus and metabolic syndrome.
- Increases bone density.
- Slows the loss of bone density.
- Reduces pain associated with arthritis.

Health Promotion

Exercise…

- Improves muscle strength and flexibility.
- Helps maintain physical functioning status.
- Improves cognitive function.
- Improves quality of sleep.
- Reduces depression and anxiety.
- Releases endorphins, resulting in increases in feeling good (could become addictive if exercise is extreme).
- Reduces body mass index and core body fat.
- Increases endurance, leading to improved sustainability of independent execution of activities of daily living.
- Reduces the risk of cardiovascular disease, type 2 diabetes, metabolic syndrome, and some forms of cancer.
- Improves strength and balance, reducing the risk for fall and injury.
- Increases longevity; people who are physically active for 7 hours a week have a 40% lower risk of early death.

From Centers for Disease Control and Prevention. (2020). *Benefits of physical activity.* Retrieved September 13, 2020, from https://www.cdc.gov/physicalactivity/basics/pa-health/

positive health behaviors (e.g., reminding clients of how they felt before they started the health promotion plan).

According to Prochaska, Redding, and colleagues (1994), some of the most frequently replicated strategies and techniques to help clients modify behaviors include:

- Consciousness raising
- Self-reevaluation
- Environmental reevaluation
- Self-liberation
- Social liberation
- Helping relationships
- Stimulus control
- Counterconditioning
- Reinforcement management

During the contemplation stage of behavior change, consciousness raising occurs as the individual seeks information. Nurses can help this process by providing informational resources so that the individual can make informed decisions and consider incentives for and barriers to change. In addition, nurses can help assess the knowledge and interest of family members (significant others) to ensure support for the client about to make a lifestyle change. It may also be helpful for the individual to talk with others who have successfully made the contemplated changes.

As movement occurs toward the preparation and action stages of change, individuals assess and evaluate themselves and their environments. They consider how the current behavior (negative or problem) affects their physical well-being, interpersonal relationships, and personal values and aspirations. Questions that might arise include "Will I like myself better as a (thinner, nonsmoking, less stressed) person?" "Is my environment supportive of the proposed changes?" and "Do I believe that I am able to make and continue the changes needed?" The assumption is that changes will not occur unless they are congruent with a person's self-concept. For some people, introduction of a new lifestyle change produces anxiety and they may turn to nurses for guidance and support.

A strategy that can assist with self-liberation and social liberation is cognitive restructuring. Cognitive restructuring involves changing one's thoughts, images, and attitude about the self as well as the ability to see the capability of making desired changes. The nurse's role is to help clients clarify the messages clients give themselves about their health and health-related behaviors. Certain beliefs can be irrational. Positive affirmations and imagery repeated several times daily can assist clients in believing and thinking more positively about their power to make desired lifestyle changes.

Helping relationships with family members, friends, colleagues, or health care professionals can be critical

in assisting individuals to progress through the preparation, action, and maintenance stages of change. For some people, self-help groups have been instrumental in modeling, supporting, and reinforcing desired behavior.

Controlling stimuli that precede previous behavior and newly acquired desired behavior helps the action and maintenance stages of change. These activities must be personally relevant for the individual client, such as a postcard, text message, or email reminder for a mammography screening; a personal call or electronic message from the nurse to encourage continued exercise; or a scheduled group meeting (face-to-face or virtually) to practice relaxation. Consistency of setting, context, and time facilitates the development of a new habit. For example, the client can be encouraged to exercise in a consistent place, early each morning before starting other daily activities.

Counterconditioning to break an undesirable association between a stimulus and a response can be desirable during the latter part of the action stage and during the maintenance stage. Undesirable associations that create a negative emotional response to the new behavior can occur. For example, many people indicate that exercising can become boring. The nurse can encourage a varied routine, walking outside when the weather permits, going to a fitness center, and exercising with a partner to counteract boredom.

Reinforcement management is an effective strategy, especially during the preparation and action stages of change. Positive messages or rewards for desired behaviors increase the likelihood that the behavior will be repeated. When negative messages or undesired consequences occur, the individual is less likely to repeat the behavior. Immediate reinforcement of the desired behavior is important, especially in the early phases of change. Personal devices that monitor a person's number of steps provide immediate feedback for walkers, joggers, and runners. Sometimes personal monitoring devices can be a source of instant reinforcement for individuals who have issues with deconditioning or hypertension. However, personalized attention and positive verbal feedback are also helpful. Eventually, a desirable consequence of the behavior can become an intrinsic reward. For example, a weekly scale reading indicating decreasing weight can be a reward in itself for continuing a weight reduction diet.

The objective of these strategies is to decrease barriers and increase incentives to change behavior. Table 5.1 summarizes barriers and incentives to change.

The nurse and the client should base the choice of appropriate strategies on fostering incentives and reducing barriers, thereby promoting behavior change. Concepts in Practice, "Weight Management Success for Night Shift Nurses," demonstrates how one group of nurses applied these strategies to their own behaviors.

TABLE 5.1   Changing Behavior

Barriers	Incentives
Inaccurate knowledge	Expectation of benefit
Perceived lack of skills or abilities	Sense of personal responsibility
Perception of control	Enjoyment of the activity
Lack of access to facilities	Previous experience
Failure to acquire needed materials	Guilt
Inability to set clear goals	Support from family, peers, and/or professionals
Lack of social support	Willingness to and capability of acquiring new attitudes and required resources to change
Lack of time	Carving out time for change
Lack of motivation	Being motivated

From Leddy, S. K. (2006). *Health promotion: Mobilizing strengths to enhance health, wellness, and well-being.* F.A. Davis; Leddy, S. K., & Fawcett, J. (1997). Testing the theory of healthiness: Conceptual and methodological issues. In M. Madrid (Ed.), *Patterns of Rogerian knowing.* National League for Nursing; Murdaugh, C. L., Parson, M. A., & Pender, N. J. (2019). *Health promotion in nursing practice* (8th ed.). Pearson; Clark, C. C., & Paraska, K. K. (2014). *Health promotion for nurses, a practical guide.* Jones & Bartlett Learning.

Concepts in Practice   IDEA → PLAN → ACTION

Weight Management Success for Night Shift Nurses

Four nurses, Maria, James, Carol, and Rachel, have worked the night shift for 2 years together with nursing assistants Derek and Chris. They established a monthly potluck to celebrate holidays and birthdays. The monthly festivity involves everyone bringing their favorite foods. On other days, one of them makes a trip to the hospital cafeteria at 5:30 a.m. to get everyone breakfast. Since working together, all of them have gained at least 20 lb each.

Maria and James, who have gained the most weight, report that they are having difficulty sleeping during the daytime. Derek and Carol each have two young children at home resulting in frequent sleep interruptions. One night, Rachel complained that she was going to have to purchase another even larger set of work clothes. The others mentioned that they were going to have to do this too.

After analyzing what they had been doing, the six of them decided to stop the monthly potluck and take turns bringing in one dessert rather than everyone bringing something. They also agreed that on days off, each of them would start some type of exercise program. Rachel created a spreadsheet for weekly weigh-ins and compliance to exercise. By the end of 6 months, each of them lost at least 5 lb.

This section has addressed models and strategies for health promotion consistent with the interaction worldview of health. In the next section, models and strategies for health patterning consistent with the integration worldview for health are discussed.

Take Note!

Modifying simple lifestyle habits, incorporating health-protecting and health-promoting behaviors, and an individual's "health strengths" can increase the length and improve the quality of life. Family members, friends, colleagues, or health care professionals can provide critical support in this process.

■ QUESTIONS FOR REFLECTION

1. Take a moment to think about your lifestyle habits during the past month. What are your current health promotion strategies? What are some of your less healthy habits?
2. Outline a plan to improve one of your identified unhealthy habits.

HEALTH PATTERNING

Models for Health Patterning

For centuries, the concept of vital life energy, or chi, has been a part of some Eastern religions and cultures. For example, the ancient Chinese originated the belief that chi circulates through invisible channels called meridians that can be blocked by stressors or by living excesses. A blockage in energy flow results in energy imbalances and areas of the body with energy deficits, producing symptoms or disease. **Health patterning** involves interventions aimed at targeting any energy source or multiple energy sources within the body, mind, or spirit to promote optimal health and healing (Leddy, 2004, 2006).

Leddy's (2004, 2006) practice theory of energy (see Chapter 7, "Nursing Models and Theories") proposed that consciousness or focused attention by the nurse can pattern client–nurse energy by clearing (transforming); conveying (carrying); coursing (reestablishing free flow); conserving (decreasing disorder); converting (amplifying resonance); or connecting (promoting synchronization to promote harmony) energy.

Rogers introduced the concept of the person as an energy field interacting with an environmental energy field (see Chapter 7, "Nursing Models and Theories"). She theorized that health patterning of the human energy field occurs simultaneously and mutually with changes in the environmental energy field. The nurse (part of the environmental energy field) can influence the client's health by redistributing energy and thus repatterning the client's energy field. Nurses work with manifestations of health patterns (Leddy, 2003). Viewing individuals as energy fields provides a rationale for nontraditional healing modalities that enhance health patterns.

Health-Patterning Modalities

Leddy (2003, 2006) identified integrative nursing interventions to promote health and healing. The following interventions act on the human energy field and can be used by nurses in clinical practice:

- To release bound energy: Herbal preparations and aromatherapy
- To reestablish energy flow: Physical activity, tai chi, qigong (chi gung), and aerobic and strengthening exercises
- To release blocked energy: Touch, massage, acupressure, reflexology, applied kinesiology (touch for health), jin shin do, self-massage, the Alexander technique, the Feldenkrais method, the Trager psychophysical integration, and structural integration (Rolfing)
- To reduce energy depletion: Meditation, autogenic training to elicit the relaxation response, progressive muscle relaxation, deep breathing exercises, yoga, biofeedback, and guided imagery
- To regenerate optimal nutrition: Vitamin and mineral supplements, a high-fiber diet, ingestion of phytonutrients (e.g., those from soy, garlic, onions, deep-colored fruits and vegetables), and antioxidants (e.g., vitamins A, C, and E, selenium, coenzyme Q 10, beta-carotene)
- To restore energy field harmony: Centering, chromotherapy (color therapy), music therapy, polarity therapy, prayer, Reiki, and therapeutic touch

Other complementary interventions aimed at strengthening or restoring energy harmony include feng shui and life energy therapies such as yoga and chakra cleansing, strengthening, and healing. Healing modalities using interventions to balance, release, or restore energy have been used for centuries in Eastern cultures (Fig. 5.1). Feng shui works on the assumption that individuals have emotional energy fields running through and around their bodies, thereby creating an external aura and concentrated internal energy centers called chakras. Chakras within the human body flow with energy outside the human body. Personal ideas,

FIGURE 5.1 The balance of hot and cold energy fields represented by the yin–yang symbol is an example of viewing health from an energy field perspective and provides the basis for many complementary health-promoting and curing practices.

thoughts, and feelings mix with the world, and the energy fields interact and become one. Feng shui incorporates chi, which is vital energy than runs through all things conveying information from one thing to another (Shumsky, 2019; Tchi, 2019). Tchi (2019) and Shumsky (2019) explain that the chi in the seven chakras relates to the aspects of a person's character. The locations of the chakras are presented in Table 5.2 along with colors that may be used for the strengthening or healing of each chakra (Shumsky, 2019; Tchi, 2019). People also have auras or outer energy fields that project the energy within the inner body, thereby enabling the life energy within to connect with the world and engage with and use the vast array of cosmic information (Shumsky, 2019).

Chi has two opposing but complementary forms: yin and yang. Yin is slower, cooler, and more dispersed, whereas yang is hotter, faster, and more compressed. Most of the time, it is healthy to be more of one form than the other. However, if one form becomes too dominant, an imbalance occurs that results in health problems. Chi energies interact with each other in a positive or negative manner. In feng shui, complex interactions (e.g., a person's position, the location of objects within the physical environment, and the magic nine patterns of chi [the magic square determines the flow of chi]) serve as the basis for timing events, arranging a home or work space, decorating, and remediating personal

TABLE 5.2 The Seven Chakras

Name	Location	Color	Influences
Crown	Top of head	Pale violet	Spirituality, peace, bliss, and enlightenment
Brow or midbrain	Between the eyebrows	Indigo	Intelligence, inspiration, intuition, insight, and wisdom
Throat	Throat	Blue	Expression in all forms, integrity, creativity, and listening
Heart	Center chest	Green	Emotional feelings, giving and receiving love, empathy, compassion, acceptance, and forgiveness
Solar plexus or stomach	Midway between the chest and navel	Yellow	Responsibility, motivation, power, prosperity, and gut feelings
Sacral or abdomen	8 cm (3 in.) below the navel	Orange	Vitality, sexual pleasure, generation of new ideas, flexibility, and ability to give and receive nurturance
Root or reproductive organs	Spinal base near genitals	Red	Survival, stability, assertiveness, self-worth, good judgment, desire, and grounding

From Shumsky, S. (2019). *The big book of chakras and chakra healing: How to unlock your seven energy centers for healing, happiness, and transformation.* Weiser Books.

problems (Shumsky, 2019). Concepts in Practice, "Using the Human Energy Field," demonstrates how awareness of your energy field can affect your daily life and may help you accomplish your goals.

Concepts in Practice IDEA ⟶ PLAN ⟶ ACTION

Using the Human Energy Field

Geena, a nursing student, is trying to start a written assignment for a class but is experiencing writer's block. Using information about the chakras, she pushes her chair back from her computer, closes her eyes, and visualizes her throat chakra. During the visualization, Geena sees the chakra turn from a pale to a vivid, iridescent peacock blue. She speaks aloud the idea generated immediately after the chakra changed colors and then types what she said into the computer. After reviewing what has been entered, Geena is pleased with the results and continues working on the assignment until it is completed.

Geena's fellow nursing student, Minh, uses a different technique when she has a difficult writing assignment. Minh always makes certain that she is facing north as she writes. According to feng shui, facing north is a good position to access deep creativity and to produce individualistic, original work.

Many of the interventions that act on the human energy field have yet to be scrutinized through double-blind controlled scientific studies. In 2007, the National Institutes of Health's Center for Complementary and Alternative Medicine reported that 38% of American adults and 12% of American children used some form of complementary or alternative medical therapy. Because of the prevalence of use, the National Institutes of Health National Center for Complementary and Integrative Health (NCCIH) provides research grants for basic and applied research to substantiate the use of complementary healing modalities. In 2020, the NCCIH funded one study that reported that acupuncture reduces general systemic inflammation and another study that reported the helpful effects of Kundalini yoga for adults living with general anxiety disorder (NCCIH, 2020b). One grant-funded study found that mindfulness mediation reduces pain levels while bypassing human opioid receptors (Chen, 2016). According to the NCCIH (2020a), more than 30% of adults and approximately 12% of children use some form of complementary or alternative strategies other than mainstream medical care to manage health issues or promote health. Because of the vast numbers of complementary and alternative health practices, the NCCIH no longer collects generalized data about the use of all practices. Their aim now is to scientifically substantiate specific health practices (NCCIH, 2020b).

Additional published studies contain increasing evidence that noninvasive complementary therapies, especially those that require the client's active participation, have tangible and highly desirable outcomes for health and healing. In fact, nursing licensing examinations in Europe contain information about the safe use of herbs and essential oils. Before using complementary interventions with clients, however, the nurse must be educated about how each may affect physiology and their potential adverse effects (Dossey, 2016). In the future, nurses will be increasingly expected to incorporate patterning methods as an integral part of clinical practice.

Take Note!
A focus on client energy fields provides a rationale for nontraditional healing modalities that enhance health patterns.

IMPLICATIONS OF THE NURSE'S VIEW OF HEALTH FOR ROLE PERFORMANCE

A positive model of health emphasizes personal strengths and power that are resources for health, wellness, and well-being. Personal strengths include having meaning, goals, and connections (with other persons and/or a higher being) in life. Personal power includes self-perceptions of capability, control, choice, and the capacity to cope with life challenges with confidence (Leddy, 2006). The integrative worldview supports the belief that nurses work with people who all display areas of strength and weakness in health pattern manifestations at any specific time. The effects of the nurse on client manifestations of patterns are complex and nonlinear. Individuals entrenched in reductionism or who espouse an interaction worldview may find this approach confusing and perhaps even nonscientific.

In trying to improve the quality of health of clients and the self, the nurse is obligated to fulfill roles that incorporate promoting health, systematically and strategically planning changes, and using the strengths displayed by the client. Note that the term "promotion and maintenance of health" was missing. "Maintenance" is an obsolete concept because wellness (health) is an active process in which life moves forward, and the client is always evolving. The nurse may promote well-being and may restore perceptions of well-being, but the process of health does not permit the status quo that the term "maintenance" implies.

If health is a process and if nurses believe that nursing focuses on the person's responses as a whole to the environment and to a perception of well-being, then nurses have a basis for a variety of professional roles when clients perceive a sense of harmony, vitality, and ability; when they can learn most effectively how to enhance their personal strengths and gain greater control of their lives; and when they perceive a lack of harmony, feel consumed by weakness, and feel vulnerable (the illness state).

SELF-CARE OF THE NURSE

This chapter has described strategies the nurse can use to help promote or protect the health of the client. In the next section, the emphasis is on self-care strategies nurses can use to promote their own health and personal and professional well-being.

Professional Well-Being

In 2019, the National Academy of Medicine and National Academies of Science, Engineering, and Medicine assembled a 17-member committee representing all members of the interprofessional health care team to examine the known scientific evidence regarding the causes and consequences of clinician burnout and to identify actions that would support professional well-being. Committee members reviewed over 4,000 articles and drafted a report. The report was then subjected to peer review. It developed a roadmap for promoting professional well-being and to reduce the incidence of burnout of all members of the health care team. The committee combined definitions to arrive at a definition of well-being as a multifaceted concept (National Academies of Sciences, Engineering, and Medicine, 2019). They used the definition of "worker well-being" developed by Chari and colleagues (2018) that defined this as "an integrative concept that characterizes the quality of life with respect to the individual's health, and work-related environmental, organizational, and psychosocial factors." "Well-being" is the "experience of positive perceptions and the presence of constructive conditions at work and beyond that enables workers to thrive and achieve their full potential" (p. 590). Chari and colleagues also included factors like being satisfied with work, finding meaning in work, having a high-quality work life, feeling engaged at work, and finding professional fulfillment in work.

The committee used a systems approach to develop a model of contributors to **professional well-being**. They identified work system factors of the external environment, the health care organization itself, and interactions associated with frontline care delivery as contributors to professional well-being.

Because each health team member is an individual, the model specifies that there are mediating factors that influence the outcomes of professional well-being. The study identified the following mediating factors that contribute to or deflate professional well-being: personality and temperament, individual coping strategies, and strength of personal relationships and support systems. When work system factors become imbalanced, they can either contribute to professional well-being or result in clinician burnout.

Stress and Burnout

A stressful work environment in nursing is often due to the pressure that is put on nurses by the external organizational forces that determine work conditions. The health care system contributes to nurse burnout through multiple regulations, inadequate staffing, heavy workloads, mandatory overtime, simultaneous competing tasks, reimbursement issues, inadequate professional input into work processes, and lack of perceived administrative and interprofessional team support. Sometimes, a nurse may feel as though client care is occurring similar to assembly line work with the goal of moving clients in and out of the system as quickly as possible to reduce costs. Client care protocols that streamline care and reduce chances for error leave little room for person-centered care. Little time is available to develop therapeutic client relationships and do the small things for clients that make big differences. With reduced client contact, nurses frequently cannot see the outcomes of nursing interventions. Nurses sometimes compromise values and beliefs about what constitutes safe, high-quality, effective care because of pressure to focus on employer financial agendas (especially in for-profit organizations). Nurses become distressed when they cannot deliver the type of care they want to provide. If left alone, the distress becomes the state of emotional and physical apathy and exhaustion known as **burnout**.

The more conscientious nurses, who have an intrinsic need to give their best, are most vulnerable to burnout. These nurses sometimes strive for perfection in their practice, increasing the likelihood of compromised mental wellness. When unable to provide the care that they want to give, the nurse will either leave the profession or the current position, lower their standards and approach care apathetically, or continually revolt against the system that fails to place nursing care as a priority (National Academies of Science, 2019).

Nurses share three burnout risk factors with other caregiving professionals. The first is denial exhibited by minimizing or avoiding naming the stresses encountered in daily practice. The second is self-blame when the nurse fails to recognize the dysfunctional aspects of health care delivery and fails to acknowledge what is outside of their span of control. The third is the discouragement that occurs when nurses fail to meet personal professional goals, especially if they are related to a care error, failure to detect a subtle change in a client's condition that evolves into a life-or-death situation, or caring for a person who is dying (Wicks & Laskowski-Jones, 2020).

A person becomes overstressed when demands exceed perceived resources. Some stress is inevitable and may be positive when it results in energizing the person. However, more stress than can be managed is associated with physical, mental, emotional, and behavioral symptoms in people, including health care providers. Some of the more common symptoms of unhealthy stress in nurses and other practitioners include:

- Sleep disturbances and fatigue
- Appetite changes; increases or losses
- Reduced abilities to think and concentrate
- Frequent tardiness or absences from work
- Substance abuse
- Sudden mood swings
- Deep resentment of clients (National Academies of Science, 2019)

If a nurse is constantly exposed to a situation in which demands exceed resources, the nurse's energy gradually becomes depleted, culminating in burnout. Stressful events may be perceived as either challenges that lead to positive growth or threats that can lead to negative consequences. Escalating and continual emotional overload is a common factor in burnout. When nurses experience constant exposure to clinical practice situations that demand continual work in overloaded and stressful conditions, they experience reduced efficiency, irritability, a sense of constant pressure against time, diminished motivation, poor judgment, accidents, and care errors (National Academies of Science, 2019). In professional nursing practice, care errors may sometimes be fatal. The threat of potentially making a fatal error exacerbates stress levels in clinical practice.

During the COVID-19 pandemic, many nurses worked in situations in which they could not provide the type of nursing care they wanted. For nurses working directly with individuals infected with COVID-19, they saw many of their clients deteriorate and die. Visitor limitations to prevent further spread of the virus meant many clients died without the presence of family and significant others. Nurses frequently filled this void. The constant exposure to human suffering and death along with being required to compromise one's values and actions related to the quality of nursing care took a toll on nurses and significantly increased nurse and care provider burnout.

The best time to think about burnout is before it happens. Answers to questions such as "Do I feel little enthusiasm for doing my job?" "Do I feel tired even with adequate sleep?" and "Do I have too much to do and too little time in which to do it?" can help the nurse identify symptoms and sources of job stress and signs of impending burnout (Davis et al., 2019). Box 5.3, Learning, Knowing, and Growing, "Managing Job Stress," provides suggestions for the ways to manage nursing job stress. Many of the strategies require that the nurse take time to assess current working conditions, determine possible actions, and make attitudinal and/or behavioral changes.

Techniques to Enhance Well-Being

Some nurses have innate or learned resilience. **Resilience** is a personality characteristic that helps people adapt to change and bounce back repeatedly after exposure to multiple, stressful situations. For nurses, resilience also enhances the ability to evolve into a more mature and deeper person and professional nurse (Wicks & Laskowski-Jones, 2020). Characteristics of resilient nurses include an internal locus of control, more socially interactive with others, high levels of empathy, positive self-image, and an optimistic approach to life (Turner & Kaylor, 2015). Methods to develop resilience are also health-enhancing techniques that can be used to avoid burnout, promote health and well-being, and reframe stressors into challenges. These techniques include mindfulness (which can include meditation),

stress management, affirmations, refuting irrational ideas, social support, values clarification, and taking care of oneself.

The practice of **mindfulness** is another technique to enhance well-being. Mindfulness is focusing exclusively on the present moment, and when thought strays away from it, a conscious effort is expended to bring oneself back to the present. Meditation is a practice that centers this idea. When being mindful, individuals become aware of how they are reacting to current life situations and challenges. They can identify negative thoughts, distress, or unhelpful reactions that may arise. By practicing mindfulness, nurses (and all others) can develop self-compassion, "the capacity to love ourselves unconditionally" (Mariolle, 2020, p. 1). Nurses who have compassion for themselves possess self-awareness and self-acceptance, and they approach themselves with kindness, understanding, and forgiveness when mistakes occur. This facilitates the ability to set realistic expectations, learn from unsuccessful attempts, display patience, recognize that many things in life take time, and persevere when encountering difficult challenges.

Stress Management

In life (and nursing practice), perfection is impossible. However, given that stressors are an inevitable part

---

5.3 Learning, Knowing, and Growing

Managing Job Stress

- Identify sources of job stress.
- Set realistic goals and priorities.
- Avoid procrastination.
- Say "no" when offered special projects or opportunities.
- Remove workplace clutter.
- Develop and maintain trusting, mutual, and meaningful collegial relationships with coworkers (and people outside the work setting).
- Adopt an attitude that change is a challenge rather than an inconvenience.
- Cast off the perception that nurses are victims.
- Inject fun and humor in the work setting.
- Create a positive environment by looking at the bright side of adversity.
- Take control over nursing work processes.
- Participate in decision making.

- Schedule time to eat a healthy meal or snacks each day while at work.
- Consume a healthy diet (a balanced diet with moderation in refined sugars).
- Take responsibility for successes and failures.
- Take a 15- to 20-minute mini-vacation daily while on the job by going to a quiet place to relax (e.g., progressive relaxation, deep breathing exercises, meditation, or prayer with your pager and/or cell phone turned off).
- Confront work issues directly with the individuals involved.
- Engage in a daily regimen of enjoyable physical exercise.
- Take vacations and personal days when needed.
- Get adequate sleep (7–8 hours per night for most people).
- Balance your work and personal life.

From Davis, M., Eshelman, E. R., & McKay, M. (2019). *The relaxation and stress reduction workbook* (7th ed.). New Harbinger Productions, Inc.; Anselmo, J. (2016). Relaxation. In C. C. Barrere, M. A. Blasko-Helming, D. A. Shields, & K. Avino (Eds.), *Holistic nursing, a handbook for practice* (7th ed.). Jones & Bartlett Learning; Mariolle, T. S. (2020). *Mindful self-compassion practical strategies to cultivate self-awareness and nurture emotional well-being*. Rockridge Press.

of personal and professional interactions, a number of techniques have been proposed in the literature as positive ways to build strength, avoid burnout, and promote well-being (National Academies of Science, 2019). First, it is necessary to identify sources of stress and be aware of tension buildup and situations that are likely to prove stressful. Nurses should try to get in touch with their bodies and learn their bodily reactions to and manifestations of stress (e.g., sweaty palms, tightening of back and neck muscles, dry mouth). If signs of stress are recognized early, it is possible to start stress-relieving exercises that can keep the effects of stress from increasing (see Box 5.4, Learning, Knowing, and Growing, "Stress Reduction and Supportive Noninvasive Modalities").

It is important for nurses to take care of themselves first before attempting to meet someone else's needs (Turner & Kaylor, 2015). Optimal time management allows people to focus on their most important goals (see Box 5.5, Learning, Knowing, and Growing, "Time Management Strategies to Achieve Goals"). Goal achievement requires setting time aside to set realistic goals, determining an

---

5.4 Learning, Knowing, and Growing

Stress Reduction and Supportive Noninvasive Modalities

- Make the environment conducive to relaxation rather than overstimulation by adjusting the noise, room temperature, and lighting.
- Follow good health practices by eating nutritious foods; avoiding excessive caffeine, simple carbohydrates ("junk food"), and food additives; and taking supplemental vitamins (A, C, E, and the B-complex group).
- Engage in regular physical activity (exercise).
- Get ample and regular rest and sleep.
- Instead of coffee and cigarette breaks, enjoy short relaxation exercises, recline in a quiet area, or listen to relaxing music.
- Adopt and care for a pet.
- Practice mindfulness and relaxation.
- Get in touch with nature.

- Build leisure activities into the day, such as engaging in a hobby.
- Take vacations and breaks from routine work.
- Use alternative therapies, such as therapeutic massage, guided imagery, progressive relaxation, meditation, yoga, herbs, or aromatherapy.
- Use herbs (e.g., Echinacea, ginseng) to protect the immune system.
- Learn how to center yourself. "The skill of relaxing in the face of stress, taking a deep breath, loosening some of the tension in your neck and shoulders, and quieting your mind for a few moments is called centering. Centering is simply regaining your physical, mental, and emotional balance in order to proceed with the task at hand" (Achterberg et al., 1994, p. 62).

5.5 Learning, Knowing, and Growing

Time Management Strategies to Achieve Goals

- Control situations as much as possible; plan your schedule to avoid too many changes or events happening at the same time.
- Organize your time to accomplish the most important goals; identify values and goals and set daily priorities accordingly.
- Set limits and be assertive.
- Say "no" to unrealistic and low-priority demands; imagine yourself protected inside a bubble.
- Reduce tasks into smaller parts to allow mastery and feelings of competence.
- Delegate responsibilities and enlist the assistance of others; never try to be "all things to all people."
- Differentiate between time urgencies that are valid and others that are needlessly created; overinvolvement leaves little time for fulfillment of personal needs and often leads to resentment and blame (Wells-Federman, 1996).

Enhancing self-esteem is another way to avoid burnout and promote well-being. Increasing self-awareness of one's positive characteristics can enhance self-esteem. Additional strategies for preventing burnout include assertive expression of thoughts and feelings, sharing with others, accepting personal shortcomings and imperfections, and maintaining a positive and tolerant attitude toward others and the world at large. One way to do this is to change the way a stressor is viewed by putting it in proper perspective to help make the stressor manageable.

To help avoid worrying, it may be helpful to practice the serenity prayer, authored by a medieval monk, St. Francis of Assisi: "God grant me the serenity to accept the things I cannot change, the courage to change the things I can, and the wisdom to know the difference." In addition, it is helpful for the nurse to try to reduce the "shoulds" and "should nots." It is reasonable, legitimate, and

(continued)

5.5 Learning, Knowing, and Growing (*continued*)

Time Management Strategies to Achieve Goals

healthy for clients to express their needs and do what is best for themselves; why do nurses perceive themselves as being different (Eliopoulos, 1999, p. 311)?

Box 5.4, Learning, Knowing, and Growing, "Stress Reduction and Supportive Noninvasive Modalities," presents stress reduction strategies that can be helpful in achieving balance and relieving stress. Many of these modalities fall within the realm of health-promoting behaviors and require that the nurse ask for help from others.

Strategies to Balance Threatening and Challenging Stress

- Develop a sense of balance among physical, mental, and spiritual dimensions.

- Get personal and social support during times of stress and distress; develop personal support systems at work.
- Find ways to maintain interest, enthusiasm, and knowledge at work by remaining alert to new ideas, learning new things, attending conferences and discussing your practice with others, giving honest positive feedback to colleagues, and hearing and accepting praise from clients and colleagues.
- Leave work behind when you go home.
- Set limits and have priorities other than work.
- Develop interests and learn new things.
- Avoid unfulfilling or burdensome relationships; minimize contact with the people who add more stress, rather than joy, to your life.
- Risk failure.

---

action plan, using personal values to determine priority goals, and delegating tasks to others.

Affirmations

Use of **affirmations**—positive declarations that facilitate identification of personal value and enhancement of self-esteem (Anselmo, 2016)—can serve as healthy alternatives to negative self-talk. An affirmation is simply a positive thought, a short phrase, or a saying that has meaning for the person. It can help change assumptions and beliefs that have negative consequences. Affirmations can be important in reinforcing new ways of thinking and behaving from moment to moment (Davis et al., 2019; Mariolle, 2020). They are statements that can be selected to reaffirm new intentions, increase the clarity of goals, and help the nurse assume responsibility for actions. When starting to feel upset, anxious, frustrated, sad, or

overwhelmed, the nurse can stop and examine their internal monologue and simply challenge that monologue with language that is more affirming, such as:

- I can ask for what I need.
- I can take care of myself.
- I'm doing the best I can.
- I can find alternatives to problems.
- I can meet my needs.
- I care for myself, and I care for others.

Initially, using affirmations may seem superficial and uncomfortable, but as the internal monologue is changed, you will begin to notice changes in behavior and in the environment (Mariolle, 2020). Negative thought patterns of others may derail efforts of effective affirmation use. Box 5.6, Learning, Knowing, and Growing, provides guidelines for the use of affirmations for personal and professional growth.

5.6 Learning, Knowing, and Growing

Guidelines for the Use of Affirmations

1. Find a calm, quiet location away from the hectic environment. Turn off all portable electronic devices. Take three to five deep breaths, breathing slowly with maximal inspirations and blowing out through pursed lips. Use the statements to name, claim, frame, and aim one's roles/concerns/issues. It is critical to use the first person singular pronoun "I" in all generated statements.
   - Naming (identifying roles/concerns/issues)
     - What occurred that triggered the negative reaction of stressful situation?

   - What is the issue precisely?
   - "I am a good, kind, compassionate nurse with special knowledge and skills to share with others."
   - "I can remain calm and in control when I disagree with others."
   - Claiming (clarifying role/concerns/issues)
     - "By taking care of myself, I can provide better care to the people I serve."
     - "By confronting issues that impact the quality of nursing care, I am a better nurse."

5.6 Learning, Knowing, and Growing

Guidelines for the Use of Affirmations

- "My loving kindness to others is a sign of personal and professional strength."
- Framing (specifying the importance of what you do)
  - "I provide essential services to clients, colleagues, and other health team members."
  - "My contributions are as important as everyone else's."
  - "I provide great value to all care situations."
  - "I am a valued member of the health care team."
- Aiming (positive action to attain the desired target outcome)
  - "I am becoming more comfortable in acknowledging the strengths I bring to the table as a team member."
  - "It is easier for me to see the differences that I make in the lives of others."

- "I am able to do my job/fulfill my role at a high level with ease."

2. Select one of the affirmations and say it to yourself or write it 10 to 20 times daily while listening to your internal gut response to it.
3. Carry your chosen affirmation with you (e.g., on video, in your smart phone, on an index card, posted on your car dashboard, formatted into your computer screensaver) so that you can read it throughout the day.
4. Build in a healthy, personal reward for using the affirmations on a daily basis.
5. Do not become frustrated by unrealistic expectations for positive results because effective use of affirmations takes much time and practice.
6. You can substitute any personal role for your role as a professional nurse.

From Clark, C. (1996). *Wellness practitioner: Concepts, research and strategies* (2nd ed.). Springer; Clark, C. C., & Paraska, K. K. (2014). *Health promotion for nurses, a practical guide.* Jones & Bartlett Learning; Anselmo, J. (2016). Relaxation. In C. C. Barrere, M. A. Blasko-Helming, D. A. Shields, & K. Avino (Eds.), *Holistic nursing, a handbook for practice* (7th ed.). Jones & Bartlett Learning; Jackson, C. (2012). Ballistic holistic nurses: Developing ourselves as healers. *Holistic Nursing Practice, 26,* 117–119. https://doi.org/10.1097/HNP.0b013e318252e6e0

Take Note!
Constant exposure to situations in which demands exceed resources will culminate in burnout. Practicing self-care through stress reduction, life balance, affirmations, and other modalities can mitigate the risk of burnout.

Refuting Irrational Ideas

In a system called rational emotive therapy, Ellis and Harper (1961) proposed that emotions are not caused by actual events. In between the event and the emotion, they identified realistic or unrealistic self-talk that produces negative or irrational emotions. Accordingly, the person's own thoughts, directed and controlled by the individual, are what create anxiety, anger, and depression. However, irrational self-talk can be changed, and the stressful emotions change with it (Davis et al., 2019).

At the root of all irrational thinking is the assumption that things are done to someone. Statements that interpret experience as catastrophic (e.g., a momentary chest pain is a heart attack) or absolute (e.g., I "should," "must," "ought," "always," or "never") are examples of irrational thinking. Other examples are presented in Box 5.7, Learning, Knowing, and Growing, "Examples of Irrational Ideas."

5.7 Learning, Knowing, and Growing

Examples of Irrational Ideas

- It is possible to please everyone all of the time.
- Complete competence and perfection are possible in everything.
- Things can always be as I want them to be.
- Misery comes from external factors.
- The unknown, uncertain, and potential dangers instill great fear in me.
- I need to rely on others at all times.
- Avoiding life's difficulties and responsibilities is easier than facing them.
- The past directs the present and the future.
- Constant relaxation and leisure lead to happiness.

- I am the only one capable of doing the job properly.
- Life situations and other people are the source of the pressure I feel.
- It is possible to have it all, all the time.
- I am responsible for everything that happens.
- Genetics dictate my reactions and life outcomes.
- It is impossible to control my emotions.
- Just getting over things is easy.
- Contributions I make to the world are unimportant.
- All my problems are my fault.
- There is one single best approach to life.

From Davis, M., Eshelman, E. R., & McKay, M. (2019). *The relaxation and stress reduction workbook* (7th ed.). New Harbinger Productions; Jones & Bartlett Learning; Mariolle, T. S. (2020). *Mindful self-compassion practical strategies to cultivate self-awareness and nurture emotional well-being.* Rockridge Press.

Irrational ideas can be disputed and eliminated through a process of rational thinking that includes the following:

- Writing down the objective facts of the event
- Writing down self-talk, rational and irrational
- Focusing on your emotional response
- Questioning the rational support (e.g., evidence) for and against an irrational idea
- Identifying the worst and best things that could happen
- Substituting alternative self-talk (Davis et al., 2019)

Social Support

Colleagues can provide the insights and perspectives necessary to cope with commonly shared experiences. Acknowledging emotional pain and seeking support from one's professional colleagues who understand are effective coping strategies. Practicing collegiality builds valuable social support networks, shows coworkers that your value their opinions, enhances teamwork, and fosters positive working relationships (National Academies of Science, 2019). The following are possible ways of developing and enhancing coworker collegiality and strengthening a professional support network:

- Acknowledge colleagues for the contributions they make to the team.
- Expect the best from yourself and those with whom you work.
- Model the values you believe.
- Take responsibility for your health and well-being, and encourage others to do the same.
- Establish a mentoring or buddy system.
- Make decisions based on solid evidence and the profession's ethical values.
- Establish a support group to help deal with the feelings that can arise from professional practice.
- Be supportive, but refer colleagues to professional support when needed.

Values Clarification

It may be helpful to consider why, despite the drawbacks, nursing can be so rewarding. Editors at Nursing 2020 magazine (Nursing Top Ten Rewards, 2000) compiled the following list of 10 values, or "qualities that make nursing great," based on the interviews with 20 seasoned nurses. These values remain relevant today:

- A way to make a difference
- The human connection
- Flexibility
- The chance to use all of yourself
- Long-term security
- The chance to mentor
- A connection between technology and humanity
- Respect

- Personal growth
- Personal rewards

A process known as **values clarification** can be used to try to identify the values that are most significant for an individual (Clark, 1996, p. 19). Being able to practice nursing without compromising personal values fosters satisfaction for many nurses (National Academies of Science, 2019; Turner & Kaylor, 2015). Spending time clarifying personal and professional values enables nurses to identify self-care priorities.

1. Prizing and cherishing
   - Learn to set priorities, become aware of what you are for or against, begin to trust your inner experiences and feelings, and examine why you feel as you do.
   - Clearly communicate personal values and actively listen to others as they share theirs.
2. Choosing
   - Choose freely by examining values that others have imposed on you.
   - Choose thoughtfully between alternatives by examining the process by which you choose and by considering the possible consequences of each choice.
3. Acting
   - Try out the value choice by developing a plan of action and implementing it.
   - Evaluate what happened when you took action, and make plans to reinforce actions that support your values.

Taking Care of Oneself

Nurses have a responsibility to take care of themselves because they can be in a position to give only when their own needs have, at least to some extent, been acknowledged and satisfied. The American Nurses Association (ANA) recognized the importance of nurses taking care of themselves and declared 2017 as the Year of the Healthy Nurse (ANA, 2017). Mitchell and Cormack (1998, p. 142) have suggested ways for nurses to protect themselves from burnout, including:

- Do some honest soul searching to determine whether you're the kind of nurse who needs to express creativity and excellence and who values and displays originality and enthusiasm in the work.
- Objectively evaluate your workplace and respond proactively to achieve a more positive outcome for yourself.
- Don't assume responsibility where you have none.
- Be honest about what you can and can't do in your role given the constraints on your time and resources.
- Remember that you're not on duty 24 hours a day and that nursing is only one part of your life.
- Remember that a good job doesn't love you back, and then get your priorities straight.

- Find your own outlets for creativity.
- Don't stay in a situation that consistently fails to meet your needs; give yourself permission to leave.
- Give yourself a break.
- Create support for yourself.
- Love yourself; heal your wounds.
- Use food for physical nourishment, not as a stress reliever. Although carbohydrate-rich, protein-poor foods stimulate serotonin production, a poor diet is associated with oxidative stress and inflammation, which contribute to numerous disorders.
- Get enough sleep. Chronic stress interferes with sleep, and sleep deprivation alters a person's moods and cognitive processes.
- If the problem is a feeling of helplessness, the solution is to develop personal power.
- Try approaching each task as a challenge.
- Remember that you are here to serve, not to rescue.

Focusing on the positive sides of giving care to others can be helpful. Helping others as professional nurses is highly rewarding. The work is challenging and fulfilling, especially when nurses can see the effects of interventions. Some nurses find problem solving thrilling, especially when they have success with creative methods never before used. Some nurses derive a deep intrinsic pleasure just by knowing that they helped another person. The personal pleasure becomes enhanced when clients express gratitude, and nurses see the results of efforts to reduce human suffering.

Barriers to Self-Care

One example of a barrier to self-care is the belief that "it can't happen to me," in which nurses may feel that they will not be in danger of burnout because they are too smart or too aware to let negative feelings progress to burnout. Another issue may be rooted in the altruistic nature of many nurses, in which the client or the job may take precedence over the nurse's own health and well-being.

In recent years, nurse scholars have identified and studied the concept of compassion fatigue that happens when nurses become tired of caring for others. **Compassion fatigue** is a state of emotional, physical, social, and spiritual exhaustion that consumes a person, resulting in a pervasive decline in the desire, ability, and energy to care for others. Compassion fatigue occurs when health care professionals consistently care for traumatized individuals and arises as a vicarious trauma in which the care provider shares in the psychological and spiritual distress of the client. When compassion fatigue arises, nurses lose their ability to feel and display genuine concern for others (Clifford, 2014). A tool measuring compassion fatigue contains items related to burnout and secondary traumatic stress (Sacco et al., 2015).

In contrast, the concept of **compassion satisfaction** has recently emerged. Compassion satisfaction is a sense of fulfillment that health care professionals experience after helping persons through traumatic events (Sacco et al., 2015). To understand the magnitude of compassion satisfaction and compassion fatigue in professional nursing, Sacco and colleagues (2015) conducted a study on the incidence of compassion satisfaction and compassion fatigue in intensive care nurses (see the Focus on Research box, "Compassion Fatigue and Compassion Satisfaction in Critical Care Nurses").

FOCUS ON RESEARCH

Compassion Fatigue and Compassion Satisfaction in Critical Care Nurses

The investigators were interested in the incidence of compassion fatigue and compassion satisfaction among practicing critical care nurses in a large tertiary medical center. Participants included intensive care unit (ICU) nurses who responded to a survey that consisted of items inquiring about nurse demographic and organizational characteristics, and the Professional Quality of Life (ProQOL) tool, an instrument that measures compassion satisfaction and compassion fatigue.

The investigator compared mean scores on the ProQOL with nurse age, gender, educational level, type of critical care unit, and organizational characteristics. They found statistically significant differences in compassion satisfaction scores in several areas. Female nurses had higher compassion satisfaction scores than male nurses. Nurses between the ages of 40 and 50 years had lower compassion satisfaction scores than nurses of other ages. Nurses working in ICUs devoted to a single specialty had higher compassion satisfaction scores compared to nurses employed in multispecialty ICUs. Lower compassion satisfaction scores were found in nurses who had experienced a recent managerial change. Nurses with associate or master's degrees in nursing had higher compassion satisfaction scores compared to nurses with

(continued)

FOCUS ON RESEARCH (*continued*)

baccalaureate degrees. Nurses aged 40 to 49 years working on mixed-acuity units had higher burnout rates and higher secondary traumatic stress scores than other nurses in the study. Finally, nurses aged 50 or older had the highest compassion satisfaction scores and lower scores on burnout and secondary traumatic stress scales than nurses in other age groups.

The investigators suggested that the older nurses' higher compassion satisfaction and lower compassion fatigue scores could be the result of them being better equipped to cope with the challenges of critical care nursing because they have more life and professional nursing experience. They also proposed that managerial change is a key factor in the development of burnout of staff within a unit and may be a contributing factor to compassion fatigue. Major systems or practice change may be contributing factors to compassion fatigue.

The investigators outlined the following study limitations: (1) the cross-sectional nature of the study and the possibility that nurses completed surveys when they were having a bad day; (2) low survey response rate (38%) and low reliability of the secondary trauma subscale of the ProQOL for this sample.

The investigators outline the several clinical implications for the study. Personal nurse circumstances and the populations for which they provide care directly affect professional nurse burnout, compassion satisfaction, and compassion fatigue. Therefore, nursing administration should examine workplace environments to see what can be changed to facilitate the work of nurses as well as to recognize nurses for the work that they perform. Nurses should be given a voice in professional practice issues in which they are directly involved. Efforts should be made to create a healthy work environment in which there is effective communication among all interprofessional health team members, increased authentic collaboration, no tolerance of intimidation, provision of safe staffing patterns, meaningful recognition of nurses, and leaders who promote a caring culture, professional development, individual nurse recognition, and debriefing.

From Sacco, T. L., Ciurzynski, S. M., Harvey, M. E., & Ingersoll, G. L. (2015). Compassion satisfaction and compassion fatigue among critical care nurses. *Critical Care Nurse, 35*(4), 32–44. http://doi .org/10.4037/ccn2015392

Take Note!

Nurses must take care of themselves first. By doing so, they will be better able to continue to deal with the stresses of the work environment and advocate for the needs of their clients.

Summary and Significance to Practice

In American society, responsibility for illness has been delegated to health care professionals who have been prepared and are rewarded for delivering care to the sick. Short-term incentives and rewards to maintain health are rare for the recipients of such care; in addition, the health care system is not organized to reward health care providers for keeping clients well.

Clients must be encouraged to assume an increased concern and responsibility for their health potential. Nurses can support, facilitate, and encourage those positive skills, qualities, and plans that will promote health. The client and the nurse, based on goals and a timeline determined by the client, can then collaboratively devise interventions.

In addition, nurses need to take responsibility for self-care. Approaches to managing job stress and techniques such as stress management, affirmations, mindfulness, refuting irrational ideas, social support, values clarification, and taking care of oneself are positive techniques that can be used to avoid burnout, reframe stressors into challenges, and enhance well-being.

REAL-LIFE REFLECTIONS

Think about Nadine and Michael from the beginning of the chapter and identify the factors in their work environment that are not health-promoting. What are the stressors in your school or work environment? Why is having a colleague to share common experiences important for promoting health? What steps can you take in the short term to alleviate stress in your life? What long-term strategies can you employ to ensure you don't experience burnout in your career?

From Theory to Practice

1. Identify the factors within your lifestyle that fall into the categories of health promotion and health protection. What are the consequences of a lifestyle focused on health protection rather than health promotion?
2. Did you find some of the tips for caring for yourself helpful? If so, which ones do you plan to use? If not, why not?

Nurse as Author

Use a mobile app or https://www.supertracker.usda.gov/ to track your food and activity level for a week. Also, make a record of your social and spiritual activities for the same week. Take time and reflect on your psychological behavior for the same week, paying close attention to when you may have felt bad about yourself, gotten angry at others, experienced stress (at work and at home), felt excited or happy, and experienced a sense of calmness and tranquility. Based on your personal assessment, create a holistic plan to improve your health and well-being (you may use the Neuman System Model dimensions of health—physiologic, psychological, sociocultural, developmental, and spiritual—or another nursing theory that addresses health from a holistic perspective).

Your Digital Classroom

Online Exploration

American Heart Association: **www.heart.org**. Visit this site to learn the latest on cardiovascular disease, and refer clients and their families to this client-oriented site.

The American Holistic Nurses Association: **https://www.ahna.org**.

American Institute for Cancer Research: **https://www.aicr.org/**. Consult this site for research-based information for the prevention of cancer and healthy lifestyle information.

Association for Applied and Therapeutic Humor: **https://www.aath.org/**. Tickle your funny bone by visiting this website, and link to other health care humor sites to lift your spirits.

Healthy People 2030: **https://health.gov/healthypeople**.

National Center for Chronic Disease Prevention and Health Promotion: **https://www.cdc.gov/chronicdisease/index.htm**. Learn the latest about the prevention of communicable diseases along with

health promotion information to reduce the incidence of chronic diseases.

National Institute of Health Center for Complementary and Integrative Health: **https://nccih.nih.gov/**.

National Institutes of Health: **https://www.nih.gov/**. Read about the latest government-sponsored health research along with opportunities for funding health promotion research.

National Health Information Center: **https://health.gov/our-work/health-literacy/resources/national-health-information-center**. Learn about special days to increase awareness about important health topics.

U.S. Department of Health and Human Services Office of Health Promotion and Disease Prevention: **https://health.gov/**. Get information about food and nutrition, physical activity, health literacy, and check health care quality in the United States.

Expanding Your Understanding

1. Visit the American Holistic Nurses Association (AHNA) website and read the "About AHNA" section. Would you be interested in joining the AHNA? Why or why not?
2. Search online for one of the nursing interventions for the human energy field identified by Leddy (2003, 2006). Prepare for a class discussion about the information you find. Do you think other health team members would agree that the identified intervention would be beneficial to clients? Why or why not?

Beyond the Book

Visit the Point® at **www.thePoint.lww.com** for the activities and information to reinforce the concepts and content covered in this chapter.

REFERENCES

Achterberg, J., Dossey, B., & Kolkmeier, L. (1994). *Rituals for healing: Using imagery for health and wellness*. Bantam.

American Nurses Association. (2017). *2017—The year of the healthy nurses*. Retrieved March 26, 2017, from http://www.nursingworld.org/MainMenuCategories/ThePracticeofProfessionalNursing/2017-Year-of-Healthy-Nurse

Anselmo, J. (2016). Relaxation. In C. C. Barrere, M. A. Blasko-Helming, D. A. Shields, & K. Avino (Eds.), *Holistic nursing: A handbook for practice* (7th ed., pp. 239-268). Jones & Bartlett Learning.

Antonovsky, A. (1987). *Unraveling the mystery of health*. Jossey-Bass.

Chari, R., Chang, C.-C., Sauter, S. L., Petrun Sayers, E. L., Cerully, J. L., Schulte, P., Schill, A. L., & Uscher-Pines, L. (2018). Expanding the paradigm of occupational safety and health: A new framework for worker well-being. *Journal of Occupational and Environmental Medicine*, 60(7), 589–593. https://doi.org/10.1097/jom.0000000000001330

Chen, W. (2016). *Mindfulness meditation reduces pain, bypasses opioid receptors*. NIH Research Blog. Retrieved April 2, 2016, from https://nccih.nih.gov/research/blog/mindfulness-meditation-pain

Clark, C. (1996). *Wellness practitioner: Concepts, research and strategies* (2nd ed.). Springer.

Clifford, K. (2014). Who cares for the careers? Literature review of compassion fatigue and burnout in military health professionals? *Journal of Military and Veteran's Health*, 22(3), 53–63. https://jmvh.org/article/who-cares-for-the-carers-literature-review-of-compassion-fatigue-and-burnout-in-military-health-professionals/

Cohen, S., & Wills, T. A. (1985). Stress, social support and the buffering hypothesis. *Psychological Bulletin*, 98(2), 310–357. https://doi.org/10.1037/0033-2909.98.2.310

Crawford, G. (1982). The concept of pattern in nursing: Conceptual development and measurement. *Advances in Nursing Science*, 5(1), 1–6. https://doi.org/10.1097/00012272-198210000-00004

Davis, M., Eshelman, E. R., & McKay, M. (2019). *The relaxation and stress reduction workbook* (7th ed.). New Harbinger Productions, Inc.

Dossey, B. M. (2016). Nursing: Holistic, integral and integrative-local to global. In C. C. Barrere, M. A. Blasko-Helming, D. A. Shields, & K. Avino (Eds.), *Holistic nursing, a handbook for practice* (7th ed., pp. 3–52). Jones & Bartlett Learning.

Dossey, B. M., & Luck, S. (2016). Self assessments. In C. C. Barrere, M. A. Blasko-Helming, D. A. Shields, & K. Avino (Eds.), *Holistic nursing, a handbook for practice* (7th ed., pp. 703–716). Jones & Bartlett Learning.

Dubos, R. (1978). Health and creative adaptation. *Human Nature*, 1, 74–82.

Dunn, H. H. (1977). What high-level wellness means. *Health Values*, 1, 9–16. https://pubmed.ncbi.nlm.nih.gov/13818678/

Eliopoulos, C. (1999). *Integrating conventional and alternative therapies: Holistic care for chronic conditions*. Mosby.

Ellis, A., & Harper, R. (1961). *A guide to rational living*. Wilshire Books.

Fawcett, J. (1993). *Conceptual models of nursing* (3rd ed.). F.A. Davis.

Hall, B. A. (1981). The change paradigm in nursing: Growth versus persistence. *Advances in Nursing Science*, 3(4), 1–6. https://doi.org/10.1097/00012272-198107000-00002

Hravnak, M. (1998). Is there a health promotion and protection foundation to the practice of acute care nurse practitioners? *AACN Clinical Issues*, 9(2), 283–289. https://doi.org/10.1097/00044067-199805000-00012

Janz, N. K., & Becker, M. H. (1984). The health belief model: A decade later. *Health Education Quarterly*, 11(1), 1–47. https://doi.org/10.1177/109019818401100101

Jensen, L. A., & Allen, M. N. (1994). A synthesis of qualitative research on wellness-illness. *Qualitative Health Research*, 4(4), 349–369. https://doi.org/10.1177%2F104973239400400402

Kobasa, S. C. (1979). Stressful life events, personality and health: An inquiry into hardiness. *Journal of Personality and Social Psychology*, 37(1), 1–11. https://doi.org/10.1037//0022-3514.37.1.1

Lazarus, R. S., & Folkman, J. (1984). *Stress appraisal and coping*. Springer.

Leddy, S. K. (2003). *Integrative health promotion: Conceptual bases for nursing practice*. Slack.

Leddy, S. K. (2004). Human energy: A conceptual model of unitary nursing science. *Visions: The Journal of Rogerian Nursing Science*, 12, 14–27. https://www.thefreelibrary.com/Human+energy:+a+conceptual+model+of+unitary+nursing+science.-a0161397669

Leddy, S. K. (2006). *Health promotion: Mobilizing strengths to enhance health, wellness, and well-being*. F.A. Davis.

Logan, A. C. (2007). *The brain diet revised and expanded*. Cumberland House.

Mariano, C. (2013). Holistic nursing: Scope and standards of practice. In B. M. Dosey & L. Keegan (Eds.), *Holistic nursing, a handbook for practice* (6th ed.). Jones & Bartlett Learning.

Mariolle, T. S. (2020). *Mindful self-compassion practical strategies to cultivate self-awareness and nurture emotional well-being*. Rockridge Press.

McElligott, D. (2013). The nurse as an instrument of healing. In B. M. Dosey & L. Keegan (Eds.), *Holistic nursing, a handbook for practice* (6th ed.). Jones & Bartlett Learning.

McWilliam, C. L., Stewart, M., Brown, J. B., Desai, K., & Coderre, P. (1996). Creating health with chronic illness. *Advances in Nursing Science*, 18(3), 1–15. https://doi.org/10.1097/00012272-199603000-00002

Mitchell, A., & Cormack, M. (1998). *The therapeutic relationship in complementary health care*. Churchill Livingstone.

Murdaugh, C. L., Parson, M. A., & Pender, N. J. (2019). *Health promotion in nursing practice* (8th ed.). Pearson.

National Academies of Sciences, Engineering, and Medicine. (2019). *Taking action against clinician burnout: A systems approach to professional well-being*. The National Academies Press. https://doi.org/10.17226/25521

National Center for Complementary and Integrative Health. (2020a). *Complementary, alternative, or integrative health: What's in a name?* Retrieved March 22, 2021, from https://www.nccih.nih.gov/health/complementary-alternative-or-integrative-health-whats-in-a-name

National Center for Complementary and Integrative Health. (2020b). *Selected research results by date*. Retrieved March 22, 2021 from https://www.nccih.nih.gov/research/research-results

Newman, M. A. (1992). Prevailing paradigms in nursing. *Nursing Outlook*, 40(1), 10–13, 32. https://pubmed.ncbi.nlm.nih.gov/1570217/

Newman, M. A. (1994). *Health as expanding consciousness* (2nd ed.). Mosby.

Nursing Top Ten Rewards. (2000). *Nursing 2000*, 30(5), 42–43. https://journals.lww.com/nursing/Citation/2000/30050/Guide_to_NURSING_ORGANIZATIONS.32.aspx

Office of Disease Prevention and Health Promotion. (2017). *About Healthy People 2020*. U.S. Department of Health and Human Services. Retrieved March 26, 2017, from https://www.healthypeople.gov/2020/About-Healthy-People

Office of Disease Prevention and Health Promotion. (2020a). *Healthy People 2030, framework*. U.S. Department of Health and Human Services. Retrieved September 11, 2020, from https://health.gov/healthypeople/about/healthy-people-2030-framework

Office of Disease Prevention and Health Promotion. (2020b). *Healthy People 2030, leading health indicators*. U.S. Department of Health and Human Services. Retrieved December 27, 2020, from https://health.gov/healthypeople/objectives-and-data/leading-health-indicators

Office of Disease Prevention and Health Promotion. (2020c). *Healthy People 2030, social determinants of health*. U.S. Department of Health and Human Services. Retrieved September 11, 2020, from https://health.gov/healthypeople/objectives-and-data/social-determinants-health

Office of Disease Prevention and Health Promotion. (2020d). *Healthy People 2030, topics & objectives*. U.S. Department of Health and Human Services. Retrieved September 11, 2020, from https://www.healthypeople.gov/2020/topics-objectives

O'Keefe, J., & O'Keefe, J. (2006). *The forever young diet & lifestyle*. Andrews McMeel.

Parse, R. R. (1987). *Nursing science: Major paradigms, theories, and critiques*. W.B. Saunders.

Parsons, T. (1958). Definitions of health and illness in the light of American values and social structure. In E. G. Jaco (Ed.), *Patients, physicians, and illness*. Free Press.

Pender, N. J. (1996). *Health promotion in nursing practice* (3rd ed.). Appleton & Lange.

Pender, N. J., Murdaugh, C. L., & Parsons, M. A. (2002). *Health promotion in nursing practice* (4th ed.). Prentice Hall.

Prochaska, J. O., Redding, C. A., Harlow, L. L., Rossi, J. S., & Velicer, W. F. (1994). The transtheoretical model of change and HIV prevention: A review. *Health Education Quarterly*, 21(2), 471–486. https://doi.org/10.1177/109019819402100410

Prochaska, J. O., Velicer, W. F., Rossi, J. S., Goldstein, M. G., Marcus, B. H., Rakowski, W., Fiore, C., Harlow, L. L., Redding, C. A., & Rosenbloom, D. (1994). Stages of change and decisional balance for 12 problem behaviors. *Health Psychology*, 13(1), 39–46. https://doi.org/10.1037//0278-6133.13.1.39

Rau, T., & Wyler, S. (2007). *The Swiss secret to optimal health*. Berkeley.

Rosenstock, I. M. (1966). Why people use health services. *Milbank Memorial Fund Quarterly*, 44(3), 94–127. https://pubmed.ncbi.nlm.nih.gov/5967464/

Sacco, T. L., Ciurzynski, S. M., Harvey, M. E., & Ingersoll, G. L. (2015). Compassion satisfaction and compassion fatigue among critical care nurses. *Critical Care Nurse*, 35(4), 32–44. https://doi.org/10.4037/ccn2015392

Shumsky, S. (2019). *The big book of chakras and chakra healing: How to unlock your seven energy centers for healing, happiness and transformation*. Weiser Books.

Smith, J. A. (1981). The idea of health: A philosophical inquiry. *Advances in Nursing Science*, 3(3), 43–50. https://doi.org/10.1097/00012272-198104000-00005

Tchi, R. (2019). *Feng shui for healing: A step by step guide to improving wellness in your home sanctuary*. Rockridge Press.

Turner, S. B., & Kaylor, S. D. (2015). Neuman Systems Model as a conceptual framework for nurse resilience. *Nursing Science Quarterly*, 28(3), 213–217. https://doi.org/10.1177/0894318415585620

Twaddle, A. C., & Hessler, R. M. (1977). *A sociology of health*. Mosby.

U.S. Department of Health and Human Services. (2000). *Healthy people 2010*. Author.

U.S. Department of Health and Human Services. (2011). *HHS releases assessment of healthy people 2010 objectives*. Retrieved January 15, 2016, from http://www.healthypeople.gov/2020/about/HP2010PressReleaseOct5.doc

U.S. Department of Health and Human Services. (2020). *Leading health indicators*. Retrieved December 27, 2020, from https://health.gov/healthypeople/objectives-and-data/leading-health-indicators

Vincent, C., & Furnham, A. (1997). *Complementary medicine: A research perspective*. John Wiley & Sons.

Wells-Federman, C. L. (1996). Awakening the nurse healer within. *Holistic Nursing Practice, 10*(2), 13–29. https://journals.lww.com/hnpjournal/Abstract/1996/01000/Awakening_the_nurse_healer_within.4.aspx

Westberg, J., & Jason, H. (1996). Fostering healthy behavior: The process. In S. H. Woolf, S. Jonas, & R. S. Lawrence (Eds.), *Health promotion and disease prevention in clinical practice*. Williams & Wilkins.

Wicks, R. J., & Laskowski-Jones, L. (2020). Resilience e in a time of crisis. *Nursing*, 50(6), 49–51. https://doi.org/1097/01NURSE0000662340.86677.ef

Yu, E., Rimm, E., Qi, L., Rexrode, K., Albert, C. M., Sun, Q., Willett, W. C., Hu, F. B., & Manson, J. E. (2016). Diet, lifestyle, biomarkers, genetic factors, and risk of cardiovascular disease in the nurses' health studies. *American Journal of Public Health*, 106(9), 1616–1623. https://doi.org/10.2105/AJPH.2016.303316

6

Patterns of Knowing and Nursing Science

Certainty

Relativity

Rationalism

Empiricism

Intuition

Historicism

Postmodernism

Intermodernism

Empirical knowing

Empirical knowledge

Aesthetic knowing

Aesthetic knowledge

Personal knowledge

Personal knowing

Ethical knowledge

Ethical knowing

Sociopolitical knowing

Emancipatory knowing

Unknowing

Nursing science

Concept

Four central concepts of nursing

Theories

Nursing conceptual models

LEARNING OUTCOMES

By the end of this chapter, the learner will be able to:

1. Discuss the evolution of three systems of thought about how to organize developing knowledge in science.
2. Describe the differences among logical empiricism, historicism, and postmodernism in their philosophical approaches to the development of knowledge.
3. Explain the differences among the patterns of knowing in professional nursing.
4. Compare and contrast concepts, theories, and conceptual models.
5. Identify the four central concepts of nursing that are the focus of scientific inquiry in nursing.

REAL-LIFE REFLECTIONS

Paul, a registered nurse for 7 years, is taking a nursing research course while working on his bachelor of science in nursing degree. He believes that knowledge from "hard science" is the only way nursing can become as respected as other health care professions. He also believes that research is only useful if it directly improves client care, and he disregards conceptual or explanatory research. Last week, one of Paul's assigned clients with pancreatitis went into shock and was transferred to the intensive care unit. His colleague Jill (a nurse with 15 years of clinical experience) happened to enter the client's room just as the client started to hemorrhage. At the end of the shift, Paul thanked Jill and asked her how she was able to detect that the client needed help. Jill replied, "I just knew. I cannot explain it other than nurse's intuition. I just get this little voice that tells me to check on clients and I do." Based on this experience, Paul decides to pursue the topic of nurse intuition for his research class.

- *How do you feel about nurse's intuition?*
- *How do you think Paul's feelings about knowledge might change after he researches intuition?*

Understanding nursing's body of knowledge is essential for competent professional practice. Knowledge can be obtained from a number of sources, including experience, reflection, and values. Science is "a unified body of knowledge about phenomena that is supported by agreed-on evidence" (Meleis, 2007, p. 36). For many years, nursing scholars have debated whether professional nursing practice is a science, an art, or both (Chinn & Kramer, 2015; Meleis, 2007, 2012; Rogers, 2005; Roy, 2007; Watson, 2007). According to Rogers (1992, pp. 28–29), "Since nursing is a learned profession, it is both a science and an art. The practice of nurses, [therefore], is the creative use of [this] knowledge in human service."

The science of nursing incorporates the study of relationships among nurses, clients, and environments within the context of health. It is also the result of interrelationships among theory, practice, research, and education. Theory provides the tools to direct nursing practice. Practice provides the professional individual with the setting to apply nursing knowledge and develop and test nursing theories. Research provides the means to test theories. Education provides the means to shape belief systems and to synthesize and disseminate knowledge.

Nursing is emerging as an autonomous, distinctive professional discipline that is valued by society. As an emerging science, the nursing profession uses and builds upon knowledge developed from many disciplines through centuries of evolution.

▌ QUESTIONS FOR REFLECTION

1. What are the benefits of establishing a base of nursing science for the profession of nursing?
2. What consequences arise for the nursing profession if it fails to generate a specialized knowledge base?
3. Do you perceive nursing as an art, a science, or both?

THE EVOLUTION OF SCIENTIFIC THOUGHT

Over thousands of years, human life has greatly progressed due in large part to advances in science. It is impossible to cover each era of human history and the entire evolution of human knowledge. Therefore, this chapter addresses three systems of thought about organizing and developing human knowledge.

Ancient people understood the world through magical beliefs; people believed they were controlled by forces beyond human understanding or control.

A second way of trying to understand the world began during the scientific revolution (around 1500 CE). Science emphasized observations, measurement, and quantification as the means for understanding the world.

With Einstein's discovery of relativity in the early 20th century, people began to accept uncertainty and focused on processes that influenced human thought. The 21st century saw a movement toward using complexity theory, which espoused nonlinear interactions, emergent phenomena, continuous and discontinuous change, and unpredictable outcomes (Nicolas & Philippe, 2015).

Ancient Civilizations

The earliest civilizations differentiated the world into two parts: me (internal) and not me (external). They viewed the external world as being populated by spirits, demons, and gods who directed good and evil in the world. Humans tried to influence gods because they believed that gods were moved to action by whims and passions.

Through trial and error, people discovered that some patterns of action led to predictable outcomes, which could be reproduced as long as the procedure was followed exactly (as one would with recipes from a cookbook). Thus, in an elementary way, humans observed life phenomena sufficiently to gather many isolated facts, which were then used to make decisions about what to do. The earliest "nurses" functioned primarily from protocols and procedures based on tradition.

Because diseases, aches, and pains were assumed to be caused by gods and evil spirits, early medicine was associated with religion or magical beliefs. However, time and attention to cause and effect led to practical approaches and logical sequencing of steps for treatment. Hippocrates (460–377 BCE) was followed by Aristotle (384–322 BCE), who emphasized classification of signs and symptoms. Increasing attention was paid to exploring the mechanisms of the human body (Spradlin & Porterfield, 1984).

▌ QUESTIONS FOR REFLECTION

1. What superstitions have you encountered in your personal or professional life?
2. How do these superstitions affect your life? How might they affect your professional practice?
3. What would be the potential consequences if you allowed superstitions to guide you in professional practice?

The Search for Certainty

The evolution of mathematics and the ability to count made relationships appear more logical and the world more predictable. By 1500 CE, interest in the scientific study of humans and nature was increasing, and the philosophy of logical positivism was driving the search for **certainty** (undisputed truth). Logical positivism was based on a belief that the world was like a simple machine, but only God understood the laws by which it operated. Time and space were absolute. Time flowed smoothly and uniformly. A reductionist approach was used to identify causes to predict effects. Scientific scholars

> became engulfed in a spiral of logic and increasing certainty about quantification of relationships among absolute entities that led to concepts of truths that could be validated. . . . We could, with the use of observation, measurement, and logical reasoning, know the laws of nature. . . . All the entities that composed the whole of nature could be reduced to their smallest parts, studied and understood, and rebuilt (Spradlin & Porterfield, 1984, p. 106).

The reduction of humans into separate psyche and soma (Cartesian dualism), both of which could be measured physically, was advanced by Descartes (1596–1650), who saw humans as machines ruled by the same laws as all of nature (Spradlin & Porterfield, 1984, p. 108). The separation of mind from matter (body) and the emphasis on the person as the sum of minute parts dominated medical and nursing science for centuries until the advent (or perhaps re-emergence) of a holistic approach to health in the 20th century.

Four basic assumptions about humans and the universe are inherent in this kind of mechanistic worldview: determinism, quantity, continuity, and impersonality. Leaving no room for uncertainty, the principle of determinism reflects the belief that "nature proceeds by a strict chain of events from cause to effect, the configuration of causes at any instant fully determining the event in the next instant, and so on forever" (Ware et al., 1966, p. 127). The ability to predict comes from this principle, whereas lack of predictability and the presence of uncertainty represent ignorance.

The quantitative principle expresses the exact nature of science. It reflects the belief that science consists of "measuring things and setting up precise relations between the measurements" (Ware et al., 1966, p. 129). In this view, humans and the universe are described by numbers (e.g., spatial coordinates, time, position, amounts, and locations) that quantify physical properties, and by relations among these quantitative characteristics.

Continuity, the third principle, is concerned with the "transitions of nature from one state to another [and] express[es] the sense, deeply engrained in the outlook of the age, that the movements of nature are gradual" (Ware et al., 1966, p. 129). This principle reflects the belief that the processes involving humans and the universe are continuous.

In the fourth principle, impersonality, the scientist is viewed as an instrument, not a person. The scientist uses observation rather than imagination, passively finds order in phenomena rather than creating it, and does not permit personal influence on the phenomena under observation (Ware et al., 1966, p. 129).

Belief in these four principles led Galileo (1564–1642) and Sir Isaac Newton (1642–1727) to develop the scientific method based on a particular method of reasoning—logic. Logic encompasses principles of reasoning applicable to any branch of knowledge. Because logic is based on reason and sound judgment, it can be convincing.

The scientific method starts with asking questions. Inquiry is a technique of science. It seeks truth, information, or knowledge to solve problems. A problem is any question or matter involving doubt, uncertainty, or difficulty that needs solution. A problem can be solved by finding the answer or explanation. The most extensive investigative process of science is the systematic inquiry of research.

▮ QUESTIONS FOR REFLECTION

1. How do logic, science, and inquiry affect your daily life or professional practice?
2. What are the consequences of using logic, science, and inquiry in the nursing profession?

The Relative World of Process

By the 20th century, scientists realized that the physical world consisted of matter and forces that interact with matter, such as gravity, magnetism, and electricity. By exploring the cell, genetic mechanisms and mechanisms that influenced cellular structure and function were explained. It appeared that "the immutable laws which governed the world" were being discovered.

In the early 20th century, Albert Einstein demonstrated that the world was composed not of events, but of observations, which were relative to the place and velocity of the observer; this was the essence of his theory of **relativity**. "Any absolutes or cause-and-effect sequences [are] illusions . . . testable only in a retrospect organization of events" (Spradlin & Porterfield, 1984, p. vi). Heisenberg's (1971) and Bertalanffy's (1968) work in quantum physics led to the postulation that mass, energy, time, and space coordinates are interchangeable. All systems were considered interrelated and interdependent on a continuum of relativity and probability, and thus uncertainty.

Relativism is a theoretical approach that specifies that truth, values, and judgments differ according to circumstances and personal perceptions. Truth may only become apparent when humans have a social structure and accepted methods to allow it to emerge. Thus, what is discovered and known about science relies heavily upon the structure and processes outlined by the scientific process. Moral relativism provides the foundation for tolerance of divergent viewpoints as in the cases of when life begins, when life should end, and all other morally charged issues. New relativism focuses on the context in which events occur, thereby paving the way for different views and actions for doing what is right (Baghramian & Adam, 2016).

The implications of this different conceptual system were enormous. Continuity was replaced by discontinuity, and probability (determined statistically) replaced certainty. Emphasis was placed on patterning rather than on discrete entities, and on interactions rather than on isolated events. The scientist was no longer an isolated objective observer of events. "Man came to be seen not as a detached observer but as an irremovable part of his observations" (Ware et al., 1966, p. 148). In addition, awareness of the limitations and biases of individual perception increased, implying that truth and meaning were not absolute but were relative to history and context. Nonetheless, "while physicists have become increasingly concerned with . . . a relative world of process, biologists have until recently tended to be even more involved in the reductionistic approach to life" (Spradlin & Porterfield, 1984, p. 189).

Complexity Science and Theory

Stephen Hawking called the 21st century the "Century of Complexity." Complexity science values both the quantitative and qualitative approaches to generating knowledge (Linberg et al., 2008). As early as the 1980s, multiple disciplines noted that similar observations and discoveries were occurring in their respective fields. There appeared to be some self-organizing framework in nature and human systems; small changes to one thing seemed to affect the whole; systems engaged in complex adaptation without predictable results; interrelated nonlinear

dynamics surfaced; and complex response processes resulted in response to changes. Everything in the world appeared to be one. Nicolas and Philippe (2015) provide evidence that there are underlying computations that may indeed mathematically explain the nature of the complexity within the universe. Thus, there is a combination of both relativism and determinism that forms the nature of the universe.

QUESTIONS FOR REFLECTION

1. Which theory—relativism or complexity—do you think best applies to the profession of nursing?
2. How do the theories of relativism and complexity apply to your daily life?
3. What future impact do you foresee these theories having on professional nursing practice?
4. How does relativism affect nursing practice? How have you used relativism to justify some of your own personal or professional nursing actions?
5. What are the consequences of the use of relativism for clients, for you as a person and as a nurse, and for the nursing profession?

PHILOSOPHY OF KNOWLEDGE

Because one's belief system is critical to determining sources and methods of discovering knowledge, an understanding of the differing philosophical approaches that currently influence nursing science is critical.

Based on Plato's concepts, knowledge is considered to be the belief that has been justified through reason (Rosen et al., 2018). What constitutes adequate justification is one concern of philosophy. Philosophy considers questions such as whether there is such a thing as truth and how one can be certain that something is true. It is necessary to accept that some things can be true in order to question the truth or falseness of any particular thing. But must certainty be beyond all possible doubt, or is certainty sufficient if it is beyond logical and reasonable doubt? How does an individual acquire knowledge? What are the roles of intellect, perception, and intuition in the process of knowing?

Processes of Knowing

The three primary processes of knowing are rationalism, empiricism, and intuition. **Rationalism** involves belief in the possibility of knowing truth by thinking and by use of reason that is *a priori*, or independent of experience. **Empiricism** involves belief that the only source of certainty about knowledge is immediate experience. However, because raw experience is subject to individual perception, the emphasis must be on verification and on confirmation or refutation of observations. **Intuition** is sometimes described as "just knowing" or a "gut feeling." The source of the knowing is internal to the individual and is often perceived as occurring independently of experience or reason. It is subjective and personal in origin, though it can be validated through experience and interaction with others.

Approaches to Knowing

Logical Empiricism

Logical empiricism, a philosophical approach to the development of knowledge accepted since the 16th century, is based on the following assumptions:

1. A body of abstract, general, and universal facts and principles that explain the way the world operates is waiting to be discovered. Theories provide alternative explanations for how the body of facts and principles is ordered and systematically unified.
2. Cause-and-effect (linear) relationships can be established by using deductive processes and experimental methodology. The results are context-free generalizations that can be applied to all individuals. Truth is achieved through sensory data and controlled experiments.
3. It is necessary to control values and biases to achieve "objective" knowledge; therefore, the observer must be separated from the observed world. Science is value free. Social relevance is unimportant.
4. Theoretical reduction is an important scientific goal. It is assumed that the ultimate character of reality is best explained using the logic and simplicity of the fewest possible theoretical concepts and laws.
5. The whole is the sum of its parts. Circumscribing (reducing) observations to small parts of the whole gives better control of the data and stronger explanatory power.

Logical empiricism is synonymous with logical positivism. Logical empiricism provides guidelines for scientific process and criteria for scientific rigor. Under logical empiricism, the goal of science is "to predict, explain, and control" world events, situations, and occurrences. To identify "pure facts," scientists must remain value free while engaging in scientific methods. Nursing knowledge based on the "hard sciences" has its roots in logical empiricism (Rogers, 2005).

REAL-LIFE REFLECTIONS

Think of Paul, from the beginning of the chapter. Explain how Paul's belief in nursing knowledge based on "hard science" relies on the assumptions of logical empiricism. What classes in your nursing program curriculum are based in logical empiricism? How is the content used in these courses applicable to daily life and professional practice?

Historicism

Advanced since the 1930s under the influence of concepts such as relativity and process, **historicism** is based on the following assumptions:

1. Because "truth" is dynamic and constantly changing, what is important is the effectiveness of a theory for solving problems.
2. The whole is more than the sum of its parts. Reducing the whole to parts is counterproductive. Interrelationships and interactions are part of what must be studied.
3. An individual or a phenomenon must be studied as a whole in a natural setting. The observer is part of the setting, so interactions between the observer and the setting should be described, rather than controlled. Emphasis is on process rather than fact.
4. Multiple research traditions are desirable (e.g., theories from psychology, physiology, education) to explain different dimensions of the same phenomenon. Synthesis and development of multiple theories are encouraged.
5. Knowledge is related to context. Values, subjectivity, intuition, history, and tradition are useful for discovery.

Unlike logical empiricism, historicism emphasizes the "importance of the context and processes in which scientific activity takes place" (Rogers, 2005, p. 99). Truth and knowledge are related to context, and multiple approaches can be used to generate knowledge. Instead of being rigid and stagnant, theories become dynamic (Rogers, 2005; Sitzman & Watson, 2014; Watson, 2007); they are flexible and can be adapted to remain relevant. In professional nursing, historicism specifies that to understand the evolution of nursing knowledge and practice, one must learn about the history of the profession. Interpretation of history relies on the person who reads historical documents and examines artifacts of a specific era. Kuhn's (1970) perspective of science as a way to "solve puzzles" and Laudan's (1981) perspective of science as a means to "solve problems" provide a practical approach to the generation of nursing knowledge. For example, a complete client family history served as the standard for determining client risk for specific diseases prior to the completion of the human genome project. For individuals with no access to genetic testing, perhaps a detailed family history may be beneficial in determining future risk of disease.

Postmodernism

Postmodernism is a social movement and a philosophy that originated in Europe in the 1960s (Reed, 1995). Postmodern perspectives on knowledge development are based on the following assumptions:

1. The focus is on understanding multiple meanings and ways of knowing reality rather than "a single, transcendent meaning of reality" (Reed, 1995, p. 71). As a result, conceptual models and grand theories are considered irrelevant.
2. Because "multiple truths" are accepted, knowledge is considered to be uncertain and provisional (Holmes & Warelow, 2000). Contradictory positions have value for generating alternative meanings.
3. Statements "reflect a concern for context rather than universality, specificity rather than generalization, uniqueness rather than sameness, and relativism rather than absolutism" (Holmes & Warelow, 2000, p. 90).
4. The emphasis of knowledge development shifts "from concern over the truth of one's findings to concern over the practical significance of the findings" (Reed, 1995, p. 72).
5. Problems are not "solved" but rather "deconstructed," which means that efforts are made to disentangle or separate concerns from underlying values and beliefs. Language is analyzed for the meanings of words and assumed power structures.
6. With lack of concern about generalization, there is a shift toward lived experience and toward "creativity, flexibility, uniqueness, and local value" (Holmes & Warelow, 2000, p. 96). Instead of probable "truth," relevance and usefulness for practice and the potential to generate additional study are the criteria for research.

There is no single definition for postmodernism. Structuralism, a subset of postmodernism, strives to analyze the basic properties of a system. For example, structuralism recognizes the role that language, rituals, social structures (including gender roles), and traditions play in influencing the discovery of what it means to be fully human. Poststructuralism challenges the dominant thoughts of unity, uniformity, and oneness (Rogers, 2005; Sitzman & Watson, 2014; Watson, 1999). Deconstruction aims to reverse hierarchies and acknowledges the importance of power in relationships. From a poststructuralist view, people have no subjective identity but reveal themselves through various forms of communication along with their actions and behaviors. In postmodernism, "a belief in a single reality that provided a unifying and stable center is discarded" because "it is indefensible" (Rogers, 2005, p. 135).

Postmodernism also embraces relativism and pluralism. Relativism proposes that knowledge is not absolute and relies upon the limited nature of the human mind and the condition of knowing (Mish, 2020, p. 1050). In relativism, there is no single truth, agreed-upon values, and multiple ethics. Pluralism espouses that there are multiple realities, and truth, values, and ethics vary depending upon what the person or group of people experience. The pluralistic view results in formation of special interest groups (Mish, 2020). According to a postmodern perspective, everyone has different perspectives and experiences about the world (Rogers, 2005; Watson, 1999).

Until recently, nursing research and theory were dominated by logical empiricism and positivistic philosophy. However, beginning with Rogers (1970) and increasing in the 1980s, nurse scientists incorporated principles of historicism and relativism into theory, research, and practice. In the mid-1990s, principles of postmodernism began to appear in the nursing literature.

Intermodernism

A debate about the appropriate methods for developing nursing knowledge has raged in nursing literature. In support of qualitative methods, Campbell and Bunting (1991, p. 2) maintained that "human behaviors cannot be isolated and quantified and that the attempt to do so results in misleading and dehumanizing outcomes rather than in knowledge that is useful for nursing practice." Others suggested that quantitative and qualitative methods can be used at different times to serve different purposes. Meleis (1997) advocated development of a worldview (Weltanschauung) that includes an integration of norms emanating from all different theories of truth. By combining the rigorous science with personal intuition, information becomes both objective and subjective. Clinical data can be directly observed, but the interpretation of the data relies on the knowledge and values of the health care professional. Thus, the door is opened for nursing to become simultaneously an art and a science.

Such a synthesis of philosophical approaches would encourage various methods for the development of nursing science, thereby capturing the complexity of the discipline of nursing. Beginning in the late 20th century, Reed formulated the concept of **intermodernism**, an unorthodox view of nursing knowledge development that blends nursing science, theory, and practice. In the intermodern approach to knowledge development, all factors entering into the nursing profession (personal values, experiences, worldviews, professional expertise and experiences, and socioeconomic conditions) enrich the knowledge of nursing. Intermodernism differs from postmodernism because it avoids radical extremes and places less emphasis on political philosophy while fostering diversity of ideas and maintaining important shared

values, such as freedom, justice, humanism, and personal autonomy. Reed (2018) uses the acronym "INTERMODERN" to describe the 11 initial tenets of the intermodern perspective (Table 6.1). From an intermodernist perspective, all things are amenable to change.

PATTERNS OF NURSING KNOWLEDGE

Chinn and Kramer (1999, pp. 1, 7) described knowing as "ways of perceiving and understanding the self and the world.... Nursing's patterns of knowing are interrelated and arise from the whole of experience."

Different Ways of Knowing

Different people use different ways of thinking and different frameworks for knowledge organization. Frameworks for knowledge organization help persons make sense of what they learn and are frequently used unconsciously. Perry (1970) outlined four ways of knowing:

TABLE 6.1	Tenets of Intermodernism
Tenet	**Brief Description**
In-between-ness	Working outside of traditional methods in between modernism and postmodernism, "between extremes and contradictions" (p. 16)
Nursing	Considers nursing's scientific knowledge and the artistic nature; nursing as a practice discipline and a scientific body of knowledge
Truth	Coordinated, multiple theoretical approaches aimed at addressing similar problems
Empiricism	Nursing evidence that includes subjective and objective data and approaches as well as a network of human, non-human, and hybrid elements that constitute the formation of knowledge
Reality	An underlying pattern, diversity, and innovation not totally within or outside the thinker's mind; it emerges through interactions, actions, and knowledge development
Methods	Systematic and chaotic approaches used to discover and generate nursing knowledge (randomized clinical trials, synthesis, and personal professional practice and life experiences)
Openness	The state of being amenable "to critique, self-correction, and change" along with an "ongoing personal reflection on one's theory and practice . . . congruent with the open, self-organizing nature of human systems in process with their environments" (p. 17)
Discovery	Multiple ways of knowing that include the use of dynamic situations and influences that extend empirical knowing; knowledge is constructed out of something such as an experience and combines inductive and deductive logic
Epistemology	The partnership of science and practice for knowledge creation; combines being and doing, thinking and reflecting, technology, and culture, thereby creating a holistic knowledge view
Romanticism	The human quest for goodness, beauty, and meaning; the part of humans that is difficult to explain or study
Nightingale	The symbol of a scholarly practitioner who generated the first nursing-specific knowledge base, proposed the unitary approach of individuals and environments, recognized the inner healing capacity, emphasized the importance of caring and vocation, and looked at the entire human lifespan

From Reed, P. G., & Crawford Shearer, N. B. (Eds.). (2018). *Nursing knowledge and theory innovation: Advancing the science of practice* (3rd ed.). Springer Publishing.

1. *Basic dualism*: Authorities hand down the truth, and subordinates are passive. Choices are perceived as either right or wrong, black or white, good or bad, and "we" or "they."
2. *Multiplicity*: A personal opinion is acceptable and may be valid. Everyone's opinions may be valid.
3. *Relative subordinate position*: Evidence is sought for opinions. The emphasis is on analysis and evaluation of information.
4. *Full relativism*: Truth is relative. The meaning of knowledge depends on its context.

Perry suggested that the positions occur in a linear sequence with each position an advance over the previous one. The feminist researchers Belenky et al. (1986) identified another five ways for knowledge organization when examining how women tend to organize knowledge:

1. *Silence*: Individuals are subject to the whims of an external authority and perceive themselves to be mindless and voiceless.
2. *Received knowledge*: External authority is all knowing. Individuals are capable of receiving and reproducing knowledge, but not creating it.
3. *Subjective knowledge*: Truth and knowledge are personal, private, and subjectively known or intuited.
4. *Procedural knowledge*: The individual is invested in learning and in applying objective procedures for obtaining and communicating knowledge.
5. *Constructed knowledge*: Individuals experience themselves as knowledge creators. They view knowledge as contextual and value both objective and subjective strategies for knowing.

Knowledge is power. Because higher education and medicine have historically been dominated by men, Perry's (1970) ways of knowing tend to be considered superior to the other ways of knowing. Gender has been linked to the distribution of power and privilege in society (Marecek, 1995). Doering (1992, p. 26) stated that knowledge reinforces and supports existing power relations that "subtly support male dominance and reinforce female submissiveness." "When the male model is assumed to be the human model, women are viewed as the 'other,' deviant from the male norm or prototype" (Doering, 1992, p. 31). However, Doering continued, "since power is always exercised in relation to a resistance" (p. 31), ways of knowing (such as intuitive knowing and contextual, phenomena-centered knowledge) that are not based on a male worldview "may alter the balance of the nursing–medicine power relation" (p. 32).

> ### REAL-LIFE REFLECTIONS
>
> *Think about Paul and Jill from the beginning of the chapter. In what ways do they use the different ways of knowing? How does Paul's scientific approach to clinical issues affect client care? How does Jill's intuition affect client care? Which approach to client care do you feel is better? Why? Is there room for different ways of knowing in clinical practice? Why or why not?*

In 1978, Carper identified the following four ways of knowing in nursing: empirical, aesthetic, ethical, and personal. Depending upon a nurse's area of clinical practice, different ways of knowing dominate. Even nursing journals prefer publishing articles addressing one pattern of knowing over others (Kearney, 2015). For example, *Nursing Research and Research in Nursing and Health* prefers empirical knowledge, whereas *Nursing Ethics* tends to publish articles addressing ethical and personal knowing. Nurses have published articles on how they use the patterns of knowing in clinical practice by sharing case studies (Carnago & Mast, 2015).

Empirical Knowledge

The pattern of **empirical knowing** constitutes the science of nursing. It "encompasses publicly verifiable, factual descriptions, explanations, and predictions based on subjective or objective group data" (Fawcett et al., 2001, pp. 115–116). "Empirical data, obtained by either direct or indirect observation and measurement . . . are formulated as scientific principles, generalizations, laws, and theories that provide explanation and prediction" (Carper, 1992, p. 76) or enrich understanding through interpretation or description (White, 1995). **Empirical knowledge** is obtained through the senses, can be verified, is credible, and is used to impart understanding (Fig. 6.1). Processes related to creating empirical knowledge include explaining and structuring (Chinn & Kramer, 1999, 2015).

Aesthetic Knowledge

Aesthetic knowing in nursing "is that aspect of knowing that connects with deep meanings of a situation and calls forth inner creative resources that transform experience" (Chinn & Kramer, 1999, p. 183). This knowledge is not universal but is uniquely experienced and expressed and has subjective meaning (Fig. 6.2).

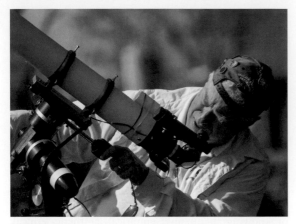

FIGURE 6.1 An amateur astronomer setting up a solar telescope, April 2012. Astronomy and all other forms of hard science and research findings constitute empirical knowing.

FIGURE 6.2 Painting and all other forms of art are examples of aesthetic knowing.

Aesthetic knowing involves the creative processes of rehearsing and envisioning (Chinn & Kramer, 1999, 2015). **Aesthetic knowledge** involves the appreciation and understanding the role that creative expression plays in the human experience.

"Art begins with the assumption of a common, generalizable human experience . . . and seeks expression of the infinite creative possibilities for experiencing or responding to the human experience" (Chinn, 1994, p. 30). Intuition, defined as "an immediate apprehension, or the power of gaining knowledge without evidence of rational thought" (Mitchell, 1994, p. 2), can be an important component of aesthetic knowledge in nursing practice.

Benner and Tanner (1987) discussed six aspects of intuitive judgment previously identified by Dreyfus and Dreyfus (1985). These aspects are not sequential but rather are used in combination by the practitioner:

1. *Pattern recognition* is the ability to recognize patterns and relationships without prior consideration of the separate components.
2. *Similarity recognition* is the ability to see similarities and parallels among client situations, even when there are marked dissimilarities in objective features.
3. *Commonsense understanding* is "a deep grasp of the culture and language, so that flexible understanding in diverse situations is possible. It is the basis for understanding the illness experience, in contrast to knowing the disease" (Benner & Tanner, 1987, p. 25). It is a way of "tuning in" to the client and grasping the client's experience.
4. *Skilled know-how* is based on a combination of knowledge and experience that permits flexibility of actions and judgment.
5. *A sense of salience* makes it possible to differentiate what is particularly significant in a situation.
6. *Deliberative rationality* involves the use of analysis and past experience to consider alternative interpretations of a clinical situation.

Carper (1978) emphasized the importance of integrating aesthetic knowledge into nursing. The experience of helping and caring "must be perceived and designed as an integral component of its desired result rather than conceived separately as an independent action imposed on an independent subject" (Carper, 1978, p. 17). The result is a richness and appreciation of the practice of nursing as an art as well as a science.

Personal Knowledge

Personal knowledge involves a "person's individualized and subjective ways of learning, storing, and retrieving information about the world" (Rew, 1996, p. 96). **Personal knowing** is "the quality and authenticity of the interpersonal process between each nurse and each [client]" (Fawcett et al., 2001, p. 116). Both the nurse and the client are considered to be "integrated, open system(s) incorporating movement toward growth and fulfillment of human potential" (Carper, 1978, p. 19). In the process of mutually establishing a nurse–client relationship, efforts must be made toward "receptive attending" (Moch, 1990, p. 155) and engagement, rather than detachment and a manipulative impersonal orientation. The result is an authentic knowing of an individual apart from the category of nurse or client. The creative processes of personal knowing include opening and centering (Chinn & Kramer, 1999, 2015).

Because personal knowing "concerns the inner experience of becoming a whole, aware, genuine self" (Chinn & Kramer, 1999, p. 5), the individual needs to accept ambiguity, vagueness, and discrepancies in what is essentially a subjective and existential process. No specific methodology can be used consistently. The individual must be open to experience and intuitive feelings, be honest with themselves, and make efforts to acknowledge the responses of others. This is an ongoing process because the self is constantly changing.

Belenky and colleagues (1986) stated that educators can help individuals develop their own authentic voices if they emphasize connection over separation, understanding and acceptance over assessment, and collaboration over debate; if they accord respect to and allow time for the knowledge that emerges from firsthand experience; if instead of imposing their own expectations and arbitrary requirements, they encourage students to evolve their own patterns of work based on the problems they are pursuing (p. 229).

Moch (1990, pp. 156–159) described three overlapping components of personal knowing:

1. *Experiential knowing* involves becoming aware through participation in which the knower learns through self-observation, by observing others, through feeling, and through sensing.
2. *Interpersonal knowing* is increased awareness through connectedness or interaction, which can involve intense attending, opening oneself to another, and conveying feelings to another.
3. *Intuitive knowing* involves the immediate knowing of something without the use of reason. The knower often describes this as a "hunch" or a "feeling about something."

Moch (1990, p. 159) believed that personal knowing can be viewed only from within a context of wholeness that "includes a process of encountering, passion, commitment, and integrity; and entails a shift in connectedness at the conscious or unconscious level." Moch saw implications for personal knowing for research and knowledge development but also recognized key assumptions underlying the capture and transmission of personal knowing. Key assumptions include the following:

1. All perceptions are involved in data gathering.
2. The process of the experience may be more important than the product of knowing.
3. Validation of the product of knowing uses both internal and external validation criteria.
4. Attempts to reproduce the process or the product are futile because each situation is unique.

"The processing may consist of any combination of human and environmental interaction, rational intuiting, appraisal, active comprehension, and personal judgment" (Sweeney, 1994, p. 917).

Ethical Knowledge

Ethics in nursing focuses on an obligation or "what ought to be done" (Chinn & Kramer, 1999, 2015, p. 5). Sarvimaki (1995) described four types of **ethical knowledge** that represent different ways of organizing and expressing moral knowledge:

1. *Theoretical or ethical knowledge* "stands for an intellectual conception of what is good and right. It is organized into concepts and propositions that are formulated into judgments, rules, principles, and theories" (Sarvimaki, 1995, p. 344).
2. *Moral action knowledge* means "having the skill necessary for performing the act as well as having good judgment. . . . Values and principles are manifested in action" (Sarvimaki, 1995, p. 345).
3. *Personal moral knowledge* "refers to the way in which morality is organized in the person, that is, in his motives, inclinations, emotions, and commitments" (Sarvimaki, 1995, p. 346).
4. *Situational knowledge* "means being aware of the moral significance of the situation and being able to identify its morally significant traits" (Sarvimaki, 1995, p. 347).

Biomedical ethics are derived from models of what is good for the client, rights-based notions of autonomy, or the social contract of medical practice (Fry, 1989). However, it has been argued that nursing ethics should be based on an ethic of caring and must consider the nature of the nurse–client relationship (Fry, 1989; Sarvimaki, 1995; White, 1995). A caring orientation is based on the moral ideal of doing what is good, rather than that which is just. Mutuality, not autonomy, is foundational (White, 1995). Chinn and Kramer (1999, 2015) specify clarifying and valuing as the creative processes of ethical caring. Thus, **ethical knowing** blends the concepts of biomedical ethics with the ethic of caring, enabling nurses to focus on making optimal decisions within the entire context of client care situations.

Other Ways of Knowing

White (1995) proposed that a fifth way of knowing, **sociopolitical knowing**, needs to be added to the original patterns identified by Carper (1978). "The pattern of sociopolitical knowing addresses the 'wherein'"

(White, 1995, p. 83), a broader context that includes the context of nurse and client (including cultural identity) as well as the context of nursing as a practice profession. White stated that "a sociopolitical understanding in which to frame all other patterns of knowing is an essential part of nursing's future in an increasingly economically driven world" (p. 85).

Chinn and Kramer (2011, p. 64) outline a sixth way of knowing, **emancipatory knowing**, which they defined as "the human ability to recognize social and political problems of injustice or inequity, to realize that things could be different, to piece together complete elements of experience and context to change a situation as it is to a situation that improves people's lives." When nurses engage in emancipatory knowing, they become aware of undesirable conditions in practice, analyze who benefits or profits from them, question what is considered knowledge, look for freedom from constraints of current knowledge and conditions, acknowledge that conditions can be improved, demystify the conditions, identify the impediments to freedom, and identify needed changes and what resources would be required to attain and sustain a new desired state. Critical reflection is used to guide action and practice. Formal expressions and creative processes raise critical questions and foster the development of required changes.

In addition, Munhall (1993) proposed **unknowing** as another pattern of knowing in nursing. She argued that the state of mind of unknowing is a condition of openness and "a decentering process from one's own organizing principles of the world" (p. 125). The intent is to "come to know the patient's world" (Munhall, 1993, p. 126), which will "lead to a much deeper knowledge of another being, of different meanings, and interpretations of all our various perceptions of experience" (p. 128).

Garrett and Cutting (2014, pp. 101–102) propose still other ways of knowing. Along with empirical knowing, they suggest additional forms of knowing in nursing and in health care:

- *Hallowed knowing*: The knowledge revealed to a person via the ancient sacred texts
- *Esoteric knowing*: Knowledge beyond human comprehension that occurs when a person cannot explain it to another
- *Coming to know*: Learning things from a natural curiosity that provides foundation for discovery learning
- *Visionary knowing*: The knowledge generated when a person learns something in a dream while sleeping

- *Supernatural knowing*: Knowledge gained from participation in magic or other mystical processes such as mediation
- *Satellite knowing*: Discovered when viewing something or a situation from a great height
- *Other knowing*: Any other form of knowledge failing to fall in either of the other eight categories

Although some of these ways of knowing may seem farfetched, some of the new ways of knowing have application to clinical practice.

■ Questions for Reflection

1. What ways of knowing have you used in your personal life?

2. How did these ways of knowing guide your personal actions?

3. What ways of knowing have you used in clinical practice?

4. How did these ways of knowing guide your professional nursing actions?

The Concepts in Practice box, "How Nurses Use the Patterns of Knowing in Clinical Practice," provides examples of how professional nurses use the patterns of knowing in clinical practice. Many years of practice may be needed to develop competence and confidence in using all of the patterns of knowing.

Paradigms for Developing Nursing Knowledge

Three different perspectives, each described as reflecting a different point of view (paradigm) of the way to develop nursing knowledge, have been identified (Newman et al., 1991, p. 4):

1. *Particulate-deterministic perspective*: Phenomena are viewed as "isolatable, reducible entities having definable properties that can be measured." Knowledge includes facts and universal laws that can be used to predict and control change.

2. *Interactive-integrative perspective*: Phenomena are viewed as having multiple, interrelated parts. Reality is assumed to be multidimensional and contextual. Relationships may be reciprocal (rather than linear and causal), and knowledge may be context dependent.

3. *Unitary-transformative perspective*: Each phenomenon is viewed as a unitary self-organizing field embedded in a larger self-organizing field. It is identified by pattern and by interaction with the larger whole. Change is unpredictable.

Concepts in Practice

IDEA → PLAN → ACTION

How Nurses Use the Patterns of Knowing in Clinical Practice

Empirical Knowing
- Administering medications and intravenous (IV) therapy safely
- Following isolation procedures for infectious diseases
- Using evidence-based strategies for preventing hospital or treatment complications
- Abiding by principles for hand hygiene
- Adhering to protocols for clinical nursing procedures

Aesthetic Knowing
- Individualizing care for all clients
- Adapting standard procedures to fit specific clinical situations
- Detecting significant client pattern changes
- Creating environments to soothe clients and families
- Using art and music as nursing interventions

Personal Knowing
- Using experiential know-how in novel or complex care situations
- Connecting deeply with clients and their families
- Opening the self to others
- Relying on intuition

Ethical Knowing
- Doing what is best for the client
- Doing what is right and just
- Safeguarding client rights
- Possessing an altruistic motive when caring for others
- Valuing the self and others
- Being aware of moral issues surrounding client situations

Sociopolitical Knowing
- Understanding legal implications of professional nursing practice
- Using health care resources prudently
- Involving oneself in the political and legislative processes
- Supporting efforts to provide effective health care for all

Emancipatory Knowing
- Raising critical questions
- Noticing undesirable practice situations
- Reporting unsafe and undesirable practice situations
- Working as an equal member of the health care team
- Changing systems for better health care
- Participating in nursing shared governance systems

Unknowing
- Being open to learning
- Quieting oneself to listen
- Learning about the client's entire story
- Connecting deeply with others to deepen understanding about them
- Acknowledging limitations of one's current knowledge and skills

Hallowed Knowing
- Finding meaning in work from studying sacred text
- Using revealed messages from a sacred text to direct work as a nurse

Esoteric Knowing
- Using intuition in practice
- Inexplicably identifying patterns or taking prompt action in any given nursing situation

Visionary Knowing
Heeding information recovered from a dream when sleeping to guide actions and decisions

Supernatural Knowing
Permitting or using various religious or cultural healing ceremonies in clinical practice

Satellite Knowing
- Taking a step back to analyze a clinical situation using a global perspective
- Thinking about health care delivery from a macro rather than a micro viewpoint

Knowledge is personal and involves pattern recognition. Both the viewer and the phenomenon are involved in a process of "mutuality and creative unfolding."

Patterns as ways of knowing are not mutually exclusive; rather, they "are interrelated and arise from the whole of experience" (Chinn & Kramer, 1999, p. 7). Different ways of knowing are not judged against one another. Each of the ways of knowing and of creating knowledge is useful. Because each pattern adds only one specific component, none alone is a sufficient source of knowledge for nursing science. "Nursing depends on the specific knowledge of human behavior in health and in illness, the aesthetic perception of significant human experience, a personal understanding of the unique individuality of the self, and the capacity to make choices within concrete situations involving particular judgments" (Carper, 1978, p. 22).

Take Note!
Comprehensive nursing knowledge must be based on an integration of all the ways of knowing.

REAL-LIFE REFLECTIONS

In attending to Paul's client with pancreatitis, which of the ways of knowing did Jill demonstrate? Which ways of knowing might have aided Paul?

THE DEVELOPMENT OF NURSING SCIENCE

Because of the complexity of the discipline of nursing and competing worldview perspectives (particular-deterministic, interactive-integrative, and unitary-transformative), defining nursing science poses a challenge. However, attaining a clear definition of **nursing science** would provide a foundation for the profession's unique body of knowledge.

Specialized branches of science develop knowledge and theories. First comes the ideas and theories. Scientists then test and refine the ideas and theories. Nursing contributes uniquely to health care delivery, but failure to articulate exact contributions may place the profession at risk.

Identification of Concepts

For a discipline to have growth of knowledge, the concepts that are important for the discipline must be identified, and there must be a shared acceptance of conceptual definitions. Fawcett (2005) defined the term **concept** as "a word or phrase that summarizes ideas, observations, and experiences" (p. 4). She also identified **four central concepts of nursing** that address the key elements of the profession:

1. Human being: An individual nurse or client, a family, a group, or a community
2. Environment: Alive or inanimate
3. Health: Well-being and illness
4. Nursing: All the interactions among the nurse, client, and environment in the pursuit of health, as well as what nurses do.

These four concepts represent the metaparadigm of nursing that encompasses all phenomena of interest in a value-neutral way to identify a distinctive domain for the nursing profession (Fawcett, 2005; Fawcett & DeSanto-Madeya, 2012).

Since the metaparadigm's creation, various nurse scholars have proposed additional concepts that should be included, such as the concepts of caring. Newman and colleagues (1991, p. 3) even asserted that "nursing is the study of caring in the human health experience." However, others have expressed concern that "caring is relatively underdeveloped as a concept, has not been clearly explicated, and often lacks relevance for nursing practice" (Morse et al. 1991, p. 119). Watson (2011) conceptualized caring as a value and ideal that also encompasses a "philosophy of action" (p. 32).

At least five conceptualizations of caring have been identified: a human trait, a moral imperative, an affect, an interpersonal interaction, and a therapeutic intervention (Morse et al., 1991). Caring seems to be part of content and relationship (Knowlden, 1991) and associated with varying outcomes, such as the client's physical response and the client's or nurse's subjective experience (Morse et al., 1991). When effective, some concepts (including care) can be directly measured using empirical indicators that take the form of clinical practice tools (Fawcett & DeSanto-Madeya, 2012), such as the McGill pain rating scale, or research instruments.

Meleis (2007, 2012) offered a different approach to the nursing paradigm and proposed the following seven central concepts:

1. Nursing client: Recipient of professional nursing services
2. Transitions: Changes in health status, role relationships, expectations, or abilities
3. Interaction: Instrument for assessment and constructing relationships
4. Nursing process: Steps that nurses use to deliver services, including assessment, diagnosis, planning, implementation, and evaluation
5. Environment: Not well defined, but relates to the setting, context, and properties or dimensions of the world that affect human health (see Chapter 7, "Nursing Models and Theories," for various nursing approaches to this concept)
6. Nursing therapeutics: Deliberate nursing activities and actions nurses use while caring for clients
7. Health: Goal of nursing services but not limited to the absence of disease (see Chapter 7, "Nursing Models and Theories," for various nursing approaches to this concept)

Because of their abstract nature, concepts can pose problems within a single discipline or across disciplines. Other issues arise when a particular phenomenon is incompletely understood or lacks procedures to explain or measure it (Fawcett & DeSanto-Madeya, 2012; Meleis, 2007; Rogers, 2005). Because the profession of nursing is highly complex and has various specialty areas of practice, attaining a "single" definition for nursing concepts is extremely difficult. At present, in the absence of a consensus on definitions for the concepts of human beings, environment, health, and nursing, multiple definitions coexist (see Chapter 7, "Nursing Models and Theories").

Theories and Theoretical Frameworks

A theoretical or conceptual framework has been defined as "a logical grouping of related concepts or theories" (Chinn & Kramer, 1999, p. 258). A model is composed of abstract and general concepts and propositions that are linked together in a distinctive way. Fawcett (2000, p. 16) stated that a conceptual model "provides a unique focus that has a profound influence on individuals' perceptions." Theoretical frameworks provide guidance and direction for nursing research endeavors (Meleis, 2007, 2012). Rogers (2005) distinguished theoretical frameworks from theories in that the theoretical framework is broader than a theory and typically has not been validated through scientific testing. Theoretical frameworks tend to address phenomena that are more global in nature. Developing theoretical frameworks for nursing ensures practice that considers the complex nature of profession. Nurses who use theoretical frameworks in professional practice typically have some sort of method to provide holistic care rather than just focusing on the client's physiologic issues.

Theories communicate links or relationships among concepts in an organized, coherent, and systematic way and vary in levels of abstraction and scope (Fawcett & DeSanto-Madeya, 2012; Meleis, 2012). Theories symbolize reality and can either be discovered or invented (Meleis, 2012). Meleis (2007, p. 37) specified that theories can describe, explain, predict, or prescribe phenomena, including relationships, events, situations, responses, or conditions. Fawcett (2005) explained that propositions are statements that either define or describe a concept (nonrelational) or specify a relationship or linkage between multiple concepts. Grand theories for professional nursing provide a broad characterization of the profession and are typically highly abstract. Thus, they fail to provide specific information to guide research and clinical practice (Fawcett, 2005; Meleis, 2007, 2012; Rogers, 2005; Walker & Avant, 2019). When theories become able to describe, explain, or predict certain relationships between or among concepts, nursing scholars categorize them as middle-range theories, which serve as theoretical frameworks for nursing research and practice (Fawcett & DeSanto-Madeya, 2012; Meleis, 2012; Rogers, 2005; Walker & Avant, 2019). Sometimes, theories can be used for a specific clinical practice situation or to guide a particular research project. Because of the narrow focus in these situations, some nurse scholars refer to these theories as clinical practice theories or microtheories (Peterson & Bredow, 2017). Theories help nurses understand how and why the phenomena of nursing are associated with one another. For example, the gate theory of pain proposes that there is a progression of nerve impulse transmissions from a noxious stimulus outside or within the body that must occur prior to the ability of a person to perceive pain. The impulse transmission may be interrupted if the nerve pathways cannot receive the painful stimulus. A nurse using this theory recognizes that the application of cold or heat to a body part can interrupt the nerve transmission thereby reducing or perhaps even eliminating the client's perception of pain.

Theories in nursing may be unique to the discipline of nursing or borrowed from or shared with another discipline that has interest in similar human phenomena (Fawcett, 2000; Meleis, 2007, 2012; Peterson & Bredow, 2017). For example, the concept of self-esteem is borrowed from the field of psychology but plays a key role when nurses establish therapeutic relationships with clients and interprofessional relationships with members of the health care team (see Chapter 4, "Establishing Helping and Healing Relationships"). Before questioning a physician's order, the nurse must have the self-esteem to have confidence in their knowledge of pharmacology in order to avoid a serious event for a client. After successfully confronting the situation, the nurse's self-esteem becomes enhanced because they did the right thing.

Effectiveness in practice is directly related to the ability to understand, describe, explain, and anticipate human responses concerning health. Theoretically based professional practice enables nurses to anticipate client complications before they occur and determine the best approaches to use in specific client care situations.

Models for Nursing

Several nurse scientists have proposed individual and distinctive models about the interrelationships of concepts that form the nature and processes of nursing. Each nurse scholar who has proposed a conceptual model has based the model on empirical observation, intuitive insights, or deductive reasoning "that creatively combine[s] ideas from several fields of inquiry"

(Fawcett, 2000, p. 16). Although they may present diverse views of nursing phenomena, each conceptual model is useful for professional nursing because of the organization it provides for thinking, observing, and interpreting in nursing practice. Some nursing conceptual models provide an illustrative diagram to depict relationships among concepts (see Fig. 1.1 in Chapter 1, "The Professional Nurse" and Chapter 7, "Nursing Models and Theories" for a discussion of selected conceptual models). **Nursing conceptual models** identify the interventions that nurses use in practice while explaining the four central concepts of nursing: human beings, environment, health, and nursing (Fawcett, 2005; Fawcett & DeSanto-Madeya, 2012; Meleis, 2007, 2012; Rogers, 2005; Walker & Avant, 2019).

Summary and Significance to Practice

Because of the complexity of client care, nurses use a variety of methods of knowing when they provide professional nursing services. Nursing science encompasses more than the physiologic aspects of client care. Most nurses encounter practice situations in which they rely on personal and ethical knowing to make effective clinical judgments and decisions. Understanding and appreciating the patterns of knowing in nursing sharpen the cognitive skills of professional nurses as they engage in daily practice.

Most nursing scholars have a general agreement on the central concepts of the discipline of nursing. The central concepts help describe the phenomenon of professional nursing practice and guide nurses in clinical practice, research endeavors, and educational programs. Clarification of the central concepts and tenets of professional nursing remain a challenge because of the various approaches to patterns of knowing available to nurses in the postmodern era.

> ### REAL-LIFE REFLECTIONS
>
> *Remember Paul, from the beginning of the chapter. What suggestions would you give him as he explores the phenomenon of nursing intuition as the topic of his class research project? How do you think Paul would respond to each of your points? What are the consequences of having a narrowly defined perception of what constitutes nursing knowledge?*

From Theory to Practice

1. How do you use the empirical, aesthetic, personal, and ethical ways of knowing in your professional practice? How do your attitudes about the ways of knowing affect your professional practice? Why are the ways of knowing important for professional nurses?
2. How has reading this chapter affected your views about nursing science and nursing theory?

Nurse as Author

Write an essay about six ways of knowing in your clinical practice. Define each identified way of knowing before you convey information about how you use it in practice. Specify the advantages of using various forms of knowing in your professional or student nursing practice.

Your Digital Classroom

Online Exploration

The Sigma Repository: **https://www.sigmarepository.org/**. In the search box, type in any topic related to nursing that interests you and see what you find.

International Journal of Nursing Knowledge: **https://onlinelibrary.wiley.com/journal/20473095**

Expanding Your Understanding

Go online, and read: Hall, A. (2005). Defining nursing knowledge. *NursingTimes.net*, *101*(48), 34. **https://www.nursingtimes.net/roles/nurse-educators/defining-nursing-knowledge-29-11-2005/**. Answer the following questions and bring the answers to these questions along with your own questions to class.

1. What constitutes nursing knowledge?
2. How is nursing knowledge used in nursing practice and education?
3. How are nurses held accountable for nursing knowledge?
4. Provide two examples of how theoretical knowledge differs from practice knowledge.
5. What was done to this article prior to its publication that makes this a reliable, professional reference?

Beyond the Book

Visit thePoint® at **www.thePoint.lww.com** for activities and information to reinforce the concepts and content covered in this chapter.

REFERENCES

Baghramian, M., & Adam, C. J. (2016). Relativism. In E. N. Zalta (Ed.), *The Stanford encyclopedia of philosophy* (Spring 2016 Edition). Retrieved September 14, 2020, from http://plato.stanford.edu/archives/spr2016/entries/relativism/

Belenky, M. F., Clinchy, B. M., Goldberger, N. R., & Tarule, J. M. (1986). *Women's ways of knowing: The development of self, voice and mind.* Basic Books.

Benner, P., & Tanner, C. (1987). Clinical judgment: How expert nurses use intuition. *American Journal of Nursing, 87*(1), 23–31. Retrieved March 23, 2021, from https://www-jstor-org.lib.rockhurst.edu/stable/3470396?seq=1#metadata_info_tab_contents

Bertalanffy, L. V. (1968). *General system theory.* Braziller.

Campbell, J. C., & Bunting, S. (1991). Voices and paradigms: Perspectives on critical and feminist theory in nursing. *Advances in Nursing Science, 13*(3), 1–15. https://doi.org/10.1097/00012272-199103000-00004

Carnago, L., & Mast, M. (2015). Using ways of knowing to guide emergency nursing practice. *Journal of Emergency Nursing, 41*(5), 387–390. https://doi.org/10.1016/j.jen.2015.01.011

Carper, B. A. (1978). Fundamental patterns of knowing in nursing. *Advances in Nursing Science, 1*(1), 13–23. https://doi.org/10.1097/00012272-197810000-00004

Carper, B. A. (1992). Philosophical inquiry in nursing: An application. In J. F. Kikuchi & H. Simmons (Eds.), *Philosophic inquiry in nursing.* Sage.

Chinn, P. L. (1994). Developing a method for aesthetic knowing in nursing. In P. L. Chinn & J. Watson (Eds.), *Art and aesthetics in nursing.* National League for Nursing.

Chinn, P. L., & Kramer, M. K. (1999). *Theory and nursing: Integrated knowledge development* (5th ed.). Mosby-Year Book.

Chinn, P. L., & Kramer, M. K. (2011). *Integrated theory and knowledge development in nursing* (8th ed.). Elsevier Mosby.

Chinn, P. L., & Kramer, M. K. (2015). *Integrated theory and knowledge development in nursing* (9th ed.). Mosby.

Doering, L. (1992). Power and knowledge in nursing: A feminist poststructuralist view. *Advances in Nursing Science, 14*(4), 24–33. https://doi.org/10.1097/00012272-199206000-00005

Dreyfus, H., & Dreyfus, S. (1985). *Mind over machine: The power of human intuition and expertise in the era of the computer.* Macmillan Free Press.

Fawcett, J. (2000). *Analysis and evaluation of contemporary nursing knowledge: Nursing models and theories.* F.A. Davis.

Fawcett, J. (2005). *Contemporary nursing knowledge: Analysis and evaluation of nursing models and theories* (2nd ed.). F.A. Davis.

Fawcett, J., & DeSanto-Madeya, S. (2012). *Contemporary nursing knowledge: Analysis and evaluation of nursing models and theories* (3rd ed.). F.A. Davis.

Fawcett, J., Watson, J., Neuman, B., Walker, P. H., & Fitzpatrick, J. J. (2001). On nursing theories and evidence. *Journal of Nursing Scholarship, 33*(2), 115–119. https://doi.org/10.1111/j.1547-5069.2001.00115.x

Fry, S. T. (1989). Toward a theory of nursing ethics. *Advances in Nursing Science, 11*(2), 9–22. https://doi.org/10.1097/00012272-198907000-00005

Garrett, B. M., & Cutting, R. (2014). Ways of knowing: Realism, non-realism nominalism and a typology revisited with a counter perceptive for nursing science. *Nursing Inquiry, 22*(2), 95–105. https://doi.org/10.1111/nin.12070

Heisenberg, W. (1971). *Physics and beyond.* Harper & Row.

Holmes, C. A., & Warelow, P. J. (2000). Some implications of postmodernism for nursing theory, research, and practice. *Canadian Journal of Nursing Research, 32*(2), 89–101. Retrieved March 23, 2021, from https://www.researchgate.net/publication/12177053_Some_Implications_of_Postmodernism_for_Nursing_Theory_Research_and_Practice

Kearney, M. (2015). Ways of knowing: A guide to the journal and clinical discipline needs. *Research in Nursing & Health, 38*(2), 97–99. https://doi.org/10.1002/nur.21649

Knowlden, V. (1991). Nurse caring as constructed knowledge. In R. M. Neil & R. Watts (Eds.), *Caring and nursing: Explorations in feminist perspectives.* National League for Nursing.

Kuhn, T. (1970). *The structure of scientific revolutions* (2nd ed.). University of Chicago Press.

Laudan, L. (1981). A problem solving approach to scientific growth. In I. Hacking (Ed.), *Scientific revolutions.* Oxford University Press.

Linberg, C., Nash, S., & Linberg, C. (2008). *On the edge: Nursing in the age of complexity.* Plexus Press.

Marecek, J. (1995). Gender, politics, and psychology's ways of knowing. *American Psychologist, 50*(3), 162–163. https://doi.org/10.1037//0003-066x.50.3.162

Meleis, A. (1997). *Theoretical nursing: Development and progress* (3rd ed.). Lippincott.

Meleis, A. (2007). *Theoretical nursing: Development & progress* (4th ed.). Lippincott Williams & Wilkins.

Meleis, A. (2012). *Theoretical nursing: Development & progress* (5th ed.). Wolters-Kluwer Health/Lippincott Williams & Wilkins.

Mish, F. C. (Ed.). (2020). *Merriam-Webster's collegiate dictionary* (11th ed.). Merriam-Webster, Inc.

Mitchell, G. J. (1994). Intuitive knowing: Exposing a myth in theory development. *Nursing Science Quarterly, 7*(1), 2–3. https://doi.org/10.1177/089431849400700102

Moch, S. D. (1990). Personal knowing: Evolving research and practice. *Scholarly Inquiry for Nursing Practice, 4*(2), 155–170. Retrieved March 23, 2021, from https://pubmed.ncbi.nlm.nih.gov/2237001/

Morse, J. M., Bottorff, J., Neander, W., & Solberg, S. (1991). Comparative analysis of conceptualizations and theories of caring. *Image, 23*(2), 119–126. https://doi.org/10.1111/j.1547-5069.1991.tb00655.x

Munhall, P. L. (1993). "Unknowing": Toward another pattern of knowing in nursing. *Nursing Outlook, 41*(3), 125–128. https://pubmed.ncbi.nlm.nih.gov/8346052/

Newman, M. A., Sime, A. M., & Corcoran-Perry, S. A. (1991). The focus of the discipline of nursing. *Advances in Nursing Science, 14*(1), 1–6. https://doi.org/10.1097/00012272-199109000-00002

Nicolas, T., & Philippe, B. (2015). Propositional dynamic logic. In E. N. Zalta (Ed.), *The Stanford encyclopedia of philosophy* (Spring 2015 Edition). Retrieved September 25, 2016, from http://plato.stanford.edu/archives/spr2015/entries/logic-dynamic/

Perry, W. G. (1970). *Forms of intellectual and ethical development in the college years.* Holt, Rinehart and Winston.

Peterson, S., & Bredow, T. (2017). *Middle range theories application to nursing research and practice* (4th ed.). Wolters Kluwer.

Reed, P. G. (1995). A treatise on nursing knowledge development for the 21st century: Beyond postmodernism. *Advances in Nursing Science, 17*(3), 70–84. https://doi.org/10.1097/00012272-199503000-00008

Reed, P. G. (2018). The spiral path to nursing knowledge. In P. G. Reed & N. B. Crawford Shearer (Eds.), *Nursing knowledge and theory innovation: Advancing the science of practice* (pp. 1–19). Springer Publishing.

Rew, L. (1996). *Awareness in healing*. Delmar.

Rogers, B. L. (2005). *Developing nursing knowledge philosophical traditions and influences*. Lippincott Williams & Wilkins.

Rogers, M. E. (1970). *An introduction to the theoretical basis of nursing*. F.A. Davis.

Rogers, M. E. (1992). Nursing science and the space age. *Nursing Science Quarterly, 5*(1), 27–34. https://doi.org/10.1177/089431849200500108

Rosen, G., Byrne, A., Cohen, J., Harman, E., & Shiffrin, S. (2018). *The Norton introduction to philosophy* (2nd ed.). W. W. Norton & Co.

Roy, C. (2007). Advances in nursing knowledge and the challenge for transforming practice. In C. Roy & D. Jones (Eds.), *Nursing knowledge development and clinical practice*. Springer.

Sarvimaki, A. (1995). Aspects of moral knowledge in nursing. *Scholarly Inquiry for Nursing Practice, 9*(4), 343–358. Retrieved March 23, 2021, from https://pubmed.ncbi.nlm.nih.gov/8820594/

Sitzman, K., & Watson, J. (2014). *Caring science, mindful practice, implementing Watson's human caring theory*. Springer Publishing Company, LLC.

Spradlin, W. W., & Porterfield, P. B. (1984). *The search for certainty*. Springer-Verlag.

Sweeney, N. M. (1994). A concept analysis of personal knowledge: Application to nursing education. *Journal of Advanced Nursing, 20*(5), 917–924. https://doi.org/10.1046/j.1365-2648.1994.20050917.x

Walker, L. O., & Avant, K. C. (2019). *Strategies for theory construction in nursing* (6th ed.). Pearson.

Ware, C. F., Panikaar, K. M., & Romein, J. M. (1966). *History of mankind, cultural and scientific development: Vol. 6. The twentieth century*. Harper & Row.

Watson, J. (1999). *Postmodern nursing and beyond*. Churchill Livingstone.

Watson, J. (2007). *Nursing human science and human care: A theory of nursing*. Jones & Bartlett.

Watson, J. (2011). *Nursing: Human science and human care*. Jones & Bartlett.

White, J. (1995). Patterns of knowing: Review, critique, and update. *Advances in Nursing Science, 17*(4), 73–86. https://doi.org/10.1097/00012272-199506000-00007

Nursing Models and Theories

KEY TERMS AND CONCEPTS

Metaparadigm

Conceptual model

Nursing models

Theory

Grand theories

Middle-range theories

Practice theory

Stability model of change

Systems theory

King's systems interaction model (theory of goal attainment)

Neuman's systems model

Roy's adaptation model

Growth model of change

Caring

Orem's self-care deficit theory

Watson's human caring science, theory of nursing

Complexity theory

Rogers's science of unitary human beings

Parse's human becoming theory

Newman's theory of health as expanding consciousness

Leddy's human energy model

Watson's human caring science

LEARNING OUTCOMES

By the end of this chapter, the learner will be able to:

1. Explain the key differences among rote, stereotypical, and theoretically based nursing practice.
2. Compare and contrast systems, adaptation, caring, and complexity theories.
3. Identify assumptions in the various nursing models presented in the chapter.
4. Outline differences in how nursing's metaparadigm concepts are defined in each of the nursing models presented.
5. Provide an example of how each nursing model and theory might be applied to a clinical practice situation.
6. Select a nursing model or theory that best aligns with your personal view about the world for use in clinical practice.

REAL-LIFE REFLECTIONS

Nicole and Brianna are two nurses working the night shift. Tonight, Ms. Green uses the call light every 5 minutes because she cannot sleep. Her nurse, Nicole, asks Brianna for help because Brianna always seems to know just what to do. Ms. Green is asleep after Brianna spends 5 minutes with her. Nicole asks, "How do you always know how to help restless clients?" Brianna shares her knowledge about Parse's human becoming theory, emphasizing being truly present with clients. Brianna also summarizes key concepts and approaches presented by other nursing theorists that she learned in her undergraduate nursing program. She mentions that although she prefers to use Parse's model, she finds that other nursing models help in different client care situations.

The discipline of nursing is highly complex. A **meta-paradigm** may be defined as a recognizable pattern or model that provides a foundation for a particular discipline used as an overarching framework to describe key organizing concepts related to the field. Over the years, most nursing scholars have adopted the following four key concepts to serve as a metaparadigm: human beings (recipients of nursing care); environment (physical and social); health (a process or state); and nursing (goals, roles, and functions) (Fawcett, 2005). Hardy (1978) introduced the idea of paradigms to the nursing profession as a means to offer a comprehensive description and possibly a method of unifying the profession (Fawcett, 2005; Meleis, 2018; Rodgers, 2005; Roy, 2007).

All existing nursing models and grand theories address these four concepts. In fact, four of the models presented in this chapter contain the word "human" in their titles. Each model also takes a different philosophical view of the world. Although nursing models and theories vary according to philosophical worldviews, all flow from the metaparadigm of professional nursing.

Take Note!
Most nursing scholars have adopted the following four key concepts to serve as a metaparadigm of professional nursing: human beings (recipients of nursing care); environment (physical and social); health (a process or state); and nursing (goals, roles, and functions).

NURSING MODELS

Prior to 1950, the writings of Florence Nightingale served as the primary source of nursing theory, and nursing science was derived principally from social, biologic, and medical science theories. Nursing science began to emerge as a part of the profession in the 1950s and continues to flourish today. Some nursing theories and models arose when nurses tried to generate a clear, concise definition of nursing; others arose from the need to demonstrate that what nurses do makes a difference in client outcomes.

A model provides a way to visualize reality and simplify thinking. For example, a spaceship model provides a representation of a spaceship. A **conceptual model** gives structure to and shows how various concepts are interrelated. Conceptual models serve as

a foundation for theory development; they can also apply theories to predict or evaluate consequences of alternative actions. According to Fawcett (2000), a conceptual model "gives direction to the search for relevant questions about the phenomena of central interest to a discipline and suggests solutions to practical problems" (p. 16). **Nursing models** tend to be more abstract than nursing theory.

Nursing Theory

Theories are abstract concepts that are ideas. Abstract concepts are intangible ideas. Caring and compassion are two examples of abstract concepts. Professional nurses apply concepts, principles, and theories from many disciplines. For example, nurses use physics when placing cardiac electrodes, pharmacology when monitoring results of administered medications, psychology when providing emotional support, microbiology when using aseptic technique, family theory when assessing effective mother–infant bonding, and human development theory when caring for clients of all ages. However, these borrowed theories and principles fail to capture the essence of professional nursing. Theories create a different way of looking at a particular phenomenon by interrelating concepts in a logical manner and provide a framework for describing, explaining, and predicting practice. They also provide a relatively simple yet generalizable view for testable hypothesis development. Once validated through research, theories expand discipline-specific knowledge while identifying other questions for future investigation. Sometimes, research provides evidence for nursing scholars to revise conceptual models and theories. In addition, new advances in clinical management of disease may be the stimulus for refinement of current models and theory or for the development of new ones.

Many nurses base their practice on traditions, experience, or "how I learned it in nursing school." These methods lead to rote and stereotypical practice. Nurses rely on memorization and habit when engaging in rote practice. Rote practice enables nurses to provide care while in an "autopilot" or robotic mode. When nurses use long-standing traditions and incorporate the expectations of others in practice, they engage in stereotypical practice. In the stereotypical practice mode, nurses try to fulfill expectations others may have of them, such as following physician orders without question or willingly assuming the role of the self-sacrificing "angel of mercy."

However, practice based on models or theories allows for hypotheses about practice, which make it possible to derive rationales for nursing actions. When using a specific nursing model or theory, nurses use concepts and relationships to direct client assessments and interventions. Testable theories provide a knowledge base for the science of nursing. As the science of nursing develops, nurses are able to understand and explain events more accurately and provide a basis for predicting and controlling future events. In addition, practice based on science fosters the recognition of nursing as a professional discipline. Looking at the philosophical differences that underlie nursing models and theories helps explain why they vary in approaches to professional practice.

■ QUESTIONS FOR REFLECTION

1. How do you rely on family traditions and personal experience when you fall ill or care for a family member?
2. How do you rely on traditions and personal experience when you practice nursing?
3. What consequences have resulted when you used traditions to guide your nursing practice?
4. What is your attitude toward nursing models and theories? Why do you feel this way?

Categories of Nursing Models and Theories

Nursing models and theories represent the depth and breadth of how they are used to guide practice, education, and research. Theories may either predict or explain phenomena. Nursing theories can also be classified according to their level of abstractness, with the most abstract representing the broadest level of theory. When a set of interrelated concepts are linked together and form a visual diagram or picture, a conceptual model has been developed. The Hood Professional Nurse Contributions Model and the Massachusetts Nurse of the Future Nursing Core Competencies are examples of conceptual models (see Chapter 1, "The Professional Nurse").

Grand theories in nursing articulate attempts to provide a perspective to guide or unite the entire nursing profession. Typically, they address the profession's nature, missions, and goals (Meleis, 2018). Peterson and Bredow (2017) and Meleis (2018) describe middle-range nursing theories as possessing a narrower scope, addressing fewer but more specific concepts and propositions, connecting to a particular or limited perspective of nursing, having enough structure to be empirically tested, and being concrete and specific enough to provide explanations to clinical phenomena and for use in clinical practice. Nursing scholars have generated numerous **middle-range theories** through deduction (fusing theoretical concepts and relationships from a grand theory to generate a more specific theory to guide practice); induction (analyzing what occurs in a practice setting and identifying key concepts and their relationships that is frequently done during qualitative research; see Chapter 10, "Professional Practice Based on Nursing Research and Best Evidence"); generation by combining ideas, concepts, and relationships from other disciplines of study (e.g., psychology, medicine, sociology); synthesizing research findings around particular nursing phenomena; and building theory from clinical practice guidelines (Peterson & Bredow, 2017).

Practice theory has been described as micro theory or situation-specific theory in the nursing literature. Practice theory is more concrete than the other forms of theory and frequently provides a theoretical approach to a specific clinical practice situation or a research study. It provides guidance for nurses encountering culturally diverse situations and specific clinical practice issues (Meleis, 2018; Peterson & Bredow, 2017). Table 7.1 provides examples of some commonly used grand, middle-range, and practice-specific theories by professional nurses as they engage in clinical practice and nursing research.

This chapter presents the work of nine nursing theorists that provide a foundation for professional practice for individual nurses, nursing research studies, and nursing departments in many health care organizations (Fawcett, 2005; Meleis, 2018; Watson, 2007, 2018). The original works of these nurse theorists are presented, so some references appear dated, but these are the primary sources. The works selected present a multiplicity of philosophical worldviews to capture reader interest and stimulate dialogue about the essence of professional nursing. To distinguish differences among them, the models and theories have been classified according to the following criteria:

1. The worldview of change reflected by the model (growth or stability)
2. The major theoretical/conceptual classification with which the model seems most consistent (systems, stress/adaptation, caring, or growth/development)

TABLE 7.1 Examples of Nursing Conceptual Models: Grand, Middle-Range, and Practice Theories Commonly Used by Nurses

Conceptual Models	Grand Theories
Johnson's Behavioral System Model (1959, 1990)	Nightingale's Environmental Model of Nursing (Chapter 2)
King's Systems Interaction Model (1968, 1981) (Chapters 7 and 8)	King's Theory of Goal Attainment (1981, 1996, 1997) (Chapters 7 and 8)
Levine's Conservation Model (1969, 1991)	Leininger's Theory of Culture Care and Universality (1978, 1988, 1995) (Chapter 11)
Neuman's System Model (1982, 1995) (Chapters 7 and 8)	Newman's Theory of Health as Expanding Consciousness (1990, 1994, 1997) (Chapters 7 and 8)
Rogers's Science of Human Beings (1980, 1984) (Chapters 7 and 8)	Orem's Self-Care Deficit Theory (1983, 1987, 2000) (Chapters 7 and 8)
Roper–Logan–Tierney Model of Nursing (1983, 1996)	Parse's Theory of Human Becoming (1981, 1987, 1992, 1998) (Chapters 7 and 8)
Roy's Adaptation Model (1971, 1999) (Chapters 7 and 8)	Watson's Human Caring Science, a Theory for Nursing (Chapters 7 and 8)
Hood's Professional Nurse Contributions Model (2010, 2014) (Chapter 1)	Peplau's Theory of Interpersonal Relations (Chapter 4)
Leddy's Human Energy Model (2003, 2004, 2006) (Chapters 7 and 8)	Pender's Health Promotion Model (Chapter 5)
Middle-Range Theories	**Practice Theories**
Mercer's Maternal Role Attachment—Becoming a Mother Model (1986)	Baird's theory of well-being in refugee women during cultural transitions (2012)
Reed's Self-Transcendence Theory (1989)	Brennan's situation-specific theory for crisis emergencies for individuals with severe, persistent mental illness (2012)
Eake, Burke, and Hainsworth Theory of Chronic Sorrow (1998, 2004, 2008)	Broussard's empowerment grounded theory in school nursing practice (2007)
Swanson's Theory of Caring (1991) (Chapter 7)	Bull and McShane's family caregiver perspectives for adults transitioning to adult day care services (2008)
Kolcaba's Theory of Comfort (1994, 2001, 2004)	Clingerman's situation-specific theory of migration transitions for migrant farmworker women (2007)
Beck's Postpartum Depression Theory (1993)	Hopia, Paavilainen, and Åstedt-Kurki's practice theory on promoting health for families of children with chronic conditions (2004)
Mishel's Uncertainty in Illness Theory (1988, 1990, 1991, 1999)	
Ray's Theory of Bureaucratic Caring (1989)	Im's situation-specific theory of the Asian cancer pain experience (2008)
The American Association of Critical Care Nurses' Synergy Model for Patient Care (1998)	Im, Stuifbergen, and Walker's situation-specific theory of midlife women's attitudes toward physical activity (2010)
	Riegel and Dickson's situation-specific theory of heart failure self-care (2008)

Adapted from Masters, K. (2015). *Nursing theories a framework for professional practice* (2nd ed.). Jones & Bartlett Learning; McEwen, M., & Wills, E. (2014). *Theoretical basis for nursing* (4th ed.). Wolters Kluwer Health/Lippincott Williams & Wilkins; Meleis, A. (2018). *Theoretical nursing: Development & progress* (6th ed.). Wolters Kluwer; Peterson, S., & Bredow, T. (2017). *Middle range theories application to nursing research and practice* (4th ed.). Wolters Kluwer.

Many nurses fail to appreciate nursing models and theories. Learning the essence of each model or theory from the original sources as much as possible fosters an appreciation of the similarities and differences among them and identifies points of congruence with the worldviews on which each is based. Some nurse theorists coin words, define familiar words in different ways, and develop new concepts. This chapter examines the models rather than critiquing them or selecting a single best model or theory for use. The selection of a nursing model or theory to guide practice is an individual decision. Interpretations of the professional nursing processes based on these models are presented in Chapter 8, "Professional Nursing Processes."

Take Note!

Nurses make individual decisions when selecting a nursing model or theory to guide their clinical practice.

Growth and Stability Models of Change

Two basic philosophical worldviews exist about the nature of change. Although change remains constant, perceptions of change differ among people. Fawcett (1989) posited two worldviews, each based on its perceptions of change. One worldview recognizes change as continuous, a desired opportunity for growth to attain maximum human potential. The other worldview is persistence, which maintains that humans strive for stability and that endurance results from "a synthesis of growth and stability" (Fawcett, 1989, p. 12). The persistence worldview focuses on continuing and maintaining patterns by emphasizing balance and equilibrium. Although the worldviews differ, they are not mutually exclusive. The selected nursing models in this chapter approach change differently, which provides a means to classify them.

▮ QUESTIONS FOR REFLECTION

1. Which worldview seems more compatible with your personal philosophy—change or persistence? Why?
2. Is it possible to embrace both worldviews? Why or why not?

THE STABILITY MODEL OF CHANGE

The **stability model of change** proposes that the natural order of things revolves around consistency. Although change is inevitable and may be undesirable, it forces adaptation. Once the adaptive adjustment is complete, a state of stability results. Stability means that the organism attains a new and stable equilibrium.

Systems Theory as a Framework

Systems theory addresses elements and interactions among all the factors (variables) in a situation. Interactions between the person and the environment

occur continuously, thereby creating a complex, constantly changing situation. Systems theory provides a way to understand the many influences on the whole person and the possible impact of change on any part of the whole. This theory can help nurses understand, predict, and control the possible effects of nursing care on the client system and the concurrent effects of the interaction on the nurse system and environment.

Auger (1976) defined a system as "a whole with interrelated parts, in which the parts have a function and the system as a totality has a function" (p. 21). Within the systems framework, single systems (subsystems) form more complex systems (suprasystems) (Fig. 7.1). Subsystems may be smaller than the tiniest cell of an organism. Suprasystems extend beyond what humans know as the universe.

Humans are composed of cells, organs, and physiologic systems. These subsystems are continuously interacting and changing. For example, as a person eats, the blood supply to the gastrointestinal organs increases. Absorption of carbohydrates increases the blood glucose level, which results in increased insulin secretion. Simultaneously, changes in the blood circulation and blood glucose level affect the person's attention level and the feeling of hunger. The person may feel satisfied and contented.

The whole person is the suprasystem for multiple interacting subsystems. The person's internal environment consists of interacting subsystems that are contained within bodily boundaries. The person, in turn, will have membership in a subsystem called family (which is a suprasystem of the person, which is a subsystem of the community system, and so on). Subsystems may be isolated for study, but humans are more than and different from the sum of their parts (Rogers, 1970).

A person cannot be characterized by describing physiologic, psychological, and sociocultural subsystems. A person's behavior is holistic, a reflection of the person as a whole. The focus of systems theory is on understanding the interaction among the various parts of the system, rather than on describing the function of the parts themselves (Auger, 1976). Systems analysis assumes that structure and stability can be measured during an arbitrarily frozen period.

Factors from the environment impinge on the system across the system boundary. These factors cause tension, stress, strain, or conflict that may upset system balance. The system seeks equilibrium, or a steady state, in which a balance exists among the various forces operating within and on the system. Change is a process

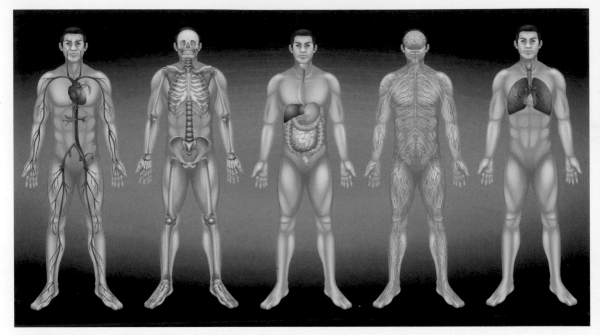

FIGURE 7.1 The human body with its multiple interactive systems provides an example of systems theory.

of tension reduction and dynamic equilibrium, which restores a new position of system balance after a disturbance (Chin, 1976).

Because they are open systems, people exchange matter, energy, and information with the environment (Sills & Hall, 1977). A human being's internal environment interacts constantly with an ever-changing external environment. Changes occurring in one affect the other. For example, walking into a cold room (change in the external environment) affects various physiologic and psychological subsystems of the internal environment, which in turn reduces blood flow to the periphery, the ability to concentrate, and the feeling of comfort. Similarly, a person's angry outburst (change in the internal environment) may have a demonstrable effect on the moods of others. It is this openness of human systems that makes nursing intervention possible. Under general systems theory, nurses interact with clients to help them attain homeostasis, defined as the constancy of the internal environment caused by the action of regulatory mechanisms. Constancy does not mean that the internal environment is static but rather that it is constantly changing to maintain its equilibrium. This relative equilibrium is maintained by homeodynamics (Cannon, 1932).

Energy, information, or matter provides system input. The system "transforms, creates, and organizes input in the process known as throughput, which results in a reorganization of the input" (Sills & Hall, 1977, p. 21). Thus, each system modifies its input. Simultaneously, energy, information, or matter is given off into the environment as output. When output is returned to the system as input, the process is known as feedback (Fig. 7.2).

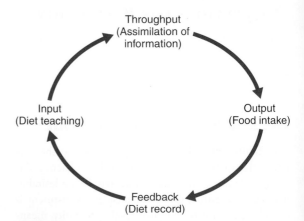

FIGURE 7.2 In this example of systems interaction, information about a therapeutic diet the nurse gives to a client is system input for the client system. What the client eats would be one type of system output, based on the throughput related to assimilation and acceptance of the information originally given. The nurse, using the client's reported food intake as feedback, can help reinforce or modify the client's future behavior.

A person can be viewed as "an interrelated, interdependent, interacting, complex organism, constantly influencing and being influenced by (the) environment" (Sills & Hall, 1977, p. 24). Because the person is in constant interaction with the environment, many interrelated factors, including the nurse, affect the person's health status. The person's response, in turn, results in environmental change. Thus, a change in any part affects the entirety of the human–environment system.

Using systems theory to guide nursing process directs assessment of the relationships among all variables that affect the client–environment interaction, including the influence of the nurse. While intervening, the nurse must anticipate the system-wide impact from change in any part of the system and appreciate the simultaneous, rather than cause-and-effect, nature of change in open systems.

Imogene King's Systems Interaction Model (Theory of Goal Attainment)

In her nursing model based on systems theory, King (1981, 1987, 1989) stressed interactions and mutuality. King developed her model when she was trying to outline essential content for a new graduate nursing program (King, 2001). According to **King's systems interaction model (theory of goal attainment)**, the purpose of nursing is to help people attain, maintain, or restore health, primarily by mutual goal setting. King described the nurse–client interaction as transactional, involving nurse–client mutual understanding of events, mutually set goals, and agreement on means to achieve the goal.

King's (1989) model has its roots in sociology and focuses on "individuals whose interactions in groups within social systems influence behavior within the systems" (p. 152). King defined humans as "open systems interacting with environment" (King, 1981, p. 10) and as "rational, sentient, reacting, social, controlling, purposeful, time-oriented, and action-oriented" (King, 1987, p. 107). The human "perceives the world as a total person" (King, 1981, p. 141), resulting in environmental interactions to which they must constantly adjust. King (1981) delineated the environment as internal (within the body/person) and external. King proposed that the personal system underlies each person as a whole system who interacts with one or more persons, thereby creating interpersonal systems. When interpersonal systems expand to include large groups of people, social systems are developed. King (1999) emphasized that the three systems (personal, interpersonal, and social)

interact with each other and "represent organized wholes in constant interaction in one's environment" (p. 292).

- In personal systems, perception is the comprehensive concept. It is "a characteristic of a human process of interaction and along with communication provides a channel for passage of information from one person to another" (King, 1989, p. 153). Concepts of self, growth and development, learning, body image, time, and space also relate to individuals as personal systems.
- In interpersonal systems, interaction is the comprehensive concept. Related concepts include communication, transactions, roles, stress, and all the concepts identified in personal systems.
- In social systems, organization is the comprehensive concept. Related concepts include power, authority, status, decision making, and control (King, 1989).

As people interact with their environment, their perceptions influence their behavior and health. Nurses interact with clients to facilitate achievement of mutually determined health-related goals.

Take Note!
According to King's systems interaction model (theory of goal attainment), the purpose of nursing is to help people attain, maintain, or restore health, primarily by mutual goal setting.

Health assumes achievement of maximum potential for daily living and an ability to function in social roles. It is the "dynamic life experiences of a human being, which implies continuous adjustment to stressors in the internal and external environment through optimum use of one's resources to achieve maximum potential for daily living" (King, 1981, p. 5). "Illness is a deviation from normal, that is, an imbalance in a person's biologic structure or in his psychological makeup, or a conflict in a person's social relationships" (King, 1989, p. 5).

"Nursing's domain involves human beings, families, and communities as a framework within which nurses make transactions in multiple environments with health as a goal" (King, 1996, p. 61). Nursing care is accomplished within goal-oriented nurse–client interactions "whereby each perceives the other and the situation, and through communications, set goals, explore the means to achieve them, (and) agree to the means, and their actions indicate movement toward goal achievement" (King, 1987, p. 113).

King (1987, pp. 109–110) identified 10 concepts relevant to understanding the dynamic interacting systems delineated in her model:

1. Interaction: A process of perception and communication between person and environment and between person and person, represented by verbal and nonverbal behaviors that are goal-directed
2. Perception: Each person's representation of reality
3. Communication: A process whereby information is given from one person to another
4. Transaction: An observable behavior of human beings interacting with their environment in which valuation is a component of human interaction
5. Role: A set of behaviors expected of individuals occupying specific positions in their social systems
6. Stress: A dynamic state whereby a human being interacts with the environment to maintain balance for growth, development, and performance
7. Growth and development: Continuous change in individuals at the cellular, molecular, and behavioral levels of activities
8. Time: A continuous flow of events in successive order that implies change, a past, and a future
9. Self: A personal system defined as a unified, complex whole
10. Space: Existing in all directions and the same everywhere

In King's theory (1995), these concepts are interrelated in a number of propositions and hypotheses that indicate "the nature of nurse–client interactions that lead to goal attainment" (p. 27). Decision making (including goal setting) is "a shared collaborative process in which client and nurse give information to each other, identify goals, and explore means to attain goals; each moves forward to attain goals." This is identified in the theory as a critical independent variable called "mutual goal setting" (King, 1989, p. 155). From the theory, a transaction process model has been designed to lead to goal attainment when practiced (King, 1999). Examples of testable hypotheses generated from King's theory include the process of mutual goal setting with clients, the strengths of mutual goal setting, and role conflict between client and nurse in nursing situations (King, 1987).

King's model and the theory of goal attainment provide a "theoretical base for applying the traditional nursing process … aimed at maintaining or restoring health" (Magan, 1987, pp. 129, 132). King's model has provided the theoretical foundation for international nursing practice, nursing departments,

■ TABLE 7.2	Major Concepts as Defined in King's Model
Human being	A personal system that interacts with interpersonal and social systems
Environment	A context "within which human beings grow, develop, and perform daily activities" (King, 1981, p. 18)
Health	"Dynamic life experiences of a human being, which implies continuous adjustment to stressors in the internal and external environment through optimum use of one's resources to achieve maximum potential for daily living" (King, 1981, p. 5)
Nursing	A process of human interaction

nurse empowerment, and client satisfaction (Fawcett, 2005). Studies using King's model have been conducted internationally and include the areas of client decision-making processes, effectiveness of client education, relationships among family coping (including caregiver stress) and health, and effectiveness of nursing and interdisciplinary interventions (Alligood, 2010). King's model also serves as a theoretical foundation for nursing education (undergraduate and programs) and for nursing service departments (Fawcett, 2005). Table 7.2 presents the major concepts of this model. Despite being originally conceptualized more than 25 years ago, King's model offers a systems approach that is compatible with the perception of health care delivery as a system with the goal of helping others attain optimal health status while coping with internal and external stressors by using available resources. When working with individuals recovering from substance abuse or receiving rehabilitation for an injury resulting in permanent disability, King's model provides a theoretical foundation for practice. The following Real-Life Reflection box provides an example of how a nurse might use King's model.

REAL-LIFE REFLECTIONS

Ms. Green, the client at the opening of this chapter, has just learned from her physician that she has multiple myeloma (malignant tumor of the bone marrow resulting in abnormal production of plasma cells) and is devastated. She received the news alone and is terrified to break the news to her husband and adult son. Nicole goes to check on Ms. Green to see if she got her lunch and how she is eating. Ms. Green says that any time she attempts to eat or drink, she chokes because she starts to cry. Nicole offers her an antianxiety pill, but Ms. Green tearfully refuses it and her lunch tray. A few minutes later, Brianna stops by to visit with Ms. Green. Ms. Green shares all of her concerns with Brianna. Brianna expresses concern about Ms. Green's refusal to eat or drink and informs her if she does not at least drink, then she will have to receive intravenous hydration. Brianna asks Ms. Green if she has a favorite food and discovered that she enjoys eating vanilla ice cream. Brianna suggests that Ms. Green should try and eat a small cup of ice cream and promises to get her all the ice cream that she can eat. Ms. Green laughs and agrees to eat some ice cream, but only if Brianna will stay with her in case she starts to cry. Brianna gets the ice cream and visits with Ms. Green as she eats an entire 4-oz cup.

- *What goals can you identify in these nurse–client interactions?*
- *What goals were attained and why were they attained?*

Betty Neuman's Systems Model

Betty Neuman also used systems theory to provide a foundation for her nursing model, known as Neuman's systems model. Neuman developed her model while attempting to help nursing students organize their thinking and look at clients holistically when teaching mental health nursing (Neuman, 2002). **Neuman's systems model** specifies that the purpose of nursing is to facilitate optimal client system stability by reducing the impact of environmental stimuli or stressors.

Neuman described human beings as having a core that is protected by buffering systems. Four key concepts describe the interaction of human beings with environmental stressors that determine health status:

1. Central core: The basic structure and energy reserves of the human that make life possible
2. Flexible lines of defense: Adaptive responses that fluctuate and protect the core from stressor penetration
3. Normal line of defense: A conscious adaptation response usually used by an individual to protect the core from stressor penetration

4. Lines of resistance: Protection factors, usually unconscious in nature, activated when stressors have penetrated the normal line of defense

Neuman's model focuses on stress reduction, the impact of stress, and how stress and the individual's response to stress affect the development, maintenance, and restoration of health. People are composites of physiologic, psychological, sociocultural, developmental, and spiritual variables that act harmoniously and simultaneously when encountering stressors from either the internal or external environment. Neuman defined clients as individuals, families, groups, or communities who interact constantly with the environment.

Take Note!
Neuman's systems model specifies that the purpose of nursing is to facilitate optimal client system stability by reducing the impact of environmental stimuli or stressors.

The environment includes "all internal and external factors or influences surrounding the identified client or client system" (Neuman, 2002, p. 18).

- The internal environment is composed of interacting elements within the human body.
- The external environment consists of anything outside the human body.
- The created environment encompasses individual perceptions of the internal and external environments.

People constantly encounter stressors from the internal, external, or created environment. Stressors are tension-producing stimuli that have the potential to disturb a person's equilibrium or normal line of defense. This normal line of defense is the person's "usual steady state." It is the way in which an individual typically deals with stressors. Stressors may be positive (eustress) or negative (distress). Stressors may be of three types: intrapersonal (arising from within the person), interpersonal (arising between two or more people), or extrapersonal (arising from the external environment rather than other people).

According to Neuman (1982, 2002), a person's basic structure and energy resources need protection from encountered stressors. Reactions and resistance to stressors are provided by lines of defense. Neuman (1982, 2002) called the outermost line of defense the flexible line of defense. This dynamic protective buffer consists of physiologic, psychological, sociocultural, developmental, and spiritual variables affecting a person at any given moment. These variables may include a person's current physiologic state, mood, beliefs, cognitive state, nutritional status, spiritual beliefs, developmental state, and cognitive ability. If the flexible line of defense is no longer able to protect the person against a stressor, the normal lines of defense work to buffer the effects produced. The normal lines of defense encompass the usual response used by the person, such as exercise, health habits (e.g., basic hygiene), relaxation strategies, and conscious coping methods.

The final protections for the core are the lines of resistance. Examples of lines of resistance include immunologic responses and unconscious emotional defense mechanisms. Obvious reactions to stress become visible when lines of resistance are penetrated.

The reaction to stressors may lead to restoration of balance or to death. Three factors influence a person's reaction to and recovery from encountered stressors: the number and strength of the stressor(s) affecting the person, the length of exposure to the stressor(s), and the meaningfulness of the stressor(s) to the person.

Neuman (1996) intended for the nurse to "assist clients to retain, attain, or maintain optimal system stability" (p. 69). Thus, health (wellness) seems to be related to dynamic equilibrium of the normal line of defense, where stressors are successfully overcome or avoided by the flexible line of defense. Neuman (2002) defined illness as "a state of insufficiency with disrupting needs unsatisfied" (p. 25). Illness appears to be a separate state when a stressor breaks through the normal line of defense and causes a reaction with the person's lines of resistance.

Nurses use primary, secondary, or tertiary prevention to help clients attain optimal wellness. Primary prevention covers interventions to promote health. Secondary prevention occurs once a stressor has penetrated the normal lines of defense or lines of resistance (e.g., pain medication). Tertiary prevention focuses on restoration of balance (e.g., rehabilitation). When restoration is complete, nursing interventions return to primary prevention.

Neuman's systems model is compatible with the traditional medical model. It has been widely used internationally, especially by nurses in the Americas, Pacific Rim, and Europe. The model serves as the framework for the World Health Organization project "Nest of Love" and for delivery of mental health services in Holland (Lowry, 2004). The Neuman Systems Model Organization and Neuman Trustee Group promote utilization of the Neuman's systems model. Table 7.3 summarizes major concepts as defined in Neuman's

▪ TABLE 7.3	Major Concepts as Defined in Neuman's Model
Human beings (client system)	A composite of physiologic, psychological, sociocultural, developmental, and spiritual variables in interaction with the internal and external environment
Environment	All internal and external factors of influences surrounding the client system
Health	A continuum of wellness to illness
Nursing	Prevention as intervention

model. By offering a systems approach, looking for ways to reduce the impact of stressors, and using prevention as intervention, the Neuman health care systems model remains a relevant approach to professional nursing practice. For example, stress has been identified as a major factor contributing to illness and inhibiting healing. Even some nursing students identify high levels of stress as a factor affecting academic performance. The Neuman's systems model provides ways for nurses to examine the level of stress in the lives of care recipients (and themselves) and look for ways to reduce it as well as develop interventions to promote effective habits to strengthen the normal lines of defense. The following Real-Life Reflection box provides an example of how a nurse might use the Neuman's systems model in clinical practice.

REAL-LIFE REFLECTIONS

After seeing Brianna's success in using nursing theories as a foundation for her clinical practice, Nicole remembers learning about Neuman's systems model of nursing. The next day, Brianna is off and Nicole is assigned as Ms. Green's nurse. Upon entering Ms. Green's room, Nicole notices that Ms. Green has been crying and her hands tremble as she takes her scheduled medications. As she reviews the medical and nursing care plans for the day, Nicole asks Ms. Green if she has any concerns. Ms. Green specifies that she continues to sleep poorly at night and states that she just wants to get a couple of hours of uninterrupted sleep. Nicole thinks of ways to create a quiet physical environment to help Ms. Green nap. Nicole's plan involves keeping the door closed, placing a note on the door for anyone who wants to enter the room to speak first with Nicole, telling individuals who want to enter the room to return in 3 hours after Ms. Green's nap, providing soft music in the room, and informing staff to be quiet when they are close to Ms. Green's room. Nicole remembers how lack of sleep weakens the flexible and normal lines of defense and believes this is affecting Ms. Green's ability to cope with her cancer diagnosis. Ms. Green takes an uninterrupted 3-hour nap and then orders a large lunch that she finishes. She also confides in Nicole about how she might lose her job because of her illness and that she is afraid of dying because her mother died at the same age that she is now.

- *In this situation, how did Nicole use the Neuman's systems model to plan and implement nursing care for Ms. Green?*
- *Were there any unintended benefits that occurred in this nursing situation?*
- *What additional nursing interventions might Nicole consider for Ms. Green?*

Stress/Adaptation Theory as a Framework

In contrast to systems theory, stress and adaptation theories view change in terms of accommodation. People adjust to environmental changes to avoid disturbing a balanced existence. Adaptation theory provides a way to understand both how equilibrium is maintained and the possible effects of disturbed equilibrium. This theory has been widely applied to explain, predict, and control biologic (physiologic and psychological) responses of individuals and serves as traditional medical therapy.

Under stress/adaptation theory, persons' regulatory systems operate by way of compensation. Any change in the internal environment automatically initiates a response to minimize or counteract the change. For example, when the blood glucose level drops, the endocrine system responds with increased cortisol secretion, which decreases the rate at which cells use glucose and stimulate the conversion of amino acids into glucose. These compensatory actions cause the blood glucose level to increase. If it should increase above acceptable limits, insulin secretion would increase the rate of glucose uptake by cells, thus reducing the blood glucose level.

Compensation occurs continuously as the body adjusts to stimuli that tend to disturb equilibrium.

A stimulus may be anything that creates change in the internal environment and thus places demands on the body to compensate. Examples of stimuli include changes in environmental temperature or sleep patterns, hunger, joy, and infection. Whether stimuli are beneficial or harmful, all require the body to adapt.

A person's ability to adapt to changes in life events may determine their potential for health or disease. One way people adapt is through coping mechanisms that aim "to master conditions of harm, threat, or challenge when a routine or automatic response is not readily available" (Monat & Lazarus, 1977, p. 8). Some regard coping methods primarily as psychological barriers when stimuli are perceived as threats. Thus, a person's reaction to stimuli involves cognitive appraisal and psychological coping methods in addition to physiologic reactions. One of the best-known nursing models that uses adaptation theory is the model developed by Sister Callista Roy.

Callista Roy's Adaptation Model

Sister Callista Roy developed her adaptation model as a graduate nursing student when confronted with the challenge of defining nursing (Meleis, 2018; Roy, 2002). Although initially concerned with the focus and target of and indications for nursing care, the model has evolved to incorporate Roy's religious views (Meleis, 2018). In 2008, Roy (2008, 2011) specified that the philosophical view underlying her model is cosmic unity, which proposes that humans and the earth have three common patterns—"unity, diversity, and self-identity" (2011, p. 346)—and "integral relationships" (p. 139). She also incorporated the concept of veritivity, defined as "a common purposefulness of human existence," which translates into people finding meaning in life (Meleis, 2018). Roy viewed purposefulness as meaning that "all persons and the earth have both unity and diversity; all are united in a common destiny; people find meaning in mutual relations with each other and the created world, and most often in acknowledging a creator or God-figure that is the common destiny or final union of all" (Roy, 2011, p. 346). **Roy's adaptation model** outlines the purpose of nursing as promoting a human being's adaptation in four adaptive modes.

Roy used five key terms in her model:

1. Stimulus: Point of interaction of the human system and environment; stimulus produces a response.
2. Adaptive modes: Ways in which people adapt (i.e., through physiologic needs, self-concept, role function, or interdependent relations)

3. Classes of stimuli: Focal (immediately confronting the person), contextual (all other stimuli present), and residual (nonspecific stimuli, such as beliefs or attitudes)
4. Adaptation level: Range of a person's ability to adapt and create changes in the integrated, compensatory, and compromised environments
5. Coping: Ways of responding to the changing environment

Roy organized her model around adaptive behaviors that encompass the set of processes by which humans adapt to environmental stimuli. The human being as a unified system is viewed as a "set of parts connected to function as a whole" (Roy & Andrews, 1999, p. 36) through homeostatic and homodynamic systems. Humans constantly interact with an ever-changing environment, and their ability to respond positively reflects their level of adaptation.

Environmental stimuli affect the human being. A focal stimulus is an environmental change that requires an immediate adaptive response from the person. Accompanying the focal stimulus are contextual stimuli (all other stimuli present) and residual stimuli (other relevant factors such as nonspecific stimuli), which mediate and contribute to the effect of the focal stimulus.

The pooled effect of the three classes of stimuli establishes a person's adaptation level. In turn, each individual's adaptation level determines a zone that indicates the range of additional stimulation that will have a positive or adaptive response. If additional stimuli fall outside the zone, the person cannot respond effectively and compromised adaptation ensues. Effective adaptation results in free energy available for use in subsequent adaptation to stimuli.

According to Roy and Roberts (1981, p. 56), "Coping refers to routine, accustomed patterns of behaviors to deal with daily situations as well as to the production of new ways of behaving when drastic changes defy the familiar responses." The two major coping mechanisms for individuals are the regulator subsystem, composed mainly of automatic neural, endocrine, and chemical activity, and the cognator subsystem, which includes cognitive–emotive channels and provides for perceptual and information processing, learning, judgment, and emotion (Andrews & Roy, 1986, p. 7).

In 2008, Roy redefined adaptation as the "process and outcome whereby thinking and feeling persons, as individuals or in groups, use conscious awareness and choice to create human and environmental integration"

(p. 138). Roy (1987, 2011) identified the following dimensions of human adaptive modes: physiologic–physical, self-concept–group identity, role function, and interdependence. The desired result is a state in which conditions promote the person's goals, including survival, growth, reproduction, mastery, and personal and environmental transformations.

Health "is viewed in light of human goals and the purposefulness of human existence. The fulfillment of this purpose in life is reflected in becoming integrated and whole" (Roy & Andrews, 1999, p. 54). Thus, health is viewed as both "a state and a process of being and becoming an integrated and whole human being" (Roy & Andrews, 1999, p. 54).

The goal of nursing is "to promote adaptation in the four adaptation modes contributing to health, quality of life, and dying with dignity" (Roy, 2011, p. 346). Nursing assessment and intervention foster the goal of adaptation with the client's active participation. The criteria for goal attainment generally encompass any positive response by the individual that creates free energy that can be used for responding to other stimuli (Riehl & Roy, 1980).

Take Note!
Roy's adaptation model outlines the purpose of nursing as promoting a person's adaptation in the four adaptive modes: physiologic needs, self-concept, role function, and interdependent relations.

Roy's model provides a classification system for stimuli that may affect adaptation, as well as a system for classifying nursing assessment. The model "has been useful in supporting the traditional concept of nursing practice within the medical model perspective" (Huch, 1987, p. 63). Roy's model has been widely used internationally, revealing its transcultural appeal. The Roy Adaptation Association has chapters in Japan, Colombia, and Mexico. Nurses use Roy's model as a framework for nursing education in baccalaureate and higher degree programs, as a foundation for health assessment in clinical practice, and as guidance for application in nursing service departments. Roy also advocated the use of the model by other health care professionals (Fawcett, 2003; Roy, 2002). It has been used as a theoretical framework for the development of tools for research and clinical practice, including a foundation for electronic health documentation, development of nursing interventions to promote empowerment,

TABLE 7.4	Major Concepts as Defined in Roy's Model
Human beings (human system)	"A whole with parts that function as a unity for some purpose" (Roy & Andrews, 1999, p. 31) that shares the patterns of "unity, diversity, and self-identity" (Roy, 2011, p. 346) with the earth. "Each individual contributes to the universe" (p. 346). Human systems include the family, organizations, communities, and global society (Roy, 2011).
Environment	"The world within and around humans as adaptive systems" (Roy & Andrews, 1999, p. 51) and any condition, situation, and influence that affect human behavior and development as an adaptive system
Health	"A state and process of being and becoming an integrated and whole human being" (Roy & Andrews, 1999, p. 54)
Nursing	Manipulation of stimuli to foster successful adaptation in physiologic needs, self-concept, role function, or interdependent relations

enhanced spirituality, reduced child pain, and factors that influence adaptation and coping; determination of effective coping strategies with impaired activities of daily living; and quality of life in the older population (Roy et al., 2009).

Table 7.4 summarizes the major concepts defined in Roy's model. Because of its global nature, Roy's adaptation model applies across nearly all nursing practice areas, especially when the nurse wants to address recipient needs from a holistic perspective. One example of how a nurse might use the model in practice would be considering the hospitalization of a single parent with small children. Because of Roy's emphasis on role function, the nurse would analyze the impact of the hospitalization on the parenting role and offer special support (assessing child care needs, initiating social service consultation early, and making special arrangements so that the children might be able to visit the parent).

THE GROWTH MODEL OF CHANGE

Unlike the models discussed so far, which focus on achievement or restoration of stability, nursing models based on the **growth model of change** tend to focus on helping people grow to realize and attain their full potential. The models of nursing that espouse the growth model of change tend to use caring theory or complexity theory as an underlying framework.

Caring Theory as a Framework

Nursing practice focuses on caring for and about others. No single, universally accepted definition exists for **caring** in the nursing context, as it can be used as a verb or noun (e.g., "The nurse cared for the client" and "Nursing care was given"). Morse et al. (1990,

p. 2) found that the literature includes references to care or caring as actions performed (as in to "take care of") as well as concern demonstrated (as in "caring about"). A literature analysis reveals at least five perspectives or categories of caring, including caring as a human trait (Benner & Wrubel, 1989; Gaut & Leininger, 1991); caring as a moral imperative (Watson, 2018); caring as an interpersonal relationship (Parse, 1987); caring as a therapeutic intervention (Orem, 1980); and caring as an affect (Morse et al., 1990).

Clients perceive caring as "those nursing ministrations that are person-centered, protective, anticipatory, physically comforting, and that go beyond routine care" (Swanson, 1991, p. 161). Kyle (1995, p. 509) concluded that there is a "marked difference between the patients' and nurses' perceptions of caring, with the nurses focusing on the psychosocial skills and the patient on skills that demonstrate professional competency." Caring outcomes may be demonstrated in terms of either subjective experiences or objective client outcomes.

The concept of caring permeates the nursing literature and appears in many nursing models. Table 7.5 compares Swanson's and Koldjeski's theoretical components of caring. Orem's self-care deficit theory uses the term "care" primarily as action, while Watson used the term to describe an attitude or display of compassion that is a moral imperative for nurses.

▍ QUESTIONS FOR REFLECTION

1. What characteristics do you identify when you have been the recipient of a caring interaction?
2. What results from a caring interaction between two people?
3. Why is caring an important aspect of professional nursing?

TABLE 7.5   A Comparison of Components of Caring

Swanson's Caring Processes (1991)	Koldjeski's (1990) Five "Essences" of Caring
1. Knowing: Striving to understand an event as it has meaning in the life of another	1. Interpersonal valuing and involvement
2. Being with: Being emotionally present for another	2. Being there for and experiencing with another
3. Doing for: Doing for others as they would do for themselves if it were possible	3. Instilling faith
4. Enabling: Facilitating another's passage through life transitions and unfamiliar events	4. Concern and love for another
5. Maintaining belief: Sustaining faith in another's capacity to get through an event or transition and face a future with meaning	5. Actualization

Dorothea Orem's Self-Care Deficit Theory

According to **Orem's self-care deficit theory** (1980, 1985, 1990, 1995, 2001), the purpose of nursing is to help people meet their self-care needs. The theory focuses on individuals "in society affected by human or environmental conditions associated with their states of health or their requirements for health care that result in inability to provide continuously for themselves the amount and quality of self-care they require" (Orem, 2001, p. 20). When the situation involves children, the nurse provides education and support to parents or guardians. Basically, Orem proposes that nurses do for others what they cannot do for themselves. She observed nurses as they engaged in clinical practice to develop the theory. Orem's theory uses five key concepts:

1. Self-care: Learned behaviors that a person performs for themselves (when able) that contribute to health
2. Self-care deficit: A relationship between actions that a person should take for healthy functioning and the capability for action
3. Self-care requisites: Needs that are universal or associated with development of or deviation from health
4. Self-care demand: Therapeutic actions to meet needs
5. Agency: Capability to engage in self-care

The essence of Orem's three-part nursing theory "focuses on a human being in relations. The theory of self-care focuses on the self, the I; the theory of self-care deficit focuses on you and me; and the theory of nursing systems focuses on we, human beings in community" (Orem, 1990, p. 49). Orem's theory integrates each of these theories (Orem, 1995, 2001).

Orem (1995) defined self-care as the "voluntary regulation of one's own human functioning and development that is necessary for individuals to maintain life, health, and well-being" (p. 95). People learn self-care activities as they mature. Culture, society, and family customs play key roles in determining individual self-care activities. Age, developmental state, or health status can affect the ability to perform self-care activities (e.g., parents or guardians must provide continuous care for infants and toddlers).

Orem (1980) specified that nursing is concerned with the individual's need for self-care action to "sustain life and health, recover from disease or injury, and cope with their effects" (p. 6). In Orem's view, nursing care may be offered to individuals and groups. However, Orem emphasized that only people have self-care requisites. The nurse cares for, assists, or does something for the client to achieve client-desired health outcomes or to meet basic human needs (Orem, 1980, 1985, 1990, 1995, 2001).

Take Note!
According to Orem's self-care deficit theory, the purpose of nursing is to help people meet their self-care needs.

Orem (1985) asserted that health is "a state of a human being that is characterized by soundness or wholeness of developed human structures and of bodily and mental functioning" (p. 179). Orem proposed that individual perception (well-being) affects health. In the self-care deficit theory, human health is a holistic concept.

Orem addressed the physical, psychological, interpersonal, and social aspects of health but indicated that they are inseparable in the human being: "Health describes the state of wholeness or integrity of human beings" (Orem, 1995, p. 96). "If there is acceptance of the real unity of individual human beings, there should be no difficulty in recognizing structural and functional differentiation within the unity" (Orem, 1980, p. 180). Orem viewed individuals as moving "toward maturation and achievement of the individual's human potential" (Orem, 1985, p. 180) rather than as organisms seeking a steady state.

Orem suggested that some people may have self-care requisites associated with development or health deviations. Self-care requisites are essential enduring needs, while other needs may surface because of internal or external conditions that alter the ability to care for oneself. Orem (1980) identified the following universal self-care requisites (p. 42):

1. Maintenance of sufficient air, water, and food intake
2. Provision of care associated with elimination processes and excrements
3. Maintenance of a balance between activity and rest and between solitude and social interaction
4. Prevention of hazards to life, functioning, and well-being
5. Promotion of human functioning and development within social groups in accord with potential, known limitations and the desire to be normal

Identified self-care requisites require actions known as "therapeutic self-care demands." Therapeutic self-care demands can be determined by:

1. Identifying existing or potential self-care requisites
2. Developing methods for meeting self-care requisites by considering basic factors (e.g., developmental state, general health status, living patterns) that "condition the values of patients' self-care agency and therapeutic self-care demands as well as the means that are valid for meeting self-care requisites and in regulating self-care agency at particular times" (Orem, 1985, p. 78)
3. Designing, implementing, and evaluating a plan of action; Orem tended to use nursing process as a way to develop a system of nursing.

The theory of nursing systems involves "an interpersonal unity at a particular time–space localization. This unity is formed by nurses, persons who have entered into an agreement to accept and participate in nursing, and the relatives or persons who are responsible for the individuals who require nursing" (Orem, 1990, p. 54). Thus, candidates for nursing care are clients who have insufficient current or projected capability for providing self-care. "It is the need for compensatory action (to overcome an inability or limited ability to engage in care) or action to help in the development or regulation of self-care abilities that is the basis for a nursing relationship" (Orem, 1980, p. 58). Other concepts and theories that have been derived from the self-care deficit theory include self-care agency, dependent care, and dependent care agency (Taylor et al., 2000).

Orem's theory, which is compatible with the traditional medical model, has been widely used in international nursing practice, education, and research (Orem & Taylor, 2011). The International Orem Society publishes the *Self-Care and Dependent Care* nursing journal to promote and validate the use of the model. Table 7.6 summarizes the major concepts defined in Orem's model. Unlike many of the nursing models and theories, Orem incorporates traditional medical approaches while carving out a unique place for nursing in health care delivery. In practice, Orem's nursing theory has been used as a framework for guiding nursing departments in acute and chronic care settings and health care utilization review programs (Meleis, 2018). Because Orem emphasizes that the nurse does for the person what they cannot do for themselves and teaches the client and/or caregiver how to care for the person, Orem's model fits nicely in practice settings in which nurses care for comatose clients, rehabilitation settings, and following any hospital or outpatient visit during which a procedure was performed (educating clients and caregivers about how to monitor for complications and when to consult health care providers following the visit). The following Real-Life Reflection box provides an example of how a nurse might use Orem's self-care deficit theory.

■ TABLE 7.6	Major Concepts as Defined in Orem's Theory
Human being (client)	A person under the care of a nurse
Environment	Physical, chemical, biologic, and social contexts (including the family) within which human beings exist
Health	"A state characterized by being structurally or functionally sound" (Orem, 2001, p. 96)
Nursing	An art by which practitioners provide specialized assistance to persons with disabilities who require special needs for self-care while participating in the medical plan of care outlined by physicians

Ms. Green has finished receiving her first round of chemotherapy and is going to be dismissed from the hospital. She and her husband need to learn about the potential complications of chemotherapy so that they can contact the oncologist if complications arise. Ms. Green's current occupation is manager of a retail clothing store. Using knowledge of basic management skills, Nicole offers suggestions for Ms. Green to chart her daily weight, temperature measurements, food and fluid intake, skin checks for bruising, and scales for rating pain, nausea, sore mouth, mood, and anxiety. Because Ms. Green has a computer at home, Nicole proposes that she develop a flow sheet to record these key assessments for chemotherapy-induced complications. Nicole also proposes that Ms. Green could record results of outpatient lab test results on the flow sheet. She provides the Greens with medication cards about each of the chemotherapy agents administered; a list of currently ordered medications outlining actions, reasons, and potential side effects; and a dismissal information form specifying activity level, dietary restrictions, and the date for her outpatient follow-up with the oncologist. After reviewing all the information with Ms. Green, Nicole validates Ms. Green's understanding by having her answer a series of questions about medications, activity level, dietary restrictions, and when to contact the oncologist. Ms. Green gives Nicole a hug as she leaves and thanks her for giving her everything that she needed as an inpatient and as a person returning home.

- *Do you think Nicole was aware that she could be practicing nursing using Orem's self-care deficit theory? Why or why not?*
- *Outline the factors for self-care covered in this nursing situation. Can you think of other things Ms. Green might need for safe, effective self-care?*

Jean Watson's Human Caring Science, Theory of Nursing

Jean Watson developed Watson's human science and human care theory while writing a book about a bachelor of science in nursing (BSN)–integrated nursing curriculum (Fawcett, 2005; Watson, 2002b). Her work blends Eastern philosophy while representing phenomenological, existential, and spiritual orientations. Watson proposed that the purpose of nursing is "to help persons gain a higher degree of harmony that fosters self-knowledge, self-reverence, self-caring, self-control, and self-healing processes while allowing increasing diversity" (Watson, 2012, p. 61). In 2012, Watson recognized that her human care theory seemed to be more of a science rather than a nursing theory. Key concepts of **Watson's human caring science, theory of nursing** are the phenomenal field (the totality of past, present, and future influences on each human being); "carative" factors (what to do); "carative" processes (how to do); and transpersonal caring (a moral ideal and art). Transpersonal caring occurs when the caregiver and care receiver engage in "a human-spirit-to-spirit connection" (Watson, 2012, p. 85), during which occurs "a special kind of human care relationship—a connection/union with another person, a high regard for the whole person, and their being-in-the-world" forms (Watson, 2012, p. 75). Outcomes of the transpersonal caring interaction include "movement toward greater harmony, spiritual evolution, and omega point/perfection" (Watson, 2012, p. 83).

Watson (2007) stated: "Human life … is defined as (spiritual–mental–physical) being-in-the-world which is continuous in time and space" (p. 47). Although the soul, mind, and body are explicitly identified as spheres of the human being, they are viewed as integrated and inseparable until the time of death, when the soul transcends and continues to exist (Watson, 2012).

Watson's human science and human care theory proposed that the purpose of nursing is "to help persons gain a higher degree of harmony that fosters self-knowledge, self-reverence, self-caring, self-control, and self-healing processes while allowing increasing diversity."

Watson (2012) described health as "a subjective experience; it can refer to unity of body-mind-spirit" (p. 60). She expanded health to include congruency between the perceived self and the experienced self, and summarized health as "I = Me—Health (harmony, 'in right relation,' with self-world and open to increased diversity)" (Watson, 2012, p. 61). Illness is not always a disease, but rather a "subjective turmoil or disharmony within a person's inner self or soul at some level or disharmony with the person" (Watson, 2012, p. 62). Illness may cause disease. Diseases can be cured, but illness requires healing.

Watson viewed each human being as having a unique phenomenal field that encompasses "the totality of human experience as one's being-in-the-world" (Watson, 2007, p. 55). Although not equivalent to human consciousness, the phenomenal field is the entire constellation of internal and external factors that shape all human experiences (past, present, and future). She described human behavior as being goal-directed with the aim of seeking harmony within body, mind, and soul, resulting in self-integration, enhancement, and actualization. When two or more individuals come together, they share a phenomenal field and experience a transpersonal event. For a caring event to occur, the nurse and client must each make a choice to enter the relationship. The nurse enters the experience of the client, and the client enters into the experiences of the nurse.

Watson (2018) used the word "nurse" as a noun (a person caring for another) and a verb (actions related to caring for another). She described caring as "the moral ideal of nursing" (p. 54) consisting of "transpersonal human-to-human attempts to protect, enhance, and preserve humanity by helping a person find meaning in illness, suffering, pain, and existence; to help another gain self-knowledge, control, and self-healing wherein a sense of inner harmony is restored regardless of the external circumstance" (Watson, 2012, p. 72).

Caring is "a moral ideal, rather than an interpersonal technique" (Watson, 2007, p. 58), which can be demonstrated through the carative factors (nursing interventions) that "allow for contact between the subjective world of the experiencing persons" (Watson, 1989, p. 227). The following "carative" factors are all presupposed by a knowledge base and clinical competence (Watson, 2012, p. 47):

1. Humanistic–altruistic system of values
2. Faith–hope
3. Sensitivity to self and others
4. Helping–trusting, human care relationship
5. Expressing positive and negative feelings
6. Creative problem-solving caring processes
7. Transpersonal teaching–learning
8. Supportive, protective, and/or corrective mental, physical, sociocultural, and spiritual environment
9. Human needs assistance
10. Existential–phenomenological–spiritual forces

During the human care process (nursing), the nurse and person engage in a mutual endeavor, a specific level of space and time. The nurse and client together embark on a journey to discover new meanings and understanding that require "serious study, reflection, and action" (Watson, 2007, p. 29). The nurse uses the "carative" factors to facilitate the human care process.

Watson's theory provides one framework for the study of caring that has served as the foundation for many nursing research studies across the world. Watson (2018) proposed that descriptive phenomenology along with transcendental or depth phenomenology and poetic results may be the most effective ways to generate evidence and knowledge about specific caring processes for professional nursing practice. Despite the abstract nature of caring, 18 instruments have been designed using the human science and human care theory as a theoretical approach to measure caring in studies related to client satisfaction, nursing student perceptions of caring, intercollegial relationships among professional nurses, and caring behaviors of nursing faculty (Watson, 2002a). Smith (2004) outlined four categories addressed by nurse researchers using Watson's theory: the nature of nurse caring, client and nurse perceptions of the nurse caring experience, human experiences, and human caring needs. Nurses use Watson's theory to measure caring behaviors, attitudes, and efficacy; in practice across various specialty areas; and in nursing education research (Smith, 2004). The University of Colorado hosts the Center for Human Caring, where nurses study and practice the human science and human care theory. The Watson Human Caring Science Institute serves as the source of an international consortium for her human science and human care theory. The consortium provides consultations to health care organizations for the implementation of her model and theory in practice settings. Human science and human care theory provides a theoretical foundation for nursing service departments, nursing research studies, and nursing educational programs worldwide (Fawcett, 2005). Watson's theory might be used by nurses in any nursing care situation during which a nurse desires to establish a deep, meaningful personal relationship with the persons to whom they provide care. Table 7.7 summarizes the key concepts defined in Watson's theory.

COMPLEXITY THEORY AS A FRAMEWORK

Like stability theory, **complexity theory** assumes that reality changes continually. However, change occurs with irregularity and cannot be predicted. Complexity theory "emphasizes change over time, long-term unpredictability, and openness to the environment with mutual simultaneous interactions … The complexity perspective seeks to understand patterns of phenomena as wholes within their contexts" (Maliski & Holditch-Davis, 1995, p. 25). In complexity theory, change occurs spontaneously when many individual

TABLE 7.7	Major Concepts as Defined in Watson's Theory
Human beings	Unities of mind, body, soul, and environment with souls that are not confined to the physical world but exist following physical death
Environment	Referred to as the world, described as all universal forces that affect a person, including the person's immediate environment and situation, "be they internal, external, human, human-made, artificial, natural, cosmic, psychic, past, present, or future" (Watson, 2007, p. 56)
Health (healing)	"Unity and harmony with in the mind, body, and soul" that is congruent with the person's perceived and experienced self; "health is I = me" (Watson, 2007, p. 48; 2012, p. 61)
Nursing	A transpersonal process of "human-to-human attempts to protect, enhance, and preserve humanity by helping a person find meaning in illness, suffering, pain, and existence; to help another gain self-knowledge, control, and self-healing within; a sense of inner harmony is restored regardless of the external circumstances" (Watson, 2007, pp. 53–54; 2012, p. 72)

factors interact interconnectedly and interdependently. Change becomes dynamic and unpredictable and co-evolves with the environment (Leddy, 2006). Unlike systems theory, interacting systems cannot be separated because they are one.

Complexity theory replaces the metaphors of separation and interaction (reductionistic) with the metaphor of participation (holistic) (Porter, 1995). The whole cannot be known from the sum of the parts, nor can the sum of the parts be more than the whole because everything is unitary.

Assumptions of complexity theory include:

1. Nonlinear change over time
2. Long-term unpredictability
3. Openness to the environment
4. Mutual, simultaneous interactions
5. Continual fluctuations that reveal patterns
6. Variable patterns that appear at critical points

Because the theory assumes mutual change in people and the environment, which provides potential for restructuring in new patterns, linear cause and effect is difficult to infer. The theory suggests that multiple, dynamic, mutual relationships, rather than enduring "causes," influence change. Thus, change of an individual, because it is related to initial conditions, is not generalizable.

Nursing models and theories with complexity theory as their foundation emphasize how individuals become more fully human ("human becoming") in terms of potential for change. Some nurses find models based on complexity theories difficult to understand because complexity theory challenges them to think in multiple dimensions.

Martha Rogers's Science of Unitary Human Beings

Martha Rogers developed the science of unitary human beings while searching for a specific and unique body of knowledge for nursing during the late 1970s (Barrett et al., 2003). In **Rogers's science of unitary human beings**, the purpose of nursing is to foster health potential. Rogers incorporates three key concepts in her model:

1. Unitary human being: An irreducible, indivisible, pandimensional energy field identified by pattern
2. Unified energy field: A pandimensional nonlinear domain without spatial or temporal attributes
3. Mutual process: Changes within the human and environmental fields that occur simultaneously

Rogers's model builds on an assumption of the human being as a unified energy field that continuously exchanges energy with an environmental energy field. Rogers proposed that "man is a unified whole possessing his own integrity and manifesting characteristics that are more than and different from the sum of his parts" (Rogers, 1970, p. 47). Physical, biologic, psychological, social, cultural, and spiritual attributes are merged into behavior that reflects the total human being as an indivisible whole. Rogers believed that it is impossible to describe humans by combining attributes of each of the parts. Only as the parts lose their particular identity is it possible to describe the human being.

Take Note!
In Rogers's science of unitary human beings theory, the purpose of nursing is to foster health potential.

The human being is an organized energy field that has a unique pattern. The continuous mutual process of energy field with environmental energy field results in continuous pattern manifestation changes in both the person and the environment (Rogers, 1970). This results in increasing complexity and innovativeness of the human being. Rogers believed that this life process "evolves irreversibly and unidirectionally along the space–time continuum" (Rogers, 1970, p. 59). She conceptualized this unidirectionality as a spiral with self-regulation "directed toward achieving increasing complexity of organization—not toward achieving equilibrium and stability" (Rogers, 1970, p. 64). The human being is also characterized by "the capacity for abstraction and imagery, language and thought, and sensation and emotion" (Rogers, 1970, p. 73).

Rogers believed that health serves as an "index of field patterning" (Maliski & Holditch-Davis, 1995, p. 27). Health and illness are not separate states, good or bad, or in a linear relationship. "Ease and disease are dichotomous notions that cannot be used to account for the dynamic complexity and uncertain fulfillment of man's unfolding" (Rogers, 1970, p. 42). Thus, observable manifestations are all "manifestations of patterning (that) emerge out of the human/environmental field mutual process and are continuously innovative" (Rogers, 1990, p. 8).

Rogers conceptualized nursing as both an art and a science. Nursing science includes knowledge specific to the domain of nursing that has an abstract nature and has been generated by scientific research and logical analysis. The art of nursing encompasses how nurses creatively use knowledge in professional practice (Fawcett, 2005; Rogers, 1992). Nursing intervention is aimed toward promoting the betterment of humans wherever they may be (Rogers, 1992). Rogers also specified that nurses must address health promotion with consumers because disease and pathology may always be a potential manifestation of human patterns. Rogers (1992) viewed caring in nursing as "simply a way of using knowledge" (p. 46).

Rogers (1990, p. 333) described three principles that explain change: integrality, helicy, and resonancy.

1. The principle of integrality emphasizes that the human energy field and the environmental energy field are continuous and must be perceived simultaneously. The relationship is one of constant interaction and mutual simultaneous change. In other words, "they are reciprocal systems in which molding and being molded are taking place at the same time" (Rogers, 1970, p. 97).
2. The principle of helicy predicts that change occurs as a "continuous, innovative, unpredictable, increasing diversity of human and environmental field patterns" (Rogers, 1990, p. 8). The human field becomes increasingly diverse with time. As the person ages, behavior may not be repeated but may recur at evermore complex levels.
3. The principle of resonancy indicates that change in pattern and organization toward increased complexity of the field occurs by way of waves, "manifesting continuous change from lower-frequency, longer wave patterns to higher-frequency, shorter wave patterns" (Rogers, 1980, p. 333).

Rogers believed that an understanding of the mechanisms that affect the life process in humans makes it possible for the nurse to purposefully intervene to affect client pattern manifestations in a desired direction. In the process, the nurse is also changed. Rogers saw the future as "one of growing diversity, of accelerating evolution, and of nonrepeating rhythmicities" (Rogers, 1992, p. 33). Her emphases on holism and on the simultaneity and mutuality of humans and the environment are concepts that have been widely accepted in nursing. Rogers proposed that the science of unitary human beings would serve as a foundation for future theory development to make this abstract science applicable to practice (Fawcett, 2003, 2005). Parse (1987), Newman (1986), and Leddy (2004, 2006) have used the science of unitary human beings as the foundation for practice. Barrett and colleagues developed a theory of power using the science that nurses use to guide nursing service departments (2003).

Nurses use Rogers's theory as a foundation for using complementary and alternative health practices (e.g., therapeutic touch, guided imagery, other energy therapies). The science of unitary human beings has also been used by nursing scholars to generate practice theories. The Focus on Research box, "Moving Beyond Dwelling in Suffering: A Situation-Specific Theory on Men's Healing from Childhood Maltreatment," provides an example of how the science of unitary human beings has been used to generate a new practice (situation-specific or micro) theory.

Table 7.8 presents major concepts as defined in Rogers's model. Despite its complexity, the science of unitary human beings provides a theoretical foundation for undergraduate and graduate nursing education programs, guidelines for administration of nursing services in health care organizations, knowledge for the development of clinical practice guidelines, and a foundation for research instrument development. Instruments have been developed for nursing research and clinical practice using the science of unitary human beings (Fawcett, 2005). The Society of Rogerian Scholars offers nursing symposia, networking, and support for nurses who base their scholarly activities on Rogerian science.

FOCUS ON RESEARCH

Moving Beyond Dwelling in Suffering: A Situation-Specific Theory on Men's Healing From Childhood Maltreatment

The investigators used hermeneutical–phenomenological techniques to uncover the deep personal meaning of the lived experiences of men who survived childhood maltreatment. Following Institutional Review Board approval, 52 men with a history of childhood maltreatment (neglect or physical, emotional, or sexual abuse) and who perceived that they had experienced healing were interviewed by a psychiatric mental health nurse. The first interview question asked about the lived experience of healing from their past experiences and they inquired about how each of them moved from living in suffering to a state of well-being. The interviews yielded rich data.

Using an iterative process, the investigative team listened to audiotaped interviews and read interview transcripts. Each member reflected on and then coded the data. The team then engaged in discussion and revised the codes and initial findings. They identified key themes related to healing and then verified their findings with eight of the study participants.

Key themes that were identified were linked to major concepts of the science of unitary human beings theory and a specific practice theory was generated for nurses to use to facilitate healing for male childhood maltreatment survivors. They described the findings in terms of pattern manifestations. The first pattern manifestation is the situation that reflected societal view of male childhood maltreatment and how little is known about the phenomenon compared to that of female childhood maltreatment. The second pattern manifestation was the specific maltreatment event experienced by each participant. Common pattern manifestations occurred for all the participants who had experienced healing.

The first pattern represented helicy and was identified as "moving beyond suffering" (p. 59). The investigators identified the following five dimensions of this pattern: "breaking through the masculine veneer, finding meaning, choosing to live well, caring for self by using diverse healing methods, and engaging in a mutual process perceived as humanizing" (p. 59). The second pattern manifestation desiring release from suffering reflects resonancy and was described as "openness to change, mindfulness, intentions, perseverance, and optimism" (p. 60). The participants' reports of experiences in healing were equated with the principle of integrality. For this aspect of healing, the participants reported experiencing compassion, peace, a mutual process of being one with the universe, and finding a meaning and purpose in their lives.

The situation-specific model generated for the process of male survivor movement from beyond suffering to experiencing well-being proposed that dwelling in suffering has either a negative or no effect on the movement and that desiring release from suffering has a positive effect on the movement toward experiencing well-being. Nurses can use a variety of health patterning modalities such as guided imagery, meditation, rhythmic movement (dance therapy), energy methods (chakra therapy, therapeutic touch), artistic methods for expression (art or music therapy), and creation of a calm, therapeutic environment to facilitate healing in male victims of childhood maltreatment. The researchers recognize that the theory may not apply to other groups of male victims of childhood maltreatment because purposive sampling was used and each participant acknowledged that they had been healed and moved from dwelling in suffering to experiencing well-being.

Willis, D., DeSanto-Madeya, S., & Fawcett, J. (2015). Moving beyond swelling in suffering: A situation-specific theory of men's healing from childhood maltreatment. *Nursing Science Quarterly, 28*(1), 57–63. https://doi.org/10.1177/0894318414558606

TABLE 7.8   Major Concepts as Defined in Rogers's Theory

Human being	A unitary energy field with a unique pattern
Environment	An energy field in mutual process with the human being
Health	An expression of the complexity and innovativeness of patterning of the energy field that is the person
Nursing	Compassionate concern for human beings by using independent science and practice art in which nurses intervene to improve pattern manifestations and the environment to achieve maximum health potentials

Rosemarie Parse's Human Becoming Theory

Like Rogers, Parse suggested that the purpose of nursing is to improve quality of life for both the client and the nurse. In **Parse's human becoming theory**, she coined three words to describe the essence of nursing:

1. Coconstitution: Development of patterning through human–environment interaction
2. Coexistence: Dynamic mutual processes between the human and the environment
3. Situated freedom: Freedom of choice in a situation

Parse's model incorporates a combination of Rogers's principles and building blocks "with the tenets of human subjectivity and intentionality and the concepts of coconstitution, coexistence, and situated freedom from existential–phenomenologic thought" (Parse, 1987, p. 161). The emphasis is on the meaning and values that influence a person's active choices of behavior. "The human being constructs his or her own meaning" (Parse, 1996, p. 57). The model honors human dignity and freedom (Parse, 2010).

Parse defined the human being as "an open being, more than and different from the sum of parts in mutual simultaneous interchange with the environment who chooses from options and bears responsibility for choices" (Parse, 1987, p. 160). As a person interacts with the environment, patterns of relating are established that provide insight into their patterning and values at that moment. Health is viewed as a "nonlinear entity," a constantly changing process of becoming that incorporates values. Because it is not a state, health cannot be contrasted with disease. "The human becoming nurse's goal is to be truly present with people as they enhance their quality of life" (Parse, 1998, p. 69).

Take Note!

Parse's human becoming theory suggests that the purpose of nursing is to improve quality of life for both the client and the nurse.

Parse described her key concepts in a highly paradoxical manner (Parse, 1998, pp. 29–51):

1. Human becoming: Human participation with the environment to create health and quality of life
2. Meaning: Human interpreted, linguistic, and imaged content of something
3. Rhythmicity: The paradoxical patterning of the human–universe mutual process
4. Transcendence: "Reaching beyond with possibility—the hopes and dreams envisioned in multidimensional experiences and powering the originating of transforming" (p. 30)
5. Imaging: Reflective—prereflective coming to know that which is "explicit-tacit-all-at-once"
6. Valuing: Confirming—not confirming cherished beliefs in light of a personal worldview
7. Languaging: Signifying valued images through speaking—being silent and moving—being still
8. Revealing–Concealing: Disclosing—not disclosing all-at-once
9. Establishing–Limiting: Living the opportunities—restrictions present in all choosings all-at-once
10. Connecting–Separating: Being with and apart from others, ideas, objects, and situations all-at-once
11. Powering: The pushing–resisting process of affirming—not affirming being in light of nonbeing
12. Originating: Inventing new ways of conforming—nonconforming in the certainty—uncertainty of living
13. Transforming: Shifting the view of the familiar–unfamiliar, the changing of change in constituting anew in a deliberate way

Parse (1998) combined these 13 concepts into three principles:

1. Structuring meaning multidimensionally is cocreating reality through the languaging of valuing and imaging (p. 35).
2. Cocreating rhythmic patterns of relating is living the paradoxical unity of revealing–concealing and enabling–limiting while connecting–separating (p. 42).
3. Contrascending (being one) with the possibilities is powering unique ways of originating in the process of transforming (p. 46).

Parse (1996) stated that "the way of living the belief system is through true presence" (p. 57), "which is a nonroutinized, unconditional loving way of being, within which the nurse witnesses the blossoming of others" (p. 57). Practicing within this model, the nurse would provide an empathic sounding board for clients and families to express and therefore uncover the meaning of thoughts and feelings, values, and changing views. In the process of expression through language and movement, and in "dwelling with" the rhythm of the client and family, new possibilities for change in quality of life would become apparent. "The new insights shift the rhythm and all participants move beyond the moment toward what is not yet. This is mobilizing transcendence" (Parse, 1989, p. 257). In this model, the nurse connects with clients through focused interactions rather than doing things for them

(Phillips, 1987). Therefore, Parse blended caring with Rogers's science of unitary human beings.

Parse (1998) also developed a phenomenological–hermeneutic research methodology to test relationships suggested by the model. The methodology uses "dialogical engagement," a researcher–participant encounter, to uncover the meaning of the live experience being studied (Parse, 1989, p. 256) and serves as the research methodology for many qualitative nursing studies. Parse (2003) expanded her model by introducing the following community change concepts (again using paradoxes): (1) moving–initiating, (2) anchoring–shifting, and (3) pondering–shaping. She perceived that human becoming could be done at a community level in addition to the individual level.

Parse's theory emphasizes the importance of the meaning that underlies behavior and provides a structure for the identification and clarification of "manifestations of whole people as they interrelate with the environment" (Phillips, 1987, p. 188). Hansen-Ketchum (2004) specified that outcomes for nursing practice using Parse's theory include opportunities for multidimensional client healing, enhanced personal growth (for the client and the nurse), and continued professional growth (for the nurse). Table 7.9 summarizes the major concepts defined in Parse's theory.

Parse's human becoming theory enables nurses to practice differently because it uses a multidimensional approach, incorporates the use of paradoxes, and fosters deep connections among nurses and nursing care recipients. Parse's theory provides a theoretical framework for undergraduate and graduate nursing programs, for individual nurses, and in descriptive applied research projects (Fawcett, 2005). The International Consortium of Parse Scholars offers networking opportunities and support services for nurses interested in Parse's human becoming theory. Parse is also the founder and editor of *Nursing Science Quarterly*, a nursing journal devoted to the advancement of nursing science. When using Parse's human becoming theory, nurses working in all areas of practice would aim for achieving deep, personal relationships with people receiving care with the aim of helping them attain their maximal human potential.

REAL-LIFE REFLECTIONS

Remember Nicole and Brianna, from the beginning of the chapter? In what ways might Brianna have applied Parse's human becoming theory in helping Ms. Green sleep?

TABLE 7.9 Major Concepts as Defined in Parse's Theory

Human being	An open being, more than and different from the sum of its parts
Environment	In mutual process with the person
Health	Continuously changing the process of becoming
Nursing	Use of true presence to facilitate the becoming of the participant

Margaret Newman's Theory of Health as Expanding Consciousness

Like Parse, Newman uses principles from Rogers's science of unitary beings in her theory. **Newman's theory of health as expanding consciousness** states that the purpose of nursing is to promote a higher level of consciousness in both the client and the nurse. Newman used the concept of consciousness as the capacity of the system (human being) to interact with its environment, the informational capacity of the system in her nursing model.

Newman's theory incorporates Rogers's concept of a unitary human being as a center of energy in constant interaction with the environment. Human beings are characterized by patterning that is constantly changing. According to Newman (1994), "The focus of nursing is the pattern of the whole, health as pattern of the evolving whole, with caring as a moral imperative" (p. 19).

"The total pattern of the human being–environment can be viewed as a network of consciousness" (Newman, 1986, p. 33) that is "expanding toward higher levels: the patterns of interaction of human being–environment constitute health … Health is the expansion of consciousness" (Newman, 1986, pp. 3, 18), and "health and the evolving pattern of consciousness are the same" (Newman, 1990, p. 38). "Consciousness is defined as the information of the system: the capacity of the system to interact with the environment" (Newman, 1994, p. 38).

Health is viewed as a process that encompasses both disease and "nondisease." Instead of the familiar linear relationship between health as good and disease (or illness) as bad, Newman conceptualized disease as a meaningful component of the whole and a possible facilitator of health. "Sickness can provide a kind of shock that reorganizes the relationships of the human being's pattern in a more harmonious way" (Newman, 1994, p. 11). As the person interacts with the environment, "the fluctuating patterns of harmony–disharmony can be regarded as peaks and troughs of the rhythmic life process" (Newman, 1986, p. 21).

Newman posited four major ways in which human being–environment patterning manifests: movement, time, space, and consciousness. Consciousness is expressed in patterns of rhythmic movement toward higher levels that can be described in time and space. Manifestations of these patterns include exchanging, communicating, relating, valuing, choosing, moving, perceiving, feeling, and knowing (Newman, 1986, p. 74). The task for nursing intervention is to recognize patterning and relate to it in an "authentic" (genuine) way.

Take Note!
Newman's theory of health as expanding consciousness states that the purpose of nursing is to promote a higher level of consciousness in both the client and the nurse.

The new paradigm is relational. The professional enters into a partnership with the client with the mutual goal of participating in an authentic relationship, trusting that in the process of its evolving, both will grow and become healthier in the sense of higher levels of consciousness (Newman, 1986, p. 68). Nursing facilitates the process of evolving to higher levels of consciousness by "rhythmic connecting of the nurse with the client in an authentic way for the purpose of illuminating the pattern and discovering the new rules of a higher level of organization" (Newman, 1990, p. 40).

Newman's theory contributes to the development of a body of knowledge about manifestations of healthy patterning of unitary human beings. Newman has described a methodology for using practice as the basis for research within the model. Nurses have used this theory in research studies addressing nurses as cancer survivors, effectiveness of nursing spiritual interventions, empowerment of clients with cancer, nurse–family relationships with medically fragile children, family caring, and the perceived health of men with human immunodeficiency virus (HIV).

Table 7.10 lists the major concepts defined in Newman's theory. Along with providing a theoretical framework for graduate and undergraduate nursing programs, Newman's theory can be used, for example, to guide professional nursing practice in substance abuse settings, pattern recognition for members of faith congregations, and pattern assessment in women with hyperthyroidism. Nurses using Newman's theory strive to help others to understand the holistic impact of a health-related situation. Application of the theory

■ **TABLE 7.10**	**Major Concepts as Defined in Newman's Theory**
Human beings	"Unitary and continuous with the undivided wholeness of the universe" (Newman, 1994, p. 83)
Environment	"Undivided wholeness of the universe" (Newman, 1994, p. 83)
Health	Expansion of consciousness
Nursing	Facilitating repatterning of the client to higher levels of consciousness

has been useful in the following clinical situations: school-aged children with insulin-dependent diabetes mellitus, the older adult living alone, family caregivers, and individuals with cancer (Fawcett, 2005). Nurses who use the model in nursing practice, education, and research can find resources from the Health as Expanding Consciousness Organization.

Susan Leddy's Human Energy Model

Leddy's human energy model was influenced by Rogers's science of unitary human beings, Eastern philosophy, and quantum physics and complexity theories. Leddy (2004) explained that the environment serves as the context, in which persons are embedded and persons are one with the environment. She conceptualized the universal essence environment as a dynamic rhythmic pattern that constantly changes with continuous transformations of matter, information, and energy that constitutes an undivided whole. In the human energy model, Leddy (2004) proposed that the purpose of nursing is to facilitate the harmonious pattern of the universal essence environmental fields of both the client and the nurse. Leddy (2004) used five key concepts in her model:

1. Self-organization: The structure of the human being demonstrated by pattern and its manifestations
2. Energy field: A dynamic web of energy interactions
3. Awareness: An energy that links humans with the environment
4. Energy: Manifested by movement and change
5. Pattern: A web of relationships

Leddy (1998, p. 192) viewed the human being as "a unitary energy field that is open to and continuously interacting with an environmental universal essence field" that can only be understood as a whole. "Sensitivity to complementary facets and vantage points for observation provides a view of the whole from different perspectives" (Leddy, 1998, p. 192; 2003, p. 68). "Self-organization distinguishes the human energy field from the environmental field with which it is inseparable and intermingled" (Leddy, 2003, p. 68). "Self-organization is a synthesis of continuity and change that provides identity while the human evolves toward a sense of integrity, meaning, and purpose in living" (Leddy, 1998, p. 192). Humans also have awareness that enables the development of self-identity, the construction of meaning, and the capability to influence change by making choices (Leddy, 2004).

Take Note!
Leddy's human energy model proposes that the purpose of nursing is to facilitate the harmonious pattern of the essence fields of both the client and the nurse.

Leddy (2004) viewed the environment as the context in which the human is embedded. People are one with the environment. Change can be partially predicted and is partially unpredictable. She explained that the universal essence environment is ordered and has a rhythmic pattern while constantly changing "through continuous transformation of matter and information" (Leddy, 2004, p. 14). However, change "is also influenced by the inherent order of the universe" (Leddy, 2003, p. 68). History, pattern, and choice also shape change.

Leddy (2003) defined health as being "the pattern of the whole" (p. 68). This pattern is rhythmic, varying in quality and intensity over time. Health is characterized by a changing pattern of harmony and dissonance.

Under Leddy's theory, knowledge-based consciousness in a goal-directed relationship with the client is the basis for nursing. "A nurse–client relationship is a commitment characterized by intentionality, authenticity, trust, respect, and genuine sense of connection. The nurse is a knowledgeable, concerned facilitator. The client is responsible for choices that influence health and healing" (Leddy, 1998, pp. 192–193).

Leddy (2004) derived three theories from her human energy model: the theory of healthiness, the theory of participation, and the theory of energetic patterning.

In the theory of healthiness, healthiness is defined as a manifestation of a health pattern. It is a process characterized by purpose, connections, and power to attain goals. The theory proposes that healthiness acts as a resource that influences the ongoing patterning that is reflected in health (Leddy & Fawcett, 1997). Leddy derived her theory empirically. The pattern of healthiness consists of a constellation of connection, purpose (challenge viewed as change, goals, meaningfulness, choice–possibilities, confidence–competence,

and control), and power (choice–creativity, capability, capacity, change–curiosity, and confidence–assurance). The theory emphasizes the importance of goals and meaningfulness in life (Leddy, 2006).

The Leddy Healthiness Scale (LHS) includes items that measure meaningfulness, connections, ends, capability, control, choice, challenge, capacity, and confidence (Leddy, 1997). In studies using the LHS (Leddy, 1997, 2006; Leddy & Fawcett, 1997), healthiness has been found to be moderately and negatively related to fatigue and symptom experience in women with breast cancer, and moderately and positively related to mental health, health status, and satisfaction with life in a sample of healthy people.

In the theory of participation, participation is defined as the experience of continuous human–environment mutual processes. Leddy (2004) defined participation as the experience of expansiveness (fullness and activity) and ease (smoothness and calmness of the mutual process of the human and environmental fields). The Person–Environment Participation Scale (PEPS) (Leddy, 1995) measures expansiveness and the ease of participation. In studies with PEPS to date, participation has been found to be moderately and positively correlated with healthiness, a sense of coherence (Antonovsky, 1987), and power (Barrett, 1990) and moderately and negatively correlated with fatigue and symptom experience in healthy people.

The theory of energetic patterning proposes that nursing interventions to facilitate the harmonious pattern of both the client and the nurse are accomplished through health pattern appraisal, recognition of patterns, and energy-based nursing interventions (Leddy, 2004, 2006). Nursing healing interventions promote healing by surrounding, supporting, or penetrating the human body. The six domains of energetic patterning are:

1. Coursing: Reestablishing free flow of energy
2. Conveying: Fostering redirection of energy away from areas of excess to depleted areas
3. Converting: Augmenting energy resources
4. Collecting: Reducing energy depletion
5. Clearing: Facilitating the release of energy tied to old patterns
6. Connecting: Promoting harmony within the human field and with the environmental field

A number of interventions are consistent with this theory, including nutrition, exercise, touch modalities, bodywork, light therapy, music, imagery, relaxation, and stress reduction (Leddy, 2003, 2004).

TABLE 7.11	**Major Concepts as Defined in Leddy's Theory**
Human being	A unitary, self-organized field of matter, energy, and information that constantly interacts with an environmental universal essence field
Environment	A dynamic, ordered, connected web in continuous transformation of energy, matter, and information with the human being (environmental universal essence)
Health	The rhythmic pattern of harmony/dissonance of the whole
Nursing	Knowledge-based consciousness involved in a mutual, connected, and goal-directed relationship with clients

Leddy's conceptual model offers a unique and modern perspective for nursing; however, because it is a newer model, its usefulness for practice and research remains to be demonstrated. Table 7.11 presents major concepts defined in Leddy's model. Leddy's model and theories have yet to be empirically tested; however, they show great promise for providing a framework to guide future research on healthiness and energetic patterning. Professional nurses might use Leddy's model when engaging with persons as individuals or as communities for promoting health and well-being.

NURSING MODELS IN RESEARCH AND PRACTICE

Use of Nursing Models in Nursing Research

Most published nursing research studies fail to use conceptual nursing models as their foundation. Currently, three kinds of research related to nursing models are being conducted: testing the relationships predicted by a model; using a model as a framework for descriptive analysis; and attempting to modify nursing care through use of a model.

For example, Leddy and Fawcett (1997) interpreted the results of a study to explain relationships among theoretical variables (participation, change, energy, and healthiness) derived from the human energy model as being supportive of the model. In another example, Sitzman (2017) discovered that caring processes outlined by **Watson's human caring science** applied to online nurse–client interactions. Maki and Devon (2018) determined that Rogers's science of unitary human beings applied to genetic and epigenetic nursing research.

Models also have been used as frameworks for descriptive analysis. For example, Parse's human becoming theory was used to describe the role of doctors dressed as clowns working in pediatric hospitals in Australia (Brockenshiren et al., 2018) and to describe facilitators for developing person-centered care environments (Timlin et al., 2018). Parse's model was also used by Wagner et al. (2019) to describe British practitioner experiences when working with adult victims and perpetrators of intergenerational domestic violence. Mitsugi (2019) used Newman's concept of a caring partnership to describe a transforming process that occurs at the end of life. In their study of African American daughter caregivers, Cannon and Fawcett (2018) identified correlations of physical and psychological health outcomes using Neuman's systems model of health.

Recent studies evaluating the effects of nursing interventions that propose modifications of nursing care have been based upon several nursing models. Byrne Notte et al. (2019) as well as Clouse et al. (2017) used King's theory of goal attainment to reduce the rate of individuals with mental health concerns not coming to their first scheduled appointments at an outpatient mental health facility. Byrne Notte et al. (2016) used Rogers's science of unitary human beings to show positive effects of Reiki therapy on individuals who had undergone knee replacement therapy. This science was also used by Dunn et al. (2019) to develop an educational program that fostered the development of resilience in family and community caregivers of older Native Americans experiencing memory loss and cognitive decline.

Use of Nursing Models in Nursing Practice

As more nurses receive BSN degrees and undertake graduate nursing education, the use of models in practice may become more prevalent. Nursing models and theories provide guidance to nurses engaged in practice for holistic assessments, rationales for various nursing interventions, and delineation of professional nursing roles in health care delivery. Some hospitals identify a particular theory as a basis for the use of nursing process. For example, nurses at St. Luke's Hospital in Kansas City, Missouri, and the University of Missouri Medical Center in Columbia, Missouri, use Orem's self-care deficit theory as a foundation and guide for nursing practice. The University of Colorado Health Sciences Medical Centers in Aurora and Denver, Colorado, employ Watson's human caring science to guide nursing practice. The American Nurses

Association requests that nursing departments specify the nursing model and theory used by the organization as part of the magnet hospital application process.

Nevertheless, the use of nursing models or theories in professional practice seems irrelevant to some nurses. Do models make real differences in nursing care delivered to clients? Does it matter if the client need is called a "noxious influence" affecting a behavioral subsystem, a "self-care deficit" leading to a "self-care demand," or a "focal stimulus" that is a stressor? How is the care given any different if its purpose is labeled to "limit self-care deficits," "reduce stressors," or "foster coping?" Why does the profession need specific nursing models and theories?

Although nursing science remains in an early stage of development, nursing scholars agree on categories of concepts (human beings, environment, health, and nursing) that are central to nursing knowledge. Nursing science must attain distinction from medical science. Much discussion about whether there should be one model for nursing has taken place, but the popularity of a growing number of models within different paradigms and frameworks indicates that disagreement still exists about how professional nursing should be described and how its goals can best be achieved.

Professional nursing continues to progress in defining nursing, identifying the unique nursing contributions to health care, developing nursing theory, and using nursing models and theories in practice. As health care evolves, nursing must demonstrate an ability to articulate its important and unique contribution to client care, and perhaps new models and theories may be needed.

▌ QUESTIONS FOR REFLECTION

1. What is your attitude toward nursing models and theories? Why do you feel this way?
2. Has your attitude changed since reading this chapter?

3. Do you think multiple approaches and definitions are advantageous or disadvantageous to the profession of nursing? Provide examples to support your response.
4. What might be the consequences of your attitudes toward nursing models and theories?

Summary and Significance to Practice

The nursing models discussed in this chapter use the metaparadigm concepts of human beings, environment, health, and nursing. Philosophical differences between the change as a stability paradigm and the change as a growth paradigm are pronounced. Professional nurses have the freedom to select which models to use in clinical practice based on personal philosophy and worldviews. Sometimes, one particular nursing model may fit a clinical situation better than others. Nursing models do not compete with each other but provide a variety of approaches and explanations for the phenomena associated with professional nursing practice.

Table 7.12 compares concepts among select theories. The major differences and similarities among the models are outlined in Tables 7.13 and 7.14. More research is needed to see if the models provide an effective description of nursing and make differences in client care outcomes.

REAL-LIFE REFLECTIONS

Consider Brianna and Nicole. Do you believe that Brianna is a better nurse than Nicole because Brianna uses theory to guide her nursing practice? Why or why not?

TABLE 7.12	**Comparison of Concepts in Select Theories**			
Theory	Human	Human–Environment Interaction	Health	Examples of Nursing Implications
Systems	Multiple interacting subsystems that form the human system	Simultaneous change in both systems	Tendency toward increased complexity	Nurse system and client system are mutually affected
Stress and adaptation	Multiple subsystems that share an internal environment	Humans cope and compensate for environmental change	Constancy of the internal environment within normal parameters	Support coping mechanisms of client
Complexity	Unitary whole	Mutual simultaneous interaction; nonlinear	Pattern of the whole	Stimulate repatterning

■ TABLE 7.13   Similarities and Differences of Conceptualization in Nursing Models Within the Change as Stability Paradigm

| Model | Person | | | | Nursing | |
	Goal	Composition	Health	Environment	Nature	Purpose
King	Functioning in social roles	Open system	Dynamic state of well-being	Internal and external stressors	Goal-oriented interaction	Attainment, maintenance, or restoration of health
Orem	Constancy	Whole with physical, psychological, interpersonal, social aspects	Meeting self-care needs	External forces	An art with systems that address self-care requisites	Help people meet self-care needs
Roy	Become integrated and whole	System with biopsychosocial components	Adaptation	External and internal conditions	Manipulation of stimuli to foster coping	Promotion of adaptation
Neuman	Balance	Composite of physiologic, psychological, sociocultural, developmental, and spiritual variables	Equilibrium	Internal and external stressors	Stress-reducing activities	Promotion of equilibrium

■ TABLE 7.14   Similarities and Differences of Conceptualization in Nursing Models Within the Change as Growth Paradigm

| Model | Person | | | | Nursing | |
	Goal	Composition	Health	Environment	Nature	Purpose
Peplau	Equilibrium	System with physiologic, psychological, and social components	Forward movement of the personality	Significant others	Therapeutic interpersonal process	Helping people meet needs and develop
Watson	Sense of inner harmony	Integrated and inseparable spiritual, mental, and physical spheres	Unity and harmony	Energy field external to the person	Transpersonal caring	Promoting harmony
Rogers	Increased complexity of pattern	Indivisible energy field	Increasing innovativeness of patterning	Contiguous, continuously interacting energy field	Promotion of repatterning	Facilitating health potential
Newman	Expansion of consciousness	Center of energy	Patterns of person–environment interaction expanding toward higher levels	Energy field in continuous interaction with the person	Repatterning partnership	Promoting higher level of consciousness
Parse	Process of becoming	Open being	Process of becoming	Energy field in continuous interaction with the person	Interpersonal processes	Improving quality of life
Leddy	Harmony, integrity, meaning, and purpose	Unitary energy field	Pattern of the whole	Energy field and person are one	Goal-directed relationship	Facilitation of harmonious health patterning

From Theory to Practice

1. Which of the nursing models or theories presented in this chapter appeals to you the most? How would you incorporate this model or theory into your professional practice?
2. What are the challenges to using a nursing model or theory to guide professional practice?
3. How important is it for all nurses working together in a practice setting to understand and use the same theories when providing care?
4. What strategies would you use to get a group of nurses to select and use the same nursing model or theory in a practice setting?

Nurse as Author

Select one of the nursing models or theories presented in the chapter. Outline the key concepts and propositions of the selected nursing model or theory. Apply the selected model and theory to a clinical nursing situation.

Your Digital Classroom

Online Exploration

Clayton State University School of Nursing's Nursing Theory Link Page: **https://www.clayton.edu/ health/nursing/nursing-theory/index**

Health as Expanding Consciousness on currentnursing.com: **http://currentnursing.com/ nursing_theory/Newman_Health_As_Expanding_ Consciousness.html**

International Orem Society: **http:// oreminternationalsociety.org**

King International Nursing Group: **https://king .clubexpress.com/**

Neuman System Model: **http://www .neumansystemsmodel.org/**

International Consortium of Parse Scholars: **www .humanbecoming.org**

Roy Adaptation Association: **https://www .msmu.edu/about-the-mount/nursing-theory/ roy-adaptation-association/**

Scroll to the bottom of the downloaded page to watch the theorist Sister Callista Roy talk about how she developed the Roy adaptation model: **https://www.msmu.edu/about-the-mount/ nursing-theory/roy-adaptation-model/**

Society of Rogerian Scholars: **www .societyofrogerianscholars.org**

Watson Caring Science: **www .watsoncaringscience.org**

Expanding Your Understanding

Visit one of the nursing theory websites listed above or found on the Clayton State University Nursing Theory website and answer the following questions:

1. Which nursing theory are you investigating?
2. Can you contact the nursing theorist?
3. Who maintains the nursing theory website?
4. What materials are available on the website to explain the nursing theory?
5. Where can you go to find additional information about the nursing theory?
6. Would you recommend the website to a colleague interested in the selected nursing theory? Why or why not?

Beyond the Book

Visit thePoint® at **www.thePoint.lww.com** for activities and information to reinforce the concepts and content covered in this chapter.

REFERENCES

Alligood, M. (2010). Family healthcare with King's theory of goal attainment. *Nursing Science Quarterly, 23*(2), 99–104. https://doi.org/10.1177/089431841032553

Andrews, H. A., & Roy, C. (1986). *Essentials of the Roy adaptation model*. Appleton-Century-Crofts.

Antonovsky, A. (1987). *Unraveling the mystery of health: How people manage stress and stay well*. Jossey-Bass.

Auger, J. R. (1976). *Behavioral systems and nursing*. Prentice-Hall.

Barrett, E. A. M. (1990). A measure of power as knowing participation in change. In O. L. Strickland & C. F. Waltz (Eds.), *Measurement of nursing outcomes*. Springer.

Barrett, E. A. M., Malinski, V. M., Ann, M., & Phillips, J. R. (2003). The nurse theorists: 21st-century updates–Martha E. Rogers. Interview by Jacqueline Fawcett. *Nursing Science Quarterly, 16*, 44–51. https://doi.org/10.1177/0894318402239066

Benner, P., & Wrubel, J. (1989). *The primacy of caring: Stress and coping in health and illness*. Addison-Wesley.

Brockenshire, N., Newall, F., Chenhall, R., & Shoemark, H. (2018). Clowning around: Understanding the role of clown doctors at the royal children's hospital Melbourne (RCH). *International Journal of Integrated Care (IJIC), 18*, 1–2. https:// doi.org/10.5334/ijic.s1165

Cannon, W. B. (1932). *The wisdom of the body* (Rev. ed.). Norton.

Cannon, S., & Fawcett, J. (2018). Correlates of psychological and physical health outcomes among African American caregiving daughters. ABNF Journal, 29(3), 86–97. Retrieved March 26, 2021, from https://web-a-ebscohost-com.lib.rockhurst .edu/ehost/pdfviewer/pdfviewer?vid=5&sid=68736862-b07c -42e4-8830-e7169077d461%40sdc-v-sessmgr02

Chin, R. (1976). The utility of systems models and developmental models for practitioners. In W. G. Bennis, K. D. Benne, K. E. Corey, & R. Chin (Eds.), *The planning of change* (3rd ed.). Holt, Rinehart & Winston.

Clouse, K. M., Williams, K. A., & Harmon, J. M. (2017). Improving the no-show rate of new patients in outpatient psychiatric practice: An advance practice nurse-initiated telephone engagement protocol quality improvement project. *Perspectives in Psychiatric Care, 53*(2), 127–134. https://doi.org/10.1111/ppc.12146

Dunn, D. J., Schwartz, A., Teufel-Shone, N. I., & Meyer, L. A. (2019). Educational program to promote resilience for caregivers, family members, and community members in the care of elderly native Americans who are experiencing memory loss and cognitive decline. *Visions: The Journal of Rogerian Nursing Science, 25*(2), 1–16. Retrieved March 26, 2021, from https://www.thefreelibrary.com/Educational+Program+to+Promote+Resilience+for+Caregivers%2C+Family...-a0583693719

Fawcett, J. (1989). *Analysis and evaluation of conceptual models of nursing* (2nd ed.): F. A. Davis.

Fawcett, J. (2000). *Analysis and evaluation of contemporary nursing knowledge: Nursing models and theories*. F. A. Davis.

Fawcett, J. (2003). Conceptual models of nursing: International in scope and substance? The case of the Roy adaptation model. *Nursing Science Quarterly, 16*, 315–318. https://doi.org/10.1177/0894318403256980

Fawcett, J. (2005). *Contemporary nursing knowledge: Analysis and evaluation of nursing models and theories* (2nd ed.). F. A. Davis.

Gaut, D., & Leininger, M. (1991). *Caring: The compassionate healer*. NLN Press.

Hansen-Ketchum, P. (2004). Parse's theory in practice. *Journal of Holistic Nursing, 22*(1), 57–72. https://doi.org/10.1177/0898010103261120

Hardy, M. E. (1978). Perspectives on nursing theory. *Advances in Nursing Science, 1*, 37–48. https://doi.org/10.1097/00012272-197810000-00006

Huch, M. H. (1987). A critique of the Roy adaptation model. In R. R. Parse (Ed.), *Nursing science: Major paradigms, theories, and critiques* (pp. 47–66). W.B. Saunders.

King, I. M. (1981). *A theory for nursing: Systems, concepts, process*. Wiley.

King, I. M. (1987). King's theory of goal attainment. In R. R. Parse (Ed.), *Nursing science: Major paradigms, theories, and critiques*. W. B. Saunders.

King, I. M. (1989). King's general systems framework and theory. In J. P. Riehl-Sisca (Ed.), *Conceptual models for nursing practice*. Appleton & Lange.

King, I. M. (1995). The theory of goal attainment. In M. A. Frey & C. L. Sieloff (Eds.), *Advancing King's systems framework and theory of nursing*. Sage.

King, I. M. (1996). The theory of goal attainment in research and practice. *Nursing Science Quarterly, 9*, 61–66. https://doi.org/10.1177/089431849600900206

King, I. M. (1999). A theory of goal attainment: Philosophical and ethical implications. *Nursing Science Quarterly, 12*, 292–296. https://doi.org/10.1177/08943189922107205

King, I. M. (2001). The nurse theorists: 21st-century updates–Imogene M. King. Interview by Jacqueline Fawcett. *Nursing Science Quarterly, 14*, 311–315. https://doi.org/10.1177/089431840101400407

Koldjeski, D. (1990). Toward a theory of professional nursing caring: A unifying perspective. In M. Leininger & J. Watson (Eds.), *The caring imperative in education*. National League for Nursing.

Kyle, T. V. (1995). The concept of caring: A review of the literature. *Journal of Advanced Nursing, 21*, 506–514. https://doi.org/10.1111/j.1365-2648.1995.tb02734.x

Leddy, S. K. (1995). Measuring mutual process: Development and psychometric testing of the person-environment participation scale. *Visions: The Journal of Rogerian Nursing Science, 3*, 20–31. Retrieved March 26, 2021, from https://www.thefreelibrary.com/Measuring+mutual+process%3a+development+and+psychometric+testing+of+the...-a0161555262

Leddy, S. K. (1997). Incentives and barriers to exercise in women with a history of breast cancer. *Oncology Nursing Forum, 24*, 885–890. Retrieved March 26, 2021, from https://www.researchgate.net/publication/14017093_Incentives_and_barriers_to_exercise_in_women_with_a_history_of_breast_cancer

Leddy, S. K. (1998). *Leddy & Pepper's conceptual bases for professional nursing* (4th ed.). Lippincott.

Leddy, S. K. (2003). *Integrative health promotion*. Slack.

Leddy, S. K. (2004). Human energy: A conceptual model of unitary nursing science. *Visions: The Journal of Rogerian Scholarship, 12*, 14–27. Retrieved March 26, 2021, from https://www.thefreelibrary.com/Human+energy%3a+a+conceptual+model+of+unitary+nursing+science.-a0161397669

Leddy, S. K. (2006). *Health promotion: Mobilizing strengths to enhance health, wellness and well-being*. F. A. Davis.

Leddy, S. K., & Fawcett, J. (1997). Testing the theory of healthiness: Conceptual and methodological issues. In M. Madrid (Ed.), *Patterns of Rogerian knowing*. National League for Nursing.

Lowry, L. W. (2004). Conceptual models of nursing: International in scope and substance? The case of the Neuman systems model. *Nursing Science Quarterly, 17*, 50–54. https://doi.org/10.1177/0894318403260470

Magan, S. J. (1987). A critique of King's theory. In R. R. Parse (Ed.), *Nursing science: Major paradigms, theories and critiques*. W. B. Saunders.

Maki, K. A., & DeVon, H. A. (2018). A nursing theory-guided framework for genetic and epigenetic research. *Nursing Inquiry, 25*(3), 1. https://doi.org/10.1111/nin.12238

Maliski, S. L., & Holditch-Davis, D. (1995). Linking biology and biography: Complex nonlinear dynamical systems as a framework for nursing inquiry. *Complexity and Chaos in Nursing, 2*, 25–35. Retrieved March 26, 2021, from https://scholars.duke.edu/display/pub721883

Meleis, A. (2018). *Theoretical nursing: Development & progress* (6th ed.). Wolters Kluwer.

Mitsugi, M. (2019). A transforming process based on Newman's caring partnership at the end of life. *International Journal for Human Caring, 23*(1), 40–50. https://doi.org/10.20467/1091-5710.23.1.40

Monat, A., & Lazarus, R. (Eds.). (1977). *Stress and coping: An anthology*. Columbia University Press.

Morse, J. M., Solberg, S. M., Neander, W. L., Bottorff, J. L., & Johnson, J. L. (1990). Concepts of caring and caring as a concept. *Advances in Nursing Science, 13*, 1–14. https://doi.org/10.1097/00012272-199009000-00002

Neuman, B. (1982). *The Neuman systems model: Application to nursing education and practice*. Appleton-Century-Crofts.

Neuman, B. (1996). The Neuman systems model in research and practice. *Nursing Science Quarterly, 9*, 67–70. https://doi.org/10.1177/089431849600900207

Neuman, B. (2002). The Neuman systems model. In B. Neuman & J. Fawcett (Eds.), *The Neuman systems model* (4th ed.). Prentice Hall.

Newman, M. A. (1986). *Health as expanding consciousness*. Mosby.

Newman, M. A. (1990). Toward an integrative model of professional practice. *Journal of Professional Nursing, 6*(3), 167–173. https://doi.org/10.1016/s8755-7223(05)80148-6

Newman, M. A. (1994). *Health as expanding consciousness* (2nd ed.). National League for Nursing.

Notte, B. B., Fazzini, C., & Mooney, R. A. (2016). Reiki's effect on patients with total knee arthroplasty: A pilot study. *Nursing, 46*(2), 17–23. https://doi.org/10.1097/01.nurse.0000476246.16717.65

Orem, D. E. (1980). *Nursing: Concepts of practice* (2nd ed.). McGraw-Hill.

Orem, D. E. (1985). *Nursing: Concepts of practice* (3rd ed.). McGraw-Hill.

Orem, D. E. (1990). A nursing practice theory in three parts, 1956–1989. In M. E. Parker (Ed.), *Nursing theories in practice*. National League for Nursing.

Orem, D. E. (1995). *Nursing: Concepts of practice* (5th ed.). Mosby.

Orem, D. E. (2001). *Nursing: Concepts of practice* (6th ed.). Mosby.

Orem, D. E., & Taylor, S. G. (2011). Reflections on nursing practice science: The nature, the structure and the foundation of nursing sciences. *Nursing Science Quarterly, 24*(1), 35–41. https://doi.org/10.1177/0894318410389061

Parse, R. R. (1987). *Nursing science: Major paradigms, theories, and critiques*. W. B. Saunders.

Parse, R. R. (1989). Man-living-health: A theory of nursing. In J. P. Riehl-Sisca (Ed.), *Conceptual models for nursing practice*. Appleton & Lange.

Parse, R. R. (1996). The human becoming theory: Challenges in practice and research. *Nursing Science Quarterly, 9*(2), 55–60. https://doi.org/10.1177/089431849600900205

Parse, R. R. (1998). *The human becoming school of thought*. Sage.

Parse, R. R. (2003). *Community: A human becoming perspective*. Jones & Bartlett.

Parse, R. R. (2010). Human dignity: A human becoming ethical phenomenon. *Nursing Science Quarterly, 23*(3), 257–262. https://doi.org/10.1177/0894318410371841

Peterson, S., & Bredow, T. (2017). *Middle range theories application to nursing research and practice* (4th ed.). Wolters Kluwer.

Phillips, J. R. (1987). A critique of Parse's man-living-health theory. In R. R. Parse (Ed.), *Nursing science: Major paradigms, theories, and critiques*. W. B. Saunders.

Porter, E. J. (1995). Non-equilibrium systems theory: Some applications for gerontological nursing practice. *Journal of Gerontological Nursing, 21*, 24–31. https://doi.org/10.3928/0098-9134-19950601-07

Riehl, J. P., & Roy, C. (1980). *Conceptual models for nursing practice*. Appleton-Century-Crofts.

Rodgers, B. L. (2005). *Developing nursing knowledge: Philosophical traditions and influences*. Lippincott Williams & Wilkins.

Rogers, M. E. (1970). *An introduction to the theoretical basis of nursing*. F. A. Davis.

Rogers, M. E. (1980). Nursing: A science of unitary man. In J. P. Riehl & C. Roy (Eds.), *Conceptual models for nursing practice*. Appleton-Century-Crofts.

Rogers, M. E. (1990). Nursing: Science of unitary, irreducible human beings: Update 1990. In E. A. M. Barrett (Ed.), *Visions of Rogers' science-based nursing*. National League for Nursing.

Rogers, M. E. (1992). Nursing science and the space age. *Nursing Science Quarterly, 5*, 27–34. https://doi.org/10.1177/089431849200500108

Roy, C. (1987). Roy's adaptation model. In R. R. Parse (Ed.), *Nursing science: Major paradigms, theories, and critiques*. W. B. Saunders.

Roy, C. (2002). The nurse theorists: 21st-century updates–Callista Roy. Interview by Jacqueline Fawcett. *Nursing Science Quarterly, 15*, 308–310. https://doi.org/10.1177/089431802236795

Roy, C. (2007). Advances in nursing knowledge and the challenge for transforming practice. In C. Roy & D. Jones (Eds.), *Nursing knowledge development and clinical practice*. Springer.

Roy, C. (2008). Adversity and theory: The broad picture. *Nursing Science Quarterly, 21*, 138–139. https://doi.org/10.1177/0894318408316407

Roy, C. (2011). Research based on the Roy adaptation model: Last 25 years. *Nursing Science Quarterly, 24*(4), 312–320. https://doi.org/10.1177/0894318411419218

Roy, C., & Andrews, H. A. (1999). *The Roy adaptation model* (2nd ed.). Appleton & Lange.

Roy, C., & Roberts, S. L. (1981). *Theory construction in nursing: An adaptation model*. Prentice-Hall.

Roy, C., Whetsell, M., & Frederickson, K. (2009). The Roy adaptation model and research. *Nursing Science Quarterly, 22*(3), 209–211. https://doi.org/10.1177/0894318409338692

Sills, G. M., & Hall, J. E. (1977). A general systems perspective for nursing. In J. E. Hall & B. R. Weaver (Eds.), *Distributive nursing practice: A systems approach to community health*. Lippincott.

Sitzman, K. (2017). Evolution of Watson's human caring science in the digital age. *International Journal for Human Caring, 21*(1), 46–52. https://doi.org/10.20467/1091-5710-21.1.46

Smith, M. (2004). Review of research related to Watson's theory of caring. *Nursing Science Quarterly, 17*(1), 13–25. https://doi.org/10.1177/0894318403260545

Swanson, K. M. (1991). Empirical development of a middle range theory of caring. *Nursing Research, 40*, 161–166. https://doi.org/10.1097/00006199-199105000-00008

Taylor, S. G., Geden, E., Isaramalai, S., & Wongvatunyu, S. (2000). Orem's self-care deficit nursing theory: Its philosophic foundation and the state of the science. *Nursing Science Quarterly, 13*, 104–110. Retrieved March 26, 2021, from http://ovidsp.ovid.com/ovidweb.cgi?T=JS&PAGE=reference&D=ovftd&NEWS=N&AN=00006236-200004000-00004.

Timlin, A., Hastings, A., & Hardiman, M. (2018). Workbased facilitators as drivers for the development of person-centred cultures: a shared reflection from novice facilitators of person-centred practice. *International Practice Development Journal, 8*(1), 1–7. https://doi.org/10.19043/ipdj81.008

Wagner, J., Jones, S., Tsaroucha, A., & Cumbers, H. (2019). Intergenerational transmission of domestic violence: Practitioners' perceptions and experiences of working with adult victims and perpetrators in the UK. *Child Abuse Review, 28*(1), 39–51. https://doi.org/10.1002/car.2541

Watson, J. (1989). Watson's philosophy and theory of human caring in nursing. In J. P. Riehl-Sisca (Ed.), *Conceptual models for nursing practice*. Appleton & Lange.

Watson, J. (2002a). *Assessing and measuring caring in nursing and health science*. Springer.

Watson, J. (2002b). The nurse theorists: 21st-century updates–Jean Watson. Interview by Jacqueline Fawcett. *Nursing Science Quarterly, 15*, 214–219. https://doi.org/10.1177/08918402015003007

Watson, J. (2007). *Nursing human science and human care: A theory for nursing*. Jones & Bartlett.

Watson, J. (2012). *Human caring science, a theory of nursing* (2nd ed.). Jones & Bartlett.

Watson, J. (2018). *Unitary caring science: Philosophy and praxis of nursing*. University press of Colorado.

Professional Nursing Processes

KEY TERMS AND CONCEPTS

Critical thinking
Nursing process
Assessment
Nursing diagnosis
Planning
Implementation
Evaluation
Goals
Outcomes
Nursing Outcomes Classification (NOC)
Nursing interventions

Nursing Interventions
  Classification (NIC)
Concept mapping
Intuition
Reflection
Reflection-in-action
Reflection-on-action
Research-based model of
  clinical judgment
Interpersonal processes
Psychomotor processes
Patterning nursing
  processes

LEARNING OUTCOMES

By the end of this chapter, the learner will be able to:

1. Outline the cognitive processes that nurses use in clinical practice.
2. Specify the steps of nursing processes.
3. Discuss variances in the use of nursing process when practice is based on a selected nursing model.
4. Appraise the strengths and weaknesses of using nursing process in practice.
5. Distinguish between linear and integrated cognitive nursing processes. Compare and contrast critical thinking, intuition, and reflection.
6. Differentiate among the stages of the novice-to-expert model of clinical practice. Discuss interpersonal nursing processes consistent with selected nursing conceptual models.
7. Outline psychomotor processes for patterning of health.

REAL-LIFE REFLECTIONS

Carol, a nurse employed in a university-based health clinic, serves as a preceptor for community health nursing students from a local baccalaureate nursing program. Today is her first day working with Jane, a senior nursing student. Carol receives a telephone call from the university campus police informing her that they are bringing in an obese student who fell and has a swollen ankle. Before the student arrives, Carol asks Jane, "What is the first thing we should do when the injured student arrives?" Jane replies, "We should find out their name and how the accident happened." Carol responds, "OK. What other information do we need?" Jane becomes nervous and answers, "I never had a client with an orthopedic problem, so I really don't know where to begin. I always get confused in the clinical setting about what I should do first. Maybe I shouldn't be a nurse."

Remembering the uncertainty she experienced as a nursing student, Carol replies, "Once I understood nursing process, it seemed as though what to do in the clinical setting fell into place for me when I was a nursing student. Can you tell me the steps of nursing process and what nursing theory you use?"

(continued on page 204)

"I get the steps of nursing process confused all the time, and the program has us use Rogers's nursing theory," replies Jane.

Carol sighs and thinks to herself, "How can a nursing student get this far in her education without understanding how to use nursing process? What can I do to help Jane master the nursing process quickly?" Carol instructs Jane to observe while she handles the injured student and tells Jane that the two of them will talk about nursing process and Rogers's nursing theory later.

Questions for registered nurse (RN) students:
- *How should Carol explain the nursing process to Jane?*
- *Why is the nursing process important to practice?*

Questions for bachelor of science in nursing (BSN) students without RN experience:
- *How well do I know the steps of nursing process?*
- *How have I used nursing process when caring for clients during clinical learning experiences or in a clinical simulation?*
- *How would I guide another nursing student who needs help understanding and using nursing process?*

Beliefs about nursing shape the way nurses practice. When nurses engage in practice using the medical model, they pay more attention to disease processes, pharmacology, and surgical and other invasive procedures. A medically oriented approach to nursing is common in acute care settings. The physician does the assessment, determines the diagnosis, and issues orders. To provide safe, effective client care, nurses use knowledge from other disciplines (e.g., pharmacology, medicine, social work, rehabilitation) while also considering the physical, mental, social, and spiritual aspects of the client's response to illness.

Nursing practice focuses on human responses to health status and the medical plan of care. Nurses practice autonomously by diagnosing and treating human responses to protect, promote, and optimize a client's well-being, health, and abilities. Nurses focus on injury and illness prevention, alleviating suffering, assessing for adverse effects of prescribed therapies, and advocating for individuals, families, communities, and populations (American Nurses Association, 2021). Nursing knowledge includes detailed understanding of the client as a whole person, health and the factors that promote it, the environment and its impact on health, the mutual and ongoing interaction between humans and the environment, and the purpose and functions of nursing. Nurses perform their own client assessments, gathering information about each client's well-being, including:

1. Health status
2. Demographics
3. Quality of life
4. Social determinants of health
5. Environmental hazards exposures (home or work)
6. Health disparities
7. Physical, psychological, cognitive status
8. Spiritual health and well-being
9. Sexual orientation and preferences
10. Family and support systems
11. Cultural values and preferences

Because nurses view clients holistically and consider themselves key partners in an interdisciplinary health care team, they also have knowledge about the care regimens of other providers, such as physicians, pharmacists, and physical therapists. Understanding care regimens outlined by other health team members helps nurses appreciate the global health care plan and acknowledge its impact on the whole client. By sharing knowledge about the plan, nurses help clients assume mutual and equal responsibility for setting health-related goals and participating as equal members of the health care team.

The model of nursing accepted by the nurse projects knowledge that provides the basis for all nursing processes. Skill in the integrated use of cognitive, interpersonal, and psychomotor processes in client care is basic to the practice of professional nursing. This chapter emphasizes the relationship between nursing processes and the practice of professional nursing according to the nursing models discussed in Chapter 7, "Nursing Models and Theories."

CRITICAL THINKING

Many definitions of critical thinking appear in the nursing and higher education literature (Table 8.1). Although they vary somewhat, some elements are common to most definitions of critical thinking.

- **Critical thinking** is a highly complex thinking pattern that requires higher-order thinking.
- People who think critically take time to examine situations in terms of content and context instead of jumping into action to make personal judgments and clinical decisions or to solve problems.
- Critical thinkers take time to examine the consequences of anticipated actions.
- Critical thinking demands that the thinkers have solid, logical reasons for judgments and actions.
- Reflective thought enables critical thinkers to look for ways to improve their thinking.

Scholars debate whether critical thinking is a general life skill, an art, or a combination of both. If viewed as a general life skill, everyone must learn critical

thinking to survive. Fortunately, both skills and arts can be learned; both need to be practiced before they are mastered.

All experts agree that critical thinking occurs within a specific situation (context) (Brookfield, 2017; Ennis, 2015; Facione, 2020; Paul & Elder, 2020). When a nurse encounters a person without a pulse or respirations, spending time critically thinking about the situation would cause great harm; instead, immediate action is warranted. After the emergency has been handled, the nurse may spend some time engaged in critical reflection about why the arrest occurred, how it could have been avoided, and the effectiveness of professional actions.

Certain personal traits are associated with the ability to think critically. Before individuals can engage in regular critical thinking, they must value truth-seeking; open-mindedness; analyticity (recognizing potential problems, anticipating results, and prizing the use of reason); systematicity (the orderly, focused approach to inquiry); inquisitiveness (natural

TABLE 8.1	**Commonly Used Definitions of Critical Thinking**
Author(s)	**Definitions**
Alfaro-LeFevre (2020)	"Important thinking" that nurses "need to do in various situations" (p. 3) "A complex process that changes depending on context (circumstances)" (p. 7) "Knowing how to focus your thinking to get the results you need (includes applying logic, intuition, standards, and evidence-based practice)" (p. 7)
Bandman and Bandman (1995)	"The rational examination of ideas, inferences, assumptions, principles, arguments, conclusions, ideas, statement, beliefs, and action" (p. 7)
Brookfield (1987)	"Reflecting on the assumptions underlying our and others' ideas and action and contemplative alternative ways of thinking and living" (p. 18); reflective skepticism
Ennis (2015)	"reasonable, reflective thinking focusing on what to believe or do" (p. 32)
Facione (2006)	"The process of purposeful, self-regulatory judgment which results in interpretation, analysis, evaluation, and inference as well as explanation of the evidential, conceptual, methodological, criteriological, and contextual considerations upon which that judgment is based. CT is an essential tool of inquiry, … liberating force in education, … and a pervasive and self-rectifying human phenomenon" (p. 27)
Kurfiss (1988)	"An investigation whose purpose is to explore a situation, phenomenon, question, or problem to arrive at a hypothesis or conclusion about it that integrates all available information and that, therefore, can be convincingly justified" (p. 37)
McPeck (1981)	"The propensity and skill to engage in an activity with reflective skepticism" (p. 8)
Paul and Elder (2020)	"The art of analyzing and evaluating thought processes with a view of improving them" (p. 9)
Scheffer and Rubenfeld (2000), Rubenfeld and Scheffer (2015)	"In nursing … an essential component of professional accountability and quality nursing care" that displays "confidence, contextual perspective, creativity, flexibility, inquisitiveness, intellectual integrity, intuition, open-mindedness, perseverance, and reflection" Critical thinkers use "the cognitive skills of analyzing, applying standards, discriminating, information-seeking, logical reasoning, predicting, and transforming knowledge" (p. 7)
Watson and Glaser (1990)	Problem definition; decision making about pertinent information for problem solving; identifying and recognizing overt and covert assumptions; hypothesis formation and selection; drawing valid conclusions and judging validity of inferences (p. 1)

curiosity); with self-awareness of one's assumptions and biases while having the maturity to make honest, reflective judgments and self-confidence in reasoning processes (Brookfield, 2017; Ennis, 2015; Facione, 2020; Paul & Elder, 2020). This view of critical thinking fits well with Benner's novice-to-expert model (Benner, 1984, 2000), which illustrates the idea that experts develop certain characteristics related to practice (confidence, competence, and maturity) that enable them to quickly make correct clinical judgments that seem to simultaneously spring into action. Critical thinking is integrated throughout the cognitive nursing processes.

COGNITIVE NURSING PROCESSES

Clinical Decision Making

Nurses make numerous clinical decisions when engaging in professional practice. The scope of professional nursing practice requires nurses to make safe and prudent clinical decisions. They are also held legally accountable for their decisions. Whenever nurses encounter situations that require them to select from several courses of action to manage a clinical situation, they engage in clinical decision making. Before settling on a final course of action, nurses consider the personal, environmental, and contextual elements of each specific clinical situation. Clinical decision making contains the following key attributes: "intuition, analysis, heuristics, experience, knowledge, clinical reasoning, and critical thinking" (Johansen & O'Brien, 2015, p. 43). After making clinical decisions, nurses have to accept the decisions that were made, the consequences that resulted, and reflect on the processes used and the outcomes. Reflection-on-action enables nurses to determine if they made optimal decisions. Reflection also provides nurses the opportunity to improve their knowledge and skills in the clinical decision-making process.

Nursing Process

Clients rely on nurses to make effective clinical decisions. Kataoka-Yahiro and Saylor (1994), Banning (2006), Huckabay (2009), Shoulders et al. (2014), and Turkel (2016) suggest that the **nursing process** as a method for problem solving and decision making in nursing practice represents a discipline-specific version of critical thinking. Huckabay (2009) proposed that the critical thinking elements embedded within nursing process and clinical judgments are (1) identifying purposes, goals, and objectives for care; (2) identifying a problem to solve or question to answer; (3) sorting and distinguishing relevant from irrelevant information; (4) considering conceptual dimensions underlying a nursing situation (concepts, principles, and theories); (5) examining different points of view; (6) identifying assumptions; (7) making interpretations and inferences; and (8) considering implications and consequences of various action options (see Box 8.1, Professional Building Blocks, "Steps of the Nursing Process").

The nursing process was established in the late 1950s and mirrors the scientific method. In its early stage it was a four-step process (assessment, planning, implementation, and evaluation) for nurses to use to identify and solve client problems. Using a standardized process for nursing gained momentum in the 1960s. By the 1970s, the nursing process became a pivotal part in the scope and standards of professional nursing, and the professional nursing licensure examination contained test items to verify that program graduates could use it effectively.

Effective problem solving relies on extensive data collection for proper problem identification. Nurses assess clients holistically to determine actual and potential health-related problems or strengths (nursing diagnoses). Problem solving, the scientific method, and the nursing process incorporate planning as a key step.

 8.1 Professional Building Blocks

Steps of the Nursing Process

Step 1. Assessment: Collect comprehensive data regarding the factors related to client health status.
Step 2. Diagnosis: Identify actual or potential client health strengths and weaknesses.
Step 3. Planning:
    a. Determine health-related goals (or outcomes).
    b. Specify a series of actions to be taken to attain the identified goals.
Step 4. Implementation: Execute the action plan outlined in Step 3.
Step 5. Evaluation: Determine the effectiveness of the implemented action plan to either make needed revisions or restart the process with Step 1.

When determining ways to solve a problem, test hypotheses, or deliver individualized nursing care, people generate action plans consisting of a desired goal and steps for attaining that goal. After executing action plans, nurses use problem solving, the scientific method, and the nursing process to evaluate the effectiveness of the action plans in meeting the desired outcome (goal).

The nursing process provides a logical and rational way for the nurse to identify actual and potential problems and make decisions to resolve them. Nurses use critical thinking skills in all steps of the nursing process to:

- collect relevant data from a variety of sources, sift out irrelevant data, determine which data are important, and validate the meaning of data with others if uncertain.

- organize data into meaningful patterns, determine if more data are required, compare data patterns with norms and known theories, examine assumptions about the client situation, and identify the major client health concerns to arrive at a nursing diagnosis.

- set safe care priorities and realistic care outcomes, determine appropriate nursing interventions, and generate a rationale for interventions while considering client needs and concerns.

- apply knowledge for intervention performance, test the efficacy of interventions, update and revise care plans as needed, noting changes in client status, and determine when to consult other health team members.

- evaluate the effectiveness of the care plan, determine alternative approaches and interventions, monitor the quality of care delivered, track client progress toward desired outcomes, and revise the plan as needed.

Although the nursing process has its roots in the scientific process, nurses execute it in a sensitive and caring manner when working collaboratively with people. Nurses consider individual client needs and preferences when providing care. Nurses use creativity to individualize nursing care for clients. Thus, the nursing process is both an artistic and a scientific process.

Take Note!
Nursing process steps come from the steps of the scientific process, but when nurses individualize client care, the nursing process becomes artistic in nature.

FIGURE 8.1 An interactional approach to the nursing process. All parts of the process are interrelated and influence the whole.

Invariably, the nursing process is presented as a series of four or five phases with a number of steps within each phase. The net effect is a procedure that appears linear (or, at best, overlapping or circular) and cumbersome. However, all parts of the process are interrelated and influence the whole. The steps or phases of the nursing process occur sequentially, but they are not linear. Planning may lead to interventions for implementation or outcomes for evaluation. However, nurses continually assess clients when using all steps of the nursing process and make needed changes based on assessment findings. Figure 8.1 depicts the nursing process viewed from an interactional perspective. The following discussion presents an overview of each step of the nursing process.

Step 1: Assessment

During **assessment**, nurses collect cues (subjective and objective data) about the client's health status. Subjective data (e.g., the presence of pain, its location, its intensity, aggravating and alleviating factors) are provided by the client or caregiver. Objective data can be directly measured or observed (e.g., test results, increased blood pressure, pulse, respiratory rates). Nurses collect cues systematically and verify the accuracy with clients. If unable to collect the desired data, nurses use critical thinking to determine the reasons for obstacles and devise alternative approaches to collect it. When working with clients, nurses continuously collect and analyze client cues to make nursing decisions. Nurses document the data collected to provide a legal record of their surveillance activities so that members of the interprofessional health care team have access to it.

Before nurses can begin collecting data, clients must trust them. Usually nurses initiate client relationships. When possible, nurses and clients work together as partners to outline specific care goals and specify responsibilities and ways to tailor nursing care to meet individual client needs. Nurses use critical thinking to evaluate client responses and determine ways to facilitate communication.

Most nurses use an organized process for data collection. They decide which data are desirable and significant to collect in a particular situation and determine what sources and methods would be best to obtain these data. First, the nurse must know who the client is, why the client needs nursing care, and what factors currently influence the client's health status. Therefore, the nurse must collect key data such as the client's name, age, gender, marital status, occupation, social determinants of health, existing knowledge about health–illness status, and family attitudes toward health care. Second, to individualize care, the nurse collects data regarding the client's personal habits, communication styles, cultural influences, growth and development status, learning capacity, supports and resources, previous experience with the health care system, medical diagnosis and regimen, coping patterns, personal values, spiritual beliefs, and desired changes. Finally, the nurse uses a preferred conceptual nursing model to guide and organize data collection using the suggestions outlined in Table 8.2.

As data are collected, the nurse validates the findings with the client and other sources and clarifies any discrepancies. Nurse evaluation of the data should consider accuracy and whether all relevant factors have

been included. As data collection continues, the organization and analysis of patterns within the data proceed concurrently, which may identify additional data collection needs. Nurse-collected data should supplement, rather than duplicate, data collected by other health care professionals (e.g., history) and should focus on information needed for nursing care. During data collection, nurses review all data to determine if more information is needed. If more information is needed, data collection is continued until the nurse decides that all relevant information has been collected. After deciding that the assessment is completed, the nurse moves to the second step of the nursing process.

Step 2: Diagnosis

Nurses derive nursing diagnoses from collected client data. Nurses analyze the client cues and cluster related ones into meaningful categories. Some nurses use a nursing model to categorize the cues while others use a framework such as bodily systems or functional health patterns. When looking at the clustered cues, the nurse then interprets what the data reveal about the client. Effective data analysis and synthesis require that nurses remain

TABLE 8.2	Implications for Data Collection in Select Nursing Models Organized by Theoretical Frameworks
Nursing Model	**Implications for Data Collection**
Systems Theory	
King	Perceptions of self, level of growth and development, stress level, abilities to function in usual role, make decisions, and communicate
Neuman	Stressors, indications of disruption of the lines of defense, resistance factors
Stress/Adaptation	
Roy	Adaptation level (related to three classes of stimuli), coping in relation to modes of adaptation, position on the health–illness continuum
Caring	
Orem	Therapeutic self-care demand, presence of self-care deficits, ability of clients to meet self-care requisites
Watson	Phenomenal field (self within life space and motivational factors for health), values, needs for information, problem-solving abilities, developmental conflicts, losses, feelings about the human predicament
Complexity	
Peplau	Physiologic and personality needs, illness symptoms, relationships with significant others, influences on establishment, and maintenance of the nurse–client relationship
Rogers	Characteristics of patterning, health potential, rhythms of life, simultaneous states of the individual and environment
Parse	Thoughts and feelings about the situation, the synchronizing rhythms in human relationships, personal meanings, ways of being alike and different, and values
Newman	Person–environment interactions, patterns of energy exchange, client's responses to symptoms, transforming potential, client's feelings and what they do because of those feelings, patterns of life
Leddy	Characteristics of human universal essence field and environmental essence field

objective, engage in thoughtful deliberation, make sound judgments, and discriminate relevant from irrelevant information. Nursing diagnoses represent the professional nurse's judgment about human responses within a contextual situation that may either threaten or strengthen health and well-being. Nursing diagnoses exclusively address care situations for which the professional nurse has responsibility. Although nursing practice may vary across state and national boundaries, nurses make independent judgments when clustering data to formulate nursing diagnoses. Professional nursing responsibility means that the nurse has the legal qualifications and accountability to take action. Nursing diagnoses may apply to individuals, families, or communities (Carpenito-Moyet, 2010; Herdman & Kamitsuru, 2018).

The concept of nursing diagnosis started in professional nursing practice in the early 1970s (Webber, 2008) in North America and has now expanded to all continents. A **nursing diagnosis** is a nurse-identified issue that becomes a key element of the nursing care plan. A nursing diagnosis can be an actual problem that needs resolution, a potential problem for close monitoring or preventive interventions, or a possible recommendation for a way to enhance client wellness.

The North American Nursing Diagnosis Association International (NANDA-I) most recently established a list of 244 approved nursing diagnoses. To be a NANDA-I-approved nursing diagnosis, it must be submitted for organizational review. NANDA-I-approved nursing diagnoses sometimes appear in standardized clinical care pathways followed by nurses at the bedside. However, not all nursing diagnoses must adhere to strict NANDA-I formatting guidelines. A diagnosis is accepted for publication and inclusion in the NANDA-I taxonomy when it has a label definition, clearly articulated defining characteristics, and related factors or risk factors and references. NANDA-I nursing diagnoses may be revised or removed when they become inconsistent with current literature or lack substantial evidence for continued use (Herdman & Kamitsuru, 2018). NANDA-I also identifies the presence of syndromes, but these are few in number. Possible nursing diagnoses may present, but they are called diagnostic hypotheses and more data need to be collected to substantiate them before use (Herdman & Kamitsuru, 2018). Herdman and Kamitsuru (2018) identified three types of nursing diagnoses: problem-focused, risk, and health promotion.

1. When defining characteristics of a problem-focused nursing diagnosis are present, nursing diagnoses are written using a three-phrase clause: the client problem, followed by the words "related to," then the etiology. NANDA-I formatting of actual nursing diagnoses forbids the use of disease names or surgical procedures as the related-to clause.

2. Risk nursing diagnoses are used when a particular person, group, or community has an increased likelihood of the appearance of an undesirable human response.

3. Wellness diagnoses occur when a person, family, group, or community experiences a desire to transition to a higher level of wellness.

4. Nurses use a syndrome diagnosis when a particular clinical situation results in a predictable cluster of commonly encountered actual or risk nursing diagnoses. A syndrome enables nurses to plan care effectively when nursing diagnoses overlap and some nursing interventions to address the group of nursing diagnoses may be similar or identical.

When nurses monitor for possible complications from medications or an invasive procedure, they use collaborative problem statements (Carpenito-Moyet, 2010; Herdman & Kamitsuru, 2018). The number of clauses in a nursing diagnosis varies according to its classification. Table 8.3 offers definitions, specific formats, and examples of the various classifications of nursing diagnoses and also includes an example of a collaborative problem statement.

Ideally, nurses develop nursing diagnoses in collaboration with clients. When nurses involve clients in generating nursing diagnoses, clients validate that the nurse has the complete story, become more aware of the goals, and have the opportunity to determine the desired outcomes of nursing care. Human response patterns, functional health patterns, and health perceptions provide different ways for nurses to collect and organize data to compile a nursing diagnosis. Gordon's (1995) 11 functional health patterns provide an internationally coherent method to classify nursing diagnoses (Herdman & Kamitsuru, 2018):

1. Health perception—health management
2. Nutritional—metabolic
3. Elimination
4. Activity—exercise
5. Sleep—rest
6. Cognitive—perceptual
7. Self-perception—self-concept
8. Role—relationship
9. Sexuality—reproduction
10. Coping—stress tolerance
11. Value—belief

TABLE 8.3   Definition, Format, and Examples of Nursing and Collaborative Diagnoses

Nursing Diagnosis Classification	Definition	Format	Examples
Problem-focused	A clinical judgment identifying a problem with major defining characteristics being present with identified contributing factors influencing the health status change	Three clauses: 1. The human response 2. Etiology (or contributing factors) 3. Clinical signs and symptoms	Malnutrition (1) related to persistent nausea and vomiting (2) as evidenced by no food intake for 1 week, refusal to eat, (3) weight loss of 4.53 kg (10 lb) within 2 weeks, prealbumin of 14.8 mg/dL, and complaints of "I feel tired all the time" and statement "I am afraid to eat because I will throw up"
Risk	A clinical judgment identifying a potential problem because of increased vulnerability to developing it	Two-clause statement designating the potential human response and the etiology	Risk for infection related to compromised host defenses from the potentially immunosuppressive effects of chemotherapy and the presence of a central venous catheter
Syndrome	A clinical judgment identifying a health-altering situation resulting in the likely presence of multiple nursing diagnoses	One-clause statement designating the type of altered health	Battered child syndrome
Collaborative problems and diagnostic statements	Potential complications arising from a disease process or medical interventions	Two-part phrase including the words "potential complication"	Potential complication: hemorrhage secondary to cardiac catheterization

Adapted from Carpenito-Moyet, L. J. (2010). *Nursing diagnosis application to clinical practice* (13th ed.). Wolters Kluwer Health/Lippincott Williams & Wilkins; Herdman, T. H., & Kamitsuru, S. (Eds.). (2018). *NANDA International Nursing Diagnoses: Definitions & classification, 2018–2020* (11th ed.). Thieme.

NANDA-I adapted the functional patterns outlined by Gordon to refine the taxonomy (classification system) of their nursing diagnoses. The domains include:

1. Health promotion: Health awareness and health management
2. Nutrition: Ingestion, digestion, absorption, metabolism, and hydration
3. Elimination and exchange: Urinary, gastrointestinal, integumentary, and respiratory function
4. Activity/rest: Sleep/rest, activity/exercise, energy balance, cardiovascular/pulmonary responses, and self-care
5. Perception/cognition: Attention, orientation, sensation/perception, cognition, and communication
6. Self-perception: Self-concept, self-esteem, and body image
7. Role relationship: Caregiving roles, family relationships, and role performance
8. Sexuality: Sexual identity, sexual function, and reproduction
9. Coping/stress tolerance: Posttrauma responses, coping responses, and neurobehavioral stress
10. Life principles: Values/beliefs, action congruence
11. Safety/protection: Infection, physical injury, violence, environmental hazards, defensive processes, and thermoregulation
12. Comfort: Physical, environmental, and social comfort
13. Growth and development: Physical growth and development (Herdman & Kamitsuru, 2018, pp. 87–95)

Although the more commonly used nursing diagnoses in acute care settings tend to be problem-oriented only, nurses also identify nursing diagnoses for enhancing client wellness and to prevent potential health complications. For example, a hospitalized person with a new diagnosis of insulin-dependent diabetes has many problems to confront in order to manage and cope with the change in health. Immediate concerns include learning how to administer insulin injections and to comply with recommended dietary changes. The client also needs to know the long-term complications associated with the disease.

Because nurses may also work with well individuals in the community, nursing diagnoses may focus on enhancing wellness. These wellness nursing diagnoses enable nurses to identify ways to enhance wellness and prevent potential health problems in risk clients (e.g., individuals with an inherited risk to develop diseases such as cardiovascular disease or cancer). Most wellness diagnoses enable nurses to focus on client strengths and use them to improve client health.

Nursing diagnoses have created a unique language for professional nurses. However, recent client safety and interprofessional team collaboration initiatives emphasize the importance of all health team members speaking a common language when discussing client care issues. Current NANDA-I publications focus exclusively on independent nursing diagnoses. Many times, professional nurses care for clients who have potential complications from surgical and diagnostic procedures as well as specific disease processes. Earlier works by NANDA-I identified these as potential complications and provided a standardized way to state them (Carpenito-Moyet, 2010). Box 8.2, Professional Building Blocks, "Strengths and Limitations of Using NANDA-I Nursing Diagnoses in Clinical Practices," outlines reasons for and against using NANDA-I nursing diagnoses in clinical practice. To date, there is no research-based evidence

that demonstrates that the use of nursing diagnoses improves client outcomes. However, recent research by Akbulut and Akpinar (2017) suggests many nurses believe NANDA-I nursing diagnoses should be used in clinical practice, but there are some issues using them in clinical practice (see the "Focus on Research" box).

Take Note!

Safe effective health care requires clear, concise communication among all health team members so that everyone understands the client situation.

▌ QUESTIONS FOR REFLECTION

1. How do you think nurses might best communicate the client's actual and potential problems with each other?
2. Why do you think this method would be best?
3. What has been your nursing education or professional experiences with nursing diagnoses?

8.2 Professional Building Blocks

Strengths and Limitations of Using NANDA-I Nursing Diagnoses in Clinical Practices

Strengths

- Provides a common language for nurses to communicate the actual and potential problems to the client
- Improved client–nursing assessments (Müller-Staub et al., 2006)
- Increased continuity of nursing care among members of the nursing care team during client handoffs when shifts change
- Increased client satisfaction
- Improved documentation of assessments
- Provides a possible organizational system for nursing documentation on electronic health records
- Provides a taxonomy that could be used for charging for professional nursing services

Limitations

- Rigid formatting of diagnostic statements increase the time to write them.
- Other health professionals, especially physicians, find nursing diagnostic terminology confusing and impede effective interprofessional communication in and across health care settings (Finkelman & Kenner, 2007; Gordon, 2005; Webber, 2008).
- Failure of interprofessional health team members to understand each other may delay emergent medical intervention (Finkelman & Kenner, 2007).
- Increased risk for errors (sometimes fatal ones) (Finkelman & Kenner, 2007)
- Exclusive use of NANDA-I-approved nursing diagnoses may limit nurse's individualized thinking when a client situation falls outside of a typical clinical situation.
- NANDA-I terminology is difficult to understand across cultures (Gordon, 1995).
- A diagnosis should be a true problem and cannot be a potential one (Zanotti & Chiffi, 2015).
- Nursing diagnoses are based exclusively on clusters of data and are not confirmed or justified by actual diagnostic testing (Zanotti & Chiffi, 2015).
- Not all nurses have adequate knowledge to generate nursing diagnoses and use them effectively (Akbulut & Akpinar, 2017).

FOCUS ON RESEARCH
Knowledge Gaps Among Nurses Regarding Nursing Diagnoses

Akbulut and Akpinar wanted to determine the level of nurse cognizance and knowledge of nursing diagnoses of the most frequently encountered nursing diagnoses in outpatient clinics and inpatient units in a large Turkish academic medical center. After receiving institutional review board approval, they conducted face-to-face interviews with 100 nurses to complete an investigator-developed survey to collect demographic data and assess nurse knowledge and understanding of frequently encountered nursing diagnoses.

One hundred nurses participated in the study. All were over the age of 18. Education level varied: high school graduation (32%), vocational school (16%), university graduation (46%), and postgraduate degree (6%). Of the nurses, 79 were female, and 47% had worked fewer than 5 years in the institution. Of the nurses, 31% worked in an internal medicine clinic, 18% worked in a surgical clinic, and 51% worked on an inpatient, specialized unit.

The researchers analyzed data using percentages and chi-square analysis. The findings revealed that 81% of the nurses thought that they must use nursing diagnoses in their clinical practice, but 33% of them had never received any formal or institutional education in identifying, generating, and using them. Only 11% of the 62 nurses who had received education reported that their formal education had been sufficient. Five nurses could not recall if they had received education about nursing diagnoses. The only nursing diagnoses that were correctly identified by more than 50% of the participants were constipation and diarrhea (61%). Less than 25% of the nurses could identify the following nursing diagnoses: impaired skin integrity, activity intolerance, knowledge deficit, self-care deficit syndrome, impaired communication, ineffective role performance, and risk for trauma. Less than 10% correctly identified the following nursing diagnoses: fatigue, impaired swallowing, spontaneous ventilation, risk

for self-mutilation, diversional activity deficit, risk of aspiration, grieving, and disturbed personal identity. Nurses who had graduated with college degrees correctly identified more nursing diagnoses than those without this level of education ($p < .05$). The length of employment in the current work setting was not significant to their knowledge of frequently encountered nursing diagnoses. To remedy their lack of education, 25 nurses reported wanting to receive information about nursing diagnoses in the forms of a seminar or conference and 9 nurses wanted printed information available in the clinic or unit to use when needed. Of the nurses, 85 reported that low nurse staffing levels affected their ability to use nursing diagnoses in practice.

The investigators concluded that the current state of nursing education in nursing diagnoses received by nurses working in this Turkish academic medical center was inadequate and that when nurses have to work short-staffed, they cannot take the time to identify and generate nursing diagnostic statements. They recommended employers create systems to promote use of nursing diagnoses in clinical practice and conduct in-service education on them.

The clinical significance of this study is that education on nursing diagnoses may vary among nurses and across nations. Nurses without college degrees are less prepared to identify and generate accurate NANDA-I nursing diagnoses. In the United States and Canada, legal scope and standards decree that care planning creation falls within the scope of professional nursing practice, though use of NANDA-I is not the only way to generate nursing diagnoses. There has been no recent research related to nurse knowledge and utilization of nursing diagnoses in clinical practice in North America. Nursing faculty and textbook authors need to provide practical application on how to use nursing diagnoses (whether NANDA-I formatted or not) in educational strategies and materials to facilitate utilization in clinical practice.

Akbulut, G., & Akpinar, R. B. (2017). Determining nurses' knowledgeability of nursing diagnoses. *International Journal of Caring Sciences, 10*(3), 1129–1135.

Step 3: Planning

Once a comprehensive list of nursing diagnoses has been generated, nurses develop a plan of care to communicate specific client care needs to other nursing personnel so that desired outcomes are attained. Care plans guide and direct client care efforts to ensure continuity of care when different nurses assume care responsibilities. In addition, care plans designate specific interventions to meet client care goals. Finally, nursing care plans outline contributions that nurses make to client health care delivery.

Nurses follow certain guidelines to generate effective nursing care plans. When **planning** client care, nurses establish a set of nursing diagnoses in priority order, designate desired nursing goals and client outcomes, and prescribe specific nursing interventions. Nurses set priorities based on preserving client functional status (except in the terminally ill), promoting client comfort, and meeting mutually agreed-upon client goals.

Because of the need to streamline care and improve client outcomes, some nurses rely on standardized care plans. Standardized nursing care plans provide less variance in care delivered to clients with similar health problems and theoretically improve quality. They address all critical assessments and customary interventions for medical therapies, invasive procedures, and diagnostic tests. When nurses follow standardized care plans, care sometimes loses its person-centered focus, resulting in a task-oriented approach to practice.

The nursing care plan includes the priorities and the prescribed nursing interventions to achieve the desired **goals** (the global desired state) derived from the nursing diagnoses. Ideally, nurses and clients work together to develop the desired goals and outcomes of nursing care. Once the goals are defined, specific outcomes can be generated. **Outcomes** are end results that, when measured, determine client progress toward resolution of the nursing diagnosis. These expected outcomes

must be realistic and stated clearly and concisely as they provide the basis for evaluating nursing care plan effectiveness. Table 8.4 presents broad guidelines for goal setting in selected nursing models. Because nursing models vary, the foci of nursing goals differ.

Nursing Outcomes Classification

Nurses must demonstrate that what they do makes a difference in client outcomes and find ways to determine the effectiveness of nursing care. The **Nursing Outcomes Classification (NOC)**, developed by nurse researchers at the University of Iowa in 1988, offers an approach for developing measurable client outcomes. Currently, the NOC provides nurses with 540 scales to measure client outcomes directly affected by nursing care. Each outcome is defined and has a list of key indicators for use in evaluation, a target outcome rating, a place to identify each data source, a scale to measure client status, and a list of references that provides evidence substantiating the validity and reliability for each identified outcome (Moorehead et al., 2018). For example, the NOC has a scale to measure personal safety behaviors. A nurse can use this scale to identify client risk for injury. After educating the client about, for example, personal safety or correction of metabolic disorders, the nurse can reassess the client using the scale to determine if improvement in behavior has occurred.

NOC facilitates the development of computerized information systems for tracking nursing care outcomes

---

■ TABLE 8.4   Broad Guidelines for Goal Setting in Select Nursing Models Organized by Theoretical Frameworks

Nursing Model	Broad Guidelines for Goal Setting
Systems Theory	
King	Achieve goals and solve problems related to personal, interpersonal, and social systems.
Newman	Maintain or restore dynamic equilibrium by reducing stressor penetration or strengthening the normal line of defense.
Stress/Adaptation	
Roy	Promote adaptation from successful coping.
Caring	
Orem	Restore external and internal constancy.
Watson	Meet human needs and solve problems in a caring interpersonal relationship.
Complexity	
Rogers	Help people design ways to attain optimal rhythmic patterns.
Parse	Illuminate meaning, synchronize rhythms, and mobilize transcendence.
Newman	Transform patterns of life and facilitate evolving consciousness.
Leddy	Mutual process to define meaningful goals to attain an optimal pattern of the whole.

across health care settings. NOC also facilitates comparable data collection, substantiates nursing care contributions, creates uniform nursing data sets, provides nurses with outcome measurement tools, facilitates electronic documentation of client care, improves reimbursement for nursing services, and standardizes the ways nurses can evaluate nursing care innovations. Through the process of determining measurable, standardized outcomes, nurses clearly articulate the contributions they make to client care while developing a unique body of nursing knowledge (Moorehead et al., 2018).

Not all nurses use the NOC in clinical practice. However, the planning phase requires long-term goals and desired outcomes (short-term or immediate goals) to be determined within the client plan of care. After goals and outcomes have been established, priorities must be set. When survival is threatened, physical needs must take precedence. Cost, available personnel, and resources (including time) may influence priorities. The theory or model being used to organize care can also influence the determination of priorities. For example, the use of Maslow's (1962) theory would assign higher priority to physiologic, safety, and security needs and lower priority to love, self-esteem, and self-actualization needs. In addition, the client must be closely involved in priority setting, as always.

Once the priorities among goals and outcomes have been determined, alternative options for care can be generated and their probability for success predicted. The possible solutions or approaches are heavily influenced by availability of resources and by factors in the client's lifestyle and cultural background. The NOC provides a standardized method to track client progress toward care objectives across inpatient, community, and home settings (Moorehead et al., 2018) (see Concepts in Practice, "Nursing Outcomes Classification in Action").

Concepts in Practice IDEA → PLAN → ACTION

Nursing Outcomes Classification in Action

NOC aids nurses with the challenge of delineating client goals and outcomes, including setting priorities, identifying potential barriers, and choosing interventions that have the best likelihood of success. Consider, for example, the client whose story opened this chapter: an overweight teenager who has a broken leg. Although weight loss may be considered an important goal for this client, the more important goal is immediate mobility. Therefore, teaching the client how to use crutches safely is a higher priority. Once

that is accomplished, the goal of weight loss can be addressed. This goal could be achieved by 2 weeks of residence at a clinic or a self-monitored weight reduction program consisting of weighing portions of food, keeping a diary of food intake, and following a prescribed exercise program. However, financial constraints may make the clinic trip unfeasible, and time and lifestyle constraints may influence the desirability of the exercise or food-weighing approach. With NOC, nurses working with the client would look at adherence to the outlined dietary regimen, knowledge and use of health-promoting behaviors, knowledge about the prescribed diet, specific weight control behaviors, and weight reduction measurements to help this client meet their weight loss goal once their leg has healed.

Today's nurses care for clients with increasingly higher levels of acuity, spend much of their time documenting care rendered, and pay close attention to safety considerations. Time pressures prevent nurses from developing multiple approaches to address client situations. As a result, nurses may quickly generate a plan of care without taking the time to analyze interventions for appropriateness and likelihood of success in a particular clinical situation.

Nurses must make a conscious effort to avoid choosing a prescribed "cookbook" approach to delineating care outcomes. To preserve nursing as a collaborative partnership with clients, the nurse and the client together must determine goals and select interventions that have the best likelihood of success. The individualized and collaborative approach can then be translated into specific actions, the desired frequency of the actions, who will be assigned to carry out those actions (e.g., the nurse, the client, or other health team members), and the timetable for expected achievements.

Along with establishing goals and outcomes (or objectives) for nursing care, the nursing care plan outlines specific nursing interventions. **Nursing interventions** are the actions nurses take to attain care goals and outcomes. Frequently, nursing students find written nursing care plans challenging and complex. Unlike the care plans written by practicing nurses, student care plans usually require written rationales for proposed nursing interventions. However, even experienced nurses must conscientiously take time to reflect and recall the rationales behind clinical interventions. Nurses determine priority lists for each identified nursing diagnosis, determine expected outcomes and goals, and prescribe specific interventions (with established frequencies and time for each action). Computerized

software for care plan generation offers nurses a series of checklists to complete individualized care plans. When nurses override the usual nursing interventions and frequency of actions, individualization of care is enhanced. However, software programs must possess this feature and nurses expend time and energy to individualize care plans.

As part of the care plan, the nurse can prescribe independent interventions (those not requiring a physician's order, such as using a pillow under a client's foot to keep the heels off the mattress), designate collaborative interventions (those requiring a physician's order, such as the administration of prescription medications), and outline specific interventions to screen for potential complications associated with medical or surgical treatments. Ideally, other nurses should be able to follow the care plan exactly as written by the nurse who developed it. Nurses can find published care plans in books and journal articles, in computer programs, and on evidence-based websites on the internet.

Take Note!
Nursing interventions are actions nurses take to attain care goals and outcomes.

Nursing Interventions Classification

In 1987, the University of Iowa developed the **Nursing Interventions Classification (NIC)** system as a means to standardize all possible nursing interventions. The NIC contains 5,655 standard nursing interventions and outlines approximately 13,000 nursing activities. Most interventions contain 10 to 40 (though a few contain more) specific activities that include information related to client assessment, safe care, environment maintenance, health education strategies, psychological and spiritual support techniques, interprofessional consultations, and client and family referrals. The NIC facilitates nursing professionalism by standardizing nursing treatment nomenclature; strengthening links among nursing knowledge, diagnoses, interventions, and outcomes; facilitating electronic documentation of nursing care; assisting in determining costs and resources needed for nursing interventions; providing a theoretical foundation to help beginning nurses learn clinical decision making; and increasing nursing-specific knowledge (Butcher et al., 2018). Concepts in Practice, "Nursing Interventions Classification in Action," applies the use of the NIC as it pertains to the overweight client with the broken leg presented at the outset of this chapter.

Concepts in Practice IDEA → PLAN → ACTION

Nursing Interventions Classification in Action

The NIC uses the label "weight reduction assistance" for the nursing intervention for the following nursing diagnosis—alteration in nutrition: more than body requirements related to reduced activity secondary to nonbearing weight status for fractured leg. There are 33 nursing interventions outlined that could be used to assist a client with weight reduction.

Nursing Activities for the Intervention

- Assess client desire and motivation for weight loss and mutually set weight loss goals.
- Use the term "excess weight" rather than "fatness," "excess fat," or "obesity."
- Set realistic weight loss goals with the client.
- Post a weekly weight loss plan in a strategic location.
- Weigh client weekly and chart weight weekly, placing this in a strategic location.
- Assess internal and external factors for eating.
- Review food intake log and reward the client for making healthy food choices.
- Develop weekly diet plans and exercise plans with the client.
- Identify client triggers for unhealthy eating patterns and offer a substitute activity.
- Create a daily exercise program to meet the challenges of non–weight-bearing status.
- Encourage the use of sugar substitutes.
- Explore support options for weight loss such as face-to-face meetings, online weight loss programs, use of activity tracking and food logging devices, and have the client select a desirable option.

Teaching Activities for the Intervention

- Instruct the client to maintain a daily food intake and exercise log using paper, online tracking program, or a mobile app.
- Discuss foods that meet nutritional needs to promote fracture healing without increasing caloric intake.
- Instruct the client to consume low-calorie and low-fat foods rich in fiber such as fruits, vegetables, whole grains, low-fat or fat-free dairy products, lean meats, fish, beans, and eggs.
- Teach the client how to read food labels and to calculate caloric and fat content in food.
- Provide examples of foods with little or no nutritional value (e.g., junk food, alcohol).

(continued)

Desired Client Outcomes

- Food selections stay within a predetermined daily caloric limit when eating out or participating in social gatherings.
- Weight loss of 1 to 2 lb per week takes place for a total loss of 20 lb.

Other optional interventions would be to discuss setbacks in weight loss with the client, referral to a physician to secure a prescription for a weight loss medication, instruction on how to eat when going to social events or restaurants, and posting reminders or encouragement to engage in healthy eating and exercise in strategic locations. Because the NIC designates a framework for nursing interventions that can be computer-coded (and clients can be charged for them), NIC use in clinical practice has become standard in some health care organizations. Evaluation of the care plan occurs by using NOC (Butcher et al., 2018).

Concept Mapping

Some nurse educators have replaced traditional nursing process papers (including written care plans) with **concept mapping**, which enables students to use creative and critical thinking processes to draw connections among assessment data, multiple nursing diagnoses, pathophysiology, nursing interventions, and desired client outcomes (Alfaro-LeFevre, 2020; Rubenfeld & Scheffer, 2015; Schuster, 2016). Concept mapping was started in the 1960s by Dr. Joseph Novak at Cornell University as a way to promote meaningful learning, which requires well-organized, relevant knowledge structures and a personal commitment to integrate new with existing knowledge (Novak & Cañas, 2008). A concept map is a diagram resulting from analytical thought that depicts relationships among important pertinent concepts related to a clinical situation. Creating a concept map incorporates multiple areas of the brain, including areas for affect, motor function, and memory (short-term, long-term, and working) (Novak & Cañas, 2008). Concept maps may be generated by using a prescriptive template or developed freely with few guidelines. The center of the map typically specifies the major concept of interest (central concept). The nurse (or student) then identifies supporting data and the relationships between that data and the central concept. Many concepts in professional nursing can serve as a central concept (e.g., client strengths or weaknesses, a medical or nursing diagnosis, a desired outcome). Figure 8.2 provides

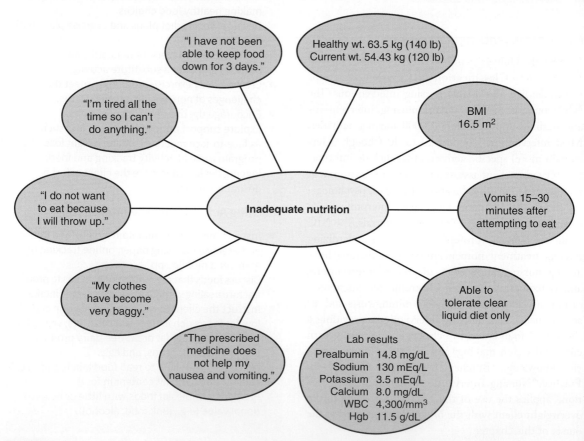

FIGURE 8.2 Sample concept map showing the relationship between assessment data and nursing diagnosis.

a sample concept map. Computer software programs and online resources are available for generating concept maps. Nurses rarely use concept mapping in clinical settings unless they are explaining complex processes to nursing students. Nevertheless, concept mapping may have value in facilitating client understanding of diseases and health management regimens.

Take Note!
Concept mapping enables students to make connections among assessment data, multiple nursing diagnoses, pathophysiology, nursing interventions, and desired client outcomes.

Client Care Paths

Since the 1990s, client care paths have outlined standardized care plans for commonly encountered illnesses, surgeries, and procedures in outpatient and inpatient health care settings. Client care plans address nursing diagnoses, outline evidence-based interventions, and specify observations for and prophylactic treatment of potential complications. Standardized client care paths reduce variation in nursing care received by clients with the same clinical problem, streamline care to reduce costs, reduce care errors and oversights, and decrease care documentation (paths frequently contain checklists, instead of requiring nurses to write detailed narrative notes). Clients receive a copy of the care path so they know what to expect, learn about how they can facilitate care, have written instructions for self-care, and can track their own progress toward health restoration. Most care paths accommodate instances when care delivery fails to follow the path exactly because of an unexpected client response. Criticisms of care paths include reduced individualization of client care plans and decreased critical thinking because of the perceived pressure to follow the path exactly as outlined.

Step 4: Implementation

During **implementation**, nurses execute proposed nursing care plans. Nursing actions support and complement the medical plan of care. Ideally, professional nurses use interventions based on scientific evidence. Nurses use the following skills for successful care plan implementation: teaching clients (and caregivers), managing others, facilitating group process, resolving conflicts, performing technical skills, and, above all, communicating effectively.

All client–nurse interactions should be goal-directed and purposeful. As nursing actions are performed, nurses collaborate with the clients and their family members and/or caregivers to involve them appropriately in the care. Nurses perform interventions with sensitivity to the client's feelings and individual preferences. Conceptual models play a role in the organization of nursing care. Table 8.5 outlines how conceptual

Nursing Model	Implications for Nursing Interventions
■ TABLE 8.5 Implications for Nursing Interventions in Select Nursing Models Organized by Theoretical Frameworks	
Systems Theory	
King	Emphasis is on exploration of the situation, shared information, mutually set goals, and explored means to resolve problems, achieve goals, and move forward
Neuman	Emphasis is on primary, secondary, or tertiary prevention to reduce stressors or strengthen the lines of defense
Stress/Adaptation	
Roy	Emphasis is on increasing, decreasing, or maintaining focal, contextual, or residual stimuli
Caring	
Orem	Emphasis is on self-care actions for or with the client if the client is unable to perform them for themselves
Watson	Emphasis is on caring that reflects interpersonal teaching–learning, mutual formulation of the problem, joint appraisals, shared need for problem solving, joint planning, provision of cognitive information, and evaluation of helpfulness for learning and coping
Complexity	
Rogers	Emphasis is on mobilization of the client's resources and repatterning of the human–environment interaction
Parse	Emphasis is on guidance to relate the meaning of the client's situation, to share thoughts and feelings with one another, and to change the meaning of the situation by making it more explicit
Newman	Emphasis is on the process of growth in which the nurse focuses on the client's evolving capacities, diversity, and complexity in the process of expanding consciousness
Leddy	Emphasis is on the mutual process of transforming energy to create change

models may be used to organize care along with possible implications for nursing interventions.

An important part of implementation is the documentation of nursing interventions and their results. Documentation provides a means to track client progress toward desired outcomes as well as a legal record of rendered health care services. More importantly, documentation serves as a key method for communication among interprofessional health team members. Nurses continually assess clients to determine responses to nursing and medical interventions. When interventions are determined to be ineffective, the nurse revises the nursing care plan. Changes in a client's condition may mean an alteration in the frequency of prescribed interventions, modification of the current interventions, prescription of new interventions, or consultation with other health care professionals. The process of intervention is integrally involved with the final phase of the nursing process—evaluation.

Step 5: Evaluation

During **evaluation**, nurses and clients collaborate to determine whether progress is being made toward the attainment of desired health-related goals. Processes in the evaluation of care include reassessing, reviewing, and reordering (if necessary) care priorities; establishing new goals; and revising the care plan. Evaluation occurs continuously throughout each phase of the nursing process. However, the main purpose of evaluation is to compare changes in client behavior or health status with the determined goals or expected outcomes specified in the nursing care plan. Results of evaluation may reveal one or a combination of the following:

- *Goals and outcomes were fully met*, and the determination of future client contacts is needed to reaffirm that the health status change remains permanent.
- *Goals and outcomes were partially met*, revealing that the health problem or the desired health status change has not been resolved. However, progress continues. Continued monitoring is warranted; more time may be needed with the current plan before considering modification.
- *Goals and outcomes were not met*. The client has little or no evidence of change in health status or health problem since the initial assessment. The care plan needs revision.
- *New problems have emerged*, and the entire care plan needs to be revised to address them.

Not all client-related health goals are amenable to quantification, so nurses sometimes have difficulty finding valid and reliable tools to objectively measure progress. It may be helpful to consider what appropriate tools are available to measure progress toward goals when the goals are established. For example, weight loss and blood pressure reduction are easily validated. However, it is difficult to assess improved self-concept or attitudes toward a more healthful lifestyle. Sources for instruments to measure progress may be found in the NOC, journal articles, websites, and instrument handbooks.

Because the nursing process is systematic, logical, and goal-directed, nurses assume that adherence to the process should result in desired goal attainment. When evaluation indicates that the problem is not resolved, other possible reasons must be considered through collaborating with clients, their families and caregivers, nursing colleagues, and other interprofessional health care team members.

If the goals have been met and no new ones have emerged, the nurse and the client may terminate the relationship, which may be difficult for both parties. Clients may be unsure of their ability to independently maintain the changes in health behavior or well-being status. The nurse may have ambivalence about not being needed any longer. Being aware of and openly sharing these feelings can lead to satisfaction in having accomplished the desired goals and acceptance of the need to end the relationship.

Take Note!

Nursing process provides a logical, sequenced, and rational way for nurses to identify potential and actual client problems, develop a plan to address them, and then evaluate the effectiveness of nursing actions on achieving desirable client outcomes.

Despite the extensive attention given to the nursing process, many experienced nurses continue to intervene using standardized procedures based on medical diagnoses. Efforts to standardize client care have resulted in the development of client care paths. In many institutions, professional nurses helped develop client care paths that incorporate nursing assessments and interventions to address commonly encountered nursing diagnoses for specific health problems.

The use of client care paths can lead nurses to engage in rote practice. However, when nurses use nursing models to guide care, they engage in critical thinking because models provide solid reasoning behind clinical practice. In the following section, two brief examples illustrate that nurses can approach the nursing process differently when they use conceptual nursing models to guide practice.

Take Note!
Nursing process provides an organized way of thinking about client care and fosters deliberate nursing actions.

▮ QUESTIONS FOR REFLECTION

1. Based on the information you have read related to nursing process, list and define each step. How do you think the nursing process will help you as you engage in clinical practice as a nursing novice?
2. How does your clinical practice setting promote or discourage the use of the nursing process?
3. What are the barriers to developing individualized nursing care plans for clients in your current practice setting?
4. Why do you perceive these as barriers?
5. How can you change your practice setting to facilitate individualization of client care?
6. What are the consequences of not individualizing client care in practice?

Conceptual Models Emphasizing the Nursing Process

Roy and Neuman addressed the nursing process specifically in their nursing models. Instead of keeping with the five-step process, however, they refined it. Roy and Andrews (1999) kept the nursing process focused on nursing practice while Neuman and Fawcett (2002) proposed the use of the nursing process for all health care professionals because it is based on the scientific method.

The Roy Adaptation Model

In the Roy adaptation model, the goal of the nurse is to manipulate stimuli to move the client in the desired direction of change toward adaptation. The process of nursing is described as a six-step problem-solving method (Roy & Andrews, 1999):

1. First-level assessment: Examine client behaviors in the four adaptation modes and make judgments about whether the behaviors are adaptive or ineffective.
2. Second-level assessment: Analyze stimuli that influence ineffective behaviors and determine nursing care priorities.
3. State problem areas as nursing diagnoses.
4. Determine specific goals.
5. Determine interventions.
6. Evaluate as behavior changes and modify as needed.

The Neuman Systems Model

In the Neuman systems model, the purpose of nursing action is "to best retain, attain, and maintain optimal client health or wellness using the three preventions as intervention to keep the system stable" (Neuman & Fawcett, 2002, p. 25). Client stability depends on the depth of stressor penetration. Nurses assess for actual and potential effects of environmental stressors before making judgments or taking action. Neuman proposed a modification of the nursing process to incorporate the following three steps:

1. Determine a nursing diagnosis.
2. Establish nursing goals.
3. Determine nursing outcomes with interventions classified as primary (wellness retention), secondary (attainment of health), or tertiary (maintenance of health) prevention.

Benefits and Criticisms of the Nursing Process

The American Nurses Association, the National Council of State Boards of Nursing, and other nurse specialty organizations incorporate the five phases of nursing process in professional nursing practice standards. Many professional nurses use the nursing process daily in clinical practice, and many organizations have documentation forms based on the steps of the nursing process. The nursing process provides an organized way of thinking about client care and fosters deliberate nursing actions.

Nevertheless, some nurses report that they do not use the nursing process in daily practice (Webber, 2008). Benner (2000) suggested that many nursing experts do not follow the steps of nursing process as they engage in professional nursing practice. Henderson (1987), Lindsey and Hartrick (1996), Rew (1996), Varcoe (1996), and Webber (2008) offered the following concerns that the nursing process:

- is inconsistent with real-world practice because it is a linear, rational problem-solving process.
- is focused on problems rather than client strengths and potential.
- is time-consuming and requires elaborate nursing jargon.
- prefers rules over interactions.
- is antithetical to a holistic approach to client care.
- labels clients by nursing diagnoses.
- minimizes disallowance of nursing intuition.
- is a questionable approach for expert nursing practice.

The formulaic structure of the nursing process has been useful to teach rules to novice learners, and the

National Council of State Boards of Nursing Licensing Examination uses it as a means for demonstrating minimal competence to begin a professional nursing career. However, many nurses treat the nursing process as if it were the only process in nursing practice. Research has demonstrated that the nursing process is inadequate "when sensory data are changing rapidly or are ambiguous, uncertain, or conflicting" (Rew, 1996). Benner et al. (1996) found that clinically proficient and expert nurses use intuitive cognitive processes, rather than rule-based thinking, to make clinical judgments. Turkel et al. (2012) stated that the current labels for the steps of nursing process fail to embrace the unitary-transformative approach to nursing practice. They propose renaming the steps as follows:

- **Recognizing:** Incorporating deeper assessment that involves intentional listening to recognize the health issue being encountered by the client
- **Connecting:** Expanding planning to integrate the client, client patterns, and client meaning into the plan and involving the client's significant others in determining what could be done
- **Partnering:** Including a process in which the nurse and the client work collaboratively while they connect to live out a mutual process in which both parties constantly recognize issues and address new ones as they arise
- **Reflecting:** Where evaluation becomes a collaborative process between the nurse and the client to verify that the implemented interventions were successful

Integrated Models for Clinical Judgment

Along with the nursing process, nurses use other models to make clinical judgments. Benner and colleagues (1996, p. 1) suggested that "the clinical judgment of experienced nurses resembles much more [the] engaged, practical reasoning … than the disengaged, scientific, or theoretical reasoning … represented in the nursing process." Experienced nurses tend to bypass some steps of nursing process, while novice nurses comply with each of the five steps.

Intuition

Studies of expert clinical practice have identified intuition, knowing the client, and reflection as important characteristics. **Intuition** has been described as "another way of knowing wherein facts or truths are known or felt directly rather than arrived at through a linear process of rational analysis" (Rew, 1996, p. 149)

(see Chapter 6, "Patterns of Knowing and Nursing Science"). In a study that supported the novice-to-expert model, Polge (1995, p. 8) found that "as the level of nursing proficiency increases from advanced beginner to expert, there is a significant increase in the use of intuitive critical thinking to make clinical nursing judgments." Young (1987) proposed that intuition is multidimensional. The functional dimension of intuition is composed of cues and judgment in which actions do not have a logical link with data. Intuition as a personal way of knowing relies on direct client contact, self-receptivity, experience, energy, and self-confidence. Many nurses have saved lives by acting on intuitive feelings. In some cases, physicians have been known to come and see hospitalized clients because the nurse identified intuition as the reason for contacting the physician.

■ QUESTIONS FOR REFLECTION

1. How have you used intuition to guide personal or professional actions? What were the consequences?
2. What advice would you give to someone about using intuition to guide action?
3. Would the advice you give be different for a professional colleague than for a friend? Why or why not?

Reflection

Reflection is a process of thinking about the concerns associated with an experience. Reflection develops the affective domain of learning and allows nurses to relate to the aspects of their experience that are the most profound at the time. Consequently, reflection has the potential to provide for personal growth. Reflective learning is multidimensional and may be triggered by a sense of inner discomfort. When things do not go according to plan, nurses engage in reflection to identify and clarify concerns surrounding a clinical situation. Effective reflection requires that the nurse be open to new information that may arise from non-empirical sources. Sometimes reflection results in the resolution (or "a-ha moment") of confounding situations or with the feeling that one has learned something that is personally significant. Reflection may result in profound changes in attitudes or behaviors.

The Pew Health Professions Commission (1998) identified reflection as one essential skill that health professionals must be able to perform along with critical thinking and rational problem solving. Health care professionals need to develop skills in reflective and critical thinking to identify and respond to new situations and practice dilemmas. Professionals also use reflection during practice and afterward to evaluate professional performance.

Schon (1987) identified two ways in which professionals use reflection: reflection-in-action and reflection-on-action. During **reflection-in-action**, health care practitioners think about the purposes and reasons behind the actions being performed. **Reflection-on-action** is a self-evaluative process in which practitioners analyze personal performance in a given clinical situation, think of what could have been done better, and determine plans to improve performance the next time a similar clinical situation is encountered.

Take Note!

Health care professionals need to develop skills in reflective and critical thinking to identify and respond to new situations and practice dilemmas.

Brookfield (2017, p. 9) proposed that reflection becomes critical when it questions "assumptions and practices" as well as seeks to understand the power forces behind current practice. Reflection also provides opportunities for professionals to find meaning in practice (Brookfield, 2017; Schon, 1987). Reflection takes time to master, especially in today's fast-paced society (see Box 8.3, Learning, Knowing, and Growing, "Developing Skills in Reflection," for actions you can take to improve your skills).

8.3 Learning, Knowing, and Growing

Developing Skills in Reflection

A variety of tools can help you to develop your skills in reflection:

- Write your autobiography.
- Keep professional logs.
- Self-audit your performance.
- Construct criteria for role model profiles.
- Develop survival advice memos.
- Record yourself in professional action.
- Undergo peer evaluations.
- Identify critical incidents.
- Engage in meaningful dialogue with others.

Brookfield, S. (1995). *Becoming a critically reflective teacher*. San Francisco: Jossey Bass.

Clinical Judgment

Tanner (2006) reviewed over 200 studies that addressed clinical judgments made by nurses in practice that substantiate the use of intuition and reflection by professional nurses. According to Tanner, what nurses bring to practice situations may be more important than the objective data available to the nurse when clinical judgments are made. Tanner developed a **research-based model of clinical judgment** as follows.

Professional nurses bring knowledge and experience to clinical practice situations. As nurses gain more experience, they learn to identify the patterns that indicate impending deterioration in client status requiring rapid action. Quick pattern identification occurs rapidly and sometimes intuitively. Most nurses who work in clinical settings typically reflect on what they are currently doing and the outcomes of interventions. When a situation fails to unfold as planned, many nurses review their actions (or lack of action) to see what went wrong. Thus, reflection-on-action becomes a mechanism for nurses to refine clinical practice strategies.

Within the practice context, experienced nurses notice (i.e., perceptually grasp) the global situation. Nurses interpret the situation by using reasoning, pattern identification, analysis, intuition, and personal narratives. They then respond by taking action to help clients. Immediately following action, they assess the client outcomes. The process of interpreting and responding requires reflection-in-action. The final step in the clinical judgment model is reflecting, in which the nurse reflects-on-action and solidifies the knowledge learned from the clinical experience.

INTERPERSONAL PROCESSES

As noted previously, intuition and reflection are professional nursing processes that integrate experience with cognition. Cognitive processes receive more attention during discussions related to the nursing process, intuition, and reflection.

Professional nursing practice, particularly the nurse–client relationship, requires the use of interpersonal processes. **Interpersonal processes** can be defined as interactions between two or more individuals. Without attention to interpersonal processes, nursing practice may become impersonal, dominated by technology, and self-serving. The following section provides brief examples of different approaches used by select nursing conceptual models and theories in the use of interpersonal processes.

King's Theory of Goal Attainment

In King's (1995) theory (discussed in Chapter 7, "Nursing Models and Theories"), the goal of nursing is to help individuals maintain their health so they can function in their roles. Nursing is a process of action, reaction, and interaction that results in goal attainment. Although the process proposed by King's theory is classified according to the steps in the nursing process, the emphasis is on interpersonal processes within the steps. Assessment incorporates perception, communication, and interaction of the nurse and the client. Planning includes mutual determination of goals and agreement on the means to attain them. Implementation is the process in which transactions are made. Finally, evaluation is the process in which nurses ask, "Was the goal attained?"

Peplau's Interpersonal Relations Model

In Peplau's model (Reed, 1996) (discussed in Chapter 4, "Establishing Helping and Healing Relationships"), nursing is a therapeutic, interpersonal process. Nurses use the interpersonal process as an educative instrument, a maturing force that aims to promote forward movement of the personality. The interpersonal process is the method by which nurses facilitate useful transformation of the client's energy or anxiety. The interpersonal process is based on a participatory relationship between the nurse and the client, in which the nurse governs the purpose for and the process in the relationship and the client controls the content. The process consists of four phases:

1. **Orientation:** Clients become aware of the availability of and trust in the nurse's abilities.
2. **Identification:** The nurse facilitates expression of feelings without rejection.
3. **Exploitation:** The client derives the full value from the relationship.
4. **Resolution:** The client no longer needs the professional nurse and is independently capable of meeting their own needs.

Paterson and Zderad's Humanistic Theory

In humanistic nursing practice theory, nursing is perceived as a lived experience between human beings. "Nursing is a response to the human situation. One human being needs a kind of help and another gives it" (Paterson & Zderad, 1988, p. 11). The humanistic nursing effort is directed toward increasing the possibilities of making responsible choices. The process, which is labeled the "phenomenologic method of nursology" (science of nursing), consists of five phases:

- **Phase I:** The nurse knower prepares for coming to know.
- **Phase II:** The nurse intuitively knows the "other."
- **Phase III:** The nurse scientifically knows the other by:
  1. Analyzing the situation
  2. Considering the relationships between components
  3. Synthesizing themes or patterns
  4. Conceptualizing or symbolically interpreting a sequential view of this postlived reality
- **Phase IV:** The nurse complementarily synthesizes known others by:
  1. Comparing similarities and differences
  2. Synthesizing the similarities and differences to create an increased knowing
- **Phase V:** Succession occurs within the nurse from the many to the paradoxical one—"a conception or abstraction that is inclusive of and beyond the multiplicities and contradictions" (Paterson & Zderad, 1988, p. 74).

Parse's Human Becoming Theory

In Parse's (1996) theory (discussed in Chapter 7, "Nursing Models and Theories"), the goal of practice is quality of life from the client's perspective, with the focus on the meaning constructed by the client. The nurse is present in a nonroutine, unconditional, loving way of being with the client. The full attention of the nurse is with their clients "as they move beyond the moment." The methodology in this theory consists of three processes:

1. **Explicating (illuminating meaning):** Making clear what is appearing now through languaging.
2. **Dwelling with (synchronizing rhythms):** Giving of self over to the flow of the struggle in connecting–separating.
3. **Moving beyond (mobilizing transcendence):** Propelling with envisioned possibilities in transforming.

Newman's Theory of Health as Expanding Consciousness

In the theory of health as expanding consciousness (discussed in Chapter 7, "Nursing Models and Theories"), Newman described nursing as "caring in the human health experience" (Newman, 1994, p. 139). "The responsibility of the nurse is not to make people well, or to prevent their getting sick, but to assist people to recognize the power that is within them to move to higher levels of consciousness" (Newman, 1994, p. 15). The focus of nursing in this theory is the pattern of the whole that is clarified through a praxis (practice) method. The method starts with the establishment of a partnership with the client with a mutual goal of participating in an authentic relationship that requires meeting and forming connections. The nurse and the client then form a shared consciousness that serves as the basis for increasing awareness. When client and nurse goals are met, the client and the nurse move apart. Each participant in the nursing encounter tells their story in their own way.

The nurse is free to be authentic and fully present. "Awareness of being, rather than doing, is the primary mechanism of helping" (Newman, 1994, p. 104). To develop a sequential pattern over time, the nurse organizes data in chronologic order as a narrative. Creating a chronologic log of client cues enables the nurse to understand the complete story of the client's reason for seeking health care and facilitates learning the full context.

PSYCHOMOTOR PROCESSES

In addition to cognitive and interpersonal processes, nursing care includes psychomotor processes. **Psychomotor processes** are defined as manual dexterity, coordination, and the ability to use equipment effectively while performing nursing procedures. Skill in the performance of physician-ordered, often invasive, disease- or problem-related interventions is a key part of nursing clinical practice. Associate degree programs emphasize these technical aspects of nursing, whereas baccalaureate and higher-degree programs focus on cognitive and interpersonal processes. Health care consumers and organizations expect nurses to be able to carry out complex procedures smoothly and efficiently.

PATTERNING NURSING PROCESSES

Patterning nursing processes use energy to enhance health and well-being. Patterning processes have compatibility with a unitary approach to nursing. Some complementary and alternative health care interventions incorporate manipulation of human–environment energy fields. Table 8.6 presents some noninvasive nursing interventions that promote self-patterning.

■ TABLE 8.6   Noninvasive Nursing Interventions That Promote Self-Patterning

Intervention	Example(s)
Imagery	Guided imagery in which client visualizes healing occurring
Relaxation	Progressive relaxation exercises or warm bath
Affirmations	Positive self-talk
Sound	Listening to music at 60 beats/min
Exercise	Yoga or tai chi
Wave modulation	Color or light therapy
Nutrition	Special diet or herbal, vitamin, or mineral supplements
Meaningful presence	Being with another
Humor	Laughing, sharing appropriate jokes
Authentic dialogue	Guided reminiscence
Wellness counseling	Health education
Therapeutic touch	Centering and altering energy fields
Movement therapy	Dance or imposed motions
Journaling	Diary writing or critical incident written records
Balancing	Finding balances between activity, rest, work, and fun
Bibliotherapy	Reading self-help or inspirational literature
Body therapy	Acupressure, massage, or healing touch

Rogers's Science of Unitary Human Beings

Nursing from an interaction perspective delineates structure in qualities and individuals in the environments. Rogers's science of unitary human beings proposes that separations do not exist, but rather all things form a single constellation. Rogers (1988, 1992) specified that the purpose of nursing is to create optimal health and well-being for all persons. The science of unitary human beings defines health not as a separate state or as the result of lifestyle choices or an encounter with illness but rather as "an index of field patterning" (Malinski, 1986, p. 27). "Pattern is concerned with qualities and is expressed by the map of the configuration of relationships" (Bartol, 2016, p. 225). Only manifestations of patterns can be accessed by humans (Leddy, 2004, 2006).

In Rogerian science, behavior patterns are viewed as manifestations of the human–environment field. Field manifestations may include lifestyle parameters such as nutrition, work, and play; exercise; sleep–wake cycles;

safety; interpersonal networks; and decelerated–accelerated field rhythms.

Examples of field rhythm manifestations might include diversity (from greater to lesser); motion (from slower to seemingly continuous); time (from slower to timelessness); and creativity (from pragmatic to visionary). The client is a knowing participant in change in this model. Through being aware, having choices and the freedom to act intentionally, and being involved in creating changes, the client is a mutual participant with the nurse in the patterning process. A healing relationship is characterized by certain principles:

- The focus is on strengths and skills.
- The nurse and the client are involved in creating changes and influencing outcomes.
- The nurse and the client are equal partners, but the client has the major responsibility for changing decisions.
- A balance of exchange or reciprocity occurs.
- Presence and involvement or connectednesses emerge.
- Flow and harmony exist.

The patterning process has two phases, appraisal and deliberative. The elements of appraisal in Phase I include the following:

- Using multiple modes of awareness, including recognizing, being aware, and being sensitive
- Tuning into a person's unique patterns
- Appreciating manifestations of the human field in the form of experience, perception, and expressions
- Constructing pattern knowing through synthesis
- Verifying with the client

Phase II involves the mutual deliberative patterning of behavior, which is possible because of the integral connectedness of the person–environment. Although diversity is considered a norm, patterning of each individual is unique. Each person has an intrinsic potential for growth, which can be identified by exploring the meaning of experiences for the individual. The client and the nurse are viewed as connected, and the healing milieu is as important as the treatment modality. Because change is viewed as inevitable, the challenge is to reframe problems into opportunities for positive becoming. By tuning in to the client's rhythms, the nurse can help the client free energy for self-patterning through a number of possible noninvasive interventions:

- Imagery
- Relaxation
- Affirmation

- Sound (music)
- Exercise
- Color/light (wave modalities)
- Nutrition (diet, vitamins, minerals, and herbs)
- Meaningful presence
- Humor
- Authentic dialogue (guided reminiscence)
- Wellness counseling (health education)
- Therapeutic touch (centering)
- Movement (dance, imposed motion)
- Journaling
- Balance between activity and rest
- Bibliotherapy
- Acupressure
- Bodywork (massage, touch for health)

The science of the unitary human being seems highly compatible with traditional and integrative approaches to health care. As clients become more aware of complementary and alternative health care treatments, professional nurses need the knowledge to help them make wise choices for health enhancement.

■ QUESTIONS FOR REFLECTION

1. How do you feel about using energy to promote healing and health?

2. Which of the patterning processes would you like to try to enhance your health? Why would you like to try that one?

REAL-LIFE REFLECTIONS

Remember Carol and Jane from the beginning of the chapter? If you were Carol, how would you respond to Jane's difficulty using the nursing process? Why is it so important that beginning nurses understand the nursing process?

Summary and Significance to Practice

Cognitive, interpersonal, and patterning nursing processes provide methods by which the nurse sensitively and systematically approaches practice to achieve mutually determined health goals with the client. Nurses use a variety of cognitive skills (knowledge, nursing process, intuition, and reflection) when delivering client care. Critical thinking enables nurses to effectively use nursing cognitive processes in clinical practice. Although nursing process arises out of scientific foundations, nurses can be artistic when developing individualized client care plans.

In addition to nurse cognitive processes, the nurse–client relationship facilitates data collection (assessment) and collaborative goal setting. Recent efforts to standardize nursing diagnoses, outcomes, and interventions may interfere with the ability to provide individualized client care developed in partnership with clients.

The use of interactive processes may provide enriching relationships for the client and the nurse because authenticity provides the basis for therapeutic partnerships. Patterning processes provide a complex holographic approach to nursing care, in which nurses focus on maximizing client–human potential. The various nursing models and theories presented in this chapter guide nursing practice. However, the individual nurse decides the approaches and processes used to implement nursing care effectively and in collaboration with clients and interprofessional health team members.

From Theory to Practice

1. Why is it important for professional nurses to use cognitive, interactive, and patterning processes when engaging in clinical practice?
2. Which nursing process do you use most frequently in clinical practice? Why? What assumptions underlie your most frequently used professional nursing process?

Nurse as Author

1. Obtain a clinical path (or standardized care plan) from a clinical setting. Make a list of all the steps contained within it. Analyze it for the presence of all steps of the nursing process. Outline the rationale behind all the nursing interventions. Write a brief summary of how the path or standardized care plan facilitates and hinders the delivery of client-centered nursing care. Specify how you would revise the path (or care plan) to individualize the plan for a person with special needs not included in the plan.
2. Take a moment to reflect about how you use nursing diagnoses in clinical practice. Write a brief essay about the strengths and weaknesses of nursing diagnoses using in-text citations and your personal clinical experiences. Based upon your analysis about the strengths and weaknesses of nursing diagnoses in practice, make a recommendation for its continued use or elimination as a step of nursing process.

Your Digital Classroom

Online Exploration

Foundation for Critical Thinking: **www.criticalthinking.org**

How to Construct a Concept Map (University of Delaware): **http://www.udel.edu/chem/white/teaching/ConceptMap.html**

Insight Assessment: **www.insightassessment.com**

North American Nursing Diagnosis Association International (NANDA-I): **www.nanda.org**

University of Iowa College of Nursing Center for Nursing Classification and Clinical Effectiveness: **http://www.nursing.uiowa.edu/center-for-nursing-classification-and-clinical-effectiveness**

Expanding Your Understanding

Visit the NANDA-I website and answer the following questions:

1. Browse the site to determine the cost of being a full member of the organization and what benefits the membership offers. Would you consider becoming a member? Why or why not?
2. Find the newly approved nursing diagnoses. Identify the ones that you would use in clinical practice to generate nursing care plans for your clients. Would the current care planning program in your practice support using one of these new diagnoses? If not, how would you proceed to make a clinical practice change so that you could use one of these new diagnoses?
3. Access the process for submitting a new nursing diagnosis. What do you think would be the barriers for proposing and submitting a new nursing diagnosis? Why do you think that the process is so detailed and prescriptive?

Beyond the Book

Visit the **Point** at **www.thePoint.lww.com** for activities and information to reinforce the concepts and content covered in this chapter.

REFERENCES

Akbulut, G., & Akpinar, R. B. (2017). Determining nurses' knowledgeability of nursing diagnoses. *International Journal of Caring Sciences, 10*(3), 1129–1135. Retrieved March 27, 2021, from http://www.internationaljournalofcaringsciences.org/docs/3_%201-akbulut_original_10_3.pdf

Alfaro-LeFevre, R. (2020). *Critical thinking, clinical reasoning and clinical judgment: A practical approach.* Elsevier.

American Nurses Association. (2021). *Nursing: Scope and standard of practice* (4th ed.). Author.

Bandman, E. L., & Bandman, B. (1995). *Critical thinking in nursing* (2nd ed.). Appleton & Lange.

Banning, M. (2006). Nursing research perspectives on critical thinking. *British Journal of Nursing, 15*(2), 458–461. https://doi.org/10.12968/bjon.2006.15.8.20966

Bartol, G. M. (2016). The psychophysiology of body mind healing. In B. Dossey, L. Keegan (authors), C. C. Barrere, M. A. Blasko-Helming, D. A. Shields, K. Avino, & C. Guzzetta (Eds.), *Holistic nursing: A handbook for practice* (7th ed., pp. 221–238). Jones & Bartlett Learning.

Benner, P. (2000). *From novice to expert: Excellence and power in clinical nursing practice* (commemorative ed.). Addison-Wesley.

Benner, P., Tanner, C. A., & Chesla, C. A. (Eds.). (1996). *Expertise in nursing practice: Caring, clinical judgment, and ethics.* Springer.

Brookfield, S. D. (1987). *Developing critical thinkers: Challenging adults to explore alternative ways of thinking and writing.* Jossey-Bass.

Brookfield, S. D. (2017). *Becoming a critically reflective teacher* (2nd ed.). Jossey-Bass.

Butcher, H. K., Bulechek, G. M., Dochterman, J. M., & Wagner, C. M. (Eds.). (2018). *Nursing Interventions Classification (NIC)* (7th ed.). Elsevier.

Carpenito-Moyet, L. J. (2010). *Nursing diagnosis application to clinical practice* (13th ed.). Wolters Kluwer Health/Lippincott Williams & Wilkins.

Ennis, R. H. (2015). Critical thinking. In M. Devis & R. Barret (Eds.), *The Palgrave handbook of critical thinking in higher education.* Palgrave MacMillan.

Facione, P. A. (2006). *Critical thinking: What it is and why it counts.* California Academic Press.

Facione, P. A. (2020). *Critical thinking and why it counts* (2020 update). Retrieved September 28, 2020, from https://www.insightassessment.com/wp-content/uploads/ia/pdf/hatwhy.pdf

Finkelman, A., & Kenner, C. (2007). *Teaching IOM: Implications of the Institute of Medicine reports for nursing education.* American Nurses Association.

Gordon, M. (1995). *Manual of nursing diagnosis, 1995–1996.* Mosby-Year Book.

Gordon, S. (2005). *Nursing against the odds.* Cornell University Press.

Henderson, V. (1987). Nursing process: A critique. *Holistic Nursing Practice, 1*(3), 7–18. https://doi.org/10.1097/00004650-198705000-00005

Herdman, T. H., & Kamitsuru, S. (Eds.). (2018). *NANDA International Nursing Diagnoses: Definitions & classification, 2018–2020* (11th ed.). Thieme.

Huckabay, L. M. (2009). Clinical reasoned judgment and the nursing process. *Nursing Forum, 44*(2), 72–78. https://doi.org/10.1111/j.1744-6198.2009.00130.x

Johansen, M. L., & O'Brien, J. L. (2015). Decision making in nursing practice: A concept analysis. *Nursing Forum, 51*(1), 40–48. https://doi.org/10.1111/nuf.12119

Kataoka-Yahiro, M., & Saylor, C. (1994). A critical thinking model for nursing judgment. *Journal of Nursing Education, 33*(8), 351–356. https://doi.org/10.3928/0148-4834-19941001-06

King, I. M. (1995). The theory of goal attainment. In M. A. Frey & C. L. Sieloff (Eds.), *Advancing King's systems framework and theory of nursing.* Sage.

Kurfiss, J. (1988). *Critical thinking: Theory, research, practice, and possibilities.* Association for the Study of Higher Education.

Leddy, S. K. (2004). Human energy: A conceptual model of unitary nursing science. *Visions: The Journal of Rogerian Scholarship, 12*, 14–28. Retrieved March 27, 2021, from https://www.thefreelibrary.com/Human+energy%3a+a+conceptual+model+of+unitary+nursing+science.-a0161397669

Leddy, S. K. (2006). *Health promotion mobilizing strengths to enhance health, wellness, and well-being.* F.A. Davis.

Lindsey, E., & Hartrick, G. (1996). Health-promoting nursing practice: The demise of the nursing process? *Journal of Advanced Nursing, 23*(1), 106–112. https://doi.org/10.1111/j.1365-2648.1996.tb03142.x

Malinski, V. M. (1986). *Explorations on Martha Rogers' science of unitary human beings.* Appleton-Century-Crofts.

Maslow, A. H. (1962). *Toward a psychology of being.* Van Nostrand.

McPeck, J. E. (1981). *Critical thinking and education.* St. Martin's Press.

Moorehead, S., Swanson, E., Johnson, M., & Maas, M. L. (2018). *Nursing Outcomes Classification (NOC): Measurement of health outcomes* (6th ed.). Elsevier.

Müller-Staub, M., Lavin, M. A., Needham, I., & von Achterberg, T. (2006). Nursing diagnoses, interventions and outcomes—Application and impact on nursing practice: Systematic review. *Journal of Advanced Nursing, 56*(5), 514–531. https://doi.org/10.1111/j.1365-2648.2006.04012.x

Neuman, B., & Fawcett, J. (2002). *The Neuman systems model* (4th ed.). Prentice Hall.

Newman, M. A. (1994). *Health as expanding consciousness* (2nd ed.). Mosby.

Novak, J., & Cañas, A. (2008). *The theory underlying concept maps and how to construct and use them* [Technical Report IHMC Cmap Tools 2006–01 Rev 2008–01]. Retrieved November 29, 2012, from http://cmap.ihmc.us/docs/theory-of-concept-maps.php

Parse, R. R. (1996). The human becoming theory: Challenges in practice and research. *Nursing Science Quarterly, 9*(2), 55–60. https://doi.org/10.1177/089431849600900205

Paterson, J. G., & Zderad, L. T. (1988). *Humanistic nursing.* National League for Nursing.

Paul, R., & Elder L. (2020). *The miniature guide to critical thinking, concepts and tools.* Rowman and Littlefield Publishing Group.

Pew Health Professions Commission. (1998). *Recreating health professional practice for a new century.* University of California, San Francisco Center for the Health Professions.

Polge, J. (1995). Critical thinking: The use of intuition in making clinical nursing judgments. *Journal of the New York State Nurses Association, 26*(2), 4–9. Retrieved March 27, 2021, from https://pubmed.ncbi.nlm.nih.gov/7636606/

Reed, P. G. (1996). Peplau's interpersonal relations model. In J. J. Fitzpatrick & A. L. Whall (Eds.), *Conceptual models of nursing: Analysis and application* (3rd ed.). Appleton & Lange.

Rew, L. (1996). *Awareness in healing.* Delmar.

Rogers, M. E. (1988). Nursing science and art: A prospective. *Nursing Science Quarterly, 1*(3), 99–101. https://doi.org/10.1177/089431848800100304

Rogers, M. E. (1992). Nursing science and the space age. *Nursing Science Quarterly, 5*(1), 27–34. https://doi.org/10.1177/089431849200500108

Roy, C., & Andrews, H. A. (1999). *The Roy adaptation model* (2nd ed.). Appleton & Lange.

Rubenfeld, M., & Scheffer, B. (2015). *Critical thinking TACTICS for nurses* (3rd ed.). Jones & Bartlett Learning.

Scheffer, B. K., & Rubenfeld, M. (2000). A consensus statement on critical thinking in nursing. *Journal of Nursing Education*, *39*(8), 352–359. https://doi.org/10.3928/0148-4834-20001101-06

Schon, D. A. (1987). *Educating the reflective practitioner: Toward a new design for teaching and learning in the professions*. Jossey-Bass.

Schuster, P. (2016). *Concept mapping: A critical-thinking approach to care planning* (4th ed.). F.A. Davis.

Shoulders, B., Follett, C., & Easonk, J. (2014). Enhancing critical thinking in clinical practice: Implications for critical and acute care nurses. *Dimensions of Critical Car Nursing*, *33*(4), 207–214. https://doi.org/10.1097/dcc.0000000000000053

Tanner, C. (2006). Thinking like a nurse: A research-based model of clinical judgment in nursing. *Journal of Nursing Education*, *45*(6), 204–211. https://doi.org/10.3928/01484834-20060601-04

Turkel, M. C. (2016). Describing self-reported assessments of critical thinking among practicing medical-surgical registered nurses. *MEDSURG Nursing*, *51*(4), 244–250. Retrieved March 27, 2021, from https://www.thefreelibrary.com/Describing+self-reported+assessments+of+critical+thinking+among...-a0461945694

Turkel, M. C., Ray, M. A., & Kornblatt, L. (2012). Instead of reconceptualizing the nursing process let's re-name it. *Nursing Science Quarterly*, *25*(2), 194–198. https://doi.org/10.1177/0894318412437946

Varcoe, C. (1996). Disparagement of the nursing process: The new dogma? *Journal of Advanced Nursing*, *23*(1), 120–125. https://doi.org/10.1111/j.1365-2648.1996.tb03144.x

Watson, J. M., & Glaser, E. M. (1990). *The Watson-Glaser critical thinking appraisal manual*. The Psychological Corp., Harcourt, Brace, Jovanovich, Inc.

Webber, P. (2008). Facilitating critical thinking and effective reasoning. In B. Penn (Ed.), *Mastering the teaching role: A guide for nurse educators*. F.A. Davis.

Young, C. E. (1987). Intuition and nursing process. *Holistic Nursing Practice*, *1*(3), 52–62. https://doi.org/10.1097/00004650-198705000-00010

Zanotti, R., & Chiffi, D. (2015). Diagnostic frameworks and nursing diagnoses: A normative stance. *Nursing Philosophy*, *16*(1), 64–73. https://doi.org/10.1111/nup.12074

Professional Practice in an Ever-Changing Health Care Context

Providing access to effective and high-quality health care for all people, delivering nursing care based on strong science and evidence, addressing specific cultural preferences and disparities when providing care, balancing accountability and quality of care in the era of cost containment, creating safe and healthy environments, and using technology effectively are challenges for today's professional nurses. In addition, spiraling health care costs have led to increased consumer discontent with the health care system, thus placing health care providers at risk for litigation. Current laws to improve health care access for Americans have created improved health care delivery for some while creating discontent in others. This section provides an overview of these challenges while reinforcing professional nursing's goal of doing what is best for clients.

PROFESSIONAL PRACTICE IN AN EVER-CHANGING HEALTH CARE CONTEXT

Health Care Delivery Systems

KEY TERMS AND CONCEPTS

Primary care
Secondary care
Tertiary care
National health service
  system
National health
  insurance system
Mandated health
  insurance system
Private free market
  system
Medicare
Medicaid

Children's Health
  Insurance Program
  (CHIP)
Prospective payment
Patient Protection and
  Affordable Care Act of
  2010
Interdisciplinary/
  interprofessional
  health care team
Nursing care delivery
  model

LEARNING OUTCOMES

By the end of this chapter, the learner will be able to:

1. Explain the differences among primary, secondary, and tertiary care.
2. Identify key concerns and pressures for all health care delivery systems based upon free enterprise, national health service, and national health insurance.
3. Specify the three major ways in which health care is financed.
4. Compare and contrast the American, Canadian, and Mexican health care systems.
5. Compare and contrast different settings for health care delivery.
6. Explain the roles of all members of the interprofessional health care team.
7. Identify the impact of changes in health systems on nurses.
8. Explore practical and ethical issues associated with health care delivery systems on professional nurses.

REAL-LIFE REFLECTIONS

Maria is a registered nurse employed by a hospital owned by a for-profit company. When Maria's father had hip replacement surgery, he received generic medication instead of his regular medicines during his hospital stay. He got quite upset because he was convinced that he was receiving the wrong medication. Two days after surgery, the case manager (CM) informed Maria's parents that her father would be transferred the next day to an extended-care facility for rehabilitation. Maria's parents became distraught because they had promised each other they would never put each other in a nursing home. Maria's parents bombarded her with questions about why her father did not receive the same medications that he took at home and why he had to leave the hospital before he was well enough to care for himself.

In recent years, health care delivery has undergone a radical transformation as a result of the explosion of scientific knowledge, technologic advances, emphasis on health promotion, resource limitations, and shortages of health care professionals (especially professional nurses, primary care physicians, licensed practical/vocational nurses, unlicensed care providers/personal care attendants, social workers, lab technologists and technicians. and radiation and imaging technologists) (United States Bureau of Labor Statistics [USBLS], 2020a, 2020b, 2020c, 2020d, 2020e, 2020f, 2020g). Health care delivery systems provide **primary care** for health promotion and illness prevention, **secondary care** for early detection of disease, and **tertiary care** for targeted services aimed at symptomatic diseases to prevent damage, progression, or complications of the disease and to restore the individual to optimal health. Tertiary care includes chronic disease management, acute care, and rehabilitation (Yarbrough Landry & Erwin, 2019). These changes affect access to health care for many people. This chapter explores current challenges for health care delivery, highlights certain countries that use different strategies to provide health care services, and outlines specific challenges for professional nurses in today's health care arena.

CHALLENGES OF HEALTH CARE DELIVERY IN THE 21ST CENTURY

All health care delivery systems in the world struggle to provide optimal services for the people they serve (Box 9.1, Professional Building Blocks, "Challenges for Today's Health Care Delivery Systems"). Access, cost, quality, and safety are the most prevalent issues today. Approaches to health care delivery vary across the globe because of differing values, beliefs, economic resources, histories, and politics.

Health Care Access

When the United Nations (UN) was chartered in 1945, its aim was to provide a global agency for international cooperation and collaboration. World health and the provision of health care services quickly emerged as key issues. The World Health Organization (WHO) was established as a UN unit with early efforts that included the eradication of infectious diseases and provision of health services for mothers and children (Jamieson & Sewall, 1954). In the middle of the 20th century, the WHO's focus broadened to include the provision of essential health services to all.

 9.1 Professional Building Blocks

Challenges for Today's Health Care Delivery Systems

- Ensuring access to care for all
- Operating within the confines of available health care resources
- Providing both preventive and curative services
- Attaining an effective system using governmental support and private resources
- Providing and maintaining a qualified, competent health care workforce
- Achieving a balance between health care needs and all other human needs
- Optimizing the use of technology for efficient care delivery while maintaining consumer privacy
- Providing coordinated health care delivery across inpatient, outpatient, home, and rehabilitation settings
- Coordinating public and private resources for optimal care delivery
- Responding to current and future epidemics and other potential public health threats
- Improving access to health insurance for those not covered by a national insurance plan
- Encouraging people to engage in healthy lifestyles and health promotion activities
- Improving public health systems
- Addressing inequality in health care access and outcomes
- Improving transparency and accountability in health care delivery
- Allowing consumer participation in the provision of health care services

From Kominski, G. (2014). *Changing the U.S. health care system* (4th ed.). Jossey-Bass; Elbel, E., Knickman, J. R., Yarbrough, A. Y., & Erwin, C. O. (2019). The challenge of health care delivery and health policy. In J. R. Knickman & B. Elbel (Eds.), *Jonas & Kovner's health care delivery in the United States* (12th ed.). Springer; Fried, B. J., & Gaydos, L. M. (2002). *World health systems: Challenges and perspectives.* Health Administration Press.

By the late 1970s, the need to change global health care delivery became apparent (Zakus & Cortinois, 2002). In 1978, WHO and the United Nations Children's Fund (UNICEF) issued a joint declaration that affirmed that health and health care were fundamental human rights and that social and economic development were keys to supporting health care initiatives. In 1981, the World Health Assembly expanded the initiatives to foster and coordinate social and economic efforts to promote the general health and welfare of all people (Zakus & Cortinois, 2002). WHO continues to monitor the progress of nations around the world with regard to the status of health care delivery and outcomes of health care services.

The 2010 *World Health Report* identified several leading sources of inefficiency in health care, including issues with medications (e.g., underuse of generics, use of substandard or counterfeit medications, inappropriate and ineffective use of medicines); overuse of health products, investigations, and procedures; inappropriate mix of and unmotivated health care workers; inappropriate use of health care services (such as overuse of emergency rooms and underutilization of primary care providers); and inefficiencies or inappropriate levels of health interventions (WHO, 2010). These persist along with poor data collection and reporting methods for most areas of health care, especially with regard to communicable diseases as made apparent during the COVID-19 pandemic (WHO, 2020b).

Despite international efforts to secure health care services for all, serious gaps persist. Wealthier nations tend to have fully developed health care systems, while many poorer countries lack basic infrastructures for health care delivery. The affluent can always access and receive health services because of their ability to purchase needed services. Typically, people living in rural areas in both developed and less developed nations have less access to health care services. According to the WHO (2020b), between 33% and 50% of individuals worldwide were unable to access essential health services in 2017 because of the inability to pay for them. Some could not access services because they were not available.

Countries differ in their approaches to health care access. Some nations aspire to a free enterprise, or business/market, approach that relies on an individual's ability to pay for health care services rendered. Other nations use government-sponsored programs, viewing health care as a basic human right that the government has the obligation to provide. Although access is guaranteed under this approach, health care may be delayed because of government funding shortfalls; this may occur in cases of high unemployment (decline in income tax revenue), reduced sales (or value-added) taxes, or reduced price of a government-controlled commodity (such as oil revenues in Nigeria [Lacey, 2002]). Whichever approach is used, funding is needed to provide the basic infrastructure and qualified health care professionals.

Health Care Funding

American culture values individualism, independence, innovation, and capitalism. In the United States, health care is a big business. Pharmaceutical and health care equipment vendors bombard the public with advertisements for the newest medications and therapies. Because American health care delivery has been based on a free enterprise system, some Americans believe that if the government were to control the system, the quality of and access to health care services might be compromised. In contrast, Canada and many European countries hold the belief that health care is the right of all citizens and fair access should be provided to all (Gusmano et al., 2019; Storch & Scaia, 2019).

The WHO (2019) reported that $7.8 trillion (6.6% of the global gross domestic product) was spent on health care services across the full spectrum of health care delivery including all three levels of care in 2018; over 50% of the revenue came from public sources ($4.7 trillion). Three different systems of funding health care expenditures include the national health service system, the national health insurance system, and the private free market system. Some countries use a combination of these three systems so that people with resources for health care have the freedom to use their own money to fund health care service and thus avoid delays in receiving them.

The National Health Service System

The **national health service system** guarantees access to health care services through a national health insurance plan, usually funded by general tax revenues. Sources of tax revenue include payroll, income, value-added, and corporate taxes. The citizens or government either own or control the factors for health care delivery and/or production of health care goods (Kominski, 2014). The national government contracts with insurance companies to reimburse health care providers directly. Under this system, citizens are free to purchase private health insurance. There are public hospitals available to all citizens and private hospitals available to citizens who can either pay privately for services or hold private health insurance policies. Using tax revenue enables greater health care resource distribution to the poor from the wealthy. The United Kingdom, Sweden, Norway, Finland, Spain, Portugal, Italy, Greece, and Australia are some nations that have a national health service system. In such a system, the national health service has an annual budget, and reimbursements to health care organizations are made by capitated fee schedules and pay-for-performance. Physicians and dentists work as private contractors and receive salaries (Gusmano et al., 2019; Storch & Scaia, 2019).

The National Health Insurance System

A **national health insurance system** provides universal health insurance coverage for all citizens financed primarily from general tax revenue. Tax revenue usually comes from payroll and income taxes, but Canada, for example, generates 25% of tax revenue devoted to health care from corporate taxation, and Canadian provinces and territories implement plan administration. Physicians receive reimbursement using a government-negotiated fee. Countries that use a national health insurance system include France, Japan, Russia, South Korea, and Canada. Health care services are reimbursed directly from the national insurance fund (Gusmano et al., 2019).

The Mandated Insurance System

The **mandated health insurance system** requires compulsory universal health care insurance for all citizens and sometimes all legal residents. Nonprofit insurance funds provide resources for individuals and employers to purchase health insurance (Knickman, 2019). Nations that have adopted this model include Germany, Israel, the Netherlands, and Switzerland. In Germany, for example, individuals who make €60,750 annually are required to purchase health insurance coverage. People who make less than this amount must contribute 14.5% of their annual income into a common public health insurance fund. German citizens with public health insurance carry a government-issued membership card. They present the card, pay a nominal fee when they receive health care services, and the insurance company pays the remaining balance (Visaguide. world, 2020).

The Universal Public Insurance System

Countries including Mexico, Austria, Argentina, Chile, and Turkey provide health insurance to citizens who cannot afford it. Most residents of these countries purchase health insurance plans privately, but coverage is not mandatory. For example, in Mexico, those who are employed are eligible to purchase government-funded health care insurance, and the government provides basic insurance plans for unemployed citizens. Those who can afford private health insurance purchase it since it provides access to the best health care available from private hospitals and clinics (Fried & Gaydos, 2002).

The Private Free Market System

The **private free market system** consists of voluntary health insurance coverage that relies on individuals purchasing health insurance. In this model, employment-based insurance is common. Employers provide group coverage, and employees pay part of the insurance premium (Reddy & Mythri, 2016). The United States, China, South Korea, Mexico, Nigeria, and India use this model (Fried & Gaydos, 2002).

With all the federal- and state-provided health insurance plans for older individuals, special groups, and those meeting strict income and asset guidelines, the United States practices a blend of the private free market and national health insurance systems. Citizens have the option to opt out of any of the government-provided plans, which include:

- **Medicare**, a federal program funded by income taxes that provides health care insurance for older and disabled Americans. Many older Americans also purchase private insurance known as "tie-in" plans to eliminate the gaps in Medicare coverage. Workers pay into the Medicare system during their employment years through required payroll tax deductions.
- **Medicaid**, which offers health care insurance coverage to people who qualify for federally supported, state-managed welfare programs. Individual states determine Medicaid eligibility requirements, but all states must provide coverage for families and children who receive federal aid.
- The **Children's Health Insurance Program (CHIP)**, which covers health care costs for children from low-income families who do not meet individual state guidelines to receive Medicaid.

Other tax-supported health care insurance programs cover public employees and their families, military personnel and their families, veterans, Native Americans, and Alaska Natives (Gusmano et al., 2019; Knickman, 2019). The U.S. Department of Veterans Affairs (VA) has a national network of inpatient and outpatient facilities to provide care to those who have served in the armed forces and sustained illness or injury directly related to their service as well as veterans who need routine health care.

■ QUESTIONS FOR REFLECTION

1. What experiences have you had with the different insurance models?
2. If you were designing an insurance model, what components would you incorporate and why? Would your model be feasible to implement? Why or why not?

Health Care Workforce

The WHO Global Health Observatory Data Repository documented a global shortage of health care professionals (WHO, 2020a, 2020c), including estimated critical shortages of 14 physicians and 40 nurses and midwives per every 10,000 individuals worldwide. The WHO defines a shortage as less than one clinical care provider per 1,000 citizens. The distribution of health care professionals is not equal among all nations, and some developed nations have more than an adequate supply. However, rural and less affluent localities may still have critical shortages even if their countries do not.

There is a shortage of registered nurses (RNs) in the United States. In 2019, there were slightly more than 3.096 million positions for RNs (excluding advanced practice nurses). By 2029, there will be slightly more than 300,000 new RN positions (USBLS, 2020f). American hospitals employ close to 60% of all working RNs; 18% of nurses work in outpatient settings such as physician offices or ambulatory care settings, another 7% work in long-term care facilities, and 6% have jobs in home health care or serve in government positions (USBLS, 2020f). Of working RNs, 59.2% work full-time (with 12% of these having more than one job) and 74.2% work more than 32 hours per week. Because of the projected growth in the older population, a shift to health promotion and disease prevention, and an increased number of persons with chronic conditions within the next decade, 7% additional professional nurses will be needed by 2029 (USBLS, 2020f). Even more may be needed because in 2017, the mean age of RNs was 51, and some of these nurses may want

to reduce their working hours or might opt for early retirement (National Council of State Boards of Nursing, 2018).

As a global phenomenon, the current nursing shortage differs from cyclical shortages of the past. Nursing has traditionally been considered "women's work." Since the women's rights movement, however, more career opportunities have become open to women, resulting in younger women pursuing more lucrative and respected careers. The WHO (2020c) reported that one in six nurses is over age 55 and expected to retire within the next decade. As these RNs retire, there are not enough entering the profession to replace them. The WHO (2020c) reported that the total nursing workforce consists of 27.9 million members with 19.3 million members identified as professional nurses. According to the WHO (2020c), 36 million more nurses will be needed by 2030 to meet worldwide nurse care needs. To achieve this goal, 8% more nurses must graduate from nursing education programs globally. Members of the nursing workforce include nursing associates (unlicensed assistive personnel [UAP]), licensed practical/vocational nurses, professional (registered) nurses, and advanced practice nurses.

Along with the U.S. nursing shortage, the need for American physicians is expected to grow; about 4% more physicians will be needed by 2029 (USBLS, 2020e). There are currently 752,400 practicing physicians in the United States; of these, about 22.5% practice primary care, with 15.8% engaged in general/family practice (USBLS, 2020e). Median salaries for American physicians are $213,270 for primary care compared to $615,156 for specialists and some surgeons (USBLS, 2020e). The lack of general/family practitioners and the increased need for primary care open the door for increased use of nurse practitioners (NPs) and physician assistants (PAs) for primary and specialty care services.

In most nations, well-equipped and well-staffed hospitals, when available, are located in larger urban areas. Rural areas have special challenges to overcome to attract qualified health care personnel. Some countries and states pay for the education of health care professionals and expect a tour of service in an underserved area for a designated time frame. Despite such incentive programs, health care professionals (including nurses) prefer to work in environments that offer them a voice in the decision-making processes, provide support for continued professional development, and pay a life-sustainable wage (International Council of Nurses [ICN], 2020).

Take Note!
The shortage of nursing professionals is a global phenomenon that is expected to worsen in the coming decades.

■ QUESTIONS FOR REFLECTION

1. Why do you think that there is a shortage of professional nurses and physicians?
2. What would you do to combat the national and global professional nurse shortage?
3. Do you think your plan would be feasible? Why or why not?

SELECT HEALTH CARE DELIVERY SYSTEMS

Health care delivery systems arose as people identified a need to care for the ill and injured. Societal beliefs about the nature of the world provided for early health delivery systems and guided their evolution. Because it is not feasible to cover all systems within a single chapter, select nations representing North America with different approaches to health care delivery are covered here.

The U.S. Health Care Delivery System

The health care delivery system in the United States was largely influenced by Europe because European immigrants quickly became the dominant cultural group in the United States. The evolution of the U.S. health care delivery system explains its emphasis on market competition and individualism.

The Roots of the U.S. Health Care Delivery System

In the United States in the late 18th and early 19th centuries, philanthropy and the government were the leading sources of health care funding. No organized health care programs existed because the predominant ethic of the time was that of self-sufficiency, and accepting charity was seen as a sign of grave weakness (Torrens, 1978). Thus, the seeds for the American value of independence were sown into its health care delivery system.

Most early hospitals in the United States were almshouses or pesthouses where the socially marginal members of society resided (Vogel, 1979). Because hospitals were supported by the philanthropy of the wealthy, class distinctions were considered to be justified. Hospital clients were stigmatized as dependent and somehow unworthy of society membership.

By 1873, the United States had 178 established hospitals (Jonas, 1998), and formal education in nursing began (Torrens, 1978). In the mid- to late 1800s, scientific discoveries also began to revolutionize health care. Anesthesia was introduced in 1847, and antisepsis became prevalent by 1865, leading to the need for centralized facilities to support expensive equipment for surgery. Germ theory became the accepted explanation for the transmission of infectious diseases, and the typhus vaccine became available in 1896. By 1860, the thermometer, ophthalmoscope, and laryngoscope were in use, joined by the gastroscope, cystoscope, hypodermic needle, and sphygmomanometer by 1883. X-rays were discovered in 1895. Hospitals improved hygiene measures. People went to hospitals for advanced diagnostic tests and treatment, and hospitals became places of healing rather than death (Jamieson & Sewall, 1954).

The Growth of the Health Care Industry and Insurance Systems

As urbanization increased, hospitals flourished. Hospital-owned schools of nursing provided an inexpensive source of nursing care. Hospitalized clients provided rich learning experiences for nursing and medical students. An apprenticeship approach dominated nursing and medical education. Medical education moved to university settings and developed independent prestige based on increased scientific knowledge, while nursing became associated with a medically dependent scope of practice with an apprenticeship type of education completely dominated by hospitals.

By the early 20th century, hospitals and physicians enjoyed high profits by providing services to wealthy clients who could afford them. However, "the poor and penniless, whom the institution had originally been meant to serve, became a liability" (Vogel, 1979, p. 115). A two-tier system of private and public institutions arose. Public institutions met the health care needs of the poor, while physician-dominated private hospitals met the needs of the affluent. As the nuclear family replaced the extended family, health care moved from being home-oriented and family-centered to institutionally centered. Health care became a stratified and localized system administered by municipalities (as in the British and French traditions).

In 1901, the American Medical Association (AMA) was restructured, and "doctors sought to assure their financial security and power through their own organization and reform of medical education" (Markowitz & Rosner, 1979, p. 186), thereby eliminating competition from other individuals becoming officially recognized as health care providers who could diagnose and treat illnesses and perform surgery. Private foundations supplied additional resources to the AMA, creating a central power source for medical practice and education. Efforts focused on replacing the haphazard art of medical practice with new science-based knowledge. As new treatments and technology developed, more hospitals were needed. By 1910, the number of hospitals in the United States had expanded to 4,400 (Jonas, 1998).

In 1910, concerned with the impact of illness on worker productivity, Montgomery Ward and Company provided group insurance to its employees for illness and injury. This plan is frequently regarded as the first group health insurance coverage in the United States. The Ladies Garment Workers Union provided the first union medical care services after a fatal fire that killed 146 women (Public Broadcasting Service [PBS], 2007). Between 1915 and 1920, 16 states introduced, debated, and rejected legislation mandating health insurance coverage for all (PBS, 2007). Accident and life insurance companies started offering insurance covering hospital services. In 1929, the first hospitalization insurance plan, Blue Cross, provided coverage for a group of teachers from Dallas, Texas (Scofera, 1994).

The global influenza epidemic of 1918 and pneumonia killed more soldiers than combat did. Because of contagious disease fatalities, public health efforts focused on containing and preventing infectious diseases. During this pandemic, individuals and families relied on their own personal resources to fund health care. Hospital overcrowding forced families to assume responsibility for nursing care at home, and physicians made home visits (Jamieson & Sewall, 1954). Physicians made home visits to monitor the progress of the infirmed and to prepare families for impending death.

The Great Depression of the 1930s devastated the developing American health care system. Without employment, many could not feed or clothe their families, much less think about paying for health care services if needed. Increasingly, the government assumed responsibility for providing and funding health care services, and illness prevention and health promotion became top priorities for government-sponsored health programs (Jonas, 1998). In 1935, the Social Security Act included provisions for financially supporting the people living in poverty and the infirmed older population, carving out for the first time a role for the federal government in providing health care services (PBS, 2007). In 1939, a Blue Shield plan for medical and surgical expenses was sponsored by the California Medical Society.

Prior to World War II, less than 20% of Americans had any form of health care insurance (Scofera, 1994). During World War II, the War Labor Board froze wages to divert resources to the war effort. To appease unions and workers, employers added health insurance to fringe benefit packages (PBS, 2007). To assume responsibility for war-related injuries (physical or psychological), the federal government established the VA program (Jamieson & Sewall, 1954). The VA health care system still offers extensive rehabilitation programs and health care services to all veterans.

Following World War II, workers came to expect reasonable wages and hospitalization insurance. In response to problems arising in the growing health insurance industry, the McCarran–Ferguson Act was enacted to provide state regulation of all forms of insurance (PBS, 2007). By 1951, 100 million Americans had some form of health care insurance coverage (Scofera, 1994), enabling many people to reap the benefits of newly developed medications and surgical interventions. Because of the technical skills required to administer new therapies, hospitals expanded and became places where people got well.

Health Care in the Mid- to Late 20th Century

Health care changed dramatically in the mid- to late 20th century. Increased scientific knowledge resulted in an information explosion that led to the era of specialization for health care delivery, resulting in fragmentation and increased cost (Jonas, 1998; Knickman, 2019). Deaths from infectious diseases lessened and the need for treatment for chronic diseases became more prevalent along with complex regimens to control chronic illness.

"The percentage of Americans covered by some form of health insurance rose from less than 20% prior to WWII to more than 70% by the early 1960s" (Torrens, 1978, p. 13). The increased demand for health care resulted in the passage of the Hill–Burton Act in 1946 stimulated hospital construction. The U.S. Department of Health, Education, and Welfare (now the U.S. Department of Health and Human Services) was formed in 1953 to provide a mechanism to coordinate health research and service programs. The Civil Rights Movement espoused the belief that equal health care is a basic right and encouraged the government to became more involved in health care. In 1965, Congress amended the Social Security Act to create the Medicare and Medicaid programs, thereby creating another role for the federal government in health care delivery for older individuals and those living in poverty (Jonas, 1998; Knickman, 2019).

By 1960, 120 million Americans were covered by some form of health insurance (Scofera, 1994). While the 1960s emphasized equity and cohesion of services, the 1970s concentrated on access, with tremendous growth in the number of hospitals, ancillary services, and sophisticated technology available. The emphasis on research and technology led to specialization and depersonalization, as well as rapidly escalating expenses (Jonas, 1998; Knickman, 2019). Health care expenditures went essentially unmonitored. Increased demand for services led to more hospitals, extended-care facilities, and health-related research facilities.

By the late 1970s, spiraling health care costs became impossible to ignore. The federal government established new regulations to monitor delivered services along with reductions in federal funding. The changes rewarded efficiency over equity, quality, and access. Prospective payment reimbursement of hospital expenses for Medicare clients was introduced in 1981 in an effort to reduce hospital costs. **Prospective payment** established prearranged reimbursement amounts (by diagnostic category known as diagnosis-related groups [DRGs]) that the federal government paid hospitals for care given to Medicare recipients. The hospital received a prearranged amount, regardless of accrued costs.

Under the prospective payment system, big profits could be made, resulting in a business approach to health care. Detailed documentation of medical services provided and supplies used became crucial as insurance providers looked for reasons to deny reimbursement. For-profit insurance companies and hospital chains grew. Not-for-profit hospitals invested increased profits back into expanding and improving hospital services for the community, thereby increasing consumer access to sophisticated health care. However, by the late 1980s, the federal government progressively reduced the amount of reimbursement for specific DRGs, adding financial pressure to struggling smaller (and usually rural) hospitals.

Managed care plans started in the 1970s and flourished as health care costs continued to rise. Enrollment in managed care plans rose from 2 million people in 1970 to more than 39 million people in 1992. Managed care proponents believed these plans could reduce health care costs by promoting health (Kominski, 2014; Scofera, 1994). Three models of managed care emerged: health maintenance organizations (HMOs), preferred provider organizations (PPOs), and point-of-service (POS). Table 9.1 highlights the differences among these structures.

In the economic downslide of the 1980s, many people lost their jobs and consequently their health care coverage. In 1985, the Consolidated Omnibus Budget Reconciliation Act (COBRA) was enacted. It requires that employers with more than 20 workers partially subsidize the health insurance coverage offered to former employees (and their dependents) for 18 months after termination of employment. Because of the high costs associated with COBRA, however, many of these unemployed individuals could not afford to continue health care coverage anyway (Knickman, 2019; Kominski, 2014).

Health care expenditures rose at close to twice the rate of inflation between 1990 and 1995. Between 1995 and 2000, health care costs rose on average by 3.4%. At the same time, inflation rose 2.5%. In response to increasing health care costs, President Bill Clinton's administration tried unsuccessfully to enact health care reform legislation in the early 1990s. Since 2003, expenditures for health care in the United States continue to outpace the rate of inflation and consumed $2.5 trillion (combined public and private funds) in 2009 (Centers for Medicare & Medicaid Services, 2011). The Centers for Medicare & Medicaid Services (2020) predicts that by 2028, health care expenditures will account for 19.7% of the gross national product.

Multiple efforts to contain health care costs in the late 20th century included reductions in prospective payments, consolidation of health care services, and hospital closures. Hospital costs fell because of reduced lengths of inpatient stays. Only those who were medically unstable remained hospitalized. Once stabilized, people were expected to leave the hospital. Medicare and insurance companies provided coverage for rehabilitation in extended-care facilities if clients were too weak to return home safely. When possible, family members would provide care to relatives at home. Insurance companies also shifted the burden of rising health care costs to consumers by increasing premiums, copayments, and deductibles (Kominski, 2014).

Increased competition as a cost-containment mechanism provided an opportunity for NPs to expand their provision of primary and secondary health care services despite opposition by many physicians.

Health Care Costs in the United States Today

The free market approach dominated the health care industry in the United States in the 20th century and continues to do so today (Knickman & Elbel, 2019). Many health care leaders debate the benefits of a market-driven health care system that is based on the

TABLE 9.1 Differences in Managed Care Models

Health Maintenance Organization (HMO)	Preferred Provider Organization (PPO)	Point-of-Service (POS) Plan
Group-model HMOs contract directly with a single medical group to care for members. Staff model HMOs contract with individual physicians to serve members. Network HMOs contract with a network of physicians to provide services for members.	A network of preferred health care providers contained within an insurance plan agree to follow the insurance company's utilization guidelines and accept deeply discounted fees for provided services	A network of preferred providers who contract to provide services for a managed care company and follow guidelines set by the insurance carrier while accepting discounted fees for rendered services
Open-panel HMOs permit physicians to treat non-HMO members. Closed-panel HMOs require physicians under contract to see members only.	Members can access physicians not on the list of preferred providers, but they have substantially higher copayments for services.	Members select their level of managed care services: Use of a primary care provider gatekeeper for specialist referrals Self-referral to specialists within the provider network Self-referral to specialist of choice
Cheapest of all forms for consumer because of limitations in covered services	Costs for copayments higher than those for HMOs	Graduated copayments with members using a gatekeeper having the lowest out-of-pocket expenses and members with the ability to self-refer to their specialist of choice having the highest copayment
Members must receive authorization for care from a specialist, usually a primary care physician.	Members can self-refer for specialist services.	Members can self-refer for specialist services but will have a higher copayment for services than if they would have had a referral from a primary care provider.
In the 1990s, some HMOs offered self-referral to specialists, but members had higher copays.	There are higher copays for members seeing specialists if they see a specialist within the preferred providers list, and if a specialist is not listed as a preferred provider, copayments are even higher	Lower copayments if members see a specialist within the preferred provider list, and if they see a specialist not in the approved provider listing, they may be 100% responsible for all costs.

Adapted from Kominski, G. (2014). *Changing the U.S. health care system* (4th ed.). Wiley.

premise that competition controls the costs of health care delivery. These changes have resulted in a highly complex, multifaceted health care delivery system in the 21st century, leading to a cost of 17.7% of the U.S. gross domestic product going toward health care (Centers for Medicare & Medicaid Services, 2020).

According to the Centers for Medicare & Medicaid Services, health care expenditures fall into the following categories: health-related research, facility construction, and payment for personal health care services and supplies. Costs for individual health care services and supplies supersede those of new construction or research, with hospital costs comprising the greatest single health care expense (Slavitt & Burwell, 2016). In 2018, private health insurers spent over $1.2 trillion covering their enrollees. Hospital costs in the same year were $1.2 trillion. Consumers spent $375.6 billion of their own money. Physician and clinical services

accounted for $725.6 billion, and prescription medications costs totaled $335 billion (Centers for Medicare & Medicaid Services, 2020).

Provider Costs

The late 20th century saw an explosion of technology and scientific advances. Today, American hospital costs surpass those of all developed nations. The amount of money charged for an acute care hospital patient day in the United States is more than twice that of Canada and three times higher than that of most other developed countries. Hospitalized Americans undergo more sophisticated diagnostic procedures and intensive medical regimens. The increased use of highly technical equipment and expensive medications fuels these rising costs. Because of the litigious nature of the American culture, the ever-present threat of malpractice suits adds to the costs as well (Knickman, 2019).

Physician income in the United States is on average one and a half to three times higher than that of physicians in other developed countries. The United States tends to have a surplus of specialist physicians because they earn substantially more than general practice physicians (Knickman, 2019).

Advanced practice RNs (APRNs) offer an alternative to the high costs of physician services. Despite resistance by organized medicine, in 1996 all states allowed third-party reimbursement to APRNs (Spetz & Chapman, 2019). In 2021, 24 states and the District of Columbia grant full practice authority for APRNs. The remaining states have restrictions on APRN practice (American Association of Nurse Practitioners, 2021). Services rendered by APRNs cost substantially less, and consumers report high satisfaction.

Insurance

The rate of uninsured Americans tends to fluctuate with the unemployment rate. Keisler-Starkey and Bunch (2020) reported that prior to the COVID-19 pandemic, 26.1% of Americans did not have health insurance. This is a marked improvement from 48.6 million Americans without health insurance in 2011 (DeNavas-Walt et al., 2012). The Kaiser Family Foundation roughly estimated that 2 to 3 million Americans lost employer-based health care coverage when they lost jobs during the COVID-19 pandemic as a direct result of 6.2% of Americans losing jobs. Medicaid enrollment increased by 4.3 million enrollees from February to July of 2020 (McDermott et al., 2020). In 2019, employer-based health insurance accounted for 55.4% of all health insurance policies. The annual average employee cost for health insurance for individual adult policies was $1,224 and for family policies $6,015. Employers paid an average of $5,946 for individual coverage and $14,561 for family coverage. This represented a 4% increase for individual and 5% increase for families in health insurance premiums within a single year. One in four workers could not afford to purchase employer-offered insurance (Kaiser Family Foundation, 2019).

Corporations represent the largest purchasers of private health insurance. To contain costs, companies have

- limited consumer choice of providers through HMOs or PPOs
- increased premiums, deductibles, and out-of-pocket charges
- required authorization for hospitalizations and second opinions

- substituted ambulatory and home care to reduce hospital stays
- encouraged reduced use of services

In 2018, 27.5 million Americans (8.5%) were lacking health insurance. This was up from 25.6 million (7.9%) in 2017. Uninsured rates differ among demographic groups with 6% of White Americans uninsured, 10% of Black Americans uninsured, and 18% of Hispanic Americans uninsured (Krisberg, 2019).

Patient Protection and Affordable Care Act of 2010

To address escalating health care costs, increased numbers of uninsured Americans as a result of increased unemployment, and the inability of many American workers to purchase expensive private and employer-based health insurance plans, President Barack Obama signed the **Patient Protection and Affordable Care Act of 2010** into law. Under the ACA, federal and state governments assume a larger role in providing health insurance to all Americans.

Some of the major key provision of the ACA include expanded access to health insurance; employers with more than 50 employee required to offer health insurance to workers, insurance premium, and cost-sharing subsidies to qualified individuals; increased taxes to fund health care; creation of health insurance exchanges; cost containment strategies (administrative simplification, bundled payments, increase use of generic medications, and more); incorporation of rewards for persons using wellness and disease prevention strategies, and improved health care quality.

The ACA sets new requirements on individuals and employers; requires insurance plans to include coverage for periodic screenings for diseases; eliminates the barrier of no coverage for preexisting conditions; removes lifetime coverage limits; and offers health promotion strategies. The provisions were to be fully implemented by January 2018, but this did not occur because of federal-level changes in the composition of Congress (Kaiser Family Foundation, 2017). However, federal rules and regulations identified the following essential health care services: ambulatory; emergency; maternity and newborn care; mental health services including substance use and behavioral disorder care (including treatment of behavioral health issues); devices and services for rehabilitation and activities of daily living; lab tests; prevention and wellness care (with no costs to clients); and pediatric care (medical, dental, and visual services) (Healthcare.gov, 2020). With the results of the 2020 election, the provisions of the ACA are expected to be fully implemented.

Other provisions of the ACA include creation of the federal insurance marketplace for individuals without employer coverage. The ACA also requires some restaurants to post caloric counts of menu items and compels employers to provide private spaces for nursing mothers to nurse or pump when lactating in the workplace. In addition, 38 states have expanded Medicaid services and rely on the federal subsidy to fund their programs (Goldstein, 2020).

However, a series of court challenges resulted in the delay of the full implementation of the ACA. The Supreme Court heard the case on November 10, 2020, and ruled to keep most of the provisions of the ACA in place but to eliminate the requirement for every American to purchase health care insurance coverage. At the time of publication, the formal written final ruling was being drafted for later release (U.S. Supreme Court, 2020).

The ACA has some new programs and renames others. Changes include:

- Bundled payment: A new approach to reimbursement for treatment received from a hospital or physician for a fixed amount for episodic care received over time if a person has a chronic condition (Knickman, 2019)
- Medical home: A medical practice directed by a physician that consists of a provider team with which a client has an ongoing relationship; a personal physician coordinates care (Knickman, 2019).
- Accountable Health Care Organization (AHCAO): A group of health care providers (nonprofit or for-profit) across the continuum of care that have legal agreements with each other and have aligned their incentives to provide and promote quality care while containing costs; an AHCAO may be an HMO, a PPO, or an integrated health care system (IHCS) that contracts with external insurance providers or self-insurers (Knickman, 2019).
- Insurance exchange: A marketplace administered through a government agency or nonprofit organization that consumers can use to compare health insurance plans, choose a desired plan, and purchase health insurance (Knickman & Elbel, 2019)
- Comparative effectiveness research: Studies comparing the outcomes of two or more health care technologies, services, or products (including medications) either against each other or with conventional treatment to compare their costs relative to benefits (Knickman, 2019)

Implementation of the ACA has resulted in both positive and negative outcomes for Americans. Benefits vary by state of residency, type of community (e.g., urban, rural), and annual income. Some health care organizations have reaped benefits, while others have experienced financial difficulty because of the increased complexities associated with administrative costs (Geyman, 2015; Krisberg, 2019). In addition, some small businesses have had to close because of requirements to provide health insurance coverage to employees. Within the first 5 years, costs have increased substantially for prescription medication use, administrative costs for organizations providing health care, and federal administration of required programs for law implementation (Geyman, 2015).

Health care access delivery and funding often emerge as key issues in American elections. A little over a month prior to the 2020 presidential election, President Trump signed an executive order outlining his "America-first" health care plan. The purpose was to bring quality health care to Americans, placing clients first. Included in the executive order were the following provisions:

1. Providing better and lower-priced health care, ensuring Americans with preexisting conditions could find affordable policies on the types of policies they desired
2. Giving Americans more choice in where they receive health care by expanding access and options for affordable health care
3. Lowering health care costs by approving more generic and bio-similar medications and assuring safe importation of low-cost medications from abroad
4. Ensuring consumers have meaningful price and quality data to make informed choices before receiving health care services
5. Improving the VA health care system and finding novel and improved treatments for COVID-19, Alzheimer disease, sickle cell disease, pediatric cancer, and all other health conditions that threaten the well-being of American citizens (Trump, 2020)

The order was signed without any specific information about how funding for each provision would be secured. The provision of this order may provide a foundation for any future health care legislation. However, within his first month in office, President Biden signed executive orders on January 28, 2021, Executive Order 14009 to strengthen Medicaid and the Affordable Care Act (Federal Register, 2021).

Canada's Health Care Delivery System

Like the United States, Canada enjoys significant wealth. The countries share a similar history, but different events have resulted in Canada adopting a different form of health care delivery.

Historical Development of Canada's Health Care System

The French established some of the earliest colonies in Canada. In May 1639, Madame de la Peltrie, along with Augustinian and Ursuline sisters, established a trading post infirmary. The Augustinian sisters established the Hôtel Dieu in Québec City, Québec, in 1639, where they dispensed medications and offered cheerful encouragement to ill individuals who preferred to stay at home. In 1645, Jeanne Mance established the Hôtel Dieu in Montreal as a hospital for wounded French and British soldiers during the Seven Years' War. In 1693, the Jesuits built another hospital in Canada using the support of the wealthy Duchesse d'Aiguillon, who obtained land and permission to establish a hospital (Jamieson & Sewall, 1954).

The Canadian Fathers of Confederation laid out terms of the British North America Act of 1867 that specified responsibilities of the Canadian government, which included taking a census, collecting vital statistics, determining quarantine regulations, providing hospitals for people in quarantine, and caring for Canadian natives. Along with these basic responsibilities, a section of the act provided for the establishment of provincial hospitals, asylums, and charities (Goldsmith, 2002; Storch & Scaia, 2019).

In the 20th century, as in the United States, rising health care costs became an issue in Canada, resulting in federal efforts to provide coverage for health expenditures for everyone. In 1947, the Province of Saskatchewan enacted the Hospital Insurance Act, which provided hospital insurance for all its residents. At the same time, the Canadian government offered grants to the provinces and public health agencies for hospital construction and provision of health care services. In the 1960s, Saskatchewan expanded insurance coverage to include outpatient health care, and by 1968, the Medical Care Act was enacted, providing national health insurance for all Canadians (Goldsmith, 2002; Storch & Scaia, 2019).

In the 1980s, paralleling the trend in the United States, Canada also experienced problems with skyrocketing health care costs and limited public funding.

In response, the Canada Health Care Act of 1984 resulted in provincial administration of health care programs.

All Canadians have equal access to a specific list of health care services under provincial policy plans. Additional costs cannot be incurred by citizens for services covered by these plans. Finally, the Canadian plan is portable and covers citizens if they move from province to province or travel abroad. However, nonemergency and out-of-province services require preauthorization (Storch & Scaia, 2019).

Principles of the Canadian Health Care System

Health care in Canada is directed by five key principles:

1. A public, nonprofit authority administers provincial health insurance plans and answers to the provincial government.
2. Each insurance plan covers all eligible residents using uniform terms and conditions.
3. Canadians have health insurance coverage when they travel abroad or across provinces. However, the plans have limited out-of-country coverage and provincial plan approval is required for nonemergency services when receiving care out of the province in which a citizen resides.
4. Each plan covers "all medically necessary services" citizens may need from physicians and hospitals.
5. The plans provide reasonable access to health services without discrimination. Provincial plans may require premiums from citizens, but care cannot be denied based on inability to pay for coverage (Goldsmith, 2002; Gusmano et al., 2019).

Funds for the Canadian health care system come from taxes (primarily payroll and corporate), health insurance premiums, and consumer out-of-pocket expenses. Tax credits offer relief for high out-of-pocket health care expenditures. National health insurance accounts for payment of about 70% of all health-related costs. Services not covered by government plans include vision and dental care; outpatient prescription medications; rehabilitative services; chiropractic care; private hospital rooms; and some complementary care services. The national health insurance system covers only Canadian citizens. Approximately 67% of Canadians opt to purchase private health care insurance policies. Most of the insurance companies in Canada are for-profit corporations. Employer-based plans make up 90% of private insurance, and 30%

of all health expenditures in Canada are reimbursed through private health insurance companies. (Allin et al., 2020).

Because of complaints about accessing required health care in a timely fashion, the provincial premiers agreed to the Health Renewal Accord in 2003. Principles outlined by the accord include nonstop access to a health care provider; timely access to diagnostic and treatment procedures; elimination of the need to repeat health histories or diagnostic tests for each provider seen; and access to home and community health care. Although the Canadian health care system is generally perceived as efficient, it responds slowly in addressing necessary reforms. Increased collaboration among the federal and provincial governments and the sharing of best practices based on solid evidence have resulted in improvement of Canadian health care outcomes (Storch & Scaia, 2019).

Mexico's Health Care Delivery System

Mexico has less wealth than Canada and the United States. Rapid industrialization with increasing environmental pollution, along with increasing tobacco and alcohol use, poor diet, sedentary lifestyles, and infectious diseases in crowded urban areas pose challenges to the health of Mexicans.

Not all Mexicans have equal access to health care services. Affluent citizens purchase private health insurance plans and have access to quality of care and services similar to that of Canadians and Americans. Workers are covered through a social security system or purchase employment-based health insurance, and the poor citizens rely on a public services system. The Ministry of Health manages health promotion and disease prevention for Mexican citizens. It also monitors and tests medications made by and sold in Mexico for quality, safety, and efficacy (Johnson et al., 2002).

The Mexican health care system consists of hospitals, outpatient facilities, and long-term care facilities. Modern medical centers are located in urban areas. Health care facilities in rural areas are often understaffed and rely on medical students as providers. In recent years, health care delivery to Mexicans covered by public services has become decentralized, and emphasis has been placed on a healthy municipalities program. Shifting the emphasis to health promotion rather than disease treatment for public health services has increased access to health care services for poorer populations (Johnson et al., 2002).

Comparing and Contrasting These Care Delivery Systems

Access to clean water sources, effective sanitation, and adequate food supply separate health care needs of developed and less developed nations. In developing nations, malnutrition, infant and child mortality, and communicable diseases are often major health concerns. In wealthy, developed nations, "diseases of affluence" (e.g., obesity, diabetes mellitus, degenerative joint disease) emerge as major health concerns.

National wealth also dictates the funding available to build and maintain health care facilities, along with providing the facilities with adequate human and material resources. Wealthy people have resources to spend on health care services even if they live in undeveloped countries. Conversely, not all citizens of a wealthy nation have resources to access and receive required health care services.

According to Tikkanen and Abrams (2020), the United States spent 16.9% of its gross domestic product on health care in 2019, significantly more than either Canada (11.8%) (Matej, 2019) or Mexico (5.48%) (Rios, 2020). Governmental support comes from local and state taxes. Of these three countries, the Canadian government pays the largest share of the health care bill at almost 72% (Matej, 2019) followed by the Mexican government at almost 49% (Rios, 2020). Combined government support for American health care expenditures is close to 45% (28.3% federal funding, 16.5% state and local funding) (Centers for Medicare & Medicaid Services, 2020). The United States spends $10,586 per person on health care compared to Canadian expenditures of $4,974 (McCarthy, 2019). Mexico spends approximately $1,140 annually per person on health care (Rios, 2020). Nations with a history of British or communist influences tend to approach health care delivery as a state rather than as a personal responsibility.

The number of health care professionals employed also varies according to the development and financial status of a country. The United States reported the highest concentration of physicians, pharmacists, and managerial and support staff (WHO, 2020a). Multiple layers of management and the prevalent use of complex medical therapies increase the cost of American health care delivery. The availability of nurses and midwives also varies among North American countries. The United States has the highest concentration of nurses and midwives at 145.48 nurses/midwives per 10,000 people; Canada has 97.48 per 10,000 people;

and Mexico has close to 24 nurse/midwives per 10,000 people (WHO, 2020d). The number of physicians per 10,000 people is similar, with the United States at 26.12 medical doctors, Canada at 23.11, and Mexico at 23.83 (WHO, 2020c). Although the United States and Canada offer similar health care services, albeit with different sources of funding, citizens of both nations tend to be satisfied with the services they receive.

■ QUESTIONS FOR REFLECTION

1. Think about your current health care insurance plan and coverage. How do you think coverage may change based on your reading of changes required by the ACA? What do you think would happen if the ACA was struck down entirely? What do you think might occur if only specific provisions are ruled unconstitutional by the Supreme Court?
2. What current disparities in health care access exist in your community? Outline some suggestions for ways to improve health care access in your community. Analyze each of your suggestions for feasibility. What actions would you need to take to implement one or more of your suggestions?

HEALTH CARE DELIVERY SETTINGS

In the United States, health care services can be obtained in a variety of settings (Table 9.2). Organizations offering health care services differ according to mission and philosophy. Although they all exist to offer health care services, some organizations may be proprietary (privately funded and for-profit) and governmental (publicly funded and not-for-profit), while others are

voluntary (privately funded and not-for-profit) (Jonas, 1998). For-profit organizations tend to emphasize providing services while achieving a high profit margin.

To mitigate the high costs associated with hospital-based care, individuals are able to access alternative ambulatory care systems, including diagnostic, urgent care, surgery, birthing, substance abuse, and rehabilitation centers. Health care consumers can also receive health care services in outpatient clinics and urgent care centers located in shopping malls or pharmacies. Some clinics may be affiliated with an integrated health care delivery system or hospital. Annual influenza vaccinations are now routinely made available at retail and grocery stores, pharmacies, and/or places of employment. In addition, home health agencies and hospice services provide in-home nursing care. Recognizing the need to offer more outpatient services, some hospitals have built plush outpatient centers complete with food courts and small shops. To promote health within the community, hospitals hold classes on health promotion topics, such as smoking cessation, weight reduction, safety, physical exercise, and basic lifestyle changes.

Primary Care Options and Prehospital Care

People who seek modern medical care typically consult physicians. Physicians tend to practice in either individual practice associations (IPAs) or PPOs. IPAs consist of a group of physicians who independently negotiate for set fee schedules with hospitals and insurance providers. Physicians employed in an IPA enjoy freedom to practice medicine as they desire; in contrast, physicians who work in PPOs must follow

TABLE 9.2   Settings for Health Care Delivery

Setting	Definition
Public hospital 1. Federal hospital 2. State/local hospital	Nonprofit, government-owned institution that provides inpatient care 1. Owned and operated by the U.S. government 2. Owned and operated by a state or local government
Community hospital	Locally owned institution that offers short-term services that are accessible to the public
Specialized hospital	Institution that offers services in one specialty area of health care (e.g., oncology, mental health, orthopedics, maternal–child health, children's services)
Acute care hospital	Institution that offers a full scope of short-term services, including obstetric care
Teaching hospital	Institution that provides medical education to undergraduate or graduate medical students, residents, or postgraduate medical fellows
Extended-care facility	Institution that offers long-term care, also known as nursing home (75% owned by for-profit companies)

Setting	Definition
Long-term care home	Small group home that provides a homelike setting for people with chronic mental illness or dementia
Rehabilitation center	Institution that offers services to help physically dependent individuals become independent
Chemical dependence center	Institution that offers detoxification and rehabilitation for individuals with drug or alcohol addiction
Neighborhood health center	Outpatient facility offering comprehensive primary care health services
Retail store–based health clinic	Clinic designed for episodic care of frequently occurring illnesses staffed by nurse practitioner; care recipient frequently able to purchase treatment for the illness in the store where the clinic is located
Private physician office	Comprehensive ambulatory client medical care provided by a single physician
Physician partnership office	Comprehensive ambulatory medical care provided by a pair of physicians
Group physician office practice	Comprehensive ambulatory medical care services provided by a group of three or more physicians
Managed care clinic	Comprehensive ambulatory medical care provided within the confines of an office or clinic operated by a managed care company
Public health clinic	State-, county-, or city-funded health service that focuses primarily on preventing or controlling communicable diseases
Community health center	Neighborhood center that offers integrated primary care, education, and social services using a community-oriented, culturally sensitive approach; receives federal financial support
Ambulatory surgery center	Outpatient center where minor surgical procedures are performed
Specialty care center	Outpatient office or center that offers full scope of ambulatory care services to people with specific health problems (e.g., renal failure, cancer, diabetes, pain); may have for-profit status
Emergency department	Outpatient facility linked to a hospital where life-threatening health problems can be managed; some emergency facilities have designated trauma center certification. Frequently used by people to receive health care after office or clinic hours
Urgent care center	Outpatient facility (may be linked to a hospital) where people receive medical care services for health-related problems when clinics or offices are closed or when the person does not have an established health care provider. These usually have for-profit status. Some emergency rooms may dedicate a specific location to provide urgent care for non–life-threatening health problems.
Hospital-based clinic	Outpatient comprehensive medical care service linked with a specific hospital. Many teaching hospitals hold resident clinics to provide health care to low-income individuals.
Hospital outpatient department	Ambulatory diagnostic testing or rehabilitation service that has connections to a specific hospital
Diagnostic testing center	Ambulatory diagnostic testing service; some have connections to nonprofit hospitals, and others are run by for-profit companies.
Industrial health service unit	Employment-based health service to address job-related illnesses and injuries; some units provide health promotion activities and health screenings for employees.
School health clinic	Health care service offered to students in academic settings (e.g., health rooms in primary or secondary schools or university health clinics)
Home health care	Medical care and nursing services offered for people who are homebound
Hospice	Comprehensive service to assist persons in receiving a "good" death; services may be given in the home, hospice facilities, extended-care facilities, or acute care hospitals

From Jonas, S. (1998). *An introduction to the U.S. health care system* (4th ed.). Springer Publishing; Knickman, J. R., & Elebel, B. (Eds.). (2019). *Jonas & Kovner's health care delivery in the United States* (12th ed.). Springer; McGinn, D., & Springen, K. (2007). Express-lane medicine. *Newsweek, 150*(5), 44; Sardell, A. (2012). Community health centers: Successful advocacy for expanding health care access. In D. Mason, J. Leavitt, & M. Chaffee (Eds.), *Policy & politics in nursing and health care* (6th ed.). Elsevier Saunders.

specific fee payment schedules and clinical utilization guidelines determined by the PPO. Integrated health care delivery systems employ physicians, and some may even own group practices.

HMOs were designed to focus efforts and resources on health promotion, preventive care, and consumer education to reduce health care costs. HMOs provide capitated payments (a set amount of money) for each member rather than paying only for rendered services. The traditional group or staff model HMO is a vertically integrated organization that operates its own physical facilities in various geographical locations and whose salaried physicians work solely for the HMO. A physician group may also contract services to an HMO. To increase practice revenues, some HMOs include NPs and PAs. The practice gets to keep surplus payments when care is delivered below the capitated payment (Knickman, 2019).

Freestanding urgent care locations and health clinics in retail establishments continue to increase. NPs provide health care services in clinics located in drug, grocery, and discount chain stores. NPs treat common illnesses that can be diagnosed with simple tests (e.g., strep throat, urinary tract and ear infections) following standardized care regimens. In 2005, only a handful of convenience clinics existed. In 2019, over 2,000 retail health care clinics and between 7,400 and 8,000 urgent care centers were seeing health care consumers (Mukamel et al., 2019). Consumers appreciate the convenience of securing a diagnosis and treatment in one location as well as reduced costs of securing a diagnosis and receiving treatment (Mukamel et al., 2019). Many consumers opt to receive routine vaccinations at public health departments or immunization clinics held in faith-based facilities, retail establishments, and/or shopping centers. Most insurance companies pay for routine immunizations. For immunizations not covered, local public health departments may waive fees for local residents who are unable to pay for services or if local taxes cover immunizations. Sometimes fees may be reduced if the health department has a fee schedule based on resident incomes.

The Hospital Industry

Hospitals provide acute inpatient and outpatient services. Inpatients often undergo expensive (and frequently invasive) procedures for diagnosis and treatment. Highly technical equipment and qualified nurses monitor clients to detect abnormal conditions, progress of ordered treatments, and potential complications associated with diagnostic procedures and therapies. The hospital industry employs more than 50% of RNs. Although hospital occupancy rates have been decreasing, the severity of illness of clients who are admitted to hospitals has been increasing (Knickman, 2019).

Hospitals vary in size and scope of service. Large medical centers may have hundreds or thousands of inpatient beds, while small community hospitals may have fewer than 50 beds. Hospitals may be owned by for-profit corporations, nonprofit organizations, or the government (e.g., state, military, VA). Some hospitals are part of larger integrated health care delivery systems. Along with providing inpatient care, hospitals offer emergency services for people who sustain traumatic injuries or become seriously ill. Sometimes people without health insurance or a primary care provider use emergency rooms for routine health care needs that arise. Inappropriate use of emergency rooms increases the cost of health care delivery (Knickman, 2019).

Some hospitals also offer outpatient services such as surgery and specialized diagnostic testing. Hospitals may specialize in a single service, such as cancer care, orthopedic surgery, burn care, pediatrics, or rehabilitation. Acute care hospitals provide services to people who have episodic health care needs. Quaternary care facilities are acute care hospitals that offer highly specialized, complex medical and surgical care such as advanced trauma care and organ transplantation. These services are most commonly located in academic medical centers. Subacute care hospitals care for clients who no longer need the intensity of care provided by acute care hospitals but have complex medical needs above the services offered by extended-care or rehabilitation facilities (Yarbrough Landry & Erwin, 2019). The intensity of required nursing care is less acute, but professional nursing care services are still necessary.

■ QUESTIONS FOR REFLECTION

1. Do you think the average person without exposure to delivering health care could navigate through the current system without assistance? Why or why not?

2. What are the benefits and potential conflicts of quick care health clinics based in retail establishments that also sell prescription medications?

3. Have you ever used a retail quick care health clinic? What was your experience? Would you use one again? Why or why not? If you have never received health care from a retail quick care health clinic, why have you not done so?

Integrated Health Care Delivery Systems: A Choice for Today's Consumer

Integrated health care delivery systems provide consumers with high continuity of care by offering primary, secondary, and tertiary health care services within a single health care system. The health care system combines dimensions of consumer preference, expert providers, and economic reimbursement into a single package. The system offers a variety of local health care centers that are typically linked to a large urban health care center that offers comprehensive, sophisticated therapies. Some systems may offer complementary therapies. The system may be part of a national proprietary (for-profit) chain, a national or regional nonprofit organization (frequently faith-based), or an arm of the local, state, or federal government.

To provide effective health care today, three factors are key: cost, access, and quality. In the United States, health care costs continue to rise and outpace the rate of inflation. High costs result in consumer inability to access necessary health services. Some consumers with low-paying jobs cannot afford the copayments on health insurance offered by their employers. Some health care organizations charge higher fees for rendered services when consumers do not have health care coverage. When consumers know that they bear the responsibility for full payment of medical services, they frequently hesitate to seek care until a condition becomes life-threatening, impedes their ability to engage independently in activities of daily living, or prevents their ability to work.

Take Note!
Cost, access, and quality are the three key factors in providing effective health care.

THE INTERDISCIPLINARY/ INTERPROFESSIONAL HEALTH CARE TEAM

The science behind health care is highly specialized. To best meet the physical, psychological, social, and spiritual health care needs of people who need care, a multidisciplinary approach is commonly used. Table 9.3 outlines the various members of the **interdisciplinary/ interprofessional health care team** and the contributions of each member. Sometimes, care is coordinated by a CM, who may be a nurse or social worker. Professional nurses usually coordinate care delivery in inpatient care environments.

As members of the interdisciplinary health care team, nurses provide key information for holistic client care. When clients and families become overwhelmed with the complexity of health care, nurses can guide them through the system while offering them emotional support. For example, "nurse navigator" programs have surfaced in the field of oncology nursing. The nurse navigator meets with clients on a regular basis to discuss questions about and barriers to care, provide individualized client education, offer emotional support, and facilitate referrals to needed community resources and other health care professionals. Identified strengths of nurse navigator programs include facilitation of continuity across the continuum of care, timely treatment, and prevention of complications in the delivery of health care (Bruce, 2007).

NURSING CARE DELIVERY MODELS

Management of nursing care for clients has always fallen within the purview of professional nurses. On a daily basis, nurses make decisions about how to organize client care. They consider a variety of factors when choosing the best way to deliver care to a group of clients, including client factors (acuity and specialized needs), staff factors (number of available staff, licensure status, clinical experience, and staff preferences), and organizational factors (the usual nursing care delivery system). A **nursing care delivery model** is a system used by nurses to organize and deliver nursing services to best meet client care needs. Effective nursing care delivery models match client care needs with available human resources to attain the best possible outcomes (Porter-O'Grady & Malloch, 2017).

Traditional methods of nursing care delivery models include the case method (total client care), functional nursing, team nursing, district nursing, primary nursing, case management, and client-focused (or modular) care. Table 9.4 outlines the origins and rationales behind each model, describes clinical decision making, outlines the scope of responsibility and authority, delineates team titles (when appropriate), presents the level of nurse and client satisfaction, and identifies major advantages and disadvantages of each model. Prior to industrialization and employer-based insurance, professional nurses practiced case nursing in which they performed all interventions to meet all the client's needs. The case method is still used in home health and private duty nursing as well as in clinical nursing education when faculty assign beginning nursing students to care for clients.

TABLE 9.3 The Interdisciplinary Health Care Team

Member	Role
Client (consumer or client)	Seeks out various health care services and makes decisions related to plan of care
Board of directors (or trustees)	■ Responsible for organizational mission, service quality, strategic planning, medical staff credentialing, evaluation and selection of the chief executive officer, self-evaluation and education, and financial status ■ For-profit companies report to stockholders. ■ Nonprofit organizations usually have a variety of people from the community with specialized expertise (e.g., lawyers) and philanthropists as board members.
Chief executive officer (or administrator)	Responsible for overall daily operation of the organization, including implementing board policies, addressing health care concerns within the local community, and preparing and delivering board reports
Administrative staff (managers or directors)	■ In large organizations, each department usually has someone responsible for its overall daily operations. ■ In nursing, the head of the nursing department has the title chief nursing executive or director of nursing.
Medical staff	■ Medical doctor, doctor of osteopathy, dentist, podiatrist, advanced practice nurse (nurse practitioner, certified registered nurse anesthetist, certified nurse midwife, or clinical nurse specialist), physician's assistant, clinical social worker, registered nurse, dietitian or nutritional professional; may be independent practitioners or organizational employees, and diagnoses and treats clients using medical therapies ■ To become a member of the medical staff the health care professional must go through a credentialing and approval process of the health care organization.
Nursing staff (registered nurses, licensed practical/vocational nurses [LPN/LVN], unlicensed assistive personnel [UAP; care assistants], clerical assistants [unit clerk, secretaries])	■ Responsible for execution of direct and indirect client care services ■ RNs assess clients, diagnose human responses to illness, outline a care plan, implement the plan (including the delegation of tasks to others), and evaluate the effectiveness of nursing care. ■ LPN/LVNs implement the care plan outlined by the RN, administer medications, and perform sterile procedures. ■ UAPs perform basic care tasks under the supervision of RNs or LPN/LVNs. In long-term care facilities, UAP with state certification may act as a medication technician and administer routinely ordered medication (excluding most parenteral medications). ■ Clerical assistants enter orders into computers, order supplies, and compile reports for client charges.
Case manager (for managed care organizations)	Advanced practice nurse or social worker who follows clients across the spectrum of health care settings; most start the discharge process as soon as clients are admitted to acute care facilities.
Dietitians	■ Baccalaureate-prepared nutritionists who have had internships to learn clinical nutrition, they outline specific client therapeutic diets, verify that client nutritional needs are met, and provide client and family education related to therapeutic diets. ■ Inpatient facilities have food service departments that prepare client and cafeteria meals.
Pharmacists	Prepare and dispense medications, educate other team members about medications, monitor controlled substance use, monitor client allergies, work to prevent medication errors, and monitor potential drug interactions
Paramedical personnel or technologists	■ Highly trained professionals with specialized education or training ■ Examples include medical technologist (lab tests), imaging technologist (e.g., X-ray, computerized tomography scan), and respiratory therapist (breathing therapies, ventilator management, oxygen therapy)

Member	Role
Social workers	■ Assist clients with social concerns that arise from illness, injury, or surgery ■ Help clients with financial issues resulting from disruption of work and insurance benefit gaps ■ Refer clients to community support agencies
Therapists	■ Physical therapists assess function and provide restorative therapy for body movement, ambulation, and safety. ■ Occupational therapists assess and provide restorative therapy for problems with activities of daily living as well as skills for employment. ■ Speech therapists assess for swallowing difficulties and speech problems, and provide restorative therapy related to these areas.
Medical records or health information services	Keep detailed and accurate medical records on clients
Business manager or office staff	Coordinates client appointments (outpatient settings) and keeps financial records for services rendered
Central supply or central products services	Warehouse and distribute client care products (not pharmaceuticals) per ordered request
Linen services	Provide client linen and gowns
Environmental or housekeeping services	Maintain a clean, safe physical environment
Biomedical engineering services	■ Maintain proper functioning of electronic client care machines (e.g., intravenous pumps, bedside monitors, thermometers) ■ Verify electrical safety of client care equipment
Information services	Develop integrated computer systems and provide user support services (some may offer computer and software staff education)
Quality management personnel	■ Monitor the quality of rendered services ■ Outline a plan for continuous quality improvement ■ Includes the risk management department, which monitors actual and potential client care errors and financial losses
Third-party payers	■ Pay for all or part of health care services used by the consumer. ■ Various levels of government are third-party payers for tax-supported health insurance plans. ■ Private insurance companies provide funding for plan enrollees. ■ Frequently audit client records to verify rendered services.
Utilization review	Set up in the late 1970s by the federal government to verify effective utilization of health care resources and avoid fraud
Spiritual support services (chaplain)	Inpatient settings usually have chaplain support services to provide spiritual and other support to clients and their families and significant others.
Human resources (personnel department)	■ Hires new employees, tracks employee incidents, and coordinates employee fringe benefits. ■ Payroll departments that issue employee paychecks may fall under this category.
Foundation	Nonprofit organizations usually have services to coordinate private donations to the organization.
Alternative care providers	Individuals who provide alternative and complementary therapy (e.g., chiropractors, herbalists, acupuncturists, massage therapists, reflexologists, folk healers)

Adapted from Centers for Medicare & Medicaid Services. (2011). *CMS Manual System Pub. 100–07 State operations provider certification, Transmittal 78.* Retrieved February 17, 2013, from http://www.cms.gov/Regulations-and-Guidance/Guidance/Transmittals/downloads/R78SOMA.pdf; Jonas, S. (1998). *An introduction to the U.S. health care system* (4th ed.). Springer Publishing; Knickman, J. R., & Elbel, B. (Eds.). (2019). *Jonas & Kovner's health care delivery in the United States* (12th ed.). Springer; American Hospital Association. (1999). *Welcome to the board: An orientation for the new health care trustee.* AHA Press.

TABLE 9.4 Comparison of Nursing Care Delivery System Models

Nursing Care Delivery Model	Case Method (Total Patient Care)	Functional Nursing	Team Nursing	District Nursing	Primary Nursing	Case Management	Client-Focused Care (Patient-Focused or Modular)
Date of origin and reason designed	1880s; clients were at home	1940s in response to nursing shortage	1950s in response to movement in management away from tasks to human relations	1950s–1960s to decrease the amount of leg work required for team nursing	1960s to facilitate movement of nurses toward independence and autonomous practice	1980s in response to diagnosis-related grouping (prospective payment system), budget awareness, and total quality management philosophy	1990s in response to increased efficiency with escalating costs and as a response to the nursing shortage
Clinical decision making	Done per shift	Done per shift	Shift based	Shift based	24 hours accountability of the primary nurse	24 hours accountability of the case manager	Shift based
Responsibility and authority	One or a small group of clients	Autonomous to a large group of clients	Large group of clients	Group of clients located in close proximity to each other	Autonomous for a small group of clients as a primary nurse	Coordination of care with members of the interdisciplinary health care team	Coordination with case manager common for plan of care Individual actions are autonomous and shift based for a large group of clients.
Work allocation	Total care to all assigned clients	Each member assigned specific tasks for all clients	Tasks for entire team, with some being assigned according to skills or license requirements	Same as in team nursing	Total care of own primary clients along with care of small number of clients with a different primary nurse	May serve as coordinator or actual provider of direct client care May be required to see caseloads of clients with similar health problems at more than one clinical site	Tasks assigned according to on-the-job training and licensure requirements

Nursing team title(s)	Nurse	Charge nurse Medicine nurse Treatment nurse Education nurse Admissions and discharge nurse Nurse's aide Orderly	RN becomes team leader and delegates tasks to team members. Team members: licensed practical nurses (LPNs)/licensed vocational nurses (LVNs), and unlicensed assistive personnel (UAP)	RN becomes the district nurse. Team members have the same titles as in team nursing.	Primary nurse Associate nurse No LPN or LVN nursing assistants and orderlies assigned to unit to help RNs	Case managers Care manager RNs and LPNs are nurses. UAP titles may be the same as in team nursing or client-focused care	Care pairs or care partners consisting of an RN with an UAP (who is called a client care technician) or client service associate
Professional nurse satisfaction	Yes	No	Yes	Yes	Yes	High for the case manager and nursing staff	Mixed for nurses Higher for UAP than for team
Client satisfaction	Yes	No	Yes	Yes	Yes	Mixed	Yes
Major advantages	Care received from one nurse per 8-hour shift Holistic care provided Clear lines of responsibility No complex assignment planning required	Highly cost-effective Clear lines of responsibility Development of technical experts if assigned the same tasks daily Useful with severe staffing shortages	Cost-effective and staff satisfaction with working with small client groups Comprehensive holistic care possible Development of better staff relationships	Same as with team nursing, except less exhaustion of nursing staff from reduced walking	Very satisfied nurses and clients Comprehensive holistic nursing care delivered	Cost-effective care coordinated to achieve client outcomes Holistic care orientation Continuity of care across the spectrum of health care settings Client knows whom to call for assistance	Cost-effective and clients seem to be satisfied Clients can ask anyone for help. Staff develop technical competence in a variety of skills.

(continued)

TABLE 9.4 Comparison of Nursing Care Delivery System Models (continued)

Nursing Care Delivery Model	Case Method (Total Patient Care)	Functional Nursing	Team Nursing	District Nursing	Primary Nursing	Case Management	Client-Focused Care (Patient-Focused or Modular)
Major disadvantages	No continuity of care; Very expensive by today's standards; Potential overloading of ancillary departments with multiple requests for the same supplies in a short time frame	Task-oriented system resulting in fragmentation of care; Staff boredom from repetitive work; Limited communication among staff members	Team leaders may not be available to lead the team; Poor communication may lead to tasks being omitted. Team leader needs time to supervise team members, which decreases time available for clients.	No district nurse available to lead team; Same as in team nursing	Not cost-effective to have all-RN staffing; Some primary nurses not available 7 days a week for 24-hours-a-day consultation; Not all nurses want to assume primary nursing responsibilities; Requires large numbers of RNs; Sense of loss by ancillary workers	High costs required for successful implementation; Critical pathways reduce individualization of client care. Physician resentment about being called for consultation by a nurse; Chief executive officer complaints of expenditures requested for care by case managers	Expensive to develop and provide technologic support; Blurs the distinctions of nursing roles from those of other interdisciplinary team members; Nurses may lose essential elements of nursing practice.
Areas where currently used	Home care; Private duty; Intensive care units; Nursing student assignments	Hospitals; Extended-care facilities; Rehabilitation centers; Operating rooms; Outpatient surgical centers; Physician offices	Hospitals; Extended-care facilities; Rehabilitation centers; Home health agencies	Hospitals; Extended-care facilities; Rehabilitation centers	Hospital intensive care units; Specialty centers such as dialysis, oncology, and diabetes outpatient centers; Hospice; Home care	Hospitals; Home health agencies; Health departments; Anywhere managed care is practiced	Hospitals; Home health agencies; Transport teams

Adapted from Manthey, M. (1991). Delivery systems and practice role models. *Nursing Management, 22*(1), 28–30; Sportsman, S. (2014). Care delivery strategies. In P. S. Yoder-Wise (Ed.), *Leading and managing in nursing* (6th ed.). Elsevier Mosby; Tappen, R. M. (2001). *Nursing leadership and management: Concepts and practice.* F.A. Davis.

In the functional team and district nursing care models, nursing staff members with different skills and licensure status care for a group of clients. Functional and team nursing models work well when there is a shortage of nursing staff. When either model is used, however, care may become fragmented, and without effective communication, little attention is paid to client needs for rest and privacy.

During the 1980s, job satisfaction among nurses plummeted, and nurse turnover in hospitals was high (Tourangeau et al., 2006). Increased responsibility for supervision of others for direct client care was cited as a major factor. Primary nursing emerged as a way to reconnect professional nurses with direct client care. A primary nurse for each client develops and revises the nursing care plan. In the event of the primary care nurse's absence, nursing care is delivered by another RN who is the designated associate nurse. Continuity of client care is also increased because the same nurses provide care services to the client. However, some nurses and hospital administrators frown upon using professional nurses to perform tasks that could be done by UAP.

The economic crunch of the early 1990s experienced by acute care facilities gave rise to redesigned care delivery systems. Quality improvement efforts focused on optimal client outcomes and satisfaction. Work redesign efforts resulted in a model that placed the client in the center. The model has been identified as client-focused care or modular nursing. Some institutions expanded the roles of UAP and provided them with intensive on-the-job training so they could perform sterile urinary catheterization, phlebotomy, and electrocardiograms. Professional nurses were then free to engage in holistic assessment, advanced nursing procedures, and client education. However, supervision of UAPs was also added to the professional nurse's role.

Modular nursing represents a unique form of client-focused care. In modular nursing, UAPs and professional nurses receive assignments to work continuously as "care partners." Care partners receive cross-training to perform basic respiratory therapy treatments, physical therapy, phlebotomy, and electrocardiography. Under this delivery system, clients receive almost instantaneous therapy as they do not have to wait for ancillary personnel to arrive.

Case management is a system of client care delivery that focuses on the achievement of outcomes within effective time frames and with appropriate use of health care resources. Key elements of case management involve a CM (who may be a bachelor-prepared RN, advanced practice nurse, or social worker) and a standardized method for managing a particular disease process. The predetermined path for specific care delivery (critical path, clinical path, or care map) is followed for the duration of client care. The path outlines typical interdisciplinary clinical problems with desired outcomes, maps out daily expected interventions, and specifies discharge client instructions and education. Staff nurses and the CM frequently monitor client progress toward desired outcomes. Some paths cross health care settings, enabling a seamless continuum of care. The CM assumes responsibility for matching client care needs so that appropriate services are rendered. The CM may use standardized clinical protocols, guidelines, and third-party payer criteria to ensure optimal outcomes with the most efficient use of resources.

The CM executes multiple roles that require critical thinking. As a clinician, the CM communicates effectively with the multidisciplinary health care team. The CM also coordinates care among all professionals and consultants. To ensure that economic constraints do not affect quality of client care, the CM justifies expenditures and care variances. The CM sometimes troubleshoots conflicts that might arise between health care providers, third-party payers, and consumers and acts as a client advocate. Some CMs maintain an ongoing relationship with clients using the telephone, internet, or other telehealth options.

Innovative Client Care Delivery Systems

Porter-O'Grady and Malloch (2017) specified that delivery of client care encompasses more than nursing care and proposed that the care delivery system models should encompass the entire multidisciplinary client care team. Such models have the client at the center of the circle and the interdisciplinary care team surrounding the client. The direct client caregivers (the nursing staff) constitute the first tier of service. Surrounding the nursing team and providing direct client care are nursing support systems, including nursing directors, resource nurses, rapid response teams (to support nurses with client care crisis situations), phlebotomy services, admissions staff, clinical nurse specialists, and staff development personnel. The outermost circle includes all other members of the interdisciplinary client care team.

Donlevy and Pietruch (1996) developed a model of nursing known as the connection delivery model. The connection delivery model provides an interdisciplinary team approach to chronic disease management. For acute care nurses, this model provides cross-training for them to work effectively in client homes. This model has been associated with high levels of client satisfaction because they are followed by nurses who cared for them in the hospital and are therefore familiar with their cases. Nurses also report high levels of satisfaction with the model because they follow clients across the continuum of care, establish long-term relationships with clients, and engage in independent clinical decision making outside of the hospital setting.

Nursing care delivery models affect health care delivery in several dimensions including cost, safety, efficiency, client satisfaction with care, and nurse outcomes (e.g., job satisfaction, retention, signs of burnout) (Allen & Vitale-Nolen, 2005; Donlevy & Pietruch, 1996; Fernandez et al., 2012; Havaei et al., 2019; Wells et al., 2011). In a recent study, nurses experience less emotional exhaustion when the nursing model provided them with the opportunity to work with licensed practical nurses (LPNs; see Focus on Research box, "Effects of Nursing Care Delivery Models on Registered Nurse Outcomes").

FOCUS ON RESEARCH
Effects of Nursing Care Delivery Models on Registered Nurse Outcomes

The investigators examined the effects nursing care delivery models, skill mix, and organizational characteristics would have on RN outcomes. They implemented a cross-sectional correlational study using survey findings from 416 Canadian nurses working in acute care settings in British Columbia.

The survey included the RN4CAST survey, a survey commonly used to assess hospital characteristics, nurse retention, and client outcomes. They employed the Masalach Burnout Inventory scale to assess levels of professional burnout. Both surveys were initially administered online. They provided potential participants with email reminders spaced 2 weeks apart. Finally, a second postal invitation with a paper copy of the survey was mailed to the 15,702 potential participants.

They received 416 completed usable surveys (3% return rate). Of the participants, 97% were female with a mean age of 38.4 years. Fifty-six percent of the nurses reported working fulltime, 24% part-time, and 20% casually or as needed. Seventeen percent of the nurses reported having two or more jobs. Eighty percent of the nurses reported working with acutely ill clients; 85% of these clients were moderately to very dependent upon the nurses for having personal care needs met. The nursing care delivery models reported included team nursing (76.92%) and the total client care model (23.17%). Sixty-eight percent of the nurses reported working with LPNs.

Data were analyzed using Chi square analysis, hierarchical multiple regression, and moderated regression. No statistically significant differences were identified with the model of nursing care delivery. Hierarchical regression revealed that skill mix affected RN emotional exhaustion scores (F [df 19,25] = 9.41, $p < .001$). High levels of client dependency were associated with higher levels of job satisfaction ($\beta = .12$, $p < .05$). Other significant contributors to job satisfaction included adequate staffing and resources ($\beta = .25$, $p < .001$) as well as nurse participation in hospital affairs ($\beta = .9$, $p < .01$).

The study concludes that the nursing care delivery model likely did not affect RN outcomes, but nurses who had the opportunity to work with LPNs had less emotional exhaustion because of the LPNs' contributions. They proposed reducing RN workload. Other organizational characteristics such as adequate resources and staffing along with nurse participation in hospital decisions affecting their practice may improve nurse job satisfaction. The investigators identified the following weaknesses of the study: low survey response rate, direct causation could not be determined (correlational study), and there was no unit identification used in the study.

The clinical significance of this study reveals that LPN use in acute care makes valuable contributions and helps ease the demands of RN workload. More research is needed to determine how LPNs are used in acute care facilities, client outcomes when direct care is delivered by LPNs, if the LPN scope of practice is compromised, and the effects of acute care nursing on LPNs.

From Havaei, F., MacPhee, M., & Dahinten, V. S. (2019). The effect of nursing care delivery models on quality and safety outcomes of care: A cross-sectional survey study of medical-surgical nurses. *Journal of Advanced Nursing, 75*(10), 2144–2155. https://doi.org/10.1111/jan.13997

NURSING CHALLENGES RELATED TO HEALTH CARE DELIVERY SYSTEMS

Each health care delivery system possesses different challenges for professional nursing practice. For example, nurses working in a system based on a free market encounter challenges when clients are unable to pay for rendered health care services. Nurses working in a government-based universal care system may experience challenges with adequate staffing and supplies to provide high-quality, effective care. Because professional nurses play a key role in health delivery, they encounter practical and ethical challenges on a daily basis.

Practical Challenges

Two key practical challenges encountered by nurses involve the shortage of professional nurses and changes in the structure of the work environment.

The Nursing Shortage

There are currently an insufficient number of nurses to meet the health care needs of clients, and the shortage is expected to worsen. The USBLS (2020f) reported that from 2019 to 2029, the number of professional nurses needed will rise from 3.15 to 3.3 million. Because many nurses over the age of 65 remain working, it is difficult to project exactly how many nursing positions will need to be filled within the next decade.

The supply of professional nurses also looks bleak in Canada, where a report from the McGill Nursing Collaborative for Education and Innovation in Patient- and Family-Centered Care (2019) reported that Canada has 431,769 nurses, and 303,146 of these nurses are RNs. According to the Canadian Federation of Nursing, 46.7% of registered nurses are under the age of 40, 66% of nurses plan to leave their current position within a year's time, and 20% plan to leave the profession (Reichert et al., 2021). According to the Canadian Institute of Health Information (2020), the mean age for registered nurses was 44.4 years in 2019. Stonebridge and Hemus (2017) reported that Canda will need 64,000 additional nurses by 2035 and 28,005 of these registered nurses will be in the area of geriatrics and long-term care. Many factors contribute to the current global nursing shortage, including:

- Reduced number of young people (18 to 24 years) entering the profession
- Decreased interest in a professional nursing career because of other career options for women (91% of the current nursing workforce identifies as female)
- Compressed salary and fewer promotions throughout a nursing career
- Increased labor intensity from increased client acuity and numbers of clients
- Chronic understaffing in acute and extended-care settings
- Poor collegial relationships with other health team members
- Widespread fear of contracting medication-resistant infectious diseases
- Increased chance of sustaining musculoskeletal injuries because of increased client body mass index (in the United States) and lack of enforceable policies related to lifting limitations for nursing staff
- Reduced job satisfaction
- High turnover
- Nurses leaving the profession
- Unfavorable stories about the profession being shared with potential nursing recruits
- Nursing faculty shortage
- Aging workforce

If the RN shortage persists, health care facilities will be forced to explore other staffing mix options, which may mean having RNs assume more supervisory responsibilities. Historically, the nursing shortage has been perpetuated by external factors such as problems with recruitment, retention, negative image, and poor working environments. In addition, internal factors such as job dissatisfaction, role overload, poor collegial relationships, and professional disillusionment exacerbate the shortage. The aging nursing workforce now seems to be a major factor driving the shortage.

Alleviating the nursing shortage requires that the nursing profession attack all these factors. Nurses must believe they have the power to change work environments to promote professional autonomy and safety. Empowering nurses begins with nursing education programs and continues through an entire career. All areas of nursing (practice, administration, and education) must collaborate rather than compete with each other to shape the nursing profession.

Challenges Resulting From Changes In the Structure of the Work Environment

Hospitals have implemented numerous changes over the past decades. In many facilities when a person is admitted, a hospitalist rather than the client's private physician manages the stay. Hospitalists are physicians (some of whom have direct employment status or contracts with the hospital) who manage client care in acute care settings for primary care physicians and NPs. After dismissal from the hospital, health care management is resumed by the primary care provider (physician or NP). Some acute care facilities have reported reduced inpatient length of stay and substantial cost savings since introducing the hospitalist role.

The emergence of hospitalists has created the need for professional nurses in hospitals to educate clients about the advantages of receiving medical care from a physician who specializes in the complex nature of acute care. Sometimes, clients and their significant others inquire if the physician whom they see in the outpatient setting will be seeing them in the hospital. In recent years, very few primary care physicians make hospital visits. Nurses reassure recipients of hospital care that their primary care physician will receive a detailed report about what transpired during hospitalization.

Some health systems, hospitals, and hospitalist physician groups have hired acute care NPs to follow hospitalized clients. Thus, hospitalized clients may be seen more often by an acute care NP than a physician. Health care systems, hospitalist physician groups, and hospitalist care teams use a list of evidence-based protocols that include a list of standardized orders for the management of commonly encountered reasons for and health problems arising from hospitalization (e.g., electrolyte replacement, constipation). Because of the transfer of client care to hospitalists who may be unfamiliar with the client history, nurses have experienced increased workload demands, such as medication reconciliation, as part of the routine hospital admission process. Medication reconciliation requires that the admission nurse makes certain that the list of medications a client is taking at home exactly matches or there is a specific reason to add or to discontinue a medication during the hospital stay upon admission. Because hospital nurses, acute care NPs, and hospitalists work closely with each other on a regular basis, they sometimes develop close, collaborative working relationships.

During the recent COVID-19 pandemic, some hospitals laid off staff or cut working hours of nurses because local governments issued decrees banning nonurgent surgical and diagnostic procedures to conserve personal protective equipment and prevent potential spread of infection. Nursing staff sometimes did not receive the correct face masks to protect them from possible airborne transmission of the virus. Physicians were given priority for having the masks, and nurses used lower-standard face masks and shields. Low client census resulted in some acute care NPs and hospital RNs finding themselves unemployed. Nurses working in outpatient settings also saw work hour reductions or unemployment.

Recent reductions in the length of hospitalization mean that nurses care for more acutely ill clients. Nurses must be more vigilant to notice small changes in client status that may foreshadow a catastrophic health event. They also must have detailed knowledge about potential adverse effects of complex interactions among medications. Nurses must also possess the ability to perform sophisticated procedures such as central line management, intravenous medication drips, and complicated dressings. Finally, nurses must document client care activities using electronic documentation systems; forgetting to document something may result in reduced hospital reimbursement from governmental and private health care insurance plans. New medications and technology demand increased knowledge, skills, and time.

■ QUESTIONS FOR REFLECTION

1. What changes have you seen (if you are a practicing nurse) or have you heard about (if you are a nursing student with no practice experience) in clinical nursing practice within the past 2 years? How do these changes impact your ability to provide safe, effective nursing care to clients and families?
2. What areas of professional nursing practice do you see expanding based on current changes to government funding of health care?
3. What has been your personal experience as a client or family member of a client with the current changes in hospital care?
4. What changes in professional practice do you foresee occurring as a result of increased governmental influences in health care delivery?
5. What strategies may be helpful for nurses to cope with current and future changes in health care delivery? Design a plan for helping current and future professional nurses. Determine the feasibility of this plan.

Ethical Challenges

Relatively new ethical concerns have arisen with increasing lifespans, the development of health care technology, and the increasing costs of health care delivery. For decades, the ability of people to pay for health care has determined who has access to services and the quality of service that can be obtained (Knickman, 2019; Kominski, 2014).

Because it is not possible to meet all goals of accessibility, equity, and quality given available resources, difficult choices must be made among competing values and multiple desirable alternatives. One basic issue is the relative valuing of containment of health care costs versus access to health care for everyone.

Ethical questions raised by these choices include:

- Is health care a basic right or a privilege?
- What is the basic acceptable level of health care?
- Who has priority for health care services if there are access limitations and finite resources for health care delivery?
- What governmental and/or social programs should be cut to increase health care resources for better access to health care?
- How much choice should people have in deciding from whom and where they can receive health care?
- Should people with resources for payment receive services before those who do not?
- How should rationing of health care be determined?
- Who should determine rationing criteria?
- What criteria should be used for rationing of health care services?
- Should expensive technology and advanced life support measures be made available to everyone?
- What (and when) is death?
- How much is the prolongation of life worth?
- What rights do clients have?
- Is curing disease possible and desirable?
- How do we use health care resources and personnel for the best interest of the human race?

"Treating health care primarily as a business and a commodity to be sold like cars is an impoverished notion of health care in relation to the concept of health care as a human service created by society to meet the needs of vulnerable people who are ill or at risk of becoming ill" (Aroskar, 1987, p. 65). It is critical that the voice of the nursing profession be added to that of the public in discussions of the philosophical considerations and values that will shape the decisions concerning the size, shape, and direction of all future health care delivery systems.

Summary and Significance to Practice

As a result of significant demographic, economic, attitudinal, and available manpower forces, health care delivery systems are in the process of massive structural reorganization, raising multiple ethical and practical considerations. Health care delivery systems are shaped primarily by history, cultural values, and resource availability. Nurses should assume leadership in shaping future health care delivery by using their cognitive skills and compassion so that everyone will have access to optimal health care services.

REAL-LIFE REFLECTIONS

Recall Maria and her parents from the beginning of the chapter. How should Maria explain to her father the benefits of receiving generic medication and a temporary stay in an extended-care facility on his recovery? How would you explain the complex web of health care delivery to older clients? What type of help do they need to navigate their way through the health care system?

From Theory to Practice

1. Identify the strengths and weaknesses of the American and Canadian health care delivery systems. Explain why you consider the items in your list strengths or weaknesses.
2. How can nurses work to improve health care delivery? What are the consequences if nurses do not get involved with changes in the health care delivery system?

Nurse as Author

Write a two- to three-page essay on how you think that the American health care system could be improved. For each of your key ideas, provide a reference citation from a peer-reviewed journal. Include a reference list at the end of your essay.

Your Digital Classroom

Online Exploration

Agency for Healthcare Research and Quality: **www.ahrq.gov**
American Association of Retired Persons: **www.aarp.org**
American Hospital Association: **www.aha.org**
American Medical Association: **www.ama-assn.org**

American Nurses Association: **www.nursingworld
.org/ana/**

America's Health Insurance Plans: **www.ahip.org**

Centers for Medicare & Medicaid Services: **www
.cms.hhs.gov**

International Council of Nurses: **www.icn.ch**

America's Health Insurance Plans website: **www
.healthplans.org**

Expanding Your Understanding

1. Visit the America's Health Insurance Plans website to learn about the complexities of the health insurance industry. Click on the "Issues" tab at the top of the page, and then click on the following titles at the left hand of the screen: "Employer-Provided Coverage," "Individual Coverage," and "Medicaid and Medicare Advantage." Answer the following questions:
   a. What type of health insurance coverage do you have?
   b. What would result in losing coverage under this type of plan?
   c. What did you learn about health care insurance that surprised you?
2. This website contains the latest updates on legislative efforts to reform health insurance and provides consumers with information about the types of health insurance plans and how to enroll in them.
3. Visit the AMA website to learn about issues confronting physicians in today's health care environment. While there, look for the listing of a physician you know.
4. Visit the American Nurses Association Nursing World website to learn about issues confronting professional nurses in the health care system.

Beyond the Book

Visit the **Point**® at **www.thePoint.lww.com** for activities and information to reinforce the concepts and content covered in this chapter.

REFERENCES

Allen, D., & Vitale-Nolen, R. (2005). Patient care delivery model improves nurse job satisfaction. *Journal of Continuing Education in Nursing, 36*(6), 277–282. doi:10.3928/0022-0124-20051101-08

Allin, S., Marchildron, G., & Peckham, A. (2020). *International health care systems profiles: Canada.* Retrieved January 31, 2021, from https://www.commonwealthfund.org/international-health-policy-center/countries/canada

American Association of Nurse Practitioners. (2021). *State practice environment.* Retrieved April 5, 2021, from https://www.aanp.org/advocacy/state/state-practice-environment

Aroskar, M. A. (1987). Fidelity and veracity: Questions of promise keeping, truth telling, and loyalty. In M. D. M. Fowler & J. Levine-Ariff (Eds.), *Ethics at the bedside: A sourcebook for the critical care nurse* (pp. 48–61). J. B. Lippincott.

Bruce, S. D. (2007). Taking the wheel, oncology nurses help patients navigate the cancer journey. *ONS Connect, 22*(3), 8–11. Retrieved April 5, 2021, from https://www.thefreelibrary.com/Taking+the+Wheel%3a+oncology+nurses+help+patients+navigate+the+cancer...-a0187772739

Canadian Institute of Health Information. (2020). *Nursing in Canada, 2019: A Lens on Supply and Workforce.* CIHI; 2020. Retrieved April 5, 2021, from https://www.cihi.ca/sites/default/files/document/nursing-report-2019-en-web.pdf

Centers for Medicare & Medicaid Services. (2011). *CMS Manual System. Pub. 100-07 State Operations Provider Certification, Transmittal 78.* Retrieved April 5, 2021, from https://www.cms.gov/Regulations-and-Guidance/Guidance/Manuals/Internet-Only-Manuals-IOMs-Items/CMS1201984

Centers for Medicare & Medicaid Services. (2020). *NHE fact sheet.* Retrieved September 24, 2020, from https://www.cms.gov/Research-Statistics-Data-and-Systems/Statistics-Trends-and-Reports/NationalHealthExpendData/NHE-Fact-Sheet

DeNavas-Walt, C., Proctor, B., & Smith, J. (2012). *Income, poverty & health insurance coverage in the United States: 2011.* Retrieved April 6, 2021, from https://www.census.gov/library/visualizations/2012/demo/p60-243.html

Donlevy, J. A., & Pietruch, B. L. (1996). The connection delivery model: Care across the continuum. *Nursing Management, 27*(5), 34–36. DOI:10.1097/00006216-199602030-00011

Federal Register. (2021). *2021 Joe Biden Executive Orders.* Retrieved June 13, 2021, from https://www.federalregister.gov/presidential-documents/executive-orders/joe-biden/2021

Fernandez, R., Johnson, M., Tran, D. T., & Miranda, C. (2012). Models of care in nursing: A systematic review. *International Journal of Evidence-Based Healthcare, 10*(4), 324–337. https://doi.org/10.1111/j.1744-1609.2012.00287.x

Fried, B. J., & Gaydos, L. M. (Eds.). (2002). *World health systems: Challenges and perspectives.* Health Administration Press.

Geyman, J. P. (2015). A five-year assessment of the Affordable Care Act: Market forces still trump the common good in U.S. health care. *International Journal of Health Services, 45*(2), 209–225. https://doi.org/10.1177/0020731414568505

Goldsmith, L. (2002). Canada. In B. J. Fried & L. M. Gaydos (Eds.), *World health systems: Challenges and perspectives* (pp. 227–248). Health Administration Press.

Goldstein, A. (2020, September 19). How Ruth Bader Ginsberg's death could jeopardize the Affordable Care Act. *The Washington Post.* Retrieved September 26, from https://www.washingtonpost.com/health/aca-scotus-ruth-bader-ginsburg/2020/09/19/440e7aa2-fa8b-11ea-89e3-4b9efa36dc64_story.html

Gusmano, M. K., Strumpf, E., Fiset-Laniel, J., Weisz, D., & Rodwin, V. G. (2019). Comparative analysis of health system performance in Montreal and New York: the importance of context for interpreting indicators. *Health Economics, Policy & Law, 14*(1), 101–118. https://doi-org.lib.rockhurst.edu/10.1017/S1744133118000166

Havaei, F., MacPhee, M., & Dahinten, V. S. (2019). The effect of nursing care delivery models on quality and safety outcomes of care: A cross-sectional survey study of medical-surgical nurses. *Journal of Advanced Nursing, 75*(10), 2144–2155. https://doi.org/10.1111/jan.13997

Healthcare.gov. (2020). *Marketplace health benefits & coverage: What to know*. Retrieved from https://www.healthcare.gov/blog/marketplace-coverage-essential-benefits-preventive-care/

International Council of Nurses. (2020). *Who we are*. Retrieved September 22, 2020, from https://www.icn.ch/who-we-are

Jamieson, E. M., & Sewall, M. F. (1954). *Trends in nursing history* (4th ed.). W. B. Saunders.

Johnson, A., Carillo, A., & Garcia, J. (2002). *Mexico*. In B. J. Fried & L. M. Gaydos (Eds.), *World health systems: Challenges and perspectives* (pp. 421–444). Health Administration Press.

Jonas, S. (1998). *An introduction to the U.S. health care system* (4th ed.). Springer.

Kaiser Family Foundation. (2017). *Compare proposals to replace the Affordable Care Act*. Retrieved April 1, 2017, from http://kff.org/interactive/proposals-to-replace-the-affordable-care-act/

Kaiser Family Foundation. (2019). *Employee health benefits: 2019 summary of findings*. Retrieved January 31, 2020, from http://files.kff.org/attachment/Summary-of-Findings-Employer-Health-Benefits-2019

Keisler-Starkey, K., & Bunch, L. N. (2020). *U.S. Census Bureau Current Population Reports, P60-271, Health Insurance Coverage in the United States: 2019*. U.S. Government Publishing Office.

Knickman, J. (2019). *Health care financing*. In J. Knickman & B. Elbel (Eds.), *Jonas & Kovner's health care delivery in the United States* (12th ed., pp. 257–275). Springer.

Knickman, J. R., & Elbel, B. (Eds.). (2019). *Jonas & Kovner's health care delivery in the United States* (12th ed.). Springer.

Kominski, G. F. (Ed.). (2014). *Changing the U.S. health care system: Key issues in health services policy and management* (4th ed.). Jossey-Bass.

Krisberg, K. (2019, November). Uninsurance rate jumps for first time since ACA; coverage falls in children. *Nation's Health*, *49*(9), 1–20. Retrieved April 6, 2021, from https://www.thenationshealth.org/content/49/9/1.2

Lacey, L. (2002). *Nigeria*. In B. J. Fried & L. M. Gaydos (Eds.), *World health systems: Challenges and perspectives*. Health Administration Press.

Markowitz, G. E., & Rosner, D. (1979). Doctors in crisis: Medical education and medical reform during the Progressive era, 1895–1915. In S. Reverby & D. Rosner (Eds.), *Health care in America: Essays in social history*. Temple University Press.

Matej, M. (2019). *Total health expenditure as a percentage of GDP in Canada from 1975-2019*. Retrieved September 24, 2020, from https://www.statista.com/statistics/436385/total-health-spending-as-percentage-of-gdp-canada/

McCarthy, N. (2019). How U.S. healthcare spending per capita compares with other countries. *Forbes Statistica*. Retrieved September 24, 2020, from https://www.forbes.com/sites/niallmccarthy/2019/08/08/how-us-healthcare-spending-per-capita-compares-with-other-countries-infographic/#724ea7dd575d

McDermott, D., Cox, C., Rudowitz, R., & Garfield, R. (2020). How has the pandemic affected health coverage in the U.S.? *KFF*. Retrieved January 31, 2021, from https://www.kff.org/policy-watch/how-has-the-pandemic-affected-health-coverage-in-the-u-s/

Mukamel, D. B., Ladd, H., Amin, A., & Sorkin, D. H. (2019). Patients' preferences over care settings for minor illnesses and injuries. *Health Services Research*, *54*(4), 827–838. https://doi.org/10.1111/1475-6773.13154

National Council of State Boards of Nursing. (2018). *2017 National nursing workforce study*. Retrieved September 22, 2020, from https://www.ncsbn.org/workforce.htm

Porter-O'Grady, T., & Malloch, K. (2017). *Quantum leadership: Creating sustainable value in health care* (5th ed.). Jones & Bartlett Learning.

Public Broadcasting Service. (2007). *The Online News Hour: The uninsured in America—Timeline: Insurance in the U.S.* Retrieved December 12, 2012, from http://www.pbs.org/newshour/indepth_coverage/health/uninsured/timeline/index.html

Reichert, C., René, B. & Genina, O. (2021). *Outlook on nursing, a snapshot from Canadian nurses on work environments pre-COVID-19*. Canaderian Federation of Nursing Unions. Retrieved April 5, 2021, from https://nursesunions.ca/wp-content/uploads/2020/12/CFNU_outlook_ENfinal_web.pdf

Reddy, M. S., & Mythri, S. V. (2016). Health-care Ethics and the Free Market Value System. *Indian Journal of Psychological Medicine*, *38*(5), 371–375. doi:10.4103/0253-7176.191387

Rios, A. (2020). *Mexico health spending as a share of GDP*. Retrieved Retrieved April 6, 2021, from https://www.statista.com/statistics/947944/mexico-health-expenditure-share-gdp/

Scofera, L. (1994). The development and growth of employer-provided health insurance. *Monthly Labor Review*, *117*(3), 3–10. Retrieved April 6, 2021, from https://www.bls.gov/opub/mlr/1994/03/art1full.pdf

Slavitt, A. M., & Burwell, S. (2016). Basic health program; federal funding methodology for program years 2017 & 2018. *The Federal Register*. Retrieved April 6, 2021, from https://www.federalregister.gov/documents/2016/02/29/2016-03902/basic-health-program-federal-funding-methodology-for-program-years-2017-and-2018

Spetz, J., & Chapman, S. A. (2019). The health workforce. In J. Knickman & B. Elbel (Eds.), *Jonas & Kovner's health care delivery in the United States* (11th ed., pp. 231–255). Springer.

Stonebridge, C., & Hermus, G. (2017). *Future Care for Canadian Seniors: A Primer on Nursing Supply and Demand*. The Conference Board of Canada. Retrieved April 5, 2021, from https://www.conferenceboard.ca/temp/19b73cde-c126-462e-915d-b2277c0a384b/8679_Seniors_Care_Nursing_Supply_and_Demand_EN_BR.pdf

Storch, J. L., & Scaia, M. (2019). Canadian healthcare. In C. McDonald & M. McIntyre (Eds.), *Realities of Canadian nursing* (5th ed., pp. 86–102). Wolters Kluwer.

The McGill Nursing Collaborative for Education and Innovation in Patient-and Family-Centered Care. (2019). *The global shortage of nurses*. Retrieved September 26, 2020, from https://www.mcgill.ca/nursing/files/nursing/nurse_shortages.pdf

Tikkanen, R., & Abrams, M. K. (2020). *Data brief January 2020, U.S. Health Care from a global perspective, 2019: Higher spending, worse outcomes?* Retrieved January 31, 2021, from https://www.commonwealthfund.org/publications/issue-briefs/2020/jan/us-health-care-global-perspective-2019

Torrens, P. R. (1978). *The American health care system: Issues and problems*. Mosby.

Tourangeau, A. E., Hall L. M., Doran D. M., & Petch T. (2006). Measurement of nurse job satisfaction using the McCloskey/Mueller Satisfaction Scale. *Nursing Research*, *55*(2), 128–136. Retrieved April 6, 2021, from http://www.tourangeauresearch.com/wp-content/uploads/job-satisfaction-with-MMSS.pdf

Trump, D. (2020). *Executive order: An America-First Healthcare Plan*. Retrieved April 6, 2021, from https://www.federalregister.gov/documents/2020/10/01/2020-21914/an-america-first-healthcare-plan

United States Bureau of Labor Statistics, United States Department of Labor. (2020a). *Occupational outlook handbook, Clinical laboratory technologists and technicians.* Retrieved September 1, 2020, from https://www.bls.gov/ooh/health-care/clinical-laboratory-technologists-and-technicians.htm

United States Bureau of Labor Statistics, United States Department of Labor. (2020b). *Occupational outlook handbook, Licensed practical and licensed vocational nurses.* Retrieved September 1, 2020, from https://www.bls.gov/ooh/healthcare/licensed-practical-and-licensed-vocational-nurses.htm

United States Bureau of Labor Statistics, United States Department of Labor. (2020c). *Occupational outlook handbook, Medical and health services managers.* Retrieved September 1, 2020, from https://www.bls.gov/ooh/management/medical-and-health-services-managers.htm

United States Bureau of Labor Statistics, United States Department of Labor. (2020d). *Occupational outlook handbook, Nursing assistants and orderlies.* Retrieved September 1, 2020, from https://www.bls.gov/ooh/healthcare/nursing-assistants.htm

United States Bureau of Labor Statistics, United States Department of Labor. (2020e). *Occupational outlook handbook, Physicians and surgeons.* Retrieved September 1, 2020, *from* https://www.bls.gov/ooh/healthcare/physicians-and-surgeons.htm

United States Bureau of Labor Statistics, United States Department of Labor. (2020f). *Occupational outlook handbook, Registered nurses.* Retrieved September 1, 2020, *from* https://www.bls.gov/ooh/healthcare/registered-nurses.htm

United States Bureau of Labor Statistics, United States Department of Labor. (2020g). *Occupational outlook handbook, Social workers.* Retrieved September 11, 2020, from https://www.bls.gov/ooh/community-and-social-service/social-workers.htm

United States Supreme Court. (2020). *19-1019 Texas V. California.* Retrieved April 7, 2021, from https://www.supremecourt.gov/qp/19-01019qp.pdf

Visaguide.world. (2020). *German healthcare system guide.* Retrieved September 21, 2020, from https://www.germanyhis.com/

Vogel, M. J. (1979). The transformation of the American hospital, 1859–1920. In S. Reverby & D. Rosner (Eds.), *Health care in America: Essays in social history.* Temple University Press.

Wells, J., Manuel, M., & Cunning, G. (2011). Changing the model of care delivery: Nurses' perceptions of job satisfaction and care effectiveness. *Journal of Nursing Management, 19,* 777–785. https://doi.org/10.1111/j.1365-2834.2011.01292.x

World Health Organization. (2010). *The world health report, health systems: Finding the path to universal coverage.* Retrieved April 5, 2021, from http:s://www.who.int/whr/2010/10_summary_en.pdf

World Health Organization. (2019). *Global spending on health: A world in transition.* License: CC BY-NC-SA 3.0 IGO. Retrieved September 24, 2020, from https://apps.who.int/iris/handle/10665/330357

World Health Organization. (2020a). *Global Health Observatory data repository. Medical doctors.* Retrieved September 22, 2020, *from* https://apps.who.int/gho/data/node.main.HWFGRP_0020?lang=en

World Health Organization. (2020b). *Global Health Observatory data repository. Nurses and midwifery personnel.* Retrieved September 22, 2020, *from* https://apps.who.int/gho/data/node.main.HWFGRP_0040?lang=en

World Health Organization. (2020c). *State of the world's nursing 2020: Investing in education, jobs and leadership.* License: CC BY-NC-SA 3.0 IGO. Retrieved September 22, 2020, from https://apps.who.int/iris/handle/10665/331677

World Health Organization. (2020d). *World health statistics 2020: Monitoring health for the SDGs, sustainable development goals.* License: CC BY-NC-SA 3.0 IGO. Retrieved September 22, 2020, from https://apps.who.int/iris/bitstream/handle/10665/332070/9789240005105-eng.pdf?ua=1

Yarbrough Landry, A., & Erwin, C. O. (2019). Organization of care. In *J. Knickman & B. Elbel (Eds.), Jonas & Kovner's health care delivery in the United States* (11th ed., p. 49). Springer.

Zakus, D., & Cortinois, A. (2002). Primary healthcare and community participation: Origins, implementation and the future. In B. J. Fried & L. M. Gaydos (Eds.), *World health systems: Challenges and perspectives* (pp. 39–54). Health Administration Press.

Professional Practice Based on Nursing Research and Best Evidence

LEARNING OUTCOMES

By the end of this chapter, the learner will be able to:

1. Describe how professional nurses contribute to research in nursing.
2. Differentiate qualitative and quantitative research.
3. Outline the sequential steps of the research process.
4. Debate the ethical considerations of nursing research.
5. Compare and contrast research utilization and evidence-based practice (EBP) models.
6. Identify barriers to research utilization in the clinical setting.
7. Identify strategies to facilitate clinical research utilization.
8. Specify how using nursing research affects the public image of professional nursing.

REAL-LIFE REFLECTIONS

Jessica and Malika work together on a surgical unit. Malika, who has been a nurse for 12 years, takes pride in her expertise and practices nursing "the way that I was taught." Jessica has read several research articles substantiating the effectiveness of noninvasive nursing interventions on reducing client's need for narcotics for postoperative pain control. Jessica is unsure about whether she should use these findings in practice and how Malika will react if she suggests implementing them on a unit-wide scale. Jessica also knows that current federal guidelines related to postoperative pain control specify that nurses should use other methods besides pain medication. Both nurses wonder what they might need to do to change practice on their unit. What steps should these nurses follow to validate the benefits of various, available nonpharmacologic techniques for postoperative pain control? What barriers might they encounter as they explore this practice change? Why would these be considered

(continued on page 267)

barriers? How might they go about attaining support from their manager and peers to change unit practice?

- *Does the idea of conducting research intrigue or intimidate you?*
- *What research-based interventions have you used in clinical practice?*

Interprofessional health care team members and consumers rely on research-based interventions (including medications) to help them provide safe, high-quality health care. Discipline-specific research enables a profession to develop and validate its unique knowledge base. Research also validates principles and techniques of clinical practice. Because nursing is primarily a practice discipline, nurses must understand basic research principles, critically analyze research study results, and use research findings to guide client care.

Although nursing research has been part of the profession since its inception, serious efforts to conduct research and develop theory to guide practice only began about 50 years ago, when nursing scholars drove the pursuit of establishing theoretical- and factual-based nursing practice instead of perpetuating nursing practice based on personal opinions, long-standing Nurses must realize that incorporating research findings into practice is not an optional activity in which to engage when there is time but rather a critical element of professional practice.

Science seeks the truth, and humans create science through research (Barrett, 2002). Therefore, nursing research should result in the creation of nursing science. **Research** is "a systematic inquiry that relies on disciplined methods to answer questions or solve problems" (Polit & Beck, 2021, p. 2). Nursing research focuses on generating knowledge for and solving problems within the profession and practice of nursing. Basic research is conducted to advance science and discover new information about the biologic and physiologic aspects of humans and the environment. In addition, basic research is also used to discover aspects of psychologic, sociocultural, developmental, and spiritual dimensions that affect the quality of human life. Nursing research addresses questions, concerns, and issues encountered in aspects of the nursing profession, including advancing nursing science, generating nursing theory, and improving nursing practice. Applied research examines how basic principles and procedures can be used to solve problems encountered in life. Clinical research is an example of applied research and focuses on improving the practice in various health care fields (including human and animal health). Clinical nursing research examines ways to enhance the health and well-being of clients and nurses while providing solid evidence to guide and improve all aspects of nursing care delivery. Nursing research studies may also have an educational or a theoretical focus. When research-generated nursing knowledge results in improved client outcomes, enhances the professional practice environment, or contains health care costs, the research has practical applications for client care. When new or unresolved client care or professional nursing issues arise, nurses can conduct research to solve the problem. Therefore, research guides practice, and practice generates new ideas for research.

Take Note!

Incorporating research is not optional; it is a critical part of the profession.

According to the American Nurses Association *Nursing Scope and Standards of Practice* (2021, p. 100), nurse generalists integrate research into professional practice with Standard 14: Scholarly Inquiry:

1. Generate questions in clinical practice that might be answered by through scholarly inquiry.
2. Use currently available evidence knowledge along with nursing expertise and client values and preferences to guide practice.
3. Participate in evidence-based practice.
4. Use evidence to increase knowledge and enhance nursing abilities, skills, and judgment.
5. Share peer-reviewed and relevant research findings with colleagues for practice integration.
6. Use evidence and nursing research when proposing changes and improving nursing practice quality.
7. Promote the value of research and scholarly inquiry into personal practice and health care setting policies and protocols.
8. Assure that ethical principles of research are followed in practice and health care settings
9. Critique nursing research reports for application into practice.

Baccalaureate nursing programs provide a natural forum for the incorporation of research into practice. One of the hallmarks of a bachelor of science in nursing (BSN) degree is a research course that prepares graduates for engagement in scholarly endeavors and evidence-based practice (EBP). The American Association of Colleges of Nursing (AACN, 2021) published re-envisioned essentials for BSN graduates also contain statements about nursing scholarship that includes research utilization and EBP. According to *The Essentials: Core Competencies for Professional Nursing Education* (AACN, 2021), BSN graduates are expected to "apply theory and research-based knowledge from the arts, humanities and sciences" (p. 29), "advance the scholarship of nursing" (p. 40), ... "integrate best evidence into nursing practice" (p. 41), and "promote the ethical conduct of scholarly activities" (p. 41). Typical educational activities include:

1. Reading and critiquing nursing research studies for the quality of evidence effectively
2. Finding incidences of nurses using research findings to guide practice
3. Developing a sense of inquiry about nursing phenomena
4. Participating in research projects when opportunities arise
5. Learning the processes of collecting, organizing, categorizing, and analyzing data
6. Identifying nursing research and evidence-based practice questions
7. Developing an evidence-based project
8. Disseminating information from a research study or evidence-based project with others
9. Initiating evidence-based changes in clinical practice

To use research and other forms of evidence effectively in practice, nurses should possess a solid understanding of the research process, a keen ability to critique research studies, comprehensive analysis skills, the creative capability to synthesize evidence from a variety of sources, and effective strategies to overcome obstacles to facilitate using research and other forms of evidence in practice.

THE RESEARCH PROCESS IN NURSING

The research process consists of a series of rigorous, logical steps of inquiry. Nurses must be familiar with the research process to critique nursing research studies effectively. Complete understanding of and comfort with the research process develops with time and practice.

The process starts with a nurse's query about some aspect of nursing that might arise during clinical practice or that seems interesting (Box 10.1, Professional Building Blocks, "Raising Questions for Research"). The **research process** structures the systematic investigation of that question, discovers answers, reports findings, and generates future questions on the topic. The process follows scientific methods, so that nursing research

- has an identifiable order.
- includes controls over factors not being investigated.
- includes gathering of evidence about the question.
- is built on a theoretical framework.
- operates for the purpose of applying results to improve nursing practice, generate theory, or expand nursing science.

10.1 Professional Building Blocks
Raising Questions for Research

The most significant step in the nursing research process may be the first one—the identification and articulation of a question. When nurses seek to find the best way to practice, they become accountable for asking questions that reflect the sensitivity necessary to better understand all that falls within the domain of nursing. Nurses identify potential research questions when they encounter clinical practice problems. Because nursing theory and practice are deeply intertwined, research questions may also arise when nurses identify a gap in theory and practice. Some potential areas for research studies include:

- Nursing assessments, interventions, characteristics, and responsibilities
- Facilitating factors for nurse–client relationships
- Environmental factors to promote and maintain health and well-being, health and disease trajectories, and client adjustment to illness and other life transitions

Clearly and concisely stated questions are essential to provide direction for studies. The successful execution of clinically relevant nursing research studies is most likely when clinical nurses and nurse researchers collaborate.

Take Note!
The purposes of nursing research are to improve nursing practice, generate new nursing theory, and expand nursing science.

Quantitative and Qualitative Approaches

Two research approaches to developing nursing knowledge can broadly categorize the types of studies: the quantitative approach and the qualitative approach. In the earliest years of nursing research, the high value placed on the scientific method led to the primary use of quantitative approaches. However, nurse researchers can also use qualitative approaches to develop subjective information when investigating human emotional, social, and existential responses to factors affecting well-being, such as illness, life transitions, or lifestyle changes.

Both research approaches have a common purpose—to gain a better understanding of the world. Evidence generated through research provides nurses with better reasoning behind the actions they take in clinical settings and eliminates practicing by tradition or rote memory. **Quantitative research** seeks to identify specific factors for desired outcomes or confirm theory through explanation. It focuses on objectivity and relies upon numerical operations to explain and make predictions. In contrast, **qualitative research** aims to discover, deeply understand, and find meaning in human subjective experiences. Use of personal narratives and rich, observational descriptions serve as data sources in qualitative research. The qualitative researcher analyzes words and observations to discover personal meanings, lived experiences, customs and worldviews, and new theories. Because nursing addresses both subjective and objective phenomena, both approaches contribute equally to nursing science.

The difference between the two research approaches can be categorized by the key assumptions each makes related to the nature of reality, relationships, truth, the role of values, reasoning, types of data to collect, best methods for data collection, best data analysis techniques, and the overall goals (Polit & Beck, 2021). These two approaches are further summarized in Table 10.1.

Appreciating the complexity of nursing phenomena and valuing subjective experiences as legitimate foci of nursing research, Artinian (1988) noted that nurses use various qualitative approaches, including participant observation and in-depth interviewing. Cohen and Tripp-Reimer (1988) supported ethnography as a significant qualitative research approach to help nurses understand cultural differences, stating that "ethnography is a method designed to describe a culture. The ethnographer seeks to understand another way of life from the native's point of view" (p. 226).

Qualitative research enables nurses to discover individualized and human phenomena surrounding health and illness. For example, phenomenology looks at the "lived experience" of a particular life transition, a clinical experience, or a specific illness or surgery. Grounded theory methodology is an approach that seeks to outline a basic social process or generate a theory based upon participant data. Hermeneutic inquiry seeks to find the deep, personal meaning of an experience. Historical studies examine artifacts from a particular era to determine what people did in the past that may be applicable today.

Steps in the Research Process

Whether the nurse researcher chooses a quantitative or qualitative approach, the overall steps in the research process are essentially the same. The study question determines which approach would be the best.

The process is a sequence of 11 steps during which researchers make decisions to plan and execute a study. While engaged in the research process, the investigator may not necessarily complete a step but rather may revisit it while planning and executing a study. Knowledge of the research process steps discussed in the subsequent sections will facilitate the nurse's use of findings in practice.

Step 1: Focus on the Clinical Problem Area

All nurses can identify problems in professional practice. Whenever a nurse identifies a gap between what is and what could be in practice, a clinical problem has arisen. Nursing research is one option to resolve such clinical problems.

Once a problem area has been identified, nurses can discover the state of knowledge about the problem by reviewing current practice protocols, research, and other forms of information on the identified topic. They can derive questions from the theories or conceptual models used to guide practice in their clinical settings or

◼ TABLE 10.1 Quantitative and Qualitative Assumptions in Nursing Research

Research Approach	Assumption	
	Qualitative	**Quantitative**
View of reality	Researcher focuses on multiple subjective constructed realities with an openness to understand naturalistic phenomena that can be gained through knowing that the whole is greater than the sum of all its parts.	Researcher focuses on objective reality seen as singular; the process for discovering reality uses reductionism, which proposes that knowledge of the whole can be gained through knowledge of the parts.
View of relationships	Researcher interacts with the subject and believes that a unity exists between them and that both are integral to the research process.	Researcher distances self from subjects and believes that boundaries must exist to ensure objectivity.
View of truth	Researcher sees the world as dynamic and believes that truth is discovered in the changing patterns of the world; the researcher's goals are to discover uniqueness, valuing differences as well as similarities.	Researcher sees the world as stable and predictable and believes that the truth is discovered in common laws, principles, and norms; the researcher's goal is generalization.
View of values	Researcher should remain neutral during the process and not introduce any biases or values as the goal is total objectivity in the process	Researcher acknowledges the inevitability of introducing values and biases into the process but tries to hold these in abeyance during the process and introduce them if they add value to the final results.
View of reasoning process	Researcher uses deductive reasoning and may determine hypotheses to test prior to study execution.	Researcher uses inductive reasoning and may end up generating hypotheses for future testing.
View of best data	Researcher clearly defines variables of interest, uses standardized tools to collect desired information (objective, numerical data desired), follows a prescribed collection plan, controls for contextual factors, and collects information from large samples that represent a population.	Researcher enters the research situation with no preconceived notions or set plan to collect anonymous numerical subjective data, adjusts data collection procedures as needed, makes no attempt to control contextual factors, and uses small numbers of participants who provide rich information.
View of best data analysis techniques	Researcher uses descriptive and inferential statistics.	Researcher uses narratives along with descriptions of context.
View of overall goal	Researcher aims to discover and make generalizations.	Researcher aims to discover and describe in-depth and holistic understandings.

From Gray, J. R., Grove, S. K., & Sutherland, S. (2017). *Burns and Grove's, The practice of nursing research: Appraisal, synthesis, and generation of evidence* (8th ed.). Elsevier; Polit, D. F., & Beck, C. (2021). *Nursing research: Generating and assessing evidence for nursing practice* (11th ed.). Wolters-Kluwer.

educational programs or by seeking out ideas from external sources such as faculty, peers, or the nursing research priorities published by the National Institute of Nursing Research (NINR) or other professional nursing organizations (Box 10.2, Learning, Knowing, and Growing, "Identifying Priority Areas for Research").

According to Polit and Beck (2021), the development of the research problem incorporates the following sequence of events:

1. Select a general area of interest about which you have questions.
2. Narrow and evaluate the topic with a mentor or expert.

3. Establish the benefits of the investigation. Who would benefit? What relevance and/or applications would the study have to the profession? How important would the findings be? In other words, so what?
4. Ensure that the selected problem is amenable to either quantitative or qualitative methodology (or both).
5. Verify that the problem is not primarily a moral issue.
6. Critique the feasibility of studying the problem in terms of time, subject and resource availability, and costs (actual and potential).

10.2 Learning, Knowing, and Growing

Identifying Priority Areas for Research

Many professional associations and governmental agencies have designated priority areas for research. For example:

- *Oncology Nursing Society*: Ongoing research initiatives on symptom science, health disparities, and palliative and psychosocial care; has established a research agenda for 2019 to 2022 (https://onf.ons.org/onf/46/6/research-agenda-oncology-nursing-society-2019-2022).
- *Canadian Association of Schools of Nursing*: Sets research priorities for Canadian nurses, including care of vulnerable populations, health care equity, home health and primary nursing care, care of older adults across the care spectrum, role and scope of practice, and the value of registered nurses and/or nurse practitioners to health care (https://www.casn.ca/wp-content/uploads/2018/12/Research-Priorities-2018-EN.pdf).
- *National Institute of Nursing Research*: Sets research priorities for American nurses on a variety of topics of interest (www.ninr-nih.gov) and has published research priorities in its 2016 strategic plan at https://www.ninr.nih.gov/sites/files/docs/NINR_StratPlan2016_reduced.pdf

Visiting one of these websites or those of other nursing organizations may help inspire your research efforts.

Step 2: Perform an Initial Literature Review

An initial review of the literature enables nurse researchers to obtain a broad understanding and general background on the problem to be studied. Once the researcher has raised a question, this initial review of the literature is helpful in

- identifying the major variables in the area of interest.
- finding out what is already known.
- gathering feasibility data on the needs for problem investigation.
- sharpening the focus of the problem to be investigated.

A literature review should make the researcher aware of all the possible relevant materials available regarding a problem of interest. Tips for searching for information about the problem include typing in key terms contained within the problem statement using a computerized database of scientific and research literature. Expanding the search to include literature from other disciplines besides nursing facilitates finding more relevant literature (medicine, psychology, social work, or business depending upon the nature of the problem). Nurse investigators frequently consult research librarians to assist in this step (and step 4) of the research process. Along with reading the existing literature, researchers must appraise each research study by assessing its strengths and weaknesses. A **research critique** points out the strengths and weaknesses of a study and helps researchers discover gaps in the current literature.

Helpful sources for locating resource materials include indexes from nursing, related disciplines, and popular literature; abstracting services from nursing and related disciplines; computer searches of appropriate databases; dictionaries; encyclopedias; guides; and directories. Most reference librarians can provide tremendous help to nurse researchers in locating and using these materials.

Frequently, those conducting qualitative research avoid reviewing the literature before collecting data to avoid developing preconceived ideas about the topic area. In quantitative research, such a knowledge base makes it possible for the researcher to proceed to the next stage of research: specifying the problem and defining the variables.

Take Note!
The initial literature review should answer some questions about the topic of interest, identify others who are interested in the topic, and help the researcher develop a knowledge base of what is currently known about the topic.

Step 3: Specify the Problem and the Defining Variables

Researchers must specify a problem and identify key variables or phenomena within the nursing domain to be investigated. The nurse researcher may investigate a client aspect that affects the nurse–client therapeutic relationship, a phenomenon that impacts client health, ways to enhance client care quality and safety, the effectiveness of a specific nursing intervention, any aspect of the delivery of nursing care services, environmental elements influencing health and well-being, professional practice issues, or any combination of these facets of nursing.

Clear articulation of the problem incorporates the identification of the phenomenon to be investigated. In quantitative research, a phenomenon of interest is generally called a "variable." A **variable** is a characteristic, trait, property, or condition. If a variable is purposefully manipulated by the researcher to have a direct effect on another variable, it is an **independent variable**. A variable that is observed, measured, and presumed to be influenced by or related in some special way to the independent variable is a **dependent variable**. Quantitative studies may have one or more independent and dependent variables (Box 10.3, Professional Prototypes, "Variables in Quantitative Research"). Variables do not exist in qualitative research because the purpose may be to identify key phenomena surrounding a client or nurse experience.

10.3 Professional Prototypes

Variables in Quantitative Research

Following is an example of a study with one variable that is manipulated and another that is observed and measured.

What is the relationship between specific parenting guidance by the professional nurse and the development of positive nutritional habits of the toddler? In this investigation, the independent variable is the specific parenting guidance, the dependent variable is the toddler's nutritional habits, and the approach to studying the variables is quantitative.

To make these variables measurable, the researcher must determine exactly what is meant by each variable, that is, what constitutes parenting guidance and what constitutes positive nutritional habits in the toddler. The statement of the problem may be in the form of a question or a declaration. In both the cases, this problem statement must also clearly identify who and what are to be studied.

Step 4: Establish Tentative Propositions—Hypotheses and Second Literature Review

After the nurse researcher has clarified the problem under investigation, studied the available data, and recalled observations from professional experience, they may formulate a hypothesis, a formal statement that predicts or explains the relationships between two or more variables (Polit & Beck, 2021). Not all studies require that the researcher generates a hypothesis; for example, questions of a descriptive, qualitative, and exploratory nature do not need hypotheses but instead generate questions. However, for studies requiring manipulation of an independent variable with the purpose of influencing a dependent variable, hypotheses must be stated and tested.

Nurses have excellent opportunities to form hunches about the relationships among variables they observe in practice. The hypothesis is like a bridge; it connects theory with those observations and is derived from observations, reasoning, and theoretical bases.

Hypotheses in quantitative studies are tested statistically in relation to the laws of chance. Thus, they are based on statistical probability and incur an element of risk of reaching an incorrect conclusion. How much risk can be afforded is a judgment of the investigator, but when permanent or serious consequences are involved, the investigator cannot afford to take too many risks. Because hypotheses sometimes force the investigator to infer from the sample findings an interpretation about the population, the researcher uses probability statistics (level of significance) to determine the likelihood that the relationship between the variables results from something other than chance.

When the researcher is determining hypotheses, additional review of the literature is used to evaluate testing procedures and to project a research design appropriate for investigating the variable(s). The literature review can be used to learn what investigative methods have been used, how data have been collected and analyzed, and what has and has not been successful in previous research.

Take Note!

In quantitative studies, hypotheses declare the researcher's proposition about the relationship between variables and then serve as the means for testing the proposed relationship.

Step 5: Determine a Suitable Research Design

The nurse researcher selects the type of research design suitable for the study based on the research questions or hypotheses:

- A descriptive design answers questions about the nature of presently occurring events.
- An experimental design tests the effects of manipulating one or more specific variables on other variables.
- A historical design is based on the desire to describe or evaluate past events.
- In ethnographic research, the researcher frequently acts as a member of or observes a group. Detailed interviews followed by participant validation of data serve as the means to capture the essence of an experience in phenomenology.

Step 6: Develop a Research Methodology: Data Collection Methods and Instruments

After the approach is selected for a particular study, the nurse researcher decides on the appropriate method for gathering data and then selects instruments for data collection depending on the purpose of the research. Instruments are generally categorized under three methods: observation, questioning, and measurement.

Examples of data collection instruments include critical incidents, tests, interviews, questionnaires, checklists, records, scales, and physical measurement techniques. The researcher strives to select a measurement tool that is appropriate to answer the research question, is unbiased, and has precision in measuring the variables being studied. For quantitative studies, the researcher carefully analyzes available measurement tools to determine instrument validity (the extent to which the tool actually measures the variable of interest) and reliability (consistency of variable measurement). In qualitative studies, the researcher exercises caution to eliminate any personal biases that could interfere with objective data collection. The quality of data generated for a study relies on careful selection of data collection methods.

Knafl and Webster (1988) pointed out how the researcher's data collection, analysis of those data, and reporting are likely to vary according to the purpose of the study. They described four purposes of qualitative research:

1. *Illustration*: The researcher aims to identify qualitative examples of specific quantitative variables.
2. *Instrumentation*: The researcher aims to collect data that serve as the basis for developing an instrument to describe and measure perceptions of some phenomenon of interest to nursing.
3. *Description*: The researcher aims to "translate the data into a form that would facilitate an accurate, complete description" (p. 200) of a phenomenon of interest to nursing by identifying and delineating the major themes.
4. *Theory building*: The researcher aims to conceptually explain the phenomenon under study.

Mixed-methods research studies (also called triangulated, multimethod, or integrated designs) combine quantitative and qualitative research methods within a single study. Blending quantitative and qualitative approaches emerged in the early 21st century in the field of nursing. By integrating the two approaches, researchers can capitalize on the strengths of each approach while minimizing their weaknesses. Typically, one method dominates the study when mixed methods are used (Polit & Beck, 2021). For example, a nurse studying the effects of nurse job satisfaction on client care outcomes (quantitative approach) might want to know about the lived experiences of the nurse working on a specific unit that have enhanced or reduced the nurse's job satisfaction (qualitative approach).

In addition to selecting instruments for data collection during this stage of research, the nurse must determine the composition of the sample (individuals who will participate in a study), establish a process for collecting data from the sample, and prepare a format for data collection (which may include designing specific forms), data classification, and data storage for later analysis. The criteria for inclusion in a sample must be clearly described, and the method for selecting subjects must be appropriate. The number of sample subjects must meet statistical requirements for the nurse to draw appropriate conclusions about the findings for quantitative studies.

Step 7: Ensure an Ethical Process

Research requires honesty and integrity. **Research ethics** are principles by which researchers abide to ensure truth in scientific studies, protection of the human rights of participants, balance of the risks and benefits of a study, and prevention of exploitation of vulnerable individuals. The importance of research ethics came to the forefront after reports of inhumane and unethical treatment sustained by prisoners during medical experiments in Nazi Germany. In 1949, the Nuremburg Code was established to protect human subjects in biomedical experiments. The researcher bears the responsibility for protecting the human rights of people who participate in the research study. This protection process is achieved primarily through informed consent and protection from harm.

- **Informed consent** means that the researcher provides subjects with a clear description about the study, how they meet study criteria, requirements for participation, information of study withdrawal, and potential hazards. Subjects must understand study details so that they can freely consent to participate. Even after giving informed consent, a subject can decide to withdraw from a study at any time.
- **Protection from harm** means that the investigator will not knowingly do anything that will harm or abuse the subjects. Investigators also work to preserve subject **anonymity** (keeping the identification of all subjects confidential).

Most research institutions have a formal process for approving research proposals before implementation. An **institutional review board (IRB)** meets on a regular schedule to review research proposals, verify that investigators have fully considered the ethics involved, and ensure that the study meets scientific standards. In health care settings, nurses sometimes hold IRB membership. Because they are client advocates and have holistic views of health care, nurses sometimes identify potentially harmful research treatments that other IRB members may overlook. A research study must always be subjected to IRB review. Depending on the potential for harm, coercion, and loss of anonymity, some EBP, research utilization, and quality improvement projects may also require IRB scrutiny (Melnyk & Fineout-Overholt, 2019; Polit & Beck, 2021).

To ensure truth in research, the researcher assumes responsibility for honesty when collecting and analyzing data and when reporting research findings. For-profit and nonprofit organizations frequently fund research studies. Corporations fill gaps in research funding to bring new health products to the market. The investigator bears the responsibility for using the highest standards of scientific inquiry and reporting findings honestly at all time. When extramural funding (public, nonprofit, or for-profit organizations) has

been received for the research study, the investigator has an obligation to report the source of funds within the written report (Blumenstyk, 2001; Polit & Beck, 2021).

Step 8: Collect Data

After protection of human rights and well-being for all subjects has been ensured, data collection can begin. However, before any subject associated with an institution can be approached, the researcher must have approval from appropriate agency personnel. The subjects of the research must also sign an informed consent form that they have received information about the purpose of the study, their role in study participation, how they can cease participation, and any potential ill effects from participation.

The researcher or a specified data collector orients each subject clearly and concisely to the data collection method and then administers the data collection instrument to each subject in the same manner. Throughout this implementation stage, the researcher follows the written proposal in the methodology as closely as possible. While collecting data, the researcher records the data on the prepared forms. The data are then classified and organized for analysis.

Step 9: Analyze Data and Report Findings

Once data are collected, the researcher organizes them in a manner that makes them amenable to analysis. If the researcher's goal is simply to display the data collected, no analysis other than a narrative description and display tables is needed. However, if the researcher aims to infer some characteristics about a population or to evaluate some relationship among variables, the organized data must be subjected to statistical analysis. Many researchers consult a statistician for help with this step. Computations may be required. If hypotheses have been stated, statistical testing by hand or by computer of those hypotheses must be done.

Based on accurate data analysis, the researcher reports and summarizes the findings exactly as they occurred. All data collected for purposes of testing the hypotheses must be reported. Tables, charts, and graphs used to present data should be pertinent, clear, and well labeled and should be discussed in the text of the research report. The reports of the findings are then used to draw conclusions.

Step 10: Make Conclusions and Outline Implications

For quantitative research studies, the researcher must determine the meaning of the findings, articulate their value to nursing, and link them to the theoretical foundation(s) guiding the study. Findings are analyzed first by inspecting the statistical tests performed to test the hypotheses or evaluate the data. The researcher then interprets the numerical analysis. With hypothesis testing, the findings may support the predicted relationship with demonstrated statistical significance (the findings were not attributable to chance alone), may not be in the predicted direction, may be contradictory, or may indicate an unpredicted relationship. Sometimes statistical significance has little practical significance. Practical significance indicates that the results add to the body of nursing knowledge or lead to major changes in clinical outcomes. For example, the tobacco industry has argued in the court system that the link between cigarette smoking and lung cancer is not statistically significant. However, research studies reveal a high degree of correlation (strong relationship) between smoking and the development of lung cancer.

For qualitative studies, the researcher determines the meaning of the study and its value to professional nursing by identifying the impact of the new knowledge generated by the study. The conceptual overview generated by a qualitative study may have profound importance to those working with clients with similar conditions. Qualitative studies frequently provide a foundation for hypothesis generation and research instrument development for future quantitative research studies.

Based on the analysis and interpretation of data, the researcher might make generalizations about what the data mean and whether the data can be applied to groups that differ from the sample. Generalizations should emerge only from the findings, and the researcher should not go beyond the data as a result of the excitement generated by scientific discovery.

Study implications usually relate to one of the four aspects of professional nursing: clinical practice with clients, professional education, clinical practice environments, and ideas for additional nursing research. In a section of the research study called "Recommendations," the implications for practice (i.e., how the findings affect the nursing process with clients) should be discussed. Recommendations for the education of

practitioners and for future research are also usually given. If the recommendations are clearly and concisely stated and derived logically, clinical nurses can find the study valuable and incorporate the findings in practice.

Step 11: Disseminate Findings: The Written Report and Professional Presentations

Research completed but not compiled into a report is wasted. Some experts argue that the research process is not complete until it is shared in writing or some other public medium. Characteristics of an effective research report are brevity, clarity, and complete objectivity.

Although faculty or other institutional requirements, or a particular style manual, may influence the form of the report, research reports usually follow the outline of the research process presented in this chapter. Most outlines include the problem statement, review of literature, methods of investigation, presentation of findings, discussion of analyses and conclusions, bibliographic data, and appendices. The reader is directed to a nursing research book or a writing style manual for specific guidance in developing each part of the written research report. Sometimes space limitations in journals prevent authors from including details about studies accepted for publication.

In addition to written reports, nurse researchers present study findings by giving oral presentations and presenting posters. Like the written report, posters and presentations describe the research methodology, present findings, articulate the significance to practice, and generate ideas for future study on the topic.

Take Note!
An effective research report is one that is brief, clear, and completely objective. Its recommended practice changes must stay within the confines of the data collected. A good research study outlines study limitations and suggests areas for further research on the study topic.

▌ QUESTIONS FOR REFLECTION

1. What questions do you have related to the research process and how to critique nursing research studies?

2. Referring back to the "Real-Life Reflections" vignette, do you think Jessica would be able to better convince Malika of the value of the studies she had read if they were qualitative or if they were quantitative? Why?

3. Would you be interested in starting or participating in a nursing research journal club? Why or why not? If so, how could you make journal club participation a reality?

NURSING RESEARCH UTILIZATION AND EVIDENCE-BASED PRACTICE

Nurses use many forms of evidence to guide clinical practice, including nursing research. Over the past two decades, nurses have made great progress in increasing the use of scientific evidence in clinical practice. Sherwood and Barnsteiner (2009) define **evidence-based practice** as "practice based on the best available evidence that also incorporates patient values and preferences and clinician judgment and expertise" (p. 134). Polit and Beck (2021, p. 29) and Melnyk and Fineout-Overholt (2019, p. 18) identify seven levels of evidence and rank them from the least to the most rigorous. The levels rating scale by Melnyk and Fineout-Overhold (2019) focuses on evidence for interventions and treatments. The two rating scales have similarities and are combined as follows rated from the least to most rigorous into nine levels of evidence:

- Level 9: Nonresearch sources like media reports, expert opinions (individuals or committees), internal evidence (e.g., quality improvement data), or case studies

- Level 8: Single descriptive, qualitative or physiologic studies (nonexperimental research)

- Level 7: Systematic reviews of descriptive or physiologic studies or metasyntheses of qualitative studies

- Level 6: Single correlational, case control, cohort, or observational studies (nonexperimental research)

- Level 5: Systematic reviews of correlational, case control, cohort, or observational studies

- Level 4: Nonrandomized clinical trials (quasi-experimental research)

- Level 3: Systematic reviews of nonrandomized clinical trials

- Level 2: Single randomized or nonrandomized clinical trials

- Level 1: Systematic reviews or meta-analyses of all relevant randomized clinical trials

Polit and Beck (2021) do not specify professional nurse and client opinions as a level of evidence. Nurses sometimes base care strategies on client preferences or the successful past use of a nursing assessment or intervention. Table 10.2 compares and contrasts the processes of nursing research utilization and EBP. Nursing research utilization is used only in nursing, while EBP ideally includes all interprofessional team members.

A clinically relevant question initiates the processes of EBP and research utilization. Melnyk and

TABLE 10.2	**Comparison of Nursing Research Utilization and Evidence-Based Practice**	
	Nursing Research Utilization	**Evidence-Based Practice**
Purpose	Establish nursing practice based on scientific evidence	Establish best practice guidelines for various clinical problems
Participants	Professional nurses	Interdisciplinary health team
Sources of evidence	Quantitative research study findings Qualitative research study findings	Research study findings Quality improvement data Retrospective and concurrent chart audits Risk management data Infection control data Local, national, and international standards Pathophysiology of clinical problem Cost-effectiveness data Benchmarking data Expert opinions Logical reasoning Clinical experience Individual client situations Client preference data

(continued)

TABLE 10.2   Comparison of Nursing Research Utilization and Evidence-Based Practice (*continued*)

	Nursing Research Utilization	Evidence-Based Practice
Processes	Critiques of research reports of topic of interest Integrative review of research reports Innovation subjected to a planned change process Evaluation of results of care innovation	Group meetings of one component of the health care team for issues related to a specific discipline Group meetings of interdisciplinary health team members to develop critical paths or other care pathways Interdisciplinary review of current clinical needs, practices, established guidelines, and care principles Extensive systematic review of published research on issue to be addressed from all health care disciplines if the guideline will be interdisciplinary or from one health care discipline if guideline will be specific to a special group Guideline review by experts, clinicians, and clients Guidelines tested for effective clinical use Guidelines subjected to continuous review
Outcomes	Improved client outcomes Improved professional practice Research-based nursing care and clinical practice protocols	Improved client outcomes Clinical guidelines for client care based on solid evidence that yields the most benefit for the least possible cost
Dissemination of information	Agency newsletter Letters to staff Staff email Electronic or printed agency clinical policy manual Staff in-services Nursing publications Nursing specialty organization websites	Agency newsletter Staff email Electronic or printed agency policy manuals Professional publications Websites of professional organizations, large health care agencies, Agency for Healthcare Research and Quality, the National Guideline Clearinghouse, American Medical Association, American Association of Health Care Plans

From Gray, J. R., Grove, S. K., & Sutherland, S. (2017). *Burns and Grove's, The practice of nursing research: Appraisal, synthesis, and generation of evidence* (8th ed.). Elsevier; Jennings, B. M., & Loan, L. A. (2001). Misconceptions among nurses about evidence-based practice. *Journal of Nursing Scholarship, 33,* 121–127.

Fineout-Overholt (2019) propose a standardized question format that will result in retrieval of the most compatible information when conducting a literature search on a clinical topic. This format uses the acronym "PICOT":

- *P*atient population
- *I*ntervention or issue of interest
- *C*omparison intervention or status
- *O*utcome
- *T*ime frame for the "I" to achieve the "O." (p. 759)

In most research utilization and EBP projects, the goal is to improve client outcomes, professional nurse work environments, or cost-effectiveness of care delivery.

Research Utilization

Research utilization is a systematic process to incorporate research study findings into clinical practice. Polit and Beck (2021) view research utilization as a narrow term and define it as "the use of findings from a study in a practical application unrelated to the original

research" (p. 802). However, nurses have been using research findings in practice for decades (Box 10.4, Professional Prototypes, "The Origins of Nursing Research Utilization").

10.4 Professional Prototypes

The Origins of Nursing Research Utilization

Florence Nightingale instituted utilization of nursing research more than a century ago. Using a systematic approach, Nightingale collected data and presented detailed results in bar graphs, pie charts, and color-coded tables to highlight how improving sanitation and using trained nurses reduced mortality of ill and wounded soldiers during the Crimean War. She presented her findings, published in *Notes on Nursing* (Nightingale, 1860) to the British government, which subsequently increased funding for the care of soldiers so that Nightingale's methods could be implemented (McDonald, 2001).

Every medication that nurses administer on a daily basis is an example of research utilization. The U.S. Food and Drug Administration requires that the efficacy of a medication has been substantiated through a series of randomized clinical trials. A randomized clinical trial is a research design in which subjects are randomly assigned to experimental (to receive the investigational drug) and control (to receive a placebo) groups, with stringent control of variables outside the study to determine whether a medication produces its stated therapeutic effects. Medical devices also undergo a series of scientific tests. Because health care is a scientifically based discipline, all health care team members use research on a daily basis. To stay abreast of practice changes, professional nurses must read the current nursing research literature and apply new findings to their practice as appropriate (Box 10.5, Professional Building Blocks, "Benefits of a Research Bases for Clinical Nursing Practice").

Research utilization may be as simple as one nurse changing individual practice based upon what they read in a research article or as complex as changing nursing practice standards. Research findings are often delayed in dissemination because they need to be reviewed by experts, and sometimes journals decide to have issues focused on a specific topic related to nursing. In addition, there are barriers for research utilization in practice settings (see Concepts in Practice, "Making a Case for Research Utilization in Practice").

Research findings can be used in many ways in professional practice. An individual nurse could read a qualitative nursing research article exploring fatigue

Concepts in Practice [IDEA] ──▶ [PLAN] ──▶ [ACTION]

Making a Case for Research Utilization in Practice

Tony works on a rehabilitation unit with many clients who, when first admitted, cannot turn themselves. Over the past year, he and several of his coworkers have experienced increased back pain as a result of lifting and turning immobile clients. Tony decides to conduct a literature review to see if any new equipment might be available to facilitate turning immobile clients in bed. He discovers that new slider sheet systems (sheets made of slick, parachute-like material) have the potential to reduce muscular and perceived nurse effort while turning clients in bed (Theou et al., 2011). When Tony suggests using the slider sheets to see if they reduce back strain on the unit, his colleagues tease him and call him "professor." His work setting does not permit him time to prepare a proposal for using research-based findings on the job.

- What barriers to research utilization do Tony face?
- How might he address the situation to ameliorate the issue of back pain among the health care team?

  Later in this chapter, we will revisit Tony and see how implemented research utilization and EBP resolve the issues he faces.

in people who receive hemodialysis and incorporates the finding by being more attentive and sensitive to increased needs for uninterrupted rest periods when planning and implementing care with these clients. Nurses also perform quality improvement studies within health care organizations using new research findings (see Chapter 18, "Quality Improvement: Enhancing Patient Safety and Health Care Quality"). Many nurses opt to use published models for research utilization and EBP. A review of the literature for this chapter revealed over 50 models for research utilization and EBP, with some solely nursing-focused and others taking an interprofessional approach. Some models can be readily accessed on the internet and others require user registration and fees. Box 10.6, Professional Building Blocks, "Models for Nursing Research Utilization and Evidence-Based Practice," provides a brief list of models for professional consideration. Research utilization, EBP, and quality improvement all begin with the identification of actual or potential clinical problems or issues.

10.5 Professional Building Blocks

Benefits of a Research Bases for Clinical Nursing Practice

- A solid, sound, scientific foundation for practice
- Enhanced self-confidence, autonomy, critical-thinking skills, and professional self-concept
- Cost-effective client care
- Increased client and job satisfaction and quality of care
- Improved client outcomes
- A stimulus for collaborative practice, retention, and recruitment
- An improved image of nursing
- An ever-increasing scientific nursing knowledge base

10.6 Professional Building Blocks

Models for Nursing Research Utilization and Evidence-Based Practice

- ACE STAR Model of Knowledge Transformation (Academic Center for Evidence-Based Practice, 2009)
- Advancing Research and Clinical Practice through Close Collaboration (ARCC) Model (Melnyk & Fineout-Overholt, 2019)
- Diffusion of Innovations (Rogers, 1995)
- Iowa Model of Evidence-Based Practice to Promote Quality Care (Titler et al., 2001)
- Model of Evidence-Based Practice Change (Larabee, 2009)
- Clinical Scholar Model (Schultz, 2008)
- Stetler Model of Evidence-Based Practice (Stetler, 2010)
- Disciplined Clinical Inquiry (Malloch & Porter-O'Grady, 2006)
- The Johns Hopkins Nursing Evidence-Based Practice Model (Dearholt & Dang, 2012)

Evidence-Based Practice

EBP has become a standard mode of care delivery. Evidence-based medicine, evidence-based physical therapy, evidence-based nutrition, and evidence-based nursing provide mechanisms for the delivery of best practices for health care. Nursing research provides nurses with the opportunity to supply their own body of evidence for clinical practice guidelines. However, the support for EBP does not rely solely on research findings but includes clinical experience, quality improvement data, logical reasoning, recognized authority, and client satisfaction, situations, experiences, and values (Melnyk & Fineout-Overholt, 2019; Polit & Beck, 2021).

Some health care organizations encourage and support nurses in implementing evidence-based nursing projects. Malloch and Porter-O'Grady (2006) outlined a model of disciplined clinical inquiry to guide the process of evidence-based patient care (EBPC). The EBPC model, which is client-centered, resource-efficient, knowledge-driven, and clinically appropriate, includes the following five phases (Malloch & Porter-O'Grady, 2006, p. 37):

- Phase 1: Needs assessment and environmental scan
- Phase 2: Learning and knowledge generation
- Phase 3: Knowledge assimilation
- Phase 4: Knowledge application
- Phase 5: Appraisal/evaluation

Melnyk and Fineout-Overholt (2019, p. 10) outlined a different approach to EBP consisting of seven critical steps. Melnyk and Fineout-Overholt's process requires a highly refined question to be answered. The question must contain a population (P), intervention (I), comparison (C), outcome (O), and optional timing (T). Here is an example of a PICOT question: In new graduate nurses (P), what is the effect of nurse residency programs (I) on retention rate (O) compared with no nurse residency program participation (C) for the first 2 years? The steps to this approach are:

- Step 1: Cultivate a spirit of inquiry.
- Step 2: Ask the burning clinical question in PICOT format.
- Step 3: Search for and collect the most relevant, best evidence.
- Step 4: Critically appraise the evidence (i.e., rapid critical appraisal, evaluation, and synthesis).
- Step 5: Integrate the best evidence with one's clinical expertise and client preferences and values in making a practice decision or change.
- Step 6: Evaluate outcomes of the practice decision or change based on evidence.
- Step 7: Disseminate the outcomes of the EBP decision or change.

Both approaches appear to be congruent with the steps of problem-solving strategies. Malloch and Porter-O'Grady (2006) emphasized the importance of creating an organizational culture that supports nurses as they embark on learning how to assess evidence and execute EBP clinical practice changes.

Proponents of EBP view it as a means to solve clinical practice problems by making the best possible decisions related to care based on client reports, clinician observations, and research data. Systematic review of all research literature on a particular health topic provides the best form of evidence for clinical practice (Melnyk & Fineout-Overholt, 2019; Polit & Beck, 2021). Clinical practice guidelines fall into this category. In the United States, the Agency for Health Care Research and Quality (AHRQ) created the National Guideline Clearinghouse (NGC) in 1998 to offer interprofessional health team members a rich source of evidence-based clinical practice guidelines. NGC publishes free guidelines on disease management and prevention that have been generated through synthesis of recent, valid research findings along with expert commentary for each guideline. Some health care insurance companies use NGC as a basis for reimbursement (NGC, 2008).

The Cochrane Collaboration is an international organization that also provides information for health care providers based on systematic integrative reviews of controlled clinical trials. The Cochrane Collaboration charges a fee to access evidence based solely on disease management.

Currently, many health care professionals use EBP guidelines developed by the AHRQ for the treatment of urinary incontinence, low back problems, pain, depression, and prevention and treatment of pressure injuries (Malloch & Porter-O'Grady, 2006). When research data are not available on a specific clinical problem, experts who specialize in a specific area develop practice guidelines by consensus. EBP also enables health care providers to use objective and subjective ways of knowing when making client care decisions and revising clinical procedures.

EBP opponents in medicine and nursing suggest that the development of clinical practice guidelines, critical care pathways, and protocols entices practitioners to adopt a "cookbook recipe" approach to client care. The basic tenet of quality improvement initiatives specifies that elimination of variation in practice decreases the chance for error and improves quality. However, quality improvement has its roots in industrial production, and such standardization may not be as desirable in the health care setting because clients have unique characteristics and needs that may be overlooked when practitioners adhere strictly to clinical practice guidelines. In addition, consumers and third-party payers may hold health care providers accountable for actions in addition to or for not strictly following established clinical practice guidelines.

Health care organizations and individual health team members hold the key to the successful implementation of EBP. Organizations must display commitment to developing evidence-based care pathways and provide health care team members with the time and required resources. Up to 6 months may be required for the development of a single evidence-based pathway (Malloch & Porter-O'Grady, 2006).

QUESTIONS FOR REFLECTION

1. What forms of evidence do you use as a basis for clinical decision making?
2. How are client care policies, protocols, and pathways developed where you engage in clinical practice?

Models to Guide Research Utilization and Evidence-Based Practice

Since the 1970s, professional nurses have used models to guide the movement of research and evidence into practice. Some of the successful models have been borrowed from the corporate world (Rogers's diffusion of innovations theory), developed by nurse researchers (Stetler model for evidence-based practice and advancing research and clinical practice through close collaboration), or designed using interprofessional collaboration (Ottawa model of research use). Some nursing research utilization models, such as the Iowa model, contain paths for nurses to follow when they cannot find adequate research on which to base practice changes (Melnyk & Fineout-Overholt, 2019; Polit & Beck, 2021; Rycroft-Malone & Bucknall, 2010). Because no single model fits each practice setting and needs, nurses can find a variety of models for use in nursing research textbooks, in professional journals and publications, and in postings from nursing specialty organizations, academic health centers, hospitals, and corporate websites.

The following key elements appear in most of the nursing research utilization models:

1. Identifying a gap in the desired outcome
2. Articulating the clinical problem clearly and concisely
3. Reviewing research literature
4. Preparing a comprehensive report outlining key research findings
5. Selecting from one of the research-based innovations found in the literature review
6. Developing specific practice outcomes for the proposed innovation
7. Establishing an implementation plan for the innovation
8. Creating an evaluation plan development to assess the effects or practice outcomes of the innovation
9. Implementing the innovation within a practice setting
10. Evaluating the clinical effects of the innovation

Concepts in Practice, "Nursing Research Utilization in Action," returns to the example of Tony and his colleagues and shows how these elements may be implemented.

Concepts in Practice IDEA → PLAN → ACTION

Nursing Research Utilization in Action

Recall Tony and his colleagues, who experienced back pain from turning immobile clients in the rehabilitation unit. The following list illustrates the key elements specified by many nursing research utilization models and how Tony might use them to help institute new evidence-based guidelines on the unit.

1. Identify a gap in desired outcome (skin integrity maintenance).
2. Articulate the clinical problem clearly and concisely (increased back strain and perceived nurse effort when turning clients in bed).
3. Review research literature (secure, read, and critique the literature based on nurse and unlicensed assistive personnel risk factors for back strain).
4. Prepare a comprehensive report outlining key research findings (prepare a table outlining the research findings from literature reviewed on risk factors for back strain and available turning devices, along with drawing conclusions and forming clinical implications for the rehabilitation unit).
5. Select from one of the research-based innovations found in the literature review (select the slider sheet system for reduction of back strain and increased perception of effort to turn clients while in bed).
6. Develop specific practice outcomes for the proposed innovation (incidence of back strain will be reduced by 50% within 1 month of using the slider sheet system to turn clients).
7. Establish an implementation plan for the innovation (educate staff on the use of the slider sheet system, and secure staff acceptance of the system).
8. Create an evaluation plan to assess the effects or practice outcomes of the innovation (keep daily staff logs documenting incidences of back strain).
9. Implement the innovation within a practice setting (use the slider sheet system to turn clients at all times for 1 month).
10. Evaluate the clinical effects of the innovation (compare incidences of back strain before and after implementation of the slider sheet system).

Once the effectiveness of the innovation has been demonstrated, agency policy and procedures may be revised to make using the innovation standard practice.

Many nurses looking to facilitate change and innovation in practice find theories and models of research utilization helpful.

Rogers's Theory of Diffusion of Innovations

According to Rogers (1983), **diffusion** "is the process by which an innovation is communicated through certain channels over time among the members of a social system" (p. 5). Rogers defined **innovation** as "an idea, practice, or object that is perceived as new" (p. 11). In the example of Tony and his colleagues used earlier in this chapter, changing the method that nursing personnel would use to turn clients in bed (the slick sheet system) would be considered an innovation.

Rogers (1983) suggested that diffusion of innovations is useful for deciding whether to adopt an innovation (something perceived as new by those who are considering adoption). **Diffusion of innovations** is a five-stage process:

- Stage 1—Knowledge: Becoming aware of the existence of the innovation
- Stage 2—Persuasion: Forming an attitude toward the innovation
- Stage 3—Decision: Making the choice for adoption or rejection of the innovation
- Stage 4—Implementation: Using the innovation
- Stage 5—Confirmation: Seeking reinforcement of the decision

Reversal of the decision can occur at any time during the implementation and confirmation stages. Concepts in Practice, "Rogers's Diffusion of Innovations Process in Action," returns to the example of Tony and his colleagues and shows how these elements may be implemented.

Concepts in Practice IDEA → PLAN → ACTION

Rogers's Diffusion of Innovations Process in Action

Tony incorporates Roger's diffusion of innovations theory in his quest to determine whether the slick sheet system will help relieve the back pain that results from turning immobile clients:

- *Knowledge*: Tony becomes aware of the slick sheet system, a research-validated method for client turning.
- *Persuasion*: Tony asks his colleagues what they would think about trying the slick sheet systems for turning for a month.
- *Decision*: Tony's staff decides to give the slick sheet system a try to see if it makes a difference.
- *Implementation*: Staff members use the slick sheet system and keep a log about how their backs feel at the end of each shift.
- *Confirmation*: Staff reports a reduced incidence of back strain.

For an individual to consider adoption of an innovation, they must be aware of the innovation. Rogers (1983) used the term *diffusion* to describe the dissemination of an innovation. The theory proposes that diffusion of an innovation is enhanced by face-to-face and mass media communication channels, time, and interaction within the social system. Adoption of an innovation is enhanced by persuasion by a peer or by influence from opinion leaders within the social system. An outside change agent may also facilitate diffusion and adoption of an innovation.

The perceived characteristics of the innovation affect favorable or unfavorable attitudes toward adoption. The probability and speed of adoption are enhanced if the staff perceives the innovation as being superior to current practice; the innovation is consistent with current values, experience, and priorities; the innovation is easy to learn, understand, or use, or can be tried out on a limited basis with the option of returning to previous practices; and the innovation causes visible results.

The Stetler Model of Evidence-Based Practice

Although Rogers's theory addresses the structure of diffusion of any innovation, including research findings, Stetler and Marram were early developers of models for incorporating research into clinical practice and in 1976 developed the original Stetler/Marram research utilization model. This model provided a decision tree for nursing students and nurses to follow before using research findings in practice (Stetler, 1994, 2001, 2010). The latest version of the model, which has been renamed the **Stetler Model of Evidence-Based Practice** (Stetler, 2010), refers to a five-phase critical-thinking and decision-making process to assist the individual practitioner in using published research (Fig. 10.1).

Stetler (2010) describes considerations for each phase in her model as follows:

- *Phase I—Preparation*: Determine purpose, context, and sources of evidence for an identified clinical issue or problem.
  - Potential issues/catalysts: A problem, including unexplained variations; less-than-best practice; routine update of knowledge; validation/routine revision of procedures, etc.; or innovative program goal
  - Affirm/clarify perceived problem(s), with internal evidence regarding current practice (baseline).
  - Consider other influential internal and external factors (e.g., timelines).

- Affirm and focus on high-priority issues.
- Decide if you need to form a team, involve formal stakeholders, and/or assign a project lead/facilitator.
- Define desired, measurable outcome(s).
- Seek out systematic reviews/guidelines first.
- Determine the need for an explicit type of research evidence if relevant.
- Select research with a conceptual fit.

- *Phase II—Validation*: Determine the credibility of evidence and potential for/detailed qualifiers of application.
  - Critique and synopsize essential components, operational details, and other qualifying factors per the source.
  - See instructions for use of utilization-focused review tables (Stetler et al., 1998), with evaluative criteria, to facilitate this task; fill in the tables for group decision making or potential future synthesis.
  - Critique (Stetler et al., 1998) systematic reviews and guidelines.
  - Reassess the fit of individual sources.
  - Rate the level and quality of each individual evidence source with a "table of evidence."
  - Differentiate statistical and clinical significance.
  - Eliminate noncredible sources.
  - End the process if there is clearly insufficient, credible external evidence that meets your need.

- *Phase III—Comparative evaluation/decision making*: Synthesize the evidence gathered, and make decisions/recommendations applicable to the setting.
  - Synthesize the cumulative findings:
    - Logically organize and display the similarities and differences across multiple findings with the common aspects or subelements of the topic under review.
    - Evaluate the degree of substantiation of each aspect/subelement; reference any qualifying conditions for application.
  - Evaluate degree and nature of other criteria: Feasibility (r, r, r = risk, resources, readiness); pragmatic fit, including potential qualifying factors to application; and nature of current practice, including the urgency or risk of current issues and needs (Stetler et al., 2006).
  - Make decision whether and what to use:
    - Can be a personal, practitioner-level decision or a recommendation to others.
    - Judge strength of decision; indicate if primarily "research-based" (R-B) or per use of supplemental info, "E-B;" note level of strength of recommendation(s) per related

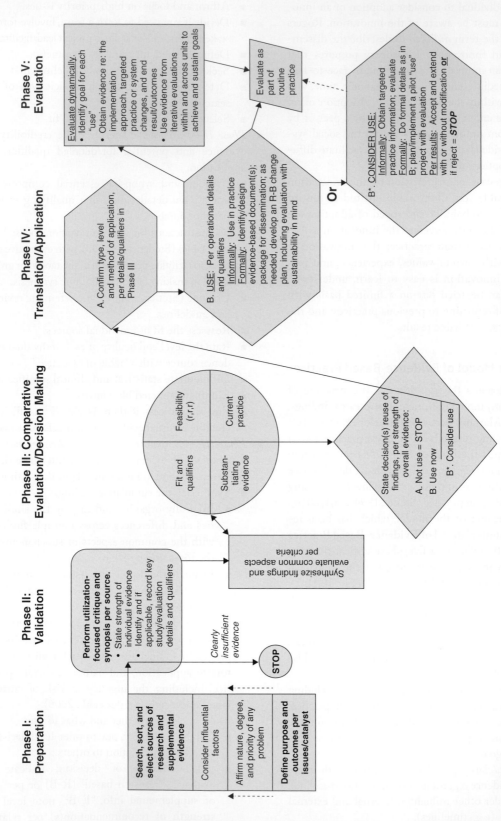

FIGURE 10.1 The Stetler model of evidence-based practice. (From Rycroft-Malone, J., & Bucknall, T. (Eds.). (2010). *Models and frameworks for implementing evidence-based practice: Linking evidence to action* (1st ed.). Sigma Theta Tau International and Wiley-Blackwell. © Reprinted with permission from Cheryl Stetler.)

table; note any qualifying factors that may influence individualized variations (Stetler et al., 1998).

- If the decision is to "not use" research findings:
  - May conduct own research or delay use until additional research is done by others
  - If the decision is still to act now (e.g., on evidence of consensus or another basis for practice), consider the need for similar planned change and evaluation.
- The decision to "use/consider use" can mean a recommendation for or against a specific practice. Table 10.3 presents considerations for examining the fit, flow, and feasibility of reported research that fit with phases II and III.
- *Phase IV—Translation/application*: Determine exactly how to use the evidence for making clinical practice changes.
  - Types of use: Cognitive/conceptual, symbolic, and/or instrumental

- Methods for action or use: Informal or formal; direct or indirect
- Levels of use or action: Individual, group, or department/organization
- Direct instrumental use: Change individual behavior (e.g., via assessment tool or prescription intervention options); or change policy, procedure, protocol, algorithm, program, etc.
- Cognitive use: Validate current practice; change personal way of thinking; increase awareness; better understand or appreciate condition(s) or experience(s).
- Symbolic use: Develop position paper or proposal for change or persuade others regarding a way of thinking.
- CAUTION: Assess whether translation/product or use goes beyond actual findings/evidence. Research evidence may or may not provide various details for a complete policy, procedure, etc.; indicate this fact to users, and note differential levels of evidence.

TABLE 10.3	Considerations for Preliminary Evaluation of Nursing Research for Use in a Particular Clinical Setting	
Fit to Clinical Setting	**Flow of Research Study**	**Feasibility of Adoption**
The purpose of the study fits the clinical area where findings may be adopted.	Research questions or hypotheses flow from the study's stated purpose.	The proposed innovation is legally permitted by the state nurse practice act.
The study sample represents clientele of the clinical setting.	Researcher follows all steps outlined in the research process.	The innovation is ethical practice.
Sample size is appropriate.	Variables are well defined.	Costs are acceptable to clients, third-party payers, or the institution.
The study enhances the fulfillment of the clinical area's mission.	Measurements for the variables make sense. Validity and reliability of variable measurements are presented. Efforts are made to control factors that might affect the results. Data are presented accurately. The correct statistics are used to answer the research question(s) or test the hypothesis(es): ■ Research purpose ■ Number and type of variables ■ Level of measurement for each variable The sample size is large enough to support the statistical test or researcher reports power level. Weaknesses of the study are reported. The study generates logical and accurate conclusions. Implications for practice logically flow from findings.	There is enough staff and time to fully execute the proposed innovation. The innovation is congruent with the nursing philosophy of the organization or unit. Risks to clients, nurses, and organization are considered. Necessary resources are obtained. Staff is ready to adopt the proposed innovation.

Note: Do not change practice on the basis of the findings of one study. Similar findings from multiple studies indicate that the findings were more likely not to be the result of chance.
From Gray, J. R., Grove, S. K., & Sutherland, S. (2017). *Burns and Grove's, The practice of nursing research: Appraisal, synthesis, and generation of evidence* (8th ed.). Elsevier; Liehr, P., & Houston, S. (1993). Critiquing and using nursing research: Guidelines for the critical care nurse. *American Journal of Critical Care, 2,* 407–412.

- Formal dissemination and change strategies should be planned per relevant research and local barriers:
  - Passive education is usually not effective as an isolated strategy. Use diagnostic analysis (Stetler et al., 2006) and an implementation framework to develop a plan (Green & Krueter, 1992; Rycroft-Malone & Bucknall, 2010). Consider multiple strategies (e.g., opinion leaders, interactive education, reminders, audits).
  - Focus on context (Stetler & Caramanica, 2007) to enhance sustainability of organizational-related change.
- Consider need for appropriate, reasoned variation for a particular setting.
- With formal use, may need a dynamic evaluation to effectively implement and continuously improve/refine use of best available evidence across units and time.
- Before making a final decision about the evidence, determine where the decision was made for considering using the evidence in practice, and determine the practicality of using the evidence in practice.
  - With formal consideration, do a pilot project.
  - With a pilot project, must assess if need IRB review per relevant institutional criteria.
- *Phase V—Evaluation*: Alternative evaluation to verify that the use of the research would benefit the clinical setting
  - Evaluation per type, method, level (e.g., consider conceptual use at individual level; Stetler et al., 2006)
  - Consider cost–benefit of change plus various evaluation efforts.
  - Use research utilization as a process to enhance credibility of evaluation data.
  - For both dynamic and pilot evaluations, include:
    - Formative, regarding actual implementation and goal progress
    - Summative, regarding identified end-goal and end-point outcomes
- Note: Model applies to all forms of practice (i.e., educational, clinical, managerial, or other).

Concepts in Practice, "Stetler Model of Evidence-Based Practice in Action," returns to the example of Tony and his colleagues and shows how these elements may be implemented.

Concepts in Practice [IDEA] → [PLAN] → [ACTION]

Stetler Model of Evidence-Based Practice in Action

Tony can also use Stetler's model to determine whether the slick sheet system will help relieve the back pain that results from turning immobile clients.

- Phase I: Tony identifies the problems of increased back strain, reviews reasons for it within his institution, networks with nurses who work elsewhere, clarifies the problem and surrounding factors, decides that reducing back strain is a high priority, forms an EBP team that includes coworkers, conducts a literature search, and selects relevant sources to review and critique.
- Phase II: Tony's team analyzes acquired resources, critiques the research studies, and based on the findings, identifies the slick sheet system as a feasible way to reduce back strain as staff turns clients in bed.
- Phase III: Tony and the team prepare a proposal to administration to support the evidence-based way to move clients differently. The manufacturer of the slick sheet system agrees to provide a unit demonstration and several sheet systems for the staff to use during the evidence-based project.
- Phase IV: Tony and his team decide that the slick sheet system should become the policy when turning clients in bed. The manufacturer provides six slick sheet systems for the unit to use in its pilot project and educates the staff on safe, effective use of the product. The team develops a daily log for the staff to complete regarding how frequently they turn clients with and without the slick sheet system and their level of back strain after turning clients. Before implementing the project, they submit a proposal to the IRB, which expedites the process because it identifies no potential harm to clients. The pilot study is implemented.
- Phase V: Tony and the team have unit staff use the slick sheet system for 2 months and provide data. They analyze the data and discover that when staff uses the slick sheet system for turning bedridden clients, they report a 50% reduction in back strain. The decision is made by the nurse manager to extend the pilot study to other units of the hospital to see if similar results occur before implementing the process of changing clinical practice policies and procedures through the established shared governance processes.

Facilitators of Research Utilization and Evidence-Based Practice

The process of research utilization is a continual one. Advances in the health science arena mean nurses must stay abreast of changes in their clinical practice areas. New theoretical developments in nursing result in different approaches to client assessments, nursing interventions, and outcome evaluation. Nursing research utilization success relies on a variety of factors that facilitate use of research findings in practice.

Many factors influence the utilization of nursing research in clinical practice. **Research utilization and evidence-based practice facilitators** are any factors that promote the use of research-based knowledge and other forms of evidence in clinical practice.

Individual nurse and employing organization factors can facilitate research utilization and EBP in the clinical practice setting. Estabrooks et al. (2003) identified six categories of possible individual nurse factors that promoted research utilization and EBP from a review of 22 studies. An additional facilitator more recently identified is the willingness and ability to seek out a mentor for guidance (Fineout-Overholt & Melnyk, 2019; Table 10.4).

In 2007, Estabrooks and colleagues developed a three-tier model to predict research utilization and again noted that individual nurse factors contributed to research utilization. Cultivating these characteristics in all professional nurses remains a challenge for the profession. They also discovered that nurses employed in larger hospitals tended to use research more

TABLE 10.4   Individual Nurse Facilitators for Research Utilization and Evidence-Based Practice

Main Category	Facilitator
Beliefs and attitudes toward nursing research	Positive attitude toward nursing research Self-expectation to use nursing research in practice Interest in nursing research Lower levels of emotional exhaustion
Involvement with research activities	Perceived availability of research findings Current collaboration or past participation on a research project Collecting data for other researchers Participation in a research study as a subject or participant Previous use of nursing research Experience with the research process
Information-seeking behaviors	Reading nursing journals as the top information source to stay current in practice Regular reading of professional journals (e.g., *Nursing Research, American Journal of Nursing*) Subscribing to professional journals More time spent studying while off duty Use of nursing school as a resource for nursing research materials and information Increased use of the internet
Education level	Education preparation in the research utilization process Attendance at professional nursing conferences Attendance at more staff in-services BSN or higher degree Perception of being well prepared in the education process Completion of a research and/or statistics course
Professional characteristics	Perceived organizational support for research utilization activities Perception of an organizational policy for research use Increased number of years' experience in a nursing specialty area or clinical unit Nursing leadership or advanced practice nursing role Membership in the American Nurses Association Specialty nurse certification Autonomy to make nursing practice changes Support from peers, administrators, and other members of the health care team Willingness and ability to seek out a mentor
Socioeconomic factors	Younger age

Adapted from Estabrooks, C., Floyd, J., Scott-Findlay, S., O'Leary, K., & Gushta, M. (2003). Individual determinants of research utilization: A systematic review. *Journal of Advanced Nursing, 43*, 506–520; Estabrooks, C., Midodzi, W., Cummings, G., & Wallin, L. (2007). Predicting research use in nursing organizations: A multilevel analysis. *Nursing Research, 56*(4, Suppl. 1), S7–S23. Younas, A. (2020). Identifying international barriers and facilitators to research utilization. *Nursing, 50*(7), 63–67. https://doi.org/10.1097/01.NURSE.0000668460.98211.39

than nurses employed in other settings (Estabrooks et al., 2007). These characteristics seem to remain relatively unchanged (Dang et al., 2019; Malloch & Porter-O'Grady, 2017; Melnyk & Fineout-Overholt, 2019; Younas, 2020).

Organizational factors also serve as facilitators to research utilization. Research utilization efforts are time-intensive and require use of human and financial resources. Nursing research utilization also requires organizational commitment. The following strategies to facilitate research utilization and EBP in nursing departments have been used with some success:

- Clear expectation of research utilization as part of a job description
- Staff educational programs on the process of research utilization
- Incentives, such as promotions or salary increases
- Formation of nursing research/research utilization committees
- Provision of time for nurses to read research reports while on duty
- Clinical career ladders requiring research utilization as criteria for promotion and maintenance of organizational positioning
- Established mentorship programs for nursing EBP
- Autonomy of nurses to change nursing procedures and practices
- Organizational support to defray expenses for research utilization projects
- Formalized collaboration between nursing service and academia
- Library services for nurses to use to perform computerized literature searches and access needed materials
- Nursing unit–based libraries and nursing journal subscriptions
- Formation of a nursing research journal club
- Sponsorship of nurses to attend professional nursing conferences

Characteristics of published research studies also serve as facilitators of research utilization and EBP in nursing. Because many nurse researchers may not engage in clinical practice on a regular basis, performing clinically relevant studies may be challenging. However, nothing captures the interest of professional nurses better than a study that demonstrates substantial improvements in client outcomes or working environments. A well-written research study using clear, concise language enhances the ability of all nurses to read and understand published nursing research studies.

Barriers to Research Utilization and Evidence-Based Practice

Research utilization and evidence-based practice barriers are any factors that block or impede the use of research findings in clinical practice. Abrahamson et al. (2012), Rutledge et al. (2004), and Funk et al. (1991) identified a number of barriers to research utilization and EBP, including barriers from researchers, practicing nurses, and the health care agency administration. These researchers developed an instrument to measure 28 items addressing the following categories of barriers: personal barriers, organizational barriers, innovation barriers, and research accessibility and communication. This instrument has been widely used in research examining facilitators and barriers to research utilization. The same barriers exist today (Dang et al., 2019; Malloch & Porter-O'Grady, 2017; Younas, 2020; Focus on Research, "Identifying International Facilitators and Barriers to Research Utilization").

Researchers

Barriers to research utilization, which result from the nature of disseminated research studies, include:

- Insufficient current research with solutions to address today's complex clinical problems
- Failure of replicated research studies
- Research reports that are difficult to read
- Many unpublished or nondisseminated research reports (especially studies done to meet graduate and postgraduate program requirements)
- Lack of a central repository for nursing research studies

Nursing practice should not be changed on the basis of a single study because of potential confounding factors that may have caused the study results. Unfortunately, few replication studies appear in the nursing literature. Either nurses are not performing replication studies or they are not being accepted for publication when they are submitted.

Practicing Nurses

Barriers to research utilization and EBP based on characteristics of practicing nurses include:

- Lack of education in how to read, critique, conduct, and use research
- Negative attitudes among practicing nurses about using research findings in practice
- Not enough time or commitment to implement research utilization projects

FOCUS ON RESEARCH

Identifying International Facilitators and Barriers to Research Utilization

The investigator wanted to identify barriers and facilitators to research utilization in nursing practice on an international scale. She conducted an integrative review of the literature of 42 published studies that were published in peer-reviewed journals in English language, having been published between January 2017 and November 2017.

The descriptive findings concluded that 36 used a cross-sectional design, three were integrative reviews, and there was one each of a grounded theory study, mixed-methods study, and secondary data analysis. Of the studies, 21 were conducted in Asia and the Middle East, 11 were conducted in Europe, five were conducted in the United States, three were conducted in Africa, and two were conducted in Australia. Study sample sizes ranged from 21 to 1,301. Half the studies had participation rates of 50% or higher with the lowest participation response rate at 3.6%. Clinical settings included emergency departments, critical care units, community health, geriatric care, oncology, pediatric, medical-surgical units, primary care, burn centers, and traditional and complementary practices. Some of the studies included more than one type of setting.

The reviewed studies used a variety of data collection instruments, some of which had established validity and reliability (e.g., BARRIERS scale) while five did not use established instruments. Sixteen studies used mailed or electronically distributed surveys. The investigator rated the quality of the studies as "strong" in 6, "moderate" in 28, and "weak" in 7.

The commonly encountered organizational barriers included insufficient time to read research reports (30% to 97% of study participants); inadequate resources for implementation (19% to 95%); not enough time to implement findings (32% to 85%); unsupportive nurse administrators and physicians (29% to 95%); and lack of authority to revise client care procedures (32% to 82%).

Barriers to research accessibility and communication included problems with literature access and compilation (13% to 88% of study participants); study findings not generalizable to their clinical practice area (28% to 91%); and inability to comprehend statistical analyses (26% to 88%). Personal barriers included insufficient knowledge of research and proposal writing (25% to 94% of participants) and poor awareness of current research findings (11% to 94%).

The following research utilization facilitators were consistently identified: increased education and awareness of research utilization and how it improves client care (6% to 88% of study participants); managerial and organizational support to conduct research projects (15% to 87%); and support from peers, colleagues with research and nursing expertise, and other health care professionals (10% to 85%).

The researcher drew several conclusions. Facilitators included organizational support while lack of it was a barrier reported internationally. The lack of authority to change practice was most common in the American studies while the lack of access to research literature was more common in African studies. Time and required resources for implementing research utilization were also reported as global issues. Facilitators such as peer support, increased education about understanding and using research findings, and increased access to the internet and peer-reviewed published articles were also identified as facilitators internationally. The most common barriers and facilitators have not changed much over the years since research utilization has become a desired nursing practice. Younas also indicated that future research addressing these issues should be conducted to determine the perception of these barriers among health policy makers, health care organizations, nursing associations, and regulatory bodies so that actions can be taken to provide necessary resources to facilitate nurses engaging in effective research utilization.

The clinical significance of this study is that nurses around the world experience similar facilitators and barriers to research utilization and EBP. Despite the documented improvement in client outcomes when research utilization and EBP interventions are used, there needs to detailed proposals written to submit to organizational administrators to get the required resources for effective research utilization in clinical practice. Future research, such as an international nursing research studies to identify current facilitators and barriers to research utilization and nursing EBP needs to be undertaken, and the results of this study could be submitted to health policy makers at the state or territorial, national, and global levels to provide public support for nursing research utilization endeavors.

From Younas, A. (2020). Identifying international barriers and facilitators to research utilization. *Nursing, 50*(7), 63–67. https://doi.org/10.1097/01.NURSE.0000668460.98211.39

- Failure of nurses to read nursing research articles or journals
- Inability of nurses to understand statistical analyses contained within studies
- Comfort with practice based on tradition, which is difficult to change, even if it is ineffective
- Difficulty determining whether studies are well designed and scientifically sound
- Isolation from knowledgeable colleagues who could assist them in understanding research studies

Nursing research utilization and EBP require much time and deep commitment. In today's society, many nurses assume multiple roles that compete for their attention. Even though practice based on sound science is preferred, changing personal attitudes and the status quo remains difficult.

The Nurse Researcher

Barriers arising from the nurse researcher perspective include:

- Submission of studies for publication to journals not read widely by most nurses
- Use of research jargon in publications that is not understood by practicing nurses
- Failure to offer realistic implications for clinical practice because of either lack of client care experience or current clinical experience
- Presentation of findings in a format not conducive to clinical implementation

Failure to understand statistics serves as another barrier to research utilization and EBP. Researchers sometimes manipulate statistics to distort the truth (Abrahamson

et al., 2012; Best, 2001). Because the average nurse does not comprehend statistical tests presented in a research study, the nurse accepts the studies' reported findings, even though the authors might have made implausible claims.

A common misconception related to statistics is that they "prove" something. A critical approach to statistics avoids the extremes of naïve acceptance and cynical rejection. When reading statistics, the research consumer must realize that researchers choose variable definitions, instruments for data collection, and samples for a variety of reasons (Best, 2001). Reported statistics represent a compromise among various choices that researchers make during a study (see Box 10.7, Professional Building Blocks, "Analyzing the Reliability of Research Study Data").

Take Note!
Statistics found in research reports must be analyzed critically before they are accepted as truth.

Health Care Agency Administration

Barriers to research utilization and EBP from the health care agency administration include:

- Minimal value placed on research by administrators and managers
- No provision made for resources such as time, financial support, and education
- Lack of nursing autonomy within a bureaucratic structure to implement data-based solutions to problems
- Lack of incentives for nurses to participate in research utilization activities

10.7 Professional Building Blocks

Analyzing the Reliability of Research Study Data

To determine whether the findings of a research study are reliable, ask yourself the following questions about the statistics used:

- Do they answer the question or issue outlined in the purpose of the study?
- What is the level of measurement of the research variables contained in the study?
- How many independent and dependent variables appear in the study?
- Is the sample size large enough to effectively use the statistical test?
- What instruments were used to collect data, and what is the level of measurement that these instruments generate?

- How might the sampling techniques affect the study results?
- Are comparisons appropriate if comparisons are being made?
- How have the figures been generated, and have any techniques been used to alter the appearance of the data?
- What stakes does the researcher have if the statistical tests used are not significant?

Instead of being awestruck or overwhelmed by complex statistical tests found in research reports, nurses should read for logical, feasible, and appropriate findings. Many advanced practice nurses find great rewards in helping staff nurses understand research reports.

- Reliance on established policy and procedures, rather than openness to change
- Lack of support for implementation of research findings by physicians and other staff

Strategies to Facilitate Research Utilization and Evidence-Based Practice

In BSN programs, students are exposed to the basic steps of the research process and how to effectively critique studies for use in clinical practice. Most BSN graduates have a basic understanding of research terminology, and some (though not all) can read and understand published research reports containing basic statistical analysis techniques. Nursing students and professionals gain confidence and expertise in reading and understanding research with continual practice. Graduate nurses focus on acquiring clinical competence and spend little or no time reading nursing research reports. Rutledge and colleagues (2004) found that when oncology nurses received formal education in research utilization, they could master the process well enough to design and implement nursing research utilization projects in clinical settings.

Researchers should make an effort to write for practicing nurses and to emphasize the meaning of the findings for practice in language that is understandable by most nurses. Consultation with a nurse holding a master's or doctorate degree serves as a useful method for understanding and interpreting complex statistical analyses. Some clinical agencies employ a nursing research facilitator for staff consultation. Nursing faculty and graduate students may also be a source of research consultation

services. A team of nurses could work together with a consultant in locating and interpreting relevant literature to address a clinical issue or to answer a PICOT question. Finally, some institutions have implemented a clinical scholar program that pairs staff nurses with research mentors to develop and implement nursing research studies or research utilization and EBP projects.

To use research findings, practicing nurses must read professional journals, including academic research journals (Box 10.8, Professional Building Blocks, "Nursing Journals that Emphasize Research"). Other means of finding research articles pertinent to one's areas of nursing practice is to use electronic databases such as Medline or the Cumulative Index of Nursing and Allied Health Literature (CINAHL). Many hospitals have a basic medical (or health sciences) library that includes a core collection of nursing journals. Nurses may also visit local college, university, or public libraries. To save time, nurses should look for integrative reviews or meta-analyses that review a number of studies and provide information about the quality of the results.

Nurses can also obtain access to research findings through research bulletin boards, newsletters, or research grand rounds, but these strategies need to be organized, maintained, and supported. Many institutions have a research committee that can take responsibility for coordinating the review of literature, exploring ideas, pilot-testing innovations, and developing and disseminating research-based protocols and policies.

Nurses may also find the nursing staff development department useful when seeking to establish nursing practice based on research. Master's-prepared clinical educators could evaluate and synthesize knowledge

---

10.8   Professional Building Blocks

Nursing Journals that Emphasize Research

The following publications are excellent sources of nursing research and associated content.

Research Findings and Methodologic Issues

- *Nursing Research*
- *Western Journal of Nursing Research*
- *International Journal of Nursing Research*

Publication of Research and Nursing Theory

- *Journal of Nursing Scholarship*
- *Journal of Advanced Nursing*
- *Nursing Science Quarterly*
- *Advances in Nursing Science*

Evidence and Research for Clinical Nursing Practice

- *Nursing in Research and Health*
- *International Journal of Nursing Studies*
- *Clinical Nursing Research*
- *Applied Nursing Research*
- *Evidence-Based Nursing*

General Nursing Journal with Research as a Regular Feature

The American Journal of Nursing (official publication of the American Nurses Association) across studies and provide direction for clinicians. Some agencies offer nurses continuing education on research processes; developing a research, research utilization, or EBP project; performing effective literature searches; evaluating the quality of research; understanding data analysis; and determining the relevance of research findings for EBP nursing policies and procedures.

Even where resources are readily available to nurses, agency managers and administration must create an atmosphere where nurses are encouraged and supported to question and evaluate current practice protocols, to use research study findings as a basis for protocol revisions, and to be valued (and even rewarded) for using research in practice. Without a supportive environment, nurses who use research in practice may become discouraged and rely on agency traditions, or they may leave the work setting for an agency that supports research utilization. Managers and administrators who use research and current literature in their positions serve as role models for research utilization and EBP.

When research utilization and EBP become valued as a way of knowing, positive attitudes and tangible resources for research utilization become standard practice. To show that they value research utilization and EBP, managers and administrators must provide the resources to nurses to develop and conduct studies. Required resources depend upon the type of study to be conducted. Nurses planning and conducting studies need access to computerized databases, financial support for consulting with nurse researchers and statisticians, and release time from client care duties. Incentives and rewards for risk taking and creativity promote research utilization. Fostering peer collaboration and networking with other colleagues also provide impetus for research use in practice. Most of all, the atmosphere must be one of respect and encouragement for professional practice and delegation of authority so that nurses control nursing practice.

In the final analysis, the clinician has to value the use of research as the basis for practice enough to put forth the time and effort required for research utilization activities. Only when a significant number of nurses value scholarship enough to participate in its creation, dissemination, and utilization will nursing be viewed as a true profession.

CREATING A PUBLIC IMAGE OF THE NURSE AS SCHOLAR

A **scholar** is an intellectual who has undertaken advanced study in a given field. Public perceptions of nurses tend toward the nurse as a person with technical

expertise, a subordinate to physicians, and as one who cares for others. However, a visit to a college or university today reveals the strides the nursing profession has made in developing a unique research base and expert researchers.

Advanced technology offers great support for today's nurse researcher. The storage, retrieval, and analysis of data afforded by computer support make conducting research much faster and more achievable by nurses. Many professional nursing journals are published in print and electronic versions. In most educational and practice settings, a researcher should not have to manage data manually. Computer programs can be used to manipulate numbers, facilitating almost unlimited analysis of data and the ability to use research findings to a fuller capacity. Laptops, smart phones, and the internet facilitate the rapid sharing and dissemination of research findings with those in practice.

Take Note!

Nurses who value conducting and using research findings and best evidence appreciate how much time can be saved by using technology.

Nurses have not traditionally been viewed as scholars. Some nurses fail to acknowledge the advanced education of colleagues. Some health care agencies refuse to place academic credentials on nurses' employment name badges. The public perception of nursing is highly affected by individual experience with nurses. With approximately 60% of nurses having less-than-BSN preparation, nurses remain among the least educated members of the interdisciplinary health care team. Nurses and clients tend to value clinical practice over nursing scholarship. However, when (and if) nurses communicate to others the contributions of nursing research to health outcomes, the nursing profession will attain recognition as a scholarly rather than exclusively practice discipline.

As nursing has developed its own theory base during the past 50 years, nurses have begun to value nursing scholarship. Most nurses today probably would agree that a practice based on research is desirable. Capitalizing on that consensus, the profession can begin to present a different image to the public. To help actualize the motivation to base nursing practice on research, educational programs need to prepare students in scientific inquiry while preparing them to apply theory in professional practice.

In 1993, the **National Institute of Nursing Research (NINR)** was established, replacing the National Center for Nursing Research. Separating the NINR from the National Institutes of Health and making it a freestanding institute acknowledges the unique contribution of nursing science and research to the health of American citizens.

"The mission of the NINR is to promote and improve the health of individuals, families, communities, and populations. The institute supports and conducts clinical and basic research and research training on health and illness, research that spans and integrates the behavioral and biological sciences and that develops the scientific basis for clinical practice" (NINR, 2016, p. 6). The NINR identifies nursing research priorities, distributes grants to nurse researchers, and disseminates nursing research findings to health professionals and the public.

Current focus areas for research for the NINR include symptom science, personalized health strategies, health promotion and illness prevention, self-management of chronic illness to enhance quality of life, and end-of-life and palliative care. In addition, the NINR conducts research related to the current nursing workforce. The NINR is also investigating the science of compassion (NINR, 2016). Health promotion, disease prevention, quality-of-life improvement, health disparities elimination, and directions for end-of-life research are other nursing research priorities (NINR, 2016). Funding for the NINR has risen steadily since its inception. The NINR is funded through Section 301, Title IV of the National Public Service Act. For fiscal year 2020, the NINR received $140,301 million in federal funding, a reduction of $6 million related to the recession caused by the COVID-19 pandemic. The 2021 budget allocation is for $156,804,000 (United States Department of Health and Human Services, 2020). Public funding of nursing research acknowledges the valuable contributions it makes to all Americans.

As nurses begin to feel and act like scholars, the public will acknowledge the scholarly side of nursing. If the profession nourishes this scholarship in nurses, it will undoubtedly help change the image of the nurse. Because scholars accept that research is a vital component of nursing, the development of scholars will increase the supply of researchers to better serve the profession and the public.

▮ QUESTIONS FOR REFLECTION

1. How can you promote the image of nurses as scholars?
2. What are the potential consequences of changing the image of the nurse from caregiver to scholar?

Summary and Significance to Practice

From the 1960s to 1990s, many researchers and scholars generated clinically relevant research for use in practice. Nurses gradually saw the benefits of using research findings in practice. By the early 21st century, nurses began to routinely incorporate research findings and other forms of evidence to improve client outcomes and contain costs. The use of nursing research findings and evidence-based practice has resulted in improved client outcomes. Nurses use multiple cognitive skills to navigate the vast web of information and decide how to use available research findings and various forms of evidence in clinical practice. With practice, nurses gain confidence in their ability to analyze, critique, and decide how and when to use evidence in clinical practice. Qualitative and quantitative research findings provide evidence that captures the complex, holistic nature of clients, nurses, and health care delivery. Recent public funding of nursing research initiatives shows that the public values nursing research. As nurses assume the roles of researcher and scholar, they make discoveries, generate evidence, and determine how to incorporate the best possible evidence to guide and change clinical practice in today's complex and sometimes chaotic health care delivery systems.

REAL-LIFE REFLECTIONS

Recall Jessica and Malika from the beginning of the chapter. What strategies would you suggest for Jessica to use in her attempts to integrate research-based knowledge about alternative forms of pain control on her unit? Outline a research utilization project for Jessica to follow.

From Theory to Practice

1. What forms of evidence are used as a foundation for current clinical policies and procedures in your area of clinical practice?
2. Has your perception as a nursing student changed about the profession of nursing now that you have read about all the evidence and research behind clinical practice? Why or why not?
3. How would you differentiate research utilization from EBP?
4. In addition to your instructor, who might you turn to for help or what resources might you use if you had difficulty making sense of a published research study?

Nurse as Author

Identify a clinical problem that you have encountered in practice. Using the PICOT format presented in the chapter, generate a question for an EBP project. Perform a literature search using a digital database, and enter the search terms by combining the terms outlined in your PICOT question. Write a one-page paper describing the literature search terms that you entered, which computerized literature database that you used, and how many articles you obtained when you completed the search.

Your Digital Classroom

Online Exploration

Agency for Healthcare Research and Quality: **www.ahrq.gov**

   American Nurses Foundation: **https://www.nursingworld.org/foundation/**

   Canadian Foundation for Healthcare Improvement: **www.cfhi-fcass.ca/Home.aspx**

   Midwestern Nursing Research Society: **www.mnrs.org**

   National Guideline Clearinghouse: **guideline.gov/**

   National Institute of Nursing Research: **https://www.ninr.nih.gov**

   Nursing Health Services Research Units: **https://nursing.mcmaster.ca/research/research-units**

   Southern Nursing Research Society: **www.snrs.org**

   The Cochrane Collaboration: **www.cochrane.org**

Expanding Your Understanding

1. Visit the NINR website, and read about the group's mission and strategic plan. Identify the research priorities of the NINR and bring them to class for discussion.
2. Visit the Cochrane Collaboration. Read the top two articles on the right-hand side under "Latest Cochrane Evidence," and answer the following questions.
   a. Do you belief the content presented? Why or why not?
   b. What is the level of evidence used to draw the conclusions for suggesting clinical action?
   c. Do you agree with the author's conclusions? Why or why not?

3. Visit the Office for Research Integrity at https://ori.hhs.gov/integrity-scientific-research-videos, and answer the following questions about Videos 3 and 4.
   a. What ethical violations occurred in each of the videos?
   b. How would you handle these situations?
   c. What would be potential consequences for the actions that you might take?
4. Read one of the misconduct case studies from the Office of Research Integrity at https://ori.hhs.gov/case_summary. Identify the case study, and summarize the key issues involved and the penalties incurred. Do you think they were fair? Why or why not?

Beyond the Book

Visit **thePoint** at **www.thePoint.lww.com** for activities and information to reinforce the concepts and content covered in this chapter.

REFERENCES

Abrahamson, K., Fox, R., & Doebbeling, B. (2012). Facilitators and barriers to clinical practice guideline use among nurses. *American Journal of Nursing, 112*(7), 26–35. doi:10.1097/01.naj.0000415957

Academic Center for Evidence-Based Practice. (2009). *ACE star model of knowledge transformation*. Retrieved April 8, 2021, from https://www.uthscsa.edu/academics/nursing/star-model

American Association of Colleges of Nursing (2021). *The Essentials: Core competencies for professional nursing education*. Retrieved April 8, 2021, from https://www.aacnnursing.org/Portals/42/AcademicNursing/pdf/Essentials-2021.pdf

American Nurses Association. (2015). *Nursing scope and standards of practice (3rd ed.)*. Author.

Artinian, B. A. (1988). Qualitative modes of inquiry. *Western Journal of Nursing Research, 10*, 138–149. doi:10.1177/019394598801000203

Barrett, E. A. M. (2002). What is nursing science? *Nursing Science Quarterly, 15*, 51–60. doi:10.1177/089431840201500109

Best, J. (2001). Telling the truth about damned lies and statistics. *The Chronicle of Higher Education, 47*, B7–B9. Retrieved April 8, 2021, from http://www.statlit.org/cp/2001bestchronicle-highered.pdf

Blumenstyk, G. (2001). A new web site details the corporate ties of some researchers. *The Chronicle of Higher Education, 47*, A25. Retrieved April 9, 2021, from https://search-ebscohost-com.lib.rockhurst.edu/login.aspx?direct=true&AuthType=cookie,ip,url&db=a9h&AN=5455567&site=ehost-live

Cohen, M. Z., & Tripp-Reimer, T. (1988). Research in cultural diversity: Qualitative methods in cultural research. *Western Journal of Nursing Research, 10*, 226–228. DOI: 10.1177/019394598801000210

Dang, D., Melnyk, B. M., Yost, J., Cullen, L., Cyach, M., Larabee, J. H., Rycroft-Malone, J., Schultz, A. A., Stetler, C. B., & Stevens, K. R. (2019). Models to guide implementation and sustainability of evidence-based practice. In B. Melnyk & E. Fineout-Overholt (Eds.), *Evidence-based practice in nursing and healthcare: A guide to best practice* (4th ed., pp. 378–427). Wolters-Kluwer.

Estabrooks, C., Floyd, J., Scott-Findlay, S., O'Leary, K., & Gushta, M. (2003). Individual determinants of research utilization: A systematic review. *Journal of Advanced Nursing, 43,* 506–520. https://doi.org/10.1046/j.1365-2648.2003 .02748.x

Estabrooks, C., Midodzi, W., Cummings, G., & Wallin, L. (2007). Predicting research use in nursing organizations: A multilevel analysis. *Nursing Research,* 56(4, Suppl 1), S7–S23. doi:10.1097/01.nnr.0000280647.18806.98

Fineout-Overholt, E., & Melnyk, B. M. (2019). ARCC evidence-based practice mentors: The key to sustaining evidence-based practice. In B. Melnyk & E. Fineout-Overholt (Eds.), *Evidence-based practice in nursing and healthcare: A guide to best practice* (4th ed., pp. 514–526). Wolters-Kluwer.

Funk, S. G., Champagne, M. T., Wiese, R. A., & Tornquist, E. M. (1991). Barriers to using research findings in practice: The clinician's perspective. *Applied Nursing Research, 4,* 90–95. DOI: 10.1016/s0897-1897(05)80062-x

Knafl, K. A., & Webster, D. C. (1988). Managing and analyzing qualitative data: A description of tasks, techniques, and materials. *Western Journal of Nursing Research, 10,* 195–218. doi: 10.1177/019394598801000207

Malloch, K., & Porter-O'Grady, T. (2006). *Introduction to evidence-based practice in nursing and health care.* Jones & Bartlett.

Malloch, K., & Porter-O'Grady, T. (2017). Innovation and evidence: A partnership in advancing best practice and high-quality care. In B. Melnyk & E. Fineout-Overholt (Eds.), *Evidence-based practice in nursing and health care. A guide to best practice* (3rd ed., pp. 255–273). Wolters Kluwer Health.

McDonald, L. (2001). Florence Nightingale and the early origins of evidence-based nursing. *Evidence-Based Nursing, 4,* 68–69. Retrieved December 15, 2012, from http://ebn.bmjjournals. com/content/vol4/issue3/

Melnyk, B., & Fineout-Overholt, E. (2019). *Evidence-based practice in nursing and healthcare: A guide to best practice* (4th ed.). Wolters-Kluwer.

National Guideline Clearinghouse. (2008). *Help & about.* Retrieved December 15, 2012, from http://guideline.gov/ about/index.aspx

National Institute of Nursing Research. (2016). *The NINR Strategic Plan: Advancing science, improving lives.* Retrieved October 6, 2020, from https://www.ninr.nih.gov/sites/files/docs/ NINR_StratPlan2016_reduced.pdf

Nightingale, F. (1860). *Notes on nursing.* Appleton.

Polit, D. F., & Beck, C. (2021). *Nursing research: Generating and assessing evidence for nursing practice* (11th ed.). Wolters-Kluwer.

Rogers, E. (1983). *Diffusion of innovations* (3rd ed.). Free Press.

Rogers, E. (1995). *Diffusion of innovations* (4th ed.). Free Press.

Rutledge, D., Mooney, K., Grant, M., & Easton, L. (2004). Implementation and refinement of a research utilization course

for oncology nurses. *Oncology Nursing Forum, 31,* 121–126. doi:10.1188/04.ONF.121-126

Rycroft-Malone, J., & Bucknall, T. (Eds.). (2010). *Models and frameworks for implementing evidence-base practice: Linking evidence to action.* Sigma Theta Tau International and Wiley-Blackwell.

Sherwood, G., & Barnsteiner, J. (2009). *Quality and safety in nursing a competency approach to improving outcomes.* Wiley-Blackwell.

Stetler, C. B. (1994). Refinement of the Stetler/Marram model for application of research findings to practice. *Nursing Outlook, 42,* 15–25. DOI: 10.1016/0029-6554(94)90067-1

Stetler, C. B. (2001). Updating the Stetler model of research utilization to facilitate evidence-base practice. *Nursing Outlook, 49,* 272–279. doi: 10.1067/mno.2001.120517

Stetler, C. B. (2010). Stetler model. In J. Rycroft-Malone & T. Bucknall (Eds.), *Models and frameworks for implementing evidence-base practice: Linking evidence to action* (pp. 51–82). Sigma Theta Tau International and Wiley-Blackwell.

Stetler, C., B., & Caramanica, L. (2007). Evaluation of an evidence-based practice initiative: outcomes, strengths and limitations of a retrospective, conceptually-based approach. *Worldviews on Evidence-Based Nursing,* 4(4), 187–199. doi-10.1111/j.1741-6787.2007.00097.x

Stelter, C. B., Legro, M. W., Wallace, C. M., Bowman, C., Guihan, M., Hagedorn, H., Kimmel, B., Sharp, N. D., & Smith, J. L. (2006). The role of formative evaluation in implementation research and the QUERI experience. *Journal of General Internal Medicine, 21* (Supplement 1). doi:10.1007/s11606-006-0267-9

Stetler, C. B., Morsi, D., Rucki, S., Broughton, S., Corrigan, B., Fitzgerald, J., Giuliano, K., Havener, P., & Sheridan, E. A. (1998). Clinical methods. Utilization-focused integrative reviews in a nursing service. *Applied Nursing Research,* 11(4), 195–206. Retrieved April 8, 2021, from https://www.science-direct.com/science/article/pii/S0897189798803297

Theou, O., Soon, Z., Filek, S., Brims, M., Leach-Macleod, K., Binsted, G., & Jakobi, J. (2011). Changing the sheets: A new system to reduce strain during patient repositioning. *Nursing Research, 60,* 302–308. https://doi.org/10.1097/ NNR.0b013e318225b8aa

Titler, M., Kleiber, C., Steelman, V., Rakel, B. A., Budreau, G., Everett, L. Q., Buckwalter, K. C., Tripp-Reimer, T., & Goode, C. J. (2001). The Iowa model of evidence-based practice to promote quality care. *Critical Care Nursing Clinics of North America, 13,* 497–509. doi:10.1016/S0899-5885(18)30017-0

United States Department of Health and Human Services. (2020). *National Institutes of Health National Institute of Nursing Research 2021 fiscal year budget.* Retrieved October 6, 2020 from https://www.ninr.nih.gov/sites/files/docs/NINR-Budget-FY-2021-508c.pdf

Younas, A. (2020). Identifying international barriers and facilitators to research utilization. *Nursing,* 50(7): 63–67. https://doi .org/10.1097/01.NURSE.0000668460.98211.39

Multicultural Issues in Professional Practice

KEY TERMS AND CONCEPTS

Culture
Transcultural nursing
Multicultural nursing
Intercultural nursing
Culture-universal care
Cultural relativism
Culture-specific care
Culturally congruent
  care
Ethnocentrism
Cultural competence

Cultural assessment
Health disparity
Folk illnesses
Variations in physical
  appearance
Variations in physiology
Multicultural nursing
  profession
Culture shock
Gender identity
Sexual orientation

LEARNING OUTCOMES

By the end of this chapter, the learner will be able to:

1. Discuss diversity and assimilation issues in a shrinking world.
2. Differentiate between transculturalism and multiculturalism.
3. Compare and contrast theoretical frameworks addressing cultural competence in nursing practice.
4. Specify strategies to address the cultural needs of nursing care consumers.
5. Outline strategies to foster a multicultural nursing profession.
6. Specify ways to enhance working relationships among multicultural health team members.

REAL-LIFE REFLECTIONS

Judy, a hospital nurse administrator, is having trouble getting U.S.-born nurses to work in the small rural hospital where she is employed. The hospital has decided to send her and a group of nurses to the Philippines to recruit Filipino nurses. Although she has reservations about hiring Filipino nurses and paying them for relocation, education, and licensure expenditures, Judy knows that she needs more registered nurses (RNs) to provide effective client care. Judy wonders how her current RNs will respond to having to work with nurses from another country, especially after they discover that the hospital has spent a lot of money to attract and hire the Filipino nurses. She also worries about the potential language and cultural barriers that might surface.

- *How do you think Judy should address the concerns about her staff working with the Filipino nurses?*
- *What might Judy do to ensure that the Filipino nurses feel welcome in the hospital and in the local community?*

Technology and transportation systems create opportunities for people to experience the world. Technology enables instant communication despite vast differences in locale. Modern transportation systems allow people to travel halfway around the world in a day, allowing individuals from different nations and cultures to meet each other easily and break down cultural barriers.

Health care in the United States is highly consumer-driven. In 2000, the Office of Minority Health published the first National Standards for Culturally and Linguistically Appropriate Services for Health Care (the national CLAS standards) in response to the increasing diversity of the American people. They quickly became a key standard for accreditation of health care organizations by The Joint Commission. The standards have undergone two revisions, with the last in 2013 (U.S. Department of Health and Human Services Office of Minority Health, n.d.-a). The revised standards strive to balance access to health care services, provide culturally sensitive care (including to those who are not fluent in English), and eliminate health disparities. These requirements for health care organizations to provide culturally sensitive health care include having foreign language interpreters for people who do not speak English or have limited proficiency. In addition, health care organizations must also periodically survey the communities they serve and attempt to employ health care providers who mirror the local community demographics. The national CLAS standards also hold health care organizations accountable for educating staff about culturally sensitive care, posting signs in the languages of frequently encountered clients, working toward promoting people from diverse backgrounds into leadership positions, and monitoring the effectiveness of culturally sensitive care and interpreter services. These standards also set criteria for the involvement of people from local cultural groups to assist in designing and implementing cultural and linguistic services. Health care organizations are required to inform the culturally diverse consumer about available language interpretation services, including written materials about available services, and how to initiate conflict resolution and grievance processes if culturally insensitive care or inappropriate situations should arise (U.S. Department of Health and Human Services Office of Minority Health, 2013). Effective nursing care includes meeting the unique cultural care and language needs of clients.

The U.S. Department of Health and Human Services Office of Minority Health (n.d.-b) conducted an evaluation of the implementation of the national CLAS standards. The standards appear to have aligned health care quality and health care equity, but more work is necessary. Participating health care organizations reported spending large amounts of money collecting databases of language used by their clients and providing highly qualified medical interpreters. Health care employees viewed CLAS standards positively after receiving education on the specific standards and how they could implement them. Organizational changes since implementation included increased linguistic and cultural staff competence, improved responsiveness to specific language and cultural needs, increased organizational capacity to serve culturally diverse clients,

and improved client experience reports. Health care organizations also noted a need for more resources for facilitating implementation of the national CLAS standards. The government responded with the creation of an online library with journal articles, videos, and fact sheets as well as online educational offerings for members of the health care team, including continuing education programs for nurses.

Take Note!
Meeting the cultural care and language needs of clients is essential for effective nursing care.

DIVERSITY AND ASSIMILATION IN A SHRINKING WORLD

American culture values unity and equality. The United States consists of many immigrants who assimilated into a blended American culture. Some people outwardly display their cultural heritage whereas others tend to try to fit in by identifying themselves in other terms, like economic status, the work they perform, and the areas in which they live. However, sometimes as people lose their original ethnic identity, they yearn for it more. Some people from immigrant backgrounds often speak their native languages when they are at home, when they are with people from the same cultural background, and when they encounter stressful situations.

Historically, people from all parts of the world have sought refuge or a new home in the United States. In the first half of the 20th century, immigrants fled from religious persecution and economic and political turmoil in Eastern Europe, often hiding their ethnic roots by anglicizing their names. After World War II, many people from Eastern Europe and the Soviet Union came to the United States to escape communism. The American withdrawal from Vietnam also resulted in increased immigration from some Southeast Asian nations.

In recent years, people from Mexico and South America have sought economic refuge in the United States. Figure 11.1 outlines the cultural diversity in the United States according to the U.S. Census Bureau (2019). From 2010 to 2019, the populations of all non-White groups grew in the United States, with those identifying as Latinx/Hispanic experiencing the fastest growth rate (47.7%) and the White/non-Hispanic population experiencing a decline of 5.6%. Growth in all other groups accounted for this proportional loss. The Black/African American population experienced a 27% growth, the Asian population

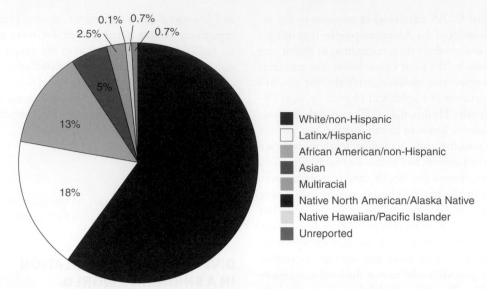

Legend:
- ■ White/non-Hispanic
- □ Latinx/Hispanic
- ▨ African American/non-Hispanic
- ■ Asian
- ▨ Multiracial
- ■ Native North American/Alaska Native
- ▨ Native Hawaiian/Pacific Islander
- ▨ Unreported

0.1% 0.7%
2.5% 0.7%
5%
13%
18%

FIGURE 11.1 Cultural diversity in the United States, 2020. (Adapted from U.S. Census Bureau (2019). *Quick facts. Population estimates, July 1, 2019 (V2019)*. Retrieved September 6, 2020, from https://www.census.gov/quickfacts/fact/table/US/PST045219)

experienced 16% growth, and those who identify as multiracial experienced 9.6% growth. The Native North American/Alaska Native population grew by 0.2%, and the Native Hawaiian/Pacific Island population grew by 0.04%. According to the U.S. Census Bureau (2021), there is one birth every 9 seconds, one death every 10 seconds, and one international migrant entering the nation every 605 seconds, resulting in a net gain of one person in the United States every 52 seconds.

The cultural backgrounds of health care providers does not mirror the demographics of American residents. In recent years, strides are being made to improve the cultural diversity of health care professionals. The Sullivan Commission on Diversity in the Healthcare Workforce identified that only 9% of nurses, 6% of physicians, and 5% of dentists came from diverse cultural groups (2004). Wilber et al. (2020) reported that 6% of medical school graduates were Black/African American and 5% were Hispanic/Latinx. Only 7.4% of physician assistant program graduates were Hispanic/Latinx and 5% were African American (Wilber et al., 2020). According to the 2018 *National Workforce Survey of Registered Nurses* conducted by the U.S. Department of Health and Resources and Services Administration, 73.3% of all American RNs are White; the remainder are 10.2% Hispanic/Latinx, 7.8% Black/African American, 5.2% Asian, 2.6% multiracial, and 0.9% Native North American/Alaska Native/ Native Hawaiian/Pacific Islander. The survey results also reported that 9.6% of RNs are male (a 2.5% increase from 2008 data), and

5% of employed nurses received their initial education outside of the United States (50% from the Philippines, Canada, and India) (U.S. Department of Health and Human Services, Health Resources and Services Administration, National Center for Health Workforce Analysis, 2019). Because many people feel more comfortable among people like themselves (especially when sharing sensitive information), the nursing profession must find ways to recruit and retain people from different cultural backgrounds. The goal is for the profession to attain a cultural profile that mirrors population demographics. Until that happens, nurses must understand cultural and ethnic factors when providing care to clients from many diverse cultures.

 Take Note!
Ideally, the cultural profile of the nursing profession should match that of the population being served.

Basic Terminology to Understand Culture

In 1871, British anthropologist Sir Edward Taylor first used the term *culture* to refer to the complex whole, including knowledge, belief, art, morals, law, custom, and any other abilities and habits people acquired as societal members. In 1935, anthropologist Margaret Mead expanded the definition of culture to include technologic systems, political practices, and habits of daily life. **Culture** serves as a guide for determining the values, beliefs, and practices of individuals or groups of people.

Transcultural nursing uses the Latin prefix "trans," which means *across*, thereby referring to nursing across cultures. **Multicultural nursing** uses the Latin prefix "multi," which means many, denoting nursing of many different cultures. Finally, **intercultural nursing** uses the Latin prefix "inter," which means between, denoting nursing between cultures (Andrews & Boyle, 2016). Box 11.1, Professional Building Blocks, "Understanding the Terminology of Culture," defines additional terms critical to this discussion.

11.1 Professional Building Blocks

Understanding the Terminology of Culture

- Acculturation: Blending of two cultures while adapting to the dominant one
- Cultural accommodation: Taking on facets of a new culture in public while maintaining aspects of a native culture in private
- Cultural assimilation: Adoption of group culture by a member or members of a different culture
- Cultural blindness: Ignoring cultural differences or acting as if they do not exist
- Cultural competence: Integration of knowledge, attitudes, and skills that enable effective and appropriate communications and behaviors when working with people from one or more cultures different from one's own; individual cultural competence focuses on the individual, and organizational cultural competence focuses on organizational leadership and the organization itself.
- Cultural diversity: Differences within and among groups
- Cultural empathy: Expressive concern and the ability to see experiences as the client sees them
- Cultural group: Two or more people sharing the same ancestry, nationality, values, beliefs, identity, or behaviors
- Cultural humility: Lifelong learning mindset aimed at providing the utmost respect for others while recognizing imbalances and attempting to remedy them.
- Cultural identity: Professed membership within a group
- Cultural imposition: Forcing cultural beliefs, values, and patterns onto someone from a different background
- Cultural lifeways: Group beliefs and behaviors related to activities of daily living and inherited traits
- Cultural maintenance: Continued practice of specific cultural norms and behaviors
- Cultural negotiation: Working with a person from another culture to determine what cultural practices can be used without jeopardizing effects
- Cultural norms: Acceptable behaviors and practices
- Cultural pluralism: Maintaining cultural differences after being assimilated into another culture
- Cultural preservation: Continued practice of a specific culture's norms and behaviors
- Cultural relativism: Acknowledging that other ways of doing things are different but not wrong or inferior

- Cultural repatterning (or restructuring): Changing unhealthy cultural behavior patterns to promote better health
- Cultural self-assessment: An exploration and critical reflection of one's own culturally based values, beliefs, attitudes, and practices
- Culture shock: State in which one feels totally disconnected from a group because of cultural differences
- Cultural values: Prevalent, powerful forces that provide meaning and direction to group actions, decisions, and lifeways
- Culture: An integrated pattern of socially transmitted behaviors, including all products of human work and thoughts specific to a group of persons, that guides formulation of worldviews and decision-making processes
- Emic perspective: An insider's view
- Enculturation: The acquisition of aspects of a culture different from one's own
- Ethnicity: Sharing the same ancestral, physical, racial, and national origins along with the same language, lifestyle, religion, or other characteristics
- Ethnocentrism: Evaluating other cultures guided by preconceptions from one's own culture
- Etic perspective: An outsider's view
- Generalization: Oversimplified assumption about a group of persons
- Prejudice: An unfavorable opinion toward another group, often originating from generalization and stereotyping
- Racism: The belief that inherent aspects of one race produce an inherent superiority in another
- Rituals: Routine practices
- Stereotype: Oversimplified idea, opinion, or belief about all members of a particular group
- Taboo: A practice that is absolutely forbidden by a group
- Transcultural nursing: Providing physical, psychological, and spiritual nursing care to clients from different cultural backgrounds while considering each client's cultural beliefs and practices
- White privilege: Advantages or benefits automatically bestowed upon people with light skin
- Worldview: Personal perception of the universe that provides a foundation for values and beliefs about the world and life

Adapted from American Association of Colleges of Nursing. (2021). *The essential core competencies for professional nursing education*. Retrieved May 27, 2021, from https://www.aacnnursing.org/Portals/42/AcademicNursing/pdf/Essentials-2021.pdf; Andrews, M. M., Boyle, J. S., & Collins, J. W. (Eds.). (2020). *Transcultural concepts in nursing care* (8th ed.). Wolters Kluwer; Giger, J. N. (2017). *Transcultural nursing assessment and intervention* (7th ed.). Elsevier/Mosby; Leininger, M. (1995). *Transcultural nursing* (2nd ed.). McGraw-Hill; Leininger, M., & McFarland, M. (2006). *Cultural care diversity and universality: A worldwide theory for nursing*. Jones & Bartlett; Purnell, L. D., & Frankl, E. A. (2021). *Textbook for transcultural health care: A population approach cultural competence concepts in nursing care* (5th ed.). Springer.

A culture may include large numbers of people, as in the global or national culture, or it may incorporate small numbers of people, such as a single-family unit or a gang. Culture can also be differentiated by age (youth culture) or sexual orientation and gender identity. Cultural analysis enables health care providers to understand the impact of lifeways (a way of life distinctly different in anthropology from lifestyle), rituals, and taboos when providing care.

Madeline Leininger, a nurse with advanced education in anthropology, started the transcultural nursing movement. Leininger (1995, p. 4) defined transcultural nursing as "a formal area of study and practice in nursing focused upon comparative holistic cultural care, health, and illness patterns of individuals and groups with respect to differences and similarities in cultural values, beliefs, and practices." The goal of transcultural nursing is "to provide culturally congruent, sensitive, and competent nursing care to people of diverse cultures" (Leininger, 1991, p. 4). Leininger's writing justifies transcultural nursing by saying that people have rights and expectations to have their cultural values and beliefs respected and that nurses are obligated to meet clients' cultural needs. Leininger asserts that being kind, relying on common sense, and ignoring prejudices do not foster culturally relevant care to clients. She proposed that nurses should receive formal education in transcultural nursing that begins with an analysis of one's own cultural values and beliefs.

Transcultural nursing blends nursing and anthropology in theory and practice. A provision of culture-specific care and culture-universal care serves as the aim of transcultural nursing. "Care" refers to providing nursing services with consideration to particular values, beliefs, and behavior patterns unique to a specific group. These tend not to be shared with people from other cultures. **Culture-universal care** denotes the commonly shared values, behaviors, and life patterns that appear among most cultures (Andrews et al., 2020; Leininger & McFarland, 2006). Examples of culture-universal care include the formation of family, the socialization of children into society, and basic physical survival needs.

Culture-Specific and Culturally Congruent Care

Most people use a culture-based health practice before entering the formal health care system (Andrews et al., 2020; Giger, 2017; Leininger, 1995). Professional nurses must understand the concept of **cultural relativism**, which encompasses a profound respect for all cultures, an acknowledgment that all cultures are equal, and an understanding that what is ethically and morally correct for each person is determined by their culture. **Culture-specific care** includes the practices unique to a particular cultural group. Culture-specific care practices may be similar across groups, but each group has slight differences in either the manner in which practices are implemented or the meaning behind them. **Culturally congruent care** incorporates aspects of a specific cultural group's practices while adding other remedies or healers that do not conflict with a culture's morals beliefs and practice.

An example of these concepts is individuals from many cultural groups using folk remedies and healers before or in conjunction with seeking care from the health care system. A culture-specific practice would be inviting a shaman of a hospitalized Native American client to perform a specific healing ceremony immediately following surgery. An example of culturally congruent care would be the nurse serving "hot" and "cold" foods and beverages to a Chinese woman (cultural health practices) who is hospitalized for a cervical radiation implant (a culturally acceptable medical intervention for cancer). Table 11.1 summarizes the culture of the American health care system, then lists examples of traditional culturally based healers and folk remedies for various populations.

Great differences may occur across various ethnic groups. Health care practitioners frequently impose their own cultural values, beliefs, and practices on clients receiving care. However, competent transcultural care blends culturally based practices with empirically based medical practices. When these practices conflict with each other, the nurse (or other health care provider) works with the client from another culture to accommodate cultural practices with the medical plan of care so that the combination of remedies does not cause harm (Andrews et al., 2020; Giger, 2017).

■ QUESTIONS FOR REFLECTION

1. Have you used folk healers or healing practices to enhance your health or recover from an illness or injury? How did you learn about these practices?
2. Have you ever encountered a folk healer in your professional practice? How did you react? How would you react if one of your clients (or a client's family member) insisted that a folk healer practice folk medicine as part of their treatment?
3. What are the policies related to the use of folk healers in your clinical practice setting?

TABLE 11.1   Examples of Traditional Cultural Healers and Folk Remedies

Cultural Group	Healers	Folk Remedies
American health care system	Physician Nurse practitioner Nurse Physical, occupational, and respiratory therapists Social worker Chaplain	Scientifically validated medication and therapies Complex technologic equipment for diagnosis and treatment Some reliance on intuition Effectiveness based on cost–benefit ratio High degree of concern for timeliness of treatments and appointments Spiritual needs of clients usually referred to chaplain
Amish	Brauch or brauch-doktor Lay midwife	Combination of many modalities, including manipulation of body parts, massage, herbs, herbal teas, reflexology, and other folk healing remedies Midwife provides prenatal, birthing, and postpartum care
Caribbean and African	Extended family members, friends, and neighbors Old lady (experienced woman who successfully raised a family) Folk practitioners Faith healer (spiritualist) Houngan (voodoo priestess or priest)	Health clinic and physician visits occur when all folk remedies have been exhausted. Herbal remedies, potions, applications of heat and cold, crystals, massage, meditation, oils, powders, tokens, rites, and ceremonies Oils, candles, soaps, and aerosolized sprays are used to repel evil forces.
Chinese (traditional)	Physician Acupuncturist Herbalist	Physician diagnoses health problems by listening, questioning, and palpating, including feeling quality of pulse and sensitivity of body parts. Acupuncture Herbal preparation (have used close to 6,000 documented herbs)
Asian Indian	Ayurvedic healer	Remedies used come from vegetable and mineral raw materials Yoga Meditation Herbal preparations
Filipino	Family traditions Folk healer	Based on hot/cold theory that requires people to consume hot foods for a cold illness and cold foods for a hot illness Widely use herbal remedies May be quiet and passive when seeking health care
Japanese	Kampo practitioners Family members	Kampo is a holistic approach to illness and uses acupuncture, herbal medicines, moxibustion, and spiritual exercises For colds, use of ginger, sake, and egg; herbal teas for "cure-all;" headaches are treated by rubbing the head with sesame or ginger oil; finger massage and exercise are used to stay well. Hot/cold (yin and yang) theory applies to health-related situations.
Mexican	Family member Curandera Sobadora (massage and bone and joint manipulation specialist) Espiritualista (spiritualist) Yebero (herbalist)	Curanderismo is an eclectic, holistic, and syncretic compilation of beliefs from the Mesoamerican Spanish, spiritualistic, homeopathic, and modern medical beliefs. System is based on herbal preparations, Spanish prayers, altered states of consciousness, and healing rituals that blend indigenous traditions and Catholic rituals. Herbal teas, ingestion or application of powdered substances, massage with warm oils, and skin popping on the small of the back
Native American and Alaska Native	Shaman Singer or chanter (highest position in the Navajo tribe) Crystal gazer, hand trembler, or diagnostician (one step below singer in the Navajo tribe) Singer for healing ceremonies Medicine man (Hopi tribe) Herbalist Nuclear and extended family (Muckleshoot tribe, some Northwest Native Americans, and Alaska Natives)	Sweating and purging usually done in a lodge Herbal remedies from local environment Healing ceremonies using the medicine wheel, sacred hoop, and singing (Lakota, Dineh, and Navajo tribes) Stargazing and hand trembling for diagnosis (Navajo) Herbalist prescribes herbs for symptomatic relief while members await healing ceremony (Navajo) Mothers, grandmothers, and aunts may be key sources of health information related to pregnancy, birth, and childhood illnesses. Health care decisions may be made by familial consensus.

(continued)

TABLE 11.1   Examples of Traditional Cultural Healers and Folk Remedies (*continued*)

Cultural Group	Healers	Folk Remedies
South and Central American	Curanderismo	Foods with qualitative (not literal) properties of "hot" and "cold" People with "hot" diseases should receive "cold" foods and vice versa to restore a balance of hot and cold
South African	Medicine man Isangoma (diagnostician) Inyanga (healer) Midwife Herbalist	Ukincinda (licking), ukubhema (inhalation of snuffing substances), ukuhlanza (emetics), ukuchatha (enemas), ukuguma (steaming), and ukugcaba (incisions made and medicine rubbed into them) are forms of traditional healing methods. Herbal preparations Spiritual ceremonies and sacrifices to spirits Goal of health is to achieve a balance with nature.
Southeast Asians	Shaman	Shaman serves as the mediator between people and the spiritual world to prevent, diagnose, and treat health problems Principles of yin and yang (hot and cold) Infections are hot and should be treated with a cold food such as fruit; cancers are cold and should be treated with hot food such as chicken soup. Strong herbal teas that may be dangerous if concurrently used with Western medicine Dermabrasion, massage, acupressure, acupuncture, and moxibustion Spiritual healing rituals (more commonly used by Vietnamese)
Puerto Rican	Santiguadora Spiritual healers	Herbal teas Massage with warm oils Spiritual rituals

From Eipperle, M. K., & Andrews, M. (2020). Influence of cultural and health belief systems on health care practices. In M. M. Andrews, J. S. Boyle, & J. W. Collins (Eds.), *Transcultural concepts in nursing care* (8th ed., pp. 105–123). Wolters Kluwer; Dayer-Berenson, L. (2011). *Cultural competencies for nurses, impact on health and illness*. Jones & Bartlett; and Purnell, L. D., & Paulanka, B. J. (1998). *Transcultural health care: A culturally competent approach*. F. A. Davis.

ESTABLISHING CULTURAL COMPETENCE

Attainment of cultural competence is a lifelong journey that requires the elimination of **ethnocentrism** (evaluating other cultures with preconceptions from one's own) and an unconditional acceptance of cultural diversity unless the practice places another person in harm's way. Establishment of cultural competence requires continuous contact and interaction with people from other cultures.

Underrepresented, Marginalized, and Exploited Populations

Many Americans do not enjoy high levels of power, status, and wealth. In the United States and other western cultures, racism (a belief that one race is superior to others) permeates society and has resulted in privilege, a set of unearned benefits and advantages automatically given to members of the White race. These benefits are built into social, political, and institutional structures, making it difficult for White people to immediately recognize the advantages they enjoy.

Inequality produces intentional and unintentional divisions among citizens. "Although individual members tied to dominant western cultures may be 'against' racism, they still benefit from a system that privileges their group" (Alexis et al., 2019, p. 29). People who do not identify with the dominant cultural group may be underrepresented (fewer in number), marginalized (perceived as being unimportant or powerless), and/or exploited (used menially or unfairly for the advantages of another) (Mish, 2020). Perceptions of reduced status (being less than a full person who deserves respect, dignity, and equality) may cause the dominant group to exclude others unlike themselves from full participation in society both intentionally and unintentionally.

Those with power, status, or wealth may frequently be viewed as being worthy of receiving health care services. In American culture, the ability to pay defines who has access to health care services. Some health care providers may view disadvantaged individuals who are employed as more worthy of health care than people who do not have jobs because employment indicates contributions to beneficial services to society as well as taxes.

Health care providers often expect culturally diverse clients to adapt to the established norms and policies of the institution, rather than the institution adapting to the needs of the client. Most health care institutions that provide routine services require clients to make appointments, arrive on time, and cancel the scheduled appointment as needed. Some providers do not fully grasp the issues that some clients may have in securing transportation and following prescribed regimens. To become culturally inclusive, health care institutions must ensure their professionals learn about the social organizations and processes of all culturally diverse populations to whom they provide service.

Steps to Acquiring Cultural Competence

Becoming culturally competent does not happen overnight but rather takes time and commitment. Burchum (2002) defined **cultural competence** as a developmental process that builds continuous increases in knowledge and skill development in the areas of cultural awareness, knowledge, understanding, sensitivity, interaction, and skills. The following six steps outline a process for nurses to follow to acquire cultural competence:

Step 1: Examine Personal Values, Beliefs, Biases, and Prejudices

The journey to cultural competence begins with an examination of attitudes, which reflect personal values, beliefs, biases, and prejudices. Attitudes result from evaluative judgments that may have developed over time, either during childhood or from life experience. A variety of self-report tools can be used to measure cultural sensitivity (the degree to which someone has awareness and demonstrates positive responsiveness to cultural differences). Lin et al. (2017) identified three common scales used in the literature to assess cultural awareness, *The Cultural Awareness Scale, the Cultural Competency Assessment Instrument*, and the *Inventory for Assessing the Process of Cultural Competence among Healthcare Professions, revised*. People are often unaware of their own values, beliefs, biases, and prejudices, as well as those of the dominant culture. For self-report tools to be effective, the people completing them must be honest in their answers rather than answering the questions items only in a socially acceptable manner. Once a person identifies areas for attitudinal and/or behavioral change, even long-standing negative attitudes and beliefs may be changed. However, sometimes a personal experience with one or more people from a cultural group may be required to eliminate individual biases and prejudices (Giger, 2017; Purnell & Frankl, 2021).

Step 2: Build Cultural Awareness

To multiple transcultural nursing specialists, cultural awareness serves as an antecedent toward obtaining specific communication strategies and knowledge about other cultures (Andrews et al., 2020; Giger, 2017; Purnell & Frankl, 2021). Results of the self-report methods presented in Step 1 provide a means for people to become more aware of values, beliefs, biases, and prejudices that may be culturally relevant. Nurses who understand how their cultural beliefs affect care delivery can change their behavior and attitudes toward clients from other cultures.

In order to build cultural awareness, nursing students typically provide inpatient client care for people from different cultures in clinical settings. Other opportunities to increase cultural awareness for students include clinical experiences such as providing health screenings and education in a neighborhood community center, administering injections at a health department–sponsored immunization clinic, and participating in national or international mission trips. Nursing students can also interact with classmates, clinical agency staff, and school employees who have cultural backgrounds different from their own.

Step 3: Learn Culturally Specific Communication Strategies

Once health team members are aware of key cultural differences, they can develop specific communication strategies to tear down barriers and provide culturally and linguistically appropriate health care. Learning and implementing culturally specific communication strategies affirm respect for diversity and is the third step toward attainment of cultural competence. Verbal and nonverbal communication patterns are a key part of understanding cultural nuances when serving people from different cultural backgrounds (Andrews, 2020a; Leininger, 1995). For example, principles of therapeutic communication suggest that making direct eye contact facilitates client assessment, shows genuine compassion, and cues people engaged in a conversation when it is each person's turn to speak. However, some cultures (e.g., Asian, Native North American) believe that making direct eye contact is rude and demonstrates a lack of respect.

A key way to foster communication with clients from other cultures is to approach them in a manner that displays authentic empathy and deep respect. Some organizations provide nurses with information about various cultural groups in print (books, pamphlets) or digital (software programs or access to online information) format. The nurse's body language also plays a big role in displaying confidence when working with people from other cultures. A calm, cheerful, unhurried approach displays a sense of concern across most cultures. When nurses hurry while working with clients from other cultures, clients may perceive that the nurse is indifferent to or biased against them.

Speaking even a few words in the client's native language conveys cultural awareness and respect. Sometimes, the nurse can learn from the client and improve foreign language proficiency by asking simple questions. Some nurses find using gestures, pantomimes, and simple questions in the client's language to be an effective way to complete nursing assessments and provide basic nursing care.

Step 4: Interact With People From Different Cultures

Interacting with people from different cultures is the fourth step in cultural competence. This requires risk taking. People sometimes avoid others who differ from themselves. This practice minimizes or denies differences that exist across various groups, such as race, class, nationality, or gender (to name a few broad differences). Such avoidance enforces the invisibility of sensitive issues (Kavanagh & Kennedy, 1992). Respectful engagement during interactions with members of another culture or group provides an opportunity to develop the personal and professional expertise needed to work effectively with culturally diverse clients and colleagues.

Most people from different cultures send cues to each other during interactions. If heeded, the cues can guide the transcultural interaction, and errors can be avoided (Andrews et al., 2020; Giger, 2017). Asking questions before acting also serves as a useful tool. For example, personal space needs to be respected when working with all people. The definition of personal space varies across cultures, with people from North American backgrounds requiring the most distance. In contrast, people from Middle Eastern, Latin American, and Japanese cultures feel quite comfortable being close to others, and the closeness indicates interest and concern. Nurses who are uncertain whether a client's cultural mores permit touching by someone other than a family member should ask the client's permission before touching them.

Some nurses and health team members may consider themselves to be bilingual or multilingual. However, the true extent of the provider's language proficiency may be more appropriate to social conversational use than a health care conversation. Some nurses may speak enough of the client's language to perform a physical assessment and meet the client's basic care needs.

Occasionally, professional nurses and other health team members rely on families, friends, or nonprofessional members of the health care team who speak the client's language to explain medical procedures to non–English-speaking clients. However, reliance on people who do not have the educational background to fully comprehend the implications of complex health care tests and interventions limits full disclosure of potential complications and accurate client education. The national CLAS standards require the use of a qualified medical interpreter rather than a translator when clients and health care providers speak different languages (U.S. Department of Health and Human Services Office of Minority Health, 2013). To avoid legal and ethical issues related to protected health information and privacy concerns, family members and friends may be used as interpreters only with client permission.

▌ QUESTIONS FOR REFLECTION

1. In either your practice or your daily activities, how much opportunity do you have to interact with those from other cultures? How do you usually handle communicating with those who do not speak English or whose cultural norms differ from yours? Do you think you conduct yourself in a culturally competent manner in such interactions? Why or why not?
2. In interacting with individuals from different cultures in clinical or other settings, what resources, policies, and procedures might you draw upon?

Step 5: Identify and Acknowledge Mistakes

Mistake identification and acknowledgment serve as the fifth step toward cultural competence. Because literature on culturally diverse practices places people into various groups resulting in large clumps of cultural categories, errors of similarities may occur with devastating effects (Andrews et al., 2020; Leininger, 1995). For example, demographics related to Pacific Islanders represent 40 different cultural groups who speak 23 languages (Farella, 2001). Within this cultural group, health practices and taboos differ greatly.

Along with errors of similarity, errors of assumption are common. People assume things about others based on outward appearances. Racial profiling results when people assume that individuals who look alike share specific traits and behaviors. The U.S. population is a melting pot, and citizens may refer to themselves as African American, Japanese American, Italian American, Native American, Mexican American, or some other "American" designation. A person's physical appearance, however, is not an accurate indicator of beliefs or practices. Further, second- or third-generation immigrants may or may not abide by the cultural practices of their ancestral homelands (Andrews et al., 2020). Likewise, as people learn about health practices from other cultural groups, culturally based folk practice may become intertwined with traditional Western medicine, resulting in an inability to know what individuals do to achieve and maintain health. For example, an American of Latin American or Asian descent may or may not abide by the hot and cold food theory for illness treatment, though this is common practice among these cultural groups. The best way to avoid errors of similarity and assumption is to perform a detailed, individually focused client health assessment.

Most people accept sincerely offered apologies when health care providers inadvertently commit a cultural faux pas. Valuable lessons can be learned from such communication and behavioral mistakes. Concepts in Practice, "The Value of an Apology," provides an example of how effective a professional apology can be when an error occurs.

Concepts in Practice [IDEA]━━▶[PLAN]━▶[ACTION]

The Value of an Apology

Alice is a professional nurse who works in a cardiac unit. During a busy day, she was assigned to provide care to an older Chinese man with a suspected heart attack. Following her usual client care routine, she entered the room and made complete eye contact as she introduced herself. Alice proceeded to speak English as she shared her intentions to perform a head-to-toe assessment before the client went for an invasive cardiac procedure. As she moved to touch the man, he grabbed her hand and stopped her. Startled, Alice realized that the man did not understand English and that this action was his way of protecting himself. She immediately apologized and then dialed the phone to reach the language interpreting services. Once the services of a Chinese interpreter were secured, she explained the situation, requested that the interpreter apologize to him for her, and then gave the telephone to the man. After speaking with the interpreter, he smiled and chuckled while baring his chest so that Alice could listen to his

heart. Alice used the interpreter during her nursing assessment. The man went for his cardiac procedure.

Upon return to the unit following his procedure, the man asked for Alice by name. Alice entered the room and the man immediately threw off his blanket, motioned for Alice to come to his side, showed her the pressure dressing on his groin, and pantomimed for Alice to touch the dressing. Alice called the interpreter to translate postprocedure care to the man. The man gave the telephone to Alice so that the interpreter could tell her that the man was very pleased with her nursing care and that he only wanted her to care for him because she displayed great respect toward him. The interpreter also told Alice that should the man offer her some food, Alice should take it and eat it in front of him because sharing food with another person would be the utmost compliment for his subcultural group.

Along with errors of assumption, nurses and other health care providers must understand that they hold membership in the American (or other national) health care provider culture. In the United States, health care delivery organizations value efficiency, quality, and empirical evidence. This culture often expects consumers to hold the same (or similar) values (Andrews et al., 2020; Giger, 2017). Some clinics that serve diverse client populations hold clients to standards determined by the values of health care providers. Health care provider expectations for clients frequently create power imbalances. When providing care with cultural humility, providers should acknowledge that mistakes occur, engage in honest self-critiques for them, work to equalize relationships, and strive toward demonstrating the utmost respect for all persons they serve (Abualhaija, 2021).

▮ QUESTIONS FOR REFLECTION

1. Do the health care settings in which you have worked or received care reflect the cultural values of the populations they serve? Provide examples of how they are or might become culturally sensitive.

2. What policies have you encountered in health care settings that reflect a foundation of the American health care system values? How do such policies obstruct the provision of culturally sensitive care?

Step 6: Remediate Cultural Mistakes

Remediation for cultural mistakes serves as the final step toward cultural competence. Correcting mistakes requires communication between individuals as well as groups. Genuine dialogues result in the development of ideas for cultural accommodation and preservation. Because nursing focuses on client comfort, culture-specific nursing interventions enhance client comfort by fostering maintenance of client cultural identity. When members of a cultural group receive culturally sensitive care, they may share this information with other members of their group, resulting in positive advertising for a particular health care organization.

Hallmarks of Culturally Congruent Care

Once transcultural communication has been established, nurses and other health care providers can expand their knowledge related to culture-specific care practices. Andrews (2020a) identifies psychomotor skills useful for when nurses engage in transcultural nursing care activities. The identified areas include assessment, communication, hygiene, activities of daily living, and religious practices. A brief overview of each is provided.

- Assessment: Nurses must consider biologic variations in signs of illness and health, avoid potential cultural taboos in routine activities like measuring the heads of infants, modify childhood developmental screening tools, and use respectful methods to conduct gynecologic examinations of women from various cultures.
- Communication: Transcultural communication skills include speaking in the client's native language, providing health care information in the client's native language, and providing a trained, medical interpreter for clients.
- Hygiene: Nurses must be cognizant of specific hair and skin care needs of clients of various ethnic backgrounds.
- Activities of daily living: Nurses must be aware and capable of coaching clients who have special needs for activities of daily living (such as eating with chopsticks or using special assistive devices such as the West African "chewing stick" for oral hygiene). Nutrition also plays a key role in health care. Providing hot and cold foods to clients whose cultures abide by this practice instills trust between nurses and clients.
- Religious practice: Permitting clients to engage in their religious practices enhances spiritual well-being. Some religious ceremonies include the anointing of the sick (e.g., among Roman Catholics), the reciting of prayers for healing (e.g.,

among those of the Jewish faith), and cleansing before daily prayer (among practicing Muslims).

Nurses are members of the culture of health care providers; thus, value conflicts frequently occur between nurses and health care consumers (Andrews et al., 2020; Leininger, 1995; Spector, 2012). At times, nurses may be unaware of cultural issues surrounding a client care situation. Failure to acknowledge and incorporate culture into client care increases the likelihood of distrust on the part of the health care consumer and antagonism on the part of the health care provider. Conversely, the client's trust and comfort increase when nurses consider cultural preferences during client care. However, transcultural care considerations should not supersede the need for safe, effective client care (Andrews et al., 2020).

Assessment

Identification of cultural nursing considerations begins with the nursing assessment. An individualized cultural assessment prevents the nurse from making cultural errors based on client appearance and provides the nurse with the opportunity to learn about the client's way of life. Elements of the **cultural assessment** include family and kinship systems, social life, political systems, language, traditions, perceptions of the world, values orientation, cultural norms, religious and health beliefs, and health practices. Table 11.2 presents information on each of these elements and suggests ways for nurses to collect data that may be relevant for nursing care. While performing a cultural nursing assessment, nurses must observe clients for cues that indicate misunderstanding or discomfort with any questions asked. Before involving family members in health care communications, the nurse should receive permission from the client to involve family members. Family involvement may be necessary when a particular family member serves as the leader who makes health care decisions for a family. However, to verify complete understanding of questions, use of a specially educated medical interpreter is the best course of action.

Along with verbal communication, the nurse can scan the environment for clues related to culture. At home and also in inpatient settings, many people display symbolic objects to signify their beliefs. Sometimes, items such as charms or religious medals are worn; such items should not be removed without first asking permission of the client. Displayed objects, such as statues, prayer beads, shrines, or special candles, may provide clues to nurses that special cultural health needs may

TABLE 11.2 Elements of Cultural Assessment

Cultural Element	Description	Suggestions for Data Collection
Biologic variations	Inherited factors based on ancestry	Inspection for obvious cultural or ethnic distinctive features Ask specific questions about family history of diseases, particularly those experienced at higher rates by the client's cultural group (e.g., diabetes, hypertension, sickle cell anemia, cardiovascular disease, lactose intolerance).
Family and kinship system	Family structure, roles, and relationships	Describe your family to me. Who lives in your home? Describe the role of each family member. Observe the client as they interact with family members.
Cultural group affiliations	The cultural groups to which the person claims membership. Many people belong to more than one cultural group.	To what civic, ethnic, cultural, or religious groups do you feel you belong? Are there any special gender-related issues associated with your group? How strictly do you follow the cultural beliefs and practices?
Social life	Daily routine and recreation	Describe your typical day or week. How do you spend your free time?
Political systems	Government, organizational, and economic affiliations	What support systems do you use outside the home? Describe your work environment. Describe any legal concerns you may have. Do you feel valued and respected by members of your local community? Do you feel safe in your community? Do you have an economic concerns regarding seeking health care?
Language	Language spoken inside and outside the home	What is your native language? Do you speak more than one language? What language do you speak at home?
Traditions	Nonverbal communications, personal space, and other rituals that may have been passed down from previous generations	Is there anything I should share with other health team members with regard to your personal space or other aspects of communication? Do you have any rituals or habits that we need to consider in providing health care to you?
Perceptions of the world	Viewpoints on the meaning of existence and how the world operates	How do you view the world and your place in it?
Values orientation	What the person considers the most important things in life	What things in life matter most to you? How can we ensure these aspects are preserved for you?
Cultural norms	Cultural attitudes about food, time, work, and leisure	What do you define as food? What do you usually eat? Do you have any special dietary considerations? How do you obtain and prepare food? Describe the work you do and how satisfying you find it. Describe your ideas about time. What do you think about time and being on time? What things do you like to do when you have free time?
Religion	Spiritual beliefs, including special beliefs and rituals surrounding life, health, illness, and death	Do you have any special spiritual needs related to your life, health, or illness? If you were to have a terminal illness, do you have a living will or advance directive?
Health beliefs	Group attitudes about health and illness	What are your beliefs about health and illness?
Health practices	Behaviors and rituals surrounding health and illness, including the use of folk healers and remedies	Tell me about the things you do at home to maintain your health. What type of measures did you take to cope with this health problem before you sought health care?

From Boyes, J. S., & Andrews, M. M. (2020). Appendix A: Transcultural nursing assessment guide for individuals and families. In M. M. Andrews, J. S. Boyle, & J. W. Collins (Eds.), *Transcultural concepts in nursing care* (8th ed., pp. 429–435). Wolters Kluwer; Boyles, J. S., & Andrews, M. M. (2020). Appendix B: Transcultural assessment guide for families, groups and communities. In M. M. Andrews, J. S. Boyle, & J. W. Collins (Eds.), *Transcultural concepts in nursing care* (8th ed., pp. 453–457). Wolters Kluwer; Purnell, L. D., & Frankl, E. A. (2021). *Textbook for transcultural health care: A population approach cultural competence concepts in nursing care* (5th ed.). Springer; Dayer-Berenson, L. (2011). *Cultural competencies for nurses, impact on health and illness*. Jones & Bartlett.

surface. Polite inquiries related to unfamiliar objects may begin a dialogue about culture (Grossman, 1996).

Sometimes a nurse and client may share the same religious beliefs but come from different cultural groups. For example, an Irish Roman Catholic nurse performing spiritual assessments on clients of Hispanic or African descent might discover that although they come from different cultural backgrounds, they share common religious beliefs. In this example, clients who know that their beliefs are acknowledged and understood may feel more at ease when receiving care (see Concepts in Practice, "Shared Beliefs"). Institutional chaplains serve as invaluable resources for information regarding religious differences and accessing services for various religious rites and practices.

Concepts in Practice IDEA ⟶ PLAN ⟶ ACTION

Shared Beliefs

Juanita is a night nurse who practices Roman Catholicism. Frequently, she notices various religious artifacts that clients bring to the hospital. Juanita received a report about an older woman of German descent who has a terminal condition and does not respond to questions. Upon entering the woman's room, Juanita notices that the woman has her eyes closed and is moving her lips while touching beads. Juanita recognizes the beads as a rosary. She decides to join the woman in her prayers. As Juanita speaks the word of one of the prayers, the older woman opens her eyes and smiles. Juanita asks the woman if she is having pain. The older woman says no and reaches out to Juanita. Juanita takes the woman's hand and gently squeezes it. Juanita asks the woman if she needs anything. The woman replies, "I would like to see a priest." Juanita makes a call to the Roman Catholic priest on call. Upon learning this, the older woman relaxes and asks Juanita to stay and pray until the priest arrives.

Provision of Culturally Congruent Care

Once the assessment is complete, the nurse proceeds with planning culturally congruent care. This may require referring to resources related to specific cultures and detailed information about the medical plan of care. Sometimes, traditional folk remedies (especially herbal ones) may interfere with ordered medications. When this occurs, the nurse must find ways to work with clients so that they understand the hazards of using folk remedies along with prescription medications. By engaging in respectful conversations, nurses and clients work together to make decisions related to accommodating lifeway practices with health care treatments.

Linguistically appropriate care serves as the final hallmark of culturally congruent care for clients who do not speak the language of health care providers. When possible, interpreters should be used for health teaching unless the provider is fluent in the client's language. Conversational foreign language provides the nurse with an ability to meet the client's basic needs. Most people who speak English as a second language find comfort with providers who speak to them in the primary language. However, mistakes can be made by the provider, so interpreters are essential when sharing critical information. If an interpreter happens to know the client or is part of a small, local community, preservation of client confidentiality might become an issue.

International Nursing Opportunities

Nurses can enhance their cultural competence by taking advantage of nursing opportunities outside of their home countries. Governmental, private, and religious organizations offer opportunities for international nursing practice. The United Nations has nursing opportunities in various areas, including refugee support, immunization programs, AIDS prevention and treatment, and health promotion in developing countries. The Peace Corps offers nurses an opportunity to improve health in developing countries under the sponsorship of the U.S. government. The U.S. Public Health Service offers assignments abroad. Private organizations, such as Doctors Without Borders, CARE, Catholic Relief Services, and Project HOPE, seek the services of professional nurses for long- and short-term programs. The International Red Cross offers worldwide disaster relief for which nursing services are also needed. Various organized religions offer opportunities for missionary nursing as well.

The nursing shortage in the United States is shared with other countries. Saudi Arabia frequently recruits professional nurses from around the world. Nurses must be aware, however, that when accepting employment for a foreign assignment, they become bound by the host country's laws, cultural values, and norms. Therefore, before embarking on an international nursing experience or career, the professional nurse (or student) should read extensively about the culture, politics and economics, religions, health care system, and laws of the destination country. Scholarly journals and popular media provide sources for this information. If possible, the nurse should meet with host country residents to learn more about the culture. Some nurses find it useful to develop fluency in the country's language(s) and visit the country as a tourist.

Upon arrival at the host country, the nurse should visit their native country's embassy or consulate (Herberg, 2008). Lack of knowledge serves as no excuse for breaking laws, and in some cases, nurses have been subjected to corporal punishment for failure to abide by laws related to dress and for being in public without escorts.

STRATEGIES AND CHALLENGES FOR MULTICULTURAL NURSING PRACTICE

Nurses who care for clients from multiple cultural backgrounds must treat each person as an individual with unique personal needs. Some people become assimilated to the culture of the nation in which they reside whereas others do not. Not only are there international differences, but there also may be geographic differences within a country. Differences also may occur within a state (or province), county, or city. Taking time to listen to clients as care is delivered and having a broad knowledge base of cultural preferences enable the nurse to increase client comfort.

Health Disparities

Healthy People 2030 (U.S. Department of Health and Human Services Office of Disease Prevention and Health Promotion, 2020) provides five domains for social determinants of health. The program defines determinants of health as environmental conditions that occur "where people are born, live, play, work, worship, and age that affect a wide range of health functioning, quality of life, and risk" (para. 1). The five categories are economic stability, neighborhood and built environment, social and community context, and access to and quality of education and health care. When social determinants of health are compromised (e.g., violent neighborhoods, discrimination, racism, low income, lack of access to nutritious food, low literacy, poor education, low-quality health care), health disparities occur.

Healthy People 2030 defines a **health disparity** as "a particular type of health difference that is closely linked with social, economic, and/or environmental disadvantage. Health disparities adversely affect groups of people who have systematically experienced greater obstacles to health based on their racial or ethnic group; religion; socioeconomic status; gender; age;

mental health; cognitive, sensory, or physical disability; sexual orientation or gender identity; geographic location; or other characteristics historically linked to discrimination or exclusion." (U.S. Department of Health and Human Services Office of Disease Prevention and Health Promotion, 2020). The initiative lists 355 core objectives to improve the health, well-being, and quality of life for all Americans, identifying over 50 health disparities that need to be reversed.

Attitudes and Behaviors Toward Health Care

As noted through this chapter, health beliefs vary across cultures. Many marginalized cultural groups in the United States report different attitudes and experiences with health care that may be associated with the following:

- General distrust of health care providers and systems
- Stigma based on race, low income, and smoking status
- Discrimination based on race, ethnicity, gender identity, and age
- Rejection of traditional or spiritual healing practices
- Lack of being an active participant in determining plans for disease prevention, health promotion, and treatments
- Perception that providers likely receive benefits for prescribing specific medications
- Overreliance on using medications (Freeman et al., 2017; Hong et al., 2018; Lago et al., 2017)

Burggraf (2000), Hong et al. (2018), and Lago et al. (2017) also noted that language barriers may be a deterrent to seeking health care in populations of older Hispanic individuals and older adult Asian women. Some groups of older women tend to rely on folk and spiritual healing practices before entering the health care system (Burggraf, 2000; Hong et al., 2018). Young immigrant women receiving obstetric care services in Canada have experienced issues with maternity care because of language barriers and lack of social support from their extended families who stayed in their homelands. Specific challenges to them are presented in the following "Focus on Research" box. The United States and Canada frequently receive immigrants from politically unstable countries that may result in immigrant recipients of health care services avoiding criticizing health services rendered. Nurses need to tailor client health assessments to collect all culturally relevant data for use in planning, implementing, and evaluating care.

FOCUS ON RESEARCH

Cultural Care Considerations for Nurses Working With Immigrants

Using individual and focus group semi-structured interviews, the investigators wanted to discover what issues immigrants were encountering in accessing and receiving health care services. Data were collected over a time frame of 2.5 years from 34 immigrant women who received obstetric care, 29 health care providers, and 23 social workers. They used purposive sampling techniques for each group included in the study.

The immigrant participants perceived personal barriers to access to effective maternity services that included communication barriers (not fluent in English or French); lack of social support (extended family not available to help the new mother); incongruent cultural beliefs (e.g., childbirth as a natural process not requiring medical care services); and lack of information about available services. The immigrant participants identified inadequate health care and high cost of prescription medications as structural barriers to services. Factors that reduced satisfaction with rendered care services included experiencing culture shock; feeling of being stereotyped; being discriminated against by health care providers; dismissal from the hospital too soon; visits with health care providers that were too short; misunderstanding the process of informed consent; and listening to health care providers violate confidentiality.

Some health care providers expressed concern about the immigrant women not fully understanding client education and treatment plans. Other health care providers expressed disdain for some immigrant women who expected medical care to be provided like concierge services in a hotel. The cultural dissonance between childbirth as a medical versus a natural event proved to be a source of distress for some health care providers as well. Cultural clashes also occurred during prenatal care (diet and exercise expectations); postnatal care (early hospital dismissals versus a 72-hour stay); and newborn care (infant staying in mother's room).

Generalizing the study findings to other situations must be done with caution because of limiting factors that include being conducted in only one Canadian province; poor language fluency on the part of the immigrant women; varying stages of the immigration process among immigrant women; and the possible reluctance of some immigrant participants to criticize services because of a previous history of civil strife in their homelands.

This study has clinical and health policy implications. In a health care system that strives for equality for all, people who are different may experience discrimination and receive care based on stereotypes of a particular ethnic group. Personal attributes of health care providers may reduce the adequacy and acceptability of care. Health information education material must be provided in multiple languages and media based on the population service by a particular organization. Health care providers caring for diverse populations should be educated about cultural competence, monitored for culturally sensitive delivery of care, and evaluated for their performance. Programs to ameliorate system and personal discrimination need to be developed and maintained.

Higginbottom, G. M., Safipour, J., Yohani, S., O'Brien, B., Mumtaz, Z., & Paton, P. (2016). An ethnographic investigation of the maternity healthcare experience of immigrants in rural and urban Alberta, Canada. *BioMed Central Pregnancy and Childbirth, 16*, 20. https://doi.org/10.1186/s12884-015-0773-z

Despite cultural differences regarding perceptions and beliefs about body parts and certain types of illness, all humans have similar biologic structures and basic physiology, and some aspects of nursing care can be considered culturally neutral care.

Folk Illnesses

In addition to different risks for specific illnesses based on ethnicity, some cultures have **folk illnesses** that may require the use of culturally based healers. For example, *empacho* is a gastrointestinal condition that individuals from Mexico believe occurs in infants. The belief is that empacho results in a backup of food and other matter within the walls of the stomach or intestines. Empacho is believed to occur if the child swallows too much saliva during teething or when parents change formulas that do not mix well with each other. Symptoms include abdominal distention, pain, poor appetite, perceived stomach lump, and diarrhea. Infants are placed on a regimen of clear liquids and herbal teas to "refresh the stomach" (Pachter, 1994, p. 692). If the infant loses too much weight, the parents may consult a physician to avoid being perceived by others as neglectful.

Culturally competent care blends conventional medical therapy with folk remedies. For example, some people with medical illnesses go to physicians but may seek the advice of a folk healer to discover why the illness occurred. Some people view medical illnesses as the result of an evil spell and need to seek treatment from a spiritual healer to be fully well (Andrews & Boyle, 2016; Giger, 2017; Pachter, 1994).

Physical Assessment Challenges

Along with increased specific health risks, people from different ethnic backgrounds have **variations in physical appearance** (Andrews, 2020a; Giger, 2017). The transculturally competent nurse considers variations in physical appearance when performing health assessments. A general appearance scan reveals information related to gender, age, skin color, body structure, consciousness level, facial features, clothing, and behavior. Initial interaction with the client permits the nurse to collect information regarding orientation, speech patterns, facial expression, mood, and cognition. Clothing choice shows the nurse whether the person is able to select appropriate clothing for the weather and social situation. Although grooming is often a matter of personal preference, it can provide the nurse with cues related to the client's culture.

Clothing styles vary widely across cultures. For example, Amish women usually wear solid-color dresses held together by pins or snaps and a bonnet. Mennonite women wear similarly styled clothing, but the dresses may be of printed material and have buttons. Islamic women may wear clothing to cover all extremities and their hair, and they sometimes cover their faces with a veil or scarf. Islamic men sometimes wear a cloth headdress and a long robe. Depending upon the sect of Islam, clothing may be all black or of high fashion. Some Indian women wear saris. In certain instances, cultural and religious clothing may be concealed, as in the case of special white undergarments known as "temple garments" that are worn by members of the Church of Jesus Christ of Latter Day Saints (Mormons) (Andrews & Boyle, 2016). Roman Catholics often wear religious medals or pictures of Jesus and the Virgin Mary encased in plastic around their necks (scapulars). When providing physical care to clients, the nurse should ask permission before removing specific items of clothing or jewelry. Attention should be paid to problems presented by caregiver's gender with alternate staffing arrangements made when feasible.

Skin color varies among everyone and depends on melanin concentrations. When assessing for skin changes, the nurse must determine what the usual healthy shade is for the individual, rather than for the ethnic group. Specific skin variations for various ethnic groups may be found in physical assessment and transcultural nursing textbooks. Table 11.3 provides a brief summary of some key aspects for nursing assessments related to variations related to ethnic descent. If the nurse relies on assessment data based on the skin color of those who present as White, critical errors could occur.

Physiologic Variances

In addition to skin color, genetic traits result in **variations in physiology** across ethnic groups, such as the adjustment in "normal" reference laboratory values

TABLE 11.3 Nursing Assessment Considerations Based on Ethnicity

Ethnic Group	Assessment Considerations
African	Mongolian spots and vitiligo more common Higher carotene levels in sclerae may give them a yellow appearance. Pallor appears as ashen or gray. Erythema difficult to see, but inflammation is more detectable by palpation for warmth, edema, and hardness. Hard and soft palates may be the best place to see a macular rash. Petechiae cannot be seen in some cases, and if seen, can be found on the buccal mucosa, conjunctiva, abdomen, buttocks, and volar forearm surface. Hair and scalp tend to be dry. Copper-colored hair in children is an indication of severe malnutrition. Less susceptible to noise-induced hearing loss Increased incidence of oral hyperpigmentation in older age Increased periodontal disease Highest bone density of all groups

(continued)

TABLE 11.3	Nursing Assessment Considerations Based on Ethnicity (*continued*)
Ethnic Group	**Assessment Considerations**
Native Americans and Alaska Natives	Mongolian spots and vitiligo more common Pallor appears yellow-brown. 18% have cleft uvula Alaska Native populations have the largest teeth. 30% of Navajo women have longitudinal vascular pattern on chest. Alaska Native populations have lower bone density than White.
Asian	Mongolian spots and vitiligo more common Areola and genitalia are darker Pallor appears as pasty or nearly white Hair usually silky, black, and straight Delayed hair graying Highest incidence of myopia (Japanese and Chinese) 10% have cleft uvula Lower bone density than White
European	Individuals of Mediterranean descent frequently have bluish lips, thereby negating reliance on circummoral cyanosis as a reliable indicator of poor oxygenation. Pallor appears pasty or nearly white. Skin wrinkles appear at a younger age. Tend to have more moles than other groups Hair turns gray at an earlier age. Smallest teeth, resulting in more tooth loss
Pacific Island	Higher carotene levels in sclerae may give them a yellow appearance. Pallor appears yellow-brown.
Middle Eastern	Vitiligo more common Pallor appears yellow-brown.
Hispanic	Pallor appears yellow-brown. Hair may have more natural oils.

From Andrews, M., Boyle, J. S., & Collins, J. W. (Eds.). (2020). *Transcultural concepts in nursing care* (8th ed.). Wolters Kluwer; Purnell, L. D., & Frankl, E. A. (2021). *Textbook for transcultural health care: A population approach cultural competence concepts in nursing care* (5th ed.). Springer.

for blood tests. For example, the hemoglobin levels of African Americans tend to be lower than those of their African counterparts; Native, Japanese, and Hispanic Americans have higher blood glucose levels than do European Americans. African Americans tend to have higher baseline levels of high-density lipoproteins (HDLs) than do people of European descent, and Hispanic Americans have lower HDL levels. The source of these variations may be genetic and/or environmental. The federal government has identified medical research across gender and ethnic groups as a research priority (Jarvis, 2016; U.S. Department of Health and Human Services, 2010).

Pharmacogenetics (or pharmacogenics) is the field of study that describes metabolic variations that result in different responses to pharmacologic agents. Some of the known responses are summarized in Table 11.4. Some variations result from an inherited enzyme deficiency, whereas the sources of other variations remain unknown. When providing care for a culturally diverse client population, professional nurses should be aware of differing responses to medications to anticipate potential adverse effects and different therapeutic responses that may require dosage alterations (Andrews, 2020b).

Take Note!
When performing health assessments, culturally competent nurses take into account variations in cultural beliefs, physical appearance, and physiology among specific ethnic groups.

Variations in Gender Identity and Sexual Orientation: Gender-Affirming Care

Precise health care needs and preferences sometimes rely on health care professionals to know the gender identities and sexual orientations of the clients they serve. **Gender identity** is determined by each person; and only that individual can identify themselves as male, female, or nonbinary. Gender identity may or may not correspond to the sex assigned at birth. **Sexual**

TABLE 11.4 Cultural Variations in Response to Pharmacologic Agents

Cultural Group	Pharmacologic Agent	Variations
African Americans	Analgesics	Reduced sensitivity to therapeutic effects Increased gastrointestinal adverse effects, especially with acetaminophen
	Antihypertensives	Blood pressure responds better to single-agent therapy. Less responsive to beta-blockers and angiotensin converting enzyme inhibitors Increased mood responses to thiazide diuretics
	Mydriatics	Less pupil dilation
	Psychotropics	Increased risk for extrapyramidal side effects
	Steroids	Increased risk for steroid-induced diabetes (especially with methylprednis-olone in renal transplantation)
	Tranquilizers	15%–20% poorly metabolize diazepam.
Arab Americans	Antiarrhythmics	Some dose reduction may be needed.
	Antihypertensives	Some dose reduction may be needed.
	Neuroleptics	Some dose reduction may be needed.
	Opioids	Higher doses may be required because this group may have diminished ability to metabolize codeine to morphine.
	Psychotropics	Some dose reduction may be needed.
Alaska Natives	Muscle relaxants	May have prolonged muscle paralysis with succinylcholine administration during surgery and may need mechanical ventilation for respiratory support.
Chinese Americans	Narcotic analgesics	Less sensitive to respiratory depressant and hypotensive effects Have a higher clearance of morphine
Asian Americans	Antihypertensives	Best response with calcium antagonists
	Neuroleptics	May need reduced dosage
	Psychotropics	May need reduced dosage and up to one half the normal dose for tricyclic antidepressants and lithium
	Fat-soluble drugs	Increased dosages of fat-soluble drugs needed because of reduced percentages of body fat (especially vitamin K for warfarin reversal)
Hispanic/Latinx Americans	Psychotropics	May need to reduce dosage because this group frequently has a higher incidence of adverse effects with tricyclic antidepressants
Americans of Mediterranean descent with glucose-6-phosphate dehydrogenase deficiency	Oxidating medications	Precipitation of a hemolytic crisis with primaquine, quinidine, thiazolsul-fone, nitrofurazone, furazolidone, naphthalene, toluidine blue, phenyl-hydrazine, chloramphenicol, and aspirin
Jewish American of Ashkenazi descent	Psychotropics	20% experience agranulocytosis with clozapine treatment for schizophrenia.

From Andrews, M. (2020). Cultural competence in the history and physical examination. In M. M. Andrews, J. S. Boyle, & J. W. Collins (Eds.), *Transcultural concepts in nursing care* (8th ed., pp. 55–104). Wolters Kluwer; Munoz, C., & Hilgenberg, C. (2005). Ethnopharmacology: Understanding how ethnicity can affect drug response is essential to providing culturally competent care. *American Journal of Nursing, 105*(8), 40–48.

orientation refers to the gender or genders to which a person is sexually attracted.

The tracking of gender identity and sexual orientation relies on self-reported data. According to Conron and Goldberg (2020), there are approximately 11,343,000 people who identify themselves as being lesbian, gay, bisexual, transgender, and/or queer (or questioning) (LGBTQ+) living in the United States (Meyer, 2019). Newport (2018) and Meyer (2019) reported that the number of self-identified LGBTQ+ individuals in the United States has risen from 3.5% in 2012 to 4.5% in 2017 according to a Gallup poll.

According to Newport (2018), the greatest proportion of LGBTQ+ individuals is in the millennial generation (8.1%) when compared to those in Generation X (3.5%), baby boomers (2.4%), and those in the Traditionalist (Silent) Generation (1.4%). The same survey results demonstrated that the incidence of LGBTQ+ identification was highest among Hispanics/Latinx (6.1%) and lowest among White/non-Hispanics (4%). Of individuals who earn less than $36,000 annually, 6.2% reported identifying as LGBTQ+ compared to 3.6% of people who earn $90,000 or more annually (Newport, 2018). There was no major difference in reports of being LGBTQ+ according to completed levels of education (Newport, 2018).

To establish cultural competence and to deliver gender-sensitive care, nurses must assess their own level of awareness and comfort when working with members of the LGBTQ+ community. The process starts with examining one's personal values and biases toward people with different gender identities and sexual orientations. Table 11.5 provides an overview of gender identity and sexual orientation terminology clients may use when seeking health care. LGBTQ+ individuals may consider themselves members of an LGBTQ+ cultural

TABLE 11.5 Sexuality-Related Terms for Providing Gender-Sensitive Care

Term	Definition
Asexuality	A lack of sexual attraction
Autosexuality	Sexual attraction to oneself
Biphobia	Fear, hatred, or stigma toward people who identify as bisexual
Biromantic	Romantic feelings toward people of one's own or the opposite gender without an interest in sex
Bisexuality	Sexual attraction toward individuals of one's own or the opposite gender
Cisgender ("cis")	Gender identity matches the sex assigned at birth; "cishet" is an abbreviation for a person who is cisgender and heterosexual
Demiromantic	Romantic feelings for another only after the development of an intense bond or emotional connection
Demisexuality	Sexual attraction that only develops once a strong emotional bond is formed
Gay	Someone who is sexually attracted to another who was assigned the same sex at birth; often used to describe men but may also be used to describe women
Gender binary	The classification of gender into male and female; excludes those who do not identify as one or the other
Gender-fluid	A person whose gender identity fluctuates; gender is not fixed
Gender identity	How a person perceives their own gender
Heterosexuality	Sexual attraction toward individuals who were assigned the opposite sex at birth from one's own
Hypersexuality	An obsession with sexual thoughts and behaviors that interferes with daily life
Intersex	Term used for someone with chromosomes, sexual organs, or genitals at birth that do not fall within the typical definitions of "male" or "female"
Lesbian	A person who identifies as female and is sexually attracted to others who identify as female
LGBTQ+	Acronym for lesbian, gay, bisexual, transgender, bisexual, questioning/queer, and the plus sign includes intersex, asexual, and other gender and sexual identities
Nonbinary or genderqueer	An umbrella term that indicates a person does not identify as either male or female identity or does not solely identify as male or female
Orientation or sexual orientation	To whom someone is sexually attracted; gender is not a determining factor
Pansexuality	Sexual attraction not limited by sex assigned at birth, gender, or gender identity
Queer	An umbrella term for those who are not cisgender or heterosexual
They, them, theirs, themselves	Gender-neutral pronouns nonbinary individuals may prefer
Transgender or trans	A person whose sexual identity does not match their sex assigned at birth

Adapted from Saint Thomas, S., & Andres T. (2020). *23 sexuality-related terms you need to know*. Retrieved October 11, 2020, from https://www.cosmopolitan.com/sex-love/a24442815/sexual-orientation-list-definitions/; University of Wisconsin-Milwaukee Lesbian, Gay, Bisexual, Transgender, Queer Plus (LGBTQ+) Resource Center. (2020). *Gender pronouns*. Retrieved October 11, 2020, from https://uwm.edu/lgbtrc/support/gender-pronouns/; Mish, F. C. (2020). *Merriam-Webster's Collegiate Dictionary* (11th ed.). Merriam-Webster.

group. Misgendering a person by using an incorrect pronoun is considered disrespectful. Some people may prefer gender-nonspecific pronouns like "they" and "them" rather than "he" or "she." The best practice is to ask the client what they prefer and, whenever possible, refer to the client by name (University of Wisconsin-Milwaukee Lesbian, Gay, Bisexual, Transgender, Queer Plus [LGBTQ+] Resource Center, 2020). The Centers for Medicare and Medicaid Services require that participating health care organizations have policies of non-discrimination in place that address gender identity and sexual orientation (Brous, 2019).

Social determinants of health are compromised for LGBTQ+ people because they often experience discrimination when obtaining health insurance, accessing affordable housing, obtaining employment, and marrying and adopting children. They may also experience issues related to retirement benefits for their partners. LGBTQ+ youth frequently experience bullying in the school setting. There is a lack of appropriate social programming for LGBTQ+ people in all age groups. Few health care providers are knowledgeable and able to provide culturally competent care targeted at their special needs (Office of Disease Prevention and Health Promotion [ODPHP], 2020)

Some health issues for members of the LGBTQ+ community revolve around complications following gender affirmation surgery (e.g., the prostate is not removed when a male undergoes a female affirmation procedure). Some LGBTQ+ people take prescribed hormones routinely, which increases the risk for cardiovascular disease, stroke, thrombi, and embolism. In addition, many common prescription and over-the-counter drugs can interfere with spironolactone, a medication that can reduce excess hair growth (Brous, 2019).

As a marginalized group, members of the LGBTQ+ community may experience many health disparities. The ODPHP (2020) has identified the following health disparities commonly encountered by the LGBTQ+ community:

- LGBTQ+ youth are two to three times more likely to commit suicide.
- LGBTQ+ youth experience higher levels of homelessness.
- Lesbian women are less likely to seek out preventive cancer services.
- Lesbian and bisexual people experience higher rates of overweight and obesity.
- Gay men have an increased risk of HIV infection and other sexually transmitted infections (STIs).

- Transgender individuals are less likely to have health insurance but are at higher risk for HIV and other STIs, victimization, mental health issues, and suicide.
- Members of the LGBTQ+ community have a higher incidence of tobacco, alcohol, and illicit drug use.
- Older adult LGBTQ+ members experience more social isolation, lack social services, and have minimal access to culturally competent care providers.

Because of discrimination and marginalization, many LGBTQ+ people delay seeking health care services. Issues arise with finding safe places for victims of domestic partner violence. Members of the LGBTQ+ community may also be targeted and become the victims of hate crimes (especially when an individual is a member of additional marginalized groups). Sometimes, injuries require immediate treatment in the emergency setting that can result in further physical injury or psychological distress if sensitive care is not provided. The constant stress of discrimination and marginalization sets the stage for the development of hypertension, diabetes, cardiovascular disease, and other stress-induced and stress-exacerbated illnesses (ODPHP, 2020).

The Polaris Project (2019) identified the following risk factors for human trafficking: recent relocation or migration, illegal substance use, runaway or homeless youth, mental health concerns, and involvement with the child welfare system. LGBTQ+ youth are estimated to account for 40% of the homeless youth population, placing them at a higher risk for becoming victims of human trafficking (Brous, 2019). The U.S. Department of Health and Human Services Office on Trafficking in Persons offers education for first responders to identify and intervene on behalf of victims of human trafficking. They devised the acronym "SOAR":

- *S*cope: Awareness of the problem of human trafficking
- *O*bserve: Looking for verbal and nonverbal indicators of human trafficking
- *A*pproach: Identifying and interacting with the person suspected using a victim-centered approach
- *R*espond: Acting effectively to assist the victim of human trafficking to get out of the situation

Knowledge, skills, and attitudes play key roles in providing culturally competent care to the LGBTQ+ community. As client advocates, nurses must strive to protect and safeguard members of this community. Health care organizations and providers must be cognizant of the intricacies of providing care to them; a provider is legally accountable if their care results in physical harm or psychological distress (Brous, 2019).

CREATING A MULTICULTURAL NURSING PROFESSION

To offer health care services to a diverse population, a **multicultural nursing profession** must be created. Attracting people from different cultural backgrounds to the nursing profession remains a challenge. Nursing competes with other professions for the same students. Unfortunately, many bright students prefer to enter other professions because nursing is sometimes perceived by outsiders as an oppressed profession that holds a status subservient to physicians. Adding membership to one more oppressed group may be more than a person can bear.

In addition to the perception of nurses as less powerful members of the health care team, White women have traditionally dominated nursing. This dominance brings with it values, beliefs, and practices that reflect the socialization of White women. Current efforts to increase cultural diversity in the nursing profession include minority nursing scholarships, grant programs, and targeted recruitment efforts. According to the American Association of Colleges of Nursing (AACN, 2019), nationwide initiatives to promote diversity in nursing include Health Resources and Service Administration Nursing Workforce Diversity grants, the Robert Wood Johnson Foundation's Doctoral Advancement in Nursing, and the AACN's own diversity, equity, and inclusion group. The AACN group offers consultation services to the federal government, provides resources to promote diversity and inclusion to member organizations, and keeps detailed records of nursing student and program graduate diversity. The Campaign for Action sponsored by the American Association of Retired Persons and the Robert Wood Johnson Foundation provides support for increasing diversity in the nursing profession, one of the recommendations from the initial *Future of Nursing* report. *The Future of Nursing: Campaign for Action's* Equity, Diversity and Inclusion Steering Committee "works to identify leaders and advocates to implement policies, programs, and best and promising practices to ensure a diverse cadre of nurses, and to promote health equity and address systemic and institutional racism and other inequities for historically marginalized populations" (Campaign for Action, 2020, para. 2). The National League for Nursing (NLN) offers a diversity and inclusion toolkit for nursing programs to use to promote diversity and inclusion in their nursing programs (NLN, 2017). Individual states and specific nursing education programs also offer grants and scholarships for promoting members of underrepresented populations to pursue nursing educational endeavors. Many specialized professional nursing organizations offer scholarships and grants for underrepresented group members to pursue nursing careers, including the Asian American Pacific Islander Nurses Association, Native Alaskan Native American Indian Nurses Association, National Association of Hispanic Nurses, National Black Nurses Association, and Philippine Nurses Association of America. According to the Campaign for Action (2021), graduation rates for professional nursing programs in 2019 revealed that 33.5% of new graduates were members of an underrepresented population (11.8% Hispanic/Latinx; 10.7% African American; 6.4% Asian; 2.8% multiracial; 0.8% international students; 0.6% Alaska Native/Native American; and 0.4% Native Hawaiian/Pacific Islander).

Once accepted into a nursing program, some minority nursing students experience **culture shock** (feelings of alienation, difficulty in relationships, loss of excitement, and a general dislike of the nursing program). This is exacerbated when some programs do not have a culturally diverse student body. Some minority students may become isolated because of an inability to interact with others like themselves or feel uneasy when interacting with students who are not like themselves. Most nurse educators come from the dominant group of nurses (White) and students of color may have difficulty connecting with them and finding professional role models who look like them.

Health care system and professional nursing values align with those of middle class, European-based values such as assuming responsibility for one's actions, being proactive rather than reactive, assuming the "Protestant work ethic," meeting deadlines, and arriving on time. Nursing programs expect students to abide by these traditional cultural values of nursing. For example, punctuality is a highly valued work practice in nursing and education. Students sometimes receive a grade penalty for arriving to class late or submitting assignments late, especially when faculty fail to explore reasons for a late assignment or neglect to explain the reasons why punctuality is valued.

Faculty may make errors when working with students from various cultural groups. Nursing students from different cultures may use different nonverbal behaviors than their instructors expect when conversing with people in positions of authority. For example, students from Asian cultures may not make eye contact when conversing with teachers, supervising staff nurses, physicians, and older persons. Although for the student this practice is a way of conveying respect, some faculty and staff may label the student as being cold and distant and question the student's ability to practice nursing with genuine compassion.

Upon graduation from a nursing program, nurses from perceived minority or "foreign" cultures may fall victim to racism and stereotyping, especially in stressful working relationships (Farella, 2001). Leininger (1995) and Farella (2001) reported incidents in the 1980s in which Filipino nurses who accepted offers of employment in the United States were subject to racial slurs and stereotyping. Clients and relatives may falsely accuse health team members from ethnic backgrounds different from their own of theft of personal belongings. Professional nurses have an obligation to be hospitable to nurses and other health team members who are from different ethnic backgrounds.

Platz and Wales (1999) outlined various methods to make others feel welcome. First, culturally competent nurses make all clients and colleagues feel cared for and appreciated. Second, standards for business etiquette include greeting everyone in each encounter; respecting the time of others; being prompt for meetings and appointments; calling to inform others if delayed for more than 5 minutes; sending thank you notes; listening actively to others; respecting the religions and cultures of others; and considering the privacy of others and the right to a neat, clean, and safe working environment.

Strategies for Working in Multicultural Health Care Teams

The influx of people from other cultures into each health care team is expected to increase as cultural diversity increases in the general population. Lack of adequate representation of various cultural groups within health care teams has been linked to disparities in access to care services and health care outcomes. Culturally diverse people have a key role to play in filling the projected vacancies in the health care team of the future. Professional programs, especially nursing programs, need to recruit culturally diverse students, commit to admitting them, and offer services to facilitate program success.

Effective health and nursing care requires a multidisciplinary effort and includes work efforts of licensed professionals and technicians. Unlicensed assistive personnel frequently perform the less mentally challenging and more physically demanding work associated with inpatients in acute or long-term care facilities. Many professional nurses encounter different cultural groups as they work with various members of the health care team. Principles of cultural competency used with clients foster effective teamwork.

As noted earlier in this chapter, the majority (73.3%) of practicing professional nurses in the United States are White with members of culturally diverse groups underrepresented in the profession (U.S. Department of Health & Human Services, 2019). Unlicensed care providers and licensed practical/vocational nurses frequently hail from more diverse backgrounds. Technical education programs frequently attract people who cannot afford a 4-year college education. Therefore, nurses from a middle-class, White cultural background find themselves supervising nursing care delivered by members of different cultural groups. Box 11.2, Learning, Knowing, and Growing, "Guidelines for Working Successfully with Health Team Members from Other Cultures" provides suggestions for easing this process.

11.2 Learning, Knowing, and Growing

Guidelines for Working Successfully with Health Team Members from Other Cultures

Cultural Issue	Suggested Guidelines
English as a second language (ESL)	Have direct caregivers repeat instructions back to validate that they understand what needs to be done. Have physicians, nurses, and other health professionals repeat what was said to validate that they understood what was reported to them. Learn a few phrases to converse with team members in their native languages. Inform team members of the importance of speaking English in clinical practice areas unless the client and family speak the same language as the team member.

(continued)

11.2 Learning, Knowing, and Growing (*continued*)

Guidelines for Working Successfully With Health Team Members From Other Cultures

Cultural Issue	Suggested Guidelines
Cultural group membership that differs from the professional nurse's cultural group	Become aware of your own biases and prejudices. Deal with personal biases, prejudices, and stereotypes openly. Get to know each team member as an individual rather than a member of a specific cultural group. Learn about cultural group values and practices of all team members. Organize and hold cultural celebrations of all team members. Offer to work for team members when they want to take time for cultural holidays or religious celebrations. Develop deep, meaningful relationships with health team coworkers while client care is executed.
Internationally educated nurses	Learn about professional nursing practice in each nurse's country of origin. Orient the nurse to state professional nursing practice laws and institutional practice guidelines. Trust the nurse to provide safe, effective client care. Correct social and nursing care errors with sensitivity. Invite the nurses to attend a local professional nursing organization meeting. Invite the nurses to participate in facility governance meetings when available. Offer to work on days when national holidays are celebrated in the internationally educated nurse's homeland. Inquire about life in the nurse's home country. Plan and hold social events for internationally educated nurses. Provide emotional support during times of homesickness. Develop deep, meaningful working relationships while client care is implemented.

■ QUESTIONS FOR REFLECTION

1. What are the benefits of having people from different cultural backgrounds and identities serving on the health care team?

2. What are the values promoted by the health care system in terms of work habits? Do you see a potential conflict with these values based on your cultural background? Why or why not?

Summary and Significance to Practice

As the U.S. population grows more diverse, professional nurses need knowledge and skills to provide culturally relevant care. Some professional nurses cling to personal biases and misconceptions related to cultural differences when providing health care services to culturally diverse populations. The reluctance to abandon negative attitudes toward people who differ from the care provider creates a climate of distrust and discrimination that increases the likelihood of negative health care outcomes.

Genetic differences and predispositions among various cultures increase the complexity of medical decision making and mandate that careful consideration be given to optimal strategies for health promotion and disease prevention as nurses encounter culturally diverse clients.

In addition to the challenges of working with culturally diverse populations, the nursing profession faces challenges in developing a workforce that mirrors the population demographics of the clients served.

To establish cultural competence in clinical practice, professional nurses must first become cognizant of personal biases; this requires the cognitive skill of honest self-reflection. Establishing cultural competence requires an attitude of genuine caring toward all humankind as well as personal commitment to make the time to learn about client cultural care considerations. Nurses should take the time to ask questions related to cultural preferences, listen to individuals, consider cues given to them by people from different cultures, and analyze the benefits (or hazards) of generic (or folk) health practices before outlining care plan strategies. Interacting with people from cultural backgrounds different from their own sometimes means that nurses must take risks, but nurses can learn from their mistakes. Nurses who practice with cultural humility engage in a lifelong process of self-reflection to improve their personal cultural awareness, cultural knowledge, communication skills, and professional behavior to promote equity for all.

REAL-LIFE REFLECTIONS

Recall Judy from the beginning of the chapter. What do you think Judy could do to facilitate the teamwork for a multicultural nursing care team? Why is it important that team members of diverse cultural groups understand each other?

From Theory to Practice

1. Think of a time when you worked with someone who belonged to a different cultural group. What did you learn from this person? Did your encounters with this person result in any changes in your thoughts, values, or beliefs? Why or why not?
2. Outline a plan of how you might resolve a dispute in a clinical situation with either a client or co-worker. How would your plan change if the person were from a background different from your own?

Nurse as Author

Think about your own level of cultural competence. Write a short essay about your level of cultural competence. Include information about your strengths and your areas for further growth to become a cultural competent professional nurse.

Your Digital Classroom

Online Exploration

International Council of Nurses: **www.icn.ch**
MinorityNurse.com: **www.MinorityNurse.com**
National Association of Hispanic Nurses: **http://www.nahnnet.org**
The American Folklife Center: **https://www.loc.gov/folklife**
The National Black Nurses Association, Inc.: **https://www.nbna.org**
Transcultural Nursing Society: **https://tcns.org**
U.S. Department of Health and Human Services Office of Minority Health: **https://www.thinkculturalhealth.hhs.gov**

Expanding Your Understanding

1. Read the national CLAS standards at https://thinkculturalhealth.hhs.gov/assets/pdfs/EnhancedNationalCLASStandards.pdf. Compile a list of the ones that apply to professional nursing practice. Read your current employer's or clinical site's policies related to the delivery of culturally and linguistically appropriate services. Based upon your observations and the established policies in your clinical setting, what actions do nurses need to take to meet these standards and organizational policies?
2. Search the term, "Living in (specify the country or countries of your heritage)," and read a description of the daily life and any legal or cultural issues that you might encounter if you lived or visited there. Note any specific laws you would have to follow. Bring these to share with your classmates.
3. Visit the National Black Nurses Association website at www.nbna.org. Click on "Read the latest Newsletter" near the bottom of the page. Select one or two articles to read. Identify three things from each article that you learned. Write down three ways in which you will incorporate this information into your professional practice. Bring these ideas to share in class or in an online class discussion forum.

Beyond the Book

Visit the**Point**® at **www.thePoint.lww.com** for activities and information to reinforce the concepts and content covered in this chapter.

REFERENCES

Abualhaija, N. (2021). Clarifying Cultural Competence in Nursing: A Concept Analysis Approach. *Journal of Cultural Diversity, 28*(1), 3-14.

Alexis, C., White, A. M., Thomas, C., & Poweski, J. (2019). Unpacking reactions to white privilege among employees of an academic medical center. *Journal of Cultural Diversity, 26*(1), 28–37. Retrieved April 26, 2021, from https://web-b-ebscohost-com.lib.rockhurst.edu/ehost/pdfviewer/pdfviewer?vid=8&sid=11b735a5-e9da-45a1-b36e-b4bb6981d044%40sessionmgr103

American Association of Colleges of Nursing. (2019). *Fact sheet: Enhancing diversity in the nursing workforce.* Retrieved February 20, 2021, from https://www.aacnnursing.org/Portals/42/News/Factsheets/Enhancing-Diversity-Factsheet.pdf

Andrews, M. M. (2020a). Culturally competent nursing care. In M. M. Andrews, J. S. Boyle, & J. W. Collins (Eds.), *Transcultural concepts in nursing care* (8th ed., pp. 31–54). Wolters Kluwer.

Andrews, M. M. (2020b). Cultural competence in the history and physical examination. In M. M. Andrews, J. S. Boyle, & J. W. Collins (Eds.), *Transcultural concepts in nursing care* (8th ed., pp. 55–104). Wolters Kluwer.

Andrews, M. M., & Boyle, J. S. (Eds.). (2016). *Transcultural concepts in nursing care* (7th ed.). Wolters Kluwer.

Andrews, M. M., Boyle, J. S., & Collins, J. W. (Eds.). (2020). *Transcultural concepts in nursing care* (8th ed.). Wolters Kluwer.

Brous, E. (2019). Legal issues with sexual and gender minority patients in the emergency department. *Journal of Legal Nurse Consulting, 30*(2), 30–37. https://doi.org/10.30710/jlnc.30.2.2019.30

Burchum, J. (2002). Cultural competence: An evolutionary perspective. *Nursing Forum, 37*, 5–15. https://doi.org/10.1111/j.1744-6198.2002.tb01287.x

Burggraf, V. (2000). The older woman: Ethnicity and health. *Geriatric Nursing, 21*, 183–187. https://doi.org/10.1067/mgn.2000.109570

Campaign for Action. (2020). *Equity, diversity, and inclusion steering committee.* Retrieved February 20, 2021, from https://campaignforaction.org/about/equity-diversity-inclusion-steering-committee/

Campaign for Action. (2021). *New RN graduates by degree type, by race/ethnicity.* Retrieved February 20, 2021, from https://campaignforaction.org/resource/new-rn-graduates-degree-type-raceethnicity/

Conron, K. J., & Goldberg, S. K. (2020). *Adult LGBT population in the United States.* The Williams Institute, UCLA. Retrieved October 12, 2020, from https://williamsinstitute.law.ucla.edu/wp-content/uploads/LGBT-Adult-US-Pop-Jul-2020.pdf

Farella, C. (2001). How we hurt our own. *Nursing Spectrum, 2*(2), 12–13.

Freeman, R., Viorst Gwadz, M., Silverman, E., Kutnick, A., Leonard, N. R., Ritchie, A. S., Reed, J., & Martinez, B. Y. (2017). Critical race theory as a tool for understanding poor engagement along the HIV care continuum among African American/Black and Hispanic persons living with HIV in the United States: A qualitative exploration. *International Journal for Equity in Health, 16*, 1–14. https://doi.org/10.1186/s12939-017-0549-3

Giger, J. N. (2017). *Transcultural nursing assessment and intervention* (7th ed.). Elsevier/Mosby.

Giger, J. N., & Davidhizar, R. E. (2008). *Transcultural nursing assessment and intervention* (5th ed.). Mosby.

Grossman, D. (1996). Cultural dimensions in home health nursing. *American Journal of Nursing, 96*, 33–36. https://doi.org/10.1097/00000446-199607000-00031

Herberg, P. (2008). Perspectives on international nursing. In M. M. Andrews & J. S. Boyle (Eds.), *Transcultural concepts in nursing care* (5th ed.). Lippincott Williams & Wilkins.

Hong, H. C., Lee, H., Collins, E. G., Park, C., Quinn, L., & Ferrans, C. E. (2018). Factors affecting trust in healthcare among middle-aged to older Korean American women. *BMC Women's Health, 18*(1). https://doi.org/10.1186/s12905-018-0609-x

Jarvis, C. (2016). *Physical examination and health assessment* (7th ed.). Elsevier.

Kavanagh, K. H., & Kennedy, P. H. (1992). *Promoting cultural diversity: Strategies for health care professionals.* Sage.

Lago, R. R., Peter, E., & Bógus, C. M. (2017). Harm reduction and tensions in trust and distrust in a mental health service: A qualitative approach. *Substance Abuse Treatment, Prevention & Policy, 12*, 1–9. https://doi.org/10.1186/s13011-017-0098-1

Leininger, M. (1991). *Transcultural nursing.* McGraw-Hill.

Leininger, M. (1995). *Transcultural nursing* (2nd ed.). McGraw-Hill.

Leininger, M., & McFarland, M. (2006). *Cultural care diversity and universality: A worldwide theory for nursing* (2nd ed.). Jones & Bartlett.

Lin, C., Lee, C., & Huang, M. (2017). Cultural competence of healthcare providers: A systematic review of assessment instruments. *Journal of Nursing Research, 25*(3), 174–186. https://doi.org/10.1097/jnr.0000000000000153

Meyer, I. H. (2019). *How do you measure the LGBT population in the United States?* Retrieved October 12, 2020, from https://news.gallup.com/opinion/methodology/259457/measure-lgbt-population.aspx

Mish, F. C. (Ed.). (2020). *Merriam-Webster's Collegiate Dictionary,* (11th ed.). Merriam-Webster Inc.

National League for Nursing. (2017). *NLN diversity & inclusion toolkit.* Retrieved February 20, 2021, from http://www.nln.org/docs/default-source/professional-development-programs/diversity_toolkit.pdf?sfvrsn=6

Newport, F. (2018, May 22). In U.S., estimate of LGBT population rises to 4.5%. *Gallup News.* Retrieved October 12, 2020, from https://news.gallup.com/poll/234863/estimate-lgbt-population-rises.aspx

Office of Disease Prevention and Health Promotion. (2020). Lesbian, gay, bisexual, and transgender health. *Healthy People 2020.* U.S. Department of Health and Human Services. Retrieved April 26, 2021, from https://www.healthypeople.gov/2020/topics-objectives/topic/lesbian-gay-bisexual-and-transgender-health

Pachter, L. M. (1994). Culture and clinical care: Folk illness beliefs and behaviors and their implications for health care delivery. *Journal of the American Medical Association, 271,* 690–694. https://doi.org/10.1001/jama.271.9.690

Platz, A., & Wales, S. (1999). *Social graces: Manners, conversation and charm for today.* Harvest House.

Purnell, L. D. (2014). *Transcultural health care: A culturally competent approach* (4th ed.). F. A. Davis.

Purnell, L. D., & Frankl, E. A. (2021). *Textbook for transcultural health care: A population approach cultural competence concepts in nursing care* (5th ed.). Springer.

Purnell, L. D., & Paulanka, B. J. (2008). *Transcultural health care: A culturally competent approach* (3rd ed.). F. A. Davis.

Spector, R. E. (2012). *Cultural diversity in health and illness* (8th ed.). Pearson Prentice Hall.

Sullivan Commission. (2004). *Missing persons: Minorities in the health professions, a report of the Sullivan Commission on diversity in the healthcare workforce.* Retrieved April 25, 2021, from https://campaignforaction.org/resource/sullivan-report-diversity/

The Polaris Project. (2019). *2019 U.S. National Human Trafficking Hotline Statistics.* Retrieved October 12, 2020, from https://polarisproject.org/2019-us-national-human-trafficking-hotline-statistics/

University of Wisconsin-Milwaukee Lesbian, Gay, Bisexual, Transgender, Queer Plus (LGBTQ+) Resource Center. (2020). *Gender pronouns.* Retrieved October 11, 2020, from https://uwm.edu/lgbtrc/support/gender-pronouns/

U.S. Census Bureau. (2019). *Quick facts. Population estimates, July 1, 2019, (V2019).* Retrieved September 6, 2020, from https://www.census.gov/quickfacts/fact/table/US/PST045219

U.S. Census Bureau. (2021). *U.S. and world population clock.* Retrieved February 19, 2021, from https://www.census.gov/popclock/

U.S. Department of Health and Human Services. (2010). *Healthy People 2020 [brochure].* Retrieved December 21, 2012, from https://www.healthypeople.gov/sites/default/files/HP2020_brochure_with_LHI_508_FNL.pdf

U.S. Department of Health and Human Services, Health Resources and Services Administration, National Center for Health Workforce Analysis. (2019). *Brief summary results from the 2018 National Sample Survey of Registered Nurses, Rockville, Maryland.* Retrieved April 26, 2021, from https://data.hrsa.gov/DataDownload/NSSRN/GeneralPUF18/nssrn-summary-report.pdf

U.S. Department of Health and Human Services Office of Disease Prevention and Health Promotion. (2020). *Healthy People 2030, Social determinant of health.* Retrieved October 13, 2020, from https://health.gov/healthypeople/objectives-and-data/social-determinants-health

U.S. Department of Health and Human Services Office of Minority Health. (2013). *National standards for culturally and linguistically appropriate services (CLAS) in health and health care.* Retrieved October 8, 2020, from https://thinkculturalhealth.hhs.gov/assets/pdfs/EnhancedNationalCLASStandards.pdf

U.S. Department of Health and Human Services Office of Minority Health. (n.d.-a). *Awareness, knowledge, adoption, and implementation of the national CLAS standards in health and health care organizations evaluation project: Summary of key findings.* Retrieved October 9, 2020, from https://thinkculturalhealth.hhs.gov/assets/pdfs/clas-ncs-evaluation-project.pdf

U.S. Department of Health and Human Services Office of Minority Health. (n.d.-b). *Health equity timeline.* Retrieved October 8, 2020, from https://thinkculturalhealth.hhs.gov/clas/health-equity-timeline

U.S. Department of Health and Human Services Office on Trafficking in Persons. (2019). *SOAR to health and wellness training.* Retrieved October 12, 2020, from https://www.acf.hhs.gov/otip/training/soar-to-health-and-wellness-training

Wilber, K., Snyder, C., Essary, A. C., Reddy, S., Will, K., & Saxon, M. (2020). Developing workforce diversity in the health professions: A social justice perspective. *Health Professions Education, 6*(2), 222–229. https://doi.org/10.1016/j.hpe.2020.01.002

Professional Nurse Accountability

LEARNING OUTCOMES

By the end of this chapter, the learner will be able to:

1. Differentiate accountability from autonomy and authority.
2. Relate current standards of professional nursing practice to accountability.
3. Identify some of the positive outcomes of nurses becoming accountable to clients, the profession, the health care team, the employing institution, oneself, managed care networks, and third-party payers.
4. Identify the essential questions the professional nurse must answer to be accountable to the client and public.
5. Evaluate oneself on professional accountability using the checklist provided.

REAL-LIFE REFLECTIONS

Carol is a charge nurse on a neurology unit. Mr. Jones, a frail 90-year-old, has been admitted for altered level of consciousness. Mrs. Jones wants absolutely everything done to make her husband well. She insists that the nursing assistant, Gloria, give him food and fluid to drink. When Gloria refuses, Mrs. Jones insists on seeing the charge nurse. Carol is busy and cannot talk to Mrs. Jones immediately. Mrs. Jones grows impatient and fixes coffee for her husband, then holds the cup to his mouth for him to take sips. Mr. Jones chokes violently. Carol runs into the room and finds that there are no suction catheters for the wall unit suction apparatus. As she delivers multiple abdominal thrusts to Mr. Jones, she sends Gloria to the supply cart to get suction catheters; none are found there. Mr. Jones stops breathing, and Carol "calls a code." Unfortunately, Mr. Jones dies.

- *List the mistakes made in this scenario and who made them.*
- *What are the potential consequences of Mr. Jones's death?*
- *How would you feel if a similar situation happened while you practiced nursing?*

In early writings about the nursing profession, the term *responsibility* meant duty. In *Notes on Nursing* (1946, 1859), Florence Nightingale frequently outlined the responsibilities of professional nurses, from the state of the sick room to the need for careful observation on the part of the nurse to avoid client accidents. She also noted, "I have often seen really good nurses distressed because they could not impress the doctor with the real danger of their patients" (p. 68).

In the early 1900s, private-duty nursing represented the epitome of nursing accountability to clients: a nurse took a "case," lived with the client, and remained until the client no longer needed nursing services. The nurse assumed responsibility and was held accountable for the client's life, space, and nursing care.

As the notion of accountability evolved, it involved nurse assuming responsibility for the action of themselves and others because they assumed supervisory functions in clinical practice. Frequently, accountability became tied to negative situations and carried a punitive connotation. Although often unaware, nurses were legally liable for their actions or their lack of action. Many nurses believed that the ultimate liability remained with the institution, which would "cover" them in the event of a lawsuit.

Accountability in the professional sense did not exist until the 1970s, when nurses' and society's view of nurses as holding subservient roles and merely following physician orders began to change. True professional accountability in nursing surfaced in the late 1970s (Clifford, 1981).

DEFINITION OF ACCOUNTABILITY AND RELATED CONCEPTS

To assume accountability, nurses must understand its definition. As an adjective, the word *accountable* means being required to explain actions or decisions to another party or being required to be responsible for the outcomes of actions and decisions (Mish, 2020). Therefore, **accountability** is the state of being responsible or answerable for one's decisions and actions. In contrast, to be responsible can describe the person who caused something to happen or "to able to answer for one's conduct and obligations: trustworthy" (Mish, 2020, p. 1062); **responsibility** can also mean a task or duty that someone is expected to accomplish, or a moral, legal, or ethical requirement (Mish, 2020). Accountability and responsibility differ in that responsibility arises within the nurse, and accountability comes from others (e.g., employers, clients, society). For example, a professional nurse assumes responsibility for providing safe effective, client care, and society holds the nurse accountable for actions taken or not taken while providing that care.

Although not part of its definition, the term *accountability* carries a negative connotation in today's business environment because the question "Who's accountable or responsible?" tends to surface only when things go wrong, resulting in looking to blame someone for making mistakes or not meeting standards

(Hwang & Han, 2020; Weber, 2018). Pegg (2020) provides an excellent example of how to clarify three terms, explaining that good workers have an effective balance between autonomy (freedom to act), authority (power to act), and accountability (knowing the exact expected results for which to be held answerable). Nurses have the freedom to use their clinical judgment to make decisions related to setting care priorities, decide when to intervene on behalf of clients, organize their daily tasks, and develop and revise nursing policies and procedures (autonomy). In addition, they have the power to perform nursing-related activities based on the nurse practice acts of their states (authority). As health professionals, nurses must explain and provide answers for the outcomes of their care (accountability).

Accountability

By dividing the term *accountability* into two parts, Dethmer (2006a) simplified its definition. Even though this approach to accountability was identified early in the 21st century, it remains applicable. Dethmer's first aspect of accountability incorporates the concept of responsibility, which means "to account for what has been done" (p. 46). Accountability for an outcome is assessed by the questions "Who did it?," "Who participated in it?," and "Who started it?." In contrast, the term *responsibility* means "to be able to respond" (Dethmer, 2006a, p. 50). Dethmer (2006a) took the concept of accountability one step further and devised the term *radical responsibility*, which is to take full responsibility for whatever happens in one's life rather than blaming others, while being committed to learning from each personal experience. The beauty of this interpretation of accountability is that people must take credit for both successes and failures.

The second aspect of Dethmer's (2006b) conceptual approach to accountability includes making and keeping agreements that he calls "impeccable agreements." He defined an agreement as anything people say they will or will not do. An impeccable agreement involves a deep personal commitment to doing what the person wants to do, fully aligned with the person's values, completely connected to something over which the person has control, personal acknowledgment of importance, and detailed record keeping to document completion. Whenever an agreement is made, people are to keep it or renegotiate it should something interfere with its execution because "broken agreements damage trust" (Dethmer, 2006b, p. 80).

Clear agreements involve facts (exactly what the agreement contains), feelings (emotional reactions to agreeing), and reasons (the specific rationale behind the agreement). Renegotiating a deadline involves just giving plain, simple facts and works best if the renegotiation occurs prior to the deadline. When an agreement is broken, all involved parties must acknowledge that the agreement was broken and communicate it to all involved people. The person breaking the agreement needs to take responsibility for the action without providing excuses, justifications, or explanations and also listen to the responses of the affected individual(s). The person breaking the agreement should inquire about what can be done to address the consequences of the broken agreement. Finally, when agreements are broken, all involved parties should take the time to analyze what happened, learn from it, and not repeat the same mistake (Dethmer, 2006b).

Thus, accountability is the state of being responsible for agreements and answerable for the behaviors and their outcomes that fall into the realm of one's professional role. The American Nurses Association's (ANA's) *Nursing Scope and Standards of Practice* (2021) and all nurse practice acts (NPAs) consider that a binding agreement has been made when a nurse establishes a relationship with a person to provide professional nursing services. Nurses become accountable for implementing these established agreements with clients. They also become accountable to employers when providing nursing services to clients. When working for an agency, professional nurses agree to abide by the agency's policies and procedures. Nurses are accountable to interprofessional colleagues for reporting changes in the physical and mental conditions of clients that they note when providing nursing care services. They are accountable to each other when working as a team to provide care to client groups. Nurses are also held accountable for their social media posts. In fact, some nurses and nursing students have lost positions for posting confidential client information, photos of themselves with clients, and negative comments about employers. Finally, society holds nurses accountable for harmful acts that occur during clinical practice.

Responsibility and Answerability

Ethical codes for nurses published by national and international nursing organizations contain information related to professional accountability (ANA, 2015; International Council of Nurses [ICN], 2012). Under these, accountability continues to retain its original meaning of responsibility but has an added dimension, **answerability**, which is the requirement to offer answers, reasons, and explanations to certain others. As the ANA *Code of Ethics for Nurses* defines,

accountability is "being answerable, or to give an account or defense to oneself or others for one's own choices, decisions and actions as measured against a standard…" (Fowler, 2015, p. 59). Examples of standards to which nurses are held accountable include the *ANA's Nursing Scope and Standards of Practice*, the ANA and ICN Codes of Ethics for Nurses, state NPAs, and standards determined by specialty professional nursing organizations (e.g., American Association of Critical Care Nurses, Oncology Nursing Society, etc.).

In 2010, the ANA revised its *Nursing's Social Policy Statement*, which specified that a social contract provides the basis for the authority of professional nursing practices (2010). The contract gives the nurse professional rights and responsibilities for all actions taken while engaged in clinical practice, such as following the scope and standards for professional and specialty nursing practice; using the best evidence to provide safe, high-quality care; abiding by legal rules and regulations for practice designated by the state or national professional organizations; following institutional policies and procedures; and making independent decisions for self-determination about practice situations. Protection of the public from unscrupulous and unsafe nurses is afforded by legal mechanisms, including civil and criminal laws and penalties, as well as various laws that govern professional nursing licensure. In the United States, state governments set rules and regulations for professional nursing licensure and practice. Nursing regulations make the nursing profession and its members accountable to the public (Brous, 2021). Currently, discussions of accountability for professional nursing revolve around client assessments, interventions (nursing care), outcomes (results), and costs (expenditures). Because of legal, accreditation, third-party payer, and managed care requirements, documentation frequently serves as evidence that nurses either performed or did not perform specific nursing assessments and interventions.

The health care delivery industry has higher error rates today than other industries do. According to the World Health Organization (WHO), one in 10 hospitalized clients in high-income countries is harmed when receiving care and 50% of these outcomes could have been prevented. Four in 10 clients are harmed in primary care and outpatient care settings. The most commonly reported care errors in outpatient settings are errors in diagnoses and prescriptions along with mistakes in medication administration. The WHO estimates that 2.6 million people die annually as a result of care errors (WHO, 2019). Makary and Daniel (2016) estimated that 250,000 Americans die from health care errors annually, accounting for 9.5% of all deaths. The Institute for Healthcare Improvement (IHI) reports that American deaths from preventable errors may be as high as 400,000 (2020b). Heron (2019) reported that accidents and unintentional injuries were the third leading cause of death in the United States in 2019, and these include health care errors.

Early initiatives aimed at improving client safety that started in the early 21st century remain in effect. The Joint Commission (TJC) revises its annual National Patient Safety Goals and has a "Leading the Way to Zero" program with the goal of causing no harm to clients (TJC, 2020). The IHI established the "10,000 Lives Campaign" in 2005 (McCannon et al., 2006) and now has a "100 Million Healthier Lives Campaign" (IHI, 2020a). The IHI (2020b) also sponsors an annual Patient Safety Awareness Week. Starting in 1996, the Institute of Medicine (IOM) published the "Quality Chasm" series of reports that outline ways to improve the safety and quality of health care and to design a health care system for the 21st century. In 2015, the IOM became the National Academies of Science, Engineering, and Medicine (Dzau et al., 2017). In 2017, they published another report entitled *Vital Directions for Health and Health Care* as a way to continue this valuable work. Additionally, the U.S. military implemented the Partnership for Patients Initiative to improve client safety in the military's health care system. This program resulted in a reduction of 500 incidents of client harm over a 10-year period, a 15.8% reduction in hospital-acquired conditions, and cost savings of $13.5 million.

Because nurses play a key role in health care safety, nurses designed the Quality and Safety Education for Nurses (QSEN) that increases nurse awareness of client safety needs. QSEN developed competencies, knowledge, skills, and attitudes for undergraduate nursing education initially and later added graduate education competencies. QSEN has evolved and is now known as the QSEN Institute. It is managed by a faculty team at Case Western Reserve University and offers free educational resources to nurses and nursing faculty that require no user account (QSEN Institute, 2020). Findings from these initiatives have been incorporated into the Patient Protection and Affordable Care Act of 2010 (see Chapter 9, "Health Care Delivery Systems"). The expectation of higher-quality, safer health care based on scientific evidence may result in increased areas of professional nurse accountability. Professional nurses display accountability each time they answer questions about the reasons behind actions, document interventions, and outcomes of delivered care, and participate in clinical competency programs.

Take Note!
Accountability is the state of being responsible and answerable for actions and client outcomes that fall under the scope of one's professional role.

Autonomy and Authority

Although related to the concept of accountability, the concept of autonomy is distinct as it refers to independence of functioning. **Autonomy** means that one can perform one's total professional function on the basis of one's own knowledge and judgment and that one is recognized by others as having the right to do so. Autonomy is related to accountability because a person who functions autonomously must be accountable for their own behavior (Holden, 1991; Hylka & Shugrue, 1991).

Another term closely related to yet distinct from accountability is *authority*. **Authority** can be defined as being in a position to make decisions and to influence others to act in a manner determined by those decisions. Authority is related to accountability because those who are in authority are accountable for the decisions they make and for both their own actions and those of others who act on the basis of their decisions. Authority also relates closely to autonomy, because those in authority often act autonomously in performing all or part of their respective roles.

Professional autonomy has been incorporated as an essential element of a magnetic work environment for nurses. According to Kramer et al. (2008), "Autonomy is the *freedom* to act on *what you know*, to make independent clinical decisions that *exceed standard nursing practice* in *the best interest of the patient*." Freedom is about trust and organizational sanction for autonomous practice (Kramer et al., 2008, p. 25). Kramer and colleagues (2008) developed their definition for "clinical autonomy" using transcripts of recorded interviews with 289 nurses employed in Magnet hospitals.[1] In the 2021 version of the *ANA's Nursing Scope and Standards*

---

[1]Magnet is a special recognition accorded to hospitals by the American Nurses Credentialing Center (a subsidiary of the ANA) and designates a hospital that practices transformational leadership, provides mechanisms for structural empowerment, displays exemplary professional practice, has commitments to discovering new knowledge, practices innovations while continuously improving quality, and possesses a record of high rankings on empirical quality outcomes (ANA, 2020) (see Chapter 13, "Environmental and Global Health," for more information about the Magnet recognition program).

of Practice, autonomy is defined as "Capacity to determine one's own actions through independent choice, including demonstration of competence." (p. 109). Thus, nurse **competence** means the nurse has the essential knowledge and skills for professional practice determined by the scope of practice in the locale where nursing services are provided.

This definition of autonomy empowers nurses to act on all forms of nursing knowledge to provide optimal client care. Nurses practicing in hospitals with Magnet status are expected to use evidence-based practice as the standard for professional practice. When nurses encounter a situation that is not based on evidence or is counterintuitive, they are expected to take steps to verify that the proposed therapeutic interventions are in the best interest of their clients before proceeding. To question physician orders, nurses must have the cognitive skills to recognize a discrepancy, the solid knowledge (or evidence) to justify questions, and the confidence to know that they must consult with a physician prior to action. When nurses exercise autonomy, they become accountable for the results, whether positive or negative.

Delegation

Professional nurses need to understand that being able to provide for every single client care need by themselves is an impossibility. Understanding the division of tasks that can be accomplished by unlicensed assistive personnel (UAP) and licensed practical/vocational nurses (LPN/LVNs) enables others to assume responsibility for executing some of the most rewarding aspects of professional practice (basic hands-on physical care). Delegating tasks enables professional nurses to focus on care coordination and education of clients and their families (White et al., 2015). **Delegation** is the act of transferring a task that one would do (if time permitted) to another person who is capable of performing the task.

Because professional nurses frequently delegate nursing responsibilities to UAPs and LPN/LVNs, professional nurses become accountable for the outcomes of the actions of others. Delegation of tasks requires that nurses use professional judgment to decide what tasks can be performed safely by another member of the nursing team. Before delegating any task, the nurse must ascertain that the person has the competence and capability to perform the task. Most state NPAs address the delegation process. Many of the directives regarding delegation leave room for the professional nurse to decide what tasks can be safely delegated to others (Box 12.1, Professional Building Blocks, "Considering the Safety of Delegation").

In 2019, the National State Boards of Nursing (NCSBN) and the American Nurses Association (ANA) developed a national set of evidence-based guidelines for effective delegation. The delegation guidelines emphasize the importance of effective communication between delegators and delegatees, assessing the competence of the person accepting the delegated tasks, the tasks to be done, the availability of the delegator to the delegate, and ongoing education and training. Once a delegated task is accepted, the delegatee assumes accountability for the results and the responsibility for completing the task. In addition, the delegator must provide directions and

---

 ## 12.1 Professional Building Blocks

Considering the Safety of Delegation

The questions that follow can help nurses decide what tasks can be safely done by another member of the nursing care team:

1. Are there laws that support delegating the task?
2. Is the task within the scope of the professional nurse's practice?
3. Does the delegating nurse have the knowledge and skills to make competent decisions about delegation (such as determining client risk for each delegated task)?
4. Does the task meet all conditions and criteria for delegation to an unlicensed care provider (i.e., guidelines

are within the NPA; task routinely recurs in daily work, needs no modification, has a predictable outcome, and does not require ongoing assessment, interpretation, or independent decision making)?

5. Does the unlicensed care provider have the knowledge, skills, and ability to perform the task effectively?
6. Do the skills of the unlicensed care provider match with client care needs?
7. Does the agency have policies, protocols, and procedures in place for the proposed delegated task?
8. Will appropriate supervision be available during task completion?

Data from National Council of State Boards of Nursing and American Nurses Association. (2019). *National guidelines for nursing delegation.* Retrieved February 21, 2021, from https://www.ncsbn.org/NGND-PosPaper_06.pdf

communication about the task to be completed and verify that the task is completed through effective supervision and evaluation (i.e., right task, right circumstance, right person, right directions and communication, and right supervision and evaluation known as the traditional five "rights" of delegation) (NCSBN & ANA, 2019).

When UAP or an LPN/LVN accepts delegated tasks, they assume responsibility for completing them. In some instances, such as delegation of a bed bath, UAP can make simple decisions about whether to use commercially prepackaged baths or traditional soap, water, and washcloths (unless the agency has set a policy on how to perform bed baths). When administering medications, an LPN/LVN can make decisions about whether to administer unscheduled medications that are ordered as needed (e.g., pain medication). At times, nurses may opt to perform a task usually delegated to UAP or an LPN/LVN when client situations reveal a high potential for harm and quick, independent decision making is required to avert a serious complication. For example, a registered nurse (RN) may decide to feed a newly admitted client who has difficulty speaking because the nurse can assess for safe swallowing and intervene quickly should the client choke, or administer and monitor the effects of oxygen therapy and bronchodilators for a client who is experiencing respiratory difficulty.

Agencies that use UAP are responsible for verifying that the UAP received adequate education and training before assuming work duties. Part of this education includes when to report problems to nurses. Nurses who fail to respond to client problems reported by subordinates typically fail to comply with their job descriptions and may be violating their state NPA. Unit charge nurses have a duty to report any conditions that keep them from effectively performing their designated roles.

The related concepts of accountability, responsibility, and autonomy project an image of responsible, independent individuals capable of making decisions and influencing others to act on them. They answer for their own behaviors as well as the behaviors of their associates. In the professional nursing context, the nurse becomes an autonomous practitioner who brings a different perspective and fulfills a particular role in the interdisciplinary health team. The nurse assumes responsibility for professional activities (including using research-based nursing actions, maintaining clinical competence, and staying abreast of new developments) and is held accountable for the outcomes of client care. This evolving image of a professional nurse demonstrates how increased accountability for the outcome of actions moves nursing toward the status given to other health care professions.

Take Note!
Accountability, responsibility, and autonomy empower professional nurses.

■ QUESTIONS FOR REFLECTION

1. Do you agree with the definitions of responsibility, accountability, autonomy, and authority presented in this chapter? Why or why not?

2. What would you do if you saw another nurse engage in dangerous practice? What is your responsibility to the clients? To your coworkers? To your manager? To your clinical faculty member?

3. Do you feel that nurses possess the authority and autonomy to change practice protocols and policies? Why or why not?

4. As a professional nursing student, to what are you held accountable? Are these the same in the clinical setting as they are in the classroom? Outline the similarities and differences. Why do you think there are differences?

PROFESSIONAL ACCOUNTABILITY

Professional accountability means that people who possess specialized knowledge and skills in providing services to others may be required to answer for the outcomes of their actions or inactions (Oussedik et al., 2019). Most often, health care professionals are called upon to answer for negative outcomes of provided care. However, they should be asked to share and explain information about their success stories with each other and society. Accountability can be explicit or implicit. Explicit accountability occurs when a professional nurse has a contract to provide service and it is outlined by a state NPA and/or in terms of employment in a care-providing organization. Implicit accountability occurs when there is an implied expectation that nurses explain their actions. In practice, nurses explain reasons for their actions to the people whom they serve many times while providing care. Oussedik and colleagues (2019) identified controlled and autonomous accountability when developing a tool to measure professional accountability. Controlled accountability is associated with external factors requiring answers, and autonomous accountability is answering to oneself for action or inaction. Autonomous accountability occurs when people work independently and need to provide answers to themselves when engaging in practice. Oussedik and colleagues (2019) also noticed an increase in autonomous accountability when the health care professional had full autonomy in practice. Nurses who internalize accountability possess a high level of moral integrity.

Nurses with moral integrity understand the importance of being, living, and becoming a person who is honest, forthright, and trustworthy. They display the capability to consistently do the right thing despite personal consequences. They stand up for what is right despite any risk of retribution (Butts, 2020). These nurses use their morals to guide clinical practice, address inequality and ambiguity, and act compassionately to prevent harm and to do what is in the best interest of the clients they serve. Because nurses possess professional accountability, they are obligated to report substandard care and care errors. Sattar et al. (2020) reviewed literature surrounding disclosing care errors to health care consumers when they occurred resulting in divergent attitudes and expectations between care recipients and providers. Health care consumers felt they needed to know when errors occurred, expected sincere apologies, and wanted to receive promises that improvements would be made to prevent error recurrence. Health care professionals identified barriers to full disclosure that included working in a culture of blame, fear of litigation, inconsistent guidance, and lack of necessary skills to engage in full disclosure. The "Focus on Research" box describes some of the fears

FOCUS ON RESEARCH

Barriers to Reporting Errors and Adverse Events

The investigators of this study were interested in determining the barriers to nurse reporting of care errors and adverse events that occur in critical care nursing in Iran. After receiving approval for research by an ethics committee, they sent out surveys to 266 critical care nurses in seven Iranian hospitals.

The questionnaire consisted of demographic items related to personal characteristics (e.g., age, gender, marital status, education) and occupational data (e.g., employment status, work history, critical care experience) and a section with 26 items inquiring about management factors, fear of reporting, and reporting processes.

There were 251 nurses who completed the survey for a response rate of 94.36%. Most of the respondents (33.9%) had 10 to 15 years of professional nursing experience with more than 5 years' experience in critical care nursing (68.5% of respondents). Of the respondents, 49% reported having been involved in an error within the previous year, and 70.9% of these nurses said they had not reported it. More than half of the nurses (51.8%) reported that they did not attend an error reporting workshop since starting their critical care nursing position.

None of the demographic characteristics was associated with the items related to management factors, fear of reporting, and reporting processes at a statistically significant level. Factor analysis revealed that 62.7% of the variance could be explained by the following three factors: fear of reporting (26.13%), procedural barriers for reporting (19.1%), and managerial

barriers to reporting (17.4%). Thus 37% of the barriers to reporting were not identified in this study.

The findings of this study are consistent with previously conducted studies in which fear of reporting has been commonly identified as a primary barrier for reporting errors. However, not all studies found this to be the most common reason. Procedural barriers for reporting and managerial factors have also been identified as key reasons for failure to report errors. There appears to be more variance in individual characteristics in deciding whether to report errors or adverse events when they occur.

The clinical significance of this study is that barriers to reporting care errors and adverse effects appears to be consistent across the profession of nursing and does not seem to differ according to where nurses engage in clinical practice. Health care organizations must develop policies promoting a blame-free and shame-free approach for managing errors when they occur and provide nurses with clear directions on when to report care issues and what reporting processes should occur. More research is needed to determine the magnitude of care errors across all specialized and general areas of professional nursing practice. In addition, more research on the effects of adopting a blame- and shame-free culture and professional education on how to report errors and adverse events also needs to be conducted.

From Mansouri, S. F., Mohammadi, T. K., Adib, M., Lili, E. K., & Soodmand, M. (2019). Barriers to nurses reporting errors and adverse events. *British Journal of Nursing*, 28(11), 690–695. https://doi.org/10.12968/bjon.2019.28.11.690

and obstacles that prevent nurses from disclosing errors when they occur.

Moffat-Bruce et al. (2016) reported that 30% of medical errors are disclosed to clients, and only 50% of care providers believe those errors arise because of system flaws. Han et al. (2017) advocates embracing errors in order to identify flaws in work and system processes. Blaming and punishing individuals for making errors only increases the fear of reporting when errors occur. Hannawa (2009) developed a micro model for physician mistake disclosure and provided suggestions to the actual disclosure process and projected outcomes for specific information to share and relational strategies to follow. Table 12.1 uses these categories, adapts the model's suggestions, and combines information from other ethical and legal experts for use in professional nursing practice.

Ideally, all people in a living system such as a workplace assume ownership of job roles and responsibilities

▪ **TABLE 12.1**	**Professional Nurse Strategies for Disclosing Care Errors and Projected Outcomes**

Information to Share
- What exactly happened
- How and why the event happened
- Possible consequences of the event
- Future prevention efforts

Relational Strategies
- Approach the client and family calmly and with compassion.
- Refrain from any defensive behavior or blame.
- Listen intently to the client and family and ask for their expectations.
- Offer a sincere apology.
- Discuss possible restitution by referring them to the risk management department.

Informational Outcomes
- Detailed analysis of the error
- Future error avoidance
- Improved management of errors
- Reduced incidence of litigation
- Reduced error repetition

Relational Outcomes
- Forgiveness for the error from the client and family
- Increased trust in the nurse
- Reduced anger toward the nurse
- Reduced nurse guilt
- Enhanced nurse mental health
- Lower chance of nurse experiencing moral distress

From Han, J., LaMarra, D., & Vapiwala, N. (2017). Applying lessons from social psychology to transform the culture of error disclosure. Medical Education, 51(10), 996–1001; Hannawa, A. F. (2009). Negotiating medical virtues: toward the development of a physician mistake disclosure model. Health Communication, 24(5), 391–399; Moffat-Bruce, S. D., Ferdinand, F. D., & Fann, J. F. (2016). Patient safety: Disclosure of medical errors and risk mitigation. Annals of Thoracic Surgery, 102, 358–362; Pozgar, G. D. (2020). *Legal and ethical issues for health professionals* (5th ed.). Jones & Bartlett Learning.

that contribute to desired outcomes. In health care, all members of the health care team work toward providing the best care possible to attain optimal outcomes for the clients. Each person is designated to fulfill a particular role, has the authority to design their work, has clear expectations of their contributions, and strives to do their best. Through increased authority and autonomy, each member assumes accountability for outcomes of their work. Coworkers develop relationships and create meaningful partnerships with each other to fulfill specified outcomes. When health care team members have high engagement in their work and have the power to develop and revise work policies and processes, they become empowered. Health care team members strive to exceed expectations and experience higher levels of job satisfaction when they feel empowered.

Professional Standards of Practice

As nurses assume more leadership and advanced practice, additional interest in and concern with accountability has surfaced. Flexner (1915) identified accountability as a key characteristic of a profession. He also indicated that professions are likely to be more responsive to public interest than are unorganized and isolated individuals. Therefore, nurses must work together professionally to develop practice standards and policies on which all can agree.

In terms of nursing's involvement with its professionalization in the 1950s and 1960s, Bixler and Bixler (1959) specified that professions function autonomously to carve out a scope of practice, develop professional standards, and institute policies that control professional activity. McGlothlin (1961) explained that a profession undertakes tasks that require the exercising of judgment in applying knowledge to the solutions of problems and accepts responsibility for the results. To be accountable, however, a profession must know that for which it is accountable. To that end, nursing organizations have established and work to enforce professional standards. **Professional standards** outline the guidelines and principles of a specific line of work or career. The ANA, nursing's major professional organization, has done this with its *Scope and Standards of Professional Nursing*, which specifies the professional standards of nursing practice, service, and continuing education. Using the standards of practice (ANA, 2021) as a guide, nurses can identify the scope and limits of professional nursing practice, and internalize that for which they are accountable. By establishing standards, the ANA has complied with one of the functions of a professional organization—i.e., of providing the means by which members of the profession can judge the competence of its members (Merton, 1958).

The National Council of State Boards of Nursing sets standards for "safe nursing practice." Individual state boards of nursing develop standards for professional practice and monitor professional nurse performance. In addition, individual nursing service departments monitor their collective accountability through the process of peer review. For example, Nolan et al. (2010) reported that initiation of morbidity and mortality peer review conferences improved client care quality, as evidenced by the following outcomes: (1) nurse compliance with an evidence-based protocol for ventilator clients increased from 90.1% to 95.2%; (2) cases of ventilator-acquired pneumonia decreased from six cases to two cases after 2 months; and (3) nurses reported increased levels of accountability.

Take Note!

Through its standards, the ANA has contributed greatly to the ability of the nursing profession to be accountable.

Nurses' monitoring of their own practice for effectiveness has increased dramatically in recent years through the introduction of systematic nursing quality improvement activities with active participation by staff nurses in many institutions and agencies. In 1991, the Joint Commission on Accreditation of Healthcare Organizations (now TJC) moved from reactive quality assurance programs to proactive quality improvement programs as mandated criteria for health care agency accreditation. This move hastened the process of operationalizing the concept of accountability as quality assurance at the nursing service department level (see Chapter 18, "Quality Improvement: Enhancing Patient Safety and Health Care Quality"). Thus, nurses become accountable for continuously improving the quality of health care for consumers.

Nurses have another document to guide them for practice accountability. The *Code of Ethics for Nurses* (2015), also developed by the ANA, outlines terms for ethical accountability for professional nurses. **Ethical accountability** means that nurses must fulfill their moral-based obligations and duties, and provide answers for professional actions. For example, under *The Code of Ethics for Nurses* (ANA, 2015), nurses consider and base actions upon what is in the best interests of clients they serve over allegiances to their employer or other health care team members. **Nurses as client advocates** base professional decisions on what is

best for clients. The *Code of Ethics for Nurses* provides a clear framework within which nurses can seek to uphold the standards of care and protect the clients they serve. The code lays to rest any doubt about accountability of the nursing profession by directly confronting the issue. As stated in provision 4 of the code, "The nurse has authority, accountability, and responsibility for nursing practice; makes decisions; and takes action consistent with the obligation to promote health and provide optimal care" (ANA, 2015, p. 15). Other items in the code do not address the area of accountability directly, but, by discussing various factors that are necessary underpinnings for accountability, indirectly support the concept. These factors include the presumed competence of the nurse, the use of informed judgment, and the use of nursing research.

Because society holds individual nurses accountable for professional actions, the nursing profession is accountable for establishing and monitoring standards for safe practice. Only nurses can determine the definition of "safe practice" and care standards. In some states, physicians routinely testify in court proceedings that a nurse displayed unsafe practice or deviated from the standard of care. Nursing is accountable as a profession and its individual practitioners are also accountable. It has been implied throughout this discussion that nurses are accountable to the public and to the profession itself. In addition, with most nurses employed by health care agencies rather than in totally independent practice, nurses are also accountable to their employers (Pozgar, 2020). Nurses are obligated to adhere to safe practice guidelines, admit when they make mistakes, adhere to nursing professional standards, maintain professional relationships and boundaries, provide compassionate care, protect clients from harm (e.g., report client abuse and dangerous physicians or care situations), serve as client advocates, maintain professional competence, and work effectively as a health care team member. In the current climate of cost control, nurses must understand the delicate balance of being accountable to their employers (cost-containment strategies resulting in rapid client turnover or abiding by outdated care polices) and being accountable to themselves (delivering client-focused care based on current, best evidence, and blowing the whistle on substandard care).

Accountability to the Public and Clients

Although it may be personally and intellectually stimulating, gratifying, and exciting to execute professional roles and responsibilities, the ultimate reason for the existence of any profession is to provide service to the public. Thus, almost by definition, a profession must be accountable to the public. Consumers have the right to receive the safest, best possible quality of care from nurses who use a specialized knowledge base while applying sound judgment and utilizing a professional value system to make clinical decisions. To provide the best possible care, nurses must stay abreast of current best practices by remaining employed in the field, attending continuing education seminars, completing required competency tests, and reading professional literature.

As consumers become more knowledgeable about health care through formal education and access to information from many media formats, they sometimes know a great deal about what the profession is supposed to be doing. This increased knowledge empowers consumers to demand more and to make those demands openly. Nurses must be aware of increased consumer knowledge and sophistication and be prepared to respond to it in an equally knowledgeable and sophisticated manner. Instead of assuming positions of authority, nurses work collaboratively with clients to determine and attain health-related goals. Nurses must clearly demonstrate the principles and concepts on which practice is based. They also need to access current information, use problem solving to effectively evaluate outcomes of care, and revise care strategies if desired outcomes are not achieved (Concepts in Practice, "Working Collaboratively with Empowered Clients").

Concepts in Practice IDEA ⟶ PLAN ⟶ ACTION

Working Collaboratively With Empowered Clients

Josiah is a nurse who works on a cardiac unit. He cares for people who frequently receive six or more medications to control heart disease. One day, one of his clients requests not to take the ordered statin to reduce cholesterol. On inquiring the reason, the client responds, "There was a research study finding on the news today that said taking statins causes more health problems for people taking them than they do in preventing another heart attack. I am just tired of taking all these prescribed pills, racking up a large monthly pharmacy bill. I feel like the medical profession treats all patients like lab rats." Josiah mentions to his client that he has not heard about the study. He holds the client's medication per request and states that he will return with more information.

Josiah goes online and reads the study. He discovers that the study compared people receiving statins to people adhering strictly to a Mediterranean diet. He makes a copy of the research study, which was conducted in Great Britain, Ireland, Scotland, and Wales. Josiah realizes that if his client refuses to take the ordered statin, he will have to notify the cardiologist.

In addition to the study information, Josiah gathers detailed information about the Mediterranean diet for his client. After presenting all the information to his client, the client balks at learning about all of the fruits and vegetables that he would have to eat, that he would have to limit consumption of red meat, and that he would no longer be able to eat fast foods. He asks Josiah if he still has the statin for him to take.

Society holds nurses legally accountable for professional practice. Every state has a board of nursing that monitors practice according to the state's NPA. A state's NPA defines professional nursing practice, specifies the scope of practice, and distinguishes professional nursing from other health professions. Nurses must practice within their state's NPA guidelines.

State NPAs hold professional nurses to a standard of safe and prudent practice, which means that the nurse must exercise reasonable judgment and deliver reasonable care (Pozgar, 2020). Reasonable actions and judgments include being competent in the area of current practice, securing help for situations one is unqualified to manage, and fulfilling professional duties as a nurse.

Take Note!

Securing a copy of the NPA for the state(s) in which you practice is essential. You can use the internet, telephone, or postal service to secure a copy of your state's NPA.

When nurses hold professional nursing licenses, they have a duty to provide health care services (either as an employee or volunteer). Negligence occurs when a nurse omits or commits "an act that a reasonably prudent person would or would not do under a given circumstance" (Pozgar, 2020). Nursing negligence is a special form of carelessness that departs from the standards of nursing care. **Liability** is a responsibility or obligation that one person has to another person or entity. In the context of damages, it is a monetary obligation "that one has incurred or might incur through a negligent act" (Pozgar, 2020). Legal nurse scholar Anselmi (2012) describes two forms of liability:

1. **Strict liability** occurs when a person (or entity) is responsible "for damage or harm without having to prove fault" (p. 45), such as when a hospital uses explosive gases or other dangerous chemicals and an accident occurs.
2. **Vicarious liability** occurs when one person assumes accountability for the actions of another (Box 12.2, Professional Building Blocks, "Forms and Examples of Vicarious Liability").

Legal actions against nurses must contain the following elements: a breach of duty (may be an omission or incorrect action); foreseeability (a specific result should have been predicted from the action or omission); and causation (the omission or action directly resulted in injury). Recipients of inappropriate nursing services may suffer physical, emotional, or financial losses and deserve compensation when losses occur (Pozgar, 2020).

When nurses deviate from approved policies, procedures, or standards, they are at increased risk of being accused of malpractice or negligence. For example, if a nurse fails to perform routine circulation, movement, and sensation checks for a client who has returned from orthopedic surgery per standardized postoperative protocols and the person ends up with a permanent loss of function, the nurse places themselves at legal risk. However, before legal action is taken, the plaintiff (individual or group originating the legal action) must demonstrate that the event caused some form of injury.

Documentation of care delivered serves as legal evidence in the nurse's defense when legal action is taken against nurses. Meticulous documentation of events enables the nurse to present a highly professional image and serves as one of the best defense resources during legal actions. When on the witness stand, the nurse must be able to formulate and present the theoretical and scientific bases for the judgment exercised while fulfilling professional responsibilities.

In addition to legal accountability, nurses must be able to formulate and present the ethical code or value system to which they refer when making judgments and using knowledge. They must answer consumers and others without becoming defensive when asked "Why did you do that?" "How did you come to that decision?" or "What makes you believe that was the most effective course of action?" Consumers have the right to know about all aspects of their nursing care, and nurses who are true professionals have the responsibility to know and provide the answers.

As knowledgeable professionals, nurses share accountability for the nation's health care delivery system with other health team members. When nurses blame others, such as physicians, administrators, or politicians, for the state of the health care delivery system or constantly look to others to improve the system, they weaken their position and power base. By accepting an appropriate degree of responsibility for the current situation and actively pursuing ways to improve it, nurses act on a more professional level and make their claim as key stakeholders in the health care system.

12.2 Professional Building Blocks

Forms and Examples of Vicarious Liability

- *Respondeat superior* means "let the superior answer." Thus, a hospital can be held accountable for any action performed by staff nurses or UAP. For example, if a staff nurse fails to follow the policies and procedures outlined for a sterile procedure such as changing a central line dressing and the client contracts a bloodstream infection, the hospital can be held accountable for the nurse's action.
- The *most distant relationship* liability occurs between an employer and an independent contractor in a situation when the independent contractor requires no supervision when performing work duties. For example, a hospital that uses physician or advanced practice nurse contractors could be held vicariously liable because clients perceived that the contractors were part of the hospital staff.
- *Negligent entrustment or supervision* arises when supervising physicians are held liable for the actions of medical students, advanced practice nurses, or residents.
- *Joint enterprise or venture* would apply when two or more individuals "form a limited liability partnership or other protective business structure" (p. 46) for a specific business purpose or a specified time frame. All parties in the joint venture share liability. For example, two nurses set up a home infusion business and hire four nurses. As a health care entity, both nurses would be liable for any errors that cause harm.

From Anselmi, K. (2012). Nurses' personal liability vs. employer's vicarious liability. *Medsurg Nursing*, *27*(1), 45–48; Pozgar, G. D. (2020). *Legal and ethical issues for health professionals* (5th ed.). Jones & Bartlett Learning.

Nursing is also accountable to the public in guarding against any ill-prepared or apathetic UAP. During times of nurse shortages and cost containment, some hospitals provide brief (4- to 6-week) training programs for unlicensed workers to prepare them to assume complex nursing care tasks. In some cases, the quality of care becomes seriously compromised (Concepts in Practice, "Accountability").

Concepts in Practice   [IDEA]──▶[PLAN]──▶[ACTION]

Accountability

Rosetta has worked nights as a UAP for 20 years. She has heard the night nurses talk about how the level of a client's pain can be considered a "fifth vital sign." One night, Rosetta finds herself working with Georgia, an RN. Rosetta volunteers to assess all the postoperative clients for pain. Georgia thanks Rosetta and teaches her how to assess client pain using the 0 to 10 pain rating scale. By delegating this, Georgia is able to manage all the intravenous lines and perform dressing changes. Rosetta checks the pain level of all the clients who are not asleep at 2:00 AM and reports her findings to Georgia. Rosetta tells Georgia that no one needs pain medication because Rosetta perceives that clients need pain medication when they report a pain level of more than 6. After all, it is a 0 to 10 pain scale.

Take a moment and jot down if you think that Georgia made a good decision and defend the reasons for your thoughts about this situation. Once you have completed your notes, continue reading.

Considering pain as a fifth vital sign and delegating its assessment to UAP is a deviation from judicious nursing practice. Effective pain management requires assessment by a professional nurse because UAP do not have the knowledge required to conduct these assessments thoroughly. In addition, a complaint of client pain needs to be managed with some form of independent or collaborative nursing intervention. Poor pain control may result in impaired healing, other potential physical complications, and client dissatisfaction with nursing care. If clients under Georgia's care complain about poor pain management and report that Rosetta was the one who asked about their pain levels and no action was taken, Georgia would have to provide answers to questions from the physicians, nurse manager, or other nurses on the unit for substandard pain management. Georgia is accountable to her clients for effective pain management based on her professional nursing pain assessment.

Take Note!
Nurses must work collectively and cohesively to protect the public against potential harm and protect aspects of health care delivery that belong to professional nursing.

Accountability to the Profession

The nursing profession exercises accountability toward itself in the performance of its duty to formulate its own policy and control its activities. Professional nurses determine standards for nursing licensure (the National Council of State Boards of Nursing and individual State Boards of Nursing) and entry into professional groups and associations (e.g., Association of Operating Room Nurses, American Association of Critical Care Nurses). When nurses determine and monitor compliance with professional nursing standards and guidelines, professional autonomy is preserved.

In connection with this aspect of accountability, individual nurses must understand the need to be aware of and accountable for not only their own actions but also those of their colleagues. For example, a colleague with a substance abuse disorder poses a danger to clients, themselves, and coworkers. Nurses have a professional and legal responsibility to abide by the law and safeguard clients and other members of society, which means they need to report coworkers with suspected or actual substance use disorder (NCSBN Regulation Division, 2013). See Box 12.3, Learning, Knowing, and Growing, "Recognizing and Managing Possible Substance Use Disorder in a Nursing Colleague."

Forty-one State Boards of Nursing offer alternatives to disciplinary actions that typically involve legally binding programs for detoxification, treatment, peer assistance, and recovery programs that include random monitoring for signs of substance use disorder. Three State Boards of Nursing approve individual programs when presented with treatment and monitoring details for the nurse's recovery (National Council of State Boards of Nursing, 2020). When nurses police themselves, professional autonomy is enhanced.

Regular peer review programs provide another means for nurses to monitor their own profession. Benefits of peer review include increased self-awareness of practice, quality of client care, professionalism, and accountability. Peer review processes require that nurses look objectively at a colleague's performance, which sometimes can be difficult when the peer is a friend. Additionally, some nurses may feel uncomfortable pointing out deficiencies in another nurse's performance. Effective peer

12.3 Learning, Knowing, and Growing

Recognizing and Managing Possible Substance Use Disorder in a Nursing Colleague

Signs of Possible Substance Abuse in a Nurse

- Subtle changes in personal appearances that escalate with time
- Breath smells excessively of breath mints or alcohol
- Absences from the unit for extended periods of time
- Frequent bathroom breaks
- Diminished mental capabilities, especially memory lapses or episodic confusion
- Inappropriate emotional reactions or verbal responses
- Reduced levels of alertness when working
- Inconsistent stories for reasons for absences or tardiness
- Arriving consistently early or late for work
- Habitually departing late from work
- Coming to work when not scheduled
- Wearing long-sleeved garments at all times
- Excessive numbers of mistakes, especially medication errors
- Wasting controlled medications excessively
- Volunteering to administer controlled medications to unassigned clients
- Spending excessive amounts of time close to a controlled medication supply cart or computerized medication dispensing system
- Volunteering for overtime often
- Keeping inaccurate records of controlled substances
- Excessive corrections on client medication administration records
- Failing to have another person with legal ability to witness wasting controlled medications during the time the drug is being prepared and administered

- Falsifying reasons for controlled medication variances in computerized dispensing systems
- Charting on electronic health records that seems incoherent
- Signing out medications for clients who have left the unit
- Frequent client reports of ineffective pain control
- Increasing personal and/or professional isolation

Managing a Nursing Colleague With Substance Use Disorder

- Before confronting or reporting suspicions of substance abuse, nurses should keep a written log (including time and date) of suspicious behaviors.
- When confronting a colleague about suspected chemical impairment or substance abuse, the nurse should display genuine empathy and concern, be direct and open, share specific behaviors and incidents, and expect the colleague to deny allegations.
- Experts in chemical impairment management advocate interventions involving the suspected nurse, colleagues who observed behaviors, the nurse's direct supervisor, and a chemical impairment counselor.
- An intervention provides the suspected nurse with immediately available assistance should the nurse want to seek professional help for the alleged problem.
- Report the nurse to the local State Board of Nursing.
- Provide support when the nurse returns to work following successful completion of a substance abuse treatment plan.
- Follow all directions for monitoring the nurse for relapses.

From National Council of State Boards of Nursing Regulation Division. (2013). *Substance use disorder*. https://www.ncsbn.org/333.htm; National Council of State Boards of Nursing. (2018). *A nurse manager's guide to substance use disorder in nursing*. https://www.ncsbn.org/Mgr_SUDiN_Brochure_2014.pdf; United States Drug Enforcement Agency. (2005). *Drug addiction in health care professionals*. Retrieved February 6, 2013, from http://www.deadiversion.usdoj.gov/pubs/brochures/drug_hc.htm

evaluations offer constructive suggestions to remedy identified performance deficiencies. Some health care organizations incorporate peer review findings in annual performance evaluations of nursing staff.

Finally, nurses are accountable for the survival of the profession. As members of a noble and well-respected profession, nurses need to recruit new members, support them through the education process, mentor them as they enter the workforce, and support them as experienced colleagues.

Accountability to Interprofessional and Unlicensed Health Care Team Members

As a professional in the interprofessional and multidisciplinary health care team, nurses are accountable for the

unique contributions they make to client care. The nurse often spends more time with the client than any other health team member. Nurses who engage in holistic nursing care consider more than just the client's physiologic needs; they also identify psychological, sociocultural, and spiritual needs. Many times, nurses identify obstacles for client self-care by spending time in assessing, teaching, and evaluating client and family responses regarding what they need to know before discharge (Concepts in Practice, "A Nurse's Contribution Makes a Big Difference").

Professional nurses also have accountability for informing UAP of potential hazards they might encounter when providing basic care to clients with contagious diseases or to clients who have the potential for violence. The UAP need to know what actions need to be taken

Concepts in Practice IDEA → PLAN → ACTION

A Nurse's Contribution Makes a Big Difference

Marian is a professional nurse who works in a rehabilitation unit. She is getting ready to dismiss Mrs. Garcia, an older woman who needs to learn how to perform glucose self-monitoring at home. The diabetes nurse educator who provided the basic instructions documented that Mrs. Garcia could effectively perform the required tasks. However, the evening before Mrs. Garcia's discharge, Marian observes that Mrs. Garcia could not effectively use the glucose monitor because of limited manual dexterity and poor vision. Marian discovers that Mrs. Garcia lives alone and has no family members available for assistance. By documenting her assessment and informing the case manager, home health care is arranged, thereby preventing hospital readmission and reducing health care costs. Marian fulfills her obligation to the client, the organization, and interprofessional team members.

to protect themselves. Likewise, UAP have the responsibility of informing professional nurses about changes in client status that indicate a potentially infectious disease or escalation of anger into physical violence. For example, UAP should inform the nurse of a new onset of frequent stools in a client (a possible sign of *Clostridium difficile* infection) and if a client or family member is disgruntled about care. In situations such as the latter, the nurse can intervene through use of therapeutic communication techniques (see Chapter 4, "Establishing Helping and Healing Relationships") to discover and alleviate potential issues and prevent escalation of anger into an episode of verbal abuse or physical assault.

Accountability to the Employing Agency

Nurses are also accountable to their employing agencies. Employees, even those with professional status, have responsibilities and must answer for job actions. The employing agency holds nurses accountable for the quality of nursing care they provide, including job preparation and fitness for duty. Optimal physical and mental status of nursing staff is essential for safe and effective client care. Nurses have the obligation to come to work well rested for peak performance. Nurses often work overtime to finish their daily jobs or take on extra shifts (scheduled or on-call) to support colleagues when staffing shortages arise. Some nurses also work

more than one job to increase income or to practice across nurse specialty areas.

The employing agency contracts with nurses for a specific job to be done at a specific time and place for a specific wage. Nurses must uphold their end of the agreement in all of these areas. They also have accountability for monitoring peer performance, providing effective supervision of UAP, and reporting safety issues (consumer or staff) when they arise.

Although not unimportant, accountability to the employing agency rightfully takes a back seat to accountability to the client, the public, the profession, and to nurses themselves.

Accountability of Health Care Organizations to the Public and Employees: Quality and Safety

Nurse accountability to health care organizations requires that the employing agency create working conditions that foster safety and quality in nursing care delivery. Just like nurses, health care organizations are accountable to the public for the quality and safety of the care they have been entrusted to perform. The agency is responsible for creating a culture of safety so that work processes and environments do not create care errors and staff can report issues without fear of reprisal.

The IOM report, *To Err Is Human*, identified gaps in health care delivery processes that sometimes resulted in death and permanent disability in clients (IOM, 2000). In 2001, the IOM followed up on safety issues by releasing *Crossing the Quality Chasm: A New Health System for the 21st Century*, which suggested actions that health care professionals can undertake to improve the quality and safety of health care delivery. In 2003, the IOM issued *Health Professions Education: A Bridge to Quality*, a report on how to completely transform the education of the interprofessional health care team so that team members would be effectively prepared to meet quality and safety issues encountered in daily practice. Nursing leaders acknowledge that the profession needed to address concerns raised by the IOM studies (IOM, 2011; Sherwood & Barnsteiner, 2012).

The Robert Wood Johnson Foundation provided a series of nursing grants to improve efforts for educating beginning and advanced practice nurses; these grants led to the development of the **Quality and Safety Education for Nurses (QSEN) Institute**. QSEN is an ongoing program that identifies core competencies and strategies to help new health team members develop essential competencies in knowledge, skills, and attitudes for client-centered care, teamwork and collaboration, evidence-based practice, safety, quality improvement, and informatics. A full description of prelicensure and nurse generalist competencies that includes specific definitions, knowledge, skills, and attitudes can be found online at https://qsen.org/competencies/pre-licensure-ksas. The QSEN Institute website offers detailed competencies for graduate nursing education, resources for nurses and educators, and educational strategies for competency attainment (QSEN Institute, 2020).

In 2010, Sammer et al. conducted a comprehensive literature review to identify key elements that contribute to a hospital culture of client safety. They concluded that communication, teamwork, learning, evidence-based practice, justice, leadership, and client-centeredness are the hallmarks of a client safety culture (Table 12.2). This text highlights many of these hallmarks.

The employing agency administration is obligated to provide competent health care providers for the consumers of its services. Thus, the employing agency has the right to expect the nurse to be accountable to the agency. Dimensions of accountability include quality of work, unsafe practice situations, nurse attitudes toward the employing agency, and professional practice with outside agency staff. The agency must be open to suggestions from nurses to improve work processes and environment without being punitive to those who report unsafe or low-quality care situations.

Along with accountability to provide the material and human resources and a safe environment for effective care for health care consumers, the employer has the responsibility and accountability to their employees in additional areas. Health care organizations are responsible for treating employees fairly, which means freedom from discrimination and administering equal pay for equal work. As caregivers, the nurse has the right to question client care practices without fear of retribution, and, if needed, suggest that the client change physicians if the physician fails to provide required safe medical care without fear of retribution. The organization must provide a civil environment and policies to address potential violence against health care workers, bullying, and sexual harassment. Nurses and all other health care team members must be treated with dignity and respect; they must not be subjected to an abusive work environment with intimidation tactics. The employer must protect employee privacy and confidentiality (e.g., of performance reviews, personal health issues, performance improvement plans) and must have policies related to the monitoring of employee computer use and video monitoring (not permissible in locker rooms or bathrooms). The employer must also follow federal regulation guidelines for family medical leave, provision of a safe work environment, breaks during shifts, and unemployment compensation (Pozgar, 2020). During the recent COVID-19 pandemic, the

TABLE 12.2   Factors Contributing to a Culture of Client Safety

Element	Factors Involved
Communication	Transparency, structured techniques for intra- and interprofessional communication about clients and client handoffs, involvement in safety briefings and debriefings, effective feedback and conflict resolution, bottom-up approach, and clear, assertive communication patterns
Teamwork	Common mission, mission alignment among all members, referral to expert members when needed, flattened hierarchy, multidisciplinary meetings, mutual respect, valued intergenerational contributions, psychological safety, flexibility, adaptive ability, and member support
Learning	Increased awareness and information transmission, success celebrations, data-driven actions, all-member participation in educational endeavors, learning from mistakes, monitoring of outcomes using benchmarks, performance improvement programs, engagement in root cause analysis, proactive rather than reactive behaviors, and sharing of learned lessons
Evidence-based practice	Best practices followed, aim for zero defect or high reliability, driven by outcomes, practice science of safety, effective use of technology and automation, standardized protocols, policies, checklists, and guidelines
Just culture	Blame-free, open disclosure, nonpunitive reporting processes and structures, awareness of at-risk behaviors, process, or systems rather than an individual as a source of errors, and high levels of trust
Leadership	Be accountable, manage change, display commitment, make administrative rounds, encourage participative governance, engage physicians, set priorities, supply material and human resources, model desired attitudes and behaviors, be supportive, use vigilance and visibility, and determine and live values and mission
Client-centeredness	Community involvement, grassroots efforts to change policies, client and family empowerment, always focusing on the client, formal client participation in care, informed clients and families, and careful listening and paying attention to client stories

From Pozgar, G. D. (2020). *Legal and ethical issues for health professionals* (5th ed.). Jones & Bartlett Learning; Sammer, C., Lykens, K., Singh, K., Mains, D., & Lackan, N. (2010). What is patient safety culture? *Journal of Nursing Scholarship, 42*(2), 156–165; Sherwood, G., & Barnsteiner, J. (Eds.). (2012). *Quality and safety in nursing a competency approach to improving outcomes*. Wiley-Blackwell.

Centers for Medicare and Medicaid Services and the Occupational Safety and Health Administration issued waivers for hospitals that affected the safety of professional nurses (American Hospital Association, 2020). For example, national shortages of personal protective equipment resulted in nurses having to improvise with available supplies of lower quality to protect themselves from contracting the disease. Many nurses had to reuse single-use N95 masks and if appropriate masks were not available, they had to wear disposable or homemade cloth masks with plastic face shields.

Nurses also have the responsibility to inform their employers about unsafe or unethical situations in which public welfare and interest supersedes that of the organization. Many health care organizations publish detailed whistleblower policies in their compliance manuals and employee handbooks (Pozgar, 2020). Recent legislation has resulted in legal protection for nurses who report unsafe practice situations. Sometimes, the employing organization may refuse to correct what nurses perceive as an unsafe practice situation. Nurses must refuse to work in areas and situations they consider unsafe. This further fulfills accountability to the employer (as well as self) because such nurses are essentially saying, "I will not put my employer in the position of giving unsafe care." Not taking action against unsafe practices places clients at risk, and clients will likely tell family members and acquaintances about the poor care received at the nurse's employing organization. However, refusal to provide client care as designated by terms of employment may result in reprimand, demotion, and even dismissal from the agency unless the nurse is employed in a state that offers whistleblower protection.

An additional aspect of the nurse's accountability to the employer involves the attitude toward that employer that the nurse projects to clients. The attitude should be one of objectivity and honesty. Nurses who find joy in working for a particular employer may appropriately and honestly promote the health care organization's strengths. However, if confronted with an employer's shortcoming, nurses must be honest in their responses. Sometimes, when particularly taxed or following a disagreement, a nurse may denigrate a health care organization where they are employed. In this case, the nurse has not acted professionally and may not be aware of the impact of such statements on the client, visitors, or the health care organization.

Concerns have arisen recently regarding accountability to the employer because of a large and growing number of agency-employed nurses who are essentially "rented" to hospitals on a per diem basis. In most cases, agency nurses possess high levels of clinical competence. However, they may be unfamiliar with the employing institution's policies and procedures. A study by Pham and Papa (2011) revealed that emergency department temporary staff members are twice as likely as permanent staff to be involved with harmful medication errors. A seasoned emergency room nurse manager, Papa specifies that emergency rooms need to be properly staffed and believes safety can be enhanced by providing adequate nurse orientation and pairing a temporary staff nurse with a seasoned fulltime nurse employee so that questions regarding care protocols can be readily answered and guidance given for accessing agency information (Pham & Papa, 2011).

Agency nurses may have more accountability to the nursing agency, thus diminishing some of the support they might offer the hospital, or they may feel primarily accountable to the hospital's clients. When allegiance to the employing institution supersedes allegiance to the agency, nurses may run the risk of being dropped by the agency.

When nurses place their accountability to their employing agency above their accountability to all others, it detracts from a desirable image of nurses as working primarily in the public interest and instead fosters the impression of the nurse as subservient to and under the control of the employing institution. Nurses must learn to balance their accountability to clients, society, the profession, and themselves with their accountability toward the employing agency; this may be more difficult in times of economic uncertainty.

▌ Questions for Reflection

1. How do you define accountability to your employer or nursing program?
2. What would you do if you found yourself in a work or educational setting that required you to take care of more clients than you thought you could safely manage?
3. Why do you think some nurses fail to report unsafe client situations to their managers?
4. What would you do if you heard a nursing colleague (professional nurse or nursing student) criticize the place you work (or attend school)?

Accountability to Oneself

Professionals who are deeply committed to their careers can sometimes be exploited by the systems in which they work. In the early days of the nursing profession, hospitals and clients expected nurses to live on the premises in which they worked. Today, agencies no longer assume "ownership" of nurses and do not expect them to work long hours without breaks. Employers and clients see nurses as free and independent individuals with multiple facets to their lives. Studies addressing nurse overtime indicate that 10% to 25% of nurses reported working extra hours without being compensated (Bae, 2012; Turnbull, 2016).

When personal accountability is lacking, blaming, complaining, and procrastination are common. People who practice personal accountability experience healthier relationships, improved teamwork, and less stress while their employers enjoy increased productivity, greater teamwork, and improved customer service. Personal accountability begins with looking at oneself and seeing how things can be changed rather than pointing fingers at others. When things do not go smoothly, two key questions to ask are "What can I do?" and "How can I help?" These questions focus on action and include a role for the individual to make a difference (Miller, 2004).

However, some job situations may cause nurses and others to overlook these basic facts. Staff shortages may keep nurses from fulfilling their basic needs for nutrition and elimination. In addition, nurses' other life roles may affect professional performance. Therefore, nurses must be accountable to themselves for their actions both on and off the job because of the potential effects of their actions on themselves and others.

Fatigue, minor illness, exhaustion, or the effects of alcohol or drugs can make the nurse a liability rather than an asset in the work situation. Professional practice may also be hampered by nurses who put in too much overtime, allow themselves to be placed in positions far beyond their abilities and knowledge, and constantly function in a highly stressed state. These nurses may find themselves too exhausted or unprepared to function effectively in professional and personal roles.

Significant others, family, and friends cannot always be expected to have lower priority than one's work, and work cannot always be expected to take second place to social and personal relationships. Nurses need to attain a certain balance. Overdoing the amount of time and energy expended on the job often leads to burnout, with the nurse becoming incapable of or unwilling to provide effective client care. Burnout also may take a toll on nurses' personal and social lives. Likewise, if the nurse ignores family needs, the family may disintegrate.

Nurses must assume responsibility for their own physical, mental, and spiritual health by maintaining a balanced lifestyle. They must decide when to give more energy to work and when to devote more energy to other life areas. When nurses sacrifice wholeness of life, they lose the capacity for optimal functioning as professionals and people. They must function at their fullest capacity when on the job while attaining a work–life balance that ensures they can avoid compassion fatigue, despair, and exhaustion.

Nurses' accountability to themselves includes refusing to work in situations deemed unsafe. Each nurse individually defines unsafe situations. Some examples of unsafe practice situations include lack of knowledge or experience to work in an unfamiliar specialty area and insufficient staffing. Nurses must learn to see refusal to work in unsafe situations as the ultimate professional service to the consumer despite potential employer sanctions that may be applied as consequences for this action. Whistleblowing is the act of reporting unsafe or unethical situations or incompetence of another health care team member. Nurses must use professional judgment when deciding whether to report wrongdoing. Murray (2007) and Mendes (2018) offered several suggestions for self-protection for nurses who opt to "blow the whistle" on unsafe client care situations (Box 12.4, Professional Building Blocks, "Self-Protection Before Blowing the Whistle").

12.4 Professional Building Blocks

Self-Protection Before Blowing the Whistle

1. Hire an attorney for legal advice.
2. Verify the legalities of whistleblower protection at the federal and state levels.
3. Consult with the state nursing association for answers to or clarification of state laws and regulations.
4. Develop a written, accurate account of all observed events (including time, date, and incident).
5. If possible, obtain a cooperative internal witness to the observed event.
6. Store all documents in a secure location and have multiple copies of each document.
7. Follow the facility's chain of command when reporting incidents.
8. Ask for help from experts, including the state attorney general, state and federal legislative bodies, and other agencies and organizations that have an interest in reducing unsafe health care delivery.
9. Forward all documents to outside agencies using certified mail for proper verification of receipt of records and materials.
10. Maintain professionalism at all times when presenting information to the employing and outside agencies.

From Murray, J. (2007). Before blowing the whistle, learn to protect yourself. *American Nurse Today, 2*(3), 40–42; Mendes, A. (2018). Being supported to whistle while you work. *British Journal of Community Nursing, 23*(7), 360–361. https://doi.org/10.12968/bjcn.2018.23.7.360

Accountability to oneself also involves acknowledging one's own limitations and knowing when additional education or assistance from another is needed for effective client care. Questioning physician orders requires confidence and sometimes courage, but it protects both the client and the nurse. Deciding when to assume a new nursing position (such as promotion to a nurse manager) should be based on each nurse's appraisal of their personal qualifications for the job rather than on opinions of other people. Completing an academic degree (such as a bachelor's degree in nursing) does not automatically prepare all nurses to assume managerial roles. Other factors such as personality, job description, and career goals should be considered before assuming an administrative position.

Accountability to oneself involves proactive protection against financial loss should an unforeseen incident occur. Many employing agencies carry insurance policies to protect themselves when client care errors and other accidents occur. Professional nurses who rely solely on the employing agency's insurance policy must remember that the agency will be looking out for its own best interests. On the other hand, when a nurse carries their own malpractice insurance, the legal counsel will focus on the nurse's interests and defend the nurse. When an error occurs resulting in client harm, the nurse and the employing agency could easily become adversaries (Anselmi, 2012; Pozgar, 2020). Incidents when professional nurses have been used as scapegoats to protect physicians and health care agencies have occurred as well as cases in which agencies have supported professional nurses. With individual malpractice coverage, the nurse knows that resources are available for legal consultation and defense. Some states require nurses to carry individual malpractice insurance policies as a condition for licensure application (Anselmi, 2012).

Client legal suits against nurses fall into two main categories: failing to do what is expected and doing what is not expected (CNA and Nurses Service Organization [NSO], 2020; Pozgar, 2020). Lawyers carefully examine client records for signs of breaches in nursing care standards and incidents of nurse failure to respond to, report, and follow up on changes in client physical and mental status. Table 12.3 presents reasons why lawsuits are filed against professional nurses. CNA Healthcare Underwriting and the Nurses Service Organization (NSO) are two companies that work together to provide professional liability insurance. They published a report outlining the indemnity (damages) awarded to the nurses who submitted claims to these companies. From January 1, 2015 to December 31, 2019, the company closed 455 cases and paid $70,171,018 in damages to settle professional nurse malpractice claims. The average payment per case was $210,513. They also noted that the average legal costs for nurses to protect their professional nursing licenses to defend against allegations was $5,300. The top six areas of nursing practice in which suits were filed were home care (20.7%); adult medical–surgical nursing care (18.5%); gerontology, including in long-term care facilities (9.7%); emergency department/urgent care (9.7%); obstetric nursing/labor and delivery (6.2%); and critical care (5.9%). Mean damage amounts exceeding $250,000 occurred in the areas of obstetric care/labor and delivery ($588,007), postanesthesia care ($384,912), and behavioral health ($258,518). Death and pressure injury were the basis for half of the claims. Medication administration errors were the most difficult cases to defend because many nurses used work-around processes to bypass hospital policies for ensuring client safety or they failed to follow the standard facility procedures for medication administration or diverted medication (CNA & NSO, 2020). Sometimes, even a slight omission in a nurse's documentation can result in legal action when harm comes to clients under the nurse's care.

As soon as a settlement is paid by a health care provider (including registered nurses), information regarding the settlement is entered into the National Practitioner Data Bank. Each State Board of Nursing where the nurse holds professional licensure status is also contacted (Watson, 2014).

Table 12.4 presents arguments for and against purchasing individual professional liability insurance. Professional liability insurance pays for an individual nurse's legal defense costs should the nurse be named in a malpractice suit or involved in an early settlement program. Liability coverage also pays damages to an injured party if the nurse is found negligent. As supervisors and coordinators of client care, nurses may be held accountable for actions of UAP, nursing assistants, other nurses, and clerical staff (CNA & NSO, 2020). According to Tamilia (2019), the nurse generalist working in a hospital and not in a specialized unit can pay $28 annually for a claims-made policy or $100 for occurrence coverage. Advanced practice nurses (depending on their specialties) may pay up to $13,250 for liability coverage. Nurses who are self-employed and nurses working in some specialty areas (e.g., critical care, obstetrics) pay higher fees than nurses employed in medical–surgical units and extended care facilities. Nurses who work in obstetrics can expect to get claims-made coverage for $168 annually or occurrence coverage for $546 annually (Tamilia, 2019). In comparison, annual physician malpractice costs may range from

TABLE 12.3 Reasons for Nurse Malpractice Suits

Reason	Example
Failure to document	Failing to document procedures, medications, and physician interactions or not documenting events leading up to a situation resulting in client harm while events occurred (charting after the fact)
Therapy error	Administering incorrect medication or treatment
Failure to follow standards of care	Using alternative treatments or procedures and/or failing to follow guidelines outlined by institutional policy and procedure manuals
Communication failure	Not listening intently to client concerns, providing inaccurate discharge instructions, not notifying a physician in a timely manner
Omitted assessment	Not performing routine assessments for various medical conditions or procedures, or neglecting to document a required assessment
Neglecting to be a client advocate	Not questioning physician orders when needed or not providing a safe environment for the client
Breach of confidentiality	Sharing of private information with others in person, over the telephone, or on social media
Invasion of privacy	Failing to provide drapes, shut the door of the client's room, or draw curtains around the client's bed for procedures requiring physical exposure
Release of medical information without permission	Failing to get written permission from clients when sharing medical information with others
Assault and battery	Performing invasive procedures without the client's informed consent
False imprisonment	Using physical or chemical restraints inappropriately
Discrimination	Giving unequal treatment based on particular group membership or specific disease
Defamation	Harming the reputation of another person
Slander	Making false statements or misrepresentations that harm the reputation of another
Libel	Making written or oral statements or other representation published without just cause for the purpose of exposing another to public contempt
Unprofessional behavior	Violation of nurse–client boundaries
Impaired nursing practice	Working under the influence of controlled medications, illegal substances or alcohol OR being fatigued

Adapted from CNA and Nurses Service Organization. (2020). *Nurse professional liability exposure claim report (4th ed.), minimizing risk, achieving excellence.* https://www.cna.com/web/wcm/connect/f8b73780-0c25-453e-b4cf-b5343da8e374/Nurse-Exposure-Claim-Report-4th-Edition.pdf?MOD=AJPERES; Helm, A., & Kihm, N. C. (2001). Is professional liability insurance for you? *Nursing, 31*(1), 48–49; Croke, E. M. (2003). Nurses, negligence and malpractice. *American Journal of Nursing, 103,* 54–64; Pozgar, G. D. (2020). *Legal and ethical issues for health professionals* (5th ed.). Jones & Bartlett Learning; Watson, E. (2014). Nursing malpractice: Costs, trends & issues. *Journal of Legal Nurse Consulting, 25*(1), 26–31.

TABLE 12.4 Reasons For and Against Nurses Carrying Individual Liability Insurance

Reasons For	Reasons Against
Employer language may cover the facility but not individual employees.	Attitude of being not at risk for malpractice
Employer policies may be insufficient to cover all claims, leaving the nurse responsible for the amount that exceeds the facility policy limits.	Perceived adequate coverage from employer
Hospital insurer might seek indemnity from the nurse after a lawsuit is settled.	Clients may file malpractice claims several years after an incident, and the nurse may change jobs, or the facility could close or change its malpractice policy.
Personal policies provide legal defense for the nurse, and some include costs for time off work and transportation during legal proceedings.	Nurse could be caught in a facility's decision to side with a physician during legal proceedings, holding the nurse responsible for malpractice.
Facility policy may have coverage gaps.	Perception that carrying own insurance policy increases the likelihood of being sued
Most jurors assume nurses carry individual liability insurance.	
Coverage of legal costs should an allegation be made against a nurse's license	

Adapted from Helm, A., & Kihm, N. C. (2001). Is professional liability insurance for you? *Nursing, 31*(1), 48–49. CNA and Nurses Service Organization. (2020). *Nurse professional liability exposure claim report (4th ed.), minimizing risk, achieving excellence.* https://www.cna.com/web/wcm/connect/f8b73780-0c25-453e-b4cf-b5343da8e374/Nurse-Exposure-Claim-Report-4th-Edition.pdf?MOD=AJPERES

$8,274 (e.g., internal medicine in California) to $214,999 (e.g., obstetrics/gynecology in New York) (Nobity, 2021).

Coverage terms vary according to the type of policy purchased. Claims-made policies cover the nurse for the time when the plaintiff files a court claim. In contrast, occurrence policies cover the nurse for the time in which the situation occurred that resulted in litigation. Claims-made policies are less expensive than occurrence coverage policies (Tamilia, 2019). The nurse should know which type of policy they carry. When a nurse has claims-made coverage, the policy needs to be active until all chances of litigation have expired. Each state determines the time frame in which people can file legal claims against health care providers for undesirable care outcomes.

Some health care organizations have implemented early settlement programs to reduce litigation against physicians and hospitals when adverse client outcomes arise. Part of these programs includes established policies and procedures outlining exactly how appropriate disclosure is made to clients and families when an adverse event occurs. The process typically includes full apologies and early offers for compensation if deemed appropriate (Greenwald, 2008). However, no assurances have been made to professional nurses that the health care organization will not take punitive action against them should the adverse event occur because of a nursing error.

Finally, nurses are accountable to themselves to do their own personal best (Styles, 1985). Factors outside nursing can influence this aspect of accountability. Federal and state governments can support or hinder the ability of professional nurses to be accountable. Government legislative efforts result in laws and regulations that directly affect many aspects of professional practice, research, and education. Federal, state, and local governments establish health care priorities and fund health care organizations for equal access to care for all. Nurses must consider political activism as a means to self-accountability as a method of bringing public policy and the most expert care into congruence (see Chapter 19, "The Professional Nurse's Role in Public Policy").

▌ QUESTIONS FOR REFLECTION

1. If a client experiences a poor outcome and you were a part of the client's care, who would be accountable?
2. What current resources are in place in your employing institution and your nursing program for employee or student defense should a medical malpractice suit be brought against you?
3. What actions can you take to prevent client care errors in the health care setting where you practice as a nursing student or professional nurse?

THE GROUNDWORK FOR ACCOUNTABILITY

From this complex description of accountability, professional nurses must consciously prepare themselves to develop the skills and attributes that will enable its accomplishment. Nurses need to know the latest research, use theoretical bases, display competence in clinical practice, assume leadership, and engage in practice based on their personal ethical framework.

Research and the Establishment of a Theoretical Base for Nurse Accountability

One of the major factors in the movement of nursing toward professional status is the growth of its theoretical and conceptual base for practice. As the level of nursing education increases, nurses are incorporating theoretical, research-based, and other forms of evidence-based knowledge into daily practice. As evidence-based health care becomes commonplace, nurses are increasingly expected to use all forms of evidence—especially research-based evidence—when providing nursing care services.

In practice, nurses use knowledge generated through research to substantiate their actions and develop clinical practice policies and procedures. Although most nurses have access to online and printed research findings, finding time to read and analyze nursing research results poses a dilemma for many. Some nurses (especially those educated in associate degree programs) have received no formal education on how to evaluate research findings for use in practice. In addition, the dissemination of nursing research results to practicing nurses occurs slowly; sometimes it may be years before key findings are published.

With the advent of evidence-based practice and quality improvement initiatives, the use of research findings has become more desirable and acceptable. Nurses need support with accessing and understanding available research reports and applying the findings to work situations. Some health care agencies have nursing research committees and offer resources to help nurses use research findings in practice. However, until nurses and all health care organizations value the use of nursing research, some nurses will continue to practice on the basis of tradition.

Clinical and Professional Competence

The public, consumers, health care agencies, and physicians expect nurses to have clinical competence. Nurses in specialty areas of practice have specific knowledge and skills for competent practice. However, all areas of practice require that nurses understand and apply principles and techniques of asepsis, physical assessment, nursing process, pathophysiology, pharmacology, human growth and development, psychology, sociology, spirituality, and safety. Because all nurses hold their clients' lives in their hands, whatever a nurse does, it must be done well.

With many levels of nursing reflected in the composition of today's health care teams, nurses at each level should have a clear idea of the scope of practice at their level and should perform responsibly to the maximum limit of that level. A nurse's accountability may be called into question if they are performing outside of the scope of their particular level's practice. It is no more appropriate for nurses who have been educated at the baccalaureate level to restrict professional activities to those they may have exercised at the associate degree level than it is for them to assume the role of the master's-prepared practitioner.

The key to expertise in practice lies in both knowledge and skill, a somewhat artificial distinction that nevertheless allows for more clarity in this discussion. Nursing has always had a strong manual skills component. To the extent that the nurse is in a role that calls for manual skills, gentleness, quickness, and accuracy remain hallmarks of excellence. Where the skills required are in the areas of communication, teaching, leadership, management, and research (the so-called hands-off skills), the need for expertise is no less pressing.

Underlying all skills is excellence in terms of command of "nursing knowledge." Nurses can never expect to contribute significantly to health care in its assessment, planning, implementation, and evaluation aspects if they perform in a mediocre manner.

Take Note!
Competence in nursing is an absolute prerequisite for accountability.

Leadership Skills

Leadership development frequently elicits questions when first introduced to nursing students. A frequent response is "Not everyone can be a head nurse or a supervisor or wants to be an instructor. I don't want to be a leader; I just want to be a nurse." The fact is

that the elements of leadership are inherent in any nursing role.

Leadership ability is one of the most important areas in laying the groundwork for accountability. The nurse's accountability extends into all areas of health care delivery, including health maintenance and promotion and promoting self-care. The nurse is a constant catalyst for change in health care quality and delivery, especially if they are "just" a nurse.

To fulfill the leadership role, nurses must be well versed in the theory and practice of change. Nurses are leaders because they influence others, provide others with desired health-related information, participate in the formation of health care and organizational policies, serve as role models of health, and coordinate client care. Accountable nurses cannot function without leadership skills.

Personal Ethical Framework

Nurses are accountable within a personal ethical framework. They cannot be accountable in a moral vacuum. They must have their personal ethics guide standards and values in which they believe and to which they refer. To some extent, these are determined by the collective values of the profession, which in turn, are partly determined by what the public expects of that profession and partly by what the profession demands of itself.

In nursing, these professional values are formalized by the *Code of Ethics for Nurses* (ANA, 2015). However, in large measure, a nurse's ethical code is personal and highly individual, developed in the course and context of the individual's total life experience. It includes values learned in the home, in schools, from social groups, during religious training, in the work setting, and from the activities and contacts of daily life. It is influenced by the nurse's ethnic and religious background, the area of the country in which they live, and their personality.

Often, a personal ethical code is something of which people are relatively unaware. It is unconsciously used in making decisions and running one's life but is rarely explicitly scrutinized or even acknowledged as existing. It is this code that is so essential in the professional nurse. A nurse must be aware of their code, how it affects decisions and actions, and where it is congruent with or departs from standard codes of the profession. Any conflicts must be worked through and compromise sought so that the nurse can feel comfortable with and confident in the ethical basis in which their practice is rooted.

1. What do you truly value in life?
2. How do your values affect your nursing practice?

ACCOUNTABILITY IN AN ERA OF COST CONTAINMENT

As increases in health care costs continue to outpace inflation, public support for imposing controls on costs for health care increases. Prospective payment systems serve as the major reimbursement method for many health care services. In efforts to curb costs, Medicare no longer covers costs for hospital-acquired infections, complications, and errors. Thus, nurse accountability for the prevention of adverse effects of hospitalization increases.

For-profit and managed care providers consistently look for ways to provide cost-effective health care. Health care practices deemed to be effective will be increased and retained, while those determined to be ineffective will be decreased or discarded. Professional nurses must substantiate the benefits of the contributions they make to health care delivery.

All too often in health care, "effective" seems to mean "cost-effective." The idea of a universal right to top-quality care for all is being diluted to a standard of adequate care to those who meet specific criteria set by third-party payers. Nurses are now asked to be accountable for the care they give and for giving that care in the least expensive manner possible, often in a setting or time frame that severely limits the comprehensiveness of that care.

Disease management programs offer a means to enhance the ability of clients to manage chronic health conditions (e.g., end-stage renal disease, diabetes, HIV/AIDS) by offering intensive client education and home support services to keep people with these conditions in their homes rather than in the hospital or an extended care facility. As key providers of care in homes, professional nurses making home visits are held accountable for accurate client assessments, effective health education, and appropriate referrals. Because of the complexity of community interventions and algorithms present in disease management programs, Goldstein (2006) recommends bachelor degree–level preparation as the minimum for nurses working in them.

Unlicensed Assistive Personnel

Increased use of UAP and LPN/LVNs adds layers of accountability for health care delivery. UAP and LPN/LVNs have always been accountable for proper performance of assigned duties and for knowing when other workers must be consulted for situations beyond the limits of the UAP's and LPN/LVN's knowledge and training. UAP and LPN/LVNs must earn the trust of the professional nurse and vice versa. Although the legal doctrine of *respondeat superior* (let the superior answer) applies, UAP and LPN/LVNs do bear some accountability for their actions. Nevertheless, the principles that have guided nursing care for years apply; the professional nurse is still accountable for the client's overall care. Thus, the current situation requires that professional nurses broaden the scope of supervision and be more vigilant. They must be more aware of the abilities and activities of UAP and LPN/LVNs while increasing their own availability for consultation.

Managed Care and Third-Party Payers

Managed care, government health care plans, and private health insurance companies monitor access to services, strive to eliminate redundancy, look for ways to reduce overuse of services, and control health care costs. Unfortunately, in some managed care and insurance companies, people without health care experience or education make approval decisions for consumers who need or want specific health care services (including health insurance coverage).

With cost containment efforts, the nurse's role as a client advocate becomes vital. The nurse advocate pays attention to and acts in instances in which clients are being denied access to essential care or seem to be short-changed by policies and actions directed primarily at cost containment. The issue of access to care has been a legitimate one for nurses to address for years, as succinctly stated in the *Code of Ethics for Nurses* (ANA, 2015):

> The nurse assumes the responsibility and accountability for individual nursing judgments and actions... The nurse collaborates with members of the health professions and other citizens in promoting community and national efforts to meet the health needs of the public. (p. 1)

This notion has also been reiterated and emphasized by its inclusion in the ANA's *Nursing's Social Policy Statement* (2010). There can be no doubt that the nurse's accountability extends to exerting efforts to respond to the health care needs of the public in a collective sense.

Along with doing what is right for clients, nurses play a key role in reimbursement to the employing agency from managed care and other third-party payers. Meticulous documentation of all supplies and interventions provides evidence that consumers received care. Third-party payers frequently audit charts in efforts to disallow charges appearing on consumer bills.

ACCOUNTABILITY IN THE FUTURE

The future relies on current actions. The nursing profession has renewed its interest in accountability, and practice changes have occurred to increase nurse accountability.

Some nurses have assumed control of practice by adopting **shared governance** models that increase nurse participation in shaping professional practice. Nurses assume responsibility and accountability for developing unit-based and institution-wide procedures for clinical practice and quality improvement.

When adverse client events or failure of work processes arise, accountable nurses complete incident reports that are used to track reasons why errors occurred. Although incident reports are used internally to discover reasons for errors, nurses completing them admit that mistakes were made and examine the reasons why they occurred. A just culture approach to care errors uses incident reports as opportunities to identify flawed work processes and to help employees grow.

Health care delivery (especially in hospitals) relies on many team members to execute physician orders. Each member of the health care team makes a contribution, and all assume accountability for their actions. Nursing may have to learn to be accountable within a more ambiguous, multidisciplinary framework.

Advanced technology has provided the means for nursing to become more accountable. Technology can be used to clearly show what nurses do, including the care they deliver, the cost of that care, and its outcomes. Nursing must be rescued from burial in the category of "room and board" in budgets and on client bills. Once nursing services departments control their budgets, they will be empowered to make decisions and be accountable for them.

CHECKLIST FOR ACCOUNTABILITY

Preparation for accountability for action requires that nurses evaluate their actions periodically. Some nurses find it helpful to use an **accountability checklist** that provides key questions to ask themselves that address their current behaviors, attitudes, and resources required to protect everyone while engaging in clinical practice. Box 12.5, Professional Prototypes,

---

12.5 Professional Prototypes

Accountability Checklists

Accountability to the Client

- Am I providing the best care of which I am capable?
- Is that care sufficient to meet the needs of the client in this situation?
- Is this client entitled to more than I can offer, and am I turning elsewhere to obtain the needed, additional dimension?
- Am I incorporating what I know of nursing theory and research into my practice in this situation?
- Am I using my leadership skills to encourage others to function to their optimal ability in the care of this client?
- Am I acting in accordance with my own ethical code and that of the profession?
- If, by meeting the needs of this client, I am in conflict with my personal ethical code, am I seeking some alternative method or person to satisfy those needs?
- Have I given the client information they want or need about their health status while considering the effects of that knowledge on them?

Accountability to the Public

- Am I seeking to improve health and nursing care?
- Am I speaking out against abuses I see in health and nursing care?
- Am I acting as a community resource in the areas of health and nursing?
- Am I remaining an active and contributing member of the profession and to society after using public funds to finance my education?
- Am I attempting to increase the knowledge of the public to enable people to make more informed choices about health and nursing care?
- Am I recruiting others to enter the profession to have future health care needs of clients met?
- Am I sharing my knowledge and expertise about health care with elected officials to shape public policy?

Accountability to the Profession

- Am I fulfilling my professional role in accordance with the requirements of the profession?
- Are other nurses in my setting doing the same?

- If I am not performing satisfactorily, or if others are not, am I taking steps to remedy that situation?
- Am I willing to help other nurses in my work setting?
- Am I a participant in professional meetings, organizations, seminars, conferences, and so forth, so that I may express my views on nursing to those in nursing?
- Am I working within the profession to improve practice, education, or research?
- Am I complying with the ethical code of the profession?

Accountability to the Agency

- Am I performing in accordance with the job description for my position?
- If I am not satisfied with that job description, am I seeking appropriate ways to change it?
- Am I seeking to ensure that I am practicing under safe, if not optimal, conditions?
- Am I giving the institution its money's worth in terms of my work?
- Am I working in accordance with the policies and procedures of the institution?

- If I am not satisfied with those policies and procedures, am I seeking to change those using principles of leadership and change with the total mission of the institution in mind?

Accountability to Oneself

- Am I satisfied in my chosen profession?
- Am I performing my professional role in the best way I can?
- Should I seek additional preparation for that role?
- Should I withdraw from that role until I receive additional preparation?
- In areas where I am dissatisfied, am I seeking alternative modes of action or thought?
- Am I ethically comfortable with the way in which I am performing my professional role?
- Am I shortchanging my clients, my family, or myself in the way I am performing my professional role?
- Do I have adequate financial protection for myself and family if I were to be involved in a professional litigation case?
- Am I satisfied with the position this role assumes within my total lifestyle?

"Accountability Checklists," provides guidance for self-assessment of professional accountability by nurses. The list is not all-inclusive but offers a beginning tool for working the concept of accountability into one's life and work.

Because of the magnitude of the checklist provided in Box 12.5, most nurses cannot confidently claim that they fulfill all criteria. Some activities are more appropriate than others for nurses in different settings and at different times. However, nurses who are to act in an accountable manner or increase the accountability of their decisions and actions must consider these and other questions. Those who wish to call themselves professional nurses must consider these questions to live a life of accountability.

Summary and Significance to Practice

Accountability in professional nursing is a complex facet of nursing that requires nurses to look globally at how their actions affect clients, society, employing agencies, colleagues, and themselves. For a long time, nurses have assumed the responsibility of protecting clients and tending to their needs. Because of the nature of nursing practice, nurses have binding legal and ethical obligations to clients, the public, the employing agency, the profession, and themselves. Nurses need to have confidence in themselves and their cognitive skills if they are to tackle successfully situations with the potential to place clients in harm's way. Sometimes, nurses have to make tough decisions such as reporting unsafe acts by a colleague or employer. In today's rapidly changing and chaotic health care environment, nurses become accountable for staying current with new treatments, research findings, cost containment issues, and clinical skills. Because of its breadth and depth, professional accountability takes time to develop. Professional accountability expands as nurses assume more autonomous and leadership career paths.

REAL-LIFE REFLECTIONS

Recall the scenario from the beginning of the chapter. In light of what you have learned in this chapter, revisit your list of who made mistakes in the care of Mr. Jones. Do you see the need for any changes to your answers? What mistakes did they make? Who is accountable for the actions of the people involved? How could this unfortunate incident have been avoided? What steps should be taken by everyone involved to avoid repeating the same errors with a future client?

From Theory to Practice

1. Do you currently carry professional malpractice insurance? Why or why not?
2. How is student accountability addressed in your professional nursing program? How is it communicated to students? What are the consequences for a student breach of accountability?

Nurse as Author

Answer the questions contained in the accountability checklists provided in Professional Prototypes Box 12.5. Write an action plan to meet all areas for your future accountability in your personal and professional life.

Your Digital Classroom

Online Exploration

American Association of Colleges of Nursing: **www.aacn.nche.edu**

American Association of Legal Nurse Consultants: **www.aalnc.org**

American Nurses Association: **www.nursingworld.org**

Code for Nurses with Interpretive Statements: **www.nursingworld.org/codeofethics**

Medical malpractice cases and outcomes including awards to plaintiffs: **https://www.medicalmalpractice.com/lander/national-medical-malpractice-facts**

National Council of State Boards of Nursing: **www.ncsbn.org**

National League for Nursing: **www.nln.org**

Nurses Service Organization: **www.nso.com** to learn about some nurse liability insurance

Options

Quality and Safety Education in Nursing (QSEN) Institute: **www.qsen.org**

Expanding Your Understanding

1. Visit the National Council of State Boards of Nursing website. Click on "About NCSBN" and read the organization's mission, vision, and purpose. Go back to the home page, and click on "Boards of Nursing" to access your state's Board of Nursing. Find your state in the list and click on the website link to learn specific information related to professional nursing in your state, including license renewal requirements and whether the state where you practice requires that nurses carry their own liability insurance policy.

2. View a sample nurse's malpractice insurance policy on the Nurses Service Organization website. Click on "Professional Liability Insurance" and "Individuals," and select either "Nurses" or "Student Nurses." Then select your state. Click on "NSO's Professional Liability Insurance Program" to get a sample of terms of liability coverage from this professional liability insurance provider.

3. Watch the following video from the IHI, "How Do You Apologize after a Medical Error?" at http://www.ihi.org/education/IHIOpenSchool/resources/Pages/Activities/ApologizingEffectivelytoPatientsandFamilies.aspx Do you think that it is harder for physicians to apologize for errors than it is for nurses? Why or why not?

Beyond the Book

Visit **thePoint®** at **www.thePoint.lww.com** for activities and information to reinforce the concepts and content covered in this chapter.

REFERENCES

American Hospital Association. (2020). *CMS, OSHA, and others release waivers and other information on COVID-19*. Retrieved October 25, 2020, from https://www.aha.org/advisory/2020-03-16-cms-osha-and-others-release-waivers-and-other-new-information-covid-19

American Nurses Association. (2015). *Code of ethics for nurses with interpretive statements*. Author.

American Nurses Association. (2021). *Nursing scope and standards of practice* (4th ed.). Author.

American Nurses Credentialing Center. (2020). *Magnet model: Creating a Magnet culture*. Retrieved April 26, 2021, from https://www.nursingworld.org/organizational-programs/magnet/magnet-model/

Anselmi, K. K. (2012). Nurses' personal liability vs. employer's vicarious liability. *Medsurg Nursing, 21*(1), 45–48. Retrrieved April 27, 2021, from https://www.thefreelibrary.com/Nurses%27+personal+liability+vs.+employer%27s+vicarious+liability.-a0280558228

Bae, S. H. (2012). Nursing overtime: Why, how much, and under what working conditions. *Nursing Economics, 30*(2), 60–72. Retrieved April 27, 2021, from https://web-a-ebscohost-com.lib.rockhurst.edu/ehost/pdfviewer/pdfviewer?vid=3&sid=b8c18882-952e-49ff-be85-81c28dbcf5f9%40sessionmgr4006

Bixler, G. K., & Bixler, R. W. (1959). The professional status of nursing. *American Journal of Nursing, 59*, 1142–1147. Retrieved April 27, 2021, from https://www.jstor.org/stable/3416626?seq=1

Brous, E. (2021). Chapter 46, Nursing licensure and regulation. In D. J. Mason, E. Dickson, M. R. McLemore, G. A. Perez (Eds.), *Policy & politics in nursing and health care* (8th ed., pp. 381–387). Elsevier.

Butts, J. B. (2020). Chapter 3, Ethics in professional nursing practice. In J. B. Butts, K. L. Rich (Eds.), *Nursing ethics across the curriculum and into practice* (5th ed., pp. 59–95). Jones & Bartlett Learning.

Clifford, J. C. (1981). Managerial control versus professional autonomy: A paradox. *Journal of Nursing Administration, 11,* 19–21. Retrieved April 27, 2021, from https://journals.lww.com/jonajournal/Abstract/1981/09000/Managerial_Control_versus_Professional_Autonomy__A.6.aspx

CNA and Nurses Service Organization. (2020). *Nurse professional liability exposure claim report, (4th edition), minimizing risk, achieving excellence.* Retrieved October 26, 2020, from https://www.cna.com/web/wcm/connect/f8b73780-0c25-453e-b4cf-b5343da8e374/Nurse-Exposure-Claim-Report-4th-Edition.pdf?MOD=AJPERES

Dethmer, J. (2006a). Chapter 3, Accountability: Part 1. Taking responsibility. In J. Ware, J. Dethmer, J. Ziegler, F. Skinner (Eds.), *High performance investment teams* (pp. 45-66). John Wiley.

Dethmer, J. (2006b). Chapter 4, Accountability: Part 2. Making and keeping agreements. In J. Ware, J. Dethmer, J. Ziegler, F. Skinner (Eds.), *High performance investment teams* (pp. 67-92). John Wiley.

Dzau, V. J., McClellan, M., McGinnis, J. M., & Finkelman, E. M. (Eds.) (2017). *Vital directions for health & health care: An initiative of the National Academy of Medicine.* National Academy of Medicine.

Flexner, A. (1915). Is social work a profession? In *Proceedings of the National Conference of Charities and Correction* (pp. 576–590). Heldman.

Fowler, M. D. M. (2015). *Guide to the code of ethics for nurses with interpretive statements* (2nd ed.). Nursebooks.com.

Goldstein, P. (2006). Impact of disease management programs on hospital and community nursing practice. *Nursing Economics, 24*(6), 308–314. Retrieved April 27, 2021, from https://web-a-ebscohost-com.lib.rockhurst.edu/ehost/pdfviewer/pdfviewer?vid=21&sid=b8c18882-952e-49ff-be85-81c28dbcf5f9%40sessionmgr4006

Greenwald, J. (2008). Stanford's medical center mulls expanding role of captive. *Business Insurance, 42*(17), 36–37. Retrieved April 21, 2021, from https://www.businessinsurance.com/article/20080427/STORY/100024693/Stanfords-Medical-Center-mulls-expanding-role-of-captive

Han, J., LaMarra, D., & Vapiwala, N. (2017). Applying lessons from social psychology to transform the culture of error disclosure. *Medical Education, 51*(10), 996–1001. https://doi.org/10.1111/medu.13345

Hannawa, A. F. (2009). Negotiating medical virtues: toward the development of a physician mistake disclosure model. *Health Communication, 24*(5), 391–399. https://doi.org/10.1080/10410230903023279

Heron, M. (2019). *Deaths: Leading causes for 2017. National Vital Statistics Report.* Retrieved October 21, 2020, from https://www.cdc.gov/nchs/data/nvsr/nvsr68/nvsr68_06-508.pdf

Holden, R. J. (1991). Responsibility and autonomous nursing practice. *Journal of Advanced Nursing, 16,* 398–403. doi:10.1111/j.1365-2648.1991.tb03428.x

Hwang, K., & Han, Y. (2020). Exploring the sources of cognitive gap between accountability and performance. *Public Personnel Management, 49*(3), 393–420. https://doi.org/10.1177/0091026019873031

Hylka, S. C., & Shugrue, D. (1991). Increasing staff nurse autonomy. *Nursing Management, 22,* 54–55. Retrieved April 27, 2021, from https://journals.lww.com/nursingmanagement/Citation/1991/05000/Increasing_Staff_Nurse_Autonomy.14.aspx

Institute for Healthcare Improvement. (2020a). *100 million healthier lives.* Retrieved October 21, 2020, *from* http://www.ihi.org/Engage/Initiatives/100MillionHealthierLives/Pages/default.aspx

Institute for Healthcare Improvement. (2020b) *Patient safety awareness week.* Retrieved October 21, 2020, from http://www.ihi.org/Engage/Initiatives/Patient-Safety-Awareness-Week/Pages/default.aspx

Institute of Medicine. (2000). *To err is human: Building a safer health care system.* National Academies Press.

Institute of Medicine. (2011). *The future of nursing: Leading change, advancing health.* National Academies Press.

International Council of Nurses. (2012). *ICN code of ethics for nurses.* Retrieved April 27, 2021, from https://www.icn.ch/sites/default/files/inline-files/2012_ICN_Codeofethicsfornurses_%20eng.pdf

Kramer, M., Schmalenberg, C., & Maguire, P. (2008). Essentials of a magnetic work environment, Part 4. In *Nursing 2008 career directory* (pp. 36–37). Lippincott Williams & Wilkins. doi:10.1097/00152193-200409000-00039

Makary, M., & Daniel, M. (2016). Medical error—The third leading cause of death in the U.S. *British Medical Journal, 353,* i2139. Retrieved October 21, 2021, from https://www.bmj.com/content/353/bmj.i2139

McCannon, C. J., Schall, M. W., Calkins, D. R., & Nazem, A. G. (2006). Saving 100,000 lives in US hospitals. *British Medical Journal, 332*(7553), 1328–1330. doi:10.1136/bmj.332.7553.1328

McGlothlin, W. J. (1961). The place of nursing among the professions. *Nursing Outlook, 9,* 214–216.

Mendes, A. (2018). Being supported to whistle while you work. *British Journal of Community Nursing, 23*(7), 360–361. https://doi.org/10.12968/bjcn.2018.23.7.360

Merton, R. K. (1958). The functions of the professional association. *American Journal of Nursing, 58,* 50–54. Retrieved April 27, 2021, from https://www.jstor.org/stable/3461366?seq=1

Miller, J. (2004). *QBQ! The question behind the question.* G. P. Putnam's Sons.

Mish, F. C. (Ed.). (2020). *Merriam-Webster's collegiate dictionary* (11th ed.). Merriam-Webster, Inc.

Moffat-Bruce, S. D., Ferdinand, F. D., & Fann, J. F. (2016). Patient safety: Disclosure of medical errors and risk mitigation. *Annals of Thoracic Surgery, 102,* 358–362. https://doi.org/10.1016/j.athoracsur.2016.06.033

Murray, J. (2007). Before blowing the whistle, learn to protect yourself. *American Nurse Today, 2*(3), 40–42. Retrieved April 27, 2021, from https://www.myamericannurse.com/before-blowing-the-whistle-learn-to-protect-yourself/

National Council of State Boards of Nursing. (2020). *Alternative to discipline programs for substance use disorder.* Retrieved October 24, 2020, from https://www.ncsbn.org/alternative-to-discipline.htm

National Council of State Boards of Nursing and American Nurses Association. (2019). *National guidelines for nursing delegation.* Retrieved February 21, 2021, from https://www.ncsbn.org/NGND-PosPaper_06.pdf

National Council of State Boards of Nursing Regulation Division. (2013). *Substance use disorder.* Retrieved October 24, 2020, from https://www.ncsbn.org/333.htm

Nightingale, F. (1946; originally published in 1859). *Notes on nursing: What it is and what it is not.* J. B. Lippincott.

Nobity, C. (2021). *How much does medical malpractice insurance cost in 2021?* Retrieved April 27, 2021, from https://www.leveragerx.com/blog/medical-malpractice-insurance-cost/

Nolan, S., Burkard, J., Clark, M., Davidson, J., & Agan, D. (2010). Effect of morbidity and mortality peer review on nurse accountability and ventilator-associated pneumonia rates. *Journal of Nursing Administration, 40*(9), 374–383. doi:10.1097/NNA.0b013e3181ee427b

Oussedik, E., Cline, A., Su, J. J., Masicampo, E., Kammrath, L. K., Ip, E., & Feldman, S. R. (2019). Accountability in patient adherence. *Patient Preference & Adherence, 13*, 1511–1517. https://doi.org/10.2147/PPA.S213113

Pegg, M. (2020). *A is for accountability, autonomy and authority.* Retrieved October 18, 2020, from https://www .thepositiveencourager.global/clarifying-your-accountability-autonomy-and-authority/

Pham, J., & Papa, A. (2011). Study: Temporary ED staff twice as likely to be associated with medication errors that cause harm to patients. *ED Management, 23*(12), 140–141. Retrieved April 27, 2021, from https://www.reliasmedia.com/articles/132635-study-temporary-ed-staff-twice-as-likely-to-be-associated-with-medication-errors-that-cause-harm-to-patients

Pozgar, G. D. (2020). *Legal and ethical issues for health professionals* (5th ed.). Jones & Bartlett Learning.

Quality and Safety Education for Nurses Institute. (2020). *QSEN competencies.* Retrieved October 26, 2020, from https://qsen .org/competencies/pre-licensure-ksas/

Sattar, R., Johnson, J., & Lawton, R. (2020). The views and experiences of patients and health-care professionals on the disclosure of adverse events: A systematic review and qualitative meta-ethnographic synthesis. *Health Expectations, 23*, 571–583. https://doi.org/10.1111/hex.13029

Sherwood, G., & Barnsteiner, J. (Eds.). (2012). *Quality and safety in nursing a competency approach to improving outcomes.* Wiley-Blackwell.

Styles, M. (1985). Accountable to whom? *International Nursing Review, 32*(3), 73-75. Retrieved April 27, 2021, from https://www .researchgate.net/publication/19315345_Accountable_to_ whom.

Tamilia, L. (2019). *Professional liability insurance for nurses: Definition costs, features and providers.* Retrieved October 25, 2020, from https://fitsmallbusiness.com/professional-liability-insurance-for-nurses/

The Joint Commission. (2020). *Leading the way to Zero^{TM}.* Retrieved October 21, 2020, from https://www.jointcommission .org/performance-improvement/joint-commission/leading-the-way-to-zero/

Turnbull, A. (2016). *Over a quarter of staff work unpaid overtime. Independent Nurse,* 1.

Watson, E. (2014). Nursing malpractice: Costs, trends & issues. *Journal of Legal Nurse Consulting, 25*(1), 26–31. Retrieved April 27, 2021 from www.AALNC_0180214_JL-NC-Spring2014_Final_25.1%20(2).pdf

Weber, D. O. (2018). Accountability: What does it mean? How do you get it?. *Physician Leadership Journal, 5*(3), 18–23. Retrieved April 27, 2021, from https://www.physicianleaders.org/news/accountability-what-does-mean-how-you-get

White, D. E., Jackson, K., Besner, J., & Norris, J. M. (2015). The examination of nursing work through a role accountability framework. *Journal of Nursing Management, 23*(3), 604–612. doi:10.1111/jonm.12186

World Health Organization. (2019). *Patient safety, key facts.* Retrieved October 20, 2020, from https://www.who.int/ news-room/fact-sheets/detail/patient-safety

Environmental and Global Health

KEY TERMS AND CONCEPTS

Environment
Global environment
Anthropocene era
Environmental health
Ecocentric
Pollution
Environmental surprises
Discontinuity
Extinct
Synergism
Unnoticed trend

Positive feedback
Cascading effects
Multiple chemical
  sensitivity
Community environment
Work environment
Home environment
Disaster
Disaster management
  cycle

LEARNING OUTCOMES

By the end of this chapter, the learner will be able to:

1. Explain how the global environment affects human health.
2. Outline factors that can negatively impact the health of a community and its members.
3. Identify health hazards in the work environment.
4. Specify characteristics of the home environment that may negatively impact the health of individuals and families.
5. List the components of a comprehensive environmental assessment to identify potential environmental sources for health issues.
6. Explain the professional nurse's role in disaster planning, mitigation, and recovery.

REAL-LIFE REFLECTIONS

Ariana is a nursing student who lives next door to Elena, a registered nurse. They commute to the hospital together when they work the same shifts. During their commutes, they have lively discussions about how the global and community environments shape the health of their neighbors and themselves. They also share stories about some of the community and workplace issues they have encountered as members of different cultural and ethnic backgrounds. Each time they drive by the older couple's house on the corner, they express concern about the Garcias because they rarely seem to have visitors.

- *What are some of the global environmental issues you think Ariana and Elena may discuss? What actions might a professional nurse and nursing student take to improve the global environment?*
- *What are possible community environmental issues that might affect the health of themselves and their neighbors, the Garcias? What actions might Ariana and Elena take to address issues in the community that impact the health of its members?*
- *List the possible community and workplace issues they are likely encountering. What could they do in their current roles to confront workplace issues? What could their colleagues do to address each identified issue?*
- *Why does the environment play such a key role in determining human health?*

Objects, conditions, and circumstances create the **environment**. Living organisms depend on the environment for formation and survival. Not all environments have the capability of sustaining life. Multiple environmental systems must remain in balance to sustain life. For the purpose of this chapter, environment refers to "all the conditions and circumstances" that surround and influence life on earth (Mish, 2020, p. 418). The environment consists of physical domains (air, water, soil) and social domains (land use, industry, housing, transportation, agriculture). Depending on the context, environments may be miniscule or enormous. **Global environment** refers to the conditions of the entire earth. **Environmental health** refers to conditions in the environment that preserve the balance of nature. The environment belongs to all life on earth. Because humans are intelligent, thinking organisms, they have the capability to make decisions that affect environmental quality.

The current geologic era has been named the *Anthropocene era,* a term coined by Paul Crutzen, a Nobel Prize–winning atmospheric scientist from the Netherlands (Pearce, 2007). The **Anthropocene era** started approximately 250 years ago (the beginning of industrialization) and encompasses the time during which humans appear to have dominated earth. Some of the human-induced changes on earth include the release of greenhouse gases and other environmental pollutants, deforestation, urban development, and pillaging of natural resources.

Humans rely on the external environment for air, water, food, and safe shelter. Within a system's framework, interacting groups create a unitary whole. When the balance is altered, changes occur in the unitary whole experience. When those changes affect the quality of the external environment that supports life as we know it, they will affect human health. Since the early 21st century, various effects of global climate change predict intense human suffering, death, and extinction (Berners-Lee, 2019; Wallace-Wells, 2020; World Health Organization [WHO], 2018a). This chapter examines the effects of the global, local, work, and home environments on human health and offers strategies for professional nurses to create a sustainable future.

THE GLOBAL ENVIRONMENT

In Victorian times, people tended to look at local, rather than global, environmental conditions. Florence Nightingale linked the quality of the environment to the health of soldiers during the Crimean War. Her writings documented reduced mortality of and infections in injured soldiers when clean air, pure water, efficient drainage, cleanliness, and light were provided for them (Dock, 1912). After Nightingale's reforms, nurses paid close attention to the hospital environment to provide a healthy environment for clients. Nursing education textbooks provided detailed information on how to optimize the hospital environment to promote health and healing (Young & Lee, 1948).

When society became conscious of all the impact of pollution on human health and well-being, the nursing profession expanded its view of the environment. Instead of focusing on just the hospital, home, or local community environments, nurses began to address issues related to the global environment (Kleffel, 1994). Because of the role that the environment plays in human health and its importance in professional nursing practice, Fawcett (1984) included environment in the metaparadigm for nursing.

Definitions of the environment depend on the philosophical stance of each theorist. Rogers (1990), Leddy (2004), and Newman (1994) defined the environment as an energy field, whereas Watson (1999), Neuman (2002), and Roy (1987) defined the environment as an open system. Neuman further separated the environment into internal and external domains that interact with each other.

With the development of the space program and advances in scientific technology, humans came to know much more about the environment. When the world saw pictures of earth from outer space, many people understood the interconnectedness of nations and how global regulation (or the lack of it) could potentially affect everyone. As people realize the importance of the environment on human health, an **ecocentric** (the perspective of the environment as being whole, interconnected, and alive) approach to health care delivery becomes a societal priority (Kleffel, 1996).

Take Note!
The future of humanity relies on a safe and clean environment.

Ecosystem Disturbance and Environmental Surprises

Earth is a delicate planet with balanced ecosystems that provide the resources to sustain many varieties of life. Humans upset this balance through environmental **pollution** (contamination with harmful chemicals) from waste products in manufacturing, energy production, and burning wood or petroleum products; chemicals used to control pests (animals, insects, plants); and widespread use of plastic products. When the balance becomes disturbed, **environmental surprises** emerge. Bright (2000) identified three forms of environmental surprise:

1. **Discontinuity**: An abrupt shift in a trend or steady state. For example, forest habitat loss causes some animals to seek refuge elsewhere or travel to human-populated areas for food. The species (e.g., bears) becomes a menace to people by scouring human garbage cans for food; local governments spend money to control them; some people are harmed; and, in extreme cases, the species becomes endangered or **extinct** (ceases to exist).
2. **Synergism**: Simultaneous changes in several natural phenomena with greater than expected environmental effects. For example, a catastrophe with a high human death toll may result from the combined effects of a heavy rainstorm, cutting trees on a hillside, and people moving to an identified flood plain.
3. **Unnoticed trend**: An event that occurs undetected but does considerable damage to an ecosystem. For example, non-native weed invasion of fertile farm acreage in the United States displaced native plants that facilitated the balance of natural fire cycles. This resulted in the destruction of 9,884 acres of farmland during a 30-year period before it was detected (Bright, 2000).

To further complicate the maintenance of earth's balance, synergisms can produce discontinuities. For example, ozone depletion combined with acid rain and other atmospheric contaminants (particles and gases) results in increased penetration of ultraviolet radiation in water, which leads to the destruction of microorganisms essential for the survival of coral reefs and fish. Alternatively, discontinuities can produce synergisms, such as the evolution of pesticide-resistant insects carrying plant viruses that destroy crops (Bright, 2000).

Positive feedback loops can also create discontinuities. In a **positive feedback** loop, the cycle of change continues to amplify itself. Global warming provides a prime example of a positive feedback loop. The Arctic ice cap is melting as the result of global warming. Although even a thick ice cap absorbs only 10% of sunlight with the oceans absorbing the rest, as the ice mass dwindles, the ocean becomes warmer, resulting in accelerated global warming (Berners-Lee, 2019; Hawken, 2017; Wallace-Wells, 2020). Cascading

effects can also lead to environmental changes. **Cascading effects** occur when a change in one component of a system results in a change in another component, which sets up a change in yet another component, with multiple changes occurring throughout various components. Cascading effects can produce discontinuities and synergisms. The Alaskan coastline provides an example of a cascading effect. When the Alaskan perch and herring populations declined, sea lions and seals starved. As the population of sea lions and seals declined, killer whales had to find new prey to survive. The sea otter was the ideal candidate. However, because sea otters feast on sea urchin, as the sea otter population declined, the sea urchin population exploded. The sea urchins then demolished the kelp forests. Many species of fish, marine invertebrates, marine mammals, and birds that rely on kelp for food are now at risk (Berners-Lee, 2019; Bright, 2000; U.S. Global Change Research Program, 2019; Wallace-Wells, 2020).

Challenges of the 21st Century

Sachs (2008) identified six trends of the 21st century that have shaped current times and continue to shape the future:

1. The age of convergence (when the per capita income of poorer nations rises to, catches up with, and even exceeds that of rich nations)
2. Increased population growth of people with higher incomes (increased demands for goods, services, and energy)
3. Dominance of Asia in the world economy
4. More people living in urban locales as a result of migration
5. Environmental challenges (how to mitigate the effects of human environmental destruction)
6. The poverty trap (large income gaps between the rich and poor) with self-reinforcing and perpetual cycles of poverty

Population Pressures

Berners-Lee (2019), Hawken (2017), and Wallace-Wells (2020) shed more light on future environmental issues resulting from the exploding human population, such as rising global temperatures, falling water tables, declining croplands, diminishing fisheries, shrinking forests, and the overall loss of plant and animal species. As of 2020, the world population was 7.69 billion (U.S. Census Bureau, 2020); with current growth trends, the population is expected to reach 9 billion by 2025 (U.S. Census Bureau,

2018), 9.8 billion by 2050, and 11.2 billion by 2100 (United Nations, 2017). The WHO (2018a) predicts that between 2030 and 2050, there will be an additional 250,000 human deaths annually related to climate change (e.g., malnutrition, malaria, diarrhea, heat stress). The direct costs for these direct health effects are estimated to be $2 to 4 billion.

According to the Dovers and Butler (2017), estimates of the numbers of people that the earth can support vary. Reasons for the variation include individual consumption patterns of food and water along with waste production. Dovers and Butler (2017) report that Americans consume 3.3 times more food and 250 times more clean water than the average world citizen. Table 13.1 outlines how many studies estimate different amounts of people the earth can support.

The growing population creates more demand for food, water, space, and goods. China, India, North Africa, and the United States pump more water than can be replenished through snow and rain. Farmers overpump water for crops, and many industries (e.g., paper, cotton) use enormous amounts of water for production. The processing of crops and livestock and the production of consumer goods result in an increased release of nitrogen and phosphorus into the atmosphere, creating acid rain. Trees become more susceptible to disease and damage from extreme temperatures, effects of acid rain, and reduced rainfall. Intense severe storms, high winds, and hurricanes also result in tree destruction. Deterioration of dead trees results in the release of more carbon dioxide and methane into the atmosphere, leading to increased global warming (Berners-Lee, 2019; Hawken, 2017; U.S. Global Change Research Program, 2019; Wallace-Wells, 2020).

TABLE 13.1 Number of Studies That Predict Different Numbers of Persons the Earth Can Support

Number of Persons the Earth Can Support	Number of Studies
8 billion	20
16 billion	14
32 billion	6
64 billion	7
128 billion	2
More than 128 billion	3

Adapted from Dovers, S., & Butler, C. (2017). *How many people can the earth actually support?* Retrieved April 21, 2021, from https://www.science.org.au/curious/earth-environment/how-many-people-can-earth-actually-support

Climate Change

Since 1850, carbon dioxide emissions have increased by 47% with September 2020 levels measuring 415 ppm in the earth's atmosphere, an increase from 387.69 ppm in 2010 (National Aeronautics and Space Administration [NASA], 2020b). Rising levels of carbon dioxide emissions since the advent of the Industrial Age have resulted in a rise in mean global temperature from $-0.19°C$ in 1880 to $0.99°C$ in 2019 with an increase of $0.33°C$ since 2009. When temperatures increase, there is a corresponding increase in humidity that makes it more uncomfortable and potentially fatal for vulnerable people while enabling microorganisms to flourish (Wallace-Wells, 2020). Increased global temperature results in increased arctic ice melt and a decrease in land ice masses. The Arctic Sea ice has been declining at a rate of at least 13.1% per decade since 1980 (NASA, 2020a). Land ice sheet masses are declining at a volume of 427 billion metric tons annually (NASA, 2020d). As of May 2020, the sea level was measured at 95 mm, an increase from 74.48 mm in 2016. The sea level is estimated to be rising 3.3 mm annually because of melting land and sea ice (increased water volume) and water molecular expansion in response to warmer temperatures (NASA, 2020e). Because of the uncertainty and complexity of earth's ecosystem, scientists can only make projections about the impact of global warming. If greenhouse gases continue to be emitted at current rates, estimations of global warming by 2100 vary from $01.6°C$ to $4.0°C$ increase (NASA, 2020c; Wallace-Wells, 2020).

Increases in global temperatures impact human health. As global temperatures increase, infectious diseases (especially those associated with insects) typically seen in tropical climates may be encountered in more temperate zones (Cascio & Sykes, 2015). Additional human health effects of climate change also include increased incidence and intensity of respiratory diseases from increased ozone levels and particulates in the air (allergic and air pollutant–induced); adverse effects on pregnancy outcomes (e.g., preterm births, low birth weight, increased incidence of preeclampsia and eclampsia, birth defects associated with infectious diseases) (Poursafa et al., 2015); cardiovascular disease (Cascio & Sykes, 2015); massive migration of individuals from coastal areas to higher ground owing to rising sea levels; mortality from extreme heat (Berners-Lee, 2019; Veenema, 2019; Wallace-Wells, 2020; WHO, 2018a); increased foodborne and waterborne illnesses; altered density of nutrients of some plant life; and potentially increasing mercury levels in seafood (Cascio & Sykes, 2015).

Many unknowns exist among the climate change models, such as the long-term changes in weather and effects of man-made pollutants on the environment. Environmental research data and conclusions often appear to be in conflict. For example, the U.S. Global Change Research Program (2019) reported that global warming would cause extreme heat and drought in northwestern states and the Great Plains and heavy rain and flooding in the southeastern states and southern Great Plains. The same program also predicts that the northeastern and Midwestern states could also have episodic heavy rain and flooding as well as extreme heat waves and drought.

Since 1950, more than 140,000 chemicals have been created. It is estimated that 9 million premature deaths occur as a result of exposure to these chemicals that have polluted the air, soil, and water (Landrigan et al., 2018). Some of these chemicals have been ingested by people in the form of artificial food additives and medications. For example, two thirds of all antibiotics are given to livestock to stimulate growth, and some of these antibiotics are then consumed when people eat this food (Berners-Lee, 2019). The long-term effect of these food chain antibiotics is unknown. Soil and water pollution from pesticide use may also be linked to development of some cancers (National Cancer Institute, 2020).

Urbanization

Urban sprawl impinges on available cropland and results in deforestation. Burning harvested trees releases more carbon and methane into the atmosphere, which increases global warming and reduces rainfall in some areas while causing flooding in others (Berners-Lee, 2019; Wallace-Wells, 2020).

Urbanization increases the consumption of fossil fuels, which also contributes to global warming. Higher global temperatures and rising atmospheric carbon dioxide levels result in increased ocean temperatures and acidity, which compromise underwater ecosystems. From 1957 to 1997, the annual oceanic fish catch increased by 71 million tons (from 19 to 90 million tons; O'Meara, 2000). Research has demonstrated that some types of fish have resilience and have been able to reproduce at a rate fast enough to prevent extinction within the past 60 years, but many of these may be close to reaching a tipping point that will result in declining numbers (Vasilakopoulos & Marshall, 2015). Fish production for human consumption occurs when fish are caught and raised via aquaculture (i.e., fish farms). According to Shahbandeh (2020), the production

of fish using aquaculture increased from 55.7 metric tons in 2009 to 86.5 metric tons in 2019. The annual fish harvesting using traditional fishing methods was 90.2 metric tons in 2009, peaked to 93.7 metric tons in 2011, and leveled off until reaching 91.3 metric tons in 2019 (Shahbandeh, 2020). Based on this current trend, more fish will be raised via aquaculture than traditional fishing in the future. Some fish farms create additional pollution to water sources when too many fish are raised in one area and water from these areas enters the greater waterways. Fish are capable of metabolizing consumed pollutants, and some of these pollutants then appear in fish for human consumption (Shahbandeh, 2020; Wallace-Wells, 2020). Eating fish that were not farm-raised can still be problematic because 60% of the world's fish are contaminated with microplastics (Sequeria et al., 2020).

The Health Care Industry

American hospitals produce approximately 5.5 tons of medical waste per day (Anthony, 2015). Since the COVID-19 pandemic, health care waste has increased to 240 metric tons per day (Carina, 2020). According to the WHO (2018b), 85% of the waste poses no risk to human health and can be disposed of without using any special treatment or precautions. However, the remaining 15% is considered hazardous to human health and can be categorized as infectious; pathologic (human waste or tissue); sharps; chemical (cleaning products); pharmaceutical (medications); cytotoxic; and radioactive. Mercury is present in some thermometers, sphygmomanometers, flow meters, gauges, and endoscopes, and dioxin has been found in discarded polyvinyl plastic materials. Infection control guidelines require that linens made of cotton be laundered in hot water that must be heated using some form of energy (additionally, farmers use pesticides to maximize cotton production). Human pharmaceuticals (e.g., analgesics, anticonvulsants, lipid regulators, beta-blockers, antidepressants, oral contraceptives, antibiotics) have been reported to be present in water treatment effluents, surface waters, groundwater, sea water, and even drinking waters (Brausch et al., 2012; Wohlford et al., 2020). Infection control guidelines require disposal of any unused supplies for clients in specific types of isolation. Medical waste is managed by use of incineration (i.e., burning, resulting in greenhouse gas emissions); autoclaving (i.e., heating at high temperature, resulting in high energy use); and chemical sterilization (usually with bleach and contains chlorine that finds its way into wastewater and eventually the general water supply) (Wohlford et al., 2020). Other pollutants attributed to health care organizations include dead batteries, old computers, and obsolete medical equipment.

Many developed countries, including the United States, practice "toxic colonialism" or "toxic imperialism," a process by which wealthy nations pay poor, undeveloped nations to take waste. Much of American hospital waste (along with other dangerous chemical waste, discarded appliances, cell phones, MP3 players, and computer hardware) are sent to less developed, poorer nations (e.g., Nigeria, South Africa, Ghana, Tanzania, India, Pakistan, and China) where children play among heavy metals (e.g., aluminum, arsenic, cadmium, barium, chromium, lithium, mercury) and low-level radioactive and transuranic waste is added (Adeola, 2011). The Basel Convention on the Control of Transboundary Movements of Hazardous Waste and Their Disposal produced an international treaty to decrease the transport of toxic waste among nations. The United States signed the treaty, but the U.S. Congress has yet to ratify it (Lotus Arise, 2021). In countries where the provision to outlaw this practice was proposed, toxic waste trafficking remains a means to generate income (Sirleaf, 2018).

Efforts Toward Global Preservation

Environmental degradation demonstrates that earth has undergone and is currently undergoing many changes as the result of human habitation. Ancient Greeks, Romans, Asians, and Native Americans viewed the world as a living organism. Traditional Native American and Eastern philosophies still espouse this belief. The Gaia hypothesis proposes that the difference between living and nonliving things is one of graded intensity and that earth remains the sole provider of resources for humans. Many environmentalists profess a worldview of wholeness, in which each cell has equal value and is reflective of the entire cosmos. All cells within the environment interact and achieve a balance. Because everything is interconnected, all parts of the universe are equally important, and no organism should receive special status (Kleffel, 1994; Pearce, 2007). However, humans have appropriated a special status for themselves, and the environment has become the casualty.

International efforts at global preservation have been formed by governmental, international, and private organizations. Governmental agencies and nongovernmental organizations frequently exert pressure on companies to become more responsible for global preservation:

- The Kyoto Protocol sought to reduce greenhouse emissions by 5% worldwide from 1997 to 2012. The protocol carried different guidelines for nations based on their wealth. Although adopted by the rest of the world, the United States has never accepted the Kyoto Protocol because of the perceived economic hardships it would cause.

- In 2005, the Earth Institute of Columbia University sponsored a Global Roundtable on Climate Change (GRTOCC) as a means to combat global warming on an international scale. A scientific consensus statement arising from the GRTOCC specified that "global warming is real and that it is caused by greenhouse gas emissions and primarily caused by our consumption of fossil fuels" (Sachs, 2008, p. 110). The GRTOCC outlined three methods to combat the issue of global warming: "mitigation, adaptation, and research, development, and demonstration (RD&D) of new technologies" (Sachs, 2008, p. 110).

- In 2015, the UN held a Climate Change Conference in Paris, France. Participating countries agreed to limit global warming below 2°C for the entire century. The desired goal for global warming would be to keep less than 5°C above preindustrial global temperatures. Nations were to begin serious efforts at reducing global warming within 30 days following ratification of the agreement by 55% of participating countries (United Nations, 2016).

- In 2019, the UN held a Climate Change Conference in Madrid, Spain. The participants announced the formation of the Climate Ambition Alliance composed of 73 countries, 14 regions, 398 cities, 786 businesses, and 16 investors who agreed to combine efforts to achieve net zero carbon emissions by 2050 (Hartman, 2019). The United States did not initially become a member of this alliance. However following the inauguration of President Joe Biden, the United States became a member of this alliance.

In addition to formal governmental and international global efforts, nongovernmental organizations serve as environmental caretakers (Table 13.2). Global networking among environmentalists provides opportunities for global solutions to global problems.

Nurses can use information from established, reputable organizations to increase their awareness of global pollution, take steps to minimize pollution-promoting behaviors, and educate others about behaviors that may contribute to global pollution and destruction.

■ TABLE 13.2   Global Environmental Organizations and Networks

Organization/Network	Purpose	Website
Association for Progressive Communications	Links nongovernmental organizations that promote human rights and environmental concerns	www.apc.org
OneWorld	Links many websites to provide information on economic development	www.oneworld.net
United Nations Environmental Programme (UNEP)	Links with partner institutions by satellite to improve the flow of environmental data	www.unep.org
UN-Habitat	Links researchers and communities to a global network of data, statistics, and evidence-based best practices in urban management	https://unhabitat.org/
Horizon Solutions (Horizon International)	Provides case studies on solutions related to water, waste, energy, transportation, toxic pollutants, public health, industrial manufacturing, biodiversity, air pollution, and agricultural issues	www.solutions-site.org
Intergovernmental Panel on Climate Change	Studies and reports on the current scientific and technologic knowledge about climate change while examining the sociocultural and economic effects of climate change; proposes ways to mitigate the effects of climate change	https://www.ipcc.ch/
Environmental Defense Fund	Examines ways and strategies to promote environmental stewardship without compromising economic prosperity by informing the public of health hazards of chemicals used in everyday life and working to pass environment-friendly legislation	https://www.edf.org/

From O'Meara, M. (2000). Harnessing information technologies for the environment. In L. R. Brown, C. Flavin, H. French, S. Postel, & L. Starke (Eds.), *State of the world 2000*. W. W. Norton & Company; Environmental Defense Fund (2020) at www.edf.org, and the Intergovernmental Panel on Climate Change (2020) at www.ipcc.ch/.

■ QUESTIONS FOR REFLECTION

1. What do you feel is the greatest threat to the global ecosystem and why?

2. What impact do you think changes in the global ecosystem will have on the nursing profession and clinical practice?

3. What impact does your personal life have on the environment?

4. What changes could you make to either your personal or professional life that would reduce your impact on the global environment?

Global Environmental Factors Threatening Health

Many global environmental factors threaten the health of people, plants, and animals. Professional nursing practice focuses on health promotion as well as caring for those who are ill. Nurses must be aware of environmental health risks.

- Many people consume chemicals from their local water supplies.
- People living in urban locales inhale chemical vapors, which results in an increased incidence of asthma, lung cancer, and other chronic pulmonary diseases.

- Agricultural workers have an increased incidence of lymphoma and other cancers that are linked to herbicide and pesticide exposure (McGinn, 2000).
- Individuals remodeling or demolishing old buildings become exposed to asbestos and sometimes carry asbestos fibers home on their clothing.
- Miners inhale dust, resulting in the development of chronic lung diseases.

Infectious Disease

Environmental factors play a critical role in the rise and spread of infectious diseases. Many diseases have a higher prevalence in certain geographic locations. Others spread through animal migration, international travel, and the growth of the global economy.

- African mosquitoes have evolved to bite only humans, resulting in a high incidence of malaria. In areas without medication for treatment or chemically treated nets for sleeping places, malaria infects over a billion people and kills over a million, many of whom are children, annually (Sachs, 2008). Some nations use pesticides to prevent malaria outbreaks, but this in turn raises concerns of land and water contamination.
- Human Ebola virus outbreaks in the early 2000s in the Republic of Congo, Sudan, and Gabon arose

after hunters were infected by handling dead primates and subsequently spread the virus to other humans (LeRoy et al., 2004).

- The West Nile virus originated in Africa but appeared in the United States when infected birds migrated to the United States. The birds transmitted the virus to mosquitoes, which in turn passed the virus to humans. Documented cases of West Nile virus infection have since been linked to blood transfusions, organ donation, and breast milk (Bender & Thompson, 2003).

- Avian flu (H5N1) originated in China. Although not highly communicable, H5N1 spread rapidly across the globe, facilitated by the close contact of humans during air flights in 2003. Between 2003 and 2012, 605 laboratory-confirmed human cases of H5N1 were reported (WHO, 2012). More than half of those infected died (WHO, 2012).

- Starting in 2013, another human Ebola virus outbreak occurred in Guinea, Liberia, and Sierra Leone. It reached epidemic proportion in 2014. According to the Centers for Disease Control and Prevention (CDC, 2016a), 28,616 confirmed cases resulting in 11,310 deaths were reported between March 2014 and February 2016. The UN said the public health emergency was over in March 2016.

- In 2015, the Pan American Health Organization issued a health alert regarding Zika virus because of a confirmed case that occurred in Brazil. Zika viral illnesses were confirmed to have occurred in Mexico, Central America, and South America. Confirmed instances of insect-borne cases surfaced in some U.S. territories. Because the Zika virus caused mild symptoms, the virus infected people without notice. However, pregnant women infected with the Zika virus sometimes had babies with microencephaly and other congenital brain malformations. Zika virus is primarily transmitted to humans through the bite of an infected Aedes mosquito. The virus may also be spread through sexual transmission and to a fetus of an infected mother any time during pregnancy. Because of unpredictable migration patterns of infected mosquitos, cases are expected to occur in other parts of the western hemisphere including the United States (CDC, 2016b). In 2020, there were three travel-associated Zika virus cases in the United States and 57 locally acquired in Puerto Rico (CDC, 2021c).

In 2019, a novel coronavirus was identified in Wuhan, China. At the time of publication, the origin of the virus was believed to be a live seafood and animal market in the same city where the virus jumped from an animal (perhaps a bat) to a human. Incidences of severe acute respiratory syndrome being spread from person to person were reported, and the virus causing the syndrome was identified as *SARS-CoV-2 or COVID-19*. There were no traces of person-to-person transmission within the market.

COVID-19 is transmitted by respiratory droplets, and short-range inhalation of aerosols may be possible in small, closed quarters with inadequate ventilation or in crowded medical wards. Health care procedures (like endotracheal intubation, sputum induction, bronchoscopy, noninvasive and manual ventilation tracheostomy, and autopsy procedures) may have contributed to the spread of the virus to health care workers (CDC, 2020a). The virus may cause asymptomatic or mild illness or may progress to a severe respiratory illness accompanied by a cytokine storm that can result in the immediate need for mechanical ventilation and circulatory support using complex medical interventions. Some prolonged effects of infection with COVID-19 include myocarditis, pericardial dysfunction, thromboembolic events, multiinflammatory syndrome in children, mental and cognitive health issues, prolonged muscle weakness, lung dysfunction that requires supplemental oxygen therapy, renal impairment, and hepatic dysfunction (National Institutes of Health, 2020). The virus spread quickly across the globe because of its highly contagious nature and international travel and will continue to spread until there are effective prevention strategies, widespread vaccination, and development of herd immunity.

Human factors also play a major role in the rise of infectious diseases. In addition to diseases transmitted to humans by animals or insects, antibiotic-resistant bacteria (methicillin-resistant *Staphylococcus aureus* and vancomycin-resistant *Enterococcus* species) have become prevalent because of indiscriminate use of and client noncompliance with antibiotic therapy. *Clostridium difficile* sometimes causes serious outbreaks in acute and long-term care facilities. All health care workers bear the responsibility of containing the spread of infectious disease.

Along with infectious disease detection and containment, nurses and other health care providers must be aware of potential environmental health hazards such as overpopulation, soil erosion and pollution, deforestation, increasing atmospheric carbon dioxide concentrations, global warming, endangered fish population, falling water tables, ozone depletion, air pollution, malnutrition, over-nourishment, persistent organic pollutants, and plastics. Awareness of exposure to environmental toxins provides nurses with the ability to teach clients about ways to avoid long-term exposure to pollutants that sometimes result in devastating health consequences. In addition, nurses can take personal actions to remedy these environmental health hazards.

Multiple Chemical Sensitivity

No matter where they live, people may be exposed to a variety of chemicals. Some people experience severe reactions to such chemical exposure. Although many people may be somewhat sensitive to certain chemicals or environmental triggers, some people experience severe sensitivities to many chemicals, even at levels that would not trigger a reaction in the majority of the population, a condition known as **multiple chemical sensitivity** (MCS). MCS is a recognized form of physical disability (Watai et al., 2018). The National Institutes of Health describe MCS as a chronic, recurrent disorder resulting from a person's inability to tolerate a specific common environmental chemical or a class of foreign chemicals. A known cause for MCS has yet to be identified.

People with MCS often have sustained "systemic damage that causes them to react negatively to common chemicals in ambient air" (Gibson, 2000, p. 8) and typically have a heightened sense of smell (Hu & Baines, 2018). This group also has an increased incidence of noise intolerance (Micarelli et al., 2016). Reactions range from slight drowsiness or nasal congestion to potentially fatal asthmatic attacks (Hu & Baines, 2018). Box 13.1, Professional Building Blocks, "Criteria for Multiple Chemical Sensitivity Diagnosis," outlines the criteria for MCS as determined by a consensus group of 34 researchers

and clinicians who treat the condition. Reactions frequently result from exposure to solvents, pesticides, formaldehyde, fresh paint, new carpets, gas exhaust (e.g., diesel, car, propane, natural gas appliances), perfumes, scented cleaners, air fresheners, aspirin, sugar, and food additives. Even processed lumber products used in new construction and electromagnetic fields from appliances can trigger reactions (Gibson, 2000; Watai et al., 2018). According to Watai and colleagues (2018), 0.74% of all adults worldwide may have MCS.

People with MCS frequently receive psychiatric diagnoses from health care providers (see Concepts in Practice, "Recognizing Multiple Chemical Sensitivity"). However, MCS appears to have a physiologic basis. The human body becomes damaged in response to repeated chemical exposures. The following physiologic theories related to the etiology of MCS have been proposed:

- Nervous system damage as a result of repeated exposures
- Limbic kindling through the olfactory limbic system, resulting in triggered responses to repeated chemical exposure
- Depletion of or damage to enzymatic production within the body
- Repeated immunologic insults
- Airway and neurogenic inflammation
- Chronic candidiasis
- Carbon monoxide poisoning
- Altered brain chemistry, electrical activity, or neurotransmitter function

With the advent of positive emission tomography, evidence linking chemical brain changes with exposure to specific chemicals substantiates that a physiologic phenomenon occurs in people with MCS. People with MCS exhibit "different patterns of cortical and subcortical brain activation during olfactory stimulation" (Chiaravalloti et al., 2015, p. 734).

A physiologic process known as toxicant-induced loss of tolerance (TILT) may also be involved in the development of MCS. TILT is a two-stage process. The first step is initiation that occurs when a person experiences exposure to chemicals below toxic levels (e.g., indoor or outdoor pollutants, pesticides, other chemicals) that later become triggers for an MCS reaction. The second phase of TILT involves becoming hyperactive to the same or different chemicals upon exposure (Horowitz, 2014).

Some scientists and health care providers do not believe the physiologic etiology of MCS and prefer to attribute the condition to one or more psychological theories:

- Psychological and behavioral conditioning
- Odor conditioning

13.1 Professional Building Blocks

Criteria for Multiple Chemical Sensitivity Diagnosis

- Identical symptoms are reproduced with repeated exposure to the same chemical.
- Reactions are chronic.
- Low levels of exposure to the offending chemical produce manifestations of the reactive symptoms.
- When the offending chemicals are removed, the symptoms lessen or resolve.
- Reactions occur to multiple, unrelated chemical substances.
- Symptoms affect multiple organ systems.

Data from Gibson, P. R. (2000). *Multiple chemical sensitivity: A survival guide* (p. 9). New Harbinger; Hu, H., & Baines, C. (2018). Recent insights into 3 underrecognized conditions: Myalgic encephalomyelitis-chronic fatigue syndrome, fibromyalgia, and environmental sensitivities-multiple chemical sensitivity. *Canadian Family Physician, 64*(6), 413–415.

- Increased vulnerability related to preexisting anxiety and depression
- Amplification of symptoms
- Negative affectivity
- Personality disorders
- Somatization disorder
- Childhood trauma
- Excessively focused thought patterns and cognitions on chemicals

Concepts in Practice IDEA → PLAN → ACTION

Recognizing Multiple Chemical Sensitivity

Emily arrives at the emergency department of a teaching hospital with complaints of an intense headache, inability to concentrate, and slight dyspnea. Yolanda, the triage and charge nurse, asks Emily about her medical history. Emily provides a multipage list of allergies to medications, cleaning products, and foods. As the interview progresses, Emily begins to hyperventilate and can only whisper when answering questions. Yolanda becomes suspicious of Emily's many allergies and seemingly overdramatic behavior, concluding that Emily must be mentally ill. As Yolanda starts to page the psychiatric resident, Emily's allergist arrives, orders epinephrine, and states that Emily has a condition called *multiple chemical sensitivity,* a rare disorder that the allergist says is becoming more prevalent. After receiving the epinephrine, Emily's symptoms subside.

- *How would you respond if you encountered a client like Emily in your clinical practice?*
- *What advice would you have given Yolanda if she consulted with you about Emily's case?*

Practitioners who espouse a physiologic theory believe that avoidance of the offending chemicals is the only way to avoid continued health deterioration. Health care professionals who believe MCS is a psychiatric disorder argue that chemical avoidance enables people with MCS to obsess more about their disorder. However, personality disturbances and panic attacks have been documented in workers exposed to organic solvents, and these problems may be the result of nervous system injury (Gibson, 2000; Hu & Baines, 2018). Environmental medical units where clients receive gradual exposure to one offending chemical at a time have been helpful in treating individuals with MCS (Horowitz, 2014).

13.2 Learning, Knowing, and Growing

The Food You Consume

Foods humans consume, especially those in developed countries, often contain an array of additives, contaminants, and/or modifications.

- To increase crop yields, many farmers use a variety of herbicides and pesticides; farmers also genetically manipulate crops.
- To improve meat production, some farmers use feed containing growth hormone and antibiotics.
- Many preservatives protect the consumer from foodborne infections.
- People trying to lose weight consume artificial sweeteners, such as aspartame and saccharin.
- To increase the visual appeal of food, some manufacturers use artificial dyes.
- Some foods contain flavor enhancers such as monosodium glutamate.
- Although some food chemicals reduce the risk for foodborne disease, others merely create another human chemical exposure (Gibson, 2000).

Consult your local food vendors and see how much they can tell you about the food that they sell. Informed consumers have the knowledge and power to make wise food choices for themselves.

The Food Chain

The food each person eats affects their health. Many foods are supplemented with chemicals to increase their visual appeal, enhance flavor, alter texture, and extend dates for safe consumption. How much do you know about the food you eat? Do you know where it comes from and how it is produced? Consider the examples presented in Box 13.2, Learning, Knowing, and Growing, "The Food You Consume."

QUESTIONS FOR REFLECTION

1. Select your favorite packaged food and read its label to see how many chemicals or additives it contains.
2. After reading the label, are you going to think twice before consuming it again? Why or why not?

The Nurse's Role in Promoting a Healthy Global Environment

Nurses play a key role in confronting the future challenges of improving the health and well-being of all.

They possess communication and clinical skills to help people understand ways to promote a healthy global environment. Global leaders in the nursing profession have made key differences in the well-being of people around the world.

In 2006, Kim et al. (2006) identified key knowledge, skills, and attitudes nurses can use to become successful, global nurse leaders. The guidance remains applicable today:

- Remain open-minded and flexible; be willing to learn from others, and display cultural awareness, sensitivity, and interest.
- Deal with complexity effectively, set high aspirations, and show resiliency, optimism, and energy.
- Play politics effectively but with honesty and integrity.
- Display patience and give others the time they need to assume responsibility.
- Seek formal and informal education on global competencies.
- Believe in the importance of global nursing work with conviction and passion.

Musker (1994) proposed a life of voluntary simplicity—a holistic, ecology-based lifestyle—to create a healing environment. In the voluntary simplicity outlook, "less is more," and people focus on the quality of life rather than the quantity of consumer products (contrary to Western culture that largely emphasizes "more is better"). Living a life based on voluntary simplicity has become a stimulus for minimalist movements in recent times. Voluntary simplicity consists of inner and outer processes:

- The inner process, "mindfulness," requires deep self-reflection to attend to personal needs and separate them from personal desires. In this inner process, people discover their genuine, authentic selves and discard the illusion of their preconceived selves. Some people keep a journal to discover patterns of behavior.
- The outer or external process of "doing" results in responsible life behaviors that serve the world rather than pure self-interest.

As the inner and outer processes fuse, being becomes doing, and doing becomes being. Voluntary action involves making purposeful life choices by eliminating automatic choices. Simplification of life involves reducing overall consumption, purchasing durable and easily repaired products, consuming a more natural diet, pursuing work that contributes to the world while using more individual creativity and

capacities, and changing transportation habits. Simplification also means releasing physical and mental clutter, emotional baggage, useless worries, and other concerns that detract from enjoying the present.

Take Note!

Through communication and education, nurses can play a key role in promoting a healthy global environment.

As individual global citizens, professional nurses can model environment-friendly behaviors for preventing pollution and conserving resources. When possible, nurses should look for ways to reduce energy consumption, recycle discarded products, and limit purchases to reusable items.

▇ QUESTIONS FOR REFLECTION

1. What actions in your workplace or school environment may be potentially harmful to the global environment?
2. What could you do differently to change those behaviors?

THE COMMUNITY ENVIRONMENT

Multiple environmental factors affect the health of the community. Community services that enhance health include public health departments, disease prevention services, and social support services. The individual health status of community residents relies on the quality of their physical and social community environments. For this discussion, **community environment** refers to the geographic location where people live and work.

Community Environmental Factors Threatening Health

Although the local community provides services to promote health, most communities also have environmental factors that threaten the health of their citizens. Heavy traffic and industrial fumes pollute the air. Some municipalities and counties use pesticides to prevent the spread of insect-borne illnesses. High-tension power lines and power stations emit electromagnetic fields (EMFs).

Huang et al. (2018) report that some people have developed electromagnetic hypersensitivity with repeated exposure to EMFs. Sources of EMFs include mobile phones, WiFi routers, visual display units, microwaves, base stations, high-voltage power lines, and radar systems (Schmiedchen et al., 2019). Some individuals have become so sensitive to EMFs that they no longer use cellular telephones. Huang et al. (2018) found that 4.7% of adults in Taiwan report signs and symptoms of EMF hypersensitivity with a higher incidence among women (62.6%). Symptoms of EMF hypersensitivity include headache, fatigue, stress, sleep disorders, skin conditions (e.g., prickly, burning sensations, rashes), muscular aches, and pain and nausea (Huang et al., 2018; Schmiedchen et al., 2019).

Along with business and industry, the level of affluence within a community affects the health of individuals and families. Taxes on the income of citizens enable communities to maintain infrastructure and provide services to enhance health. Individuals with higher incomes typically have access to healthier food and better health care services.

However, affluence can also negatively affect health. Private passenger vehicles make it convenient for Americans to drive short distances rather than walking. According to the U.S. Department of Transportation Bureau of Transportation Statistics (2017), the average miles driven by Americans annually was 14,500 miles in 2017. Of these trips, 45% were for shopping or running errands, 27% were for social activities, and 15% were commuting. In 2018, the average American daily one-way commute from home to work and vice versa was 27 minutes. This translates into 9 days per year. Approximately 4.3 million Americans spent 90 minutes commuting each time they went to work. During rush hour, traffic jams contribute to road rage and increased pollution. Time spent commuting means less time with family, increased chance of motor vehicular accidents, road rage, and higher incidence of obesity and hypertension. People with long commutes also experience more social and emotional problems as well as increased divorce rates (Ingraham, 2019). According to the U.S. Environmental Protection Agency (2020), the 2019 model year vehicles have reduced carbon emissions to 246 g/mile, and fuel efficiency has increased to 25.4 mpg. This represents a 6.1 mpg improvement in fuel efficiency and a 214 g/mile improvement in carbon emissions since 2004 (U.S. Environmental Protection Agency [EPA], 2020). However, the prevalence of driving instead of walking or cycling results in less exercise.

Although obesity has multiple causes (e.g., genetics, metabolism, culture), for many Americans, the ease of obtaining high-calorie foods contributes to an unhealthy diet and an obesity epidemic. The CDC (2021b) defines obesity as a body mass index of 30 or more and severe obesity as 40 or more. According to the CDC (2021a), the prevalence of obesity among adult Americans increased from 30.5% in 2000 to 42.4% in 2018. The prevalence of severe obesity increased from 4.7% to 9.2% in the same time frame. The risk factors from an affluent lifestyle also contribute to the incidence of diabetes, cardiovascular disease, and stroke (CDC, 2020b).

Physical Threats

According to Ridlington et al. (2020), global ozone pollution and other fine particulate pollution were responsible for 470,000 to 2.1 million deaths worldwide in 2018. The same study also reported that in 2018, 108 million Americans lived in areas that had more than 100 days of degraded air quality, an increase from 73 million Americans in 2016. Air pollution results in shortness of breath, chest pain with inspiration, asthma attacks, increased susceptibility to respiratory infections, increased risk for pulmonary inflammation, and reduced lung capacity. It also plays a role in the development of cardiovascular disease. Indoor air pollution is a community health problem, and it affects more people when poor air quality occurs in multifamily dwellings.

Although pesticides play a key role in preventing infectious disease epidemics, they can also cause systemic, long-lasting, environmental pollution. Many pesticides are persistent organic pollutants (POPs) that are fat-soluble and resist being broken down by water. They rest in the soil for many years, and food grown in contaminated soil contains POPs. After consumption by animals, POPs accumulate in fat cells and enter the human food chain. The top 10 POP-contaminated foods are butter, cantaloupe, cucumbers/pickles, meatloaf, peanuts, popcorn, radishes, spinach, and summer and winter squash. Despite the potential negative effects of POPs, control of insect-borne illnesses justifies their use (Adeola, 2011). For example, the West Nile virus has been linked to insects that infect birds, and Lyme disease has been linked to insects that infect deer. The proper application of pesticides limits environmental fallout from their use. Responsibility for the proper use of pesticides lies with homeowners and companies that secure community contracts. Professional nurses frequently participate in the development of community education programs or community service announcements to help citizens avoid contracting insect-borne infectious diseases.

To eliminate the risk for foodborne illness, local health departments license businesses and organizations that serve food. Poor handwashing by people who handle food has led to outbreaks of hepatitis A, *Salmonella*, and *Escherichia coli* infections. Foodborne illnesses also occur when people fail to abide by guidelines for food storage and safe food preparation.

The potential for the spread of infectious illnesses, such as tuberculosis (TB), influenza, and viral or bacterial meningitis, is increased in people who are subjected to overcrowded conditions. College dormitories, schools, and day care centers also provide residence for a variety of disease-causing organisms.

Social Threats

In addition to threats to the physical integrity of communities and the people within them, social problems also threaten human health. Poverty, substance abuse, incivility, and systemic prejudice have led to a decline in communities. Violence occurs in some urban, rural, and suburban settings. According to the CDC (2020d), assault was the reason for 1.7 million emergency room visits in 2019. They also reported 18,830 homicides (5.8 deaths per 100,000 Americans). The CDC (2019b) reported that homicide accounted for 27.6% of deaths among African American men aged 20 to 44 years, making it the leading cause of death in this group. In most instances, homicide victims knew their killers. The second leading cause of death for this group was unintentional injuries (24.3%). The leading cause of death for men from other groups in the same age group was unintentional injuries followed by suicide (CDC, 2019a, 2019b, 2019c, 2019d, 2019e). In 2017, nearly 1,770 children died as a direct result of abuse or neglect (CDC, 2020c). Domestic, child, and elder abuse occur in all socioeconomic groups but is more common when families struggle to meet basic human needs (i.e., food, water, and shelter).

In addition to economic factors, the media expose people to acts of violence in movies, fictional television programs, cartoons, and newscasts, and some computer and video games use violence as entertainment. As individuals are repeatedly exposed to images of violence, victims of violent crime become depersonalized, and violence becomes a more integrated part of life.

Mass shootings have become frequent across the United States with the deadliest shooting occurring in Las Vegas, Nevada in 2017 during an outdoor concert that left 58 dead and 500 injured. Mass shootings have occurred in elementary schools, high schools, colleges, nightclubs, churches, movie theaters, businesses and factories, and outdoors in the street or parking lots. The United States accounts for 5% of the world's population but has had 30% of the world's mass shooting events (Harris & Smith, 2019). The Federal Bureau of Investigation defines mass murder as a violent event leaving four or more persons dead. In 2012, a Congressional committee defined mass shooting as a shooting resulting in three or more deaths. Another definition for a mass shooting includes the number of persons injured and defines it as a shooting in which at least four people lose their lives or are injured.

Harris and Smith (2019) identified two types of shooters that commit mass shootings. The first type is a traumatized shooter who has been the victim of physical or psychological abuse, including being bullied. The second type of shooter is a sociopathic killer who is hard, cold, and callous, possibly incapable of feeling emotion. They also reported that the youngest shooter was 11 years old, and the oldest was 64 years old. Many shooters have a desire for revenge against specific people (they know the victims), targeted locations (bad experiences in the past at the site of the shooting), or society in general. They often cite a series of events in their lives that compounds until they feel the urge for revenge. The research linking violent video games and ineffective parenting to mass shootings is inconclusive. Mental illness is associated in the profiles of many mass shooters. Stricter gun control laws are necessary because loopholes in current laws have enabled 20% of guns sold in the United States to be purchased without background checks (Harris & Sims, 2019). The permeation of violence in American society creates distrust among people and can affect social interactions.

Social interactions vary according to the type of communities in which people reside. People tend to socialize more with others who share similar life situations. In working class neighborhoods (especially when both adults in a household are employed), relationships tend to be more casual. Time constraints present challenges for maintaining relationships with neighbors. Schools and places of worship also provide opportunities for people with similar values to develop relationships.

The Nurse's Role in Promoting a Healthy Community Environment

Professional nurses play key roles in promoting a healthy community environment. Nurses assess communities for actual and potential factors that are noxious to human health and well-being. When such factors are identified, nurses can inform community members, provide community education, and take action to eliminate the factors. Reporting local health hazards, such as deteriorating road conditions or dangerous thoroughfares that need traffic signs, signals, or speed controls, helps prevent motor vehicle and pedestrian accidents. To avoid mosquito-borne illnesses, nurses can educate family, friends, and neighbors about the health hazards of standing water found in bird baths, fish ponds, and yard fountains.

Nurses can also inspire other community members to incorporate health promotion activities into their lives. For example, nurses who engage in a daily neighborhood walk or cycling trip serve as role models for daily exercise. Nurses, like all citizens, have the right and obligation to attend local governmental meetings to express concerns related to community development projects. By participating in community cleanup programs, nurses reduce the community's risk for injury from exposure to broken glass, used needles, and sharp metal objects, as well as the risk for infectious illnesses from exposure to rotting food.

Nurses can also become active participants in local school, civic, and faith-based activities to foster mental health and offer safe recreation for community members of all ages. To take a stance against societal violence, nurses can refuse to purchase products that promote violence as entertainment or from companies that advertise their products during violent television programs; they can also refuse to attend movies or plays that glorify violence. When working with teenagers, nurses should be alert to any precursors of imminent violent acts, including inappropriate angry outbursts, cruelty to animals, essays with violent themes, fascination with weapons (especially firearms), obsession with playing violent computer games, threats to harm themselves or others, vandalism (even of their own property), assumption of the victim role, involvement in fringe groups or gangs, behavior with the goal of getting suspended or expelled, and incidents of bringing weapons to show to other students.

Teaching violence awareness, stress management, self-esteem, gun safety, substance abuse prevention, and cultural diversity classes in the community serves as a means to help eliminate violence in society. In response to the December 2012 Sandy Hook Elementary School shooting incident in Newtown, Connecticut, the American Nurses Association and more than 40 other nursing organizations issued a call to action to improve access to mental health services for all Americans, increase student access to mental health professionals, and join together to ban assault weapons and to pass meaningful gun control legislation (American Nurses Association [ANA], 2013). Nurses can also serve as resources to local schools for violence prevention, violence recovery, and other health promotion programs. Finally, nurses can lobby with local, state, and federal legislative bodies to protect environmental health.

Take Note!

Awareness, observation, participation, and education are key roles for nurses in promoting a healthy community environment.

▮ Questions for Reflection

1. How would you rate the health of your local community based on the information presented in this chapter?
2. What community resources are available to you as a citizen to improve the environment of your local community? As a professional nurse?
3. What strategies could you use to promote a healthy community environment?

THE WORK ENVIRONMENT

Many people spend more time in the workplace than they do at home. The quality of the **work environment** relies on physical and cultural factors. National, state, and local laws protect worker safety. Individual organizations have policies that guide worker behaviors and inform workers of potential health hazards.

Work Environmental Factors Threatening Health

Many offices and work settings contain factors that threaten the physiologic, psychological, and spiritual health of employees and consumers. Some industries and manufacturers rely on chemicals and solvents to produce products. Some jobs require workers to perform repetitive movements. According to the U.S. Bureau of Labor Statistics (2020), there were 2.8 million incidences of workplace-related illnesses and injuries in 2019. Of these, 888,200 were nonfatal but caused the employee to miss at least a day of work. The Bureau of Labor Statistics reported that in 2019, 575,000 health care workers sustained a work-related illness or injury, and 201,500 of these workers were registered nurses. The most commonly reported injuries among health care workers were back injuries, muscle strains or sprains, tendonitis, and carpal tunnel syndrome. Other common injuries sustained by nurses in clinical practice include overexertion, falls or slips, twisting injuries, bruises or lacerations (from bumping against or being struck by objects), injuries from violent acts, harmful substance exposure, transportation accidents, repetitive motion insults, and compression injuries.

Health care professionals, including nurses, have a suicide rate of 17.4 per 100,000 persons compared to an American suicide rate of 13 per 100,000 persons. More than half of suicides by health care providers are women (McIntosh et al., 2016). In 2020, Davidson et al. reported that female nurses had a 1.395 higher rate and male nurses had a 1.205 higher rate of committing suicide compared to the general population.

Tasks required for client care performed by nurses in hospitals create an "ergonomic nightmare" (Trossman, 2000, p. 1). Many nurses work 12-hour shifts and experience repetitive movement stress from lifting and turning clients, entering data into computers, drawing up parenteral medications, pumping sphygmomanometers, resetting monitor alarms, and moving heavy equipment.

Since the federal mandate of removing powdered latex gloves from health care settings, the incidence of latex allergies among health care workers has markedly decreased. Most health care organizations have created latex-free environments, but some products used for client care still contain latex. However, the vinyl gloves that have replaced latex tend to tear more readily, and vinyl gloves release toxic substances such as dioxin. Nitrile, neoprene, and thermoplastic gloves offer protection equal to that offered by latex gloves. However, like latex, these products may trigger allergic reactions because their chemical composition is similar (Worthington, 2000).

Depending on their practice area, nurses are at risk for exposure to a number of dangerous chemicals. The Occupational Safety and Health Administration (OSHA) has published standards for safe handling of all dangerous chemicals used in the workplace. In addition, nurse specialty organizations publish guidelines for safe practice use; these guidelines are usually covered in nurse specialty certification examinations. For example, antineoplastic agents may cause birth defects, allergic reactions, and

skin, eye, and mucous membrane irritation. Radiation exposure can lead to birth defects, infertility, and increased risk of cancer in nurses. Chemicals used for sterilization and anesthesia have been associated with cancer development, birth defects, spontaneous abortion, respiratory tract irritation, central nervous system symptoms, dermatitis, eye irritation, liver dysfunction, and renal disorders (National Institute of Occupational Safety and Health, 2018).

In addition to chemical and radiation exposure, infectious diseases pose a workplace hazard to nurses and other health care workers. Nurses have the potential to contract hepatitis B and HIV from a percutaneous stick with a contaminated needle or other sharp implements. Strategies for preventing such an event include strict adherence to OSHA bloodborne pathogen standards and obtaining a hepatitis B vaccination. Nurses can encounter hepatitis A if they work in places where personal hygiene may be poor. Effective hand hygiene serves as the best method for preventing contraction of this virus.

In recent years, nurse exposures to pulmonary illnesses such as severe acute respiratory syndrome (SARS), COVID-19, and TB have increased along with the incidence of these illnesses in clients. Contributing factors for the resurgence in cases of TB include the AIDS epidemic, immigration, incarceration, homelessness, and the evolution of drug-resistant strains of TB and the novel COVID-19 virus (Tamuzi et al., 2020). Diligent attention to isolation procedures and wearing special ventilation masks decrease the chance of contracting COVID-19, TB, and SARS. Measles, rubella, mumps, and influenza also threaten the health of nurses as they engage in professional practice. Determination of immune status and offering appropriate immunizations eliminate the risk for nurses of contracting most of these diseases. Nevertheless, nurses bear the responsibility for protecting their own health by following specific isolation procedures and using protective devices when caring for clients with potentially contagious diseases.

Nurses may also come into contact with many organisms that cause nosocomial (hospital-acquired) infections. Vancomycin-resistant *Enterococcus* and methicillin-resistant *S. aureus* thrive in hospital environments. Frequently, nurses may be colonized with these organisms but because of immunocompetence, may not develop an infection. Other infections that threaten the health of nurses include herpes zoster and *C. difficile*. Diligent isolation practices, meticulous handwashing, and habits to promote immunocompetence protect nurses from contracting infectious diseases from clients or the work environment.

Violence in the Workplace

According to the International Council of Nurses (ICN, 2020), professional nurses worldwide may experience violence. The most egregious attack on nurses occurred in Mexico during the early days of the COVID-19 pandemic. Twelve nurses were taken captive, robbed, and assaulted until their families paid ransoms to have them returned safely (ICN, 2020). The ANA (2019a) reports that one in four nurses experiences assault during their professional careers. In Australia, there are reports of as high as 95% of health care workers being involved in violence on the job (Spelten et al., 2020).

Forms of workplace violence encountered by nurses include physical assault, verbal abuse, bullying, mobbing, and sexual harassment. Nurses can be assaulted physically or verbally by clients, clients' families and friends, physicians, administrators, and coworkers. On rare occasions, nurses and other health team members have been assaulted or shot by client visitors when caring for an injured party from an act of gang violence (ICN, 2020; Longo & Smith, 2011). According to Cooper and Swanson (n.d.), there has been an upswing in workplace violence during the last 15 years, especially in Europe, Australia, and North America. A Canadian study revealed that 44% of inpatient psychiatric nurses experienced physical assault, and 70% experienced emotional abuse while working (Campbell et al., 2019).

Violence against nurses has been a persistent issue. Surveys of nurses reveal that incidences of psychological abuse and sexual harassment range from 24% to 91% (ANA, 2019a; Bartholomew, 2006; Longo & Smith, 2011; Papp, 2007; Sutton, 2006). Of nurses who encounter violence in the workplace, 40% to 70% suffer posttraumatic stress disorder (ANA, 2019a). Although nurses once considered working with violent people to be part of the job, recent initiatives by health care administrators, nurses, and collective bargaining units have resulted in zero tolerance for workplace violence. In the United States, some states have passed legislation requiring health care facilities to provide a safe work environment, including provisions for rapid response teams to handle situations with a high potential to become violent. Efforts to promote a violence-free workplace include policies of zero tolerance for physical violence, sexual harassment, or verbal abuse. Staff education may include the definition of what constitutes an act of violence, triggers of violent acts, causes of violent behaviors, assessment of potentially violent situations, signs and symptoms of anger, phases of the assault cycle, conflict resolution strategies, techniques to disrupt escalating violent behavior, strategies for effective intervention for potentially violent situations, procedures for reporting acts of violence, and techniques of medical and physical restraint (as a last resort). Some health care organizations have rapid response teams to deploy during situations when basic conflict management strategies fail and nurses (or other health care providers) feel threatened. These teams consist of people with advanced education in conflict management and resolution.

Prevention is the best protection against workplace violence. However, a history of violent behavior seems to be a predictor. Therefore, flagging the charts of clients with a history of violent or disruptive behavior alerts staff to the potential for violence should conflict arise. Clearly written policies and procedures offer staff actions to take to avoid and report acts of violence. Organizations should keep records of actual and alleged acts of violence. Confidentiality of reports of violence must be ensured so that incidents involving supervisors and/or physicians will be reported. After an act of violence occurs, a debriefing session is useful to determine potential causes of the event, review steps taken, help victims cope with the effects, and determine if follow-up counseling or education is warranted (ANA, 2019b).

The Nurse's Role in Promoting a Healthy Work Environment

Before a nurse can promote a healthy work environment, they must become cognizant of actual and potential hazards in the workplace. The nurse should assess the work setting systematically to identify the quality of the work environment, paying close attention to its impact on worker physical, mental, and spiritual health. When nurses identify actual or potential health hazards, they should educate staff about them and make referrals to people who can eliminate them. The nurse has an ethical obligation to protect the health of all health team members. The nurse should validate that governmental guidelines to protect workers and clients are followed and take risks to advocate for change when needed.

Along with protecting the physical health of coworkers, nurses play a key role in promoting the mental and spiritual health of colleagues and client care team members. Health care team members sometimes encounter ethical dilemmas, especially those who work in health care organizations that emphasize profits over client care quality, when they find themselves unable to provide services to all clients, and they have to make decisions on how best to use new technology in clinical practice. These conditions create an unhealthy work environment characterized by little or no commitment, worker rebellion, deflated morale, incivility, worker disengagement, inferior problem solving, scapegoating, and sloppy client care.

Incivility is defined as "a rude or discourteous act" (Mish, 2020, p. 629). Lack of courtesy toward others is another definition of incivility. Forms of workplace incivility include rudeness, lack of inclusivity, spreading false rumors, harassment, and bullying. Health care professionals with genuine talent and accomplishments sometimes experience attacks from others because of professional jealousy. The attackers have the goal to denigrate and reduce the status of the professional. When highly competent and respected nurses courageously speak out against substandard care, they sometimes fall victim to incivility, harassment, and bullying (Glasper, 2018).

Racism among health care providers creates unhealthy work situations, another insidious form of incivility in the workplace. Disparities in health status, professional success, and inclusivity stem from racism. In a conversation with Dr. Monica McLemore, McSpedon (2020) learned how nurses can work toward dismantling racism in society and in the profession. McLemore developed the SPLIT to address systemic racism in the community and nursing profession. The *S* stands for stimulation so that nurses can have conversations among themselves without interference from employers, regulators, and professional organizations. Social media provides opportunities for unstructured dialogues and information sharing about racism.

Public health is represented by the *P* in SPLIT. Racism has been identified as a threat to one's health and well-being. Health care systems in the United States tend to revolve around middle class, Eurocentric values (see Chapter 11, "Multicultural Issues in Professional Practice"). Nurses can access the American Public Health Association's Antiracism Resources for Health Professionals and use these tools to work toward dismantling racism in client care and enhancing health care professional team effectiveness (McSpedon, 2020).

Nursing should be taking the lead (the *L* in SPLIT) and provide support and assist with educating the public about health disparities and unequal societal treatment. They can honor people who have shared the disproportionate burdens of these issues, including those who have died. Nurses can organize, lead, and participate in peaceful protests; place pressure on businesses for better standards; and meet and lobby legislatures (McSpedon, 2020). Nurses must insist on a seat at the table when health care policies and regulations are developed.

By becoming immersed (the *I* in SPLIT) in antiracism work, nurses can read, engage in conversations, and wrestle with their own long-standing views about people who are different from themselves. Nurses will have to try (and probably fail several times) sharing and incorporating new information and incorporate it into their personal and professional lives (McSpedon, 2020).

Tension (the *T* in SPLIT) is highly prevalent in today's society. Nurses are expert clinicians, but they may lack the knowledge and skills needed to adequately combat racism and racial injustice in society, health care delivery, and professional nursing. Prejudice occurs across identities, not just race, and White nurses who hold membership in other marginalized groups have knowledge and expertise to share with their colleagues in upholding antiracist values. As long as people are different, there will be tension among them. However, learning about the lived experiences of others, engaging in meaningful conversations, and recognizing that significant change may take a long time to achieve are steps in the right direction. When nurses of different cultural and ethnic backgrounds work together, they can engage in meaningful conversations about their differences, celebrate different cultures' holidays together, and become trusted friends while dismantling systemic racism.

Hierarchic relationships among different health team members (e.g., physicians, nurses, administrators, unlicensed personnel) compound the problem of unhealthy work environments, especially when power is inappropriately used to control subordinates. Harassment involves creating a hostile or unpleasant situation for another person either with verbal threats or undesired physical contact. Harassment can occur between superiors and subordinates as well as between and among peers. Longo (2012) reported that bullying is a form of abusive behavior that occurs repeatedly in nursing and that 31% to 35% of nurses have been targets of bullying. Hartin et al. (2020) report that the full extent of nurses who experience bullying and other forms of psychological abuse in the workplace remains unknown because of nurse fear of retaliation if it is reported. Recognized forms of bullying include (1) personal attacks with the intent to isolate, intimidate, or degrade another person; (2) behaviors aimed at eroding professional competence and reputation that result in deterioration of professional identity and limit career options (public criticism, unjustified blaming, gossip); and (3) personal attacks through work orders and tasks that obstruct work flow or deny due process. Factors that increase bullying include major organizational change, worker characteristics, poor workplace relationships, and undefined work systems (Hartin et al., 2020; Longo, 2012).

When people connect deeply with each other to do important work, a healthy work environment emerges. Client care in any setting is important work. When nurses and other team members focus all their efforts on what is best for their clients, they become united in purpose. Finding meaning in one's existence nourishes the human spirit (Frankl, 1963).

Efforts to create a healthy work environment require personal commitment, cooperation with others, and a courageous attitude to express genuine authenticity. Intentional movement toward creating a healthy work culture started in the late 1990s, and many of the strategies remain relevant today. Wesorick and team (1997, p. 9) have identified three characteristics to connect souls and create healthy work cultures: (1) shared meaning and purpose in work; (2) healthy relationships, and (3) meaningful conversations. Identification of shared meaning and purpose in work requires that everyone working together is aware of and agrees to what matters most in their work. Wesorick and colleagues defined healthy relationships as partnerships and outlined six basic partnership principles:

1. Intention: A personal decision to connect with another at the deepest level of humanness
2. Mission: A calling to live out something that deeply matters or is meaningful
3. Equal accountability: Mutual ownership of the mission without one person having power over or instilling fear in another
4. Potential: The human capacity of all individuals (including oneself) to continuously learn, grow, and create
5. Balance: Harmonious relationships with oneself and others required to attain the mission
6. Trust: Synchronous sense on important things or issues that matter

Wesorick and colleagues (1997) outlined meaningful conversation as the vehicle for developing healthy and meaningful relationships in work settings. Participants engaging in dialogue feel welcomed and honored while they share ideas, thoughts, and feelings. In dialogue, messages are deeply listened to and not judged. The partnership approach to clinical practice has the potential to transform a toxic work setting for all health team members into one that promotes health in body, mind, and spirit.

Take Note!
A shared purpose, healthy relationships, and meaningful conversations all help foster a healthy work environment.

Unfortunately, incivility and harassment in the work setting have created toxic workplace cultures. Many workplaces have high-conflict and high-drama environments. Holley (2019) outlines three key steps for creating a healthy workplace culture. The first step is to accurately assess and diagnose the current culture to identify areas for growth. The second step is creation of confidential reporting processes. The processes need to include early reporting (so interventions can occur to correct problematic behaviors) and to identify the scope of the identified issue. Most issues surrounding incivility and harassment go unreported because the person making the report fears retaliation. To avoid false accusations of harassment and incivility, investigations of alleged cases must occur. Investigations enable each involved person to share their perceptions of what occurred followed by a determination of what actually occurred. Ideally, a zero-tolerance policy for harassment or incivility is in place, but sometimes the perpetrator may be totally unaware of the offending behavior. The final step is managing the power dynamics within the organization. Managing power dynamics starts by empowering employees to stop any offensive behavior and empowering them to control or remove themselves from any uncomfortable situation.

Using conflict positively to attain the best possible outcome is another means of managing power dynamics. Positive use of conflict involves having individuals share their diverse opinions along with their rationales (more on conflict management appears in Chapter 17, "Leadership and Management in Professional Nursing"). Finally, managing power dynamics involves transparency, or sharing expectations, rewards, punishments, financial health, and future plans with employees. Employees feel empowered when they have key information about their organizations (Holley, 2019).

The Magnet Hospital Model

In 1983, the American Academy of Nursing embarked on identifying "Magnet" hospitals that delivered excellent client care, recruited and retained professional nurses, and provided an empowering environment for nurses. Using descriptive research methods, the American Academy of Nursing derived eight essential elements that distinguished Magnet hospitals from other hospitals:

1. Support for education
2. Working with other nurses who are clinically competent
3. Positive nurse–physician relationships
4. Autonomous nursing practice
5. A culture that values concern for the client
6. Control of and over nursing practice
7. Perceived adequacy of staffing
8. Nurse manager support (Kramer & Schmalenberg, 2004, p. 50)

In 2008, the American Nurses Credentialing Center (ANCC) revised the Magnet model, adding six new Magnet forces. The model has not since been revised, and the 14 forces of magnetism still remain embedded in the following five model components:

1. Transformational leadership (old model components: quality of nursing leadership and management style)
2. Structural empowerment (old model component: organizational structure, personnel policies and programs, community and the health care organization, image of nursing, and professional development)
3. Exemplary professional practice (old model components: professional care models, consultation and resources, nurse autonomy, nurses as teachers, interdisciplinary relationships)
4. New knowledge, innovations, and improvements (old model component: quality improvement)
5. Empirical quality outcomes (old model component: quality of care)

Kramer and Schmalenberg (2002) and McClure and Hinshaw (2007) identified that health care organizations that held Magnet status had an increased ability to recruit and retain nurses.

As of this writing, 462 health care organizations worldwide have earned Magnet status (ANCC, 2020). The majority of these are in the United States, but Magnet hospitals are also located in Australia, Lebanon, and Singapore. The ANCC outlines the following benefits of Magnet designation: ability to retain and attract the best possible nurses; improved client satisfaction, safety, and care; attainment of a collaborative work culture; advanced nursing standards and practices; and increased business and financial success. Multiple studies have found that nurses working in Magnet hospitals have higher job satisfaction, more autonomy in practice, and better work environments (Goode et al., 2011). Some nurses apply only for positions in health care organizations that hold Magnet status because these organizations value nurse contributions to health care delivery. The following "Focus on Research" box discusses how

---

FOCUS ON RESEARCH

Magnet Status and Client Hospital Experience

The research team in this study wanted to see if there was a difference in the hospital experience for clients who received care in Magnet hospitals compared to hospitals without this designation of nursing excellence. They used a retrospective, observational study design and conducted a secondary data analysis using the 2010 Hospital Consumer Assessment of Healthcare Providers and Systems (HCAHPS) survey.

The team used hospital identifiers and compared the data from the HCAHPS survey from 212 hospitals with Magnet designation and 212 hospitals without Magnet status. They used Magnet status information from the ANCC, HCAHPS survey data that measures client satisfaction with hospital and health care provider services, and the American Hospital Association Annual Survey about hospital structure, financial status, and other hospital characteristics. Only hospitals who had 300 or more clients completing the HCAHPS survey were included in the study. They matched the hospitals from the comparison groups according to bed size, occupancy rates, percentages of Medicare and Medicaid clients, teaching status, use of technology status, Catholic affiliation, payroll expenses per bed, core-based statistical area, and rural referral area (p. 1126). Results of the matching process revealed marked similarities of the Magnet and non-Magnet hospitals in these areas.

(continued)

FOCUS ON RESEARCH (*continued*)

Magnet Status and Client Hospital Experience

Data analysis was performed using least squares regression analysis following the matching. Statistically significant differences were found in the following areas: client ratings of hospital as 9 or 10 (higher scores mean higher satisfaction with hospital care); increased likelihood of a definite client recommendation to someone else to receive care at the hospital; staff-provided dismissal instructions; effective communication from nurses; effective pain control; and staff-provided explanations for administered medications.

The research team concluded that clients had better experiences when they received care at Magnet hospitals. They noted that hospitals would receive more reimbursement for care based on federal reimbursement schedules based on HCAHPS scores

and other financial benefits, making the investment in attaining Magnet designation worthwhile. Other financial benefits include higher hospital net income, lower mortality rates, and less nurse turnover.

The clinical significance of this study is that Magnet designation may improve client experience with hospital care. Nurses strive to deliver the best possible care to persons they serve. Based on the findings of this study, it may be easier to provide higher quality nursing care in Magnet hospitals. From a business perspective, hospitals with Magnet designation report higher incomes, reduced staff turnover, lower mortality rates, and possible increased market share from the increased likelihood of client recommendations to others to receive care at the hospital.

From Witkoski Stimpfel, A., Sloane, D. M., McHugh, M. D., & Aiken, L. H. (2016). Hospitals known for nursing excellence associated with better hospital experience for patients. *Health Services Research, 51(3),* 1120–1134. https://doi.org/10.1111/1475-6773.12357

hospitals with Magnet designation have improved client experiences that may impact market share and hospital reimbursement.

▌ QUESTIONS FOR REFLECTION

1. How would you rate the health of your work or educational environment based on the information presented in this chapter?

2. In what ways have you promoted a healthy work or educational environment within the past month?

3. What factors in your work or educational environment negatively affect your health and that of your colleagues?

4. What strategies could you implement to promote a healthy work or educational environment now and in the future?

THE HOME ENVIRONMENT

The **home environment** plays a key role in health. A family's home creates a haven for individual autonomy and control. Some consider their homes to be extensions of their personal identities. The quality of the physical structure, general cleanliness, storage of chemicals, and interpersonal relationships in the home affect the health of individual family members.

Home Environmental Factors Threatening Health

People seek safe living quarters. Those without homes try to find ways to stay warm and dry. People with established residences live in single- or multiple-family dwellings. Homes may be purchased or rented. A home's floor plan usually provides family members with space for privacy, sleeping, and interactions. In American culture, social status and self-esteem are linked to the home. Homeowners or landlords bear the responsibility for repairs to maintain environmental safety.

Accidents frequently occur at home. The types of accidents vary according to the ages and developmental levels of family members. The structural integrity of stairs, railings, ceilings, walls, and furniture must be assessed periodically to prevent injury. Safe storage and proper labeling of cleaning products and medications are critical in homes with young children. Homes with throw rugs create hazards for falls, especially for the older adult. Fire safety relies on periodic inspection and maintenance of household appliances, functioning smoke detectors, storage of paper and flammable materials away from furnaces or other appliances that could generate sparks, and unobstructed access to home entrances and exits. Power sources such as natural gas and electricity can pose health hazards if basic rules for each are not followed.

Appliances provide another source for accidents, especially in households where children reside. Hot water may cause burns, especially if the hot water tank is set above 140°F. Stairs and throw rugs provide opportunities for falling. Fireplaces and improper storage of paper, rags, and combustible materials may create fire hazards.

In addition to accidents, the home can be a source of illness. Problems with cleanliness and personal hygiene result in outbreaks of infectious disease. An estimated average 37 million cases of foodborne illnesses (CDC, 2018b) resulted in 228,744 hospitalizations and 2,612 deaths each year in the United States since 2006 (CDC, 2018a). *Salmonella*, *E. coli* (especially *E. coli* 0157:H7, found in raw ground beef), and *Pseudomonas aeruginosa* thrive on many kitchen counters and other food preparation surfaces. Adequate water supply, plumbing, refrigeration, garbage disposals, and general household cleaning practices reduce infections in the home. Handwashing after using the toilet and before food preparation and eating remains the most effective measure for the prevention of infectious illness in the home. Proper kitchen counter cleaning using commercially prepared disinfectants or a 10% bleach solution effectively destroys bacteria when left on surfaces for at least 30 seconds. Homemade recipes for cleaning solutions such as a combination of vinegar and baking soda fail to provide adequate disinfection (Rutala et al., 2000).

Indoor air pollution and allergens set the stage for the development of allergic disorders, especially asthma. Smoking is the main source of indoor air pollution. Sources of indoor allergens include dust mites, insect particles, pet dander, rodent dander, and mold. Limiting smoking to the outdoors and regular house cleaning help eliminate these factors that can impair respiratory health. Radon, a causative factor of lung cancer, can also seep into basements from radioactive element decay in soil. Radon test kits are widely available. If a home tests positive, the U.S. Environmental Protection Agency (2013) recommends hiring contractors certified in radon mitigation to seal foundations against radon emission and install special ventilation systems. In an effort to save energy, some homeowners tightly seal their homes, setting up the potential for high carbon monoxide levels, sometimes emitted from poorly maintained furnaces and gasoline-powered generators that are run inside or too close to a house. Air quality can be enhanced by opening windows and doors when the weather is suitable.

Pets and insect infestation may also serve as vectors for infectious diseases. To control lawn and household infestations, some people use pesticides. Organophosphate insecticides kill insects by inducing muscle paralysis.

However, organophosphates can be easily absorbed by people and pets through inhalation, ingestion, and dermal and optical contact (CDC, 2018c). According to the CDC (2018c), common symptoms associated with pesticide poisoning include increased saliva, abdominal cramps, excessive sweating, muscle weakness, muscle twitching, blurred vision, shortness of breath, and cough that can progress to respiratory distress, increased thirst, severe muscle twitching, convulsions, and loss of consciousness. In addition to problems arising from direct contact, organophosphates contaminate freshwater supplies, especially if applied too heavily.

Many potentially noxious substances can be found in the home. Household chemicals, fixtures, construction materials containing organic compounds, and carbon monoxide may contaminate the indoor environment. Benzene, a known human carcinogen, is present in synthetic materials, plastic, cleaning solutions, and tobacco smoke (CDC, 2018b). Construction materials such as particleboard and plywood emit formaldehyde, especially during the first year after construction. Most new carpeting contains a latex back, and latex carpet pads also are common. Newly poured concrete, fresh mortar, and paint emit gases (Davis, 2007; Gibson, 2000). Most commercial cleaners contain petrochemicals, fragrances, dyes, organophosphates, and/or bleach. Tap water contains pollutants such as bacterial colonies, nitrates, pesticides, particulates, and metals.

In addition to indoor pollution, people are exposed to chemicals and vapors used by neighbors. Propane cookers, gasoline-powered lawn tools, gasoline appliances, and fresh paint emit fumes (Gibson, 2000). Many people apply dangerous herbicides and pesticides on lawns to make lawns look thicker and greener.

Psychological health requires privacy. People need to have a place for emotional release, to feel independent, and to express affection toward those they love. When people have time to recharge emotionally, the threat of domestic violence is reduced. This is another facet of the home environment.

Individual, relationship, community, and societal factors contribute to intimate partner violence (IPV). The four types of IPV include physical violence, sexual violence, stalking, and psychological violence. One in five women and one in seven men report experiencing severe IPV in their lifetimes. One in five women and one in 12 men report experiencing sexual violence in their lifetimes. The economic costs, including those incurred from health care and legal services, is estimated to be $3.6 trillion annually (CDC, 2020e). Factors contributing to a perpetrator's history of IPV include a history of violent behavior; being a victim of physical or psychological abuse; witnessing IPV as a child; unemployment; strict ideas on traditional gender roles (male superiority); substance impairment; hostility; antisocial behavior; marital conflicts; unhealthy family relations and interactions; low levels of education; and cultural norms that support aggression toward others (CDC, 2020f). Because of its prevalence, health care providers are required to screen for IPV at every client encounter. In the United States, all admission and outpatient assessment forms contain direct questions to screen for physical and psychological abuse. Once violence has been confirmed, the nurse's priority is to ensure the safety of the victim and any dependents. Sometimes, immediate referrals to social workers, police departments, or domestic shelters may be needed to protect the victim(s). If there is no threat of immediate danger, the nurse should help the client outline a plan for safety if the violence escalates. In some states, professional nurses are legally required to report incidents of child and elder abuse but not IPV.

The Nurse's Role in Promoting a Healthy Home Environment

The professional nurse detects home health hazards by performing a comprehensive environmental assessment. When hazards are identified, the nurse provides education and support to help clients eliminate them. Sometimes, especially when nurses work with individuals with disabilities, community resources can be obtained to assist the clients with housekeeping and home maintenance.

Take Note!
Nurses can help promote a healthy home environment by screening for hazards, educating clients, and assisting clients with resources and referrals.

▌ QUESTIONS FOR REFLECTION

1. How would you rate the environment of your home based on the information presented here?
2. What things could you change to promote a healthier home environment?

COMPREHENSIVE ENVIRONMENTAL HEALTH ASSESSMENT

Before professional nurses can take action to promote a healthy community environment, they must identify environmental factors that affect health. Shaner (1994)

and Pope et al. (1995) outlined various elements of an environmental health history that remain applicable to current practice (Table 13.3). The age of residences (lead paint was commonly used in home construction prior to the 1970s) and their proximity to military installations and industries provide clues to potential exposure to substances and chemicals that impair health (Davis, 2007). Because people might be exposed to health hazards within work settings, information about occupations also provides clues to environmental health hazards. Workers in businesses that prepare foods for consumption (e.g., restaurants and grocery stores) may use latex gloves to prevent foodborne infections (Kim et al., 1999). Hobbies such as photography, furniture restoration, and gardening may result in exposure to hazardous chemicals. Household and lawn chemicals used on a regular basis also serve as a source of exposure to substances that may affect health. Nurses should also assess individuals for being potential perpetrators or victims of violence and assess the surrounding community for potential disasters that might occur.

THE NURSE'S ROLE IN DISASTER PLANNING, MITIGATION, AND RECOVERY

The education of professional nurses arms them with the knowledge and skills needed to help others in times of disaster. In addition, the public perceives nurses as people with knowledge and expertise who have an obligation to provide care in times of distress. Nurses have a detailed understanding of first aid principles, helping victims of trauma, and preventing the spread of contagious illnesses. Professional nurses also have well-refined teaching, organizational, and leadership skills that can be put to use in executing and coordinating care during all phases of a disaster. Finally, nurses have expertise in therapeutic communication skills to help provide psychological and spiritual support to people during times of uncertainty.

Take Note!
Professional nurses play a key role in helping people prepare for, survive during, cope with, and adapt to life after a disaster.

A **disaster** is "a sudden, calamitous event bringing great damage, loss, or destruction" (Mish, 2020, p. 355). Makwana (2020) proposes a definition of a disaster as any "high impact event that is responsible for a large number of persons to be ill, injured, or dead" (p. 5107). The International Federation of the Red Cross and Red

TABLE 13.3   Elements of a Comprehensive Environmental Assessment

Location or Activity	Key Questions
Home	Where do you live?
	What is the distance from your home to a major thoroughfare, industrial complex, or military base?
	If your home is close to an industrial complex, what type of industrial plant is it?
	What is the drinking water source for your home?
	What types of cleaning agents do you use for housework and laundry?
	What types of chemicals do you use for yard care?
	What insecticides do you use inside the home?
	How old is your home?
	How is your home heated?
	How is your home cooled?
	What is your fuel source for cooking?
	Have you tested your home for radon gas?
	Do you have a carbon monoxide alarm and smoke alarms in your home?
	Do you purify your home air or water?
	Have you recently acquired new furniture or carpeting?
	What type of paint is used on the exterior and interior of your home?
	Have you ever or recently refinished furniture or wood items in your home?
	What are the occupations of other household occupants?
	Do household occupants come into contact with chemicals as part of their employment or leisure activities?
	Does anyone living with you smoke inside the home?
Work	List your past jobs (including military experience) and whether you were exposed to any chemicals.
	Describe any work-related health problems or accidents.
	Did any of your coworkers have similar health problems or accidents?
	Where do you currently work?
	Are you employed fulltime or part-time?
	How does your employer inform you of potentially hazardous chemicals, equipment, or procedures used in the workplace?
	Describe your work safety education programs (if applicable).
	What protective devices are available for your use?
	Do you use the protective devices?
	How old is the building in which you work?
	Do you have any symptoms associated with your work setting? If so, please describe them.
Hobbies	What hobbies do you have?
	Are any chemical agents used while engaging in the hobby?
Symptom assessment	What symptoms do you currently have?
	When did they start?
	When do they occur?
	Where do they occur?
	Does anyone who works with you or lives with or near you have the same symptoms?

Adapted from Shaner, H. (1994). Environmentally responsible clinical practice. In E. A. Schuster & C. L. Brown (Eds.), *Exploring our environmental connections practice*. NLN Publication No. 14–2634. National League for Nursing; Pope, A. M., Snyder, M. A., & Mood, L. H. (Eds.). (1995). *Nursing, health, and the environment*. National Academy Press.

Crescent Society (IFRCRCS, 2020a) defines a disaster as "a sudden calamitous event that seriously disrupts the functioning of a community or society, or society's ability to cope using its own resources" (para. 1). Disasters may arise suddenly without warning (e.g., terrorist attack, plane crash, subway accident, earthquake), occur with warning (e.g., wildfire, hurricane, typhoon, flood, tornado, blizzard), or evolve over an extended period of time (e.g., drought, famine, pandemic). Disasters can be caused by nature (natural) or by humans. Disasters caused by humans fall into three broad categories: complex (e.g., multiple causation, such as a drought

leading to a famine that stimulates political unrest and relocation of large numbers of people); technologic (e.g., destruction of community infrastructure, industrial accidents, massive power failure); or human settlement (e.g., evacuation to a safe place or migration of an entire ethnic group to avoid persecution).

The magnitude of a disaster depends on its location. Disasters in highly populated areas affect more people and strain more resources than those occurring in rural, less populated areas. In 2020, multiple natural disasters occurred worldwide. Record-breaking bushfires in Australia, forest fires in India, and wild fires in California and Colorado charred millions of acres of lands, destroying buildings and displacing residents. The Philippine Islands were devastated by the super typhoon Goni and the Taal volcano eruption. Earthquakes measuring over a 6.0 magnitude hit Turkey, the Caribbean, China, Iran, and India. There were 28 named tropical depressions with hurricane potential, setting a record, and Hurricane Eta caused devastating flooding in Central America. Five hurricanes landed on the Louisiana coast, setting a record for the number of hurricanes hitting the state. Locusts swarmed in East Africa and parts of Asia. A typhoon hit Vietnam, causing flooding and landslides that destroyed over a million homes (IFRCRCS, 2020b; Thompson, 2020). A supercell thunderstorm hit Iowa and destroyed close to two thirds of summer crops. Near midland Michigan, Tittabawassee River flood waters caused breaches in the Edenville and Sanford Dams resulting in the evacuation of 10,000 residents (Thompson, 2020). Finally, the COVID-19 pandemic affected the entire world, in some places overwhelming many area health care systems. Evacuating people to avoid disasters while protecting them from catching COVID-19 posed many challenges for local and public health officials. Unfortunately, when disasters occur in remote areas, getting assistance to the disaster site may be difficult. A medical disaster occurs when a catastrophic event creates more casualties than the health care resources within a community can effectively accommodate (Veenema, 2019).

In many developed nations, most communities have disaster plans in place (see Box 13.3, Professional Prototype, "Disaster Planning, Mitigation, and Recovery"). Disaster planning, mitigation, and recovery are the steps of the **disaster management cycle**. These plans address probable disasters that might occur within each community such as an earthquake along a fault line, hurricane in a coastal region, or a blizzard in temperate climate areas. Disaster preparedness, mitigation, and recovery consume vast resources. Local and national governments pool resources to develop and maintain effective disaster plans. Note that plans best remain intact under stable governments.

Professional nurses play key roles in each phase of disaster response. Nurses who are uninjured at the disaster site offer basic first aid to victims. Some nurses, especially those working in emergency departments and as flight nurses, have special certifications in trauma nursing and find themselves assisting in the rescue of victims in the field, triaging people for appropriate treatment, and/or treating victims in first aid stations or emergency departments. Nurse administrators participate by assisting in communicating information about victims to

13.3 Professional Prototypes

Disaster Planning, Mitigation, and Recovery

Veenema (2019) and McGlown (2004) outlined a timeline for handling disasters that starts with preparation and ends with recovery.

- Phase 1 (before the disaster): In the first phase, which encompasses planning/preparedness, prevention, and warning, communities identify hazards and make attempts to remove them. If hazards cannot be removed (such as weather), then the community develops early warning systems, evacuates members at risk, institutes public awareness campaigns, performs disaster drills, develops nursing databases (mass casualty plans), and devises means to evaluate all components of the disaster response. During this phase, hospitals enact established disaster plans.
- Phase 2 (during and 72 hours after the disaster): The second phase consists of response, emergency management, and mitigation. In this phase, the disaster response plan is activated; potential and ongoing hazards are identified, and action is taken to relieve human suffering (mitigation); public health needs are anticipated; victims are triaged for effective use of available health care resources; emergency food and water distribution centers are established; and alternatives for sanitation and waste removal are established if the community infrastructure has been damaged. During this time, essential hospital personnel report to work per agency disaster policies so that enough personnel are available to provide care to anticipated victims (Adams & Berry, 2012).
- Phase 3 (beginning 72 hours after the disaster): The final phase focuses on recovery, rehabilitation, reconstruction, and evaluation. In this phase, victims receive medical and nursing care, disease surveillance continues, public health infrastructure is restored, family members are reunited, victims are monitored for long-term physical and psychological injuries, disaster responders attend debriefing and counseling sessions, and the disaster team evaluates the original disaster preparedness plan and revises it as needed (McGlown, 2004; Veenema, 2019).

From Adams, L. M., Berry, D. (2012). Who Will Show Up? Estimating Ability and Willingness of Essential Hospital Personnel to Report to Work in Response to a Disaster. *Online Journal of Issues in Nursing, 17*(2), 1. https://doi.org/10.3912/OJIN.Vol17No02PPT02; McGlown, K. (Ed.). (2004). *Terrorism and disaster management.* Health Administration Press; Veenema, T. (2019). *Disaster nursing and emergency preparedness for chemical, biological, radiological terrorism and other hazards.* Springer Publishing Co.

families. Community health nurses and Red Cross/Red Crescent volunteer nurses engage in setting up temporary shelters for people affected by the disaster. Some nurses may assume the responsibility of reuniting family members and friends who become separated during the disaster. Mental health nurses offer counseling to victims and relatives of victims. Acute care nurses may find themselves mobilizing supplies, adjusting staff assignments, and determining which clients can be discharged early to make room for other victims according to the facility's disaster plan. If the prospect of the spread of infectious disease arises, other nurses may participate in mass vaccination programs. Finally, nurses may become involved with shelter supervision.

In response to the terrorist attacks on September 11, 2001, the United States has developed the Emergency System for Advance Registration of Volunteer Health Professionals to rapidly mobilize required health care personnel. Using this system, individual states have created a nationwide database of 100,000 to 200,000 qualified volunteer health care professionals. Each state verifies its volunteers' credentials, offers access to disaster training and drilling, and develops a plan for requesting registration activation. Such a system is needed as people who volunteer spontaneously during disasters may get in the way or be denied participation in response efforts; even if used, a spontaneous volunteer's skills may not be fully deployed because of lack of verification of professional status (Veenema, 2019). Some states called upon health care professionals who had volunteered for the national health care personnel database in the early days of the COVID-19 pandemic. Some requested even more volunteers who met service criteria. For example, some required providers to have health care practice experience within the past year and be able to work 12-hour shifts. Missouri also provided pay for volunteers compatible with the average wage for each status of health care provider (ShowMe-Response.org, 2020). Nurse volunteers were deployed to the St. Louis area in the early days of the pandemic when working nurses were infected at high rates. In the event of a disaster, an incident commander could use the system to identify and mobilize health care personnel with the skills to handle specific types of incidents (Association of Public Health Nurses [APHN], Public Health Preparedness Committee, 2014; Veenema, 2019).

Effective disaster planning for nurses involves personal and professional preparation (see Box 13.4, Learning,

---

 13.4 Learning, Knowing, and Growing

Effective Disaster Planning for Nurses

Personal Preparation

Be aware of possible or potential disasters that are likely to occur in your geographic location.

Develop a personal household plan, including a 3-day to 3-week supply of food, over-the-counter and prescription medications, batteries, and water for all family members (including pets). Build a kit including a battery-powered or hand-crank radio with warning tones; flashlight; first aid kit; dust mask; extra batteries; plastic sheeting and duct tape (for sheltering in place); moist towelettes; garbage bags; wrench or pliers (to turn off utilities if needed); local maps; cell phone with charger and extra batteries; face masks; soap; hand sanitizer; personal hygiene supplies; disinfectant wipes; an extra pair of prescription glasses or contact lenses; cash or traveler's checks; fire extinguisher; important family documents; a change of clothing (for 3 days if possible); sturdy shoes for each person; sleeping bags or warm blankets for each person; matches in a waterproof container; paper and pencil (or pen); and books, games, and other items for recreation (FEMA, 2020).

Drill the family on the emergency action plan, including what to do if separated.

Professional Preparation

Obtain disaster nursing certification through a local American Red Cross chapter or university.

Provide community education about disaster preparedness, response, and recovery.

Become involved in local disaster plan development.

(continued)

13.4 Learning, Knowing, and Growing (*continued*)

Effective Disaster Planning for Nurses

Personal Preparation	Professional Preparation
Stay current on immunizations.	Participate in local disaster drills.
Keep first aid supplies and skills up to date.	Make arrangements with employer for work relief if called to serve in a disaster.
Learn about wilderness survival, especially if power plants become disabled for prolonged periods.	
Become involved in community activities, and support leaders who want to pass ordinances that protect the community against floods, mudslides, or collapses.	

From Veenema, T. (2019). *Disaster nursing and emergency preparedness for chemical, biological, radiological terrorism and other hazards* (4th ed.). Springer Publishing Co.; United States Federal Emergency Management Agency. (2020). *Build a kit*. https://www.ready.gov/kit.

Knowing, and Growing, "Effective Disaster Planning for Nurses"). Nurses can access detailed checklists for emergency preparedness from the Red Cross or the U.S. Federal Emergency Management Agency (FEMA). Many nurses realize they must report to work in the event of a local disaster, but few have detailed disaster plans in place to care for family and pets (Nash, 2015).

Following a disaster, nurses play key roles in screening and assessing community members for symptoms associated with infectious illnesses and exposure to environmental toxins (APHN Public Health Preparedness Committee, 2016; Veenema, 2019). Nurses can also offer valuable contributions to disaster debriefings to improve responses to future events (Veenema, 2019).

Summary and Significance to Practice

The relationship of the environment to human health is highly complex. Professional nurses who have solid knowledge about environmental factors affecting human health can effectively assess clients for injuries and diseases arising from various forms of exposure. Ecocentric professional nurses act to preserve the environment at the global, community, workplace, and home levels by practicing lives of voluntary simplicity. Nurses routinely assess factors that threaten health and provide education to promote environmental health for clients, each other, other health team members, and communities. Because professional nurses have specialized knowledge and skills to protect human health and promote healing, they are prepared to provide assistance in disaster preparedness, mitigation, and recovery

in the event of a natural or man-made disaster. When nurses become truly committed to improving the environment, they educate clients, coworkers, and community officials about potential hazards and advocate for change.

REAL-LIFE REFLECTIONS

Recall Ariana and Elena from the beginning of the chapter. During a blizzard, the electricity in their neighborhood stops working. After checking with each other to verify that neither of them has power, they decide to spend the day clearing the sidewalks of snow with the help of Elena's two teenagers. They wonder if they should check on the Garcias.

1. *Does a nurse have an obligation to check on older adult neighbors? Why or why not?*
2. *Why would a nurse want to check on older adult neighbors if there was an extended power failure?*
3. *Would you check on older adult neighbors if you confronted a similar situation? Why or why not?*
4. *What would you say to Ariana and Elena if you decided to check on older adult neighbors?*
5. *What aspects of the Garcias' lives would you want to assess to ensure they have the resources needed to be safe during the power outage?*
6. *What additional environmental safety assessment data might you want to collect?*
7. *What would you do if you identified that the older adult neighbor did not have the resources to remain safe?*

From Theory to Practice

1. What workplace environmental hazards can you identify in your clinical practice setting? What are the procedures for making changes in your health care organization? Why is it important to know the established policies and procedures for making changes in a workplace setting?

2. What individual behaviors could you change to promote healthier global, community, work, and home environments? What would be the consequences for making these changes?

Nurse as Author

1. Perform a home assessment using the questions related to "Home" found in Table 13.3. List areas for improvement or areas where you do not know the answers to the questions. Design a plan to improve the health of your home.

2. Write a short story of a personal or close encounter with a natural or man-made disaster. Include information about the disaster and your reaction to the disaster. Describe if you have any residual effects from the disaster. Relate how your experience with the personal or close encounter affects your ability to provide safe, effective nursing care.

Your Digital Classroom

Online Exploration

- Resources for global environmental health
- Center for International Earth Science Information, gridded population of the world: **https://sedac .ciesin.columbia.edu/data/collection/gpw-v4**
- U.S. Centers for Disease Control and Prevention: **www.cdc.gov**
- U.S. Environmental Protection Agency: **https:// www.epa.gov**
- Health Care Without Harm: **www.noharm.org/**
- National Center for Environmental Health: **www .cdc.gov/nceh**
- National Institute of Occupational Safety and Health: **www.cdc.gov/niosh**
- Toxic Release Inventory Program: **https://www .epa.gov/toxics-release-inventory-tri-program**
- Toxnet: **https://www.nlm.nih.gov/toxnet/index .html**
- University of Wisconsin Space Science and Engineering Center: www.ssec.wisc.edu/data/sst (ocean and sea surface temperature)
- Resources for workplace safety

- OSHA Ergonomics: **https://www.osha.gov/SLTC /ergonomics/**
- OSHA Workplace Violence: **https://www.osha .gov/SLTC/workplaceviolence/index.html**
- Resources for health in the home environment
- Environmental Protection Agency: **https://www .epa.gov/indoor-air-quality-iaq**
- Consumer Product Information Database: **https:// www.whatsinproducts.com/**

Expanding Your Understanding

1. Visit the U.S. Environmental Protection Agency website at https://www3.epa.gov/myem/envmap/ find.html. Type in your zip code in the location box and hit "Go." Note the air and water quality in the area where you live by clicking on the "MyAir" and "MyWater" tabs. Follow the directions to identify the top air and water polluters in your zip code and the top chemicals that cause cancer ("MyHealth"). Note if there are any businesses or locations where water is released directly into local streams. Bring this information to class to share or post this information in a class online discussion. Click on the "Environmental Topics" tab found on the right upper corner of your screen. Select one topic of interest and share the information that you found with your colleagues in class in an online course discussion.

2. Visit the National Institute of Occupational Safety and Health (NIOSH) at https://www.cdc.gov/ niosh/topics/healthcare/, and learn about the health and safety hazards of nursing. Select two of the policies and procedures regarding nurse safety where you are engaged in clinical practice and compare these to the policies published by NIOSH. Observe health team members to see how well they comply with the agency and NIOSH guidelines. Note areas of compliance and noncompliance to the policy or guideline. Develop a report and action plan to improve compliance.

3. Calculate your carbon footprint by visiting the Environmental Protection Agency's carbon footprint calculator at https://www3.epa.gov/carbon-footprint-calculator/. The calculator will offer strategies for you to reduce your carbon footprint. Was your household's carbon footprint above or below the national average? If it is above the national average, list some ways you can reduce it while reaping the benefits of lower utility bills.

4. Read about 35 ways to reduce your carbon footprint on Renee Cho's (2018) blog post, "The 35 Easiest Ways to Reduce Your Carbon Footprint" online at

https://blogs.ei.columbia.edu/2018/12/27/35-ways-reduce-carbon-footprint/. Make a list of things you do routinely that reduce your carbon footprint and things that you might do to improve it.

Beyond the Book

Visit the**Point**® at **www.thePoint.lww.com** for activities and information to reinforce the concepts and content covered in this chapter.

REFERENCES

Adams, L. M., Berry, D. (2012). Who Will Show Up? Estimating Ability and Willingness of Essential Hospital Personnel to Report to Work in Response to a Disaster. *Online Journal of Issues in Nursing, 17*(2), 1. https://doi.org/10.3912/OJIN.Vol17No02PPT02

Adeola, F. (2011). *Hazardous waste, industrial disasters, and environmental health risk local and global environmental struggles.* Palgrave Macmillan.

American Nurses Association. (2013). *A call to action from the nation's nurses in the wake of Newtown.* Retrieved April 29, 2021, from https://www.nursingworld.org/~48d9f6/globalassets/docs/anf/pressrelease_newtowncalltoaction_12_18_12_final.pdf

American Nurses Association. (2019a). *ANA: A nurse's call to action! I will protect my own life so I can protect my patients.* Retrieved November 5, 2020, from https://cdn2.hubspot.net/hubfs/4850206/198331%20End%20Nurse%20Abuse/198331%20END%20Nurse%20Abuse%20One%20Pager.pdf

American Nurses Association. (2019b). *ANA Issue Brief: Reporting incidents of workplace violence.* Retrieved November 6, 2020, from https://www.nursingworld.org/~4a4076/globalassets/practiceandpolicy/work-environment/endnurseabuse/endabuse-issue-brief-final.pdf

American Nurses Credentialing Center. (2008). *A new model for ANCC's Magnet Recognition Program.* Retrieved April 21, 2021, from https://www.nursingworld.org/organizational-programs/magnet/magnet-model/

American Nurses Credentialing Center. (2020). *Characteristics of magnet organizations.* Retrieved November 8, 2020, *from* https://www.nursingworld.org/organizational-programs/magnet/about-magnet/why-become-magnet/characteristics-of-magnet/

Anthony, S. (2015). *How much waste do hospitals generate?* Retrieved November 1, 2020, from https://www.medassureservices.com/blog/hospitals-medical-waste/#:~:text=To%20put%20it%20bluntly%2C%20a%20lot.%20According%20to,wastes%20are%20just%20a%20general%20sort%20of%20waste

Association of Public Health Nurses Public Health Preparedness Committee. (2014). *The role of the public health.* Retrieved April 29, 2021, from https://www.phnurse.org/assets/docs/Role%20of%20PHN%20in%20Disaster%20PRR_APHN%202014%20Ref%20updated%202015.pdf

Bartholomew, K. (2006). *Ending nurse-to-nurse hostility: Why nurses eat their young and each other.* HCPro.

Bender, K., & Thompson, F. (2003). West Nile virus: A growing challenge. *American Journal of Nursing, 103*, 32–40. https://doi.org/10.1097/00000446-200306000-00018

Berners-Lee, M. (2019). *There is no plant B: A handbook for the make or break years.* University Press.

Brausch, J., Connors, K., Brooks, B., & Rand, G. (2012). Human pharmaceutical in the aquatic environment: A review of recent toxicological studies and considerations for toxicity testing. *Review of Environmental Contamination and Toxicology, 218*, 1–99. https://doi.org/10.1007/978–1–4614–3137–4_1

Bright, C. (2000). Anticipating environmental "surprise." In L. R. Brown, C. Flavin, H. French, et al. (Eds.), *State of the world 2000.* W. W. Norton.

Campbell, V. L. S., Foley, H. L., Vianna, K. W., & Brunger, F. (2019). Folie du système? Preventing violence against nurses in in-patient psychiatry. *Psychiatric Quarterly, 90*(2), 413–420. https://doi.org/10.1007/s11126-019-09636-1

Carina, J. (2020). *The COVID-19 pandemic is generating tons of medical waste.* Retrieved November 1, 2020, from https://www.theverge.com/2020/3/26/21194647/the-covid-19-pandemic-is-generating-tons-of-medical-waste

Cascio, W., & Sykes, K. (2015, August 31). *Health effects of climate change. Advisory Meeting of the Surgeon General.* Retrieved October 31, 2020, *from* https://cfpub.epa.gov/si/si_public_record_report.cfm?Lab=OSIM&count=10000&dirEntryId=334630&searchall=&showcriteria=2&simplesearch=0&timstype=

Centers for Disease Control and Prevention. (2016a). *2014 Ebola Outbreak in West Africa—Case count.* Retrieved May 15, 2016, from http://www.cdc.gov/vhf/ebola/outbreaks/2014-west-africa/case-counts.html

Centers for Disease Control and Prevention. (2016b). *About Zika virus disease.* Retrieved May 15, 2016, from http://www.cdc.gov/zika/about/index.html

Centers for Disease Control and Prevention. (2018a). *Estimated annual episodes of illnesses caused by 31 pathogens transmitted by food, United States.* Retrieved November 8, 2020, from https://www.cdc.gov/foodborneburden/pdfs/scallan-estimated-illnesses-foodborne-pathogens.pdf

Centers for Disease Control and Prevention. (2018b). *Estimated annual hospitalizations and deaths caused by 31 pathogens transmitted by food, United States.* Retrieved November 8, 2020, from https://www.cdc.gov/foodborneburden/pdfs/scallan-estimated-hospitalizations-deaths-foodborne-pathogens.pdf

Centers for Disease Control and Prevention. (2018c). *Facts about benzene.* Retrieved November 8, 2020, from https://emergency.cdc.gov/agent/benzene/basics/facts.asp

Centers for Disease Control and Prevention. (2019a). *Leading cause of death, males-Hispanic-United states, 2017.* Retrieved November 5, 2020, from https://www.cdc.gov/healthequity/lcod/men/2017/nonhispanic-asian-or-islander/index.htm

Centers for Disease Control and Prevention. (2019b). *Leading cause of death, males-non-Hispanic black-United States 2017.* Retrieved November 5, 2020, from https://www.cdc.gov/healthequity/lcod/men/2017/nonhispanic-black/index.htm

Centers for Disease Control and Prevention. (2019c). *Leading cause of death, males-non-Hispanic American Indian or Alaskan Native-Unites States, 2017.* https://www.cdc.gov/healthequity/lcod/men/2017/nonhispanic-native/index.htm

Centers for Disease Control and Prevention. (2019d). *Leading cause of death, males-non-Hispanic_ Asian or Pacific Islander.* Retrieved

November 5, 2020, from https://www.cdc.gov/healthequity/lcod/men/2017/nonhispanic-asian-or-islander/index.htm

Centers for Disease Control and Prevention. (2019e). *Leading causes of death, males–non-Hispanic white–United States, 2017.* Retrieved November 5, 2020, from https://www.cdc.gov/healthequity/lcod/men/2017/nonhispanic-white/index.htm

Centers for Disease Control and Prevention. (2020a). *COVID-19 overview and infection preventions and control priorities in non-US healthcare settings.* Retrieved November 2, 2020, from https://www.cdc.gov/coronavirus/2019-ncov/hcp/non-us-settings/overview/index.html

Centers for Disease Control and Prevention. (2020b). *Prevalence of obesity and severe obesity among adults: 2017–2018.* Retrieved November 3, 2020, from https://www.cdc.gov/nchs/products/databriefs/db360.htm

Centers for Disease Control and Prevention. (2020c). *Underlying Cause of Death 1999–2018 on CDC WONDER Online Database, released in 2020. Data are from the Multiple Cause of Death Files, 1999–2018, as compiled from data provided by the 57 vital statistics jurisdictions through the Vital Statistics Cooperative Program.* Retrieved November 5, 2020, from http://wonder.cdc.gov/ucd-icd10.html

Centers for Disease Control and Prevention. (2020d). *Violence prevention. Preventing child abuse and neglect.* Retrieved November 5, 2020, from https://www.cdc.gov/violenceprevention/childabuseandneglect/fastfact.html

Centers for Disease Control and Prevention. (2020e). *Prevention intimate partner violence.* Retrieved November 8, 2020, from https://www.cdc.gov/violenceprevention/intimatepartnerviolence/fastfact.html

Centers for Disease Control and Prevention. (2020f). *Risk and protective factors for perpetration.* Retrieved November 8, 2020, from https://www.cdc.gov/violenceprevention/intimatepartnerviolence/riskprotectivefactors.html

Centers for Disease Control and Prevention. (2021a). *Overweight and Obesity. Adult obesity facts.* Retrieved March 6, 2021, from https://www.cdc.gov/obesity/data/adult.html

Centers for Disease Control and Prevention. (2021b). *Defining adult overweight & obesity.* Retrieved April 29, 2021, from https://www.cdc.gov/obesity/adult/defining.html

Centers for Disease Control and Prevention. (2021c). *Zika virus. 2020 case counts in the U.S.* Retrieved March 6, 2021, from https://www.cdc.gov/zika/reporting/2020-case-counts.html

Chiaravalloti, A., Pagani, M., Micarelli, A., Di Pietro, B., Genovesi, G., Alessandrini, M., & Schillaci, O. (2015). Cortical activity during olfactory stimulation in multiple chemical sensitivity: A 18F-FDG PET/CT study. *European Journal of Nuclear Medical Molecular Imaging, 42,* 733–740. https://doi.org/10.1007/s00259-014-2969-2

Cho, R. (2018). *The 35 easiest ways to reduce your carbon footprint.* Retrieved April 29, 2021, from https://news.climate.columbia.edu/2018/12/27/35-ways-reduce-carbon-footprint/

Cooper, C. L., & Swanson, N. (n.d.). *Workplace violence in the health sector state of the art.* Working paper WHO. Retrieved November 5, 2020, from https://www.who.int/violence_injury_prevention/violence/activities/workplace/WVstateart.pdf?ua=1

Davidson, J. E., Proudfoot, J., Lee, K. E., Terterian, G., & Zisook, S. (2020). A longitudinal analysis of nurse suicide in the United States (2005–2016). *Worldviews on evidence-based nursing/Sigma Theta Tau International, Honor Society of Nursing, 17,* 6–15. https://doi.org/10.1111/wvn.12419. Retrieved

November 5, 2020, from https://sigmapubs.onlinelibrary.wiley.com/doi/full/10.1111/wvn.12419

Davis, A. (2007). Home environmental health risks. *Online Journal of Issues in Nursing, 12*(2), 5. https://doi.org/10.3912/OJIN.Vol12No02Man04

Dock, L. L. (1912). *A history of nursing* (Vol. 3). G. P. Putnam's Sons.

Dovers, S., & Butler, C. (2017). *How many people can the earth actually support?* Retrieved October 30, 2020, from https://www.science.org.au/curious/earth-environment/how-many-people-can-earth-actually-support

Fawcett, J. (1984). *Analysis and evaluation of conceptual models of nursing.* F. A. Davis.

Frankl, V. (1963). *Man's search for meaning.* Washington Square Press.

Gibson, P. R. (2000). *Multiple chemical sensitivity: A survival guide.* New Harbinger.

Glasper, A. (2018). Protecting healthcare staff from abuse: Tackling workplace incivility in nursing. *British Journal of Nursing, 27*(22), 1336–1337. https://doi.org/10.12968/bjon.2018.27.22.1336

Goode, C., Blegen, M., Park, S., Vaughn, T., & Spetz, J. (2011). Comparison of patient outcomes in Magnet® and non-Magnet Hospitals. *Journal of Nursing Administration, 41*(12), 517–523. https://doi.org/10.1097/NNA.0b013e3182378b7c

Harris, D., & Sims J. (2019). *Mass shootings in America.* Abdo Publishing.

Hartin, P. Birks, M., & Lindsay, D. (2020). Bullying in nursing: How has it changed over 4 decades? *Journal of Nursing Management, 28,* 1619–1626. https://doi.org/10.1111/jonm.13117

Hartman, T. (2019). *COP25 climate talks: What just happened and what lies ahead?* Retrieved November 1, 2020, from https://www.weforum.org/agenda/2019/12/un-climate-change-conference-environment/

Hawken, P. (Ed.) (2017). *Drawdown: the most comprehensive plan ever proposed to reverse global warming.* Penguin.

Holley, M. (2019). *The inclusive leader's guide to healthy workplace culture.* Difference Press.

Horowitz, S. (2014). Toxicant-induced loss of tolerance, a theory to account for multiple chemical sensitivity. *Alternative and Complementary Therapies, 20*(2), 96–100. https://doi.org/10.1089/act.2014.20201

Hu, H., & Baines, C. (2018). Recent insights into 3 underrecognized conditions: Myalgic encephalomyelitis-chronic fatigue syndrome, fibromyalgia, and environmental sensitivities-multiple chemical sensitivity. *Canadian Family Physician, 64*(6), 413–415. Retrieved April 21, 2021, from https://www.cfp.ca/content/64/6/413

Huang, P.-C., Cheng, M.-T., & Guo, H.-R. (2018). Representative survey on idiopathic environmental intolerance attributed to electromagnetic fields in Taiwan and comparison with the international literature. *Environmental Health: A Global Access Science Source, 17,* 5. https://doi.org/10.1186/s12940-018-0351-8

Ingraham, C. (2019). *Nine days on the road. Average commute time reached a new record last year.* Retrieved November 3, 2020, from https://www.washingtonpost.com/business/2019/10/07/nine-days-road-average-commute-time-reached-new-record-last-year/

International Council of Nurses. (2020). *Press release June 15. ICN calls for immediate government action to end violence against nurses on all fronts, underlined by heinous attack in Mexico.* Retrieved November 5, 2020, from https://www.icn.ch/sites/default/files/inline-files/PR_31_Attacks%20on%20

nurses%20in%20Mexico%20-%20June%202020%20V2_FINAL.pdf

International Federation of the Red Cross and Red Crescent Societies. (2020a). *What is a disaster?* Retrieved November 9, 2020, from https://www.ifrc.org/en/what-we-do/disaster-management/about-disasters/what-is-a-disaster/#:~:text=A%20disaster%20is%20a%20sudden%2C%20calamitous%20event%20that,caused%20by%20nature%2C%20disasters%20can%20have%20human%20origins

International Federation of the Red Cross and Red Crescent Societies. (2020b). *List of press releases.* Retrieved April 27, 2021, from https://media.ifrc.org/ifrc/press-release/red-cross-faces-record-number-climate-related-disasters-2020/

Kim, K. T., Wellmeyer, E. T., & Miller, K. V. (1999). Minimum prevalence of latex hypersensitivity in health care workers. *Allergy and Asthma Proceedings, 20*, 387–391.

Kim, J., Woith, W., Otten, K., & McElmurry, B. (2006). Global nurse leaders: Lessons from the sages. *Advances in Nursing Science, 29*(1), 27–42.

Kleffel, D. (1994). The environment: Alive, whole and interacting. In E. A. Schuster, C. L. Brown (Eds.), *Exploring our environmental connections* (NLN Publication No. 14–2634, pp. 3–15) . National League for Nursing.

Kleffel, D. (1996). Environmental paradigms: Moving toward an ecocentric perspective. *Advances in Nursing Science, 18*, 1–10. https://doi.org/10.1097/00012272-199606000-00004

Kramer, M., & Schmalenberg, C. (2002). Staff nurses identify essentials of magnetism. In M. McClure & A. Hinshaw (Eds.), *Magnet hospitals revisited: Attraction and retention of professional nurses* (pp. 26–41). American Nurses Publishing.

Kramer, M., & Schmalenberg, C. (2004). Essentials of a magnetic work environment: Part 1. *Nursing, 34*, 50–54. https://doi.org/10.1097/00152193-200406000-00043.

Landrigan, P. J., Fuller, R., Hu, H., Caravanos, J., Cropper, M. L., Hanrahan, D., Sandilya, K., Chiles, T. C., Kumar, P., & Suk, W. A. (2018). Pollution and global health—An agenda for prevention. *Environmental Health Perspectives, 126*(8), 1–6. https://doi.org/10.1289/EHP3141

Lazarus, R. S., & Folkman, S. (1984). *Stress, appraisal and coping.* Springer.

Leddy, S. K. (2004). Human energy: A conceptual model of unitary nursing science. *Visions: The Journal of Rogerian Scholarship, 12*, 14–27. Retrieved April 29, 2021 from https://www.thefreelibrary.com/Human+energy%3a+a+conceptual+model+of+unitary+nursing+science.-a0161397669

Leroy, E., Rouquet, P., Formenty, P., Souquière, S., Kilbourne, A., Froment, J. M., Bermejo, M., Smit, S., Karesh, W., Swanepoel, R., Zaki, S. R., & Rollin, P. E. (2004). Multiple Ebola virus transmission events and rapid decline of central African wildlife. *Science, 303*, 387–390. Retrieved April 29, 2021 from https://science.sciencemag.org/content/303/5656/387.full

Longo, J. (2012). *Bulling in the workplace: Reversing a culture.* NurseBooks.

Longo, J., & Smith, M. (2011). A prescription for disruptions in care: Community building among nurses to address horizontal violence. *Advances in Nursing Science, 34*(4), 345–356. https://doi.org/10.1097/ANS.0b013e3182300e3e

Lotus Arise. (2021). *Hazardous waste and related convention—UPSC IAS.* Retrieved March 6, 2021, from https://lotusarise.com/hazardous-waste-upsc/

Makwana, N. (2020). Public health care system's preparedness to combat epidemics after natural disasters. *Journal of Family Medicine & Primary Care, 9*(10), 5107–5112. https://doi.org/10.4103/jfmpc.jfmpc_895_19

McClure, M., & Hinshaw, A. (2007). The magnetic matrix: Building blocks of Magnet™ hospitals. *American Nurse Today, 2*(12), 22–24. Retrieved April 29, 2021, from https://www.myamericannurse.com/tme-magnetic-matrix-building-blocks-of-magnet-hospitals/

McGinn, A. P. (2000). Phasing out persistent organic pollutants. In L. R. Brown, C. Flavin, H. French, et al. (Eds.), *State of the world 2000* (pp. 79–100). W. W. Norton.

McGlown, K. (Ed.). (2004). *Terrorism and disaster management.* Health Administration Press,

McIntosh, W. L., Spies, E., Stone, D. M., Lokey, C. N., Trudeau, A. T., & Bartholow, B. (2016). Suicide rates by occupational group—17 states, 2012. *Morbidity and Mortality Weekly Report, 65*, 641–645. Retrieved April 29, 2021, from https://www.cdc.gov/mmwr/volumes/65/wr/pdfs/mm6525.pdf

McLean, A. (1974). Concepts of occupational stress: A review. In A. McLean (Ed.), *Occupational stress* (pp. 1–21). Charles C. Thomas.

McSpedon, C. (2020). A conversation with Monica R. McLemore, the nurse, scientist and activist discusses how nurses can work to dismantle racism. *American Journal of Nursing, 120*, 68–70. https://doi.org/10.1097/01.NAJ.0000697676.06959.19

Micarelli, A., Viziano, A., Genovesi, G., Bruno, E., Ottaviani, F., & Alessandrini, M. (2016). Lack of contralateral suppression in transient-evoked otoacoustic emissions in multiple chemical sensitivity: A clinical correlation study. *Noise and Health, 18*(82), 143–149. https://doi.org/10.4103/1463-1741.181997

Mish, F. C. (2020). *Merriam-Webster's collegiate dictionary* (11th ed.). Merriam-Webster

Musker, K. (1994). Voluntary simplicity: Nurses creating a healing environment. In E. A. Schuster & C. L. Brown (Eds.), *Exploring our environmental connections (NLN Publication No. 14–2634)* (pp. 199–212). National League for Nursing.

Nash, T. J. (2015). Unveiling the truth about nurses' personal preparedness for disaster response: A pilot study. *Med-Surg Nursing, 24*(6), 425–431. Retrieved April 29, 2021, from https://www.thefreelibrary.com/Unveiling+the+truth+about+nurses%27+personal+preparedness+for+disaster...-a043936228

National Aeronautics and Space Administrations. (2020a). *Global climate change-Vital signs of the planet: Artic sea ice.* Retrieved April 29, 2021, from https://climate.nasa.gov/climate_resources/130/arctic-sea-ice/

National Aeronautics and Space Administrations. (2020b). *Global climate change—Vital signs of the planet: Carbon dioxide.* Retrieved April 29, 2021, from https://climate.nasa.gov/vital-signs/carbon-dioxide/

National Aeronautics and Space Administrations. (2020c). *Global climate change—Vital signs of the planet: Global temperature.* Retrieved April 29, 2021, from https://climate.nasa.gov/vital-signs/global-temperature/

National Aeronautics and Space Administrations. (2020d). *Global climate change—Vital signs of the planet: Ice sheets.* Retrieved October 30, 2020, from https://climate.nasa.gov/vital-signs/ice-sheets/

National Aeronautics and Space Administrations. (2020e). *Global climate change—Vital signs of the planet: Sea level.* Retrieved October 30, 2020, from https://climate.nasa.gov/vital-signs/sea-level/

National Cancer Institute. (2020). *Cancer prevention overview (PDQ®)-Health professional version.* Retrieved November 1,

2020, from https://www.cancer.gov/about-cancer/causes-prevention/hp-prevention-overview-pdq#_67

National Institutes of Health. (2020). *COVID-19 critical care general considerations*. Retrieved November 2, 2020, from https://www.covid19treatmentguidelines.nih.gov/critical-care/general-considerations/

National Institute of Occupational Safety and Health. (2018). *Health and safety practices survey of healthcare workers. Study findings*. Retrieved November 5, 2020, from https://www.cdc.gov/niosh/topics/healthcarehsps/findings.html

Neuman, B. (2002). The Neuman system model. In B. Neuman & J. Fawcett (Eds.), *The Neuman systems model* (4th ed., pp. 3–34). Prentice-Hall.

Newman, M. A. (1994). *Health as expanding consciousness* (2nd ed.). National League for Nursing.

O'Meara, M. (2000). Harnessing information technologies for the environment. In L. R. Brown, C. Flavin, H. French, et al. (Eds.), *State of the world 2000* (pp. 121–141). W. W. Norton.

Papp, E. (2007). *Occupational health and safety management programme for nurses*. International Council of Nurses.

Pearce, F. (2007). *With speed and violence: Why scientist fear tipping points in climate change*. Beacon.

Pope, A. M., Snyder, M. A., & Mood, L. H. (Eds.). (1995). *Nursing, health and the environment*. National Academies Press.

Poursafa, P., Keitkha, M., & Kelishadi, R. (2015). Systematic review on adverse birth outcomes of climate change. *Journal of Research in Medical Sciences, 20*, 397–402. Retrieved April 29, 2021, from https://pubmed.ncbi.nlm.nih.gov/26109998/

Ridlington, E., Weissman, G., & Folger, M. (2020). *Trouble in the air: Millions of Americans breathed polluted air in 2018*. Retrieved November 3, 2020, from https://environmentamerica.org/sites/environment/files/reports/Trouble-In-The-Air/EnvironmentAmerica_TroubleintheAir_scrn.pdf

Rogers, M. E. (1990). Nursing: Science of unitary, irreducible human beings: Update 1990. In E. A. M. Barrett (Ed.), *Visions of Rogers' science based nursing* (pp, 5–12). National League for Nursing.

Roy, C. (1987). Roy's adaptation model. In R. R. Parse (Ed.), *Nursing science; Major paradigms, theories and critiques* (pp. 45–62). W. B. Saunders.

Rutala, W. A., Barbee, S. L., Aguiar, N. C., Sobsey, M. D., & Weber, D. J. (2000). Antimicrobial activity of home disinfectants and natural products against potential human pathogens. *Infection Control and Hospital Epidemiology, 21*, 33–38. https://doi.org/10.1086/501694

Sachs, J. (2008). *Common wealth: Economics for a crowded planet*. Penguin.

Schmiedchen, K., Driessen, S., & Oftedal, G. (2019). Methodological limitations in experimental studies on symptom development in individuals with idiopathic environmental intolerance attributed to electromagnetic fields (IEI-EMF)—A systematic review. *Environmental Health: A Global Access Science Source, 18*(1), 88. https://doi.org/10.1186/s12940-019-0519-x

Sequeria, I. F., Prata, J. C., de Costa, J. P., Duarte, A. C., & Rocha-Santos, T. (2020). Worldwide contamination of fish with microplastics: A brief global overview. *Marine Pollution Bulletin, 160*, 111681. https://doi.org/10.1016/j.marpolbul.2020.111681

Shahbandeh, M. (2020). *World fish production from 2007–2019 by fishing and aquaculture*. Retrieved November 1, 2020, from https://www.statista.com/statistics/272311/world-fish-production-by-fishing-and-aquaculture-since-2004/

Shaner, H. (1994). Environmentally responsible clinical practice. In E. A. Schuster & C. L. Brown (Eds.), *Exploring our environmental connections practice* (NLN Publication No. 14–2634, pp. 42–51). National League for Nursing.

Show-Me-Response.org. (2020). *Disasters call for heroes… answer the call*. Retrieved March 6, 2021, from https://www.showmeresponse.org/

Sirleaf. V. S. (2018). Not your dumping ground: Criminalization of trafficking in hazardous waste in Africa. *Wisconsin International Law Journal, 35*(2), 326–366. Retrieved April 29, 2021, from https://papers.ssrn.com/sol3/papers.cfm?abstract_id=3161739

Spelten, E., Thomas, B., O'Meara, P., van Vuuren, J., & McGillion, A. (2020). Violence against Emergency Department nurses; Can we identify the perpetrators? *PLoS ONE, 15*(4), 1–12. https://doi.org/10.1371/journal.pone.02307

Sutton, R. (2006). *The no asshole rule: Building a civilized workplace and surviving one that isn't*. Warner Business.

Tamuzi, J. L., Ayele, B. T., Shumba, C. S., Adetokunboh, O. O., Uwimana-Nicol, J., Haile, Z. T., Inugu, J., & Nyasulu, P. S. (2020). Implications of COVID-19 in high burden countries for HIV/TB: A systematic review of evidence. *BMC Infectious Diseases, 20*(1), 1–18. https://doi.org/10.1186/s12879-020-05450-4

Thompson, A. (2020). *A running list of record-breaking disasters in 2020*. Retrieved November 9, 2020, from https://www.scientificamerican.com/article/a-running-list-of-record-breaking-natural-disasters-in-2020/

Trossman, S. (2000). Moving violations: Working to prevent on-the-job injuries. *The American Nurse, 32*(1), 12–14.

United Nations. (2016). *With Global Goals agreed, UN focuses on what it will take to achieve sustainability targets by 2030*. Retrieved May 15, 2016, from http://www.un.org/sustainabledevelopment/blog/2016/04/with-global-goals-agreed-un-focuses-on-what-it-will-take-to-achieve-sustainability-targets-by-2030/

United Nations. (2017). *News. World population projected to reach 9.8 billion in 2050 and 11.2 billion in 2100*. Retrieved October 30, 2020, from https://www.un.org/development/desa/en/news/population/world-population-prospects-2017.html#:~:text=The%20current%20world%20population%20of%207.6%20billion%20is,a%20new%20United%20Nations%20report%20being%20launched%20today

United States Bureau of Labor Statistics. (2020). *Employer-reported workplace injuries and illnesses, 2019*. Retrieved November 5, 2020, from https://www.bls.gov/news.release/archives/osh_11042020.pdf

United States Census Bureau. (2018). *Notes on the world population clock*. Retrieved October 30, 2020, from https://www.census.gov/data/data-tools/population-clock/world-notes.html

United States Census Bureau. (2020). *U.S. and world population clocks*. Retrieved October 30, 2020, from https://www.census.gov/popclock/

United States Department of Transportation Bureau of Transportation Statistics. (2017). *National household travel survey daily travel quick facts*. Retrieved November 3, 2020, from https://www.bts.gov/statistical-products/surveys/national-household-travel-survey-daily-travel-quick-facts

United States Environmental Protection Agency. (2013). *Consumer's guide to radon reduction, how to fix your home*. Retrieved November 8, 2020, from https://www.epa.gov/sites/production/files/2016-02/documents/2013_consumers_guide_to_radon_reduction.pdf

United States Environmental Protection Agency. (2020). *The 2019 EPA Automotive Trends Report: Greenhouse gas emissions, fuel economy and technology since 1975. Executive Summary. EPA-420-S-20-0001 March 2020*. Retrieved November 3, 2020, from https://nepis.epa.gov/Exe/ZyPDF.cgi?Dockey=P100YVK3.pdf

United States Federal Emergency Management Agency. (2020). *Build a kit*. Retrieved November 9, 2020, from https://www.ready.gov/kit

United States Global Change Research Program. (2019). *The climate report, the national climate, assessment—Impacts, risks and adaptation in the United States*. Melville House.

Vasilakopoulos, P., & Marshall, C. T. (2015). Resilience and tipping points of an exploited fish population over six decades. *Global Change Biology*, *21*, 1834–1847. https://doi.org/10.1111/gcb.128

Veenema, T. (2019). *Disaster nursing and emergency preparedness for chemical, biological and radiological terrorism and other hazards* (4th ed.). Springer Publishing Co.

Wallace-Wells, D. (2020). *The uninhabitable earth, life after warming*. Tim Duggan Books.

Watai, K., Fukutomi, Y., Hayashi, H., Kamide, Y., Sekiya, K., Taniguchi, M. (2018). Epidemiological association between multiple chemical sensitivity and birth by caesarean section: a nationwide case-control study. *Environmental Health: A Global Access Science Source*. 17(1), 1-9. https://doi.org/10.1186/s12940-018-0438-2

Watson, J. (1999). *Postmodern nursing and beyond*. Churchill-Livingstone.

Wesorick, B., Shiparski, L., Troseth, M., & Wyngarden, K. (1997). *Partnership Council Field Book*. Practice Field Publishing.

Wohlford, S., Esteves-Fuentes, N., & Carter, K. F. (2020). Reducing waste in the clinical setting. *American Journal of Nursing*, *120*(6), 48–55. https://doi.org/10.1097/01.NAJ.0000668744.36106.24

World Health Organization. (2012). *Influenza at the human-animal interface*. Summary and assessment as of 4 June 2012. Retrieved December 27, 2012, from www.who.int/influenza/human_animal_interface/EN_GIP_20120706CumulativeNumberH5N1cases.pdf

World Health Organization. (2018a). *Climate change and health*. Retrieved November 1, 2020, from https://www.who.int/news-room/fact-sheets/detail/climate-change-and-health

World Health Organization. (2018b). *Health-care waste, key facts*. Retrieved November 1, 2020, from https://www.who.int/en/news-room/fact-sheets/detail/health-care-waste

Worthington, K. (2000). Seeking the perfect fit. *American Journal of Nursing*, *100*, 88. https://doi.org/10.1097/00000446-200008000-00064

Young, H., & Lee, E. (Eds.) (1948). *Essential of nursing*. G. P. Putnam's Sons.

Informatics and Technology in Nursing Practice

(continued on page 368)

KEY TERMS AND CONCEPTS

Informatics

Electronic health record (EHR)

Meaningful use

Personal electronic health record (PEHR)

American Medical Informatics Association (AMIA)

Clinical research informatics

Consumer health informatics

Public health informatics

Translational bioinformatics

Clinical informatics

Alliance for Nursing Informatics (ANI)

Nursing informatics

Informatics nurse specialist

Nursing informatics innovator

Telemedicine

Telehealth

Educational informatics

Robotics

Family health history

Genomic medicine

Technology in clinical practice

Internet addiction

LEARNING OUTCOMES

By the end of this chapter, the learner will be able to:

1. Discuss the roles and implications of informatics and technology in professional nursing practice.
2. Outline the educational preparation and roles of the informatics nurse specialist.
3. Identify current technologies used in clinical practice.
4. Debate the advantages and disadvantages of complex technology used in clinical practice.
5. Identify key ethical considerations as technologic advances become standard practice in professional nursing.
6. Outline ways to balance informatics and technology in personal and professional life.

REAL-LIFE REFLECTIONS

Jorge, Susan, and Amy graduated from the same nursing program several years ago. They now work at three different health care facilities. Jorge, who works at a large university medical center, has been documenting care using a computer for many years and has worked with two different computer documentation systems. Susan, a director of nursing at a rural hospital, just introduced a computerized client care documentation system at her facility. Amy works in a home health care agency that uses laptop computers to record home visits as well as computer technology for remote client monitoring. When they meet at a college alumni event, they compare notes about the strengths and weaknesses of the current computer systems and technology they use in practice. Susan poses the following questions during their discussion: "I know that computers are wonderful, but I have some concerns about our overreliance on them. With all of the hackers out there, what types of safeguards

(continued on page 368)

do your organizations have to prevent cyber-attacks? How can we ensure confidentiality of client information with computerized medical records? What key elements need to be included in an employee policy related to computer use, safety, and confidentiality of information? How much time does it take you and your staff to complete computer documentation? What are the legal implications for nurses who use technology for remote client monitoring?"

For optimal professional practice and client care, nurses must have proficient computer skills. This chapter provides an overview of the informatics and technology used in today's nursing practice and explores the implications for professional nurses because technology plays an increasingly important role in health care delivery. Key computer competencies for professional nursing and advances in technology for clinical practice are presented. Finally, the chapter challenges students to consider the advantages, disadvantages, and ethical issues of technology use for client care.

Changes in technology occur quickly. In fact, by the time this book is published, some of the information presented in this chapter may already be obsolete. Faster, improved models of computer equipment seem to be introduced just as soon as the latest model has been purchased. New materials superior to silicon continue to make computer chips smaller and faster. In fact, purchasing a hard copy of any book (including this one) may one day be a rarity, especially with the proliferation of e-readers capable of storing hundreds of books. One day libraries may no longer provide books, journals, and newspapers, except in digital formats. Currently, most consumer health-related information is stored on computers. Nurses use computers for nearly all aspects of client care, except for hands-on skills and conversing with clients and families.

INFORMATICS AND HEALTH CARE

The average person today has access to more information online than a single person could possibly comprehend in a lifetime. **Informatics** or information science deals with the "the collection, classification, storage, retrieval, and dissemination of recorded knowledge treated both as a true and applied science" (Mish, p. 641). Because of the wide array of information available, devising effective methods for organizing and managing it is imperative. Essential information in one area of life may be irrelevant in another area.

For example, how informatics is used to generate, store, manage, and communicate information for computer gaming has little relevance to health care providers (unless a provider is working in the field of neuroscience and is studying the effects of computer gaming on memory, for example).

Take Note!

In professional nursing, informatics plays a critical role in how nurses access, enter, retrieve, manage, store, and share key knowledge essential for professional practice and client care.

Informatics and Professional Nursing

Nurses use a variety of computers in daily clinical practice. Nurses document various aspects of client care using computers, thereby creating an **electronic health record (EHR)** for each client. An EHR stores client health information digitally in a secure database. When consumers receive care from an integrated health system, EHRs can be accessed nearly seamlessly.

The federal government recognized that for effective use of EHRs, they needed to be meaningful and so "meaningful use" was defined. **Meaningful use** means "the use of certified EHR technology to achieve health and efficiency goals" (HealthIT.gov, 2014, para 1). Some examples of meaningful use include electronic prescribing of medications and making certain that certified EHR technology would connect effectively for exchanging health information for improving health care quality, including efficiency and avoiding duplicative services. The government determined objectives of meaningful use and classified them into the following client-driven domains:

- Improve quality, safety, and efficiency
- Engage clients and families
- Improve care coordination

- Improve public and population health
- Ensure privacy and security for personal health information (CDC, 2020, para 2; HealthIT.gov, 2014, para 2)

Most health care organizations use EHRs contain the following features: electronically stored health information in a standardized format, tracking of key clinical conditions using the captured electronic health information, coordinating of care using the data, reports of clinical quality measures and public health information, and engaging of clients and families in their health care.

Beginning in 2018, all eligible health care providers previously participating in the CMS's Promoting Interoperability Program (a federal program funding the new advances in health care technology and meaningful EHR use through a reimbursement process) had to start reporting quality payment program requirements to the CMS. The providers now earn points for meeting specific criteria for meeting meaningful use objectives under the following headings: electronic prescribing, health information exchange between health care organizations, provider-to-client exchange, and public health and clinical data exchange (from provider to national clinical data registries such as immunization, public health, and clinical data registries; syndrome surveillance reporting, and electronic case reporting). The goal for reporting cases to the various registries and reporting systems is to improve data collection for public health initiatives (CDC, 2020).

Electronic documentation of client care comes with benefits, barriers, and hazards. Benefits include immediate documentation as care is delivered when computer terminals are in rooms or if nurses use tablets or handheld devices; elimination of the need for duplicate documentation (once data is entered, it appears on all required forms); automatic reminders for nurses of upcoming care tasks; notification when tasks are due or overdue; reduction of issues with interprofessional communication because of use of standard terminology; transmission of information from monitoring devices for immediate entry; specialized flow sheets to be generated for identified health issues (e.g., screening for sepsis documentation); a consistent order and format to facilitate data retrieval; storage of data apart from the health record form, enabling data extraction for quality reporting and research; and enhancement of client safety and timely care delivery because of notifications of new orders, client data trends associated with deteriorating health, and eliminating the need to decipher others' handwriting. Barriers and frustrations

to EHR use include high costs, increased waiting times for computers to start, having to scroll or click multiple times to find the appropriate screen for the desired documentation, multiple clicks to complete documentation entries, cumbersome order entry, and screens that are difficult to read or disappear because of time limits for documenting medications. Electronic documentation has not reduced the time nurses spend in documenting client care (Nation & Wangia-Anderson, 2019). Hazards include system failures (computers going down, needing updating, and power outages), overly simplified charting (checking boxes for health findings and inability to document detailed notes on abnormal assessment findings), and duplicate documentation on paper for later computer entry (increases the chance for error or inconsistency of data).

Nurses frequently use paper to help organize their day. Many nurses find it useful to print and carry computerized reports. Privacy concerns arise if nurses accidently leave a report in a location with public access. Privacy issues also arise should a nurse forget to log off a computer following client care documentation or if computer screens can be read by someone other than the user.

However, when nurses realize that computerized systems provide them with messages about things that need to be done within a specific time frame, some nurses (including the text author) have abandoned the use of printed client reports when providing inpatient care. Reduction in care errors is a key element of meaningful use of EHRs. Nurses who use nursing care reminders report having fewer misses or more near misses in care delivery (Piscotty et al., 2015). The following Focus on Research box, "How Health Care Information Technology Impacts Nursing Practice" outlines how nurses believe health care information technology assists them in providing the right care at the right time to clients in daily clinical practice.

Personal Electronic Health Records

Many people keep personal health records. A computer-savvy health care consumer may keep a **personal electronic health record (PEHR)**. PEHRs emerged when people began entering their personal health information into their home computers. Some PEHRs are stored in secure electronic databases; others can be accessed using smart phones. Benefits of a PEHR include error reduction, seamless health care delivery, improved outcomes for some chronic illnesses (e.g., asthma, diabetes, HIV, hypertension,

FOCUS ON RESEARCH

How Health Care Information Technology Impacts Nursing Practice

One hundred fourteen nurses working in a large teaching hospital participated in a descriptive study to identify the nurse's perceived impact of health information technology on clinical practice and how it mediated the relationship between nurse electronic reminder use and missed nursing care events.

Using online surveys, the participants completed three surveys: the Nursing Care Reminder Usage Survey (RCRS), the Impact of Health Information Technology Scale (I-HIT), and the Missed Nursing Care Survey (MISSCARE). Data were analyzed using multiple regression equations to identify any mediating effects among the variables.

The investigators found that nurses who perceived that health information technology affected their clinical practice reported fewer incidents of missed nursing care ($t = -4.12$, $p < 0.001$) and accounted for 9.8% variance in missed nursing care. When I-HIT was present, the reminder use scores were no longer significant, but if I-HIT was not present, the reminder use increased. Thus, the investigators interpreted that I-HIT mediated the relationship between reminder usage and missed nursing care.

The researchers concluded that nurses who recognize the impact of health care information technology tend to use electronic nurse messages and have fewer incidents of missed nursing care. Nurses who discount the impact of health information technology tended not to use electronic nurse messages and reported more incidents of missed care.

This study provides evidence that health care information technology improves the safety and efficiency of nursing care. However, sometimes nurses may tend to ignore key messages related to client care if they discount the impact of technology over paper methods of keeping track of client care in daily clinical practice.

These results should be interpreted with caution because there was no documentation on the validity and reliability of instruments used to collect data, and no power analysis to determine sample size and the nurses who participated in the study; 114 out of 169 nurses may differ from the nurse nonparticipants. The study is also limited to one hospital.

More research is needed to know what specific nurse reminders are useful to nurses in clinical practice, the effects of redundant nurse reminder messages, and what nurses would prefer to have in the nursing component of EHR software to facilitate organizing all the care activities required in a day of clinical practice.

Piscotty, R. J., Kalisch, B., & Gracey-Thomas, A. (2015). Impact of healthcare information technology on nursing practice. *Journal of Nursing Scholarship, 47*(4), 287–293. doi: 10.1111/jnu.12138

and hyperlipidemia), increased consumer control of well-being, consumer convenience of requesting prescription refills, and direct communication with providers. Interactive PEHRs enable consumers to feel more empowered and to actively participate in the management of their health conditions. If they are integrated with personal health tracking applications and software, the health care provider can note additional positive or negative trends associated with the client's health. A PEHR enables a new care provider to access specific health information about a client, including diagnostic tests (including viewing digitalized radiographic films if the PEHR is linked to an integrated health care delivery system), accurate lists of currently prescribed medications, and up-to-date third-party payment information (Fylan et al., 2018).

Unfortunately, there are no universal or standardized versions of PEHRs. The American Health Information Management Association keeps records of progress toward standardization and policy development about electronic health information on its website. The "Putting Patients First" initiative from the National Health Council was the first to specify that health information should be "portable, belong to the patient, and empower the patient to make informed decisions regarding care" (Nelson, 2007, p. 27). The National Health Council also emphasized the importance of standardization of electronic platforms used for PEHRs so that when a person changes insurance coverage or health care providers, there is no loss of health information. The Affordable Care Act has also set regulations defining criteria for standardization of PEHRs (HealthIT.gov, 2010). Currently, more than 65 software programs are available for PEHRs; some offer the ability of transfer of data between software programs. Hospitals, outpatient facilities, physician offices, and integrated health care systems currently purchase computer platforms and software for keeping client EHRs, and some offer clients access to PEHR software programs. Some physician offices send annual reminders to clients to update their PEHRs.

Logue and Effken (2012, 2013) developed the Personal Health Records Adoption Model to explain why some people decide to use PEHRs. The model remains relevant for current professional practice. This model identifies four interactive factors that contribute to behavior required for PEHR adoption by health care consumers:

1. *Personal factors* encompass cognitive abilities, emotional attributes, and biologic characteristics that influence decisions for changing behaviors (intention to act and actual action).
2. *Environmental factors* include social and physical conditions that influence behavior.
3. *Technology factors* include resource availability, compatibility, and cost; perceived usefulness; perceptions of external control; ability to observe and try the system; complexity; and relative advantage.
4. *Chronic disease factors* are separated from personal factors based on the belief that self-management of and chronic diseases themselves create specific contexts and a variety of influencing factors, especially when people with chronic diseases have specific care preferences, understand the complex nature of their disease, see multiple health care providers in various settings, engage in negotiated collaboration with health team members, and prefer to self-manage their conditions.

Before people adopt PEHRs, they need to have some ability to understand and use computer technology, perceive that PEHRs would be useful and advantageous, and have the time to enter and update personal health data. The PEHR system must also have the ability to provide online support should consumers experience difficulties accessing or navigating within the program. Consumers experience frustration if support services are only available during business hours, as they may want to access their records later in the day. Nurses can assist clients directly by helping them enter data or indirectly by providing education, support, and guidance as clients develop and maintain their PEHRs. In an ideal world, consumers would be offered the opportunity to access their PEHR during each outpatient visit.

Many nurses currently use computer tablets, smart phones, wearable devices, and other electronic devices with software or apps for managing daily tasks, keeping calendars, calculating medication dosages or complex clinical calculations (e.g., body mass index, corrected serum calcium levels), and consulting clinical references (e.g., medication information and terminology, disease references, medical calculation software programs). Some health care organizations issue unit cell phones to nurses for use in the clinical setting to facilitate staff communications. Most health care organizations provide convenient ways for nurses to access and document information in client EHRs, such as having computers in every room, providing mobile, laptop, or tablet computers, or placing computers in strategic locations throughout the work setting.

Take Note!

Not only do EHRs eliminate the need for paper, but they also allow instantaneous transfer of client information to all relevant health care personnel.

Informatics Beyond the EHR

Health care informatics encompasses more than EHRs. The **American Medical Informatics Association (AMIA)** identifies four categories of medical health care informatics (Kulikowski et al., 2012):

1. **Clinical research informatics** for new discoveries about health and illnesses
2. **Consumer health informatics** for client and family use, especially in the areas of health literacy and education, with the aim of giving people valid and reliable information and resources, such as tools for identifying health risk assessments, maintaining PEHRs, and accessing all forms of health-related information in lay terminology
3. **Public health informatics** for disease surveillance and reporting, health promotion, electronic lab reporting, and coordination of outbreak responses
4. **Translational bioinformatics** for storage, analysis, and interpretation to optimize integration of new research and treatment strategies into predictive, preventive, and participatory health care, such as the use of molecular information (e.g., genomic data) into practical clinical applications

Nurses deal primarily with **clinical informatics**, which has been subdivided into specialty job positions of systems and support analysts, systems administrators, training managers, project managers and leaders, and chief information officers. To facilitate computer and information systems use for nurses, expert or nursing liaison positions have been developed. Informatics specialists design software programs and computer systems to manage information related to clients and health care. Specialists who focus on the health care delivery aspects design software and create integrated systems that facilitate health care delivery (American Nurses Credentialing Center [ANCC], 2018).

The **Alliance for Nursing Informatics (ANI)** consists of 25 nursing informatics associations, representing over 25,000 nurse informaticists. The organization is cosponsored by the Health Information and Management System Society and the AMIA who identified the need for the specialty of nursing informatics. The goal of the organization is "to advance nursing informatics leadership, practice, education, policy, and research by providing a unified voice of nursing informatics organizations" (Alliance for Nursing Informatics [ANI], 2020a, para 1). The organization provides a nursing perspective on health care informatics, addresses issues surrounding nursing practice, and focuses on nursing phenomena and incorporating the values and beliefs of professional nursing (Alliance for Nursing Informatics, 2020b).

The AMIA (2021) recognizes five subspecialties in the arena of informatics. **Nursing informatics** is a subspecialty of health care informatics that address the unique issues contained within the domain of nursing. These are clinical informatics (used for direct and indirect client care), consumer health informatics (used by clients to get health-related information), educational informatics (used for client, staff, and student education), public health informatics (used for tracking public health information), and research in nursing informatics (used to track client outcomes and the effectiveness of nursing interventions). ANI works closely with the American Nurses Association (ANA) to develop scope and standards of nursing informatics practice and to determine credentialing criteria for certification in the field of nursing informatics. ANA and ANI collaborate with the National League for Nursing and Technology Informatics Guiding Education Reform Collaborative Workgroup to determine informatics competencies across the nursing education spectrum. ANI also collaborates with AMIA and the Healthcare Information Management Systems Society so that nursing has a voice in the development of effective health care informatics and information systems. Recognizing the importance of engagement in public policy development, ANI issues position statements regarding pending legislation, drafts of regulations, and issues arising that impact the practice of nursing informatics (ANI 2020a).

Take Note!
For effective clinical practice, nurses must know how to use computers and manage enormous volumes of information.

■ Questions for Reflection

1. What are your current skills and abilities with computers and technology? How have you refined your skills and abilities to keep up with the pace of change in this area?

2. What additional skills would you like to acquire and why do you think they might be useful to you in your future nursing career?

3. What are the benefits and hazards of giving clients online access to their own EHRs from a provider's office? Why do you think that these examples are benefits and hazards?

Computer and Informatics Competencies for Professional Nurses

Computer use in health care delivery became prevalent in the early 21st century. In their pioneering efforts to determine professional nurse knowledge and skills in informatics, Staggers, et al. (2001, 2002) conducted a Delphi study that serves as the basis for today's competencies. The 2003 Institute of Medicine report, *Health Professions Education: A Bridge to Quality*, noted deficits in current education of all health professionals, including the following six core areas that needed vast improvement: client-centered care, teamwork and collaboration, evidence-based practice, quality improvement, safety, and informatics (these are also the six key areas for Quality Safety Education for Nurses [QSEN] competencies). Professional nurse leaders, educators, and informatics experts recognized the need to develop a vision for integrating informatics into practice, education, and research (Sherwood & Barnsteiner, 2012).

In 2006, the Technology Information Guiding Education Reform (TIGER) Initiative established seven key areas for nursing workforce development: management and leadership, education, communication and collaboration, informatics design, information technology, policy, and culture. The final report resulted in the TIGER Nursing Informatics Competencies Model, which addresses the basic computer competencies, information literacy, and information management skills nurses need. Listed competencies from the model have become part of most baccalaureate and higher-degree nursing programs (TIGER Summit, 2007).

In 2008, the American Association of Colleges of Nursing (AACN) revised its criteria for program accreditation to include informatics competences. The current AACN recommendations for professional nurse generalists outline the following informatics skills that nurses are expected to have:

- Use information and communication technology to document and evaluate client care, advance client education, and enhance the accessibility of care.
- Use appropriate technologies in the process of assessing and monitoring clients.
- Work in an interdisciplinary team to make ethical decisions regarding the application of technologies and the acquisition of data.
- Adapt the use of technologies to meet client needs.
- Teach clients about health care technologies.
- Protect the safety and privacy of clients in relation to the use of health care and information technologies.
- Use information technologies to enhance one's own knowledge base.

In 2009, QSEN established specific knowledge, skills, and attitudes for all professional nurses to achieve competency in nursing informatics (and in the aforementioned key areas). Key knowledge for informatics outlined by QSEN competencies include explaining the importance of information and technology skills that are essential for safe client care; identifying basic, essential information that must be contained within common databases for supporting client care; contrasting benefits and limitations of various communication technologies and their impact on the safety and quality of client care; providing examples of how technology and information management relate to client care quality and safety; and recognizing that time, effort, and skills are required for computers, databases, and other technologies before they can become effective, reliable instruments for client care delivery (Sherwood & Barnsteiner, 2012; QSEN.org, 2020).

Knowledge is not enough for safe clinical practice. Professional nurses must also display skill in the application of knowledge in clinical settings. QSEN key prelicensure nursing skills related to informatics include seeking education about health care information management before providing client care, applying technology and information management (computerized warning systems and resources) to promote safe client care, navigating the EHR documentation,

planning client care using EHR programs, coordinating client care using communication technologies, responding effectively to clinical decision-making support systems and alerts (warning systems built into the EHR to prevent errors from occurring), using information generated from information management tools to track outcomes of nursing care delivered, and utilizing high-quality electronic sources of health care information for answering questions arising from practice and for client education (Sherwood & Barnsteiner, 2012; QSEN.org 2020).

Professional nurses are people who have attitudes, values, and beliefs about the use of technology, computers, and informatics when providing client care. The key QSEN prelicensure competencies regarding informatics include appreciating the need for all health care professional to engage in lifelong, continuous learning of information and technology skills; valuing the technologies that support care coordination, error prevention, and clinical decision making (if they are valued, then they will be used); protecting the confidentiality of the client's private health information contained within her; and valuing the involvement of professional nurses in the designing, selecting, implementing, and evaluating of information technologies used to support client care (Sherwood & Barnsteiner, 2012; QSEN.org, 2020). Nurse experiences with health care informatics and technologies shape attitudes toward its use as well as identifying deficiencies within an adopted EHR program, clinical decision support systems, and communication technologies.

The Nurse of the Future Nursing Core Competencies also addresses competencies related to computer and information technology in professional nursing. Professional nurses provide a bridge for the integration of informatics into health care. Nurses use computers to document client care, find valid and relevant information for client education, access information to guide clinical actions, and use technology and information to improve the health of the people whom they serve (David, 2014).

The experienced nurse must be able to use applications for diagnostic coding, evaluate computer-assisted instruction as a teaching method, and integrate selected resources into a client file. The experienced professional should also be able to define how computerized information affects the nurse's role, assess the accuracy of health information posted on the internet, and serve as an advocate for client system users. Box 14.1, Professional Building Blocks "Checklist for

14.1 Professional Building Blocks

Checklist for Professional Nurse Competencies in the Use of Technology and Informatics

Competency	Yes	No
Explain basic concepts of computer hardware, software, and networks.		
Use computer hardware, including a keyboard, screen, signing on, and turning on the computer.		
Use computer software, including basic word processing, spreadsheet, email, and internet search programs.		
Use a computerized database to search professional nursing and other professional health care literature to access high-quality health care information.[a]		
Access dictated client reports such as histories and physicals, radiology and lab reports, surgery reports, pathology reports, and consultations.[a]		
Access telemetry, vital signs, and pulse oximetry data (all practice areas); access central venous pressure, cardiac output, pulmonary wedge pressure, and intracranial pressure (intensive care nursing areas); and access nursing and other health team members' electronic documentation (all areas of nursing practice).[a]		
Document client assessments electronically.[a]		
Document independent and collaborative nursing interventions electronically.[a]		
Document evaluation of independent and collaborative nursing interventions electronically.[a]		
Enter a basic care plan for clients electronically and update it as needed.[a]		
Take steps to ensure confidentiality of client personal health information.[b]		
Enter verbal and written orders (unless the program requires physician direct entry).[a]		
Determine safe staffing needs for assigned unit.		
Perform basic maintenance and/or calibration of handheld computer devices.		
Enter and monitor client-ordered medication dosages on IV pumps with computer chips.		
Use telecommunication devices effectively (pagers, cell phones, or online meeting applications).		
Assist clients as needed to learn how to use and maintain PEHRs.		
Develop an attitude of confidence when using technologic devices in professional practice.		
Outline strategies for continued client care in the event of a situation during which computer systems may not be available.		
Specify the advantages of using computers and telecommunication device use in clinical practice.[c]		
List disadvantages of using computers and telecommunication devices in clinical practice.[c]		
Explain how and why informatics and technology skills enhance client care safety.[c]		
Identify essential information that must be available in a common database for all health team members to use to support client care.[c]		
Describe examples of how technology and information management are related to the quality and safety of client care.[c]		
Recognize the time, effort, and skill required for computers, databases, and other technologies to become reliable and effective client care tools.[c]		
Obtain education about how information is managed in care settings before working in them.[a]		
Use electronic technology and information management tools to enhance safe-care processes.[a]		
Utilize communication technologies to coordinate client care.[a]		
Respond effectively to clinical decision-making support tools and other clinical action alerts.[a]		

14.1 Professional Building Blocks (*Continued*)

Checklist for Professional Nurse Competencies in the Use of Technology and Informatics

Competency	Yes	No
Appreciate the need for all health team members to participate in lifelong, continuous learning of new information technology skills.[b]		
Value technologies that facilitate clinical decision making, prevent errors, and foster care coordination.[b]		
Value the professional nursing involvement in designing, selecting, implementing, and evaluating all information technologies used to support client care.[b]		

[a]Covered in QSEN skill competency.

[b]Covered in QSEN attitude competency.

[c]Covered in QSEN knowledge competency.

American Association of Colleges of Nursing. (2008). *The essentials of baccalaureate education for professional nursing practice*. Author; American Nurses Association. (2015). *Nursing informatics: Scope and standards of practice* (2nd ed.). Nursebooks.org; Qsen.org. (2020). *QSEN competencies, Definitions and pre-licensure KSAS*. Available at https://qsen.org/competencies/pre-licensure-ksas/; Ellerbee, S. (2007). Staffing through web-based open-shift bidding. *American Nurse Today, 2*(4), 32–34; Lin, J., Lin, K., Jiang, W., & Lee, T. (2007). An exploration of nursing informatics competency and satisfaction related to network education. *Journal of Nursing Research, 14*(1), 54–65; and Nelson, R. (2007). The personal health record. *American Journal of Nursing, 107*(9), 27–28.

Professional Nurse Competencies in the Use of Technology and Informatics" provides a tool for nurses to verify their levels of competence with informatics and technology for general clinical practice. Nurses who specialize in nursing informatics have additional advanced competencies such as developing backup systems in the event of a computer systems failure, designing software programs applicable to clinical care settings, and troubleshooting software and computer system problems as they arise.

THE INFORMATICS NURSE SPECIALIST

The complex nature of designing, developing, implementing, and maintaining a health care clinical information system requires many experts. Therefore, numerous positions in the field of clinical informatics have emerged. Applied/professional roles focus on the design, development, execution, and maintenance of information systems (e.g., systems analyst, support analyst, systems administrator, software designer, project leader, chief information officer).

Sometimes, staff within a health care organization find themselves in the position of deciding what health care information system program would best fit their institutional needs. Informatics experts or liaisons focus on performing organizational needs assessments, helping organizations select particular hardware and software programs, implementing selected information systems, and training users on the selected programs.

Once an information system is designed and developed, nurses and other health care providers need to learn how to use it. Organizations frequently employ nursing informatics specialists to educate staff on optimal use of the information system. Other expert/liaison positions include informatics coordinator, chief nursing informatics officer, and information technology nursing advocate. Professional nurses with specialization in computer applications develop nurse-friendly computer systems to support nurses working at the bedside.

The **informatics nurse specialist** has a graduate education, advanced levels of computer and information literacy, and professional development in leadership. The informatics nurse specialist can analyze information systems and work processes to apply knowledge to client care, health care administration, nursing research, and education. The **nursing informatics innovator** holds a doctorate degree and designs new technologic systems, techniques, and conceptual models for databases and information systems. They employ advanced knowledge and experience while formulating and developing unique methods to enhance current system or design new ones. The nurse informatics innovator also evaluates the safety, effectiveness, cost, and social impact of the technologic systems and researches theoretical foundations of the specialty itself (Staggers & Gassert, 2000).

Responsibilities of the Informatics Nurse Specialist

In 2014, the ANA revised its *Scope and Standards of Nursing Informatics Practice* to address the ever-increasing complexity of health care informatics. Informatics nurse specialists and nurse informatics innovators manage projects, offer specialized systems services, consult with information technology professionals and personnel, conduct quality improvement and research studies, educate nursing colleagues, and develop products and policies (ANA, 2015). Informatics nurse specialists and nurse informatics innovators work for health care organizations, for product vendors, and for themselves as entrepreneurs. Some informatics nurse specialists manage large databases specific to a specialty area of practice. Because of rapid advances in technology, all informatics nurse specialists must engage in lifelong learning. Knowledge of computers and information systems comes through formal education (collegiate and continuing education programs) as well as practical experience (ANA, 2015).

The perspective of the informatics nurse specialist gives the technologic development team a working knowledge of the nursing profession, so client care information can be better managed. Without input of nurses, health information systems may miss critical aspects of client care and may create procedures that reduce nursing effectiveness.

Take Note!
Informatics nurse specialists have an integral role in the development of health information systems.

Education of the Informatics Nurse Specialist

Because nursing informatics is a new area of specialty practice, the educational preparation and role of informatics nurse specialists vary (Table 14.1). The

TABLE 14.1	**Educational Requirements and Role Description of the Nursing Informatics Specialist**
Educational Requirements	**Role Description**
A bachelor's degree in nursing or a relevant field At least 2 years of clinical nursing practice 30 continuing education credit hours in nursing informatics within the past 3 years One of the following: ■ 2,000 practice hours of clinical practice in nursing informatics ■ 1,000 practice hours of clinical practice in nursing informatics plus 12 credit hours in graduate-level nursing education courses from a program offering a graduate degree in nursing informatics ■ Recent graduation from a graduate nursing program in nursing informatics that required a faculty-supervised clinical practicum of a minimum 200 clock hours in nursing informatics practice[a]	Thorough understanding of clinical practice to develop, implement, and maintain information systems that are relevant to clinical nursing practice
Successful completion of the ANA Certification Examination in Nursing Informatics[a]	Provides evidence for competence in the area of nursing informatics
Foundations of professional practice[b]	Nursing informatics scope and standards of practice Professional informatics organizations that can be used for career development
Methodologies and theories[b]	Foundations of nursing informatics (e.g., computer information, and nursing science) Theories and concepts supporting practice (e.g., the data, information, knowledge, wisdom pyramid, organizational behavior, communications, learning styles, change theory, systems theory) Nursing taxonomy and nomenclature (e.g., NANDA-I, Nursing Interventions Classification System/Nursing Outcomes Classification System, Nursing Management Minimum Data Set, Omaha System, Patient Care Data Set, Nightingale Tracker) Mental models of data and information processing Nursing decision-making models and decision support systems

Educational Requirements	Role Description
Rules, regulations, and requirements[b]	Regulatory, reimbursement, and accreditation systems and requirements Legal issues Privacy, security, and confidentiality laws, rules and regulations, principles, and practices
Interprofessional collaboration[b]	Effective communication techniques and strategies Team building and working with teams Planning education, coordinating project plans, and analyzing clinical workflows Conflict management and resolution
System life cycle[b]	Informatics needs assessment Strategic planning System planning Designing and building systems (e.g., dashboards, templates, flow sheets) Implementing and testing systems Monitoring, maintaining, supporting, and evaluating systems
Data management and health care technology[b]	Data standards (e.g., nomenclatures, metadata, concepts related to technical standards) Databases (data types, warehousing data, backup systems, recovery, disaster recovery, client information portals)
Data analysis, transformation, and application[b]	Metastructures (data, information, knowledge, clinical decision-making support, wisdom from evidence-based practice) Data analytics using big data, client safety, quality measures, and risk management Transforming data into meaningful units such as surveys, core measures, graphs, charts, images, root cause analyses, close call events, failure mode and effects analysis
Hardware, software, and peripheral equipment[b]	Hardware selection for specific uses Hardware and software for health care technology trends, clinical devices, communication technologies, recommending and troubleshooting software and hardware, and applying technology to clinical simulations

[a]Certification requirements from the ANCC (2018).
[b]Topics covered the American Nurses Credentialing Center Examination (2016).
Data from Thede, L. (1999). *Computers in nursing: Bridges to the future* (pp. 289–293). Lippincott Williams & Wilkins; Turley, J. P. (2000). Informatics and education: The start of a discussion. In B. Carty (Ed.), *Nursing informatics education for practice* (pp. 271–293). New York: Springer Publishing.

informatics nurse specialist needs a thorough understanding of clinical practice in addition to detailed computer expertise.

The ANA offers certification examinations to validate competence in nursing informatics. To stay abreast of changes, the ANA requires certified informatics nurse specialists to engage in clinical practice and complete continuing education. Hours of clinical practice vary. Eligibility requirements to take the ANCC exam in nursing informatics include an unencumbered, active, registered nurse license in the United States (or an international equivalent); hold a bachelor's degree in nursing or a relevant field; a minimum of 2 years of full-time employment as a registered nurse; and completion of 30 continuing education contact hours in nursing informatics within 3 years along with one of the following criteria: 2,000 clock hours of practice in nursing informatics within the past 3 years, 1,000 hours of clinical practice in nursing informatics within the past 3 years and 12 credit semester hours of graduate-level courses in nursing informatics that are part of a graduate-level program in nursing informatics, or graduation with a master's degree in nursing informatics from a program that required a minimum of 200 clinical hours of a faculty-supervised clinical practicum in nursing informatics (ANCC, 2018). Certification in nursing informatics must be renewed every 5 years, and the nurse renewing certification must document 75 contact hours in nursing informatics to qualify for renewal (ANCC, 2018).

Role of the Informatics Nurse

Software developers and computer programmers have expertise in computer systems but lack familiarity with clinical nursing practice and health care delivery. Thus, to develop software and computer systems that are compatible with nursing care delivery and facilitate rather than hinder client care, health care systems and software companies seek nurse consultants or hire nurses with special education in nursing informatics. Nurses contribute critical information that affects client care. They also field test software programs to determine the ease of use and feasibility of implementation in client care settings.

As computer technology and complex information systems permeate health care, more informatics nurse specialists will be needed to verify that systems address key nursing practice considerations and facilitate nursing care delivery. Table 14.2 and Box 14.2, Professional Prototypes, "Clinical Informatics in Practice," outline the complex nature of health information systems currently in use. Nearly every application has

implications for professional nursing practice. As the need for automated systems to manage health care and document client health information increases, the need for computer analysts and computer support personnel is expected to rise. The U.S. Department of Labor Bureau of Labor Statistics (2020) projects that the need for professional nurses, health systems, computer analysts, and computer support specialists will grow by more than 20% between now and 2029. Nurses certified in nursing informatics have a mean income of $90,920 and typically work more than 40 hours per week. Nurses with advanced education in informatics have the ability to design nurse-friendly systems, direct nurses effectively in their use, and provide support services to other nurses when they experience problems using computer and information systems.

▪ TABLE 14.2   Components of Health Information Systems Used in Today's Health Care Institutions

Application	Function
Admission, discharge, and transfer	Tracks client demographic data, insurance information, responsible parties, medical record number, care provider, and dates of admissions, transfer, and dismissals.
Financial	Keeps records related to billing information for medical supplies and services rendered, tracking of accounts receivable, general ledger, and institutional costs for care delivery.
Physician order entry	Provides computer order entry and almost instant notification of orders to ancillary departments. Sometimes, information related to specific test preparation is sent immediately to the unit.
Ancillary department	Shares information among various departments to facilitate scheduling of entered orders. These applications also provide information related to quality control.
Documentation	Consists of pop-up screens that enable care providers to select assessment parameters, document care delivered, and evaluate client response using checklists. These also have the capability of free text entry should the need arise. Most systems offer care alerts for nurses to see when ordered care has not been documented.
Care planning	Allows the nurse to select appropriate nursing diagnoses, expected care outcomes, and nursing interventions for any client.
Scheduling	Enables client scheduling of radiographic, nuclear medicine, and other specialized diagnostic tests and surgery. Also provides a means to schedule staff. Both systems are integrated into the financial information system. Some systems allow scheduling of client appointments with care providers.
Acuity application	Provides a summary of client care needs based on the acuity of illness and, in some cases, the projected hours of nursing care in order to verify adequate staffing levels to fulfill client care needs.
Specialty practice	Provides health care providers within a specific specialty practice area to collect specific client data. Unfortunately, many of these systems fail to integrate data with other components of the health information system.
Decision support	Provides algorithmic decision making related to specific health problems, client demographics, and laboratory test results.
Communication	Provides email and internet access. Some institutions publish policies and procedures in this system component.
Critical pathways	Streamlines the efforts of the interdisciplinary health team by focusing on specific care outcomes. Because all members document on the same form, a more coordinated approach to care results. When documentation is done by computer entry, comparisons of clinical data related to intervention, outcomes, and multidisciplinary approaches become possible.

Data from American Nurses Association. (2008). *Nursing informatics: Scope & standards of practice* (2nd ed,). Nursebooks.org; Hassert, M. (1999). Information systems. In L. Q. Thede (Ed.), *Computers in nursing: Bridges to the future* (pp. 237–247). Lippincott Williams & Wilkins.

14.2 Professional Prototypes

Clinical Informatics in Practice

Clinical informatics addresses the needs of nurses and other health care providers to streamline client care documentation, keep accurate client records, and integrate various aspects of client care to improve the quality of care. For example, a physician orders a diagnostic test by entering it directly into a computer. The request is received automatically by the department that performs the test. The nurse caring for the client receives a copy of routine client preparation orders and educational materials. When the client leaves the nursing unit for the test, a chip in the client's hospital identification bracelet monitors their location. After the test is complete, computerized postprocedure orders are generated, and the client's hospital bill is updated to indicate that the test was performed and what supplies were used. In addition, the institution gathers data about the diagnostic procedure for quality improvement and electronically sends data to a registry collecting information about the procedure for research purposes. Finally, the updated bill is sent directly to the client's health insurance company.

▌ QUESTIONS FOR REFLECTION

1. How do you currently use technology in your clinical or professional practice?
2. What are the benefits of using complex technology in professional nursing practice?
3. How does the use of technology affect the nurse–client relationship?
4. What is the impact of technology on the cost and quality of health care?

CONSUMER HEALTH INFORMATICS IN PRACTICE

Many people participate actively in health-related decision making by surfing the internet for information about health promotion, illness prevention, disease management, and specific symptoms. Consumers can watch video clips of surgical and other invasive procedures, subscribe to online health promotion newsletters, and receive checkup reminder text messages. When COVID-19 vaccines became available, many consumers used online registration systems to receive notifications about vaccine availability and make reservations for vaccine appointments. However, consumers without internet access or skills to navigate the online registration and scheduling systems had difficulty securing appointments, exacerbating existing health disparities.

Consumer health informatics focuses efforts on delivering health care services to people who need or want services. Consumer health informatics services include telemedicine, telehealth, and telemonitoring.

Telemedicine

Telemedicine provides medical care services to people who are physically distant from required medical services. The term "telemedicine" first appeared in the literature in the 1960s, when telephone lines were used to transmit client information, such as test results sent via fax or electrocardiograph information sent using telephone lines. With advances in technology, telemedicine has expanded to provide people residing in areas without specialized health care services with access to those services using video technology (Institute of Medicine [IM], 2012). For example, a victim of a motor vehicle accident who is seen in the emergency room of a rural hospital can receive consultation from a trauma team at a larger urban trauma center when both centers are equipped with video technology. Physicians at the trauma center can assess the victim, review all diagnostic tests, consult with the rural emergency physician, and make suggestions about how to deliver the best possible care. If needed, the victim may be transported to the trauma center or the trauma surgeon may walk the rural physician step-by-step through a life-saving procedure.

Telehealth

Telehealth, although sometimes used interchangeably with telemedicine, refers to the use of technology for disease diagnosis and treatment of a client at a remote location by a physician. Telenursing refers to nursing care delivered to a client at a remote site. Today, a comprehensive telehealth system enables clients to interact in real time with health care providers using computer connections. Health care providers can see clients when computer cameras are used. In the process known as "store forward," images, photographs, and client records become digitized for transmission from one location to another. Telecare refers to providing nursing care by contacting clients using the telephone to provide verbal instructions for procedures, check on clients following procedures, and track client recovery after procedures (da Silva et al., 2020). With telehealth, health care professionals working in remote locations can participate in continuing education programs that occur in large urban health centers. They also can receive step-by-step instructions from specialists in how to perform complex life-saving procedures. During the COVID-19 pandemic, many states offered waivers for providers from other states to provide telehealth services so that consumers could stay at home and avoid risk of contracting the disease. In addition, many insurance companies added telehealth as part of covered services and paid providers for providing care using this technology.

Telemonitoring

Telemonitoring is another use of technology that allows client data to be transmitted to health care providers. The earliest use of telemonitoring was when clients with pacemakers sent information to cardiology offices using the telephone.

Telemonitoring systems consist of a video camera, monitor, thermometer, blood pressure cuff, and stethoscope. The nurse calls the client to connect to the system and receives real-time images and data that can be stored electronically. This system provides client access to a home health nurse on a 24-hour basis (IM, 2012; White, 2020). Telemonitoring also occurs in inpatient settings. The electronic intensive care unit (EICU) offers continuous remote monitoring and medical services for people in the intensive care unit (ICU). The EICU team is typically composed of a critical care physician and at least one critical care registered nurse who use telecommunication to provide additional monitoring of clients occupying ICU beds. The ICU staff can consult the EICU physician simply by picking up a special phone. In-room video cameras allow the nurse to send real-time video surveillance to the physician. The EICU team also contacts the critical care nurses when they notice a change in a monitored client and order early interventions. Remote monitoring improves critical care client outcomes in addition to lengthening the career spans of ICU nurses and physicians (Loustau, 2007).

Some home health organizations offer clients the option of having a video or web camera along with monitoring devices (e.g., telemetry, blood pressure monitor, fetal heart monitor). Using a high-speed internet connection, the home health nurse and the client can hold video conferences with each other. If the conference reveals no problems, the nurse does not have to make a home visit. However, if a client fails to contact the agency at the specified time or if the nurse determines during the conference that the client needs to be seen in person, the nurse makes arrangements to go see the client.

With consumer use of smart phones and computer tablets, telemonitoring using applications (apps) has

emerged as a new way to manage chronic diseases. In an analysis of nine randomized control clinical trials, Whitehead and Seaton (2016) identified that some individuals with chronic illnesses (e.g., diabetes mellitus, chronic lung disease, coronary artery disease) had improved symptom control, fewer hospitalizations, reduced outpatient medical care visits, and increased compliance to disease management regimens. Using Bluetooth technology, clients could either manually record or use direct links for data to be uploaded and shared with health care providers wirelessly. The studies reviewed also identified that client compliance to data entry were improved for morning (70% to 75%) data transfer compared to evening data transfers (50% to 56%). Most study participants used the devices more readily when the apps were combined with either an instant message or phone call from a health care provider.

Advantages to using apps for managing health care conditions includes acceptance by people who use either smart phones or tablets on a daily basis, reduced consumer time for travel to and from provider office visits, and increased client assurance that their data are constantly monitored. Costs for remote monitoring devices make the use of this technology prohibitive unless the costs are covered by a third-party payer (government or private health insurance provider). The cost for a wireless connection and fees for data transfer rest with the consumer. When this technology is used by consumers, the health care provider incurs costs for personnel used to monitor incoming data, notify clients as to what actions must be taken should abnormal data be received, provide some form of acknowledgment of data receipt, and send messages or call clients complimenting them on using the devices (Whitehead & Seaton, 2016).

Take Note!
Informatics nurses and clinical specialists develop and improve telemedicine, telehealth, and telemonitoring systems (Ozbolt et al., 2007).

EDUCATIONAL INFORMATICS

Educational informatics provides students, health care professionals, and clients with access to information. Health care professionals can earn continuing education credit by completing online courses. Nursing and other health care students have access to online collegiate courses. Students can choose from courses that are either synchronous (faculty and students meet online at the same time for classes) or asynchronous (students access course information at their own convenience).

Most programs use clinical simulations as a means to standardize student exposure to specific clinical situations without the possibility of harming a client. The clinical simulation starts with the student preparation using media to learn about the client, the health issues being covered, and specific skills required to manage the case study that will occur in the simulation lab. The client may be a high-fidelity mannequin loaded with software that makes it act like a real person or an actor may assume the role of the client. Simulations may be interdisciplinary in nature and offer students of all health professions opportunities to interact with each other or they may occur within the confines of the nursing program; students and/or faculty then assume the roles of other interprofessional team members. Documentation during the clinical scenario may occur on virtual client EHRs. The simulated experience may be simple or complex depending upon the level of the student. When a clinical simulation is used, all nursing students within a nursing program receive exposure to a common clinical practice situation (such as a birth or death), gain experience in clinical decision making (without harming anyone), and perform specific clinical nursing skills (Jeffries, 2021).

The use of high-fidelity simulation may be used for formative learning (building student clinical skills, developing clinical decision making, and learning how to interact with others as a health care team) or evaluative learning (assessing student outcomes for skill attainment, clinical decision making, specific elements of the nurse–client relationship, and interprofessional team communication). Some health care facilities are using high-fidelity simulations for orienting new graduate nurses, improving interprofessional team performance in client crisis situations (such as rapid responses and codes), skill building with newly acquired equipment for health care delivery, and facilitating team building among members of the interprofessional health care team.

Online Learning

Access to distance education is available to anyone with a high-speed connection to the internet; perhaps the course in which you are using this text is taught online. Each institution specifies required hardware

and software for online courses, and many have vendor contracts for student discounts. Students can confirm with the program's information technology expert to verify that they have all required resources to access and run the learning platform, access student email, and download required course resources. Many online education programs provide students with lists of all technologic resources required for optimal use of online learning platforms.

In addition to having the technologic resources needed (e.g., high-speed internet access, appropriate hardware and software), students must have the skills for success and verify the quality of education being offered before they enroll in an online course (see Box 14.3, Learning, Knowing, and Growing, "Is

14.3 Learning, Knowing, and Growing

Is an Online Course the Best Choice?

Although online courses can offer many advantages over in-person learning, it is imperative for students to gauge the quality of the course and understand how they learn best *before* enrolling.

The Course

Asking questions about course content, the number of times the course has been offered online, and faculty experience with online education can provide clues about the quality of the instruction. In addition, the following five factors are usually good indicators of a high-quality online course: (1) reasonable faculty electronic office hours; (2) online library resources; (3) alternative ways to interact with student colleagues beyond email; (4) secure online examinations; and (5) course content that balances passive lecture with interactive teaching techniques (Short, 2000).

The Student

Some students may not learn effectively in a virtual setting. The isolation of home study may impede learning for students who rely heavily on peer contact. Likewise, people who need structure and strict deadlines to complete course requirements do not fare well with online education (Short, 2000). Because most faculty–student and student–student interactions occur in written format in online courses, students with poorly developed writing skills may find such courses too burdensome (Mueller & Billings, 2000). Some students perceive that because they determine the time of instruction, online courses require less work than live courses, only to be surprised by the actual time commitment involved.

An Online Course the Best Choice?"). A self-assessment can reveal whether a student has the ability to connect to the class, engage in online class discussions, download complex documents, manage files, and access help. A student should ask questions related to available technical assistance and have a backup plan in place should technologic problems occur (Billings & Halstead, 2016). Some nursing programs may offer backup computers to students for home use.

Online courses can be offered synchronously (students meet with faculty online at the same time) or asynchronously (faculty post detailed learning activities including exams online and students work independently). Some courses require students to attend some face-to-face classroom sessions on campus along with online learning class sessions (hybrid format) or blend required synchronous learning sessions with asynchronous class sessions. A key benefit of asynchronous online courses is the student's ability to develop an individually tailored class schedule, which is especially important to students juggling multiple roles. Access to technical support services at all times enables students to meet program requirements based on their individual needs.

Learning activities associated with online and hybrid courses include faculty-developed online lectures, podcasts, self-pace learning modules, online discussions, online exams and quizzes, and synchronous or asynchronous chats (Billings & Halstead, 2016). The goal of online instruction is to promote student learning and professional growth. With effective faculty facilitation, learning communities can form and flourish (Billings & Halstead, 2016). Students can form online collegial relationships and friendships and engage in interactive problem solving. In hybrid courses, students learn the key concepts and concepts surrounding a course topic, and class time is spent in interactive learning activities such as solving a case study.

Educational informatics also enables practicing nurses to access continuing education programs at any time of the day. Some professional nursing associations offer online continuing education programs to nonmembers (for a fee) and their members (for free or reduced costs). Some hospitals use online educational vendors (e.g., HealthStream, eLeaP) or their own educational platform to offer employees programs for meeting annual continuing education and competency requirements (e.g., in privacy; infection control; fire, radiation, and electrical safety; age-related developmental care strategies; domestic abuse).

Most colleges have detailed websites that contain useful student information. Students can obtain registration information and register online for courses, view student policies and faculty and staff information, and obtain financial aid information, class schedules, and a list of required textbooks for courses. Along with their websites, institutions that offer online and hybrid courses often have an electronic learning management system. In the learning management system, faculty post course syllabi, online weekly lessons that outline required learning activities, course resources, and grades for exams and assignments. When learning management systems are used, there is nonstop help available to students. Students typically are required to have computer systems that have the hardware and software to use the learning management system effectively. Many colleges offer students the ability to purchase computers with all the required features. Some colleges even offer backup computers for student use in the event that a student computer ceases to function properly.

Through social networking, students can connect with other students in similar educational situations or with the same major. Students can check with other students to identify a tutor, participate in a study group, form a carpool, broadcast classes, serve as or find a student mentor, and establish social support groups. Social networking can be done using online networking tools, accessing a professional nursing organization's website, or employing a discussion board feature found on many online learning platforms (e.g., Blackboard, Web CT, Angel). Faculty must set clear guidelines for online student discussion. For example, a faculty member may use the Oncology Nursing Society's networking feature for nursing students to share thoughts and feelings about working with oncology clients. In this case, a student from another nursing program may also enter into the discussion.

Although popular, online discussions using Facebook, Twitter, or other social media have some disadvantages. It is almost impossible to remove information from the internet once it has appeared there, whether through a blog, social media, or other means. Everything posted can likely be read by almost anyone, even future employers, and may "live" on in the electronic world long after you believe it has been deleted. Any person who posts things online may have to assume legal responsibility and other consequences for these posts. The National Council of State Boards of Nursing (2011) have developed *Social Media Guidelines for Nurses*. The guidelines specify that nurses are legally accountable for any client-identifiable information posted on social media. Breaches of client-protected health information may result in formal actions by a state board of nursing against a nurse's professional license (warning, suspension, or revocation). The nurse may also be subject to legal action by a client or client's family for posting anything that can link a client to a social media posting.

Moorley and Chinn (2019) discuss untapped potential uses for social media for continuous professional development in nursing in professional practice. The first way to use social media is to share information with others about professional nursing practice. Social media is an inexpensive, readily accessible, and easily used platform to access a global platform to showcase what nurses do, resulting in the elevated profiles of individual nurses, the profession, and nursing organizations. For example, the ANA and state nurses associations implemented a "get out and vote" campaign for the 2020 U.S. general election and have shared stories of interest about nurses who left home to fill staffing vacancies in hard-hit locations during the early phases of the COVID-19 pandemic.

Another potential use for social media for professional nurses is using it to inform nursing practice. Social media is an accessible and easy way for nurses to share information, learn from each other, validate each other, revalidate their reasons for becoming nurses, and generate ideas for future nursing research studies. For example, many nurses working in COVID-19 units have shared information, success stories, and tribulations during the pandemic. When they share experiences of exhaustion, frustration, and compassion fatigue, other nurses may reply with messages of validation and support. Nurses also shared tips for skin care regarding prolonged wearing of face masks and N95 respirators.

Moorley and Chinn (2019) also propose using social media as a direct way of communicating with clients. Nurses can connect with clients and encourage clients with similar conditions to connect with each other. Nurses can use their expertise to post relevant question to large groups of people, network, and receive information from clients. Social media also offers opportunities to create films, presentations, and other media for public viewing. Tapping into this use of social media must be done with caution to avoid violating any confidentiality and security of private health information.

The final potential Moorley and Chinn (2019) identified for social media is celebrating nursing practice. Nurses can post information celebrating big moments like saving lives or smaller moments like making little differences in a client's life. Celebrating each other and professional success improves nurse morale and increasing the public's understanding of the contributions nurses make to health care world in general.

Take Note!
Social networking offers an opportunity for nursing students at all levels to connect with each other.

TECHNOLOGY IN THE ACUTE CARE CLINICAL SETTING

Effects of Technology on Direct Client Care

Technology has revolutionized client care delivery. Nurses use a variety of technologic tools in clinical practice. For client assessment, nurses use bedside and handheld monitors to collect a variety of information, including blood glucose level, clotting time, electrocardiograph rhythm, cardiac output, blood pressure, oxygen saturation of hemoglobin, and temperature. Some monitoring systems require that the client be physically connected to the device, and others require a drop or two of blood. Point-of-care testing enables nurses to receive instantaneous results for peripheral blood glucose levels for diabetic clients and activated clotting time for clients receiving anticoagulation therapy. Client monitoring systems that use wireless technology enable automatic nurse-paging capabilities when client measurements fall outside normal parameters. Pressure sensor monitors on beds also alert nurses when clients at risk for falling make maneuvers indicating that they may be getting out of bed.

Nurses also use technology for nursing interventions. Most intravenous (IV) pumps contain microprocessors for effective operation. Computerized pumps enable nurses to program administration rates for ordered medications without having to perform manual calculations. The pumps are also programmed for safe dosage limits over a specified time frame and have features for nurses to start infusions after hanging IV fluids or medications. Pumps with complex features enable nurses to program an infusion of multiple medications for specific time frames and schedules. All pumps contain alarms to warn nurses that the pump needs attention.

Many other nursing care devices use computer technology as well. Even some air mattresses use computer components and software to regulate the amount of air inflation. Implantable subcutaneous pumps deliver local anesthetic along surgical incisions and have the technology to regulate the rate of subcutaneous drug administration. Some diabetic clients use computer-programmed pumps for insulin administration.

Computerized documentation eliminates the need for nurses to shuffle through paper records. Nurses spend approximately 20% of their time documenting information on EHRs, which is about the same amount of time they spend in handwritten documentation systems (Yee et al., 2012). However, diagnostic test and assessment findings become available almost instantaneously to the entire interprofessional team as soon as the data are entered into the computerized system. With wireless technology and highly integrated wired information systems, radiologists can access digital x-rays and then dictate their findings without leaving their homes.

Computers can also be used to plan client care. Many health care institutions provide software that enables nurses to enter care plans by selecting specific nursing diagnoses. The software provides the nurse with appropriate expected outcomes and nursing interventions related to the identified nursing diagnosis. Software programs can also organize client care, store clinical forms, and house teaching protocol information. Some programs have the ability to translate client education materials into multiple languages.

Computerized medication-dispensing stations prevent nurses from making medication errors while automatically notifying the pharmacy when the stocked medications need to be replenished. These devices facilitate the work of nurses, especially when mounted on bases that enable mobility. Portable medication stations equipped with barcoding devices require that nurses scan client identification bracelets and medication prior to medication administration. This safety feature facilitates following the "five rights" of medication administration: the right medication, right dose, right route, right client, and right time. This reduces potentially costly errors. Successful implementation of computerized medication-dispensing stations relies on the system's ability to be user-friendly, efficient, and well-supplied. Some computerized stations offer information about the therapeutic action, pharmacokinetics, adverse effects, and incompatibilities of medications in device software. More sophisticated models offer features such as warning signs for potential drug interactions that require communication between physicians and pharmacists before dispensing medications (Hurley et al., 2007). Some

even require biometric identification of users such as fingerprinting.

Nurses and other health care providers have access to computerized clinical decision-making support systems. Decision-making support systems help nurses define clinical problems, generate potential solutions, and select the best solution based on the likelihood of success. Many decision-making models use spreadsheets with formulas to predict the results of specific actions in a given client care situation (Thede, 2003). Nurses also have access to decision-making algorithms when clinical practice guidelines and procedures have been entered into computer systems.

Effects of Technology on Client Education

Going online enables consumers to use interactive educational materials and self-manage illnesses and health. Interactive websites may be sponsored by proprietary companies or nonprofit organizations. Some hospitals and integrated health care systems offer online educational materials to the public. For example, a person diagnosed with early-stage breast cancer can visit the American Cancer Society to learn about treatment options, view information about breast cancer from the National Institutes of Health and the National Library of Medicine, and view actual surgical procedures and radiation devices on the websites of medical centers, university-based cancer centers, and drug and device manufacturers. Sometimes, clients may have more information about recent advances in the management of a particular disease than the health care provider, especially if the client has a rare medical condition. Access to comprehensive, detailed online information may result in client self-diagnosis and treatment based on information found online that may or may not be accurate or comprehensive.

Blogs and social media also offer consumers health-related information as well as links to others with a particular health problem. Often, health information accessed through blogs or other online resources has not been empirically tested and can be harmful for consumers.

Effects of Technology on the Nursing Professional

Some nurses use computer tablets or handheld devices with programs or apps that enable the nurse to access current information, record self-reminders, set alarms, and perform clinical calculations without having to leave the bedside. The more sophisticated information systems enable nurses to record client care information onto the device and then place the device into a docking station or transmit the information wirelessly into the client's EHR. However, clients or families have reported incidents of nurses using handheld devices for personal use, such as checking email or texting, while providing care.

When nurses connect their devices to a hospital's wireless system or use the hospital's internet network, the hospital can monitor and track all online activity. In some cases, nurses have been dismissed because they used their handheld devices for personal rather than professional reasons when on the job. Some hospitals have opted to ban nurse use of all personal handheld devices while in the clinical setting.

Some institutions make clinical practice guidelines and employee policies available on their intranets for ease of employee access.

Nurses frequently access institutional email accounts to stay abreast of organizational news, receive policy updates, and access minutes of staff meetings. Most professional nursing organizations send email messages to members routinely to inform them of new developments in clinical practice, organizational elections, and legislative issues.

Computer software is also used for staffing nursing units and making daily staff assignments. Programs can be used to determine the number of direct client care hours that are needed based on client acuity levels. Some staffing software allows nurses to look online for vacant shifts that fall outside their established schedules and then sign up to work those shifts. By allowing regular employees to sign up for extra shifts, overtime and the use of agency nurses have declined (Ellerbee, 2007).

Record Keeping and Documentation of Care Outcomes

Computer information systems enable nurses to enter, process, store, retrieve, and display data. When computer information systems include Nursing Minimum Data Set (NMDS) components, nursing care documentation encompasses all phases of the nursing process used by nurses in practice. As these phases are included in clinical documentation systems, the potential to report and merge client care information into a large multi-institutional database becomes possible. Thus, a large database may become available for use in nursing research studies and to compare the effects of nursing care across institutions and health care settings. In the United States, the NMDS includes information about client demographics (personal identification, birth date, gender, ethnicity, and residence), nursing care elements (care intensity, nursing diagnoses, interventions, and outcomes), and service components (unique agency code, client health record, admission dismissal or termination dates, client disposition when leaving the facility, and expected bill payer). In contrast, the Nursing Management Minimum Data Set compiles data regarding nursing management decisions and actions across all settings. Establishment of a large database enables the nursing profession to develop best practices based on client outcomes.

Communication

The use of cell phones and smart phones reduces the time spent by health care professionals in trying to reach each other and decreases the need for overhead paging, which can disrupt client rest. Physicians can call nurses directly. Cell phones enable staff members to inform each other of specific events or assistance needs. Some nurses provide assigned clients with their cell phone number for direct communication.

Email can also be used to send messages about clients to physician's offices or inform staff of continuing education opportunities, special institutional events, and personal messages. Clients can be notified about health care appointments via email and can email questions to their health care providers. Because of the confidentiality of health-related information, email message information about clients must be encrypted (digitally electronic coded). Encryption keeps personal health information private and accessible only to those directly involved in the client's care.

Protecting client identity in outpatient waiting rooms and hospital admission departments poses a challenge to health care providers. The use of technology fosters the protection of clients' personal identities in waiting rooms. Some facilities give clients a beeper, cell phone, or lighted handheld device that goes off when it is time to receive care. However, these devices can sometimes create confusion for older adult clients seeking health care services.

TECHNOLOGIC CHANGES AFFECTING NURSING PRACTICE AND HEALTH CARE

Robotics

In the future, some nursing tasks may be safely accomplished by machines. **Robotics** is the designing of machines to perform tasks usually done by humans.

Pharmacy robots are currently used to perform mundane tasks associated with preparing and dispensing medications. As described earlier, robots equipped with video and audio capabilities allow nurses and physicians to see, hear, and talk to clients and staff even when not physically present. Some nursing tasks performed by robots (nursing bots) include meal tray delivery, filling water pitchers, making routine rounds, and taking vital signs (Jossi, 2004). Increasingly, surgery and other invasive procedures are being performed by robots because robots have better dexterity and eliminate human error when performing delicate procedures. Nevertheless, for the robots to perform, they currently must be controlled by an experienced physician. The use of robotics increases access to sophisticated procedures for people living in rural areas. Surgeons have the ability to control a robot in an urban medical center while the procedure is performed by the robot in a local hospital. The use of robots decreases surgical costs when clients who need specialized surgery no longer need to travel to a large metropolitan medical center to undergo the procedure (Jossi, 2004; Yuh, 2013). In some surgical cases, robotic surgery is less invasive, thereby resulting in less recovery time, reduced length of inpatient care, and smaller incisions. However, surgical robots do not provide surgeons with the tactile feedback to know how much tension and force is being exerted on tissue during the procedure. Excessive forces can result in temporary or permanent tissue damage. Sometimes, signs of tissue damage may take years to surface (ECRI, 2020).

Genomic Medicine

For many years, health care providers have relied on a client's family health history for understanding and predicting many disease processes. A **family health history** tracks incidences of illnesses that have occurred in people who share ancestors. Ideally, three generations' worth of data should be collected.

In 2003, the mapping of the human genome was completed. Since then, 1,800 disease genes have been identified. Currently, there are more than 2,000 genetic tests for human conditions that can be used by clinicians to detect risk for developing specific inherited disorders. Clinical trials are currently in progress for at least 350 health-related products made possibly by the Human Genome Project (National Institutes of Health [NIH], 2018).

Advances in genetics have transformed health care delivery. **Genomic medicine** applies knowledge generated from the human genome to develop new medical treatments and determine specific regimens for clients based on their particular human genetic sequence. Initial publicized findings of the Human Genome Project revealed that humans have approximately 34,000 genes and that the genetic makeup of all people is 99.5% identical. However, the 34,000 genes have the ability to make between 500,000 and 1 million proteins. This implies genes do not cause disease, but proteins do. Implications for disease screening and therapy most likely lie with the study of proteomics (human proteins). Diseases with verified or potential genetic links include some cancers (e.g., ovarian, breast, lung, colon), mental illnesses (e.g., depression, schizophrenia, chemical addiction, bipolar disorder), birth defects (e.g., neural tube defects), preterm birth, obesity, type I and type II diabetes, cardiovascular disease, hypercholesterolemia, chronic sinusitis, immune deficiency disorders (e.g., X-linked combined immune deficiency), and neurologic diseases (e.g., Huntington chorea, Alzheimer disease, multiple sclerosis) (Califano et al., 2012; Calzone et al., 2014; Conley & Tinkle, 2007; Dolan et al., 2007; Holden, 2003; NIH, 2018; Spiegel & Hawkins, 2012). Genetic screening and genetic-based therapies have transformed many disease screening and treatment protocols (Conley & Tinkle, 2007; NIH, 2018; Spiegel & Hawkins, 2012). See the Concepts in Practice box, "It's in Your Genes."

Concepts in Practice   IDEA ⟶ PLAN ⟶ ACTION

It's in Your Genes

Genetic differences in metabolism explain variations in therapeutic responses of medications based on ancestral heritage (Holden, 2003; Marshall, 2003a). Genetic differences have been identified to explain the lack of effectiveness of angiotensin-converting enzyme inhibitors in controlling blood pressure in some people of African descent. People from India have survived famines that resulted in a "thrifty gene" presentation in approximately one third of the Indian population. This gene is linked to the development of hypercholesterolemia when Indians westernize their diets (Holden, 2003). Risky genes have been identified in people who experience long QT syndrome (an electric conduction system heart condition resulting in sudden cardiac arrest) after receiving specific medications (Marshall, 2003b). Twenty medications have warning labels specifying that fatal reactions may occur in people with inherited metabolism disorders (Conley & Tinkle, 2007; Calzone et al., 2014; Marshall, 2003a).

Genetic testing of malignant tumors is now commonplace and is used to help tailor treatment plans. Cancer is the disease for which the most progress has been made for individualization of treatment plans. Progress on being able to develop individualized health promotion, disease prevention, and individualized therapies for all diseases is taking much longer than originally anticipated after sequencing of the human genome was completed (Califano et al., 2012; Calzone et al., 2014; Spiegel & Hawkins, 2012). Eventually, physicians may be able to send a genetic sample from a client and receive a medication plan tailored to the client's genotype, resulting in better disease management. Newborns may be genetically tested and receive a lifetime plan (including when to begin taking medications designed for their genotypes) to prevent illness (Spiegel & Hawkins, 2012).

Genetic testing may be offered to people at risk for particular illnesses (Fig. 14.1). However, personal behaviors and environmental factors also play a role in disease development. Once a genetic predisposition to an illness within a family is identified, the professional nurse sometimes becomes a resource for how to tell other family members they are at risk. In 2003, the cost of testing for a single gene that affects drug metabolism or identifying a person at risk for a particular disease ranged from $100 to $1,000 (Marshall, 2003a). People can now get genetic testing for ancestry and DNA matches for as low as $59 and upgrade the testing to include personal traits and health reports for higher prices (Ancestry.com, 2020; Vitagene.com, 2021). Other DNA testing kits may provide information about diet and other lifestyle factors to optimize health. Although clients can undergo genetic testing on their own, they may not fully comprehend the meaning and implications of results, and nurses play a key role in verifying client understanding of results, reinforcing information about treatment options, and providing emotional support. Nurses who specialize in genetic counseling are frequently employed in health care facilities where genetic testing is frequently performed. In these settings, nurses provide clients with detailed information about the implications of positive and negative genetic tests.

In 2016, the ANA and the International Society of Nurses in Genetics published the scope and standards of practice for genetic/genomic nursing. Nurse generalists need to have a solid understanding of genetic and genomics so they can provide safe, effective client care and essential education and emotional support to clients who have undergone genetic testing. Some of the nurse's responsibilities related to genetics and genomics include:

- Recognize when one's personal attitudes and values about genomic medicine could affect client care
- Advocate for client access to genetic/genomic services and support groups upon request
- Analyze personal competency with genomics and genetic science and seek additional education if needed
- Include genetics and genomic science as part of routine professional practice
- Tailor client education on genetics and genomic science to the client's culture, religious beliefs, literacy level, and preferred language
- Advocate for clients as they make autonomous, voluntary, and informed choices regarding genetic testing and genomic interventions
- Engage in political advocacy to determine health policies inclusive of genetic and genomic considerations for health and well-being

Specific nurse generalist competencies related to genetics and genomics include:

- Displays an understanding of the interrelationships of relationships of genetics and genomics to health promotion, disease prevention, screenings, diagnostics, prognostics, selecting treatment, and monitoring treatment effects
- Collects client's family history for a minimum of three generations using standardized symbols and terms to construct a pedigree from a client's family history
- Uses standardized symbols and terms to construct a pedigree from a client's family history
- Assesses client's personal, health, and developmental histories inclusive of genetic, environmental, and genomic risks and influences on health and well-being

FIGURE 14.1 Genetic and genomic testing enable providers and consumers to make scientifically based decisions related to health promotion, early screenings, disease prevention, and tailored treatment plans for individuals.

- Analyzes health and physical assessment data for the presence of genetic, environmental, and genomic risks and influence on health and well-being
- Assesses and acknowledges client knowledge, perceptions, attitudes, and responses to genetic and genomic information
- Creates a holistic nursing care plan that considers genetic and genomic assessment findings

Nurses can play a key role in shaping public policy regarding access to genetic testing and therapies for all people. Nurses also need to build knowledge for evidence-based practice so that effective public and client education about genomics and proteomics can be implemented. Finally, nurses must collaborate with interprofessional team members to evaluate the effectiveness of advances in health care based on new genetic and protein information.

Take Note!
Technologic advances in health care diagnostics and treatment are changing the ways in which nurses will treat clients.

CHALLENGES IN MANAGING HEALTH-RELATED INFORMATICS AND TECHNOLOGY

The rapid introduction of **technology in clinical practice** provides a challenge to professional nurses. Just as the nurse becomes competent and confident with a new piece of client care equipment, it may seem as if the medical device manufacturer introduces a newer version. Although new generations of client care equipment usually contain features that increase accuracy or efficiency, some nurses find it challenging to adapt to constantly changing equipment.

ECRI is an independent nonprofit organization that strives to provide the safest and best health care for everyone. The organization has an independent laboratory that tests medical devices and products. It also collects data related to care errors and near misses. In 2020, ECRI compiled a report outlining the top 10 list of technology hazards in health care. This list is provided in Table 14.3. By being aware of technology hazards in the clinical practice environment, nurses and other health care professionals can exercise appropriate caution when using them.

The vast amount of available health-related information also creates challenges for health care professionals and consumers alike. The ever-increasing use of technology and computers in health care makes it imperative

that professional nurses ensure ethical use of protected health information, determine the quality of health information for use in practice, maintain data security, and struggle to stay abreast of new developments.

Confidentiality

To protect people from discrimination based on genetic testing, the United States provided legal protection through the Genetic Confidentiality and Nondiscriminatory Act of 1997. When medical and pharmaceutical research centers use biologic material and data to develop new therapies for illnesses, the donors of human tissue and cells have the right to privacy. Nevertheless, pharmaceutical companies and research centers retain the right to ownership of discoveries from human-extracted materials (Lee, 2012).

The Health Information Portability Accountability Act (HIPAA) mandates confidentiality of client medical records and certain information shared with insurance companies, physicians, hospitals, and other health care providers. Access to private health information (PHI) is limited either to people who are directly involved in the client's care or to people designated by the client (U.S. Department of Health and Human Services Office of Civil Rights, 2013). HIPAA requires health care organizations to offer education about PHI to all employees and that employees review PHI policies annually. Initial education about HIPAA occurs before employees (and nursing students) start working with clients in a clinical setting. Content for HIPAA education includes a definition of PHI, strategies to protect PHI, legal use of PHI, and consequences for misuse of PHI.

Documented consent from the health care consumer is required before health care providers can disclose PHI to anyone not involved directly in the client's care (including family members). HIPAA provides health care consumers with the following four rights: (1) to receive written notice related to PHI storage and use changes before they are implemented, (2) to access and view one's health information, (3) to obtain an account of how PHI has been disclosed, and (4) to request a correction or amendment to PHI. Violators may be fined $25,000 to $250,000 and imprisoned for up to 10 years. Most health care organizations employ privacy officers to protect PHI (U.S. Department of Health and Human Services Office of Civil Rights, 2013). Some terminate employees for accessing the PHI of anyone who is not under their direct care.

Health care organizations take extreme care to ensure confidentiality of their client's PHI. Computer screens, fax machines, and even boards containing

TABLE 14.3 ECRI's Top 10 Health Care Technology Hazards

Device	Scope of Hazards
Surgical staplers	Misuse or misfiring of the stapler has resulted in 412 deaths, and 11,181 serious injuries between 2011 and 2019. In the same time, reports of 98,404 incidents of misfirings were reported to the Food and Drug Administration (FDA).
Point-of-care ultrasound	Point-of-care ultrasound units are convenient and can result in immediate diagnosis. However, not all people operating ultrasound machines have the education to know when and how to use it effectively. Safeguards to protect the consumer have not kept pace with their adoption. Misdiagnosis and overreliance place consumers at risk when more comprehensive images should be performed by imaging specialists.
Sterilizers in medical and dental offices	Incidences of operation failure and poor maintenance have been reported. Many practices fail to have a qualified staff member or a contractor that performs routine maintenance or to educate others in the safe operation of devices to assure proper cleaning, disinfecting, and sterilizing reusable equipment used for consumer care. No periodic competency validation processes are required for users of sterilizing equipment.
Hemodialysis central venous catheters	Inpatient and outpatient dialysis facilities can effectively manage and troubleshoot central venous catheters. However, with recent federal government initiatives for home dialysis, home care providers (usually family members) do not have the knowledge and skills to maintain sterility when catheters are used, dressings are changed, and when problems arise.
Unproven robotic surgical procedures	Robots fail to provide tactile feedback to surgeons on the force of exertion to tissues involved in the procedure. A 2019 FDA report noted it may take years for complications from robotic surgery to appear. Sometimes, surgeons move from hospital to hospital following a series of unsuccessful procedures, obscuring their track records. More robust training, education, credentialing, and granting of privileges to surgeons and operating room staff is needed. Hospitals need to provide strict processes for approving new robotic surgical procedures.
Alarm, alert, and notification overload	Nurses and other direct care providers report sensory overload from the constant exposure to alarms, alerts, and notifications. This may desensitize nurses and others from attending to alarms and alerts and cause distractions as they try to decipher the urgency of multiple alarms. Sometimes, distractions can result in failure to reset alarms. Some EHRs have pop-up notifications for clinical decisions and required documentation that may also be bypassed or ignored.
Cybersecurity in the connected home care environment	Home networks fail to have protection against data flow, alteration, or degradation. A lack of cybersecurity safeguards can result in misdiagnoses or care delays.
Missing implant data	Direct harm can result if magnetic resonance imaging (MRI) is conducted when clients have implants or implanted devices containing metal. Testing delays have occurred when clients cannot recall if they have had implants. An implant list similar to an allergy list needs to be deployed in all EHRs.
Medication errors related to dose timing	Missed or delayed medications occur in EHRs when the system relies upon complex processes for providers to change a routine medication time, especially when new medications are ordered. An example of a solution would be to provide a "now" option or to easily adjust a medication administration time especially when new medications are ordered. Delays and omissions of newly ordered medications have resulted in significant clinical consequences including death or transfer to critical care units.
Loose nuts and bolts on equipment	Loose or missing nuts and bolts can result in devices collapsing, falling, or tipping. From 2018 to 2019, two dozen reports of equipment failure were submitted to ECRI. Equipment included baby scales, carts, and massive angiography systems. Staff need to be alert to unusual noises or device movements as they are warming signs of loose nuts and bolts. They should also note any missing or loose fasteners on clinical care devices.

Data from ECRI (2020). *The top 10 list of technology hazards in health care. Executive Brief.* Retrieved November 11, 2020, from https://www.ecri.org/landing-2020-top-ten-health-technology-hazards

client names are placed in locations accessible only to health care providers. All email messages containing PHI must be encrypted.

Health care institutions that use EHRs protect private data with passwords and firewalls. Many health care providers sign binding confidentiality agreements. Most health care organizations have departments devoted to information management that set policies for computer access and for managing violations of computer security policies.

Wielawski (2020) noted some health care organizations have formed partnerships with Google. St. Louis-based Ascension Health formed a partnership with Google, enabling the tech company to access health records of 10 million clients. The collaborative partnership proposes to use artificial intelligence and other sophisticated mechanized learning systems to discover disease patterns and assist clinicians in making decisions while developing treatment plans. The Mayo Clinic in Rochester, Minnesota, has also embarked on a similar partnership with Google, but has contract provisions giving the Mayo Clinic exclusive control over client data access as well as processes to conceal client identities. Benefits of health systems partnering with tech companies include state-of-the-art cybersecurity, assistance with fixing EHR inefficiencies, updates for entering data more efficiently, and improving daily operations management (e.g., staffing, communication, finances, care delivery). Microsoft and Apple also have similar plans with other health systems.

Because of the potential loss of confidentiality of protected health information, the legislatures of 25 states and Puerto Rico have introduced bills "to regulate the privacy practices of commercial entities" (Wielawski, 2020, p. 20). Similar legislative action has occurred at the federal level, but the bills have yet to be passed. California successfully enacted legislation that went into effect in early 2020 that enables consumers to review company-collected personal data and bans the selling of these data (Wielawski). Without being fully aware of potential consequences, some people may use computer software and applications to track their own indicators of health status. For example, some apps use sensor technology in wearable devices to measure blood pressure, oxygen saturation, and pulse rates. These data are uploaded onto a consumer dashboard or flow sheet stored in cloud-based systems. Sometimes, consumers form groups so that they can hold each other accountable, compete with, and support each other when working toward health promotion goals, for instance runners training for a race. These devices may cleverly provide the consumer with positive reinforcement when goals are reached. Unless they read the fine print carefully when accepting user agreements, users may not realize that they have given the app company access to their personal data and/or permission to use and possibly sell this information for marketing and advertising purposes.

Although telecommunication has progressed in recent years, no connection offers complete security, and information can be lost in cyberspace, or "broken into" by computer hackers. Computer hackers anywhere in the world have the capability of infiltrating any system containing private and personal information. Transmission of private medical data to an outside computer or server creates an opportunity for unauthorized people to access it.

Ethics and Technology

Ethical debates regarding new technology in health care are common. For example, stem cell therapy triggers debate about the definition of the beginning of human life; for instance, does life begin at conception or does it begin when the fetus becomes viable? Other ethical issues surround the cost of procedures and access to services. If insurance companies do not cover the cost (e.g., of storing umbilical cord stem cells, using genetically designed medications), then only people with adequate financial resources can reap the benefits of such technology (Korhonen et al., 2015). The Affordable Care Act does not cover every complex, expensive medical, or surgical intervention. Health care consumers with ample resources will be able to pay for expensive therapies and may be able to access care services more readily. Thus, in the future, disparities over the quality of health care for the rich and poor may widen (Korhonen et al., 2015).

Data Security

The potential loss of data (e.g., through hardware failures and system programming errors) is the biggest concern when using individual PEHRs. Data may be lost through the processes of acquisition, storage, and processing. PEHRs can be stored on personal computers, compact disks, on insurance company servers, or on private servers. Routine data backups and off-site storage protect information against natural disasters for health care institutions. Long-term storage of computerized data may be unstable. Recent observations indicate that data stored on CD-ROMs may begin to disintegrate after 5 years. Files and disks can become corrupt at any time.

Computer systems rely on quality information entry by humans. Bad information input results in poor use of technology. Computers cannot detect many of these errors, even though they are capable of performing complex mathematical operations and implementing algorithms for complicated decision making (Thede, 2003). Finally, computers rely on a power source (electricity or battery) to work. When the power source is severed, the computer stops. During a power failure, most health care organizations have backup processes that use paper copies of documents so that client care can be seamlessly delivered. Once power is restored, paper documents are scanned and electronically stored.

The Struggle to Stay Abreast of New Technologies

The success of high-technology client care devices depends on the ability of the nurse (or consumer) to operate them. If a device is shown to promote client comfort or save time, nurses tend to adopt it readily. New devices are more readily accepted by nurses if nurses participate in making the decision to use them.

One of the disadvantages of high-tech care is the inclination of nurses to focus on the machinery rather than clients. Sometimes, nurses attend to machine alarms before observing clients. This practice may result in a nurse being perceived as cold or aloof.

Informatics and technologic advancements will expand exponentially over the next 5 years (Kaku, 2011). With the vast amount of information required for effective client care, professional nurses frequently experience information overload. To provide effective client care, nurses must stay abreast of new developments in health care information and technology, be willing to admit knowledge deficits, consult others when uncertain, and stay focused on the ever-increasing importance of authentic therapeutic relationships with clients and their significant others.

Take Note!
No machine can replace the warmth of a genuine, caring human interaction.

Accessing Information

Nurses can access information through publishing guides, journal articles, and bibliographies on millions of websites. When accessing health information for professional use, nurses should check to verify sites are from reputable source as indicated by educational domains (.edu), government websites (.gov), or respectable nonprofit organizations (.org). Some nonprofit organizations post information that support their views and use their websites to fundraise. Sites of for-profit companies typically exist for the sale of products or information. Once a site has been found to be useful, the user can file it by using a bookmark or a list of favorites for easy access in the future.

Chat rooms and discussion boards connect people with similar interests. Information can be exchanged through synchronous or asynchronous postings. Many nursing programs use discussion boards for asynchronous communication and chat rooms for synchronous discussion. Some professional nursing organizations offer discussion boards and chat rooms but require users to register and log in before posting entries. When posting information on a discussion board (or forum), a good rule to follow is to not post information that you would not want broadcasted on a televised news show.

Balancing Technology with Life

For some people, computers and smart phones can become an impediment to leading a balanced life. The purchase of each new device as soon as it becomes available may be considered a status symbol for some people, but it can be a sign of an addiction to technology. Some people (including nurses) have become addicted to computer technology and spend hours on computers or handheld devices, participating in chat rooms, surfing the internet, shopping, tweeting, and playing games. Small handheld devices enable people to be constantly connected to the internet or to the job. Using technology may also lead to not interacting personally with other people. Box 14.4, Professional Building Blocks, "Criteria for Internet Addiction," presents proposed criteria from Chinese, Turkish, and American researchers for identifying **internet addiction**.

14.4 Professional Building Blocks

Criteria for Internet Addiction

Approximately 6% of the global population may be addicted to the internet with higher incidences among adolescents and university students. The incidence of internet addiction in the United States ranges from 1.5% to 8.2%. The *Diagnostic and Statistical Manual of Mental Disorders*, 5th edition, recognizes internet addiction as a mental disorder (Tural Hesapçioğlu & Yeşilova, 2020). An individual may be diagnosed with an internet addiction if they meet criteria 1 and 2 plus one additional criterion:

1. **Preoccupation with the internet:** The internet becomes the dominant daily life activity. The user has a constant strong desire to use the internet, thinks about previous activity, and anxiously anticipates the next session. They also perceive the need for increasing internet time.
2. **Withdrawal:** The user experiences dysphoric mood, anger, anxiety, irritability, or boredom if they do not use the internet for several days.
3. **Tolerance:** Increasing internet use is required to achieve personal satisfaction.
4. **Use is difficult to control:** Efforts to cut back on use are futile.
5. **Disregard for harmful consequences of excessive use:** The individual ignores personal, physical, or psychological needs, loses their job, or incurs high expenses online.

(continued)

14.4 Professional Building Blocks (*continued*)

6. **Loss of social communications, engagements, and interests:** The person has no interest in interpersonal communications, attending social events, developing friendships, and interacting with family members.
7. **Emotional outlet:** Use of internet to alleviate negative emotions and a link is made that internet use results in feeling better emotionally.
8. **Deception:** The user lies about the actual time and costs of internet use to family members, therapist, or significant others.
9. **Adverse effects of use:** Obsession with the internet negatively affects familial relationships, academic achievement, and work. In young people, there is a high incidence or depression, social anxiety, attention deficits, dysfunctional social behaviors, loneliness, and self-injurious behaviors.

Flisher, C. (2010). Getting plugged in: An overview of internet addiction. *Journal of Pediatrics and Child Health, 46*, 557–559. https://doi.org/01.1111/j.1440–1754.2010.011879.x; Tao, R., Huang, Z., Wang, J., Zhang, H., Zhang, Y., & Li, M. (2010). Proposed diagnostic criteria for internet addiction. *Addiction, 105*, 556–564. https://doi.org/10.1111/j.1360–0443.2009.02828.x. Tural Hesapçioğlu, S., & Yeşilova, H. (2020). Internet addiction prevalence in youths and its relation with depressive symptoms, self-esteem, and bullying. *Anatolian Journal of Psychiatry / Anadolu Psikiyatri Dergisi, 21*(5), 483–490. https://doi.org/10.5455/apd.72881

Some people rely heavily on cell phones. Having nearly instantaneous information related to medical emergencies and community health hazards enables nurses (especially those working in emergency departments or community health settings) to act swiftly, save lives, and prepare for victims of a disaster. However, the need to respond to a phone notification immediately sometimes impedes a person's ability to engage in deep, meaningful, face-to-face conversations. In addition, some people assume that because a nurse is issued a pager or an email account in the workplace, they are available at all times. Nurses need to have time away from the work setting and technology to cultivate personal relationships and outside interests.

Conversely, computers and other handheld technologic devices can enhance interpersonal relationships among professional colleagues, health team members, and families. Online meeting platforms and video chatting enable friend and families to remain connected while seeing each other when people need to stay at home, shelter in place, or follow quarantine guidelines. Whitmore (2005) outlined etiquette for email use and coined the term "netiquette" (Table 14.4).

TABLE 14.4   Email "Netiquette"

Technique	Rationale
State the main reasons for the message in the subject line area.	Recipients can efficiently prioritize email messages.
Consider email messages business letters.	Email has become a formal communication medium in business.
Use proper grammar and avoid using all uppercase letters.	Email is a means of professional communication, and using uppercase letters is interpreted as yelling.
Avoid use of fancy or cute decorations.	This distracts the recipient's attention from message content.
Keep messages succinct but not abrupt.	Avoid being perceived as rude when sending a message.
Treat email as a public document.	Recipients can forward, print, or photocopy any message, and messages can be retrieved from computers.
Wait until anger passes before sending an email message.	Strongly emotional messages can easily be misinterpreted because of the lack of body language and voice characteristics. Also, there is no opportunity to immediately clarify should a misunderstanding occur.
Praise people in person, or send them a handwritten note.	People usually cherish handwritten notes or greeting cards, and these forms of communication are more likely to be appreciated and saved.
Proofread messages before sending them.	Use of automated correction devices for spelling or grammar may not always be accurate, especially when potential homonyms are used within a message.
Use the "Reply All" feature only when everyone on the list requires a response.	This limits the number of emails sent and received, thereby increasing productivity.
Avoid sending multiple messages if the recipient fails to respond within your expected time frame.	If something is that urgent, contact people via phone or stop by their office. Some people check email only once daily or less.

Technique	Rationale
Respond as quickly as possible, especially to messages that are flagged as urgent.	Courtesy goes a long way in the work environment, especially when deadlines for responses are required.
Send attachments only when necessary.	Consider what is actually needed to get business done.
Less is more.	Sometimes an entire message can be sent using only the subject line, but end the line with the letters "EOM" to indicate "end of message."
Mark messages to denote whether they are urgent or just "FYI" (for your information).	Recipients can efficiently prioritize messages.
Think twice before sending unsolicited advertisements or humorous messages.	What you think might be humorous may not be humorous to others, and some organizations may enforce strict email usage policies.
Inform others when you are unavailable by using an out-of-office feature, and provide contact information if something occurs during your absence that needs your immediate attention.	Senders of messages will know of your unavailability and contact you only if absolutely necessary.

Data from Whitmore, J. (2005). Business class etiquette: Essentials for success at work. New York: St. Martin's Press.

QUESTIONS FOR REFLECTION

1. How do you balance high-tech with high-touch in your personal life? In your professional life?
2. Why is it important to strike a balance between high-tech and high-touch in client care?
3. Why is it important to strike a balance between technology and other aspects of your personal life?

Summary and Significance to Practice

Nurses must have competence in managing complex technology and must stay abreast of new advances in health care delivery. Increased technology and information have the ability to improve health care by providing early disease detection, reducing errors, and facilitating optimal use of limited resources. However, increased use of technology may threaten the therapeutic and effective relationships nurses build with others because of the loss of face-to-face human interactions.

Effective use of informatics and technology has become a critical clinical skill for nurses practicing in today's complex and chaotic world of health care delivery. However, nurses must use their cognitive skills to determine how to best incorporate and evaluate the use of new information and technology in clinical practice. Nurses need to strike a balance in providing high-tech and high-touch client care while taking time to lead satisfying personal lives.

REAL-LIFE REFLECTIONS

Recall the conversation among Jorge, Susan, and Amy from the beginning of the chapter. Based on your current use of computers and technology in clinical practice, what information would you share if you were part of this discussion?

From Theory to Practice

1. During your next shift as a practicing nurse at your work site or as a nursing student on your assigned clinical unit, keep a log of how much time that you spend documenting client care electronically. Compile a list of events that prevented you from being able to document efficiently. Compile a list of things that facilitated efficient documentation. Keep a log related to the time spent on retrieving information necessary for safe client care. How easy was it to access this information? What improvements would you like to see happen with the documentation system that was used? Bring this information to share with the class or post on an online discussion board or forum.
2. What computer safety issues can you identify in your area of clinical practice or nursing program? What safeguards are in place to prevent these safety issues?
3. What do you feel are the advantages of using computers and technology in clinical practice for nurses and consumers? Why are these advantages? What

do you feel are the disadvantages of using them in clinical practice for nurses and consumers? Why are these disadvantages?

Nurse as Author

1. Look around your clinical unit and make a list of all the technologies you use in daily clinical practice. Select one technologic device and write a five- to six-paragraph essay on how it facilitates client care quality and safety, and identify any ethical issues that could be encountered when using the device for daily client care. In your final paragraph, summarize the benefits and hazards of using the device and indicate any identified areas to improve the device for client care delivery.
2. Watch the National Council of State Boards of Nursing video "Social Media Guidelines for Nurses" at **https://www.ncsbn.org/347.htm**. Write an essay about how you use social media and what, if any, of your current practices regarding posting information related to school or work may need to change. Write your reactions to the student nurse's and professional nurse's actions as presented in the video, and discuss the penalties imposed by the nursing program or health care institution. Address what you would do if you found one of your colleagues either posting specific information about a client for whom they provided care, or posting something derogatory about a health care agency or nursing program.

Your Digital Classroom

Online Exploration

Alliance for Nursing Informatics: **https://www.allianceni.org/about-us**

American Health Information Management Association: **www.ahima.org**

American Nursing Informatics Association: **https://www.ania.org/about-us**

Mitelman Database Chromosome Aberrations and Gene Fusions in Cancer: **https://mitelmandatabase.isb-cgc.org/**

Daniel Kraft: Medicine's Future? There's an app for that: **https://www.ted.com/talks/daniel_kraft_medicine_s_future?language=en**

National Institute of Health Human Genome Project Fact Sheet: **https://archives.nih.gov/asites/report/09-09-2019/report.nih.gov/nihfactsheets/ViewFactSheete078.html?csid=45&key=H#H**

International Society of Nurses in Genetics: **https://www.isong.org/**

National Human Genome Research Institute: **https://www.genome.gov/**

Expanding Your Understanding

1. Select a topic that interests you as a professional nurse and search for it online. Identify a number of potential websites to visit. Select two or three of these websites and compare and contrast them in terms of the type of website, the fees required (if any) to use the site, when the site was last updated, and whether the information presented is credible.
2. Visit the online source for the Institute of Medicine's 2012 report, *The role of telehealth in an evolving health care environment: Workshop Summary* at www.nap.edu/catalog.php?record_id=13466. Click on "READ THIS BOOK ONLINE FOR FREE!" Scroll through the book and read Chapter 9, "Technological Developments." After reading this chapter, answer the following questions:

   What do you perceive as advantages and disadvantages with the following aspects of telehealth: remote client monitoring, increased social networking with clients and health care providers, and access to wireless health services?

   Do you think that there might be a time when a client might receive only telehealth services? Why or why not?

Beyond the Book

Visit **thePoint®** at **www.thePoint.lww.com** for activities and information to reinforce the concepts and content covered in this chapter.

REFERENCES

Alliance for Nursing Informatics. (2020). *About ANI*. Retrieved November 11, 2020, from Alliance https://www.allianceni.org/

Alliance for Nursing Informatics. (2020a). *Statements and positions*. Retrieved November 1, 2020, from https://www.allianceni.org/statements-positions

American Association of Colleges of Nursing. (2008). *The essentials of baccalaureate education for professional nursing practice*. Author.

American Medical Informatics Association. (2021). *AMIA Mission and History*. Retrieved May 9, 2021, from https://www.amia.org/about-amia/mission-and-history

American Nurses Association. (2015). *Nursing informatics: Scope and standards of practice*. 2nd ed. Nursebooks.org.

American Nurses Credentialing Center. (2016). *Test content outline, American Nurses Credentialing Center Nursing Informatics*. Retrieved November, 10, 2020, from https://www

.nursingworld.org/~490a5b/globalassets/certification/certi-fication-specialty-pages/resources/test-content-outlines/27-tco-rds-2016-effective-date-march-23-2018_100317.pdf.

American Nurses Credentialing Center. (2018). *Informatics nursing certification RN-BC*. Retrieved November 10, 2020, from https://www.nursingworld.org/our-certifications/informatics-nurse/

Ancestry.com. (20202). *Discover the things that keep you connected to family this holiday*. Retrieved November 12, 2020, from https://www.ancestry.com/dna/?clickref=1011lc69asRI-&adref=&clickref=1011lc69asRI&o_xid=01100l5eDU&o_lid=01100l5eDU&o_sch=Affiliate%2BExternal

Billings, D., & Halstead, J. (2016). *Teaching in nursing, a guide for faculty*. (45th ed.). Elsevier.

Califano, R., Landi, L., & Cappuzzo, F. (2012). Prognostic and predictive value of K-RAS mutations in non-small cell lung cancer. *Drugs, 72*(Suppl. 1), 28–36. https://doi.org/0012-6667/12/0001-0028/$55.55/0

Calzone, K. A., Jenkins, J., Culp, S., Caskey, S., & Badzek, L. (2014). Introducing a new competency into nursing practice. *Journal of Nursing Regulation, 5*(1), 40–41. https://doi.org/10.1016/s2155-8256(15)30098-3

Centers for Disease Control & Prevention. (2020). *Public health and promoting interoperability programs (formerly, known as electronic health records meaningful use) Introduction*. Retrieved November 10, 2020, from https://www.cdc.gov/ehrmeaning-fuluse/introduction.html

Conley, Y., & Tinkle, M. (2007). The future of genomic nursing research. *Journal of Nursing Scholarship, 39*(1), 17–24. https://doi.org/10.1111/j.1547-5069.2007.00138.x

da Silva Schulz, R., Santana, R. F., dos Santos, C. T. B., Faleiro, T. B., do Amaral Passarelles, D. M., Hercules, A. B. S., & do Carmo, T. G. (2020). Telephonic nursing intervention for laparoscopic cholecystectomy and hernia repair: A randomized controlled study. *BMC Nursing, 19*(1), 1–9. https://doi.org/10.1186/s12912-020-00432-y

David, D. (2014). *Informatics and technology. The Massachusetts nursing core competencies: A toolkit for implementation in education and practice settings*. Retrieved May 21, 2016, from http://www.mass.edu/nahi/documents/Toolkit-First%20Edition-May%202014-r1.pdf

Dolan, S., Biermann, J., & Damus, K. (2007). Genomics for health in preconception and postnatal periods. *Journal of Nursing Scholarship, 39*(1), 4–9. https://doi.org/10.1111/j.1547-5069.2007.00136.x

Ellerbee, S. (2007). Staffing through web-based open-shift bidding. *American Nurse Today, 2*(4), 32–34. Retrieved May 9, 2021, from https://www.myamericannurse.com/staffing-though-web-based-open-shift-bidding/

ERCI. (2020). *The top 10 list of technology hazards in health care. Executive Brief*. Retrieved November 11, 2020, from https://www.ecri.org/landing-2020-top-ten-health-technology-hazards

Fylan, F., Caveney, L., Cartwright, A., & Fylan, B. (2018). Making it work for me: Beliefs about making a personal health record relevant and useable. *BMC Health Services Research, 18*(1), 445. https://doi.org/10.1186/s12913-018-3254-z

HealthIT.gov. (2010). *Patient protection and Affordable Care Act Section 1461 recommendations*. Retrieved from March 23, 2013, www.healthit.gov/sites/default/files/rules-regulation/aca-1461-recommendations-final2.pdf

HealthIT.gov. (2014). *How to implement EHRs, Stage 5, achieve meaningful use*. Retrieved May 22, 2016, from

https://www.healthit.gov/providers-professionals/ehr-implementation-steps/step-5-achieve-meaningful-use

Holden, C. (2003). Race and medicine. *Science, 302*, 594–596. https://doi.org/10.1126/science.302.5645.594

Hurley, A. C., Lancaster, D., Hayes, J., Wilson-Chase, C., Bane, A., Griffin, M., Warden, V., Duffy, M. E., Poon, E. C., & Gandhi, T. K. (2007). The medication administration system—nurses assessment of satisfaction (MAS-NAS) scale. *Journal of Nursing Scholarship, 38*(3), 298–300. https://doi.org/10.1111/j.1547-5069.2006.00117.x

Institute of Medicine. (2003). *Health professions education: A bridge to quality*. National Academies Press.

Institute of Medicine. (2012). *The role of telehealth in an evolving health care environment: Workshop summary*. Retrieved March 23, 2013, from www.nap.edu/catalog.php?record_id=13466

Jeffries, P. (2021). *Simulation in nursing education from conceptualization to evaluation*. (3rd ed.). Elsevier.

Jossi, F. (2004). *Robostaff. Healthcare informatics online*. Retrieved July 8, 2005, from www.healthcare-informatics.com/issues/2004/04_04/jossi.htm

Kaku, M. (2011). *The physics of the future*. First Anchor Books.

Korhonen, E. S., Nordman, T., & Eriksson, K. (2015). Technology and its ethics in nursing and caring journals: An integrative literature review. *Nursing Ethics, 22*(5), 561–576. https://doi.org/10.1177/0969733014549881

Kulikowski, C. A., Shortliffe, E. H., Curie, L. M., Elkin, P. L., Hunter, L. E., Johnson, T. R., Kalet, I. J., Lenert, L. A., Musen, M. A., Ozbolt, J. G., Smith, J. W., Tarczy-Hornoch, P. Z., & Williamson, J. J. (2012). AMIA Board white paper: Definition of biomedical informatics and specification of core competencies for graduate education in the discipline. *Journal of the American Medical Informatics Association, 19*(6), 931–938. https://doi.org/10.1136/amiajnl-2012-001053

Lee, T. (2012). *Supreme Court to rule on patentability of human genes*. Retrieved March 29, 2013, from http://arstechnica.com/tech-policy/2012/11/supreme-court-to-rule-on-patentability-of-human-genes/

Logue, M., & Effken, J. (2012). Modeling factors that influence personal health records adoption. *Computers Informatics Nursing, 30*(7), 354–362. https://doi.org/10.1097/NXN.0b013e3182510717

Logue, M., & Effken, J. (2013). Validating the personal health records adoption model using a modified e-Delphi. *Journal of Advanced Nursing, 69*(3), 685–696. https://doi.org/10.1111/j.1365-2648.2012.06056.x

Loustau, L. (2007). Working to save lives—from a distance. *Kansas City Nursing News 2007 Guide to Nursing, 2*, 14.

Marshall, E. (2003a). Preventing toxicity with a gene test. *Science, 302*, 588–590. https://doi.org/10.1126/science.302.5645.588

Marshall, E. (2003b). First check my genome, doctor. *Science, 302*, 589. https://doi.org/10.1126/science.302.5645.589

Moorley, C., & Chinn, T. (2019). Social media participatory CPD for nursing revalidation, professional development and beyond. *British Journal of Nursing, 28*(13), 870–877. https://doi.org/10.12968/bjon.2019.28.13.870

Mueller, C. L., & Billings, D. M. (2000). Focus on the learner. In J. Novotny (Ed.), *Distance education in nursing*. Springer.

Nation, J., & Wangia-Anderson, V. (2019, Winter). Applying the data-knowledge-information-wisdom framework to a usability evaluation of electronic health record system for nursing professionals. *Online Journal of Nursing Informatics, 23*(1). http://www.himss.org/ojni

National Council of State Boards of Nursing. (2011). *Social media guidelines for nurses.* Retrieved November 12, 2020, from https://www.ncsbn.org/347.htm

National Institutes of Health. (2018). *Research portfolio online reporting tools (report), Human genome project.* Retrieved November 10, 2020, from https://archives.nih.gov/asites/report/09-09-2019/report.nih.gov/nihfactsheets/ViewFactSheete078.html?csid=45&key=H#H

Nelson, R. (2007). The personal health record. *American Journal of Nursing, 107*(9), 27–28. https://doi.org/10.1097/01.NAJ.0000287504.92887.de

Ozbolt, J., Nahm, E., Roberts, D., & Wilson, M. (2007). Career sphere. How about a career in nursing informatics? If you have the interest, informatics has the opportunities. *American Nurse Today, 2*(9), 34–36. Retrieved May 9, 2021, from https://www.myamericannurse.com/how-about-a-career-in-nursing-informatics/

Piscotty, R. J., Kalisch, B., & Gracey-Thomas, A. (2015). Impact of healthcare information technology on nursing practice. *Journal of Nursing Scholarship, 47*(4), 287–293. https://doi.org/10.1111/jnu.12138

QSEN.org.(2020).*QSENcompetencies.Definitionsandpre-licensure KSAS.* Retrieved November 12, 2020, from https://qsen.org/competencies/pre-licensure-ksas/

Sherwood, G., & Barnsteiner, J. (2012). *Quality and safety in nursing, a competency approach to improving outcomes.* Wiley-Blackwell.

Short, N. (2000). Online learning: Ready, set, click. *RN, 63,* 28–32.

Spiegel, A., & Hawkins, M. (2012). 'Personalized Medicine' to identify genetic risks for type 2 diabetes and focus prevention: Can it fulfill its promise? *Health Affairs, 31*(1), 43–49. https://doi.org/10.1377/hlthaff.2011.1054

Staggers, N., & Gassert, C. (2000). Competencies for nursing informatics. In B. Carty (Ed.), *Nursing informatics: Education for practice.* Springer.

Staggers, N., Gassert, C., & Curan, C. (2001). Informatics competencies for nurses at four levels of practice. *Journal of Nursing Education, 40*(7), 303–316. Retrieved May 9, 2021, from https://www.nursing-informatics.com/niassess/NIcompetencies_Staggers.pdf

Staggers, N., Gassert, C., & Curan, C. (2002). A Delphi study to determine informatics competencies for nurses at four levels of practice. *Nursing Research, 51*(6), 383–390. https://doi.org/10.1097/00006199-200211000-00006

Tao, R., Huang, Z., Wang, J., Zhang, H., Zhang, Y., & Li, M. (2010). Proposed diagnostic criteria for internet addiction. *Addiction, 105,* 556–564. https://doi.org/10.1111/j.1360–0443.2009.02828.x

Thede, L. (1999). *Computers in nursing: Bridges to the future.* Lippincott Williams & Wilkins.

Thede, L. (2003). *Informatics and nursing: Opportunities and challenges* (2nd ed.). Lippincott Williams & Wilkins.

TIGER Summit. (2007). *The TIGER initiative: Evidence and informatics transforming nursing: 3-year action steps toward a 10-year vision.* Retrieved January 23, 2013, from www.tiger-summit.com/Downloads.html

Tural Hesapçioğlu, S., & Yeşilova, H. (2020). Internet addiction prevalence in youths and its relation with depressive symptoms, self-esteem, and bullying. *Anatolian Journal of Psychiatry / Anadolu Psikiyatri Dergisi, 21*(5), 483–490. https://doi.org/10.5455/apd.72881

Vitagene.com. (2021). I need a DNA test. Retrieved May 9, 2021, from https://vitagene.com/shop/?utm_source=cj&utm_medium=affiliate&utm_campaign=Better+Impression+LTD.&cjevent=0f0e11b0255111eb839300650a240611

U.S. Department of Health and Human Services Office of Civil Rights. (2013). *HIPAA administrative simplification.* Regulation text. Retrieved May 9, 2021, from https://www.hhs.gov/sites/default/files/ocr/privacy/hipaa/administrative/combined/hipaa-simplification-201303.pdf

U.S. Department of Labor Bureau of Labor Statistics. (2020). *Occupational outlook handbook,* Computer Systems Analysts, Retrieved November 10, 2020, from https://www.bls.gov/ooh/computer-and-information-technology/computer-systems-analysts.htm

White J. (2020). A guide to Medicare's new remote patient monitoring program: Here's how to implement this into your practice. *Podiatry Management, 39*(8), 65–72. Retrieved May 9, 2021, from https://podiatrym.com/pdf/2020/10/White-1020web.pdf

Whitehead, L., & Seaton, P. (2016). The effectiveness of self-management mobile phone and tablet apps in long-term condition management: A systematic review. *Journal of Medical Internet Research, 18*(5): e97–e108. doi:10.2196/jmir.4883

Whitmore, J. (2005). *Business class etiquette: Essentials for success at work.* St. Martin's Press.

Wielawski, I. M. (2020). Are patient privacy and health data at risk? *American Journal of Nursing, 120,* 4, 19–20. https://doi.org/10.1097/01.NAJ.0000659992.21831.e2

Yee, T., Needleman, J., Pearson, M., Parkerton, P., Parkerton, M., & Wolstein, J. (2012). The influence of integrated electronic medical records and computerized nursing notes on nurses' time spent in documentation. *Computers Informatics Nursing, 30*(6), 287–292. https://doi.org/10.1097/NXN.0b013e31824af835

Yuh, B. (2013). The bedside assistant in robotic surgery-keys to success. *Urologic Nursing, 33*(1), 29–32. https://doi.org/10.7257/1053–816X.201333.1.29

PROFESSIONAL NURSING ROLES

Professional nurses assume a variety of roles—often simultaneously—as they engage in the complexities of clinical practice. Nurses consciously choose the roles they assume based on the nature of the client system, specific client needs, and the interprofessional team's efforts. Nurses provide focused and individualized care to meet the needs of individuals, families, and communities. They assume the role of teacher when providing individuals, families, and communities with crucial information for health promotion and optimal well-being, disease prevention and management, and recovery and rehabilitation. Nurses assume leadership and management roles as a part of the interprofessional health care team. These nurses aspire to provide the best quality health care by constantly assessing the clinical practice environments for ways to improve the safety and quality of health care and actively participating in organizational quality improvement efforts. By using a constellation of cognitive, communication, and interpersonal skills, nurses play a special advocacy role in shaping legislation, developing regulations, and building coalitions to advance and improve health care.

PROFESSIONAL NURSING ROLES

Nursing Approaches to Client Systems

LEARNING OUTCOMES

By the end of this chapter, the learner will be able to:

1. Define individual, family, and community as clients for professional nursing care.
2. Explain the concept and elements of person-centered and person- and family-centered care.
3. Outline how various nursing conceptual models differentiate client systems in professional nursing.
4. Compare and contrast nursing approaches in the realms of family nursing using the change/growth view and the change/stability view.
5. Articulate how nurses can define community in clinical practice settings.
6. Outline the ethical issues when making decisions while delivering nursing care to an individual as client, family as client, and community as client.
7. Explain the differences in viewing communities as aggregates of people, human systems, and human field–environmental field process.
8. Explain the concept of healthy community.
9. Outline the key differences in how nurses adapt their strategies based on their perceptions and theoretical approaches to the three-client systems.
10. Identify professional nursing career options in community health.

REAL-LIFE REFLECTIONS

Lisa is a teenager who prides herself on her skills in gymnastics, ballet, and academics. She strives for perfection in all her endeavors because she knows that her parents make great sacrifices so she can pursue her interests. Lisa's ballet teacher has been encouraging her to lose 9.07 kg (20 lb) because she carries 56.69 kg (125 lb) on her 170.18 cm (5 ft 7 in.) frame. Today, Gina, a friend of Lisa who also takes ballet lessons, collapsed during physical education class. Gina had recently lost 9.07 kg (20 lb), as requested by the ballet teacher, and secured a starring role in a local ballet production.

(continued on page 424)

On hearing about Gina, Lisa has come to the health room complaining of dizziness. Her friend Cindy helps her to the health room. Nancy, an experienced school nurse, notices that both Cindy and Lisa have sunken eyes and appear to be extremely thin. Nancy gives both girls some orange juice. Nancy suspects that the girls have eating disorders. When she asks Cindy and Lisa about their eating habits, they both say they can eat anything they want without gaining weight. Both girls fail to make eye contact with Nancy when responding to her questions.

Nancy, concerned for the health of both girls, recalls that families play a key role in eating disorders and that peer pressure sometimes makes teenagers do unhealthy things. Nancy realizes she has an opportunity to help these individual clients, their families, and the school community.

Human systems are living systems open to interactions with other systems. Interacting systems are characterized by mutual change; that is, each human system can effect change in another while also being influenced (changed) by that other system. Nurses involved in professional practice interact with client systems and the health care delivery system.

The nursing profession defines **clients** as the recipients of nursing care. In addition to being passive care recipients, clients assume the important role of active participants, or partners, with nurses when they seek the services of professional nurses. This chapter explores the professional nurse's role in client systems and differentiates between individuals, families, and communities as clients.

Recent efforts to improve quality and safety in nursing and health care emphasize the importance of **person-centered care**, during which nurses and other health care team members assess the care recipient's personal values and preferences and use this data to plan and implement holistic and integrated care to support the person's realistic health and life goals (ECRI Institute, 2019). In person-centered care, nurses provide the knowledge, resources, and support that each client needs to be involved in informed decision-making processes, assume important aspects of total self-care (if capable), and change behaviors to promote health, well-being, and the best possible quality of life. Person-centered care cannot occur exclusively for an individual because most people are parts of families. Therefore, person-centered care incorporates the family and becomes **person- and family-centered care** (PFCC).

Early efforts of PFCC started with the concept of patient- and family-centered care. The Institute for Patient- and Family-Centered Care developed many of the key concepts surrounding a consumer-centered approach to health care. The two approaches share the philosophy that the recipient of care and their significant others should be at the center and the main focus of care delivery. The key difference between client-centeredness and person-centeredness is that the term "client" assumes a slightly more dependent role on the health care team or other person. For example, in the specialty of pediatrics, the child may not be old enough to make key decisions regarding health care and relies on a parent or guardian. In PFCC, the care recipient is viewed as capable of deciding and directing all actions regarding health, well-being, and the quality of life.

Philosophical beliefs surrounding person/patient- and family-centered care include the following:

- Dignity and respect must be apparent for anyone receiving health care treatment; this includes taking into account their preferences, dislikes, values, beliefs, and abilities with an attitude of unconditional acceptance.
- Health care providers share complete and unbiased information with clients and families so that they can understand and use it to make informed decisions regarding options for health promotion, disease treatment, interventions, and recovery.
- Care is focused on capitalizing and building on the strengths of clients and families by enhancing independence and control and identifying and incorporating the person, family, and care team in health care.
- Development of policies and programs, professional education, and care delivery includes effective collaboration among clients, family members, and

health care providers; these should be disseminated among all members of the health care team and revised when improvement is necessary.

Along with these characteristics, PFCC strives to provide physical comfort, emotional support, and involvement of family and friends (Zonsius et al., 2020).

PFCC means nurses respect and honor the person's and family's values, beliefs, and preferences while placing their needs at the forefront of care delivery. The nurse assesses the holistic needs of the family, and the client and the family work as genuine partners of the health and nursing care team (Fig. 15.1). Care coordination for smooth transitions across the health delivery system is a hallmark of PFCC. Care coordination focuses on what matters most to care recipients and families while promoting the most effective use of health care resources. Outcomes of care coordination include optimally using resources (including personal time for all involved), having everything necessary in place for transitioning from one setting to another, and reducing costs of health care delivery (Institute for Healthcare Improvement, 2020).

Clients and families need and expect PFCC. National standards and regulations require that data regarding client perceptions of a hospital experience be collected and reported. The Hospital Consumer Assessment of Healthcare Providers and Systems (HCAHPS) is a survey the federal government uses to collect, analyze, and report data about consumer experiences in hospitals. Survey items address hospital cleanliness, quietness, staff responsiveness, effectiveness of communication with providers, communication about medications, quality of dismissal information, management of pain, overall hospital rating, and likelihood of recommending the facility to another person. The results of the survey are posted on the Medicare

care comparison tool at http://www.medicare.gov/hospitalcompare. Many health care consumers use this tool before selecting a hospital and physician for surgery or other invasive procedure. The Centers for Medicare & Medicaid Services (CMS) reimburses facilities for rendered services based on HCAHPS results (Centers for Medicare & Medicaid Services, 2020).

To be consistent with Fawcett's metaparadigm of nursing (see Chapter 6, "Patterns of Knowing and Nursing Science"), the conceptual models of nursing developed their views of "the person" (individual) even though nurses practice with families and communities (Fawcett & DeSanto-Madeya, 2012). In traditional practice, a person's family and community have actually been treated as context surrounding the client receiving nursing care. However, the person is integral to the family and vice versa. Because a family cannot provide for all its own physical and safety needs, groups of families pool their resources and talents to create communities. The major questions for the professional nurse are, how do I practice nursing with the individual client? With the whole family as client? With the community as client?

Take Note!

PFCC is not a new concept for professional nurses because for generations nurses have considered both the person and the family when they provided nursing care services.

Change for human beings is lifelong, natural, and evolutionary. As people move through their lives, they establish themselves as integral elements of larger and more complex systems. The individual synthesizes the concept of "me" with "my family" and "my community." At times, nurses effectively and appropriately work with "me" in professional relationships (e.g., an independent adult receiving care). In other instances, the nurse must consider that working with "the family" may be more effective (e.g., child receiving care). Finally, nurses sometimes have to work with "the community," especially when the health of a large group of people may be affected.

When nursing conceptual models were originally developed, Fawcett's metaparadigm provided the foundation. Nursing scholars equated "person"with the individual client. The models have since been refined either by the model author or by other nursing scholars to explain how the models can be applied when the family and/or community becomes the client (or

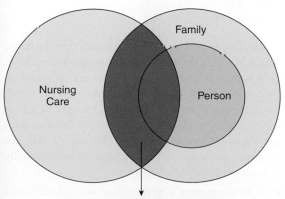

Person- and Family-Centered Care

FIGURE 15.1 The person- and family-centered care model.

care recipient) (Fawcett & DeSanto-Madeya, 2012; Kaakinen et al., 2018; McFarlane, & Anderson, 2019).

1. As a health care consumer, have you ever been in a situation in which a family member or friend needed to have care? Describe the situation. How did the nurses handle the family member or friend of the person receiving health care services? Were the strategies used effective? Why or why not?
2. Have you ever encountered a nursing situation that required more than caring for the individual as client? Describe the situation. How did you handle the situation? Were your strategies effective? Why or why not?
3. Does consulting with family members breach client confidentiality? Why or why not?
4. How can you know when a health-related issue involves more than an individual or family system?

THE INDIVIDUAL AS CLIENT

As people progress through life and interact with their environments, unique patterns evolve. This philosophical assumption espouses that such patterns of interaction determine a person's health. In general, the changes that occur in the developing human beings are characterized by higher abilities to organize and deal with more complex levels of interaction. The individual's patterns are unique and are continuously evolving from earlier life experiences, including biologic, genetic, cultural, interpersonal, and social influences, as well as current interactions and conceptions of the future.

Because the conceptual models of nursing were developed with individual people defined as the client, professional nurses derive directives for nursing practice from the discussion of nursing processes according to both the integration and interaction nursing models (see Chapter 7, "Nursing Models and Theories"). The following discussion reflects our efforts to differentiate the professional nursing care of families and communities from that of individuals.

THE FAMILY AS CLIENT

The question of what a family is evokes many definitions, from the conjugal or nuclear family (the family of marriage, parenthood, or procreation) to the extended family (the kinships of biologically related people—grandparents, aunts, uncles, and cousins). Such definitions have limited applicability in today's society. Families may be defined by legal, biologic, psychological, and social relationships (Kaakinen et al., 2018). Thus, the accepted definition of **family** is "two or more individuals who depend on one another for emotional, physical, and/or economic support. The members of the family are self-defined" (Hanson, 1996, p. 6; Kaakinen et al., 2018, p. 5).

Many terms are used to describe family nursing care, including family-centered care, family-based care, family-focused care, and, most simply, family nursing. These different terms reflect confusion about whether the family is the client (the recipient of care) or the context of care (in which the individual family member is the care recipient). Family approaches to nursing care have been standard practice in the areas of maternal–child nursing, school nursing, and mental health nursing. In the era of cost containment in health care and early hospital dismissals, families frequently assume caregiver roles. Families may also become the recipient of nursing care when they commit to caring for an aging or disabled family member in the home instead of sending the person to an extended-care facility (Gross, 2020). The importance of family as client emerges as a key component of cultural competence in professional practice (Boyle et al., 2020) (see Chapter 11, "Multicultural Issues in Professional Practice"). When providing care to terminally ill clients, nurses sometimes find themselves focusing more on the families than on the individual who is dying (Marrelli, 2018). In today's practice settings, nurses frequently view the family, including the person receiving care, as the unit of care or client.

 Take Note!
A family is any two or more people who depend on each other for support.

The **family as client** approach means that the entire family becomes the recipient of nursing services. Multiple approaches identify the indices and phenomena that represent the family as a holistic unit on which the professional nurse must focus. One approach is to view the family as a system interacting with subsystems and suprasystems. According to Artinian (1994), the following are some of the assumptions of the family systems perspective.

■ A **family system** is an organized whole; individuals within the family are parts of the system and are interdependent.

- The family system is greater than and different from the sum of its parts.
- There are logical relationships (connectedness patterns) between the subsystems. In some families, the connectedness patterns may reflect rigid and fixed structures and relationships. In other families, the connectedness patterns may reflect highly flexible structures and relationships.
- Using feedback from the environment, the family system responds (adapts) to change in ways that reduce strain and maintain a dynamic balance.

REAL-LIFE REFLECTIONS

Recall Lisa from the beginning of the chapter, who is complaining of dizziness. If the nurse focuses on the unit of care as the individual, nursing interventions would address only specific interventions for Lisa. Because of Lisa's age and the nature of eating disorders, however, a more appropriate unit of care would be the family. Why do you think this is so? What could be achieved by considering the problem from a family-centered approach? Why would these things be important for providing care to Lisa and her family?

In the systems family approach, the phenomena of interest are wholeness, relationships, belief systems, family rules, family needs, roles, and tensions between individuation and togetherness. Two theories that are congruent with the family systems model are the Calgary family assessment model (Kaakinen et al., 2018; Wright & Leahey, 1988) and the framework of systemic organization (Friedmann, 1995). Box 15.1, Professional Building Blocks, "The Family Systems Model," summarizes key concepts.

The family as client approach focuses on the family as a structural–functional social system (Artinian, 1994). The focus is the family structure and its effectiveness in performing its functions. Friedman et al. (2003) identified the following seven **family functions** that remain relevant today:

1. Affective support: Meeting the emotional needs of family members
2. Socialization and social placement: Socializing children and making them productive members of society
3. Reproduction: Producing new members for society
4. Family coping: Maintaining order and stability
5. Economic stability: Providing sufficient economic resources and allocating resources effectively
6. Providing physical necessities (food, clothing, shelter)
7. Maintaining health

The Friedman family assessment model (Friedman, 1992; Friedman et al., 2003; Kaakinen et al.,

---

15.1 Professional Building Blocks

The Family Systems Model

Overview: Focuses on interaction between members of the family system and on the family system with other systems. A change in one member of the family system influences the entire system.

Concepts: Subsystems, boundaries, openness, energy, negentropy (energy that promotes order), entropy (energy promoting chaos), feedback, adaptation, homeostasis, input, output, internal system processes.

Assumptions: The family system is greater than the sum of its parts. Subsystems are related and interact with one another, and the whole family system interacts with other systems. Family systems have homeostatic features and strive to maintain a dynamic balance.

Clinical Application: Assess, diagnose, and intervene with family according to major concepts.

Sample Assessment Questions

- How did change caused by the critical illness event affect all members of the family?
- How are members of the family system relating with one another?
- How is the family system relating to the critical care environment?
- What is the "input" into the family system?
- Is the family system internally processing the input? What is the family system output?
- How open is the family system? Does the family system have homeostasis?
- How does behavior of all family members affect the client?
- How does the client's behavior affect the entire family?

(continued)

15.1 Professional Building Blocks (*continued*)

The Family Systems Model

Interventions

- Encourage nurse–family interactions by establishing trust and using communication skills to check for discrepancies between nurse and family expectations.
- Establish a mechanism for providing family with information about the client on a regular basis.
- Foster the family's ability to get information.
- Listen to the family's feelings, concerns, and questions.
- Orient the family to the critical care environment.
- Answer family questions or assist the family in obtaining answers.

- Discuss with family members strategies for normalizing family life.
- Provide mechanisms for the client and other family members to interact with one another through pictures, videos, audio, or open visiting.
- Monitor family relationships.
- Facilitate open communication among family members.
- Collaborate with the family in problem solving.
- Provide necessary knowledge that will help the family make decisions.

Artinian, N. T. (1994). Selecting a model to guide family assessment. *Dimensions of Critical Care Nursing, 14*, 6. Used with permission of the publisher.

2018) appears congruent with a combination of the structural–functional model and the family systems model. Friedman stated that nurses must view the family in two ways when implementing family nursing: as each individual within the family context and the whole family as the unit of care. A summary of the structural–functional model presented in Box 15.2, Professional Building Blocks, "The Structural–Functional Model," summarizes key concepts.

A third approach to family as client is the family stress model. Artinian (1994) outlined the following assumptions of this model:

- The family is a system.
- Unexpected or unplanned events are usually perceived as more stressful than expected events.
- Events within the family that are defined as stressful are more disruptive than events outside the family.

- Lack of experience with a stressor leads to greater perceived stressfulness.
- Ambiguous stressor events are more stressful than unambiguous ones.

Artinian (1994) indicated that client assessment should include family resources, the meaning of the situation to the family (e.g., is it viewed as a threat or a challenge?), the level of crisis the family is experiencing, and coping mechanisms.

Patterson (1999) presented a postmodern view of a family and provided an ecologic perspective that requires nurses to think in layers. The smallest unit, the person, is in the center, with larger units extending outward from the person to include the family, social groups, the local community, and so on, until the outermost layer comprises the entire cosmos. In this model, the family is an integral part of an ecosystem, and many variations

15.2 Professional Building Blocks

The Structural–Functional Model

Overview: Focuses on family structure and family function and how well the family performs its functions

Concepts: Structural areas include family form, roles, values, communication patterns, power structure, and support network. Functional areas include affective, socialization, reproductive, coping, economic, physical care, and health care functions.

Assumptions: Family is a system and a small group that exists to perform certain functions.

Clinical Application: Assess, diagnose, and intervene with family according to major concepts.

Sample Assessment Questions

- What impact did the critical illness event have on family structure and function?
- How did the critical illness alter the family structure?
- What family roles were changed? What family functions have been affected?
- What are family members' physical responses to the illness event?

(continued)

15.2 Professional Building Blocks (*continued*)

The Structural–Functional Model

Interventions

- Assist the family with modifying its organization so that role responsibilities can be redistributed.
- Respect and encourage the family's adaptive coping skills.
- Counsel family members on additional effective coping skills for their own use.
- Identify typical family coping mechanisms.
- Tell the family it is safe and acceptable to use typical expressions of affection.

- Provide privacy for the family to allow for family expression of affection.
- Provide for family visitation.
- Encourage family members to recognize their own health needs.
- Help family members find ways to meet their health needs while helping them feel their concern for the client has not diminished.
- Assist the family in using existing support structure.

Artinian, N. T. (1994). Selecting a model to guide family assessment. *Dimensions of Critical Care Nursing, 14,* 7. Used with permission of the publisher.

in family form exist. Children receive support and protection from family members (parents, grandparents, siblings, and other relatives). The family serves as a unit of the community that encompasses schools, child care providers, faith-based groups, health care providers, workplaces, locally supportive services (police, fire, city, and county services), neighborhoods, and friends. The community is part of society, which is composed of the military, government, multinational corporations, online personal and professional networks, prisons, research institutions, courts, banks, insurers, transportation systems, media, and welfare systems. Patterson (1999) designated the following four family functions:

1. Family formation and membership: To provide a sense of belonging, personal and social identity, and meaning and direction for life
2. Economic support: To provide basic shelter, food, clothing, and other things that facilitate and enhance human development
3. Nurturance and socialization: To provide holistic development and support of members while instilling social values and norms
4. Protection of vulnerable members: To provide care for the young, disabled, ill, or aging family members incapable of self-care or at risk for harm

Patterson (1999) also proposed that each family develops specific functioning patterns that include consistent ways in which they display affection, show anger, cope with stress, deal with conflict, accomplish daily routines, discipline children, seek health care, and celebrate special occasions. The family alters these patterns as it experiences developmental transitions (birth, raising children, departing children, aging, and death). Because the familial experience is multidimensional,

Patterson suggested that assessment using only family questionnaires limits the amount of data collected by health care providers. Health care professionals should consider observing family interactions when families enter the health care system. Because a family is a system, the conceptualization of family health requires consideration of the individual health status of each member and the health of the family's functioning patterns (Patterson, 1999). Alteration in the health of one member usually results in altered family functioning patterns.

Two theories that are congruent with a combination of the family stress model and the family systems model are the family assessment and intervention model (Kaakinen et al., 2018) and the resiliency model (McCubbin & McCubbin, 1993). Box 15.3, Professional Building Blocks, "The Family Stress Model," summarizes key concepts.

Anderson and Tomlinson (1992, p. 61) identified five realms of family experience that represent elements of the approaches identified and direct professional practice:

1. Interactive processes: Family relationships, communication, nurturance, intimacy, and social support
2. Developmental processes: Family transitions and dynamic interactions between the stages of family development and individual developmental tasks
3. Coping processes: Management of resources, problem solving, and adaptation to stressors and crisis
4. Integrity processes: Shared meanings of experiences, family identity and commitment, family history, family values, boundary maintenance, and family rituals
5. Health processes: Family health beliefs, health status, health responses and practices, lifestyle practices, and health care provision during wellness and illness

15.3 Professional Building Blocks

The Family Stress Model

Overview: Focuses on stressors, resources, and perceptions to explain the amount of family disruption caused by a stressful event.

Concepts: "A"—stressful event with associated hardships; "B"—physical, psychological, material, social, spiritual, and informational resources of the family; "C"—the family's subjective definition of the stressful event; "X"—crisis, the amount of disruption or incapacitation within the family caused by the stressful event

Assumptions: Family is a system. Unexpected and ambiguous illness events are stressful. Stressful events within the family are more disruptive than stressor events outside the family. Lack of experience with a stressor event leads to increased perceptions of stressfulness.

Clinical Application: Assess, diagnose, and intervene with the family according to major concepts.

Sample Assessment Questions

- Identify the family's understanding and beliefs about the situation.
- What family hardships are associated with the critical illness event?
- What are other situational stressors for the family?

- Did the family have time to prepare for the event?
- Has the family had experience with the event?
- What resources are available to the family?
- Are the resources sufficient to meet the demands of the event?
- What are the family's perceptions of the event?
- Do they perceive the event to be a threat or a challenge?
- Does the family blame themselves for the event?
- How incapacitated is family functioning?

Interventions

- Help the family cope with imposed hardships.
- If appropriate, provide spiritual or informational resources for the family.
- Introduce the family to others undergoing similar experiences.
- Discuss existing social support resources for the family.
- Assist the family in capitalizing on its strengths.
- Assist the family in resolving feelings of guilt.
- Help the family visualize successfully handling all the hardships associated with the situation.
- If possible, encourage the family to focus on the positive aspects of the situation or cognitively reappraise the situation as positive.

Artinian, N. T. (1994). Selecting a model to guide family assessment. *Dimensions of Critical Care Nursing, 14*, 4–12. Used with permission of the publisher.

These realms remain applicable in the 21st century. Therefore, nurses need to implement the nursing process in a way that facilitates exploration of all the family realms listed rather than focusing exclusively on health processes. In all of the conceptual nursing models, the client system is viewed holistically; thus, the nurse cannot extricate the health processes from other processes (integrity, coping, development, and interaction).

Family nursing interventions depend on the clinical practice context. For example, early inpatient discharge planning requires that nurses teach and counsel families as they anticipate taking clients home. Nurses listen to families as they express concerns about the changes in the family's previous lifestyle. They give families knowledge and skills so they can safely provide care, anticipate potential complications, and know what to do should complications occur. In inpatient settings, families frequently find the ability to room-in with their loved one to be most beneficial. Nurses also assess family dynamics as families interact in all nursing care settings and intervene when needed. Gross

(2020) identified some potential family dynamics that might occur in the delivery of PFCC. These are presented in Table 15.1 along with some nursing interventions to use should family dynamics issues arise. Nurses also need to assess the family's and person's view of health status and verify that realistic health and well-being goals are set collaboratively with the family unit.

Nurses collaborate with families in many nursing care settings to design family nursing care plans when needed (Kaakinen et al., 2018). One of the most disturbing and significant changes during the COVID-19 pandemic was the drastic alterations in visitor policies in acute and long-term care facilities. Open visitation hours ceased to limit the spread of infection, resulting in increased client and resident anxiety, delirium, and depression. Families were no longer present to question actions of nurses and nursing staff, resulting in increased care errors (Owens, 2020).

PFCC aims to keep families connected as well as respecting and facilitating their preferences for care.

TABLE 15.1 Nursing Interventions for Family Dynamics That Impact Person- and Family-Centered Care

Family Dynamic and Description	Nursing Intervention
Capacity: The ability to voice participate in decision making and communicate care preferences	Therapeutic listening for optimal assessment of preferences Inquire about the durable power of attorney for health care decisions and have that person participate in proxy decision making. Abide by guidelines specified in the living will if one has been enacted. Document and share preferences in the electronic health record (EHR). Provide information for optimal decision making with the person and family.
Legal capacity: The ability of a person to manage personal and financial affairs	Inquire about who has durable power of attorney for personal and financial affairs. Social worker consultation
Family disagreements: Conflicts among family members who become incapacitated	Therapeutic listening Documentation of family disagreements when appropriate Social worker or case manager consultation and other consults for mediators and mental health care Defer to court-appointed guardians or conservators who represent the person receiving health care
Single family member decision maker: Power is consolidated, leading one family member to perceive they have the right and/or responsibility to make all the decisions.	Formal cognitive assessment of the person receiving medical care Therapeutic listening to all family members Documentation of the key decision maker if they have legal authority for making decisions Coach the single family member to consult with other family members when crucial, life-altering decisions are to be made. Inclusion of all interested family members in team meetings for planning care Case manager and social work consultations as needed
Caregiver burden: The physical, mental, and spiritual toll of caring for a loved one[a]	Social service consultation for arranging respite care (if care is given in the home) Therapeutic listening to the caregiver as they share the issues that arise with caregiving responsibilities Coach the caregiver that it is fine to ask for help, take a break, and engage in self-care activities.
Caregiver strain: The effects of caregiver burden when the caregiver feels unappreciated or underappreciated without the support required of others[a]	Social work consultation for arranging respite care Remind the person receiving care to express gratitude for care delivered by the caregiver if appropriate Case manager to arrange a family meeting and a formal mediator if family members refuse to help the caregiver
Sibling rivalry: Conflicts among offspring of the person when one of them assumes a power of attorney role or is a preferred caregiver by the person receiving care; sometimes has deep roots in family roles and situations that started when the siblings were growing up together	Therapeutic listening Documentation of any rivalry that might escalate into violence against the person receiving care, the siblings, or health care providers Social work consultation for any required legal action to protect the person receiving care Referrals to mental health services as needed
Butterfly effect: Small events get blown out of proportion and become major events	Assess the family dynamics on a daily basis. Document any issues identified. Remain calm and composed if a situation spirals out of control. Follow guidelines for violence crisis management for the facility where care is provided.

[a]Nurses may also experience this when assuming the caregiver role in clinical practice.
Data from Gross, S. L. (2020). Managing family dynamics when caring for older adults. *Nursing 2021, 50*(4), 56–62. https://doi.org/10.1097/01.NURSE.0000654040.24421.7f

Family presence during resuscitation (FPDR) exemplifies the philosophy and principles of PFCC. FPDR began taking place more than three decades ago when a Michigan hospital offered family members the facility of being in the room during resuscitation efforts (Powers & Reeve, 2020). FPDR is a common practice in intensive care units, but not as commonplace on medical–surgical units. Research on family outcomes of

FPDR reveals that 94% to 100% of family members would again want to be present at their loved one's bedside during resuscitation. Family members also reported that being there provided comfort to their now deceased loved one, they experienced less anxiety during the event, it enhanced the grieving process, and they experienced less posttraumatic stress (Powers & Reeve, 2020). The following Focus on Research box outlines facilitators and barriers to FPDR on medical–surgical units.

Practice barriers may prevent nurses from addressing all relevant realms when the family is the client. Because of laws related to client privacy, nurses must exercise caution when disclosing protected health information about individuals to their family members. Most health care organizations limit the number of people who may

FOCUS ON RESEARCH

Nurses' Perceptions of Family Presence During Resuscitation

Because of limited research on reasons why FPDR does not occur commonly on medical–surgical units, the investigators studied what personal, professional, and workplace characteristics medical-surgical nurses had contributed to limiting use of FPDR.

Using a cross-sectional research design, data were collected via a survey from nurse participants who responded to a study advertisement posted on the Academy of Medical-Surgical Nurses website. The researchers collected data on nurse demographic factors; professional factors (i.e., certification in advanced cardiac life support, certification in cardiopulmonary resuscitation [CPR], and experience with CPR); previous education related to FPDR; specialty nurse certification; and professional organizational management. A presence risk-benefit scale was used to measure nurse perceptions of the risks and benefits of FPDR. A family presence self-confidence scale measured nurse self-confidence in implementing FPDR. The investigators also provided the nurses with a survey outlining perceived barriers to implementing FPDR and asked an open-ended question to obtain personal thoughts about possible barriers. Additionally, the researchers gathered data for participants' preferences for FPDR resuscitation education.

Data analysis was done using software that summarized descriptive data to describe characteristics of the participants, self-confidence with FPDR, and the use of invitations to families for FPDR. A series of correlational analyses were performed to identify which of the professional nurse factors contributed to the most variance in nurse perceptions, self-confidence, and use of FPDR invitations.

Ninety nurses agreed to participate, but it is unknown how many nurses viewed the study advertisement, so a response rate cannot be calculated. Of the 90 nurses who participated, 50% completed all the study surveys for a 57% completion rate. The nurses were predominately female (94%) and White and non-Hispanic (88%), worked in suburban or urban settings (84%), held at least a BSN (79%), worked at the bedside (67%) with adults (84%), had advanced cardiac life support (ACLS) certification (61%), held specialty certification (55%), and belonged to a professional nursing organization (75%). Only 7% of the nurses reported having received education on FPDR, and 7% knew for certain that their employers had FPDR policies. Of the nurses, 63% reported CPR nursing experience, 37% indicated that they had never experienced FPDR, and 57% of the nurses reported having no family requests to be present. Sixty-three percent of the nurses reported never extending an invitation to families to be present during resuscitation efforts.

The regression analysis revealed that previous FPDR experiences were the most consistent predictor of positive perceptions ($\beta = 0.21$), self-confidence with FPDR ($\beta = 0.18$) and extending family invitations ($\beta = 0.74$), revealing small to moderate correlations. ACLS certification had a moderate impact on self-confidence ($\beta = 0.35$). The top barrier to FPDR was not having a staff person available for family support during the process. Other barriers included lack of a facility policy, not knowing the client's wishes, concern for family well-being, family being in the way of delivering care, and need to care for the family members. Of the respondents, 55% indicated they wanted education on FPDR, and the preferred method was computer-based/online instruction (76%).

The investigators concluded that each denied request for FPDR revealed a lack of compliance with PFCC. There was a 43% rate of denials, which is 10% higher than the finding of a similar study

FOCUS ON RESEARCH (*Continued*)

conducted on critical care nurses. The researchers concluded facilities should develop policy and practice guidelines for FPDR for nurses to follow. They noted study limitations of convenience sampling at a very small sample size that may have introduced either a positive or a negative bias to the study.

The results of this study should be viewed with caution owing to the data collection and sampling methods used. Clinical implications drawn from the result demonstrate a need for future bedside nurse education in all areas of the hospital for FPDR

education, having staffing levels to appoint a family support person for each shift in case of an unexpected client resuscitation event, and a critical need for well-developed and fully communicated policies and procedures for FPDR. In addition, national and local health care policies should include FPDR options for facility accreditation and reimbursement to support PFCC initiatives.

Powers, K., & Reeve, C. L. (2020). Family presence during resuscitation: Medical-Surgical nurses' perceptions, self-confidence and use of invitations. *American Journal of Nursing, 120*, 11, 28–38. https://doi.org/10.1097/01.NAJ.0000721244.16344.ee

---

receive client information, which sometimes creates friction among family members. Situations such as decreased length of stay in inpatient settings, inadequate staffing, poor coordination of services across the health care setting continuum, suboptimal communication among interprofessional health care providers, lack of nursing education regarding family structure and processes, and overwhelming complexity of family needs are factors in ineffective family nursing care (ECRI Institute, 2019; Institute for Healthcare Improvement, 2020). In addition, medical care supersedes nursing care in most acute care health care settings.

Nursing models presented in previous chapters explain how nursing care includes the concept of family as client and how nurses provide care to families. The following is a discussion of how the family may be understood in nursing models within the change/growth paradigm (Newman, 1983; Orem, 1983; Parse, 1996, 1998; Peplau, 1952; Rogers, 1983; Watson, 1996) and within the change/stability paradigm (King, 1983; Neuman & Fawcett, 2010; Roy, 1983).

▌ QUESTIONS FOR REFLECTION

1. How do you define family?
2. What ideas related to health and health care have you learned from your family?
3. Where and when did you seek health care services as a child?
4. Do you still use the same approach to health care services? Why or why not?
5. What obstacles to working with family as client have you experienced in your clinical practice setting? How can you create a clinical practice environment that supports family care?

The Family in the Change/Growth Models of Nursing

Nurses who use the **change/growth models** of nursing assert that families experience growth when confronted with change. Like the individual, the family possesses great potential to develop in ways that maximize health for all members.

Orem's Self-Care Deficit Model

According to Taylor and Renpenning (1995, p. 356), Orem viewed family as a multiperson care system, defined as those courses and sequences of action that are performed by the people in multiperson units for the purpose of meeting the self-care requisites and the development and exercise of self-care agency of all members of the group and to maintain or establish the welfare of the unit. The subsystems of the multiperson system are the self-care systems of the individuals.

Whall and Fawcett (1991, p. 20) indicated that Orem's self-care conceptual framework primarily "views the family as only a backdrop for individuals." In her own words, Orem (1983, p. 368) directed the nurse to "first, accept the system of family living, the physical and social environment of the family, and the family's culture as basic conditioning factors for all the family members." She stressed that the family support system needs to be explored and "adjusted as needed and then incorporated into the system of family living" (Orem, 1983, p. 368).

Family is context in self-care. Family self-care involves the creation of conditions for each family to be able to engage in actions for essential human functioning, growth, and development. Infants, children, and adolescents rely on adult family members to provide for their self-care needs. In multigenerational families, the older family members may either assist in the care of younger members or may be the recipients of care if they are incapable of caring for themselves. Both self-care and dependent care are directed toward creating and maintaining conditions that support life and integrated functions toward promoting human growth. Self-care and dependent care "are forms of deliberate action, learned behaviors, learned within the family and other social units within which individuals live and move" (Orem, 1983, p. 209). However, Orem also considered the family to be a unit, "a complex entity which can be regarded as a whole" (Taylor & Renpenning, 1995, p. 350). Thus, there is concern with the quality of interaction and the outcomes of those interactions on the family as a whole.

Two realms of family can be readily implemented in Orem's self-care model: the interactive processes, particularly the social support systems in the family, and the developmental processes, particularly in the understanding of dependent care needs at various life stages. "Conditions which justify identifying the multiperson unit include a need for protection and prevention, regulation of a hazard, need for environmental regulation, [and] need for resources" (Taylor & Renpenning, 1995, p. 366).

Lapp et al. (1991) stressed the concept of the family as a partner in health care decision making. In keeping with the self-care perspective, they see "the primary responsibility for health and life choices as ultimately resting with the client family" (Lapp et al., 1991, p. 306). Lapp and colleagues further suggested that the main responsibility of the nurse is "ensuring that those choices were made on the basis of the most complete information possible while facilitating self-discovery of strengths and resources already existing for a family" (p. 306).

Chevannes (1997) specified that Orem's three levels of care enable nurses and families to develop a caring partnership. The nurse and family collaborate to determine the care level needed to fulfill the needs of the incapacitated member. In the wholly compensatory level of care, the nurse provides care to the client while beginning to teach family members. The nurse assesses family needs for direct nursing care services and additional education as they assume a more active role in caring for the incapacitated family member. Eventually, the nurse provides episodic care to the family (partially compensatory nursing care) when they no longer need continuous nursing care services. Finally, when families assume full care responsibilities, the nurse provides support and education as needs arise.

REAL-LIFE REFLECTIONS

If Nancy practiced according to Orem's self-care deficit theory, she would assess Lisa and her family for their ability to access physical and mental health services independently and offer assistance if the family could not access services on their own, discuss treatment options for Lisa and the family, and help them select specific services and treatment plans. Once the family obtained the help they needed, Nancy would offer education and support to them.

Watson's Human Science and Human Care Model

Watson's caring model lends itself to a view of the family as client if the nurse redefines the phenomenal field to be the family within the family system's environment. The nurse assesses family values by exploring the five realms of family experience (the integrity processes) (Anderson & Tomlinson, 1992; Bell, 2009) through the following:

1. The family's shared meanings of experiences
2. The family members' identities and commitment to the family identity
3. The family history
4. The family members' shared values and rituals
5. The family's strategies for maintaining family boundaries

During care, nurses learn about the family and discover the needs for information and problem-solving abilities by identifying the family's past and current coping processes. Nurses and family members are "co-participants in becoming in the now and the future and both are part of some larger, deeper, complex pattern of life" (Watson, 2007, p. 60). Together, nurses and family members analyze interaction processes, focus on familial relationships and communication patterns, explore the meanings of various transitions occurring within the family, identify support networks, and share feelings and meanings about family life. They also observe how the family members nurture each other and express intimacy, acting as coparticipants. In the human science and human care framework, nurses relate all familial processes to the health processes, clarifying with the family specific health beliefs, responses, and practices, and the patterns of caring for each other during times of wellness and illness.

Peplau's Interpersonal Relations Model

Peplau based her nursing model on the central concepts of growth and development facilitated by relationships with significant others. This model provides the foundation for the nurse to focus on the family as the unit of care if the patterns of interaction within the family and the family developmental processes replace individual needs as the central area of concern. Forchuk and Dorsay (1995, p. 114) stated that Peplau's model and family systems nursing "both share a common focus on interactions, patterns, and interpersonal relationships."

Perhaps Peplau's greatest contribution to the family nursing process is the enumeration of the stages of the nurse–client relationship. According to Friedman (1992, p. 42), "trust and rapport-building set the stage for and are the cornerstones of effective family nursing care." In the orientation stage, if the nurse and the family are to have an effective relationship, each member of the family must be able to share their concerns so that the nurse and other family members may more fully understand the whole family and the meaning of its experience together. In the planning stage, mutual goal setting—which is jointly formulated among family members and the nurse—and ways to meet commonly derived goals are directed toward reframing the need for help in the professional relationship to be a learning and growth experience.

It is proposed that in the intervention stage (which Peplau called the exploitation stage) with families, Peplau's role behaviors originally designated as professional nursing roles could be developed as strategies for the entire family. Family needs to replace individual needs, and the roles of resource person, teacher, leader, counselor, and surrogate may be played by both the nurse and various family members. Each role performance in the family should be fully explored in such a way that the family learns about its interactive processes and the effect of those interactive processes on health processes.

Rogers's Science of Unitary Human Beings Model

Various analysts agree that Rogers's conceptual model of nursing science lends itself readily to the family as the recipient of nursing care—the client system. As Friedman (1992, p. 62) said, "Rogers' legacy is clearly associated with general systems theory, and because of this orientation there is a good fit between Rogerian nursing theory and family nursing." Rogers herself said that the family system is an energy field that serves as the focus of study and interaction. She asserted that family fields and their respective environmental fields are engaged in a continuously evolving mutual process and that patterns identify this ongoing process (Rogers, 1983, p. 226). Some patterns may represent togetherness, others may represent activity/rest, and still others may represent rhythms in the family experience.

Whall and Fawcett (1991, p. 22) suggested that in the Rogerian model, the family is "viewed as an irreducible whole that is not understood by knowledge of individual family members." Newman, Sime, and Corcoran-Perry (1991, p. 4) pointed out that from the unitary-transformative perspective (the perspective first described by Rogers), a phenomenon (any client system) is "viewed as a unitary, self-organizing field embedded in a larger self-organizing field . . . and identified by pattern and by interaction with the larger whole." Given this perspective, the family represents a unitary phenomenon embedded in the larger environmental field and a phenomenon that has patterns of energy exchange within its field and within its interactions with the larger environment.

Whall (1986) suggested that despite Rogers not being completely clear about what assessment strategies are used in the unitary model, she deserves credit for the idea that the nurse providing care must assess the family as a whole. Other nurses have developed some of the tools needed for assessing the whole family. For example, Smoyak developed the idea of using genograms and the identification of family rules of organization as approaches in the nursing process (Whall, 1986). The genogram records information about family members and their relationships over at least three generations. It involves mapping the family structure, recording family information, and delineating family relationships. According to McGoldrick et al. (2020), genograms "display information graphically in a way that provides a quick gestalt of complex family patterns" (p. 1) and provide "a rich source of hypotheses about how clinical problems evolve in the context of a family over time" (p. 1).

The genogram is one of nursing's most useful tools for studying family patterns. By mapping relationships and patterns of functioning, it facilitates clinician systematic thinking about how events and relationships in client lives relate with patterns of health, illness, and resilience (McGoldrick et al., 2020). Using the historical data obtained by completing the genogram, the nurse assesses previous life cycle transitions. This assessment helps the nurse identify important connections between the health of the family and the environment in which they arise (Jarvis, 2020). Readers are referred to McGoldrick et al. (2020) or Jarvis (2020) for additional details on constructing and interpreting the genogram as a tool for nursing assessment of the family. Genograms may also be generated using online software programs, some of which are free.

All of the family realms described by Anderson and Tomlinson (1992) and discussed earlier in this chapter represent patterns of the family as a unitary phenomenon. Thus, these realms could be used as a basis for assessment, planning, intervention, and evaluation by nurses practicing on the basis of a Rogerian philosophy of nursing.

> ### REAL-LIFE REFLECTIONS
>
> *If Nancy used Rogers's science of unitary human beings model to guide practice, she would see that the health status of both students in her office was a manifestation of the pattern of the whole. She would focus on understanding all mechanisms that affect the life process of these clients, one of which is the family.*

Parse's Humanbecoming Model

The nursing models of Parse and Newman may be considered Rogerian based. Thus, the nurse practicing within any of these models would incorporate Rogerian concepts in the caregiving process with the family.

In 2009, Parse published the humanbecoming family model in which she conceptualized the family as "an indivisible, unpredictable, ever-changing, connectedness with close others" (Parse, 2009, p. 35). A family member is defined as any person who designates themselves as a family member, thereby transcending the need for a blood or legal relationship. Parse identified cocreated patterns of relating, involving, and being together and being alone while cotranscending with endless possibilities. The ebb and flow of everyday life occurrences structures the deep personal meaning that results in seeing the familiar–unfamiliar differently. Parse (2009) identifies the following three key essences within the humanbecoming family model

1. *Revering intentions* arise "with the wellspring of laughter and tears in honoring the personal significance of joy–sorrow" (Parse, 2009, p. 307).
2. *Shifting patterns* emerge when family members have opportunities and restrictions for being alone or together when they can either attend or distance themselves.
3. *Unfolding possibilities* occur as the result of family intentions and actions and lead to transcendence toward human becoming.

> ### REAL-LIFE REFLECTIONS
>
> *Using Parse's humanbecoming model as a framework for professional practice, Nancy's approach would be similar to that of Rogers's science of unitary human beings model. However, Nancy would expend more energy to uncover the meaning that underlies the intentions and behaviors associated with eating disorders. To discover the true meanings, she would be truly present with the family as they expressed concerns that would ultimately reveal the meaning of thoughts, feelings, values, and changes that may have contributed to Lisa's condition. She would also provide a deep personal–professional relationship so that the family could express these things as they engaged in the treatment process and recover once treatment was completed.*

Newman's Theory of Health as Expanding Consciousness

Newman, who views the individual as a center of energy, views the family the same way—a center of energy in constant interaction with the environment. Newman (1983) made five assumptions about families:

1. Health encompasses family situations in which one or more family members may be diagnosed as ill.
2. The illness of family members can be considered a manifestation of the pattern of the family interaction.
3. Elimination of the disease condition in the identified ill family member will not change the overall pattern of the family.
4. If one person's becoming ill is the only way the family can become conscious of its pattern, then that is health (in process) for that family.
5. Health is the expansion of consciousness of the family. Consciousness has been defined as the informational capacity of the system, a factor that can be observed in the quantity and quality of responses to stimuli.

The nature of nursing with the family would be the repatterning of partnerships between the family and the environment that promote higher levels of consciousness. Newman (1983) said that the purpose of nursing with the family is to facilitate the development of an increased range of responses of family members to each other and to the world outside the family and to facilitate the refinement of those responses (quality). She suggests that the first task is to assess the patterns of movement, time, space, and consciousness in the family. The nurse would consider the following factors to assess movement through observation: (1) the coordinated movement of language between speaker and listener, (2) other coordinated movements (such as dancing, lovemaking, and playing sports), (3) the freedom of individual movement within the family, and (4) movement outside the family.

Time is assessed for the quantity and quality of private time, coordinated time, and shared time. Space is assessed for territoriality, shared space, and distancing. Finally, consciousness is assessed by collecting data on the informational capacity of the family system, the quantity and quality of interaction within the family, and the quantity and quality of the interaction of the family with the community.

By completing these assessments, the nurse providing care for the family would be able to analyze the patterns of energy exchange between the family and the environment and the transforming potential and life patterns of the family. These patterns will identify where the family energy is flowing and where it is blocked, depleted, or diffused and will determine whether there is overload or buildup of energy in the family. Newman (1983, p. 173) said that as these patterns emerge, the family's informational capacity will be increased in the nurse–client relationship. Assessment of these patterns will also reveal the family's evolving capacities, diversity, and complexity.

> **REAL-LIFE REFLECTIONS**
>
> *If Nancy used Newman's theory of health as expanding consciousness, she would intervene to facilitate repatterning the family into a higher level of consciousness.*

Consistent with the models of Rogers, Parse, and Newman is the fact that the family functions as a unitary, open system integrated with its environment. Family functions may be organized around Anderson and Tomlinson's (1992) five realms of family experience; thus, the assessment, planning, implementation, and evaluation of the family as client by nurses practicing from any of the change/growth nursing models should reflect interactive, developmental, coping, integrity, and health processes and the relationships among all of these processes.

The Family in the Change/Stability Models of Nursing

When nurses use **change/stability models** of nursing, they acknowledge that nursing roles focus on assisting families in solving problems. This section presents a brief discussion of how the family may be viewed as the recipient of care in the nursing models in which the changes are directed toward restabilizing the client system.

King's Systems Interaction Model

King (1983, p. 179) viewed the family as "a social system that is seen as a group of interacting individuals." Thus, the family is an interpersonal system. In King's model, a theory of goal attainment in the family emphasizes interaction between family members.

The major concepts in this theory of goal attainment are self, role, perception, communication, transaction, stress, growth and development, time, space, and interaction. Each of these concepts is assessed in the nursing process between the nurse and the family. Communication is the interrelating factor among these concepts. Nurses and families make transactions to attain goals. King said that family movement through space and time may be social (called vertical movement) or physical (called geographical mobility). She also stated that family roles are related to growth, development, and stress in the family.

According to King's perception of the family as client, the nurse assesses the family situation to identify real or potential problems. They "assist family members in setting goals to resolve problems [and] provide relevant information to help families make decisions about those factors that detract from or enhance healthy living" (King, 1983, p. 183).

REAL-LIFE REFLECTIONS

Using King's approach to professional practice, Nancy would assess the families to identify factors contributing to the suspected eating disorders and help them identify actual and potential issues and concerns regarding having a family member with an eating disorder.

Neuman's Health Care Systems Model

A stress/adaptation-based conceptual model for family nursing is Neuman's health care systems model. The nurse practicing with this model can modify assessment strategies to plan, implement, and evaluate primary, secondary, and tertiary interventions with families.

According to Neuman (1983, p. 241), "the concept of family as a system can be viewed as individual family members harmonious in their relationships—a cluster of related meanings and values that govern the family and keep it viable in a constantly changing environment." Stability is considered to represent the wellness state, instability the illness state, and transition the mixed wellness–illness state. The role of the nurse is "to control vigorously factors affecting the family, with special goal-directed activities toward facilitating stability within the system" (Neuman, 1983, p. 243). To understand influences on the stability of the family system, Neuman proposed the following points:

- The nurse must deal with the needs of each family member in terms of their developmental age, developmental state, strengths and weaknesses, and environmental influences according to their perceptions of events.

- The nurse must determine the structure and process of the family by studying the values and interaction patterns. The significant values and interaction patterns are the decision-making process (how power is distributed); coping style (how differences are negotiated in relation to stress); role relationships (the controlling or facilitating effects of roles in meeting individual and family needs); communication styles and interaction patterns (congruence of verbal and nonverbal messages and the effects of situational or entrenched defense mechanisms in the family); goals (the sharing and supporting of concerns and feelings between members); boundaries (rules that define the type of behaviors that are acceptable or unacceptable to the family); socialization process (the adequacy of resources to support cultural and structural factors in meeting family needs); individuation (the quality of individuality of each family member that defines the wellness or stability of the unit); and sharing (an index for family stability).

- The nurse must facilitate the meeting of family needs by intervening in the intrafamily stressors (all things occurring within the family unit); interfamily stressors (all things occurring between the family and the immediate environment); and extra-family stressors (all things occurring between the family and the distal or indirect external environment). These interventions occur as primary prevention, secondary prevention, or tertiary prevention.

Tomlinson and Anderson (1995) described five areas of interface between Neuman's systems model and a general family health system paradigm:

1. Complexity of the system: The "need to consider not only the individual stressor response in relation to the family but also the family's response relative to lines of defense and resistance" (pp. 138–139).

2. Conceptualization of the core of the family: "The core of the family is composed of its individual members, and assessment of the family is done in relation to the dynamics of individual member contributions to the whole within their environmental interactive context … [in comparison] the core of the family systems is viewed as the interface of its members in interaction with the environment" (p. 139).

3. Goal of family health: "Neuman's central concern is to facilitate optimal client system stability or wellness in the face of change … [in comparison] from a family health system perspective, it is most desirable to facilitate family system wellness using strengths

to reduce stressor effects and enhance family growth toward positive transformation" (p. 140).

4. Entry point in caring for families: The family becomes partners in health care. According to Neuman, "nursing functions to conserve system energy" (p. 140).
5. Nursing interaction: In the Neuman model, "the nurse role creates an explicit cooperative alliance with the client … [in comparison] based on a family systems perspective…in the family caregiving situation there may be considerable boundary ambiguity" (p. 141).

The nurse's prevention activities are the heart of Neuman's model of care. Primary preventions are the activities aimed at preventing stressors from invading the family. Secondary preventions are the protective activities that follow stressor invasion. Tertiary preventions are the activities during the family's reconstitution from stressors. All of these preventions are aimed at reestablishing stability within the family.

REAL-LIFE REFLECTIONS

If Nancy used Neuman's systems model as a foundation for practice, she would assess Lisa's family for stressors using five variables (physiologic, psychological, sociocultural, developmental, and spiritual). She would look for ways to minimize the impact of stressors associated with familial factors that may have contributed to the eating disorder, the stressors of living with a family member with an eating disorder, as well as the stressors associated with treatment.

Roy's Adaptation Model

Roy's adaptation model can be used by the nurse dealing with the family as client. Roy (1983) believed that the family as an adaptive system can be analyzed and that interventions can be organized around enhancing stimuli to the family.

Inputs for family include individual needs and changes within and among members as well as external changes in the environment. These inputs serve as focal stimuli for the family system. Processes handling the inputs are the control and feedback mechanisms. The control mechanisms—supporting, nurturing, and socializing—serve as contextual and residual stimuli to the family system. The feedback mechanisms are the transactional patterns and member control.

Outputs of the family system are the behaviors manifested. Roy (1983) has chosen three goals as the proposed output of the adaptive family system: (1) survival, (2) continuity (role function), and (3) growth (the system's self-concept). At the current stage of development, Roy (1983, p. 275) simply said that "family behavior can be observed as it relates to the general family goals of survival, continuity, and growth."

The nurse observes for the outputs of survival, continuity, and growth and for the transactional and member controls that serve as feedback to the family to signal the need to adjust the behavior of a member or the group. Nursing practice emerges from the assessment of the previously described family factors. The nursing process continues to (1) identify and validate with family members the factor that is most immediately affecting their behavior, (2) identify individual family member needs as focal stimuli, (3) make nursing diagnoses and set goals, and (4) intervene to enhance stimuli configuration in the family.

Friedman (1992, p. 61) supported Roy's suggestion that "nursing problems involve ineffective coping mechanisms, which cause ineffective responses, disrupting the integrity of the person" and suggested that "this notion could easily be broadened to the family unit, where ineffective family coping patterns lead to family functioning problems." Whall and Fawcett (1991, p. 24) acknowledged the potential contribution of Roy's model of nursing care to the care of the family as an adaptive system but noted that "theories of family adaptation and nursing practice theories of family need to be generated and tested." Family adaptation theories need to be elaborated by identifying specific and concrete inputs, processes, and outputs of the family system.

It can be clearly seen that the family as client, rather than context, is a significant new conceptual basis for nursing. Although the attribution "of wellness and illness to the family unit is a recent phenomenon" (Gilliss et al., 1988, p. 5), it is anticipated that an eclectic view of family incorporating both the nursing conceptual models and other social systems approaches will continue to be refined.

Nurses frequently integrate family approaches to clinical situations. Family theory and nursing models provide solid foundations for professional practice. Many family assessment tools exist. Most inpatient admission databases collect data surrounding family life. Although family models and theories are not specific to a particular nurse theorist, they complement many current nursing models and theories. Some cases, such as the structure provided by Anderson and Tomlinson

(1992), provide an eclectic approach when working with families as clients. The family plays a key role in its own health and the health of individual members. Current family health practices evolve from previous health practices. When a family unit forms, the health practices of the new family frequently blend health patterns that the family heads learned as children. Women tend to assume primary responsibility for family health; family members have specific health routines; and community and cultural contexts affect family health (Boyle et al., 2020; Lundy & Janes, 2014; Schumacher et al., 2007).

Take Note!
Family models and theories are not specific to any specific nurse theorist; instead, they complement many current nursing models and theories.

THE COMMUNITY AS CLIENT

This book philosophically defines **community** as a social system with open communication networks between structural and functional subsystems and the greater societal systems. Vertical bureaucratic relationships tie the community to the larger society. A community always has a sense of common identification, even if it does not exist as a common geographical location (making internet communities possible). Thus, the boundaries of a community can be determined in terms of role relationships as well as geography.

As with all open systems, the nurse influences change in the community. This change is directed toward higher levels of wellness in the system. Shuster and Geppinger (2004) specified that the community becomes the client when service providers aim to achieve what is best for the collective good of the population receiving care services instead of focusing on what is best for the individual. Nurses and community members need to work collaboratively as equal partners to identify community needs and develop programs to meet them. Nurse–community partnerships promote community empowerment. When the nurse and community members work together in partnership, efforts can focus on improving the health, well-being, and quality of life for community members. This facilitates community-centered care.

Basic concepts from community health nursing apply to the care of **community as client**. Throughout time, nursing scholars such as Neuman (1989) and

Murdaugh et al. (2019) (see Chapter 5, "The Health Process and Self-Care of the Nurse") have agreed that the following considerations are essential to professional nurses working with the community as client:

- **Health promotion:** Improving the well-being and quality of life of the community
- **Risk:** Identifying factors that increase the chance the community will either experience or be affected by a particular health problem
- **Disease prevention:** Protecting the population from diseases, disabilities, and their consequences
- **Primary prevention:** Preventing the occurrence of health problems or diseases
- **Secondary prevention:** Identifying and treating health problems and diseases
- **Tertiary prevention:** Preventing further deterioration following a health problem or restoring health and functioning after disease occurs

REAL-LIFE REFLECTIONS

Sometimes, social change is needed to address the key considerations in community health nursing. For example, Nancy may find the need to confront the societal value that it is impossible to be too thin. In addition to educating the students and their families, Nancy may find it necessary to consult with teachers, school administrators, the parent–teacher organization, other students, and the ballet teacher to inform them of the dangers and plan a community-wide program to alleviate malnutrition stemming from the desire to be thin.

Definitions of Community

Because community has been thought of primarily as a setting for care, nurses need to explore the various definitions of community to determine how they may view the community as a client for nursing services. Multiple definitions exist. Mish (2020) defines a community as a unified body of people; individuals with common interests living in a particular location; an interacting population of different kinds of people (or species) sharing a common location; a group of people possessing common characteristics or interests living together in a larger society; a body of people with common (especially professional) interests; and "society at large" (p. 251). From a nursing perspective, Hanchett (1988, p. 7) said that community can be considered as an aggregate, a system, or a human–environment field. "As an aggregate, the individual is the basic unit of the community; that is, the community is a number of separate individuals." As a system, one must consider the "relationships among the individuals or groups who constitute the community" (Hanchett, 1988, p. 8). As a human–environment field, the community represents a human field integral with its environment and "manifesting correlates of the patterning of that field process" (Hanchett, 1988, p. 8).

If the nurse views the community as an aggregate, nursing is truly organized around the concept of the community serving as a context for individuals. Clark (1999, p. 56) defined community health nursing as "a synthesis of nursing knowledge and practice and the science and practice of public health, implemented via systematic use of the nursing process and other processes, designed to promote health and prevent illness in population groups. The focus of care is the aggregate." Clark indicated that community health nursing is characterized by the following:

- Health orientation: Health promotion and prevention of disease rather than cure of illness
- Population focus: Emphasis on aggregates, rather than individuals or families
- Autonomy: Greater community control over health care decisions
- Continuity: Providing continuing, comprehensive care rather than short-term, episodic care
- Collaboration: Nurse and client interacting as equals
- Interactivity: Awareness of interaction of a variety of factors with health
- Public accountability: Accountability to society for public health
- Sphere of intimacy: Greater awareness of the reality of client lives and situations

Nurses can select from a variety of community nursing and community health models to follow when working with the community as client. Christensen and Kenney (1990) proposed a comprehensive model for implementing the nursing process focusing on the aggregate within the context of a geopolitical environment.

Take Note!
A community is a group of people who share a bond, interact with one another, and function as a unit.

Zotti et al. (1996, p. 211) differentiated between community-based nursing and community health nursing (Table 15.2). Community-based nursing uses "a philosophy of nursing that guides nursing care provided for individuals, families, and groups wherever they are, including where they live, work, play, or go to school." In contrast, community health nursing is "a systematic process of delivering nursing care to improve the health of an entire community" (Zotti et al., 1996, p. 212).

When the community becomes the client, nurses may find themselves approaching ethical issues in a different manner. Many times, ethical practice requires nurses to balance ethical considerations for the individual with those for the community. For example, protecting the community or collective becomes more important when determining the allocation of scarce resources and when the need for community information supersedes the privacy and autonomy of an individual. Professional nurses must also look for ways to ensure social justice and equal access to care services while working with culturally diverse and marginalized groups within a designated community. When serving the community, professional nurses may encounter ethical conflicts arising from roles and responsibilities outlined by the profession and employing agency as well as conflicts arising among cultural values and practices from different groups within the community. However, as with all clients, professional nurses serving the community must act with honesty, integrity, transparency, loyalty, and truthfulness (Allen & Easley, 2008; Kurtz & Burr, 2009).

If nurses view the community as a system, then they seek to introduce changes in the community systems and base interventions on their understanding of the impact of these changes on system functioning (Spradley, 1990). Christensen and Kenney (1990) also proposed a general systems assessment model for directing the nursing process with families. Considerable work on viewing the community as a system that is the recipient of nursing care has emerged from Neuman's conceptual model of nursing. Hanchett (1988) postulated that Roy's adaptation model of nursing and King's general system framework also offer nurses the opportunity to practice nursing with the community as a client system, in which the focus is on the pattern of relationships among the elements of the system.

Following are brief discussions of (1) a systems model of community as client based on Neuman's conceptual model, in which change is directed toward restoring stability to the system; and (2) a human field–environment model of community as client based on Rogerian nursing science, in which change is directed toward increasing capacities and evolving growth, and Parse's perception of community from a human becoming perspective. Despite their different approaches,

TABLE 15.2 Community-Based Nursing Versus Community Health Nursing

Component	Community-Based Nursing	Community Health Nursing
Goals	Manage acute or chronic conditions Promote self-care	Preserve/protect health Promote self-care
Client	Individual and family	Community
Underlying philosophy	Human ecologic model	Primary health care
Autonomy	Individual and family autonomy Individual rights may be sacrificed for the good of the community	Community autonomy
Client character	Across the life span	Across the life span, with emphasis on high-risk aggregates
Cultural diversity	Culturally appropriate care of individual and families	Collaboration with and mobilization of diverse groups and communities
Type of service	Direct	Direct and indirect
Home visiting	Home visitor	Home visitor
Service focus	Local community	Local, state, federal, and international

From Zotti, M. E., Brown, P., & Stotts, R. C. (1996). Community-based nursing versus community health nursing: What does it all mean? *Nursing Outlook, 44,* 212. Used with permission of the publisher.

these models tend to agree that community nursing interventions primarily address health promotion and interactions among the domains of space, human relationships, and the environment.

REAL-LIFE REFLECTIONS

If school nurse Nancy operates from a community as client perspective, her focus on eating disorders would shift. Instead of intervening with the individual students affected by the problem, she would consider how the problem affects the entire school community. She would plan and execute educational programs for students, faculty, staff, and administration on the detection and prevention of eating disorders. Along with education, Nancy would offer her time and attention to listen to concerns and counsel all people affected by the declining health of students with eating disorders.

A Systems Model of Viewing the Community as Client

McFarlane and Anderson (2019) adapted the Neuman health care systems model to provide a way for nurses to conceive of the community as the recipient of care. This adaptation synthesizes public health with nursing. In this systems approach, the community has eight subsystems: (1) recreation, (2) safety and transportation, (3) communication, (4) education, (5) health and social services, (6) economics, (7) politics and government, and (8) the physical environment.

The boundaries of a community are generally geopolitical. According to systems theory, the interactive nature of these eight subsystems results in a whole that is more than the sum of its parts. Nursing interventions for a community must address collecting targeted information related to a geographical location and/or a specific group of people (McFarlane & Anderson, 2019).

The application of Neuman's model to the development of the nursing process with the community as the recipient of care is built around the redefinition of person, environment, health, and nursing. Community nursing scholars have described communities as groups of people who share common characteristics, such as language or culture, who may or may not live in a specific geographical area (Lundy & Janes, 2014; McFarlane & Anderson, 2019). The redefined environment includes all conditions, circumstances, and influences that affect the development of the community. Health is equated with competence to function and "a definable state of equilibrium in which subsystems are in harmony so that the whole can perform at its maximum potential" (Saucier, 1991, p. 59).

Nurses participate in the care of the community by participating in community assessment, identifying and diagnosing problems amenable to nursing interventions, planning for and implementing interventions that enhance the interacting forces within the system, and evaluating the outcomes of the interventions on the community's health.

The systems model focuses on prevention:

Primary prevention strategies for the professional nurse include (1) increasing the public's awareness of health problems; (2) increasing the public's knowledge of the available community resources and services to resolve the problems; (3) preparing the public to self-refer to appropriate resources; and (4) preparing the public to become involved in preventing the factors that lead to the problem (Saucier, 1991). Informing the public of strategies to avoid an infectious illness (e.g., seasonal influenza) is an example of a primary prevention strategy.

Secondary prevention strategies include facilitating self-screenings and referral to appropriate community resources. Providing community testing for an infectious disease (e.g., COVID-19), placing people in quarantine who test positive, referring them to a local retailer to purchase oxygen saturation monitors, and then having clients go to the hospital if certain symptoms occur are examples of steps comprising a secondary prevention strategy.

Tertiary prevention strategies include lobbying for adequate services and resources to meet the particular community health problems. Developing a plan, securing adequate resources, and creating a response team in anticipation of the next infectious disease epidemic is an example of a tertiary prevention strategy.

The systems model presents a comprehensive approach when nurses serve the community as client. The systems approach uses the change stability perspective.

A Human Field–Environment Field Model of Viewing the Community as Client

The paradigm of nursing in which change is directed toward growth uses the Rogerian framework for viewing the community as client.

Hanchett (1988, p. 128) said that in this view the community is seen as an energy field in process with the environmental energy field and health is viewed as the dynamic well-being of the community–environmental process. Manifestations of these energy fields in process may be reflected in visible expressions such as motion, rhythms of quiet and activity, and the togetherness of the community's members in participating in change.

For example, motion that is observable by the nurse is the speed of people and traffic in daily life. Rhythms of quiet and activity may be seen in the sleep–wake patterns of the community. For example, sometimes people living in communities lock themselves inside their homes at night, resulting in no outdoor activity, giving the impression that the community is asleep. During daylight hours, adults and children are engaged in outdoor activities, and many cars are driving on the streets; the community is awake. Gatherings of people in community settings can be observed to analyze togetherness. Other pattern manifestations of this energy process include the "number of cultural and ethnic groups of the community, the variety of lifestyles and ideas that flourish, and pragmatic, imaginative, and visionary approaches to change evidenced by the community" (Hanchett, 1988, p. 129).

The goal of nursing is to help the community achieve maximum well-being. According to Hanchett (1988), this is done by the nurse participating in the process of change, assisting community groups to move toward well-being. Rogers's definition of health as "dynamic well-being" means that the community must become more aware of factors that maximize well-being and minimize conditions that limit actualization or realization of full potential.

This view of health as "dynamic well-being" directs the actions of the nurse in this model. The nurse's actions all center on facilitating the process of people becoming more aware of their patterns of energy exchange with the environment and the evolving outcomes of these exchanges. Manifestations of field patterning include "diversity, rhythms, motion, the experience of time, sleep–wake and beyond-waking states, and pragmatic, imaginative, and visionary approaches to conscious participation in change" (Hanchett, 1988, p. 128). The nurse attempts to facilitate evolutionary change in the human field–environmental field process from lesser diversity to greater diversity; from longer rhythms and slower motion to seemingly continuous rhythms and motion; from experiencing time as slower, pragmatic foci to experiencing time as timelessness, visionary foci; and from longer sleeping to longer waking, perhaps even beyond waking (Hanchett, 1988).

The essence of this model for community nursing is that the community as a group–environmental field process determines the health of the community. In each community, the process unfolds at a unique pace and in unique patterns. The community's health is an expression of the mutually evolving process. Nursing approaches in community health focus on enhancing the well-being of community members and their environments with the aim of promoting community well-being. Influencing public policies to provide improved shelter, food, and clothing for all people is an example of approaches to improve community well-being (see Chapter 19, "The Professional Nurse's

Role in Public Policy"). Nursing is "the science that the art of nursing uses in the conscious participation in the human–environmental field process toward the goal of maximum well-being" (Hanchett, 1988, p. 132).

In the Rogerian model of nursing, the community field–environmental field process integrates all other definitions of community; that is, it validates the community as a social system, as a place (space), and as people. The resultant health of the client system (community) is more than the sum of these identified parts. Well-being is an integral process in which human beings and the environment evolve toward greater awareness of their being. Respect for both diversity and sameness in patterns of energy exchange is essential for the professional nurse to operate out of this conceptual model of nursing.

It is evident from the general nature of the discussion of this model that much research is needed to facilitate further development of the Rogerian model. Determining manifestations of patterning of life, identifying patterns that maximize health, and developing strategies that focus on the community field–environmental field process are necessary for fuller implementation of this model in community nursing practice in which the community is the recipient of the care.

Similar to the Rogerian perspective of community, Parse (2003) espoused the interconnectedness of the community and the environment. Parse (2003) defined community as "a oneness of human-universe connectedness incarnating beliefs and values" (p. 1) that is "objective, measurable, and concerned with relationships, change, symbiosis, localism, cooperation, and the commonality of interests and goals" (p. 5). Parse (2003) further explained that the community is "an ever-changing incarnated interconnectedness correlated with all that is" (p. 21). Parse also envisioned a community that is more than just an acreage or a location. Using her consistent method of what seem to be nearly polar opposites, she identifies two key considerations for the ever-evolving community.

- *Anchoring–shifting* deals with the phenomenon of holding fast to some things while giving up others.
- *Pondering–shaping* refers to thoroughly thinking about how, dialoguing and listening to all community members, and considering all options before developing a means for change.

Parse also specified that when one barrier to change is removed, others typically appear. Parse specified that true presence serves as the core for nursing practice in the community and that nurses need courage and confidence along with the understanding of key community members in order to make changes. Cocreating rhythms occur within the community, thereby facilitating human interconnectedness that is ever-changing and creating new possibilities.

To learn how to care for communities as clients, nurses may benefit most from participating in service-learning projects or clinical experiences in community agencies. Community-based nursing experiences enable nurses to appreciate the value of being an engaged citizen in a community while learning how to provide nursing services to larger groups of people. Community-based experiences offer situations in which nurses give to the agency while they increase their repertoire of community nursing skills. When engaging in community nursing, nurses must expand their views to see how internal and external factors affect an agency while collaborating with community members to ensure that they offer relevant services (Narsavage et al., 2003). Nurses also work to build stronger communities as well as improve community health. Through role modeling, nurses can inspire community members to participate actively in the political process, increase participation in community activities, develop community goals, manage conflicts effectively, attain consensus on goal priorities and how to reach them, use resources effectively, and obtain external resources for desired programs (Head et al., 2004). Finally, and most importantly, nurses advocate for underprivileged community members so that they can gain access to health care and other basic services (McElmurry et al., 2003).

From an idealist perspective, the goal of community health nursing would be to facilitate the development of healthy, healing communities. Nurses live and work with others in communities. If a community is defined as anyone who works together to attain a common goal, then nurses could view a community from a variety of perspectives. Provision of nursing services to any community begins with a community assessment.

Community Assessment

In a community assessment, community health care nurses assess the community in terms of status, structure, and process:

- *Status assessment* includes reported statistics related to birth, death, poverty, crime, and incidence of mental and physical illness.
- *Structure assessment* includes inpatient and outpatient health care facilities, local government structures, schools, law enforcement agencies, retailers,

roads, and population demographics (e.g., socioeconomic status, gender, age).

- *Process assessment* includes factors such as member commitment, communication patterns, relationships of the community with the larger society, and how well the community voices its need for, accesses, and uses resources (McFarlane & Anderson, 2019; Rector, 2018; Stanhope & Lancaster, 2018).

In the professional nursing work setting, the nurse would consider aspects of the building structure, actual and potential health hazards, employee demographics, and incidences of work-related injuries and illnesses within the overall organization and at the nursing unit levels. For the academic setting, the nurse would look at the campus buildings, campus plan, demographics of students, faculty administration and staff, actual and potential health hazards, presence of academic support systems, and instances of campus-related violence, injuries, and illnesses. In both settings, the nurse would examine current policies and procedures for getting the work done (client care for a clinical setting or student education in an academic setting). The nurse would also look at how the institution communicates its mission and its commitments to local and global communities. Finally, the nurse would assess the frequency with which the community accesses and uses the organizational (or institutional) services and resources.

▌ QUESTIONS FOR REFLECTION

1. What additional professional skills do nurses need when the community is the client?
2. What are current health concerns within your local community?
3. What are current health concerns within your academic community?
4. What health concerns can you identify in your clinical practice community?
5. Why are the health concerns that you identify important for each community?

Hallmarks of a Healthy Community

The healthy city/community movement began in the mid-1980s in Europe. Hancock and Duhl (1986) specified that the following must be present for a community to be classified as healthy:

- A clean, safe, and ecologically stable physical environment
- Resident access to resources that promote and maintain a healthy, diverse, vital, and innovative economy

- A strong, supportive, nonexploitative community
- Basic human needs (food, water, shelter, income, and safety) met for all members
- Access to a wide variety of experiences and resources (e.g., communications, cultural events, diverse contacts)
- A connection to the community's heritage and past
- Equal access to public health and illness care services
- Good health status of citizens
- High levels of public participation in and control over decisions that affect individual citizens' lives, health, and well-being

Morse (2004) denoted characteristics of successful communities that plan for and adapt to change. Healthy communities have members who understand their relationship and responsibility to others rather than focusing solely on individual pursuits. By strategically planning for change, communities ensure their survival and enable brighter futures for members following in their footsteps. Morse identified seven key points that result in successful community adaptation to change:

1. Making the right investments/decisions the first time
2. Working together instead of as individuals or special interest groups with specific agendas
3. Building on current community strengths
4. Using a democratic process
5. Preserving the community's history
6. Growing their own leaders
7. Inventing a better and brighter future

Community-Level Nursing Interventions

Health promotion within a community encompasses collective efforts. Community nursing interventions work best when the community assumes ownership of the plan, responsibility for community health program maintenance, and control for planning future programs. Nurses use multiple strategies to help communities improve their health. They empower, collaborate with, build capacity for, and advocate for individual members and the entire community (Leddy, 2003; Lind & Smith, 2008).

Nurses empower communities by investing time and resources to enable communities to assume control over their own destinies. Some community members view the nurse as a health expert who has knowledge and expertise in developing programs and supporting others to attain better health, whereas others see the nurse as someone who plans to force sometimes culturally incompatible ways on them (Andrews et al., 2020; Leininger & McFarland, 2006; McFarlane & Anderson, 2019). Poverty-stricken communities perceive a lack of control over their futures and feel powerless because they may not be valued by others, have few or no resources, lack economic and political power, have no experience in making decisions, and have learned helplessness. Sometimes, community members have a history of fighting with each other. Nurses can serve as mediators to settle long-standing disputes so community members can determine which programs are needed. Nurses also serve as consultants, coaches, and cheerleaders as community members plan, implement, and evaluate community health programs.

Collaboration with the community requires that the nurse and community members share information and resources with each other but, above all, trust each other. Lind and Smith (2008) proposed the use of appreciative inquiry as a means to connect with the community and identify community strengths. Appreciative inquiry provides opportunities for people to share their stories and perceive that they have been heard and that their ideas are valued. Everyone involved shares ideas and listens intently. Through the use of appreciative inquiry, the community health nurse becomes familiar with traditional folk medicine, key community concerns, and community leaders. Appreciative inquiry fosters deep personal connections while encouraging the participation of everyone engaged in the development, planning, and implementation of community nursing interventions. The community and nurse work in partnership to promote health rather than to merely identify health problems.

Capacity building occurs with individual members, small groups, and the entire community. Capacity building involves building on the current strengths, resources, and abilities already present in the community. Individual capacity building involves changing personal values for health-enhancing outcomes, having a positive attitude toward collaboration, making decisions using consensus, sharing power and information, showing respect, giving support, participating in egalitarian relationships, perceiving self-efficacy, setting future goals, feeling a sense of coherence, identifying with others who have similar problems, feeling able to help others, and understanding community member roles and responsibilities. Small-group capacity building includes interacting with others to help them

assume control, fostering a sense of connectedness, establishing trust, and creating positive interactions. Capacity in building communities involves helping members and the community articulate health problems and potential solutions, providing them with access to information, supporting current community leadership, and assisting them in overcoming obstacles to action. While building capacity within a community, the nurse may act as a strategist, coach, meeting facilitator, mediator, and developer of community leadership (Leddy, 2003).

Once the community has mobilized its internal human and physical resources, the community shares a group consciousness. With a united purpose, the community becomes capable of taking social and political action to obtain additional resources for use in community building and improvement. Disenfranchised people may not have the ability to develop independently as a community. The nurse helps these individuals achieve community-building skills through role modeling, providing support, and listening to them share their problems and concerns. Nurses have the ability to service communities in multiple ways, and there are many opportunities for nurses to pursue a career in community health nursing.

CAREER OPPORTUNITIES IN COMMUNITY HEALTH NURSING

Nurses have many opportunities to engage in community nursing, including in public health departments, factories, businesses, camps, homes, homeless shelters, prisons, schools, parishes, and the armed forces. Some nurses engage in volunteer nursing. Community members who know professional nurses sometimes ask them for health advice and information outside the work setting. Nurses who give health-related advice to friends and acquaintances are practicing nursing and should assume accountability for their actions. Thus, the professional nurse should keep a record of nursing actions (including consultations with neighbors) and evaluate outcomes of health education, advice, recommended consultations, and nursing procedures.

According to Khederian (2020), the five healthiest states in the United States in 2020 were Vermont, Massachusetts, Hawaii, Connecticut, and Utah, and the five least healthy states were Mississippi, Louisiana, Arkansas, Alabama, and Oklahoma. According to the May 2019 mean wages for registered nurses (U.S. Bureau of Labor Statistics [USBLS], 2020), registered nurses in these states experienced salary disparities. In the healthiest states, the mean annual earnings for registered nurses was more than $64,840, with registered nurses earning more than $69,000 in all five states. The annual mean wages for nurses in four of the least healthy states was less than $64,000 (USBLS, 2020).

There are no updated reports on the number of registered nurses per capita in each state to verify whether this factor has an impact on the states' general health and well-being. However, in an examination of state health rankings and the 2004 National Survey of Registered Nurses, Bigbee (2008) reported that an increased nurse-to-population ratio resulted in higher state health rankings in terms of reduced motor vehicle crash deaths, crime rates, incidence of infectious diseases, childhood poverty, uninsured people, premature deaths, and time off work for poor physical and mental health. In addition, the higher ratio resulted in increases in high school graduation rates, recommended immunizations, and prenatal care. The study also revealed that higher nurse-to-population ratios resulted in an increased level of healthiness and general well-being in the community, whereas higher physician-to-population ratios resulted in improved physical health of individuals. Therefore, the study findings "suggest that more RNs per capita may be associated with healthier populations" (Bigbee, 2008, p. 250), substantiating the need for effective strategies to alleviate the current and projected future nursing shortage (see Chapter 3, "Contextual, Philosophical, and Ethical Elements of Professional Nursing").

The following discussion briefly describes selected practice areas for community health nursing. More detailed information regarding community nursing opportunities may be found by consulting website resources or references at the end of this chapter.

Public Health Nursing

Public health nurses have been serving individuals, groups, communities, and populations since 1893. The Institute of Medicine (2003) defined public health as what a society does collectively to guarantee that conditions occur so that people can be healthy. Public health nurses respond to societal health needs by focusing on promoting and protecting the health of populations. Public health nurses do not work in isolation; rather, they collaborate with interprofessional health care team members, typically within a local government agency (city or county health department). When health issues arise that concern more than the local community, public health nurses find themselves

consulting and working with national governments (e.g., U.S. Public Health Service), and even world organizations (e.g., United Nations). Health promotion and protection are the top priorities for public health nurses (DeMarco & Healey-Walsh, 2020; American Nurses Association [ANA], 2014b). Since 1999, the Quad Council of Public Health Nursing Organizations has stipulated the baccalaureate degree as the entry level for public health nursing practice. The ANA offers certification in community/public health nursing. Certification in public health nursing has intrinsic value for nurses (personal satisfaction, sign of professional growth, evidence of professional accomplishment and specialized knowledge, increased confidence, and professional credibility). However, not all nurses receive increases in salary by earning community/public health certifications. Still, this professional certification benefits nurses looking for community/public health nursing positions.

Public health nurses aim to promote and protect the health of populations through the creation of situations and provision of services to help people optimize their health. Along with using foundational nursing knowledge, public health nurses incorporate knowledge from social and public health science into practice (ANA, 2014b). Public health nurses provide services to meet government-specified health objectives as outlined in *Healthy People 2030* (USDHHS, 2020a). In 2018, The Quad Council Coalition Competency Review Task Force published core functions and competencies of community/public health nursing. The core functions of community public health nursing are (1) community assessment (health needs, health problem investigation, analysis of medical and nonmedical determinants of health); (2) engagement in policy development (advocating for resources, prioritizing and addressing community/public health needs, planning and developing policies to address the prioritized needs); and (3) assurance (managing resources, implementing planned programs, evaluating the interventions executed in the programs, informing the community about current and potential health issues, communicating available community resources).

The list of essential services offered by public health nurses include (1) monitoring the community health status to identify and solve specific problems; (2) diagnosing and investigating community health problems and hazards; (3) informing, educating, and empowering individuals about actual and potential health issues; (4) mobilizing community partnerships and actions to identify and solve community health issues; (5) developing policies and plans that support individual and community health efforts; (6) Enforcing laws and regulations that protect community/public health and safety; (7) linking individuals to needed personal and health-assuring provisions or providing services when they are not available; (8) ensuring a competent personal and public workforce; (9) evaluating the accessibility, quality, and effectiveness of available personal and public/ community-based services; and (10) using research to find new insights and innovative solutions to current and potential health problems (Quad Council Coalition Competency Review Task Force, 2018).

■ QUESTIONS FOR REFLECTION

1. Do you know how to contact your local public health department?

2. What services does your local public health department offer? Have you or has a member of your family ever made use of those services?

Community Mental Health Nursing

Promoting the mental health of citizens is important to the quality of life of a community. Many countries, including the United States, have a full array of mental health services (from acute and long-term residential programs to home health care) for people who need them. In 1963, the passage of the Community Mental Health Centers Act provided federal funding for community mental health centers, resulting in the deinstitutionalization of mentally ill people who were once confined to psychiatric inpatient facilities. These individuals became part of local communities and were no longer required to conform to the restrictions required by hospitals, shelters, and group homes.

Because of the lack of residential programs, many people with severe mental illness may live at home. In addition, many people with mental disorders cannot work, which means they frequently have no health care insurance. Many people without homes suffer from mental illness. Without support, some mentally ill people have no access to mental health services to receive the psychotropic medications necessary to function in activities of daily living. Some communities have civil ordinances against people living on the streets, some provide homeless shelters, and others rely on private agencies or faith-based organizations to provide shelter for people without homes. Some homeless shelters provide mental health services for their clients.

Community mental health nurses may find themselves working with people who may have a history of violent behavior or have been victims of violence. Some people living in high-crime areas become isolated because of their fear for their safety or the safety of their property. Community mental health nurses work in a variety of settings, such as mental health clinics, public health departments, chemical abuse programs, homeless shelters, group residential homes, prisons, and home health, to address the needs of these populations.

When working in community settings, community mental health nurses assume the following client care activities: assessing client condition and progress, managing medications, promoting health, supporting clients and families, and intervening to prevent and manage psychiatric emergencies. When signs of mental deterioration occur, community mental health nurses collaborate with physicians for emergency management and make referrals for emergency or immediate care. In life-threatening situations, community mental health nurses activate the emergency response system. Advanced practice mental health nurses may have prescriptive privileges for psychotropic medications and frequently have education and credentials to offer counseling services (ANA & American Psychiatric Nurses Association [APNA], 2015; Rector, 2018; Stanhope & Lancaster, 2018).

Community mental health nurses collaborate with and support community members as they make autonomous decisions. They also work with other health care professionals to maximize use of available resources for health promotion, such as using a social worker to help secure food stamps or vouchers (ANA & APNA, 2015). Many people with mental disorders receive mental health services from home health nurses who specialize in psychiatric-mental health care.

Not all public health departments provide mental health services for their communities. When they do, community health nurses provide mental health services to clients who seek care in public health clinics. If the public health department fails to provide mental health services, community members receive mental health services from freestanding, government-supported, nonprofit, or for-profit mental health centers. To access mental health services, community members must be informed of the location and nature of the mental health services offered by each center. They receive such information from nurses or other health care providers.

If a major event occurs within a community that has the potential to affect the mental health of its members, coordinated efforts from all facilities offering mental health services are required. For example, community mental health nurses from various mental health facilities may be consulted to support students and teachers in schools after an act of violence or student loss of life has occurred.

In *Healthy People 2030*, the U.S. government specified goals to improve and increase access to quality mental health services (USDHHS, 2020b). Because nearly half of all Americans will experience mental health issues in their lifetimes, *Healthy People 2030* emphasizes the importance of "prevention, screening, assessment, and treatment of mental health and behavior disorders" (USDHHS, 2020b, para 1). Some of the targeted mental health services for improvement include enhancing preventive services for mental health issues in schools for children and adolescents; routine screening for depression in all age groups whenever health care services are rendered (especially at primary care visits); ensuring people with substance abuse disorder receive treatment for their addictions and underlying mental health issues; preventing suicides (of all age groups and in the LGBTQ+ community), violence, and opiate addiction; improving screening and treatment for postpartum depression; increasing the number of children and adolescents getting help for depression, anxiety, attention-deficit/hyperactivity disorder, and behavioral disorders; and increasing the number of schools that employ counselors, social workers, and psychologists. The initiative also aims to improve services for adults without homes and those who have serious mental illnesses. Areas for treatment expansion for mental health and illness include (1) primary care, including screening and assessment; (2) pediatric mental health services, including routine screening for mental disorders in all schools; and (3) improving treatment services for adults, especially older adults (USDHHS, 2020a). More community mental health nurses are and will be needed to attain these goals.

Electronic Community Health Nursing

Online chat rooms, blogs, and social media create virtual gathering places for people with similar interests or conditions. When a chat, blog, Facebook page, or other social media dialogue is formed for a specific purpose, such as providing support, education, and resource information for people with similar health conditions or life situations, the purpose is consistent with the ANA's *Scope and Standards of Public Health Nursing Practice* (2014b). When nurses participate in these online interactions with the aim of promoting and protecting the health of their community members, they could be considered to be providing community nursing services. In such forums, nurses may provide social support to other members, model effective communication strategies, provide therapeutic communication, reinforce positive behaviors among group members, offer self-care or health-promoting advice, provide health-related information, and monitor group dynamics.

Before electronic community health nursing can be recognized, current international, national, and state laws require changes. The following questions about professional nursing practice must also be addressed:

- How will professional nurses receive compensation for their services (or will they)?
- What accountability will the nurse have to the members of the electronic community?
- What are the roles of the professional nurse providing e-community health nursing services?
- If the nurse shares a similar condition as other chat room participants, how will professional and personal boundaries be delineated?
- How will states and/or the federal government regulate online professional nursing practice?

Camp Nursing

Camps are temporary, small communities. "Like all communities, camps provide basic services for their members, including food, shelter, socialization, protection from harm, meaningful activity, and the other necessities of life" (Lishner & Bruya, 1994, p. 7). Although seen primarily as a form of recreation, camps offer opportunities for nurses to practice first aid skills and care for the injured and ill in more rustic settings, thereby providing practice in skills that might be required when responding to disaster situations and caring for disaster victims (Erceg & Pravda, 2009).

Camp nurses work toward attaining a healthy camp community. Depending on the type of camp, camping allows individuals of all ages to experience nature; escape the stress of a fast-paced, highly technologic society; and learn self-reliance while learning skills for survival and recreation. Camp gives people an opportunity to live with others unlike themselves and shows them how to establish a community for a prescribed time. Skills learned at camp transfer to other settings.

Professional nurses have opportunities to participate in a variety of camping experiences. Day camps provide sessions of varying lengths, with participants and staff returning home at night. Residential camps require participants and staff to live on site for a few days or up to 2 months. Residential camps assume great responsibility to ensure the safety and health of participants and staff. Travel camps typically involve some form of motorized transportation so that participants can move from site to site. Trip camps use individually guided vehicles or animals (such as horses, bicycles, or canoes). Special needs camps offer people with special physical, cognitive, or emotional needs an opportunity to reap the benefits of camp life. These camps include various members of the interdisciplinary health care team or staff to ensure that the participants' special health needs are met (Erceg & Pravda, 2009).

The Association of Camp Nurses (2020) has published practice guidelines for frequently encountered conditions and situations. Topics included in the camp nursing guidelines are as follows:

- Communicable diseases (including COVID-19)
- Medication management (including cannabidiol [CBD] oil administration)
- Allergy and anaphylaxis identification and management
- How to build a health center for a camp
- Concussions at camp
- Diabetes management
- Environmental and pest concerns (e.g., insects, snakes, mice, poison ivy, oak, sumac)
- Delegation
- Documentation

Nurses working or volunteering in camps may find themselves providing direct care to campers by administering medications, performing specialized procedures and therapies, and monitoring the effects of interventions and the camping experience on those with special needs. Camp nurses must also be aware of, develop relationships with, and secure camp contracts for emergency care with health care providers located in the camp's vicinity (Erceg & Pravda, 2009). The Association of Camp Nursing website also offers information for new camp nurses as well as strategies for hiring and orienting camp nurses. The organization also conducts research on a variety of issues regarding campers, parents, and nurses and has built a repository for studies to build a strong evidence base for camp nursing.

Occupational Health Nursing

Because employers and employees in work settings share common goals and spend time together, workplaces fit the definition of community. Occupational health nurses provide primary, secondary, and tertiary care to people in the work setting. Occupational health nurses build deep relationships with employees, empower employees to safely do their work, and provide primary and sometimes emergency care to employees. Federal guidelines for worker safety specify that employers bear responsibility for deleterious effects encountered by workers for occupational and environmental hazards; occupational health nurses can teach employees and monitor work environments to prevent work-related injuries and illnesses. Most occupational health nurses who enter this field of nursing earned bachelor degrees in nursing and have experience in public/community health nursing. Many occupational nurses have earned graduate degrees in public health, business, and advanced practice nursing (American Association of Occupational Health Nurses, 2020). Large businesses may have an occupational health department that employs many nurses; small businesses may employ only one nurse or contract with health care providers to provide occupational health services for employees.

In addition to direct care services, occupational health nurses may provide health education to employees. They also compile statistical reports summarizing the annual incidence of employee occupational illness and injuries. By law, these reports are submitted to federal, state, and local agencies and made available to employees. Commonly occurring occupational illnesses include repetitive stress injuries, allergic and contact dermatitis, respiratory disorders caused by inhalation of toxic agents, poisoning, hearing loss, low back disorders, traumatic injuries, fertility problems, and pregnancy abnormalities (American Association of Occupational Health Nurses, 2020).

In 2004, the American Association of Occupational Health Nurses (AAOHN) developed 11 standards for occupational and environmental health nursing practice, which were revised in 2019 to include a list of competent performance levels for each of the standards:

1. Assess the health status of the clients, workforce, and work environment using a systematic approach.
2. Analyze the health data from the assessment, and develop nursing diagnoses that need to be addressed.
3. Develop specific expected client outcomes to address identified nursing diagnoses.
4. Create a goal-directed plan with comprehensive interventions and therapies to achieve care outcomes.
5. Implement identified interventions to achieve desired care plan outcomes.

6. Evaluate the developed care plan systematically and continuously in response to client responses.
7. Manage and use corporate resources to support occupational health and safety programs.
8. Assume responsibility for professional self-development for enhancement of professional growth and competency.
9. Collaborate with clients and other health team members to prevent health issues while promoting and restoring health in the work environment.
10. Use research findings in and contribute to the scientific knowledge base for occupational and environmental health nursing for improving practice and advancing the profession.
11. Use an ethical framework when making practice decisions (AAOHN, 2019).

Occupational health nursing provides nurses with opportunities to improve the health of employees and the work environment. By screening employees for various health problems related to work before symptoms occur, occupational health nurses not only improve the health of workers but also reduce long-term health care costs for employers. These nurses played a pivotal role in preventing, detecting, and managing COVID-19 outbreaks in many work settings in 2020.

▌ QUESTIONS FOR REFLECTION

1. What occupational health hazards are present in your current work setting?
2. What health hazards are present in your position as a student and in the building where you attend classes?
3. How can you reduce health hazards that you find in your work or school setting?
4. Does your school or workplace offer opportunities to improve your health?

Home Health Nursing

Home health nurses provide nursing services to clients within the confines of each client's residence. Although home health nursing practice focuses primarily on individuals, the home health care nurse also considers the needs of the family and designated caregivers. Home health nursing is considered a form of community nursing because the care occurs within the community and numerous community resources are used. Home health nurses view the client, family, and designated caregivers as partners when planning and implementing nursing care. The nurse performs a detailed home assessment to determine the safety of the home for the client (ANA, 2014a; Marrelli, 2017). The nurse also assesses the community in which the client's home is located to determine access to services and availability of resources for client support. The home health nurse provides direct care; educates the client, family, and caregivers about how to independently meet health care needs; counsels the client and family; and coordinates community resources and benefits. Home health nurses continually evaluate the effectiveness of planned interventions and community resources as nursing care is delivered (ANA, 2014a; Marrelli, 2017).

The nurse–client relationship differs in home health nursing because the client (and family) considers the nurse a guest (Marrelli, 2017). This perception sets up different dynamics for the nurse–client relationship. The nurse must work diligently to ensure that they are welcome while helping the client and family assume responsibility for meeting individualized health needs. The nurse exercises special care not to offend the host or disaffirm client and family self-determination. Sometimes, the nurse must politely refuse client requests when they fall outside the arena of professional nursing practice. When such requests are made, the nurse might consider referring the client to appropriate community resources or set up visits by a homemaker or unlicensed care provider (Marreli, 2017).

Home health nurses frequently supervise visits by unlicensed care providers and coordinate the schedules of other members of the health care team and home care services so that the client has someone visiting each day of the week. Home health care nurses frequently take calls on weekends and holidays so that homebound clients have access to a nurse should health care problems arise.

Advances in technology now enable home health nurses to have daily contact with clients. Telehealth and satellite home monitoring systems enable home health nurses to check client weight, blood pressure, pulse, peripheral blood glucose, and prothrombin times remotely. Some home monitoring systems set alarms and verbally prompt clients when it is time to get connected and send physical assessment data to the home health care agency. Certain systems offer direct video monitoring and/or wireless technology to obtain results of client home monitoring. With computer technology, the home health agency can create printed records of client data using tables or graphs to detect trends toward meeting expected outcomes or to indicate deteriorating parameters. Some systems even have the capability to ask a client specific questions to assess for potential disease complications.

Home health nurses use these systems for planning the sequence of daily visits or determining whether an additional, unscheduled visit should be made. They can also call clients when they fail to perform required, daily monitoring tasks. Medicare covers home monitoring systems as long as clients have been certified for home health nurse visits. Once clients no longer need home health care, the monitoring system may be removed from the home. Some clients with financial resources elect to keep the monitoring system in their home using private funds. Home health nurses need to emphasize to clients that home monitoring systems do not replace calling 911 or an ambulance when an emergency arises.

For home health agencies to be reimbursed for services, the professional nurse maintains detailed records of home health visits. However, during the COVID-19 pandemic, federal and private health insurance companies changed policies and permitted home health nurses to "visit" clients using telephone calls or teleconferencing systems. Complete, accurate documentation of the visit serves as data for third-party payer reimbursement, validation of services rendered, and data for nursing research. The professional nurse completes approval and recertification forms to validate the need for nursing services.

Hospice and Palliative Care Nursing

Hospice and palliative care nurses visit clients where they live and assist care providers with end-of-life care issues. This may include the home or extended care or residential facilities. The goal of hospice and palliative care is to promote the best possible quality of life for terminally ill individuals and their families and significant others by alleviating suffering, promoting comfort, providing support services, and recognizing that terminally ill clients are living until they die. According to the Hospice and Palliative Nursing Credentialing Center (2020), more than 15,000 nurses have attained certification in hospice and palliative care nursing (CHPN).

The nurse generalist provides direct care to clients and families and coordinates hospice and palliative care resources. Nurse practitioners and clinical nurse specialists also offer advanced practice nursing care (including prescriptive services) in accordance with state laws (ANA & Hospice and Palliative Nurses Association, 2014). Since 1983, Medicare has covered home health services for terminally ill clients (Stanhope & Lancaster, 2018).

Nurses have a long history of caring for those who are dying. In 1950, Dr. Cicely Saunders founded the hospice movement at St. Christopher's Hospital in London. Hospice aims to add greater quality of life to each day when medical science cannot add additional time to a person's life. Hospice uses a team approach to maximize quality of life for the terminally ill client and caregivers by providing: (1) intermittent nursing services; (2) physician services aimed at alleviating human suffering; (3) medications for relieving pain, nausea, and other discomforts associated with the dying process; (4) home health aides; (5) medical equipment and supplies; (6) pastoral services for spiritual support; (7) continuous care when crises arise; and (8) follow-up bereavement services for the family for as long as a year after the client has died.

Hospice nurses receive special education on the dying process, grief, and bereavement management. To effectively care for terminally ill clients and their caregivers, hospice nurses must have confidence in their clinical skills and spiritual beliefs. Much of the nursing care focuses on helping the terminally ill and their families find meaning in their past, present, and future lives. As a team member, the hospice nurse frequently spends more time with clients and families than do other members of the hospice care team and shares comprehensive information with the team (ANA & Hospice and Palliative Nurses Association, 2014; Stanhope & Lancaster, 2018).

Nursing for People Without Homes

The National Alliance to End Homelessness (2020) reported that in 2019, there were an estimated 567,715 people without homes, an increase of more than 14,000 from 2018. Of people without homes, 49.2% were individual adults, 8.6% were families (multiple people within a family group), and 37.2% were unaccompanied youth 18 years of age or younger. Of individuals without homes, 70% are male, with 10% being young men or children 18 years of age or younger. Individuals at risk for becoming homeless are people who live in poverty; the likelihood of homelessness increases when two or more people or families living in poverty share living quarters. With losses in employment related to the COVID-19 pandemic, many more people are at increased risk for homelessness. The incidence is disproportionately higher among Pacific Islander, Native American, Black, Hispanic/Latinx and multiracial Americans. There is a national shortage of more than 200,000 beds in homeless shelters across the United

States. The highest numbers of people without homes are in New York and California; the lowest rates of homelessness are in Virginia and South Dakota. People who live without homes make up 24% of this population, and 63.4% do not have access to regular shelter (National Alliance to End Homelessness, 2020).

Individuals and families without homes lack a fixed, regular night-time residence; may use a shelter, mission, or transient hotel; or live in places not intended for human slumber (e.g., a motor vehicle, under a bridge, in a subway tunnel, in a park or a vacant house or lot). For some people, homelessness may be temporary (the person has no home, but community membership remains), episodic (several periods of having no home), or chronic (no home as a way of life). During times of economic recession, the number of homeless families increases. Reasons for homelessness include poverty, lack of affordable housing, unemployment, lack or inadequacy of government financial support, crime, violence, lack of family support, mental illness, substance abuse, and socially stigmatizing infectious diseases (McEnroe-Petitte, 2020; Stanhope & Lancaster, 2018). In American life, securing a job, societal privileges, or government-sponsored social services requires a permanent address. Accessing health care services can be difficult, if not impossible, for the homeless population. Frequently, people without homes seek health care services only when they are seriously ill and injured (often as crime victims), and they tend to use emergency rooms for treatment. Once they recover, placing these clients in safe situations where they can meet the demands of follow-up care poses a challenge to social workers and case managers (McEnroe-Petitte, 2020).

Of people without homes, 84% have preexisting health conditions such as diabetes, hypertension, foot conditions, and mental illness (National Alliance to End Homelessness, 2020). Crowded conditions in shelters facilitate the spread of communicable diseases. Malnutrition is prevalent, and oftentimes people without homes do not have access to healthy foods and may opt for consuming less expensive, high-caloric, high-fat foods (McEnroe-Petitte, 2020). Living in places without effective shelter from the weather increases the risk of frostbite and hypothermia in the winter and dehydration, heat exhaustion, and heat stroke in the summer. People living on the street may not have access to facilities for personal hygiene and elimination, resulting in ideal situations for infection.

Individuals without homes may be employed but may not earn enough or work enough hours to have health insurance benefits. Other barriers to receiving routine and follow-up care services include language barriers, low literacy, sleep deprivation, lack of transportation, and mental illness. When they do seek care, they may experience a lack of acceptance and respect in mistrust of health care providers. People without homes may be incapable of following discharge instructions owing to a lack of access to supplies and medications (McEnroe-Petitte, 2020). When routine health care is needed, some people without homes rely on free community health or homeless shelter clinics that may rely on volunteers because they cannot afford to hire staff. This can result in the lack of continuity of care. Some nurses provide health care to people without homes in soup kitchens and on the streets.

Homelessness is not confined to urban settings. Migrant workers may also experience homelessness. Rural county health departments frequently serve as the vehicle for health care for transient farm workers and people without homes seeking refuge in rural areas.

For effective nursing practice for people without homes, the community health or volunteer professional nurse must develop and maintain a realistic understanding of the realities of homelessness. Often, individuals without homes lack knowledge of available local programs and services to which they are entitled. Sometimes, people without homes become so overwhelmed in securing food and shelter that they lose hope. To survive, some individuals without homes engage in behaviors like manipulation, lying, and panhandling.

Professional nurses may play a variety of roles when working with and for people without homes. Nurses can work with clients to prevent the factors contributing to homelessness. Nurses can also lobby for legislation that increases services to people without homes and provide government officials with information about the challenges of homelessness (see Chapter 19, "The Professional Nurse's Role in Public Policy"). Nurses can provide direct care and health screening to people who seek help at public health departments, free health clinics, homeless shelters, places of religious worship, or soup kitchens. Finally, nurses can refer clients without homes to mobile treatment centers, mental health facilities, and drug and alcohol rehabilitation programs.

Nursing for Individuals Who Are Incarcerated

Nurses who work in prisons and detention centers provide physical and mental health care to people who have been convicted of committing crimes. Professional nurses engage in primary, secondary, and tertiary interventions for those who are incarcerated. Professional nurses do not participate in procedures exclusively for correctional purposes; professional nursing practice in correctional facilities emphasizes disease prevention, promotes health enhancement activities, and recognizes and treats physical and mental illnesses and injuries from accidents or acts of violence. Nurses frequently administer medications for the purpose of controlling behavior and diagnosed mental illnesses. They also evaluate the effectiveness of care and look for ways to improve health services for those incarcerated (ANA, 2020b). In prison settings, nurses make most health care decisions. They may work with medically approved care protocols for the use of physical and chemical restraints when individuals are in danger of harming themselves or others (Solell & Smith, 2019).

Solell and Smith (2019) report that there are 2.3 million people in the United States serving custodial prison sentences. Many inmates have mental health issues, smoke, and/or suffer from HIV and hepatitis infections. As prison sentences lengthen, nurses encounter older inmates who may have more than one major chronic illness. Although not common, some terminally ill inmates may be seen by prison hospice workers or volunteers (Solell & Smith, 2019).

Security systems at correctional facilities apply to health care professionals and other staff members. Security systems protect staff, volunteers, and visitors from acts of violence. Prison officials have corrections officers stand outside examination rooms and accompany nurses to cells as they deliver health care to inmates who may have histories of violence. Some inmates receive outpatient care in prison clinics, and if 24-hour nursing care is needed, most prisons have infirmaries (Solell & Smith, 2019). Prisons frequently develop partnerships with university health care centers and the private sector to obtain medical staff coverage for clinics. However, prisons often staff infirmaries with nurses and unlicensed care providers who are employed by the prison system (ANA, 2020b; Watson et al., 2004).

Forensic Nursing

The scientific study of forensics is a vital arm of law enforcement. In recent years, the application of forensic science to investigate trauma in emergency departments has created the need to secure reliable evidence and support victims of violent crimes. The practice of forensic nursing includes sexual assault nurse examiners, forensic nursing educators/consultants, nurse coroners, nurse death investigators, legal nurse consultants, nurse attorneys, correctional nurses, clinical nurse specialists,

forensic pediatric nurses, forensic gerontology nurses, and forensic psychiatric nurses. Forensic nurses use the nursing process to determine and appropriately treat the occurrences of sexual assault, homicide, physical assault, intimate partner abuse, and child abuse (International Association of Forensic Nurses & ANA, 2017).

Forensic nurses identify injuries that have forensic implications. Using strict protocols, they collect evidence when a crime has occurred. Nurses who collect evidence frequently provide expert witness testimony as to the integrity of the evidence. They also meticulously document client interactions and evidence collection because the documentation will be used in legal proceedings as evidence. Forensic nurses also interact with the victims of crimes and their families. Finally, forensic nurses may consult with other agencies and law enforcement personnel when forensic information is shared (International Association of Forensic Nurses & ANA, 2017).

Armed Forces Nursing

The branches of the U.S. armed forces work and live together for a common purpose: to protect the country. Because each branch of the military has a specific area of expertise, each branch can be considered a community. Armed forces nursing provides nurses with the opportunity to work with military personnel and their families, as well as civilians affected by warfare. The U.S. Army, Navy (whose nurses serve the Marines as well), and Air Force each have a nursing corps. Nurses serve the military by enlisting for active duty, for reserve status, or for the National Guard. Military nurses have the opportunity to practice with clients of all ages in ambulatory clinics, community hospitals, large medical centers, hospital ships, field hospitals, and aircraft. Military nurses receive comparable compensation to nurses in civilian practice settings. Branches of the armed services offer generous signing bonuses, a full array of benefits, and the option to retire with full benefits after 20 years of service. Nurses in all branches of the armed forces have the potential for upward mobility (Marquand, 2004). Professional practice responsibilities vary according to assignment.

Military nurses confront special personal and professional challenges when deployed in a combat zone. Some of the challenges include long separations from family (sometimes a year or longer), language and cultural differences, climate issues (e.g., temperature extremes, dust, tropical storms), supply shortages, severe trauma exposure, violent threats from enemy combatants or insurgents, and posttraumatic stress disorder. When serving in a combat zone, military nurses, like soldiers, receive increased pay (Spencer, 2006). Sometimes, nurses are deployed on humanitarian missions for which no extra pay is provided.

Armed forces nursing provides professional nurses with opportunities for advanced education. Nurses can earn graduate degrees in nursing, receive specialty education, and pursue graduate degrees outside the discipline of nursing. Military nurses have opportunities for teaching client care skills to corps members and leadership classes to future officers (Marquand, 2004). The branches of the armed forces also conduct nursing research related to issues of deployment, the needs of military personnel and their beneficiaries in times of war and peace, and cultural aspects of military nursing (Marquand, 2004).

Military nursing provides the opportunity for nurses to work with other health team members as equal partners. Camaraderie among health team members is high because everyone focuses on what is best for the service member receiving care. Physicians and nurses have weapons training together. In some circumstances, nurses may outrank physicians. When armed forces deploy active duty and reserve nurses during times of war, they expend energy and resources to recruit civilian nurses to fill vacancies left in stateside hospitals and clinics (Marquand, 2004).

School Nursing

Within a school, many people work together to attain the goal of imparting cognitive, affective, or psychomotor knowledge and skills to others. Thus, all levels of schools meet the definition of a community. Many people tend to view school nursing as confined to the kindergarten through high school levels, but many colleges and universities also provide health services to students, and some nurses work with college students.

Regardless of student age group, school nurses use the nursing process to guide client care activities and bear a number of specific responsibilities (see Box 15.4, Professional Building Blocks, "Responsibilities of the Professional School Nurse"). They also systematically evaluate the effectiveness of nursing practice and health care services. School nurses must abide by various regulations of the states in which they practice.

Elementary and High School Settings

The role of the school nurse remains consistent across all levels of education. However, when nurses work with children and minors, they also spend much time working with the parents of these younger clients. As a nursing specialty, school nursing aims to advance

---

15.4 Professional Building Blocks

Responsibilities of the Professional School Nurse

- Maintain competence.
- Assess, diagnose, identify outcomes, plan, implement, and evaluate student health care services.
- Coordinate student health care services.
- Provide health teaching.
- Promote student health.
- Consult with other health professionals.
- Abide by state and federal laws when using prescriptive authority, treatments, and therapies (advanced practice nurses only) in regard to knowledge and issues affecting their student populations.
- Provide ethical care.
- Use research findings and best evidence in practice.
- Conduct research studies when gaps in practice are identified.
- Engage in quality improvement processes.
- Use school resources judiciously.
- Collaborate with others to develop relevant health care services.
- Communicate effectively in all areas of professional nursing.
- Demonstrate leadership in practice settings and the profession.
- Collaborate with health care consumers, families, and others.
- Evaluate one's practice against practice standards.
- Maintain environmental safety.
- Manage student health programs.

American Nurses Association & the National Association of School Nurses. (2017). *School nursing: Scope and standards of practice.* (3rd ed.). Nursebooks.org and National Association of School Nurses. (2016). *The role of the 21st century school nurse (Position Statement).* Author. https://www.nasn.org/advocacy/professional-practice-documents/position-statements/ps-role.

student well-being, academic success, lifelong achievement, and health. School nurses work to facilitate positive student responses to normal growth and development, promote safety and health, intervene when health problems arise or are anticipated, and provide community referrals and other case management services (ANA & National Association of School Nurses [NASN], 2017).

School nurses have various roles. They provide direct health care to students who have bouts of acute physical or chronic illnesses, as well as to students with special health care needs resulting from disabilities. Professional school nurse generalists also provide first aid; administer medications; screen students for health problems, general fitness, and signs of abuse; monitor vital signs; participate in case management activities; change dressings; and perform urinary catheterizations. School nurses develop individualized nursing care and health educational plans for students with chronic illnesses or those who need to learn complex self-care skills to cope with disabilities. School nurses also engage in enhancing the wellness of teachers, administrators, counselors, and nutritional, janitorial, and clerical staff. School nurses perform periodic environmental assessments to ensure a safe and health-promoting school environment. They may also review the daily menu for school cafeterias to verify that healthy meals are being served. When specific health care needs arise, school nurses make referrals to local health care providers (ANA & NASN, 2017; Stanhope & Lancaster, 2018).

In some school systems, nurses develop the health education program in collaboration with the school administration, teachers, and parents. Health education programs may be tailored to an individual school's needs or be developed to meet the needs and concerns of a school district. Often, the school nurse teaches health education classes to students, parents, school staff, and/or community groups (ANA & NASN, 2017; Stanhope & Lancaster, 2018).

School nurses spend much time maintaining student health records. They verify that all students have received required immunizations and that students have received screening for visual, hearing, and skeletal abnormalities. When students visit the school nurse, the nurse documents the reason for the visit, interventions performed, parental contact (if needed), and referrals made as needed. Most school health programs have protocols indicating actions that can be taken by nurses without parental consent. Many schools have parents sign forms specifying particular

over-the-counter medications (e.g., acetaminophen, antibiotic or steroid ointments, antihistamines, decongestants) the nurse may administer to their children. School nurses also receive detailed information about routinely prescribed medications that students may require. Because of the prevalence of drug abuse and zero-tolerance laws in many school districts, students taking prescription medications must visit the school nurse to receive their scheduled doses (Stanhope & Lancaster, 2018).

The school nurse serves as a resource for health information for students, faculty, and staff. Sometimes, faculty and staff consult the school nurse when they suspect a potential health-related problem in a student. The nurse may develop several approaches to the problem and consult with school administration before activating a plan. Sometimes nurses work collaboratively with teachers and administrators to develop plans for students with learning disabilities and mental health problems. In some cases, the school nurse assumes responsibility for monitoring school compliance with specific portions of student disability regulation (NASN, 2016; Stanhope & Lancaster, 2018).

School nursing is a specialized area of nursing practice, and additional education beyond the baccalaureate degree is recommended for optimal clinical effectiveness. School nurses may become certified through the NASN or ANA. Many states also have certification requirements for school nursing. The Rehabilitation Act in 1973 required that public schools provide appropriate and free education for children with disabilities; this required that nurses be readily available to attend to needs of children with severe and sometimes unpredictable medical conditions (Stanhope & Lancaster, 2018). In 1990, the Americans with Disabilities Act specified that all children with any form of cognitive, physical, or social disabilities had equal rights to educational opportunities. The school nurse has the responsibility to develop and monitor student individualized health plans with other health team members to address identified student health needs. The school nurse is legally bound to write emergency individualized health plans for students with potentially life-threatening health issues (e.g., seizures, insulin-dependent diabetes, asthma, anaphylactic reactions to peanut exposure) (Stanhope & Lancaster, 2018). Some school districts offer school-based clinics that are staffed by school nurse practitioners who provide primary health care services to students (including prescriptions for contraceptives and treatment for sexually transmitted infections). School-based clinics have been credited with reducing the number of school absences for students with chronic diseases, especially asthma (NASN, 2016; Stanhope & Lancaster, 2018).

In addition to providing nursing services and health education, the school nurse participates in research, investigates cases, and delegates health-related tasks to unlicensed personnel. Unfortunately, not every school has a nurse on campus, and certain tasks must be delegated to school staff members. When this happens, the nurse must provide the staff members with education to safely accomplish health-related tasks (NASN, 2016; Stanhope & Lancaster, 2018).

College Campus Setting

College health nursing focuses primarily on the health care needs and concerns of people between the ages of 17 and 24 years. Nurses working with college students emphasize self-care and wellness. College nursing services vary in size and scope. Some college health programs offer ambulatory care services with scheduled office hours exclusively, whereas others provide an infirmary for acute care staffed by a multidisciplinary health team. The American College Health Association Review Group, in collaboration with the ANA, has published guidelines for collegiate nursing practice. Many colleges and universities provide clinics that have advanced practice nurses on staff to deliver required health services to students (ANA, 1997).

▇ QUESTIONS FOR REFLECTION

1. What are the health care services offered at the college you attend?
2. What health-promoting factors are present within the college you attend?
3. What are your major health-related concerns as a nursing student? Why are these important to you?

Faith Community Nursing

Faith community nursing provides nurses with an opportunity to practice within faith communities. Faith communities are groups of people who share common faith traditions and meet in a specific place of worship (e.g., church, mosque, synagogue) (ANA & Health Ministries Association Inc. [HMAI], 2017). In 1984, Granger Westberg started a parish nursing program at Lutheran General Hospital in Chicago. The International Parish Nursing Resource Center offered the

first continuing education program in parish nursing in 1987 (Stanhope & Lancaster, 2018). In 1998, the ANA published *Scope and Standards of Parish Nursing Practice*, thereby acknowledging parish nursing as a distinct specialized area of professional practice. These guidelines were revised in 2012 and renamed *Faith Community Nursing: Scope and Standards of Parish Practice* and underwent a subsequent revision in 2017 (ANA & HMAI, 2017).

Two models for faith community nursing exist: the congregational model and the institutional model. In the congregational model, the nurse acts autonomously, and nursing and health programs arise from the community in which the nurse serves. The nurse is held accountable to the congregation and the governing body. In the institutional model, the nurse collaborates more closely with local hospitals, medical centers, extended-care facilities, and educational institutions. Sometimes, the faith community nurse holds contracts with the collaborating agencies. The nurse works in partnership with the local health care and educational institutions to meet the needs of faith community members (Jacob, 2020; Stanhope & Lancaster, 2018).

Nurses who are members of faith-based communities frequently serve as first responders when a congregation member has a health-related problem during a service or activity. Parish nurses also engage in health ministry activities, such as visiting homebound congregation members, arranging for meals for families in times of crises, forming prayer circles or chains, serving healthy meals and refreshments at congregational activities, and volunteering for local community care groups. In some faith communities, nurses provide volunteer services. Other faith communities have formalized programs staffed by paid directors, coordinators, and nurses. Some faith community nursing programs allow the nurse to run clinics to serve poor or marginalized congregations. These clinics may be staffed by nurse practitioners (Jacob, 2020; Stanhope & Lancaster, 2018).

As a specialized area of professional practice, certain factors distinguish faith community nursing from other practice areas:

- The client spiritual dimension is the core and central dimension of faith community nursing practice.
- The faith community nurse balances knowledge of nursing science, humanities, and theology as nursing services are delivered.
- The faith community and its ministry become the focus of practice.

- The faith community nurse emphasizes individual, family, and faith community strengths.
- Spiritual health, physical health, and healing are viewed as dynamic ongoing processes (Jacob, 2020; Stanhope & Lancaster, 2018).

Nursing skills used when providing care to faith-based communities vary across programs. No two faith community nursing programs are identical, and the nursing services offered in them cannot fully meet all health needs of the community. The eight key functions of the faith community nurse have been identified as health education, personal health counseling, health care referral services, support group development, volunteer facilitation, volunteer training, faith and health integration, and health care advocacy. Westberg envisioned the faith community nurse as a part-time paid position assumed by a baccalaureate-prepared nurse (Jacob, 2020; Stanhope & Lancaster, 2018).

Education preparation for faith community nurses has evolved from a 1- or 2-day continuing education seminar into more formalized programs. Nurses can attend a 1-day continuing education program or take a formal course of study lasting several years to earn a master's degree in nursing or a graduate degree in divinity. In 1996, 50 parish nurse coordinators identified key elements of a standardized curriculum for parish nursing. Curricular content addresses the church's role in health; health theology; the history and philosophy of parish nursing; models of parish nursing practice; the teaching, counseling, referring, and educating functions of the parish nurse; the integration of faith and health; parish community assessment; health promotion and maintenance; families and faith communities as client; parish nurse self-care; working with churches and within a ministerial team; legal and ethical issues; accountability and documentation techniques; prayer and worship leadership; and how to start a faith community nursing program. Additional content for faith community nurse coordinators includes budgeting, writing grants, managing human and fiscal resources, developing spiritually, and planning continuing education for parish nurses. Advanced practice and health ministry specialty practice education along with practical experience in community health nursing enrich faith community nursing services (Jacob, 2020).

Faith community nursing offers an avenue for the development of new spiritual (or religious) community and interpersonal nursing diagnoses and interventions. Proposed new nursing diagnoses include the potential for improved acceptance, spiritual concern, altered spiritual development, spiritual isolation, altered spiritual ritual patterns, risk of cultural incongruity, ineffective boundaries, ineffective meditation skills, and communication enhancement. Spiritual nursing interventions focus on enhancing health by strengthening faith and hope while preventing religious addiction. Faith community nurses empower faith communities to engage in unified political actions on health-related legislation, support and teach each other to provide volunteer assistance to ill and frail members, and promote health by enhancing the spiritual dimensions of congregation members (Solari-Twadell & McDermott, 2006).

Volunteer Nursing

Many nurses volunteer to provide nursing services in community settings. Some nurses routinely schedule volunteer activities into life routines, such as serving on organizational or institutional boards, monthly or weekly duties at a free health clinic, and regularly scheduled community health screening activities. Other nurses may provide volunteer service for episodic events such as health fairs, camps, community service projects (e.g., Habitat for Humanity), faith community activities, and community events. When volunteering, nurses have an obligation to have adequate knowledge about actual and potential situations that may arise. For example, when volunteering in a foreign country, nurses must be knowledgeable about any specific laws that govern clinical practice as well as laws that may govern personal behaviors (ANA, 2020a).

When providing services, the nurse assumes responsibility for providing accurate health information and ensuring that those served receive the care they require. In the case of blood pressure screening, the nurse must establish guidelines for people who require emergency treatment, those with dangerously high or low blood pressure measurements, those who need medical referral for abnormal measurements, and those with borderline measurements. While engaging in blood pressure screening, nurses can teach people about blood pressure and ways to avoid hypertension. Sometimes, nurses provide clients with forms containing the client's blood pressure reading and recommended actions for various readings. The professional nurse cannot force anyone to seek immediate treatment for blood pressure problems or verify that clients participate in follow-up with referral recommendations.

Nurses who volunteer their services are legally and ethically accountable for their actions when engaging in service (ANA, 2020a). Therefore, they should have individual liability practice insurance because the insurance provided by employers will not provide legal resources should an adverse event occur that directly causes harm or if the nurse is accused of something that occurred during volunteer service.

Summary and Significance to Practice

Conceptual models of the client–environment relationship provide frameworks to guide practice with family and community clients as well as individual clients. Views of change reflected by the models underlie strategies to promote growth of the family or community or to facilitate return to stability. When working with the family or community as clients, nurses must develop the ability to think in multiple dimensions because more than one person becomes the client system. In most cases, the impact of an individual's health-related change affects a family system. The impact of a health change may also have implications for the entire community. As health care professionals, nurses must look beyond individual clients and develop strategies to provide relevant care for families and communities. There are many opportunities for nurses who want to pursue a career in community health. Nursing models provide a theoretical foundation for guiding professional nursing actions as nurses provide service with individuals, families, and communities. In an ideal world, all nurses would be able to provide person-centered, person- and family-centered, and community-centered care.

REAL-LIFE REFLECTIONS

Recalling what you have learned in this chapter, consider the following questions about school nurse Nancy and Lisa, the student she suspects has an eating disorder.

- *List the individual as client, family as client, and community as client in this school nursing scenario.*
- *Why is it important in this situation to expand the definition of client to include the family and community?*
- *What do you think is Nancy's top priority? Why do you think this issue should be addressed first?*
- *What other issues need to be addressed? Why are these important?*

From Theory to Practice

1. After reading this chapter, do you think it is possible to provide nursing care services only to individuals? Why or why not?
2. Which definition of family appeals most to you? How will you incorporate PFCC concepts into your current or future professional practice? What potential obstacles might occur when trying to include the family unit when caring for an individual client?
3. Which of the nursing models presented in the chapter would you consider using if you were providing nursing services to a community? Why do you prefer this model over the other nursing theoretical approaches to caring for communities?

Nurse as Author

1. Think of areas in which the health of your current educational community or professional practice community could be improved, and list several strategies you might use to address them. Select one of these strategies and search peer-reviewed literature, such as journal articles and books, for four to six references to support it. Develop a nursing care plan for the community or a concept map for your chosen strategy. After completing this exercise, write a four- to five-paragraph essay about your experience, what you learned about the specific health issue, and what you learned about your community's openness to tackling the health issue.
2. Most states identify professional nurses as mandatory reporters for identified instances of child abuse or neglect. Write two to three paragraphs about how you feel about becoming a mandatory reporter and what future issues you might encounter should you directly witness an incident of child abuse or neglect. Include a list of resources who might be of help should you find yourself in such a position.

Your Digital Classroom

Online Exploration

For the Individual Client

What is person-centred care and why is it important? **https://www.highspeedtraining.co.uk/hub/what-is-person-centred-care/**

Video: Person-Centered Care Guidelines produced by Cancer Care Ontario, Canada: **https://www.youtube.com/watch?v=NTYRtRNsAko**

For Family as Client

American Academy of Pediatrics: **https://www.aap
.org/en-us/Pages/Default.aspx**

Children Now: **https://www.childrennow.org/**

Children's Institute: **https://www.childrensinsti-
tute.org/**

Center for Health Care Strategies: **https://www
.chcs.org/**

Centers for Medicare & Medicaid Services:
https://cms.hhs.gov

Hospital Compare: **https://www.medicare.gov/
hospitalcompare/search.html**

March of Dimes: **https://www.marchofdimes.org/**

Child Welfare Information Gateway: **https://
www.childwelfare.gov/**

For Community as Client

Centers for Disease Control and Prevention Immunization Information: **https://www.cdc.gov/vaccines/
adults/rec-vac/index.html**

Recommended vaccines by age: **https://www.cdc
.gov/vaccines/vpd/vaccines-age.html**

Recommended vaccinations for immigrants and
refugees: **https://www.cdc.gov/vaccines/adults/
rec-vac/immigrants-refugees.html**

Healthy People 2030: **www.healthypeople.gov**

National Highway Traffic Safety Administration:
www.nhtsa.gov

Substance Abuse and Mental Health Services Administration: **www.samhsa.gov**

Expanding Your Understanding

1. Visit the Child Welfare Information Gateway at
   **https://www.childwelfare.gov/topics/respond-
   ing/reporting/how/**. Read how to report child
   abuse and write key information for a fictitious
   report. To determine whether you live in a state
   that has mandatory reporting, go to **https://www
   .childwelfare.gov/topics/systemwide/
   laws-policies/state/**. Select your state from the
   drop-down menu and read about child abuse and
   child welfare. Learn the penalties for failure to
   report and for false reporting of child abuse and
   neglect.
2 . Visit the Centers for Disease Control and Prevention
   website and read "Influenza (Flu)" at. **https://www
   .cdc.gov/flu/index.htm**. Under "POPULAR TOP-
   ICS," click on "Seasonal Flu" to read information about
   this year's influenza season and read the recommended
   vaccines by age at https://www.cdc.gov/vaccines/vpd/

vaccines-age.html. Check to see if you and your family
are protected according to CDC guidelines for infectious diseases for this year's influenza.
3. Visit the Healthy People 2030 website, "Promoting Healthy People 2030," and access a preview of
   resources for promoting Healthy People 2030 at
   **https://health.gov/our-work/healthy-people-
   2030/promoting-healthy-people-2030**. Choose
   one of the resources and explain why this resource
   appeals to you. Bring this information to class or
   share it in an online class discussion forum.
4. Access the Community/Public Health Nursing
   Competencies published by the Quad Council Coalition Competency Review Task Force (2018) at
   **https://www.cphno.org/wp-content/uploads/
   2020/08/QCC-C-PHN-COMPETENCIES-Ap-
   proved_2018.05.04_Final-002.pdf**. Look at the
   competencies required for the nurse generalist and
   complete the competency checklist found in Appendix A of the document. Make a list of areas for
   your professional growth and set three priorities.
   Outline a professional development plan for the
   top two identified areas for professional growth in
   community/public health nursing.

Beyond the Book

Visit the**Point**® at **www.thePoint.lww.com** for activities and information to reinforce the concepts and
content covered in this chapter.

REFERENCES

Allen, C., & Easley, C. (2008). Ethics and human rights. In L.
   Ivanov & C. Blude (Eds.), *Public health nursing: Leadership,
   policy and practice*. Delmar Cengage Learning.
American Nurses Association. (1997). *Scope and standards of college health nursing practice*. Nursebooks.org.
American Nurses Association. (2014a). *Home health nursing:
   Scope and standards practice* (2nd ed.). Author.
American Nurses Association. (2014b). *Scope and standards of
   public health nursing practice* (2nd ed.). Author.
American Nurses Association. (2020a). ANA position state-
   ment: Ethical considerations for local and global volunteer-
   ism. *Online Journal of Issues in Nursing, 25*(1). https://doi.
   org/10.3912/OJIN.Vol25No01PoSCol01
American Nurses Association. (2020b). *Correctional nursing:
   Scope and standard of practice* (3rd ed.). Nursebook.org.
American Association of Occupational Health Nurses. (2019).
   Occupational health nursing practice standards. http://aaohn
   .org/p/pr/vi/prodid=3
American Association of Occupational Health Nurses. (2020).
   Occupational nursing as a career. http://aaohn.org/page/
   become-an-ohn
American Nurses Association & Health Ministries Association
   Inc. (2017). *Faith community nursing: Scope and standards of
   practice* (3rd ed.). Nursebooks.org.

American Nurses Association & Hospice & Palliative Care Nurses Association. (2014). *Palliative nursing: Scope and standards of practice.* Author.

American Nurses Association & the American Psychiatric Nurses Association. (2015). *Psychiatric-mental health nursing: Scope and standards of practice* (2nd ed.). Author.

American Nurses Association & the National Association of School Nurses. (2017). *School nursing: Scope and standards of practice* (3rd ed.). Nursebooks.org.

Anderson, K. H., & Tomlinson, P. S. (1992). The family health system as an emerging paradigmatic view for nursing. *Image, 24,* 57–63. https://doi.org/10.1111/j.1547-5069.1992.tb00700.x

Andrews, M., Boyle, J., & Collins, J. (2020). *Transcultural concepts in nursing care* (8th ed.). Wolters Kluwer.

Artinian, N. T. (1994). Selecting a model to guide family assessment. *Dimensions of Critical Care Nursing,* 14, 4–12. https://doi.org/10.1097/00003465-199401000-00002

Association of Camp Nurses. (2020). *Resources.* https://camp-nurse.org/education-and-resources/resources/

Bell, J. (2009). Family systems nursing: Re-examined. *Journal of Family Nursing,* 15(2), 123–129. https://doi.org/10.1177/1074840709335533

Bigbee, J. (2008). Relationships between nurse-and physician-to-population ratios and state health rankings. *Public Health Nursing,* 25(3), 244–252. https://doi.org/10.1111/j.1525-1446.2008.00701.x

Boyle, J. S., Barid, M. B., & Collins, J. W. (2020). Culture, family and community. Chapter 11. In Andrews, M. M., Boyles, J. S., & Collins, J. W. (Eds.), *Transcultural concepts in nursing care* (8th ed., pp. 333–370). Wolters Kluwer.

Centers for Medicare & Medicaid Services. (2020). *HCHAPS: Patient perspectives of care survey.* https://www.cms.gov/Medicare/Quality-Initiatives-Patient-Assessment-Instruments/HospitalQualityInits/HospitalHCAHPS

Chevannes, M. (1997). Nursing caring for families' Issues in a multiracial society. *Journal of Clinical Nursing,* 6, 151–157. https://doi.org/10.1046/j.1365-2702.1997.00081.x

Christensen, P. J., & Kenney, J. W. (1990). *Nursing process: Application of conceptual models* (3rd ed.). Mosby.

Clark, M. J. (1999). *Nursing in the community* (3rd ed.). Appleton & Lange.

Demarco, R. F., & Healey-Walsh, J. (2020). *Public health nursing, evidence for practice* (3rd ed.). Wolters Kluwer.

ECRI Institute. (2019). *Person-centered care in aging services. Continuing Care Risk Management 2019 June 6.* https://www.ecri.org/components/CCRM/Pages/ResCare7.aspx

Erceg, L., & Pravda, M. (2009). *The basics of camp nursing* (2nd ed.). American Camping Association.

Fawcett, J., & DeSanto-Madeya, S. A. (2012). *Contemporary nursing knowledge: Analysis and evaluation of nursing models and theories* (3rd ed.). F. A. Davis.

Forchuk, C., & Dorsay, J. P. (1995). Hildegard Peplau meets family systems nursing: Innovation in theory-based practice. *Journal of Advanced Nursing,* 21, 110–115. https://doi.org/10.1046/j.1365-2648.1995.21010110.x

Friedman, M., Bowden V., & Jones, E. (2003). *Family nursing: Research theory & practice* (5th ed.). Prentice-Hall.

Friedman, M. M. (1992). *Family nursing: Theory and practice* (3rd ed.). Appleton & Lange.

Friedmann, M. L. (1995). *The framework of systemic organization.* Sage.

Gilliss, C. L., Highley, B. L., Roberts, B. M., & Martinson, I. M. (1988). *Toward a science of family nursing.* Addison-Wesley.

Gross, S. L. (2020). Managing family dynamics when caring for older adults. *Nursing,* 50(4), 56–62. https://doi.org/10.1097/01.NURSE.0000654032.78679.f1

Hanchett, E. S. (1988). *Nursing frameworks and community as client.* Appleton & Lange.

Hancock, T., & Duhl, L. (1986). *Healthy cities: Promoting health in the urban context (Healthy Cities Paper No 1.).* World Health Organization Europe. Retrieved March 18, 2021 from https://www.euro.who.int/data/assets/pdf_file/0013/101650/E87743.pdf

Hanson, S. (1996). Family assessment and interventions. In S. Hanson & S. Boyd (Eds.), *Family care nursing: Theory, practice and research.* F. A. Davis.

Head, B., Aquilino, M., Johnson, M., Reed, D., Mass, M., & Moorehead, S. (2004). Content validity and nursing sensitive community-level outcomes from the nursing outcomes classification (NOC). *Journal of Nursing Scholarship,* 36, 251–259. https://doi.org/10.1111/j.1547-5069.2004.04046.x

Hospice and Palliative Nursing Credentialing Center. (2020). *Certification.* Retrieved from https://advancingexpertcare.org/HPNA/Certification/About_Certification/HPCC/CertificationWeb/About_Certification.aspx?hkey=150e1796-0870-4556-b384-3405621cd800

Institute for Healthcare Improvement. (2020). *Person-and family-centered care overview.* Retrieved from http://www.ihi.org/Topics/PFCC/Pages/Overview.aspx

Institute of Medicine. (2003). *Health professions education: A bridge to quality.* National Academies Press.

International Association of Forensic Nurses & the American Nurses Association. (2017). *Forensic nursing: Scope and standards of forensic nursing practice* (2nd ed.). Nursebooks.org.

Jacob, S. R. (Ed.). (2020). *Foundations of faith community nursing curriculum: Participant guide, 2019 revision.* Westberg Institute.

Jarvis, C. (2020). *Physical examination and health assessment* (8th ed.). Elsevier.

Kaakinen, J. R, Coehlo, D. P, Steele, R., & Robinson, M. (2018). *Family health care nursing: Theory, practice and research* (6th ed.). F.A. Davis.

Khederian, H. (2020). *10 most and least healthy states in America for 2020. MSN Money Benzinga.* Retrieved from https://www.msn.com/en-us/money/news/10-most-and-least-healthy-states-in-america-for-2020/ar-BB16EblI

King, I. M. (1983). King's theory of nursing. In I. W. Clements & F. B. Roberts (Eds.), *Family health: A theoretical approach to nursing care.* Wiley.

Kurtz, P., & Burr, R. (2009). Ethics and health. In B. Lundy & S. Janes (Eds.), *Community health nursing caring for the public's health* (2nd ed.). Jones & Bartlett.

Lapp, C. A., Diemert, C. A., & Enestredt, R. (1991). Family-based practice. In K. A. Saucier (Ed.), *Perspectives in family and community health.* Mosby-Year Book

Leddy, S. (2003). *Integrative health promotion.* Slack.

Leininger, M., & McFarland, M. (2006). *Culture care diversity and universality: A worldwide theory for nursing* (2nd ed.). Jones & Bartlett.

Lind, C., & Smith, D. (2008). Analyzing the state of community health nursing: Advancing from deficit to strengths-based practice using appreciative inquiry. *Advances in Nursing Science,* 31(1), 28–41. https://doi.org/10.1097/01.ANS.0000311527.35446.4c

Lishner, K. M., & Bruya, M. A. (Eds.). (1994). *Creating a healthy camp community: A nurse's role.* American Camping Association.

Lundy, K., & Janes, S. (2014). *Community health nursing: Caring for the public's health* (3rd ed.). Jones & Bartlett.

Marquand, B. (2004). An Army (and Navy and Air Force) of opportunities: in both wartime and peacetime, nursing careers in the military offer exceptional opportunities to see the world, serve your country and advance to leadership positions. *Minority Nurse, 26*–30.

Marrelli, T. M. (2017). *Home care nursing: Surviving in an ever-changing care environment.* Sigma Theta Tau International.

Marrelli, T. M. (2018). *Hospice & palliative care handbook: Quality, compliance and reimbursement* (3rd ed.) Sigma Theta Tau International.

McCubbin, M. A., & McCubbin, H. I. (1993). Families coping with illness: The resiliency model of family stress, adjustment, and adaptation. In C. B. Danielson, B. Hamel-Bissell, & P. Winstead-Fry (Eds.), *Families, health, and illness: Perspectives on coping and intervention.* Mosby.

McElmurry, B., Park, C., & Buseh, A. (2003). The nurse-community health advocate team for urban immigrant primary health care. *Journal of Nursing Scholarship, 35,* 275–281. https://doi.org/10.1111/j.1547-5069.2003.00275.x

McEnroe-Petitte, D. M. (2020). Caring for patients who are homeless. *Nursing, 50*(3), 24–31. https://doi.org/10.1111/j.1547-5069.2003.00275.x

McFarlane, J., & Anderson, E. T. (2019). *Community as partner, theory and practice in nursing* (8th ed.). Wolters Kluwer Health.

McGoldrick, M., Gerson, R., & Petry, S. (2020). *Genograms: Assessment and treatment* (4th ed.). W.W. Norton & Company.

Mish, F. C. (Ed.). (2020). *Merriam-Webster's collegiate dictionary* (11th ed.). Merriam-Webster, Inc.

Morse, S. (2004). *Smart communities.* Jossey-Bass.

Murdaugh, C. L., Parsons, M. A., & Pender, N. J. (2019). *Health promotion in nursing practice* (8th ed.). Pearson.

Narsavage, G., Batchelor, H., Lindell, D., & Chen, Y. (2003). Developing personal and community learning in graduate nursing education through community engagement. *Nursing Education Perspectives, 24,* 300–305. Retrieved May 10, 2021, from https://www.researchgate.net/publication/8935190_Developing_personal_and_community_learning_in_graduate_nursing_education_through_community_engagement/link/553ebdba0cf20184050f8c2f/download

National Alliance to End Homelessness. (2020). *State of homeless: 2020 edition.* https://endhomelessness.org/homelessness-in-america/homelessness-statistics/state-of-homelessness-2020/

National Association of School Nurses. (2016). *The role of the 21st century school nurse (Position Statement).* Author. https://www.nasn.org/advocacy/professional-practice-documents/position-statements/ps-role

Neuman, B. (1983). Family interventions using the Betty Neuman health care systems model. In I. W. Clements & F. B. Roberts (Eds.), *Family health: A theoretical approach to nursing care.* Wiley.

Neuman, B. (1989). *The Neuman systems model* (2nd ed.). Appleton & Lange.

Neuman, B., & Fawcett, J. (2010). *The Neuman systems model* (5th ed.). Pearson Education Inc.

Newman, M. A. (1983). Newman's health theory. In I. W. Clements & F. B. Roberts (Eds.), *Family health: A theoretical approach to nursing care.* Wiley.

Newman, M. A., Sime, A. M., & Corcoran-Perry, S. A. (1991). The focus of the discipline of nursing. *Advances in Nursing Science, 14,* 1–6.

Orem, D. E. (1983). The self-care deficit theory of nursing: A general theory. In I. W. Clements & F. B. Roberts (Eds.), *Family health: A theoretical approach to nursing care.* Wiley.

Owens, I. T. (2020). Supporting nurses' mental health during the pandemic. *Nursing, 50*(1), 54–57. https://doi.org/10.1097/01.NURSE.0000697156.46992.b2

Parse, R. (2003). *Community: A human becoming perspective.* Jones & Bartlett.

Parse, R. (2009). The humanbecoming family model. *Nursing Science Quarterly, 22,* 305–309. https://doi.org/10.1177/0894318409344767

Parse, R. R. (1996). The human becoming theory: Challenges in practice and research. *Nursing Science Quarterly, 9,* 55–60. https://doi.org/10.1177/089431849600900205

Parse, R. R. (1998). *The human becoming school of thought.* Sage.

Patterson, J. M. (1999). Healthy American families in a postmodern society: An ecological perspective. In H. M. Wallace, G. Green, K. J. Jaros, L. L. Paine, & M. Story (Eds.), *Health and welfare for families in the 21st century.* Jones & Bartlett.

Peplau, H. (1952). *Interpersonal relations in nursing.* G. P. Putnam's Sons.

Powers, K., & Reeve, C. L. (2020). Family presence during resuscitation: Medical-Surgical nurses' perceptions, self-confidence and use of invitations. *American Journal of Nursing, 120,* 11, 28–38. https://doi.org/10.1097/01.NAJ.0000721244.16344.ee

Quad Council Coalition Competency Review Task Force. (2018). *Community/public health nursing competencies.* https://www.cphno.org/wp-content/uploads/2020/08/QCC-C-PHN-COMPETENCIES-Approved_2018.05.04_Final-002.pdf

Quad Council of Public Health Nursing Organizations. (1999). *Scope and standards of public health nursing practice.* American Nurses Publishing.

Rector, C. (2018). *Community and public health nursing: Promoting the public's health* (9th ed.). Wolters Kluwer.

Rogers, M. E. (1983). Science of unitary human beings: A paradigm for nursing. In I. W. Clements & F. B. Roberts (Eds.), *Family health: A theoretical approach to nursing care.* Wiley.

Roy, C. (1983). Roy adaptation model. In I. W. Clements & F. B. Roberts (Eds.), *Family health: A theoretical approach to nursing care.* Wiley.

Saucier, K. A. (Ed.). (1991). *Perspectives in family and community health.* Mosby-Year Book.

Schumacher, K., Stewart, B., & Archbold, P. (2007). Mutuality and preparedness moderate the effects of caregiving demand on cancer family caregiver outcomes. *Nursing Research, 56*(6), 425–433. Retrieved May 10, 2021, from https://doi.org/10.1097/01.NNR.0000299852.75300.03

Shuster, G., & Geppinger, J. (2004). Community as client: Assessment and analysis. In M. Stanhope & J. Lancaster (Eds.), *Community and public health nursing.* Mosby.

Solari-Twadell, P. A., & McDermott M. A. (Eds.). (2006). *Parish nursing: Promoting whole person health within faith communities* (2nd ed.). Sage.

Solell, P., & Smith, K. (2019). If we truly cared': understanding barriers to person-centred nursing in correctional facilities. *International Practice Development Journal, 9*(2), 1–16. https://doi.org/10.19043/ipdj.92.007

Spencer, B. (2006). Nursing care on the battlefield, how the war in Iraq is changing critical care. *American Nurse Today*, 1(2), 24–26. Retrieved May 10, 2021, from http://www.myamericannurse.com/nursing-care-on-the-battlefield

Spradley, B. W. (1990). *Community health nursing: Concepts and practice* (3rd ed.). Scott, Foresman/Little Brown Higher Education.

Stanhope, M., & Lancaster, J. (2018). *Foundations of nursing in the community, community-oriented practice* (5th ed.). Elsevier.

Taylor, S. G., & Renpenning, K. M. (1995). The practice of nursing in multiperson situations, family and community. In D. E. Orem (Ed.), *Nursing: Concepts of practice*. Mosby.

Tomlinson, P. S., & Anderson, K. H. (1995). Family health and the Neuman systems model. In B. Neuman (Ed.), *The Neuman systems model* (3rd ed.). Appleton & Lange.

U.S. Bureau of Labor Statistics. (2020). *Occupational employment statistics. Occupational employment and wages, May 2019. 29-1141 Registered nurses*. https://www.bls.gov/oes/current/oes291141.htm

U.S. Department of Health and Human Services. (2020a). *Healthy people 2030, topics & objectives*. https://www.healthypeople.gov/2020/topics-objectives

U.S. Department of Health and Human Services. (2020b). *Healthy people 2030, mental health and mental disorders*. https://health.gov/healthypeople/objectives-and-data/browse-objectives/mental-health-and-mental-disorders

Watson, J. (1996). Watson's theory of transpersonal caring. In P. H. Walker & B. Neuman (Eds.), *Blueprint for use of nursing models: Education, research, practice and administration*. National League for Nursing.

Watson, J. (2007). *Nursing human science and human care, a theory of nursing*. Jones & Bartlett.

Watson, R., Stimpson, A., & Hostick, T. (2004). Prison health care: A review of the literature. *International Journal of Nursing Studies*, 41, 119–128. https://doi.org/10.1016/S0020-7489(03)00128-7

Whall, A. L. (1986). *Family therapy theory for nursing: Four approaches*. Appleton-Century-Crofts.

Whall, A. L., & Fawcett, J. (1991). *Family theory development in nursing: State of the science and art*. F. A. Davis.

Wright, L. M., & Leahey, M. (1988). *Family nursing trends in academic and clinical settings*. Paper presented at the International Family Nursing Conference, Convention Centre, Calgary, Alberta, Canada, May 24–27, pp. 29–37.

Zonsius, M. C., Cothran, F. A., & Miller, J. M. (2020). Acute care for patients with dementia: A review of best practices for integrating person-centered care throughout the hospital stay. *AJN American Journal of Nursing*, 124(4), 34–43. https://doi.org/10.1097/01.NAJ.0000660024.45260.1a

Zotti, M. E., Brown, P., & Stotts, R. C. (1996). Community-based nursing versus community health nursing: What does it all mean? *Nursing Outlook*, 44, 211–217. https://doi.org/10.1016/S0029-6554(96)80094-7

The Professional Nurse's Role in Teaching and Learning

Teaching
Personal health literacy
Organizational health
    literacy
Functional health
    literacy
Interactive health
    literacy
Critical health literacy
Process

Experts
Learning
Client education
Core quality measures
Readiness for learning
Validation
Feedback
Client-focused teaching
Motivation

By the end of this chapter, the learner will be able to:

1. Explain the importance of providing and document-ing client education.
2. Explain the concept of health literacy and how it affects client education.
3. Compare and contrast the concepts of personal health literacy and organizational health literacy.
4. Describe the skills required for the development of functional, interactive, and critical health literacy.
5. Provide the rationale for identifying clients and nurses as "experts" in the client education process.
6. Describe each step of the traditional teaching–learning process.
7. Specify key client assessment data to collect before developing and implementing client education.
8. Specify ways to validate client learning.
9. Outline key strategies for effective client education.

Lillian works as a staff nurse in a rural community hospital. She often cares for people with poorly controlled diabetes, chronic kidney and lung diseases, and people recovering from surgery. Because of recurrent admissions to the hospital for many of the clients, she wonders about the effectiveness of client education delivered during the hospital dismissal processes. Within the past 2 weeks, Lillian counted three clients who were readmitted for complications after failing to abide by their home instructions; two were recovering from surgery and one was struggling with poorly controlled diabetes. When these clients were dismissed, they did not seem engaged when receiving client education or they did not appear to fully compre-hend what they were expected to do when they returned home. Lillian knows that improved client education will likely prevent recurrent hospital admissions. As a personal professional goal, Lillian decides to learn about teaching and learning processes and try some her newly acquired knowledge to improve the effectiveness of client education.

Client- and family-centered care focuses on developing partnerships with individuals, families, and communities to empower them with knowledge, skills, and attitudes that promote health, safety, and well-being. Since knowledge can be viewed as power, client education becomes a vehicle to manage their health issues independently and promote equity in health care access and health outcomes.

Teaching is the process of imparting or sharing knowledge and skills with another. It involves instructing, coaching, and guiding another through unfamiliar content or procedures. Without proper education, health care treatments—especially medication administration—can be dangerous.

Professional nurses have been teaching clients for decades. In 1918, the National League for Nursing Education issued a statement specifying the need to educate professional nurses to assume teaching responsibilities. In all health care settings, clients and families need the knowledge and skills about the health care issues they encounter. Historically, compliance with treatment plans has served as the main reason for client education (Falvo, 2004). Current views of client education focus on empowering clients by providing them with knowledge and skills to manage their own health.

In daily practice, nurses share a lot of information with clients. Each client encounter provides an opportunity for sharing health-related information. Clients need to have information about their health problems (knowledge), the ability to do what is needed (skill), and commitment to adhering to instructions (attitude) for recovering from surgery or acute illness, managing chronic disease, and optimizing health and well-being. In some cases, clients must make lifestyle changes to avoid and manage certain diseases. As health care professionals, nurses serve as role models of good health for their clients and communities. Optimal education for lifestyle changes improves when clients see that nurses and other health care providers follow healthy lifestyle habits (Joos & Hickam, 1990).

Take Note!
Nurses provide clients with educative experiences that increase the integration of knowledge, skills, behaviors, and attitudes that improve health.

Teaching–learning is considered a societal duty of most professions. Lawyers inform clients about the law, physicians teach clients about diseases, social workers educate clients about available community resources,

and pharmacists teach clients about medications. As part of the interprofessional health team, nurses have an obligation to educate clients so that the clients can safely and effectively manage their own health and well-being. Professional nurses extend educational efforts beyond individuals and families by providing community-based health education programs, leading support groups, and steering public discussions about necessary public health policy changes. By listening to and learning from all clients (individuals, families, and communities), nurses become capable of providing relevant information that promotes health and improves well-being.

The health education needs and wants of consumers vary. Some clients want to learn how to best promote personal health and avoid illnesses, while others do not see the value of health information until they find themselves ill and in need of health care services (Rankin et al., 2005). Many clients use the internet to access health information but may not be able to evaluate the quality of the information they obtain. Clients need to be aware of how to prevent illness and treatment options for health disorders so they can make informed choices and comply with complex treatment regimens (Falvo, 2004; Rankin et al., 2005). Topics of interest to health care consumers may include:

- Complex health care delivery systems
- Health insurance options
- Available community resources
- How to ask questions of health care providers to get desired information
- Medication safety
- Finding valid and reliable health information using the internet
- When to consult health care providers
- Safe use of assistive devices and other technology

Some clients have multiple health care providers. Nurses play a pivotal role in ensuring client safety across the continuum of care. Nurses carefully gather current client information regarding medications and complementary therapies being used, document this information, and look for any potential harmful interactions with new treatment orders. When clients and families are informed of prescribed medications and treatments, fewer errors occur (The Joint Commission, 2020a, 2020b). Shorter hospital stays coupled with ineffective client education have been linked to increased hospital readmission rates (Herzlinger, 2004).

HEALTH LITERACY

The U.S. Department of Health and Human Services defines (USDHHS) **personal health literacy** as "the degree to which individuals have the ability to find, understand, and use information and services to inform health-related decisions and actions for themselves and others" (2020, para. 4). The changes in health literacy made for *Healthy People 2030* emphasize the importance of using health information rather than just understanding it. Definition revisions also address the ability of people to be able to make well-informed decisions about their health, not just appropriate ones.

New ideas regarding health literacy specify that organizations have the responsibility for addressing health literacy. Therefore, the concept of **organizational health literacy** is defined as "the degree to which organizations equitably enable individuals to find, understand, and use information and services to inform health-related decisions and actions for themselves and others" (USDHHS, 2020, para. 4). Because personal health literacy is context-dependent, producers of health-related information, organizations have a role in improving the quality of materials so that they are more accessible, easily understood, and easier to use. Organizations are also responsible for addressing health literacy in an equitable manner (USDHHS, 2020).

Nutbeam et al. (2018) identified three skills necessary to develop effective personal health literacy. **Functional health literacy** encompasses basic skills such as reading and writing as well as the ability to find, obtain, and apply information. **Interactive health literacy** is the ability to communicate effectively with health care providers so that health care concerns can be addressed and knowledge can be obtained and applied. **Critical health literacy** involves using advanced cognitive skills to analyze and use information to make decisions to control one's health.

Factors associated with high levels of personal health literacy include high reading comprehension, well-refined vocabulary, membership in the dominant cultural group, higher income, higher levels of education, previous encounters with health care providers, being married, intact cognitive status, and possession of health insurance. Biologic women tend to have higher personal health literacy than biologic men because they traditionally manage the health care needs of the family (Ingram & Kautz, 2012; Zhou et al., 2019). Factors associated with limited or low personal health literacy include being older, being part of a disenfranchised group, low socioeconomic status, low educational skills, immigrant status, cultural barriers, limited English proficiency, and being medically underserved (Health Resources and Services Administration [HRSA], 2019). Limited or low personal health literacy levels are associated with limited knowledge about encountered illnesses and disease management, difficulty completing health care forms and surveys, decreased access to high-quality health care information, incorrect use of prescription medication, increased health care expenses, higher use of emergency rooms, depression, and problems keeping appointments and scheduling follow-up visits (Hersh et al., 2015; HRSA, 2019; Mayo-Gamble & Mouton, 2018; Pellowski et al., 2016; Zhou et al., 2019). Higher levels of health and well-being are associated with higher levels of personal health literacy, and higher numbers of chronic illnesses are associated with lower levels of health literacy (Zhou et al., 2019).

Weiss and colleagues (2005) developed a 3-minute assessment tool for use in primary care to assess individuals likely to have low health literacy. They named the tool *The Newest Vital Sign*. Clients are asked to read a nutritional label from a carton of ice cream followed by answering a list of six questions that related to the content of the label and to make decisions based upon dietary recommendations. The first question asks the person to calculate the total number of calories contained in the carton. The second question asks the amount that could be consumed in order to eat 60 g of carbohydrates. The third question asks how much saturated fat the person would consume if they stopped eating ice cream if they typically eat 42 g of saturated fat that includes a serving of ice cream. The fourth question asks the percent of calories for the day if the person consumed one serving of ice cream, assuming the person consumed 2,500 calories on a given day. The final two questions address the safety of consuming the ice cream in a scenario in which the client has certain allergies. The time to administer this tool is about 3 minutes, and getting fewer than four correct answers to the questions indicates a possibility of limited health literacy. Because the tool measures basic reading, math, and decision making sills, nurses can use the results to plan individualized client education.

In 2019, the Agency for Healthcare Research and Quality (AHRQ) identified 10 attributes of health-literate health care organizations:

1. Has leadership that makes health literacy integral to its mission, structure, and operations
2. Integrates health literacy into planning, evaluation measures, client safety, and quality improvement

3. Prepares the workforce to be health-literate and monitors progress
4. Includes populations served in the design, implementation, and evaluation of health information and services
5. Meets the needs of populations with a range of health literacy skills while avoiding stigmatization
6. Uses health literacy strategies in interpersonal communications and confirms understanding at all points of contact
7. Provides easy access to health information and services and navigation assistance
8. Designs and distributes print, audiovisual, and social media content that is easy to understand and implement
9. Addresses health literacy in high-risk situations, including care transitions and communications about medicines
10. Communicates clearly what health plans cover and what individuals will have to pay for services. (AHRQ, 2019, para. 3)

Nurses working in health-literate health care organizations should receive education in what health literacy means, their roles in ensuring health literacy, communication strategies to promote health literacy, and providing context appropriate to client education. For example, data regarding client preferences in language, learning strategies, and educational materials typically appear as items on client admission databases. Computerized documentation systems provide access to a variety of educational materials for clients to receive during hospitalization and when being dismissed. Many educational platforms in health care organizations have materials available in a variety of languages. To ensure clients receive the knowledge and skills needed for self-care (or the care of a significant other), nurses document client education into the electronic health record. When thinking about Lillian's professional goal of improving the effectiveness of her client education, she is enhancing the health literacy of the clients for whom she provides nursing care and the health literacy of her hospital.

According to an international study on educational skills, 43 million American adults have low literacy levels and struggle to follow written directions. Over 8 million American adults (4%) scored at the level of being functionally illiterate while participating in an international survey measuring international educational competencies. The study defines functionally illiterate as being unable to determine the meaning of a sentence,

to read text for a single piece of information, and to complete simple forms (U.S. Department of Education [DOE], National Center for Education Statistics [NCES], 2019). In the same study, 62.7 million American adults (9%) lacked proficiency in basic numeracy skills (e.g., counting, sorting interpreting graphs, and spatial representations) (U.S. DOE, NCES, 2020). Additionally, 8.2 million Americans could not complete the study survey due to cognitive or physical disabilities (U.S. DOE, NCES, 2019). The inability to read, follow directions, or complete surveys along with difficulty counting and sorting has serious implications for persons to manage their health at home. For example, the inability to count and read may result in a person not taking medications as prescribed.

According to the U.S. Department of Education (DOE), an estimated 90 million Americans have low health literacy levels; that is, they experience problems comprehending and acting on health information (Hersh et al., 2015). Low health literacy levels seem to increase as a person ages, possibly the result of cognitive, memory, and executive function declines associated with aging. People with lower levels of health literacy live in impoverished areas and tend to be members of marginalized groups (Hersh et al., 2015; Ingram & Kautz, 2012). The average reading level of American adults is between the seventh and eighth grade levels (U.S. DOE NCES, 2019), but 75% of health information and educational materials are written at the high school or college reading levels (Hersh et al., 2015).

Take Note!
Limited or low levels of health literacy have a detrimental effect on health, well-being, and ability to access health care.

Low health literacy has been linked to hospital readmissions. Reports estimate 2 million hospitalized Medicare clients reenter the hospital within 30 days of dismissal and cost taxpayers an additional $27 million; $17 million of these costs could have been avoided (Kauffman, 2016). Ingram and Kautz (2012) described low health literacy as a "silent epidemic" (p. 22). Teaching health care consumers health literacy basics is a challenge for all health care professionals. Information regarding how to plan and carry out client education in this chapter includes specific strategies to address low health literacy.

PHILOSOPHICAL ASSUMPTIONS ABOUT TEACHING AND LEARNING

Education can be defined as a product or as a process. As a product, education can be perceived as a commodity for purchase that yields intended results. As a **process**, the focus becomes how education is planned and implemented; the teaching–learning process considers the relationships among **experts**, thereby emphasizing the essential nature of communication. Clients are experts in how health issues affect them, and nurses are experts in the health issues encountered.

Process—Not Product

Interpersonal relationships with others deeply affect human health and well-being. Through relationships, growth can occur when a person integrates new knowledge, attitudes, and skills that lead to a more healthful and satisfying life. Teaching–learning in the nurse–client relationship is aimed toward such growth.

Education involves personal growth and development. In professional nursing, nurse–client relationships facilitate the educational process. Mish (2020, p. 708) defined **learning** as "gaining knowledge or understanding or skill by study, instruction, or experience." In the late 20th and early 21st centuries, neuroscientists identified physiologic processes in the brain for developing different types of memory for knowledge and skill acquisition. Short-term memory lasts for 30 seconds to 2 days, accepts typically up to seven items, and can be enhanced through repetitive and rehearsal exercises. Long-term memory typically takes longer than a day to develop (Collins, 2007). Lupien and McEwen (1997), as cited in Collins (2007), described the process of memory in the following three phases: acquisition (exposure to knowledge to be remembered), consolidation (transformation of short-term to long-term memory), and retrieval (recall of knowledge or skill). Without long-term memory, learning cannot be recalled. Because of the neurophysiologic processes required for learning, nurses must recognize that a client's physical health may affect the ability to learn. If the client possesses impaired cognition, then the nurse needs to delay client education efforts until full cognition returns.

Nurses who view education as a product ignore the physiologic and psychological processes required for long-lasting learning. When education is viewed as a process, the nurse limits the amount of information in each learning session, provides opportunities for clients to repeat new information and practice new skills, and allows clients time to adjust attitudes so they can be successful using the newly acquired knowledge, skills, and attitudes required for self-care and personal growth. The nurse also assesses the client for high stress levels and fatigue, which might impair the learning process. In addition, the nurse can offer information in small chunks to facilitate knowledge acquisition and consolidation (Collins, 2007). Client education culminates with the client receiving validation from the nurse that mastery of new knowledge, ideas, or skills has occurred. Teaching–learning is an interpersonal process in which both the teacher and the learner acquire and consolidate new information, experience new relatedness, and behave in new ways.

Current health care seeks to empower consumers to make informed, autonomous decisions. Many facilities strive to become centers of excellence for a particular disease, health condition, or procedure. Effective client education is a hallmark of a center of excellence. Typically, effective education facilitates learning by engaging clients in purposeful, sequenced learning activities while providing them with support and guidance for mastering required knowledge and skills. The final outcome of learning becomes apparent when clients can recall key information and independently perform skills required for self-care. Nurses can assess recall and comprehension of client education by engaging in a variety of methods. Nurses can ask direct questions about information shared, provide computerized or pencil and paper quizzes for completion, or have the client participate in a return demonstration of skills or "teach-back" (which is simply asking clients to explain what was taught and state what they plan to do when they are at home) (Miller & Stoeckel, 2019; Stewart, 2020).

When nurses believe clients have the required abilities for self-care management, they view learning as far more than discovery by their clients. Their educator role becomes focused on "learning that leads to new action and new problem-solving, which enable individuals and systems to continue to learn" (Argyris, 1982, p. 160). Thus, teaching–learning becomes an ongoing dynamic process.

If learning is to be more than the passive acceptance by the learner of information from the teacher, then nurses must commit themselves to collaborative relationships with clients to fulfill the responsibility for providing optimal client education. The nurse invites and expects clients to participate in the process, define their own strengths and problems, share information about personal preferences for teaching strategies, and construct their own meanings. Thus, teaching–learning is a collaborative process that is most effective when nurses fully engage clients as participatory learners.

Relationship Between Experts

Teaching–learning can be viewed as a relationship between experts. Experts are people who have special knowledge and skills about a particular subject derived from specialized education, training, or experience (Mish, 2020, p. 440). In the professional nursing process, nurses are the experts on health, and clients are the experts on their own health experiences and life circumstances (Stewart, 2020). In the teaching–learning process, clients and nurses view nurses as the experts on knowledge about health and the information that enables people to achieve health and clients as experts on the context of their life and the need for information and experiences to achieve their intentions to maximize health.

The Nurse: Information and Knowledge Expert

Teaching–learning may be viewed as a part of the healing process. Nurses who have reported that they believed their interventions made a difference in their clients' progress outlined several steps in that healing relationship (Benner, 2000, p. 49): mobilizing hope for the nurse as well as for the client; finding an acceptable interpretation or understanding of the illness, pain, fear, anxiety, or other stressful emotion; and assisting the client with using social, emotional, or spiritual support.

Viewing teaching as a coaching function, Benner (2000) proposed that "nurses become experts in coaching a patient through an illness. They take what is foreign and fearful to the patient and make it familiar and thus less frightening" (p. 77). The teacher also needs to have expertise in helping. Helping the learner become aware of learning and thinking processes in understanding the nature of the problems may be equally as important as providing information.

To be an expert in the teaching–learning process, the nurse must also enable the person to feel free to express opinions; react honestly to how content is presented; and assume responsibility for mastering knowledge, skills, and attitudes to change behavior to maximize potential for optimal health and well-being. Learning is facilitated when teachers treat learners as responsible people. In addition, learning empowers clients to take action and assume responsibility for their health (Miller & Stoeckel, 2019; Stewart, 2020).

In addition to coach and enabler, several other roles are proposed for the nurse–teacher (Forbes, 1995, p. 99):

- **Learning facilitator:** Breaks down barriers to learning by listening, probing, and being aware of feelings
- **Authority:** Sets up a teaching structure and rules
- **Ego ideal:** Serves as a role model for the client's "altered existence"
- **Socializing agent:** Acknowledges concerns and fears for the future
- **Person:** Relates to clients as people rather than just disease diagnoses

Each of these roles contributes to teaching–learning situations. However, knowing when to assume each role for optimal effectiveness remains unknown and provides an opportunity to be answered through nursing research studies.

Take Note!
For the teaching and learning process to be successful, the nurse may need to assume multiple roles.

▮ QUESTIONS FOR REFLECTION

1. How do you prefer to learn new things? What teaching strategies enhance your learning? How might you employ your preferred teaching strategies in the future when teaching clients, families, and communities?
2. How do you involve your clients and their families during health teaching?
3. How frequently do you teach clients, families, and communities about health promotion?
4. What education strategies do you tend to use when providing client/family/community education?
5. What factors in your current practice environment support your role as a client teacher?
6. What factors in your current practice environment prevent you from providing effective client education?

The Client: Context and Need Expert

No one knows better the meaning of their life, individual health status, and full circumstances integral to life experiences than the client (Miller & Stoeckel, 2019; Stewart, 2020). Thus, clients serve as the experts on the context in which they will be attempting to implement new health behaviors. They are the experts on their own individualized needs for information, support, and relatedness. When nurses appreciate their professional expertise and the personal expertise of the client, the teaching–learning process can truly be implemented as a mutual responsibility.

The Joint Commission (TJC) developed standards for client and family education as an essential element of nursing. According to TJC, **client education** should convey knowledge and understanding, create a different perspective or attitude, build self-care skills, and change behavior. According to McCollum (2008), TJC's 2009 educational standards include the following elements for effective client education:

1. Facilitate, plan, support, and provide client education.
2. Comprehensive learner assessment before education occurs (ability, readiness, literacy, learning style preferences, cultural or language obstacles, physical or mental limitations).
3. Age and educational level; appropriate teaching methods and materials
4. Consideration of client-preferred learning style
5. Education should be included on rights and responsibilities of being a client, all identified medical diagnoses and treatment options, meaning of signing all consent to treatment forms, the concept of pain, treatment modalities and pain control methods employed, safe and effective use of medications, medical equipment, potential food–drug medication interactions, therapeutic diets, and rehabilitation techniques. The education for each topic should be performed by the best qualified member of the interprofessional health care team.
6. Information on specific home care instructions, available community resources, and how to obtain additional treatment if needed
7. Education on client and family responsibilities for ongoing health care needs and the knowledge and skills on how to fulfill these responsibilities (e.g., ways to promote personal privacy and demonstrating respect when providing basic personal hygiene on incapacitated individuals; knowing specific signs and symptoms that require immediate medical attention)
8. Educational strategies that are interactive, provide detailed instructions, and present available and reliable resources for future use
9. Use of a medical translator when needed
10. Evidence that intended learning outcomes for education have been achieved

McCollum (2008) suggested using the TJC client education standards as a framework for nurses to follow as they plan and execute client educational activities. Starting in 2020, TJC released client safety information in a series of "Speak Up" initiatives. Currently, there are 19 "Speak Up" resources for health consumers to use to learn about and actively participate in their care. Each brochure provides an infographic display of each topic and are available on the TJC website (TJC, 2020a). TJC also offers "TakeCHARGE" information on its website to encourage clients to become full participants and advocate for themselves and others as health care is delivered. Topics included in this campaign include how to ask questions about care, compile and store health information, develop advance directives, and confront health care providers when they fail to wash their hands properly (TJC, 2020b).

Because TJC accreditation meets all requirements for federal reimbursement to organizations for delivered health care, many health care facilities use them for accreditation so they have an established structure and process for meeting all requirements. Therefore, documentation of client education is critical to demonstrating compliance to accreditation standards. During accreditation visits, TJC surveyors examine client care documentation for evidence of client education. Of all client charts (both paper and electronic), 90% should contain this evidence to avoid a citation for improvement. In addition to facilitating reimbursement and accreditation, documenting client education provides solid evidence of nursing's contributions to the interdisciplinary client care efforts.

Federal- and state-funded reimbursement programs for health care services also require proof of client education in documentation. The Centers for Medicare & Medicaid Services (CMS) identify **core quality measures** (evidence-based practice interventions) that indicate that high-quality health care services have been rendered. The core quality measures are developed and released by the National Quality Forum's Core Quality Measures Collaborative. The list areas in which measures have been released include accountable care organizations/client-centered medical homes/primary care; cardiology; gastroenterology; human immunodeficiency virus (HIV) and hepatitis; medical oncology; obstetrics and gynecology; orthopedics; and pediatrics. In 2020, plans were underway to release measures for behavioral health and neurology, but the COVID-19 pandemic stalled this work. Currently, CMS and some health insurance providers require documentation of education related to available core quality measures before reimbursing health care facilities for services. For all clients who currently smoke, education regarding smoking cessation needs to be documented. In acute care facilities, nurses and other health team members must document detailed education on the management of many specific diseases (e.g., diabetes, heart failure, HIV) and dismissal education regarding home medications (with special attention on informing clients about possible side effects), follow-up care, and other special treatments (e.g., activity limitations, dietary education) (The Core Quality Measures Collaborative, 2020). Along with external agency requirements for client education, the American Nurses Association Scope and Standards of Practice for Nursing (2021) specified that professional nurses are responsible for assessing clients and families for anticipated or actual health education needs. They recognize nurses can identify gaps in knowledge in clients for effective management of health conditions and health promotion. The standards also expect nurses to develop health education plans for clients, families, and other caregivers. Nurses bear responsibility and accountability for implementing and evaluating individualized educational plans to determine client mastery of knowledge and skills for effective self-management of health.

Communication: The Condition for Teaching–Learning

Nurses who display empathy, respect, mutuality, and genuineness while teaching are likely to create effective teaching–learning environments. By using empathy, nurses are more apt to understand client global situations and take full advantage of client expertise. Likewise, clients need to perceive that nurses are sensitive to their needs and will generate effective educational plans that include measurement of the cognitive, affective, and psychomotor domains of learning.

Some clients perceive that nurses and other health care professionals have superior status and therefore may be reluctant to ask questions. To combat this issue, the National Patient Safety Foundation in 2012 developed the "Ask Me 3" campaign. This program outlines three key questions consumers should ask during each visit to a health care provider: (1) What is my main problem? (2) What do I need to do? (3) Why is it important for me to do this? (Institute for Healthcare Improvement, 2021)

An effective teaching–learning process occurs when both nurses and clients share a mutual responsibility for the education process and experience respectful communication. Feelings of self-worth facilitate teaching and learning because teachers and learners need to see themselves as capable of effectively fulfilling their roles. Teachers believe and know they can create and execute meaningful learning experiences, and learners believe and know they have the capabilities to master the content and skills being taught.

Full exploration and analysis of the health concerns and information needed to change behaviors cannot occur unless nurses and clients perceive each other as real, and as genuinely human, open, honest, and caring in their responses to each other. Nurses must provide clients with accurate health-related information, and clients must perceive that nurses have information to facilitate health promotion, maintenance, or restoration. Although clients may display an authentic interest in the information being shared with them, the client makes the final determination of what, if, and when received information will be used.

When providing clients with printed or web-based materials, nurses should consider the client's ability to read, reading level, language preferences, and access to the internet. Published, printed, and posted internet educational materials are often written above the average fifth-grade reading level of Americans (Remshardt, 2011; Taylor-Clarke et al., 2012). The CMS has a toolkit for health care professionals to develop clearly and effectively written materials that can be printed or posted online (Centers for Medicare & Medicaid Services, 2020). Some facilities offer client educational software programs that can provide printed materials in a variety of foreign languages to meet the educational needs of clients who do not have fluency in English.

Nurses empower clients to have control over their lives when they give them information or teach them skills to care for themselves. Rankin and colleagues (2005, p. 75) outlined a four-step counseling model for empowering individual clients:

1. Identify the problem or issue (past)
2. Explore feelings and meanings (present)
3. Identify goals and choices (plan for the future)
4. Commit to action (future)

To identify the problem or issue and its impact on the client, the nurse uses holistic assessment skills. Once the issue or problem has been identified, the nurse uses the nursing process step of planning to specify goals and strategies to resolve the problem or issue in collaboration with the client. Once the client has committed to action, the change process begins.

TEACHING–LEARNING PROCESS APPROACHES

The Traditional Approach

Nurses can choose from a variety of approaches when providing client education. The traditional process has been used with success by many nurses and provides a structured approach. Similar to the nursing process, the steps of the traditional teaching–learning process are assessment; identification of learning needs; planning (including the development of learning objectives and selection of educational materials); implementation; evaluation; and documentation (Miller & Stoeckel, 2019; Rankin et al., 2005; Redman, 1993; Stewart, 2020).

Assessment and Identification of Learning Needs

The first activity on the part of the nurse–teacher is assessment: gathering facts and information that will help the nurse meet the client's or the family's learning needs. Rankin and team (2005) indicated the following four steps in the assessment process: (1) selecting the areas to be assessed; (2) gathering the data; (3) sorting and categorizing the data; and (4) writing a summary statement (nursing diagnosis). Box 16.1, Professional Building Blocks, "Purposes of Client-Centered Assessment for Education," outlines the purposes of client assessment (Health Care Education Association, 2020a, 2020b; Miller & Stoeckel, 2019; Rankin et al., 2005; Redman, 1993).

Assessment may be conducted by listening and questioning, observing, reviewing records, collaborating with the health care team, and integrating the client's verbal description with the nurse's observations. Nurses can also use formalized tools to assess learners to determine preferred learning styles and levels of health literacy. The AHRQ offers a Health Literacy Universal Precautions Tool Kit (available at http://www.ahrq.gov/professionals/quality-patient-safety/quality-resources/tools/literacy-toolkit/index.html) that helps nurses identify clients at risk for not being able to understand and use health care information. Of all these assessments, the client's perceptions of what is needed serve as the most important factor in determining educational needs. Therefore, the nurse must engage in active listening and validate professional perceptions with the client.

Nurses must consider the learner's reading ability. In 2015, a study released by the U.S. Department of Education, National Institute of Literacy revealed that

16.1 Professional Building Blocks

Purposes of Client-Centered Assessment for Education

Approach the client in an unhurried manner, and ask open-ended questions to identify:

1. Current client health issues, current knowledge, and concerns
2. What the client wants to learn
3. What the client needs to know
4. Client-preferred ways for learning (visual, auditory, kinesthetic, and materials); options may include printed, multimedia, technology, equipment for practice, one-on-one discussions, etc.
5. People other than the client who should be involved in the educational endeavors (e.g., family members, significant others, and personal caregivers)
6. Client readiness to learn (goals, priorities, and motivation)
7. Client ability to learn (cognitive and physical capabilities)
8. What the client already knows to establish a point of reference for learning (relate new information to preexisting knowledge)
9. Client's incorrect information and assumptions
10. Environmental factors that may pose barriers
11. Potential barriers to client learning (e.g., language, culture, education level, cognitive skills, reading ability, health literacy level, physical limitations)
12. What and how to evaluate the effectiveness of the educational offering(s)
13. Level of trust and rapport between the client and nurse
14. Priorities for needs, problems, and issues to be addressed by education

From Health Care Education Association (2020a). *Assessment*. Retrieved November 23, 2020, from https://www.hcea-info.org/assessment; Ingram, R., & Kautz, D. (2012). Overcoming low health literacy. *Nursing 2013 Critical Care*, 7(4), 22–27; Rankin, S., Stallings, K., & London, F. (2005). *Patient education in health and illness* (5th ed.). Lippincott Williams & Wilkins; Redman, B. K. (1993). *The process of patient education* (7th ed.). Mosby Year Book; Roett, M., & Wessel, L. (2012). Help your patient "get" what you just said: A health literacy guide. *The Journal of Family Practice*, 61(4), 190–196.

the reading level of Americans has remained consistent over the past decade. Data from this study revealed that only 13% of Americans read at a proficient level, 44% read at an intermediate level, 29% read at a basic level, and 14% read below a basic level. Of high school graduates, 19% read below a basic level. Demographics reveal that 44% Hispanic Americans, 24% African Americans, 9% White Americans, and 13% other groups read below a basic level (Statistic Brain, 2015).

Planning and Implementation

After determining the learning needs in the assessment stage, the nurse and the client collaboratively develop a plan that contains objectives or outcomes for the client's learning. These objectives and outcomes clarify what is to be taught, what is to be learned, what and how to evaluate, and what to document. An objective or outcome must be singular to be specific, inclusive of all elements of content necessary to be understood, measurable, and realistic to the extent that it can be attained by the client.

After objectives or outcomes are clarified and validated, the nurse continues planning by determining and analyzing the information to be presented. The nurse identifies the knowledge, skills, and attitudes (competencies) to be incorporated into health education and then selects presentation modalities based on the client's learning styles and preferred learning methods. Using physiology of learning principles, the nurse also strives to use presentation methods that involve the client, stimulate as many human senses as possible, and link new ideas to previous learning. Often, the nurse complements the presentation of information by using supplemental materials, such as audiovisual aids or printed materials. To verify that the client is absorbing new material, developing new skills, and changing personal attitudes during educational sessions, the nurse should frequently observe the client's reaction to the teaching–learning activities. Unfortunately, many health educational materials do not meet appropriate levels of client health literacy.

Two instruments are available for measuring the suitability and readability of health care consumer educational materials: the Fry Reading Formula (FRF) and the Suitability Assessment of Materials (SAM). The FRF determines reading grade level by plotting the syllable and sentence counts from three 100-word passages on a graph. Longer sentences and larger word syllable counts are plotted onto a graph. Reading level increases with longer sentences and more words with three or more syllables. The SAM analyzes client education materials for message content, text appearance, visual displays, layout, and design. For example, text font size should be at least 12 points; key points should be summarized at the end of each section; strategically placed learner evaluations for success should be present; visual displays should be age-appropriate, relevant, culturally sensitive, and easy for readers to follow and comprehend; key messages should be organized; no dense text blocks or large amounts of white space should be present; and the text formatting should be easy for the eye to follow. A SAM score of more than 70% indicates superior suitability; scores ranging from 40% to 69% indicate average suitability. Research studies have revealed that only 10% to 36% of free, health care consumer educational materials (print or internet) meet readability and suitability standards for use. Some of these health resources may also contain factual errors about ways to prevent and manage disease (Taylor-Clarke et al., 2012; Wiener & Weiner-Pla, 2014).

Evaluation and Documentation

As the final activity in the teaching–learning process, the nurse and client determine whether the client has achieved the identified learning objectives and outcomes. Criteria for evaluation include specifications of what the client will do and the particular behavior that the client will demonstrate, which were previously stated in each objective or outcome. To provide proof of client learning, the nurse documents what was taught and whether the client met the desired educational objectives or outcomes. A way to assess attainment of desired objectives or outcomes is to have the client teach back the information to the nurse. The "teach-back" method allows active client participation in the teaching–learning process. When nurses use the teach-back method for validating client understanding of information, they ask clients open-ended questions to get them to repeat the newly acquired information. When used for evaluating skill mastery (e.g., home injections), the nurses ask clients questions so they can share knowledge of safe equipment use, storage maintenance, and proper disposal. The client then performs a return demonstration, pretending they are teaching another person the skill. Nurses can validate that clients understood what was taught and provide reeducation if something was misunderstood or not mastered. Other benefits of the teach-back method include improved adherence to treatment regimens and mitigation of issues occurring with low health literacy. The effectiveness of the teach-back method for verifying attainment of desired objectives and outcomes of education is supported by nursing research (Scott et al., 2019). The following Focus on Research box provides an example of how this practice can improve client dismissal instructions.

If learning objectives and outcomes are not met, the nurse needs to either provide additional teaching or report to other interprofessional health team members that additional education is needed (see Concepts in Practice, "Client Education—A Collaborative Process").

FOCUS ON RESEARCH

Using the Teach-Back Method to Improve Client Discharge Teaching on an Oncology Unit

The investigators wanted to learn if the teach-back method would improve adherence to complex cancer treatment protocols and their ability to detect and prevent treatment complications in adult clients being dismissed from a 20-bed inpatient hematology–oncology unit located in an academic medical center. Clients receiving care on the unit possessed risks for low health literacy (i.e., rural counties, over age 65 years, African American and Hispanic/Latinx descent).

Nineteen nurses working on the unit attended a mandatory, 1-hour class on the teach-back method that included a client teach-back simulation. Prior to implementing the method for the research study, the nurses practiced it by using it 2 weeks prior to data collection. The nurses completed the Conviction and Confidence (C&C) scale, a previously developed and validated self-report instrument that addresses the elements of the teach-back method that they used more than 50% of the time, nurse perceptions of importance, and how often the method was used. Nurses completed the C&C scale prior to implementing the teach-back method, 1 month into its implementation, and 3 months following its implementation. Clients receiving care on the unit routinely completed Press Ganey surveys containing items addressing the hospitalization experience (including the quality of dismissal education and client satisfaction). Thirty-eight client participants completed the survey 3 months prior to data collection and 32 clients completed the survey within the 3-month data collection window.

Data were analyzed using descriptive and parametric statistics such as t-tests, analysis of variance, and chi-square tests. The investigators determined the level of statistical significance at p equal to or less than 0.05. Analysis of variance enabled investigators to determine changes between more than two data collection points, t-tests were used to compare preintervention with postintervention changes, and chi-square tests were used to detect changes in categorical variables with numerical values.

The nurses scored significantly higher on the C&C scale items related to the importance of using the teach-back method after the method was implemented. Less experienced nurses reported using the teach-back method less frequently than experienced nurses before the intervention was implemented. Confidence using the method also increased at a statistically significant level. Statistically significant gains were also noted in the use of plain, simple language for teaching, nurse assumption of responsibility for ensuring clear communication, providing reader-friendly printed materials to clients, and documentation of using the teach-back method and the client response to it.

Of clients, 43% rated their home care instructions as very good prior to the teach-back intervention, 75% of clients rated it as very good at the 1-month data collection point, and 70% rated it as very good 3 months into the study (when data collection ceased). Gains were not made in the client perceptions of feeling ready for dismissal from the medical center.

The investigators acknowledged several study limitations. They reported the study was conducted on a single nursing unit and the sample sizes for the nurse group and client groups were small. Another issue was that sometimes nurses who did not receive education in the teach-back method worked on the unit. Some nurses also might have provided socially desirable answers to items on the C&C survey. Additionally, some nurses might have been hypercritical of themselves when implementing the teach-back method, resulting in lower confidence or use of elements of teach-back method when completing C&C surveys. Finally, the low numbers of completed Press Ganey surveys might call into question the validity of using this tool to assess client satisfaction with dismissal education.

The investigators concluded that the teach-back method had no impact on client education because clients did not show improvement in being ready for dismissal. However, they reported that nurses valued using the teach-back method for dismissal instructions for their clients. They also reported that education about the teach-back method was valuable for nurses to ensure effective implementation. Finally, the researchers reported that the nurses perceived that clients had a better understanding of their home care following hospitalization, thus making the teach-back method valuable as a tool to use when providing clients with dismissal information.

FOCUS ON RESEARCH (*continued*)

The clinical significance of this study is that the teach-back method works effectively when nurses provide clients with home care instruction. The investigators concluded that the teach-back method did not impact the education clients received before going home because there were not changes in client perception of being ready for dismissal. Other factors such as fear and anxiety about possible treatment complications or treatment-induced fatigue could have been factors making clients feel that they were not ready to go home. Findings of this study need to be exercised with caution due to small sample sizes of the nurse and client groups and that the study was conducted in a single oncology unit. The findings of this study may not be generalizable to other settings. More research needs to be conducted to validate the effects of the teach-back method in client education and the effects of nurse education on the methods and effectiveness of its implementation.

From Scott, C., Andrews, D., Bulla, S., & Loerzel, V. (2019). Teach-back method: Using a nursing education intervention to improve discharge instructions on an adult oncology unit. *Clinical Journal of Oncology Nursing, 23*(3), 288–294. https://doi.org/10.1188/19.CJON.288-294

Concepts in Practice

Client Education—A Collaborative Process

Mr. H is a 75-year-old man who has been admitted to the hospital for slurred speech, right arm weakness, and right leg weakness. His wife has accompanied him and is concerned and worried. Within 18 hours of admission, his symptoms subsided completely. The neurologist sends him home on clopidogrel 75 mg and aspirin 325 mg daily.

When planning dismissal instructions, Juliana, the nurse caring for Mr. H, sets the following learning objectives for the client educational encounter:

1. Accurately describe the signs and symptoms of a stroke.
2. Explain the emergency measures to take if signs and symptoms occur (activate the emergency medical system [EMS] and get to a hospital as soon as possible).
3. List the side effects of clopidogrel and aspirin.
4. Outline ways to reduce the gastrointestinal irritation that may arise from the medications.
5. Specify when to contact the physician for adverse effects of the medications.
6. Explain the reasons for newly ordered medications, dietary and activity restrictions, and follow-up care with the primary care physician and neurologist.

Juliana provides Mr. and Mrs. H with instructions about the side effects of the medications, signs and symptoms of a stroke, and what to do if any should occur. Along with verbal instructions, Juliana provides them with a booklet about transient ischemic attacks and brain attacks (cerebral vascular accidents or strokes).

Mr. and Mrs. H repeat all of the required information correctly with the exception of what they will do if either one of them has the signs and symptoms of brain attacks. They insist that their first action would be to contact their closest family member for a ride to the hospital rather than activating the EMS.

Recognizing that transporting family members using a family member's care as a client preference, Juliana can try to figure out how to motivate them to call 911 first. However, if unsuccessful, additional teaching will be needed and this educational need should be shared with a home health nurse (if one was ordered) and/or someone in an outpatient setting where Mr. and Mrs. H will be receiving follow-up care. Juliana could also refer the couple and their family members to a community-based stroke education program.

Juliana notifies the neurologist about the need for further education. The neurologist states that this information will be retaught during the follow-up office visit. Based on the results of the response from the neurologist, Juliana provides the couple with information about the local stroke educational program and support group. Mrs. H expresses intense interest in attending these programs.

The Holistic Approach

The holistic approach to the teaching–learning process offers another avenue for nurses to use for client education. Holistic teaching–learning espouses the use of active learning principles. Holistic active learning links the concepts of experiences (doing, seeing, simulating); information and ideas (formal or informal acquisition of knowledge, learning on your own or from others, original ideas or ideas from others or resources); and reflection (taking time to think about what is being learned, either alone or with others) (Fink, 2003). The holistic approach addresses the cognitive, affective, and psychomotor domains of learning simultaneously and facilitates clients finding personal meaning in information that is needed for self-care and health promotion.

The holistic approach provides foundational knowledge for clients while paying attention to human interactions, caring, and learning how to learn while learners work toward meeting intended learning goals (Fink, 2003). Self-assessment by clients toward achieving health education–related goals instills confidence in their ability to do what is needed to care optimally for themselves or their loved ones. Taking time to reflect on what is learned facilitates the development of the implicit memory that recalls sensory, emotional, and skeletal responses along with procedural skills (Collins, 2007). However, little research is available to validate whether the holistic approach to client health education is better than the traditional teaching–learning process.

TEACHING–LEARNING AS A RESPONSIBILITY OF THE ADVOCATE

As nurses engage in the teaching–learning process with clients, they assist clients in becoming better informed about how to manage their own health. Thus, clients are able to make informed choices about the type of health care that they receive. By eliminating the "mysteries" behind navigating the health care system, medical interventions, and complementary therapies, nurses assume the role of client advocate.

The belief in advocacy as an appropriate role of the nurse has evolved in harmony with the current societal characteristics and values of consumerism, self-care, justice and human rights, equal opportunity for all, and individual accountability for health. Many people no longer believe that illness is always an event over which they have control. One of the most significant activities

of the nurse advocate is to provide informational support to assist the client to make the wisest possible decisions in the pursuit of well-being.

Take Note!
As clients begin to make informed choices for health and health care–related decisions, they look to professional nurses for support.

Functions of the Advocate in the Teaching–Learning Process

Providing the opportunity for dialogue to fully explore health concerns is the major function of the nurse acting as an advocate for clients, regardless of whether those clients are experiencing high or low levels of wellness. Within this exploration, nurses use their expertise to "not only offer information (but also) offer ways of being, ways of coping, and even new possibilities" for clients (Benner, 2000), p. 78).

Benner (2000) proposed that teaching–learning transactions take on new dimensions when the learner (client) is ill. She cited the following competencies necessary for the nurse to assume the teaching–coaching function with a client who is ill:

■ Carefully time the interventions to capture the client's readiness to learn.
■ Help the client integrate the implications of the illness and recovery into their lifestyle.
■ Elicit and respect the client's interpretation of the illness.
■ Respond fully and cogently to the client's request for an explanation of what is happening (within the limits of both the client's and the nurse's own understanding).
■ Make approachable and understandable any culturally avoided or uncharted aspects of an illness by exploring ways of being and coping for the client and the family and by identifying new possibilities.

Growth through learning is maximized if the nurse fulfills these functions with the client.

Mutuality in the Teaching–Learning Process

One of the primary characteristics of an advocate–client relationship is mutuality. Watson (2007) stressed that nurses must strive to develop client interactions that are liberating and empowering based on an understanding that nurses and clients have equal status as people. Teachers and learners should learn from each other. Learning should be mutual, characterized by anticipatory–participatory behaviors, shared power, and knowing, doing, and being to become one. Watson's model of nursing is cited as one that mandates mutuality in the nursing process and places high priority on teaching–learning as a significant intervention mode in a reciprocal nurse–client relationship.

Mutuality can be defined as "a connection with or understanding of another that facilitates a dynamic process of joint exchange between people. The process of being mutual is characterized by a sense of unfolding action that is shared in common, a sense of moving toward a common goal, and a sense of satisfaction for all involved" (Henson, 1997, p. 80). Mutuality balances power and respect, encourages accountability, and "facilitates active involvement of both nurses and clients in effectively working toward mutually identified goals" (Henson, 1997, p. 77). Mutuality is consistent with any learning theory used to guide the teaching–learning process.

▆ QUESTIONS FOR REFLECTION

1. Have you ever learned anything from a client, client's family, or community? If so, what did you learn?
2. Have you ever received health education from a nurse? How effective was the education? What key things do you remember from your experience that you might want to incorporate into your future professional practice when educating clients, families, or communities?
3. How do you feel when clients or their family members learn a new skill or grasp key information regarding self-care for the first time?
4. How do you promote active participation by clients, families, and communities in the client education process?
5. Why is active participation important in the teaching–learning process?

LEARNING THEORIES

The process by which learning occurs has been described in multiple ways. Learning theories and models explain how people learn. When nurses use models and theories to guide the client education process, they can use principles to structure meaningful client educational experiences, prevent overloading clients with information, and understand the reasons for unsuccessful client education encounters. Educational effort should be focused on learners (individuals, families, significant others, and communities). Because the vast

amount of information available on learning theories is too broad to cover in this text, the following section outlines Bruner's perspective, which encompasses five different learning models.

Bruner's Learning Models

Bruner (1986) cited five popular models of how the learner learns: empiricism, hypothesis generator, nativism, constructivism, and novice-to-expert. Empiricism is considered the oldest model. It is based on the premise that "one learns from experience" and that "such order as there is in the mind is a reflection of the order that exists in the world" (Bruner, 1986, p. 199). People need life experience for success in educational situations based on empiricism.

Unlike the rather passive view of the empiricism model, the hypothesis generator mode includes a major premise of intentionality. "The learner, rather than being the creature of experience, selects that which is to enter and possesses an active curiosity guided by self-directed projects" (Bruner, 1986, p. 199). A person is a successful learner in this model if they have a good theory from which hypotheses are generated. This perspective of learning supports the use of active learning educational strategies.

The nativism model proposes that the mind is innately shaped by "a set of underlying categories, hypotheses," both forms of organizing experiences (Bruner, 1986, p. 199). The task of the learner in this model is to develop a way of organizing perceived reality. Using the innate powers of the mind is the formula for successful learning in this model. Concept mapping facilitates the organization of concepts to be learned under the nativism model.

The constructivism model was developed primarily by Piaget, who, according to Bruner (1986, p. 199), stated that "the world is not found, but made, and according to a set of structural rules that are imposed on the flow of experience." These structural rules provide boundaries for learning. The learner goes through stage-like progressions characterized by tension between previously assimilated structural rules and changes in the rules that come in later-stage development. In accommodating these new rules, the learner is successful if their learning structure changes by moving to higher systems that subsume earlier structures. Thus, the constructivism model supports a holistic approach to teaching–learning.

The novice-to-expert model "begins with the premise that if you want to find out about learning, ask first about what is to be learned, find an expert who does it well, and then look at the novice and figure out how he or she can get there" (Bruner, 1986, p. 199). In this model, the formula for success is to be specific and explicit in taking the steps to attain expertise. The novice-to-expert model substantiates the use of collaborative partnerships in the teaching–learning process.

Bruner (1986, p. 200) suggested that there is not just one kind of learning and that we would be better served if we understood that "the model of the learner is not fixed but various." In many health care organizations, nurses use standardized teaching guides; documentation frequently consists of checking off items on a list. Nurses who use Bruner's learner models individualize client education, thereby maximizing client mastery of desired outcomes.

Types of Learning

Bevis (1988, p. 40) outlined six types of learning that may be useful in the teaching–learning process (see Box 16.2, Professional Building Blocks, "Bevis's Six Types of Learning"). She suggested that different educational approaches work best for different types of learning but noted that syntactic, contextual, and inquiry learning are necessary for change that can truly maximize the client's abilities to gain the best control of their health. Item learning, directive learning, and rational learning typically are needed for safe performance of a skill. For example, item learning generates lists or outlines procedures (think about gathering all supplies for preparing an injection and then learning the skill

of how to give an injection). Directive learning involves rules, injunctions, and exceptions to rules (e.g., do not give an injection where there is a break in the skin). Rational learning involves the use of theory and other information to make logical judgments (e.g., if an injection is given where the skin is broken, there will be an increase chance of causing an injection-site infection.).

In contrast, syntactic, contextual, and inquiry learning incorporate personal meaning, cultural considerations, and discovery in the client education process rather than approaching learning as an exercise in mastery of relationships, rules, and logic. For example, syntactic learning would result when a person with a newly diagnosed case of diabetes links improved cognitive abilities based on optimal blood glucose control or excessive urination with poor glucose control. Contextual and inquiry learning might occur simultaneously while finding ways to participate fully in family celebrations centered on special holiday foods without disrupting optimal glucose control.

Principles of Learning

Principles identified by Babcock and Miller (1994) are considered useful in any of these learner models or types of learning (see Box 16.3, Professional Building Blocks, "Babcock and Miller's Guiding Principles

16.2 Professional Building Blocks

Bevis's Six Types of Learning

1. **Item learning:** Simple relationships between separate pieces of information, as seen in mechanistic and ritualistic lists and procedures
2. **Directive learning:** Rules, injunctions, and exceptions, as seen in safety requirements
3. **Rational learning:** Use of theory to buttress action, enabling logical decision making, and logical judgments
4. **Syntactic learning:** Seeing meaningful wholes, relationships, and patterns that enable the learner to develop insights and find meaning
5. **Contextual learning:** Acceptance of culture, mores, folkways, rites, and rituals as ways of being; these learning transactions are "caring, compassionate, and positive"
6. **Inquiry learning:** Investigating, categorizing, and theorizing in a way to generate ideas and develop a vision

Data from Bevis, E. O. (1988). New directions for a new age. In National League for Nursing (Ed.), *Curriculum revolution: Mandate for change* (p. 40). National League for Nursing.

16.3 Professional Building Blocks

Babcock and Miller's Guiding Principles in the Teaching–Learning Process

1. Focusing intensifies learning.
2. Repetition enhances learning.
3. Learner control increases learning.
4. Active participation is necessary for learning.
5. Learning styles vary.
6. Organization promotes learning.
7. Association is necessary to learning.
8. Imitation is a method of learning.
9. Motivation strengthens learning.
10. Spacing new material facilitates learning.
11. Recency influences retention.
12. Primacy affects retention.
13. Arousal influences attention.
14. Accurate and prompt feedback enhances learning.
15. Application of new learning in a variety of contexts broadens the generalization of that learning.
16. The learner's biologic, psychological, sociologic, and cultural realities shape the learner's perception of the learning experience.

Data from Babcock, D. E., & Miller, M. A. (1994). *Client education: Theory and practice* (pp. 45–48). Mosby Year Book.

in the Teaching–Learning Process"). In addition, because individual learning preferences of clients vary, the professional nurse needs to understand the multiple models and types of learning to personalize the teaching–learning process effectively. Effectiveness is measured by the success of the nurse and the client in changing the client's health behaviors in a positive direction.

■ QUESTIONS FOR REFLECTION

1. How do you assess clients for preferred learning styles?
2. How do you learn best? Why is it important for you to know your preferred learning style?

IMPLICATIONS OF CHANGE THEORY ON TEACHING–LEARNING

Growth is inherent in the definition of learning. Growth implies that change occurs. Because change is the only thing that occurs constantly, change, growth, and learning happen continuously throughout life. Desired outcomes of education are changes in behavior, attitude, and psychomotor abilities (Bloom, 1974). However, in the process of learning, the human brain also experiences long-lasting changes (Collins, 2007).

Change as a Goal of Teaching: Growth

The mutually determined goal of the nurse and the client who are participating in the teaching–learning process is "becoming different than before" (Douglass, 1988, p. 226). Douglass noted that forces that influence change can be external or internal. The nurse is an intentional external force assisting the client with demonstrating different and better health behaviors.

The nurse in the teaching–learning relationship needs to follow a series of sequential steps that are consistent with planned change theory. Planned change is a deliberate process to make a desired change in a situation, knowledge, skill, or attitude (such as redecorating a room, learning to play a musical instrument, searching for information on an unfamiliar topic, or adjusting one's attitude and approach when working with a person different from oneself). Unplanned change is unanticipated and may arise from an unexpected situation such as a sudden illness, motor vehicle accident, falling and injuring oneself, or house fire (see Box 16.4, Professional Building Blocks, "Sequential Steps Consistent with Planned Change Theory") (Douglass,

16.4 Professional Building Blocks

Sequential Steps Consistent with Planned Change Theory

1. Explore the client's perceived need for change.
2. Identify the forces for change with the client.
3. Help the client state their health concerns.
4. Identify constraints and opportunities in the situation.
5. Provide the information needed to analyze both the change needs and the potential strategies to achieve the desired change.
6. Critique each of the possible change strategies on the basis of both the information understood and the situational factors.
7. Select the change strategy in partnership with others to be attempted in the effort to achieve a different and better health behavior.
8. Plan the implementation, filling in all of the informational gaps perceived by the nurse and the client.
9. Design an evaluation process to determine success in changing health behavior.
10. *Client:* Implement the planned behavioral activities. *Nurse:* Offer feedback and facilitate opportunities in the delivery system environment to promote success of the client.
11. Evaluate the overall results of the teaching–learning interaction and the specific health behavior changes on the part of the client.

Data from Douglass, L. M. (1988). *The effective nurse: Leader and manager* (3rd ed., pp. 226–232). Mosby Year Book.

1988). The steps mirror the nursing process: exploring and identifying factors for the change (assessment); determining specific knowledge gaps (diagnosis); selecting an educational strategy (planning); executing the strategy (implementation); and determining the overall results (evaluation).

Outcomes of Knowledge Acquisition

The outcome of knowledge acquisition in the teaching–learning process may not always be satisfying to the nurse and the client. Harmony within the human system results when the newly acquired information is congruent with previously integrated functions. However, if the new information is incompatible with the previously integrated functions, clients and nurses may perceive disharmony. Feelings of being unsettled, restless, and uncertain frequently accompany periods of growth. Nurses often need to help clients understand that change may not be a painless process.

To reduce the discomfort that sometimes occurs in the teaching–learning process, nurses and clients can analyze the current situation using a holistic perspective. The holistic approach would consider all aspects of the client's life, including how the change would affect the client as an individual, impact all people involved in the client's life, and alter social structures along with the client's motivation for change. Both the situational context and the motivational aspects of planned change play a significant role in the client's ability to integrate information and develop new behaviors. The holistic approach to client education is highlighted in the following Concepts in Practice Box, "Holistic Client Education."

Readiness for Learning

A central issue for nurses in implementing the teaching–learning process as a strategy for changing behaviors is the client's **readiness for learning**. Benner (2000, p. 79) noted that teaching–learning interventions are often dictated by schedules in the health care delivery environment: "Assessing where a patient is, how open he is to information, deciding when to go ahead even when the patient does not appear ready, are key aspects of effective patient teaching."

Nurses frequently find themselves pressured to implement client teaching quickly, especially when clients want to go home immediately, physicians write discharge from the hospital orders, or the dismissal from the hospital is unanticipated. Unless a preferred learning style assessment has been performed sometime during the hospital stay (many institutions include this as part of the nursing admission database), the nurse must quickly ask clients and significant others how they learn best. Nurses quickly assess clients for learning readiness, and most of the time, clients are ready to

---

Concepts in Practice

IDEA → PLAN → ACTION

Holistic Client Education

A client with newly diagnosed diabetes has multiple learning needs. In today's fast-paced society, effective control of blood sugar is challenging. Such would be the case for a single, working parent who has just found out that they have insulin-dependent diabetes while in the hospital.

1. The nurse would teach the client how to perform blood glucose checks using a handheld glucometer. Effective use of the meter involves turning on the meter; calibrating it; checking glucose strips for expiration dates and calibrating them to the meter; acquiring blood safely for accurate testing; reading and understanding meter testing results; turning off the meter; and caring for the meter.
2. In order to affirm understanding of how and when the insulin would be prepared and administered, the nurse would share information about proper storage of insulin, when insulin would become outdated, and how to safely prepare and administer insulin injections.
3. While observing the client performing all the required skills for safe home management of diabetes, the nurse would note any visual (inability to see syringe markings), literacy (inability to read or understand printed directions), psychomotor (poor fine-motor hand coordination), and psychological (extreme anxiety or denial) barriers in performing any required skills.
4. In addition to glucose testing and insulin injection administration, the nurse would review the signs and symptoms of hypoglycemia and its

management. The nurse would also provide education about signs and symptoms of hyperglycemia, the importance of managing strict glucose control, and the complications of poorly managed glucose levels.
5. The nurse would stress the importance of daily inspection of feet, daily foot hygiene, and proper toenail care and actions to take if foot problems are identified.
6. The nurse would verify that the client received effective education about current dietary needs. Typically, newly diagnosed individuals with diabetes receive special nutritional education from a dietitian. However, the nurse needs to validate client understanding of nutritional strategies to promote optimal glucose control (e.g., testing blood glucose levels before meals, eating regularly scheduled meals, counting carbohydrates consumed, knowing how to follow a sliding-scale insulin regimen).
7. For identified gaps in education, the nurse would make referrals to a specialized diabetic educator for further education. The nurse would consult a social worker to facilitate acquisition of diabetes testing and management supplies if problems securing them arose.

Unless the client understands the benefits of controlling glucose levels, they may put taking care of themselves behind caring for their children.

learn because they want to go home and many clients want to assume responsibility for their own health.

For commonly encountered surgical procedures and disease processes, many health care organizations have standardized teaching plans for nurses to follow when providing client education. Because many clients use computers and mobile phones daily, if the health care facility's policies permit, nurses can provide photos or videos for client education, especially if the client identifies video technology as the preferred learning tool (Holt et al., 2011).

Most people experiencing a newly diagnosed disease, illness, or surgical procedure experience some anxiety. Thus, learning readiness must be evaluated in terms of the degree of anxiety the client expresses. Minimal anxiety serves as a positive force for attention, alertness, or awareness, all of which are necessary for learning and integration of functions to occur. Moderate anxiety is usually associated with selective inattention and decreasing awareness; extreme anxiety is associated with lack of attention and loss of awareness. Moderate and extreme anxiety are usually an indicator of the client's lack of readiness for learning. In these two anxiety states, the nurse's focus needs to be on reducing anxiety to enable the client to regain a sense of security and repossess the energy required for attention and awareness, which are prerequisites for learning (Collins, 2007; Rankin et al., 2005).

Validating Learning: Feedback

Validation, a process of confirmation, is a necessary element of teaching–learning. In client education, **validation** means that the client understands the educational material, has mastered a particular health care skill, or uses the new information or skill effectively. For a behavioral change to become well integrated, it must be validated by people significant to the client. Nurses frequently play a significant role in clients' lives.

As teachers, nurses share their knowledge and expertise with clients. Learners appreciate feedback from teachers. **Feedback** is the transmission of information regarding how well learning outcomes are being met by learners. Frequently, constructive feedback stimulates learners to want to learn more. In client education, nurse feedback provides clients (and families) with specific information on how well they have absorbed the knowledge and skills needed to care for themselves (Miller & Stoeckel, 2019; Rankin et al., 2005).

Take Note!
Throughout life, a person requires validation through feedback from significant others to maintain the integrity of their self-system.

STRATEGIES FOR EFFECTIVE TEACHING AND LEARNING

Client-Focused Teaching

Although nurses often use standardized teaching plans, **client-focused teaching** hones in on individual client learning needs and preferences. Client education works better when nurses and clients involved in the teaching–learning process know about each other (Miller & Stoeckel, 2019; Rankin et al., 2015; Redman, 1993). As they use their repertoire of therapeutic communication skills and conduct their assessments, nurses get to know their clients. However, clients may know little about their nurses other than the information found on the nurse's employer name badge. Some health care facilities include professional licensure, earned academic degrees, and nurse specialty certifications on name badges. Some nurses carry business cards that they give to clients specifying their academic degrees, certification, and scope of practice. In addition to providing their credentials, nurses should clearly communicate their intentions in the teaching–learning process, share a clear plan of the time commitments to clients, and offer information about how a contract can be established if clients desire one.

For instructions to be effective, the nurse should know the following information about clients involved in the education process: (1) how the client perceives the health situation; (2) physical, cultural, linguistic, or psychological limitations that may impede learning (including anxiety or cognitive impairment); (3) intended learning outcomes; (4) interprofessional team members' plans for the client; (5) what the client's conscious intentions and desires are regarding health behaviors; and (6) what information the client perceives is needed to achieve their health goals. With this basic information, nurses and clients should be able to engage fully in the teaching–learning process (Miller & Stoeckel, 2019; Rankin et al., 2005; Redman, 1993).

Motivational Strategies

Many teaching strategies are available to enhance client **motivation** (stimulus) to participate in learning, but only a few are mentioned in this chapter. Additional motivational teaching strategies may be found in books devoted to teaching strategies (see the reference list at the end of this chapter).

Theis and Johnson (1995) synthesized the existing research examining teaching strategies and found "66% of subjects receiving planned teaching had better outcomes than did control group subjects receiving routine care" (p. 100). The literature also supports the effectiveness of structured approaches, reinforcement, independent study, and multiple strategies (Allen et al., 2008; Edwardson, 2007). Box 16.5, Professional Building Blocks, "Effective Teaching Strategies," suggests additional approaches (Babcock & Miller, 1994; Miller & Stoeckel, 2019; Rankin et al., 2005; Redman, 1993).

Motivation for learning is enhanced if the learner and the teacher trust and respect each other, the teacher assumes and expects that the learner can learn, the teacher is sensitive to the student's individual needs, and both the learner and the teacher feel free to learn and make mistakes in their own unique styles. Boswell et al. (1990) reinforced the idea that active participation in learning is a strong motivator. Box 16.6, Professional Building Blocks, "Effective Motivational Strategies for Learning," suggests additional motivational approaches (Bevis, 1988).

16.6 Professional Building Blocks

Effective Motivational Strategies for Learning

- Engaging the learner in active analysis by conducting a motivational interview that dispels the perception that the nurse is always right affirms the client's interests and efforts, instilling client competence, control, interest, values to learn, and social approval processes or rewards
- Nurturing and supporting the learner as attempts are made at content or skill mastery
- Finding ways to make the learning meaningful and significant for the learner
- Following the ethical ideal in giving clients all the information they need to make sound choices
- Displaying a caring attitude
- Using and encouraging creativity in the teaching–learning process
- Encouraging curiosity and the search for satisfying ideas
- Being assertive
- Desiring to engage in and seek dialogue for enhancing understanding

From Bevis, E. O. (1988). New directions for a new age. In *Curriculum revolution: Mandate for change* (p. 45). National League for Nursing; Miller, M. A., & Stoeckel, P. R. (2019). *Client education, theory and practice* (3rd ed.). Jones & Bartlett Learning.

 QUESTIONS FOR REFLECTION

1. Look back at the teaching struggles and motivational strategies presented here. Which have you experienced in your nursing education program? Were they helpful to you? Why or why not? Which have you used in clinical practice? Do you think that they were helpful when providing client education? Why or why not?

2. Can you identify additional teaching and motivational strategies for working with clients? Make a list, and indicate why you think they would be effective.

16.5 Professional Building Blocks

Effective Teaching Strategies

- Computer-based instruction
- Observation and assessment scales
- Demonstration
- Lecture/discussion
- Modeling
- Programmed instruction
- Role playing
- Group activities
- Use of media (posters, flip charts, overhead projections, videotapes, audiotapes, films)
- Games and simulations
- Concept maps

From Babcock, D. E., & Miller, M. A. (1994). *Client education: Theory and practice*. Mosby Year Book; Fink, L. (2003). *Creating significant learning experiences*. Jossey-Bass; Miller, M. A., & Stoeckel, P. R. (2019). *Client education, theory and practice* (3rd ed.). Jones & Bartlett Learning; Rankin, S., Stallings, K., & London, F. (2005). *Patient education in health and illness* (5th ed.). Lippincott Williams & Wilkins; Redman, B. K. (1993). *The process of patient education* (7th ed.). Mosby Year Book.

Take Note!

Teaching is more effective when nurses tailor the education strategy to fit client-preferred learning styles.

Contextual Constraints and Opportunities

Some contextual constraints, such as the dilemma of insufficient time and great need on the part of the client, have been mentioned. To attempt to control environmental constraints that might be imposed on the teaching–learning process, the nurse should keep the following teaching strategies in mind:

- Try to arrange learning experiences when the learner feels relatively healthy.
- Provide time for learning at a comfortable pace.
- Have sufficient grasp of the subject matter to translate concepts into different terms for different learners.
- Make sure expectations and standards are clear.

Certain clients, such as older adults, require a slower pace of instruction to allow for increased time for mental processing. The Hartford Foundation offers a vast array of resources for nurses working with older adult clients, including tips for effective teaching and learning (Fulmer, 2007).

Bruner (1986, p. 198) asserted that educators need to assist learners to perceive the value of the rich diversity in the world. He encouraged educators to view the learner as "equipped to discriminate and deal differentially with a wide variety of possible worlds exhibiting different conditions, yet worlds in which one can cope." The nurse should perhaps heed this advice and have confidence in the client's ability to mutually participate in teaching–learning and to succeed in a diverse world, rather than trying to control all the contextual constraints that might interfere with learning. Power sharing would be more likely by nurses with this type of confidence in clients. Perceived abilities and learning are more likely in such relationships.

SPECIFIC CLIENT EDUCATION ACTIVITIES

Many routine nursing activities involve client and family education. When clients enter a health care institution, they frequently need instructions related to their expected role responsibilities. Health care professionals cannot deliver effective care unless clients are willing to provide them with information related to health problems and educational needs. During an initial client encounter, the nurse may learn more about the client's needs and concerns and the client assumes the role of teacher. To plan effective nursing care, the nurse needs to understand the client's perspective of the health problem or illness. Usually, additional information related to specific care needs (special adaptive devices, cultural concerns) also surfaces during the initial encounter.

Nurses assume the role of educator when they inform clients and families of the purposes behind nursing interventions and rationales for administered medications. Educational efforts such as these enable clients to understand the reasons behind care activities and learn why they must comply with the ordered medical regimen. Most teaching related to medication administration reinforces information clients have received from physicians. However, sometimes, as in the case of a client with newly diagnosed diabetes, the physician delegates the task of teaching insulin administration to a nurse or certified diabetic educator (who is usually a professional nurse).

Sometimes the roles of educator and client advocate become intertwined. As a client advocate, the nurse frequently verifies that clients understand procedures that are about to happen. Nurses commonly obtain signatures on informed consent forms before clients undergo invasive procedures. Informed consent requires that the client is competent, has had other treatment options explained to them, understands the treatment/test and its potential adverse effects, agrees to the procedure without coercion, and consents to having the procedure performed (Miller & Stoeckel, 2019; Rankin et al., 2005). The nursing process is used to determine the multiple elements of informed consent. When assessing for the elements required for informed consent, questions related to the procedure may arise. The nurse who answers them engages in the process of client education. However, if the nurse discovers that the client does not fully understand the anticipated procedure, the role of educator is put aside and the nurse assumes the role of advocate, informing the physician of an inability to obtain a signature on a consent form because the client fails to understand the procedure's risks and benefits.

Nurses also participate in community health education. Successful community education starts with the participation of community members. Nurses secure community input when planning community education programs by performing a needs assessment. In a manner similar to that used to identify individual client learning needs, the nurse asks community members to identify community learning needs. Methods for performing a needs assessment include individual interviews, informal polls, focus groups, or written surveys. Key community leaders must also be asked to identify group learning needs to ensure successful program development and implementation. Once a learning need has been identified, professional nurses secure credible resources and financial support for the program. Financial support may be secured in the form of grants or corporate sponsorships or from the community. Involvement of community members during the program-planning process increases the chance that the program will appeal to community members.

Teaching tools that appeal to individual clients (e.g., videos, slides, flip charts) may be highly effective for community education. However, the teaching strategies must consider the projected number of people who will attend the program (Rankin et al., 2005). Commonly, health care consumers are using technology to access health care information. Computer, tablet, and smart phone applications help consumers keep records regarding health promotion efforts (e.g., dietary intake, exercise) and disease management.

Not all client education occurs in a formalized setting, such as a health care organization or community agency. Nurses reside in neighborhoods and are members of families. Family members, neighbors, and friends frequently consult nurses they know when health care concerns or questions about a health condition arise. Sometimes, the questions fall within the realm of the professional nurse's area of expertise; at other times, they do not. Directing family, friends, and acquaintances to credible resources sometimes poses a great challenge for the professional nurse. As more people use the internet as a source of health information, the professional nurse should become aware of the quality of information posted on various popular websites. Nurses have an obligation to share accurate health-related information or refer the question or concern to another health team member when unable to provide the requested information.

Miller and Stoeckel (2019), Rankin and colleagues (2005), and Smeltzer (2005) outlined several factors that distinguish credible from less reputable information for client education and care (see Box 16.7, Learning, Knowing, and Growing, "Assessing the Suitability of Sources"). The process of peer review increases the

---

16.7 Learning, Knowing, and Growing

Assessing the Suitability of Sources

How do you know if an information source is credible and suitable for health education for clients? Certain defining characteristics can help you identify suitable sources for use in your studies or with your clients. Other characteristics should be considered based on client needs.

Suitable Source Characteristics

- Peer-reviewed
- Primary source of information
- Written or developed by known experts in a field
- Editorial ideas clearly documented as such
- Governmental or higher educational sources
- Professional nursing organization
- Recognized nonprofit organizations for a disease process (e.g., American Cancer Society, American Diabetes Association, Multiple Sclerosis Society)
- Websites from government, higher education, and nonprofit organizations that are updated on a regular schedule
- Clearly delineate editorials and advertisement from objective information
- Display biographic information of all content authors (academic and professional credentials) as well as their relationship to the organization
- Disclaimer present that sends clients to physicians or other health care providers for specific use of content provided
- Open disclosures if funds from companies were used to develop the study or website

- Hyperlinks to reports of original studies or primary sources of information
- Website design easy to navigate in order to reach desired information

Unsuitable Source Characteristics

- Use of secondary sources of information
- Use of editorial ideas as facts
- Product advertisements or information for sale
- Websites that are not updated on a regular basis
- No content review by medical experts
- For-profit organizations
- Nonprofit organizations displaying narrow viewpoints
- Poorly designed websites
- Websites linked directly to advertisements (e.g., automatic pop-up ads come when site is accessed)
- No disclaimer statement to warn clients of the need to consult with a health care provider to meet specific needs

Additional Considerations Based on Client Needs

- High level of literacy required to read and/or understand content
- Print or font smaller than 12 points in size (for those with visual impairments or older adults)
- Only the English language option (for people who have limited fluency in English)

From Rankin, S., Stallings, K., & London, F. (2005). *Patient education in health and illness* (5th ed., pp. 280–282). Lippincott Williams & Wilkins; Smeltzer, S. (2005). Is that information safe for patient care? *Nursing, 35,* 54–55; Miller, M. A., & Stoeckel, P. R. (2019). *Client education, theory and practice* (3rd ed.). Jones & Bartlett Learning.

credibility of information because the information has been appraised by experts in the field. Before suggesting materials for client education, nurses must review them to verify accuracy, readability, and ease of use.

▌ QUESTIONS FOR REFLECTION

1. How do you currently evaluate the educational information that you give to clients? That you use in your own studies?
2. Why is it important for nurses to determine the suitability of client educational materials before using them with clients?

CLIENT EDUCATION AS AN INTERDISCIPLINARY PROCESS

Along with nurses, other members of the health care team make significant contributions to client education. Because nurses tend to spend more time with clients than other providers, nurses have the opportunity to assess client learning needs and responses to health teaching implemented by other team members. The nurse also has the ability to determine whether the client has the ability to absorb teaching from other disciplines. Thus, the nurse may suggest that other health team members (e.g., dietitians, physical therapists, social workers, pharmacists) refrain from educational activities until clients are physically stable and emotionally ready to benefit from detailed self-care education.

In addition to determining the best times for client education, the nurse has the responsibility to coordinate educational activities and verify that clients receive the same information from all health care team members. Documentation of teaching by all disciplines (including nursing) is key so that instructions from one discipline can be effectively reinforced. Documented teaching content may also eliminate duplicate teaching efforts, ensure continuity of content, and provide a detailed record to meet TJC standards for client education and for third-party reimbursement.

For decades, nurses have participated in the development of client care paths. Most of these care paths are integrated into client electronic health records. Care paths designate specific client educational activities so that client education does not occur haphazardly or at the last minute when the physician writes a dismissal order. Some institutions have formed multidisciplinary educational committees to develop guidelines for client education and identify continuing educational needs for the entire health care team.

Summary and Significance to Practice

Teaching–learning is presented as a complex process among experts, the teacher, and the learner, in which all acquire new information, experience new relatedness, and change behavior as a result of the interaction. The nurse–teacher is an expert on health, and the client–learner is an expert on the client's experience of health and life circumstances. As the person who bears responsibility for developing and implementing effective client education, the nurse uses communication skills to assess and collaborate with learners to develop relevant learning experiences. Cognitive skills prove useful when determining priorities, materials, and specific strategies to use during the teaching–learning process. When clients need to learn procedural skills, the nurse shares clinical skills with them. Effective teaching and learning result in increased confidence and competence for nurses and clients.

REAL-LIFE REFLECTIONS

Recall Lillian, the nurse from the beginning of the chapter. What barriers does Lillian encounter in providing effective client education? What suggestions could Lillian make to the hospital to improve client education? What potential barriers might prevent her suggestions from being implemented? How could these suggestions be financed?

From Theory to Practice

1. After reading this chapter, what ideas will you incorporate into your client education in clinical practice? Why are these ideas important?
2. What are the consequences when clients are dismissed without receiving detailed education about medications, diet, activity, and follow-up health care?

Nurse as Author

Using ideas presented in this chapter, write a three- to four-paragraph essay about key considerations that need to be made for health care consumer education. Include ideas related to the assessment of learning needs, identification of educational outcomes, development of an individualized educational plan, facilitators and barriers to plan implementation, and evaluation of educational outcomes.

Your Digital Classroom

Online Exploration

American Academy of Family Practitioners: **www.aafp.org**

American Cancer Society: **www.cancer.org**

American Heart Association: **www.heart.org**

American Medical Association: **www.ama-assn.org**

Institute for Healthcare Improvement Patient Safety Topics: **http://www.ihi.org/Topics/PatientSafety/Pages/default.aspx**

Cancer Control P.L.A.N.E.T.: **https://cancercontrolplanet.cancer.gov/planet/ Centers for Disease Control and Prevention: www.cdc.gov**

Health Care Education Association: **hcea-info.org**

The John A. Hartford Foundation: **https://www.johnahartford.org/about**

The National Library of Medicine MedLine Plus Program for Evaluating Health Information: **www.nlm.nih.gov/medlineplus/evaluatinghealthinformation.html**

National Institutes of Health: **www.nih.gov**

Centers for Medicare & Medicaid Services Toolkit for Making Written Material Clear and Effective: **https://www.cms.gov/outreach-and-education/outreach/writtenmaterialstoolkit**

Expanding Your Understanding

1. Search online for a health topic of interest to you. Scan the first 10 websites in your search results. How many of these sites are trying to sell a product? How many are nonprofit organizations? How many are sponsored by a national or local government agency? Compare the quality of each website. Which sites would you recommend to a potential client for health information? Why or why not? Which sites would you use for personal health information? Why or why not?

2. Visit one of the websites listed in the "Online Exploration" section. Print out information that you would like to use for client teaching and bring it to class. Analyze the information according to the following criteria:
   ▪ Readability
   ▪ Visual appeal
   ▪ Accuracy of information
   ▪ Use of more than one language
   ▪ Ability to sustain interest and actively engage the learner

3. What types of policies does your current work setting or assigned clinical unit have related to the distribution of internet resources for client education? Describe the materials available for client education in your current work setting. Search the internet to find teaching materials on the same topic. Compare and contrast the two resources.

Beyond the Book

Visit **thePoint®** at **www.thePoint.lww.com** for activities and information to reinforce the concepts and content covered in this chapter.

REFERENCES

Agency for Healthcare Research and Quality. (2019, reviewed 2020). *Ten attributes of health literature health care organizations*. Retrieved April 10, 2021, from https://www.ahrq.gov/health-literacy/publications/ten-attributes.html

Allen, M., Iezzoni, L., Huang, A., Huang, L., & Leveille, S. (2008). Improving patient-clinician communication about chronic conditions: Description of an internet-based nurse E-coach intervention. *Nursing Research*, 57(2), 107–112. https://doi.org/10.1097/01.nnr.0000313478.47379.98

American Nurses Association. (2021). *Nursing: Scope and standards of practice* (4th ed.). Author.

Argyris, C. (1982). *Reasoning, learning, and action: Individual and organizational*. Jossey-Bass.

Babcock, D. E., & Miller, M. A. (1994). *Client education: Theory and practice*. Mosby Year Book.

Benner, P. (2000). *From novice to expert: Excellence in power and clinical nursing (Commemorative ed.)*. Addison-Wesley.

Bevis, E. O. (1988). New directions for a new age. In *Curriculum revolution: Mandate for change*. National League for Nursing.

Bloom, B. (Ed.). (1974). *Taxonomy of educational objectives*. D. McKay.

Boswell, E. J., Pichert, J. W., Lorenz, R. A., & Schlundt, D. G. (1990). Training health care professionals to enhance their patient teaching skills. *Journal of Nursing Staff Development*, 6, 233–239. Retrieved April 10, 2021, from https://www.researchgate.net/publication/20943269_Training_health_care_professionals_to_enhance_their_patient_teaching_skills

Bruner, J. (1986). Models of the learner. *Education Horizons*, 64, 197–200. Retrieved April 10, 2021, from https://www.jstor.org/stable/1174162?seq=1

Centers for Medicare & Medicaid Services. (2020). *Toolkit for making written material clear and effective*. Retrieved April 10, 2021, from https://www.cms.gov/outreach-and-education/outreach/writtenmaterialstoolkit

Collins, J. (2007). The neuroscience of learning. *Journal of Neuroscience Nursing*, 39(5), 305–315. Retrieved April 10, 2021, from https://www.nursingcenter.com/wkhlrp/Handlers/articleContent.pdf?key=pdf_01376517-200710000-00008

Core Quality Measures Collaborative. (2020). *CQMC core sets*. Retrieved April 10, 2021, from http://www.qualityforum.org/CQMC_Core_Sets.aspx

Douglass, L. M. (1988). *The effective nurse: Leader and manager* (3rd ed.). Mosby Year Book.

Edwardson, S. (2007). Patient education in heart failure. *Heart & Lung*, 36(4), 244–252. doi:10.1016/j.hrtlng.2006.08.011.

Falvo, D. (2004). *Effective patient education: A guide to increased compliance* (3rd ed.). Jones & Bartlett.

Fink, L. (2003). *Creating significant learning experiences*. Jossey-Bass.

Forbes, K. E. (1995). Please, more than just the facts. *Clinical Nurse Specialist: The Journal for Advanced Nursing Practice*, 9, 99. Retrieved April 10, 2021, from https://journals.lww.com/

cns-journal/Citation/1995/03000/Please,_More_Than_just_the_Facts.9.aspx

Fulmer, T. (2007). How to try this: Fulmer SPICES. *American Journal of Nursing*, *107*(10), 40–49. https://doi.org/10.1097/01.naj.0000292197.76076.e1

Health Care Education Association. (2020a). *Assessment*. Retrieved April 10, 2021, from https://www.hcea-info.org/assessment

Health Care Education Association. (2020b). *Patient education guidelines for health care professionals*. Retrieved April 10, 2021, from https://www.hcea-info.org/patient-education-guidelines

Health Resources and Services Administration. (2019). *Health literacy*. Retrieved April 10, 2021, from https://www.hrsa.gov/about/organization/bureaus/ohe/helath-lieracy/index.html

Henson, R. H. (1997). Analysis of the concept of mutuality. *Image*, *29*, 77–81. https://doi.org/10.1111/j.1547-5069.1997.tb01144.x

Hersh, L., Salzman, B., & Snyderman, D. (2015). Health literacy in primary care practice. *American Family Physician*, *92*(2), 119–124. Retrieved April 10, from https://www.aafp.org/afp/2015/0715/p118.html

Herzlinger, R. (2004). *Consumer-driven health care*. Jossey-Bass.

Holt, J., Flint, E., & Bowers, M. (2011). Got the picture? Using mobile phone technology to reinforce discharge instructions. *American Journal of Nursing*, *111*(8), 47–51. https://doi.org/10.1097/01.NAJ.0000403363.66929.41

Ingram, R., & Kautz, D. (2012). Overcoming low health literacy. *Nursing Critical Care*, *7*(4), 22–27. https://doi.org/10.1097/01.CCN.0000415831.85364.cb

Institute for Healthcare Improvement. (2021). *Ask me 3: Good questions for your health*. Retrieved June 15, 2021, from http://www.ihi.org/resources/Pages/Tools/Ask-Me-3-Good-Questions-for-Your-Good-Health.aspx

Joos, S. K., & Hickam, D. H. (1990). *How health professional influence health behavior: Patient-provider interactions and health care outcomes*. Jossey-Bass.

Kauffman, B. (2016). *Readmissions and Medicare: What's the cost?* Retrieved April 10, 2021, from https://www.nic.org/blog/readmissions-medicare-whats-the-cost/

Lupien, S. J., & McEwen, B. S. (1997). The acute effects of corticosteroids on cognition: Integration of animal and human model studies. *Brain Research Reviews*, *24*, 1–27. doi: 10.1016/S0165-0173(97)00004-0

Mayo-Gamble, T. L., & Mouton, C. (2018). Examining the association between health literacy and medication adherence among older adults. *Health Communication*, *33*(9), 1124–1130. https://doi.org/10.1080/10410236.2017.1331311

McCollum, V. (2008). *Complying with Joint Commission patient education standards*. Retrieved April 10, 2021, from https://www.reliasmedia.com/articles/9548-complying-with-joint-commission-patient-education-standards

Miller, M. A., & Stoeckel, P. R. (2019). *Client education, theory and practice* (3rd ed.). Jones & Bartlett Learning.

Mish, F. C. (Ed.). (2020). *Merriam-Webster's Collegiate Dictionary* (11th ed.). Merriam-Webster, Inc.

Nutbeam, D., McGill, B., & Premkumar, P. (2018). Improving health literacy in community populations: A review of progress. *Health Promotion International*, *33*(5), 901–911. https://doi.org/10.1093/heapro/dax015.

Pellowski, J. A., Kalichman, S. C., & Grebler, T. (2016). Optimal treatment adherence counseling outcomes for people living with HIV and limited health literacy. *Behavioral Medicine*, *42*(1), 39–47. https://doi.org/10.1080/08964289.2014.963006

Rankin, S., Stallings, K., & London, F. (2005). *Patient education in health and illness* (5th ed.). Lippincott Williams & Wilkins.

Redman, B. K. (1993). *The process of patient education* (7th ed.). Mosby Year Book.

Remshardt, M. (2011). The impact of patient literacy on healthcare practices. *Nursing Management*, *42*(11), 25–29. https://doi.org/101097/01/01.NUMA.0000406576.26956.53

Scott, C., Andrews, D., Bulla, S., & Loerzel, V. (2019). Teach-back method: Using a nursing education intervention to improve discharge instructions on an adult oncology unit. *Clinical Journal of Oncology Nursing*, *23*(3), 288–294. https://doi.org/10.1188/19.CJON.288-294

Smeltzer, S. (2005). Is that information safe for patient care? *Nursing*,*35*, 54–55. https://doi.org/10.1097/00152193-200501000-00049

Statistic Brain. (2015). *Illiteracy statistics*. Retrieved April 10, 2021, from http://www.statisticbrain.com/number-of-american-adults-who-cant-read/

Stewart, M. N. (2020). *The art and science of patient education for health literacy*. Elsevier.

Taylor-Clarke, K., Henry-Okafor, Q., Murphy, C., Keyes, M., Rothman, R., Churchwell, A., Mensah, G. A., Sawyer, D., & Sampson, U. K. A. (2012). Assessment of commonly available education materials in heart failure clinics. *Journal of Cardiovascular Nursing*, *27*(6), 485–494. https://doi.org/10.1097/JCN.0b013e318220720c

The Joint Commission. (2020a). *Speak up campaigns*. Retrieved April 10, 2021, from https://www.jointcommission.org/resources/for-consumers/speak-up-campaigns/

The Joint Commission. (2020b). *TakeCHARGE*. Retrieved April 10, 2021, from https://www.jointcommission.org/resources/for-consumers/take-charge/

Theis, S. L., & Johnson, J. H. (1995). Strategies for teaching patients: A meta-analysis. *Clinical Nurse Specialist*, *9*, 100–105. Retrieved April 10, 2021, from https://journals.lww.com/cns-journal/Abstract/1995/03000/Strategies_for_Teaching_Patients__A_Meta_Analysis.10.aspx

United States Department of Education, National Center for Education Statistics. (2019). *Adult literacy in the United States*. Retrieved April 10, 2021, from https://nces.ed.gov/pubs2019/2019179.pdf

United States Department of Education, National Center for Education Statistics. (2020). *Adult numeracy in the United States*. Retrieved April 10, 2021, from https://nces.ed.gov/pubs2020/2020025.pdf

United States Department of Health and Human Services. (2020). Health literacy in healthy people. *Healthy People 2030*. Retrieved May 16, 2021, from https://health.gov/our-work/healthy-people/healthy-people-2030/health-literacy-healthy-people-2030

Watson, J. (2007). *Nursing human science and human care: A theory for nursing*. Jones & Bartlett.

Weiss, B. D., Mays, M. Z., Castros, K. M., DeWalt, M. P., Mockbee, J., & Hale, F. A. (2005). Quick assessment of literacy in primary care: The newest vital sign. *Annals of Family Medicine*, *3*(6), 514–522. https://doi.org/10.1370/afm.405

Wiener, R. C., & Winer-Pla, R. (2014). Literacy, pregnancy and potential oral health changes: The internet and readability levels. *Maternal Child Health Journal*, *18*(3), 657–662. https://doi.org/10.1007/s10995-013-1290-1

Zhou, A. Q., Lee, H. Y., & Lee, R. M. (2019). Who has low health literacy and does it matter for depression? Findings from aggregated and disaggregated racial/ethnic groups. *Cultural Diversity & Ethnic Minority Psychology*, *25*(1), 73–81. https://doi.org/10.1037/cdp0000210

Leadership and Management in Professional Nursing

LEARNING OUTCOMES

By the end of this chapter, the learner will be able to:

1. Compare and contrast the concepts of leadership and management.
2. Explain contemporary thoughts about the concepts of leadership and management.
3. Discuss ways that power is used in leadership situations.
4. Explain the role of orientation to task and relationship affect leadership approaches.
5. Specify the value of empowering others and oneself in professional nursing relationships.
6. Identify the essential habits of effective leaders.
7. Outline criteria to evaluate leadership effectiveness.

REAL-LIFE REFLECTIONS

Elena is a registered nurse (RN) who graduated from school a year ago. While attending a parent–teacher association (PTA) meeting at her son's school, Elena learns that the school does not have a fulltime nurse. At the previous meeting, many parents voiced complaints related to the school's current health education and health care services. The PTA forms a task force and elects Elena to chair it because she is an RN. Uncomfortable with her new leadership position, Elena decides she needs to read about principles of leadership and finds her nursing leadership textbook.

- *Do you think the PTA made a wise decision in selecting Elena as their leader?*
- *How would you feel if you were in Elena's position?*
- *What would be the first things you would do as the task force chair? Why?*

Distinguishing leadership and **management** is difficult because the concepts overlap and business literature often uses the terms interchangeably. **Leaders** are people who influence others. Leaders view issues globally, create visions of what might be, inspire others, tolerate chaos and ambiguity, do not fear taking risks, and work with others in connected ways. Managers usually receive the title because of an appointment to a position within an organization. **Managers** tend to focus energy and efforts to ensure a smooth workflow and the efficient use of resources to meet the objectives of the organization. Effective managers and leaders both possess expertise in working with people, understand organizations as authentic, and pursue their work with passion (Covey, 2004; Covey, 2020; Robinson-Walker, 2021).

Formal leaders are people who hold positions of power via appointments or elections in groups, organizations, or workplaces. In contrast, **informal leaders** are not formally appointed to their position; rather, they emerge when members of a group recognize that they have special knowledge, expertise, communication skills, or other personality traits that are respected and admired (Donnelly, 2003; Videbeck, 2008).

Nurses influence clients and other members of the health care team as they fulfill professional roles and responsibilities. A strong knowledge base of leadership and management skills enables nurses to influence others (including clients) to make optimal health care decisions. As leaders of the interprofessional health care team, nurses coordinate efforts and inspire others to provide the best possible client care.

Take Note!

Because they influence clients and the health care team in performing their everyday duties, all nurses are leaders.

CONCEPTUAL AND THEORETICAL APPROACHES TO NURSING LEADERSHIP AND MANAGEMENT

Leadership is a complex concept with multiple definitions but is typically defined as a process of influencing others or guiding or directing others to attain mutual goals (Mish, 2020). Leadership can be transactional (relationships based on the exchange of effort or something valued by followers) or transformational (empowering others to create and work toward achieving anything that is possible). Transactional leaders typically use strategies that exercise power over others, whereas transformational leaders use strategies that empower others (Bass & Riggio, 2005; Burns, 2003).

Perceptions of Power and Empowerment

The ideas of mutuality, empowerment, and transformation as key elements of leadership surfaced in the late 1970s (Burns, 1978). During the second wave of the feminist movement, Noddings (1984), a scholar in leadership, education, and feminist theory, noted that men and women had different approaches to leadership, with women being more apt to share power ("power with") and focus on relationships rather than dominating others ("power over") and emphasizing tasks. Table 17.1 presents some current leadership theories classified according to approaches to how power is used and the focus on the emphasis of tasks and relationships. Leaders choose how they use power and focus on how work is accomplished based on their philosophical beliefs.

Mutuality, empowerment, and transformation serve as hallmarks of contemporary leadership. In health care, the interprofessional team and unlicensed assistive personnel (UAP) work collectively toward attaining optimal client outcomes. Professional nurses assume leadership roles when coordinating care and making

Theory Name	Theory Creator(s)	Key Principles	Approaches to Power Use and How Work Is Done
-TABLE 17.1	**Use of Power and Task/Relationship Approaches to Leadership and Management**		
Leadership styles	White and Lippitt (1960)	The leader's style affects worker performance. Identifies three basic leadership styles: *Authoritarian:* Leader exercises great control to get the work done. *Democratic:* Leader and group work together to get goals accomplished. *Laissez-faire:* Leader abstains from leading and lets subordinates lead themselves.	Power over others and task oriented Power with and balanced orientation of tasks and relationships Power given to followers with no attention to either tasks or relationships
Theory X	McGregor (1960)	The manager must control, direct, and motivate workers by offering rewards or threatening punishment. Workers avoid responsibility and seek security. Workers cannot be trusted.	Power over Task oriented

(Continued)

TABLE 17.1 Use of Power and Task/Relationship Approaches to Leadership and Management (Continued)

Theory Name	Theory Creator(s)	Key Principles	Approaches to Power Use and How Work Is Done
Theory Y	McGregor (1960)	Managers can trust workers to do the best possible job. Workers value their work, are motivated by rewards, contribute to the organization, and derive satisfaction from meeting goals. Workers can solve work-related problems with their own initiative and creativity. Managers can create an environment to increase worker commitment and self-direction.	Power with Relationship and task oriented
Managerial grid model	Blake and Morton (1964)	Identifies five basic leadership styles based on balancing concern for task and concern for people: *Impoverished:* Low concern for tasks and people *Produce or perish:* High concern for tasks with low concern for people *Country club:* High concern for people with low concern for tasks *Middle of the road:* Balanced, but low concern for people or tasks *Team:* High concern for people and tasks	Power over with no attention to tasks or relationships Power over and task oriented Power with high concern for relationships but minimal concerns for task accomplishment Power balanced between power over and power with. Minimal concern for tasks and relationships Power with and highly focused on relationships and tasks
Be–know–do	U.S. Army (2004)	Leaders influence other people by providing them with purpose, direction, and motivation while operating to achieve the mission and improve the organization. Effective performance is the result of transforming human potential. To be a leader means to have values and attributes of a leader (loyalty, duty, respect, selfless service, honor, integrity, and personal courage). To know involves knowledge and mastery of interpersonal, conceptual, technical, and tactical skills. To do means to live out the values, use knowledge and skills to influence others to achieve the mission, and improve the organization by providing everyone with purpose, meaning, and motivation. There is a high level of trust among subordinates and leaders. Officers have a duty to protect their subordinates, and subordinates have a duty to follow orders issued by officers.	Power over with high emphasis on tasks and relationships, especially in the development and maintenance of camaraderie
Theory Z	Ouchi (1981)	Leaders share responsibility with workers. Leaders match work with employee strengths. Work processes are designed and work problems are solved by using quality circles in which workers and managers have equal status. Decisions are made by democracy and consensus building. However, leaders consider the long-term effects to evaluate management decisions.	Power with and high concern for tasks and equal relationships
Contingency leadership	Fieldler (1967)	A leader selects a particular leadership style to best fit a given situation that includes the nature of staff–leader relationships, formal position of the leader, and the nature of the task.	Power is exerted over others or shared according to the situation along with high focus on tasks or relationships depending on the situation

Theory Name	Theory Creator(s)	Key Principles	Approaches to Power Use and How Work Is Done
Leader participation model	Vroom and Yetton (1973)	Leaders choose from autocratic, consultative, or participative styles when making decisions. The leader uses a list of questions to analyze the environmental contingencies that may affect the quality of the decision made.	Autocratic: Power over with high emphasis on tasks Consultative: Power over with some concern for relationships in that follower's ideas are considered Participative: Power and emphasis on tasks and relationships
Transformational leadership	Burns (2003)	Identifies two types of leaders: *Transactional leaders* maintain daily operations using rewards to motivate subordinates. *Transformational leaders* inspire and empower everyone with the vision of what could be possible. The transformational leader has a high level of trust, gets others to share common values and mission, shows a committed work ethic, defines reality, keeps the dream alive, examines effects of actions, and makes adjustments as needed.	Power over and task oriented Power with and relationship oriented
Path–goal theory	House and Mitchell (1974)	Leaders coach, guide, and reward staff to select the best paths to meet organizational goals using one of the four leadership styles: *Achievement oriented:* Used to set challenging goals for competent followers *Directive:* Used to set expectations and operational methods for followers *Participative:* Used when the leader wants follower suggestions *Supportive:* Used to build follower trust and confidence	Power balanced and task oriented Power over and task oriented Power with and relationship oriented Power balanced between power over and power with and relationship oriented
Situational theory	Hershey and Blanchard (1977)	The leader selects from four leadership styles while considering the amount of direction required, specific factors about the situation, and the maturity of followers: *Telling:* High task/low relationship (leader needs to be in command in a situation with one correct response) *Selling:* High task/high relationship (leader has most of the controls but assists followers to boost confidence) *Participating:* High relationship/low task (leader and followers share decision making) *Delegating:* Low task/low relationship (leaders assume the followers are competent and capable of assuming full responsibility for the decision or task)	Power over with task orientation Power over with high levels of task and relationship orientation Power with and high relationship orientation Power with and balanced orientation toward tasks and relationships
Transforming leadership	Anderson (1998)	"Transforming leadership is vision, planning, communication, and creative action that has a positive unifying effect on a group of people around a set of clear values and beliefs to accomplish a clear set of measurable goals. This transforming approach simultaneously impacts the personal development and corporate productivity of all involved" (p. 270). Transforming leadership anticipates future trends, develops new leaders, assesses, plans, implements organization-wide leadership and self-leadership development programs, and creates a community within the organization. The leader uses communication, counseling, and consulting to create the organizational community.	Power with and a balance orientation toward tasks and relationships

(Continued)

▀ TABLE 17.1 Use of Power and Task/Relationship Approaches to Leadership and Management (*Continued*)

Theory Name	Theory Creator(s)	Key Principles	Approaches to Power Use and How Work Is Done
Authentic leadership	George (2003)	Leadership is not about style but rather authenticity. Five qualities of authentic leaders are "understanding their purpose, practicing solid values, leading with heart, establishing connected relationship, and demonstrating self-discipline" (p. 17). Leadership is more effective when the leader leads a balanced life with authenticity in each of life aspects.	Power with and higher emphasis on relationships
Servant leadership	Greenleaf (1977)	Leaders use their values to empower workers by providing them with all the needed resources and an environment that enables each one to achieve their maximum potential. The top priority for the leader is to serve others (employees, customers, and the community).	Power with and high orientation toward relationships
Quantum leadership	Porter-O'Grady first presented the idea in 1997; Porter-O'Grady and Malloch (2018)	Quantum leaders use relational and whole-systems thinking in the processes of integration and synthesis, recognize the importance of relationships and formation of partnerships, empower workers to take ownership of their contributions toward common goals, understand that work is valuable only when it fulfills a purpose, embrace and steer change, stay abreast of issues that may result in future changes, enumerate and evaluate the effectiveness of changes, demonstrate personal engagement with the creation of sustainable value, create safe environments to address the struggles and emotional pain associated with changing practices and services, and celebrate the journey and all progress attained (pp. 6, 19). Quantum leaders understand that action in one place ultimately impacts other places, realize that mutuality means authority will shift between and among people, recognize that the interactions within and among system result in mobile and fluid outcomes, realize that the value of an action is its driving force and informs its content, views relationship building as "the primary work leadership" (p. 23), trusts intuition and gut thinking, acknowledges the unique and vital contributions of others, and knows how to achieve value in processes that being present to the process and players involve being supportive of, stretching, challenging, pushing, and helping others achieve goals and expectations (p. 23). Quantum leaders have a willingness to lead and display the qualities of trust, courage, passion, energy, and self-discipline. They embrace and address problems directly, and they hold themselves and others accountable for outcomes, products, results, making differences, role execution, and sustainability. Quantum leaders have a high level of self-awareness, visible vulnerability, and creativity. They honor diversity, take rational risks, display authenticity, recognize their limitations, possess an absence of ego, trust others, feel adequate about themselves, and remain open to new ideas. Leadership can be learned and developed.	Power with and high orientation to relationships

Theory Name	Theory Creator(s)	Key Principles	Approaches to Power Use and How Work Is Done
Trait theories	Evolved in the early history of man	Leaders are born. They inherit characteristics that make them suitable as leaders.	Highly dependent on the each individual. One may exert power over, whereas another uses power with. Orientation to tasks and relationships would depend upon inherited traits.

Anderson, T. (1998). *Transforming leadership* (2nd ed.). St. Lucie Press; Blake, R., & Morton, J. (1964). *The managerial grid: Key orientations for achieving production through people.* Gulf Publishing; Burns, J. (2003). *Transformational leadership.* Grove/Atlantic; Fiedler, F. (1967). *A theory of leadership effectiveness.* McGraw-Hill; George, B. (2003). *Authentic leadership.* Jossey-Bass; Greenleaf, R. (1977). *Servant leadership: A journey into the nature of legitimate power and greatness.* Paulist Press; Hershey, P., & Blanchard, K. (1977). *Management of organizational behavior: Leading human resources* (3rd ed.). Prentice Hall; House, R., & Mitchell, T. (1974). Path–goal theory of leadership. *Journal of Contemporary Business, 3,* 81–97; McGregor, D. (1960). *The human side of enterprise.* McGraw-Hill; Ouchi, W. (1981). *Theory Z: How American business can meet the Japanese challenge.* Addison-Wesley-Longman; Porter-O'Grady, T., & Malloch, K. (2018). *Quantum leadership: Creating sustainable value in health care* (5th ed.). Jones & Bartlett Learning; U.S. Army. (2004). *Be–know–do: Leadership the Army way.* Jossey-Bass; White, R., & Lippitt, R. (1960). *Autocracy and democracy: An experimental inquiry.* Harper & Row; Vroom, V., & Yetton, P. (1973). *Leadership and decision making.* University of Pittsburgh Press.

REAL-LIFE REFLECTIONS

As a PTA task force leader, Elena analyzes the situation, the characteristics of task force members, and the people in key decision-making positions before deciding what approaches may work best. Which of the management and leadership theories in Table 17.1 might she find useful in achieving these factors?

recommendations to interprofessional team members. In an ideal world, all members of the health care team assume leadership roles when needed because of their unique expertise. Author and motivational speaker Covey (1996, 2020) proposed that today's leaders must combine personal values and visions to develop strategic pathways and align organizational resources and processes to fulfill visions and missions while empowering others. Leaders create a vision that inspires commitment and empowers people by sharing authority. Empowering leaders prefer to be transformational, thereby changing individuals, organizations, and societies.

According to Covey (1989, p. 222), the real test of interpersonal leadership is the leader's ability to permit others to validate themselves and realize that they will benefit more by working toward accomplishing goals that are shared by the leader and team members. In **transformational leadership**, there is "mutual learning, mutual influence, and mutual benefits" (Covey,

1989, p. 216). Donnelly (2003) noted that all definitions of leadership contain the following elements: "relationship, context, purpose, and accountability" (p. 40).

REAL-LIFE REFLECTIONS

Elena's leadership position means she needs to spend time building and cultivating relationships to enhance teamwork and influence people who make decisions about student health services and education. If you were in Elena's position, who would you consult in the decision-making process? Why would the input of these individuals be important? What key topics should Elena cover when talking to these key people?

▌ QUESTIONS FOR REFLECTION

1. Think of your current manager or a faculty member. Which of the leadership theories do you see this person using to motivate employees or students? Why do you think they use this theory?
2. List the pros and cons of traditionally gendered ideas of approaches to the use of power.
3. Identify separate clinical practice situations and whether a "masculine" or "feminine" approach to leadership would best fit each identified situation. Explain your choices.

Leadership as a Process of Empowerment

Perceptions of power and power relationships have changed markedly in recent years. In the past, physicians were viewed as all powerful and dominated health care because they held a monopoly on key medical information and did not share it with others. Today, many people have access to state-of-the-art information about health care advances. Health care professionals and consumers have easy access to content about health conditions and how to manage them. Online databases can be readily accessed on the National Library of Medicine website. Anyone with internet access can read information available on a variety of health care profession associations and academic medical websites. If knowledge is perceived as a power source, power is redistributed as more people gain access to it.

Porter-O'Grady and Malloch (2018) proposed that power has conflicting connotations. People can think of power in terms of either coercion and domination or influence and strength. All people have some level of power and the right to exercise that power legitimately. Instead of centralizing power to people in administrative positions or to an elite group, Porter-O'Grady and Malloch suggested that power should be shared by all (decentralized) so that all people can use their expertise in delivering client care. By sharing knowledge and expertise with others, nurses empower clients, families, each other, health team members, and communities.

Blanchard et al. (1996) conceptualized **empowerment** as a releasing of the knowledge, experience, and motivation that people already possess. They identified the following three keys to empower people within organizations:

1. Share information: Trust people with information, and they will act responsibly.
2. Create autonomy through boundaries: Clearly delineate purposes, values, images, goals, roles, structure, and systems; everyone within an organization then understands and executes their own roles to meet the mission.
3. Replace the traditional organizational hierarchy with self-directed teams: Workers assume full responsibility for entire work processes and products.

Take Note!
When knowledge is perceived as a power source, power is redistributed as more people gain access to it.

Empowering leadership gives energy to the work of nursing and allows leaders and followers to maximize personal areas of strength. Empowered people make decisions about the work they do and feel valued by the organization and leaders. Empowerment becomes an outcome of leadership. Bennis (1989, p. 23) said that empowerment is evident in the four themes shown in Box 17.1, Professional Building Blocks, "Empowerment Themes Related to Nursing Leadership." These themes have been adapted to nursing.

Empowered nurses make each person with whom they interact feel important. Nurse leaders also value the knowledge and skills that each person brings to a health care situation. Finally, clients, nurses, and health care team members collaborate to determine a preferred vision for the future, and all work together to attain optimal client care.

17.1 Professional Building Blocks

Empowerment Themes Related to Nursing Leadership

1. **People feel significant:** All feel that they make a difference and that what they do has meaning and significance. In the nursing process, the nurse and the client are equal in significance; both have meaning, and what they do together is mutually significant.
2. **Learning and competence matter:** The nurse and the client value learning and mastery. The nurse makes it clear that there is no failure, only mistakes that provide feedback and tell us what to do next.
3. **People are part of a community:** The nurse, other health care providers, and the client are experienced as a team, a family, and a unit. A person does not have to like another to feel a sense of community (striving for a common goal).
4. **Work is exciting:** The nursing process is stimulating, challenging, and fun. The nurse "pulls" rather than "pushes" a client toward a goal. This pull style of influence energizes the client to "enroll in an exciting vision of the future. … It motivates through identification, rather than through rewards and punishments" (Bennis, 1989, p. 23). The nurse articulates and embodies the ideals of health toward which both the nurse and the client strive.

Data from Bennis, W. (1989). *Why leaders can't lead: The unconscious conspiracy continues.* Jossey-Bass.

LEADERSHIP DEVELOPMENT

When nurses envision themselves as leaders, they embark on the journey of **leadership development**. Aspiring leaders need to realize that leadership does not automatically occur with position appointment but rather must be learned and developed (Barrett, 1998; Donnelly, 2003; Dotlich et al., 2004; Kouzes & Posner, 2011, 2017; Porter-O'Grady & Malloch, 2018; Van Velsor et al., 2010). Table 17.2 outlines two different approaches for leadership development and includes examples of how a nurse might experience it. Most of the approaches begin with establishing a personal leadership mission followed by self-analysis. Once aspiring leaders envision the type of leader they want to become, they engage in a process of mastering key leadership skills that fit with the desired leadership approach.

Take Note!
Leadership must be learned and developed; it is not automatically acquired when one is appointed to a leadership position.

Leaders learn from challenging assignments, education, significant people, hardship, and other unidentified situations. Van Velsor et al. (2010) specified that leadership development occurs from a variety of experiences. They proposed that through leadership development programs, aspiring leaders learn self-management capabilities (increasing self-awareness, balancing conflicting demands, learning new skills and ideas, and developing a personal set of values for leadership). Along with personal capacity for development, novice leaders learn social capabilities (building and

TABLE 17.2 Three Approaches to Leadership Development

Barrett (1998)	Leadership Passages (Dotlich et al., 2004)	Professional Nurse Experience
Becoming a facilitator by focusing on physical, emotional, mental, and spiritual balance and aligning personal mission, vision, and values with those of an organization	Joining an organization or company and learning the organizational culture	Finding a first nursing job, learning work expectations and the culture of the particular nursing department as well as the larger organization
	Moving into a leadership role that results in losing one's personal identity, losing one's status as the upcoming star, and learning how to balance tasks and people	Realizing that some enjoyable client care tasks must now be delegated to other people in order to provide efficient client care
Becoming a collaborator by developing one's emotional intelligence, learning effective interpersonal skills, building collaboration and team spirit, accessing the intuition and creativity of others, empathizing with others, and giving and receiving effective feedback	Accepting the stretch assignment resulting in the need for overcoming feeling like a victim, coping with skepticism and hostility from others, and realizing what is not known and when to seek out other trustful team members	Accepting the position of "charge nurse"
	Assuming responsibility for actions by valuing the unfamiliar, displaying resiliency despite setbacks, and accepting the paradoxical characteristics of the work	Taking responsibility when the nursing unit fails to run smoothly, realizing that more tasks need to be delegated, deciding that more knowledge and practice are needed for managing coworkers effectively, and doing what is needed to improve job performance
Becoming a servant/partner or wisdom/visionary by increasing individual role awareness, understanding the role of the organization, creating a sustainable future, partnering, forming strategic alliances to attain long-lasting success, and deepening and strengthening personal and professional growth as a leader	Dealing with significant failures one has caused or is responsible for by examining decisions that resulted in the failure; sharing experience with a trusted boss, coach, or advisor; reflecting on the failure and devising different actions for future situations; and rallying the energy needed for perseverance	Sharing personal frustrations with a trusted nurse who has more experience; developing a mentoring relationship; generating alternative actions if similar situations are encountered in the future; and keeping oneself physically, emotionally, and spiritually healthy to remain in professional nursing practice

(Continued)

◾ TABLE 17.2   Three Approaches to Leadership Development (*Continued*)

Barrett (1998)	Leadership Passages (Dotlich et al., 2004)	Professional Nurse Experience
	Coping with a bad boss or competitive co-workers by developing a strategy to manage the ineffective relationship; analyzing your reaction to the boss or peer regarding what it tells you about yourself; and defining personal values	Finding effective strategies to manage an ineffective manager or jealous coworkers and engaging in a process of clarifying one's personal values and identifying own personal weaknesses
	Dealing with losing a job or not getting an expected promotion by using the following strategies: not letting a job or event define you as a person, trying to understand what occurred by contemplation, using a support network, and devising a strategy to address "what next"	Engaging in conversations with other nurses who have survived similar circumstances, recognizing that professional nursing does not need to consume one's total being, and perhaps changing to a new area of professional practice (or leaving the profession)
	Being part of an acquisition or merger	Learning new ways of working and learning a new organizational culture (this is true especially when a nonprofit health care organization becomes part of a larger for-profit network)
	Living in a different country or culture	Learning alternative ways of living and working (some nurses may go on medical missions, travel abroad, relocate to different areas, or go to different locations to further their education)
	Finding and maintaining a meaningful balance between family and work	Achieving an effective balance between one's personal and professional lives
	Letting go of ambition by realizing that you do not have to be "the best" or "first," accepting that all people cannot be the best forever, redirecting energy to other things, and redefining a personal definition of achievement	Acknowledging that "perfection" in nursing is impossible, developing a meaningful professional practice, becoming more involved in life outside nursing, and realizing that others need to be educated to fill nursing positions as you and some of your colleagues consider retirement
	Facing personal upheaval by accepting tragedy as a means for humanization by revealing personal vulnerabilities to others, being authentic, and accepting fate and carrying on	Using personal losses and challenges to connect more effectively with clients, colleagues, and other health team members
	Losing faith in the system by finding meaning in one's life and current work, sponsoring a protégé for a leadership position, finding fulfillment with a current project, achieving new skills, reconnecting with what originally led you to your area of expertise	Being a mentor to a younger professional nurse, clarifying personal values, and finding joy and meaning with current professional work

maintaining relationships, developing effective work groups, enhancing interpersonal communication skills, and learning how to develop other people). Finally, leaders develop work facilitation capacities by learning management skills, learning how to engage in strategic thought and action, increasing their ability for creative thinking, and learning how to imitate and implement change (Van Velsor et al., 2010). Porter-O'Grady and Malloch (2018) concurred with this leadership development framework but also added that leaders must learn how to take risks.

Nurses embark on a career in nursing leadership for a variety of reasons. Some nurse leaders assume leadership positions because they displayed leadership qualities throughout life. Others view an administrative position as being less physically taxing. Some find daytime hours and salaries attractive. Nurses may find themselves in a leadership position because no other nurse in the organization would assume it, whereas others enter the profession with the intention of becoming a nurse administrator. In a qualitative research study, Bondas (2006) identified several paths to nursing leadership:

- Nurses who had a desire to seek knowledge and education followed the *path of ideals*. These nurses engaged in self-reflection and dreamed about making a professional difference. Previous positive and negative experiences with nurse leaders also influenced their career decision.
- Nurses who used personal power in making the decision to assume a leadership position because they perceived themselves to have personality traits, skills, and previous experiences to offer chose the *career path*. They also perceived themselves as self-directed, wanting desirable daytime hours, and needing to have a less physically demanding job.
- Nurses who found that a leadership position was the only available nursing job when they were seeking employment took the *path of chance*.
- Nurses who substituted for other nurse leaders and viewed the experience as a trial to see if a leadership position worked for them were using the *temporary path*.
- The nurses who developed a career plan to assume a nursing leadership position used the *path of choice*.

Nurses following the temporary path or path of chance often had no formal leadership education. The path of chance was a more passive approach in which the nurses felt that these choices were made by others.

Business scholars Kouzes and Posner (2017) spent over 30 years studying people globally in leadership positions in a variety of fields, including professional nursing. Their research revealed that characteristics of admired leaders appear to be consistent regardless of age and geographic location; the top descriptors include honest, forward-looking, inspiring, competent, intelligent, broad-minded, dependable, supportive, fair-minded, and straightforward. They also identified the importance of clarity in personal values for exemplary leadership and organizational commitment.

Exemplary leaders accomplish extraordinary things by empowering others. Kouzes and Posner (2017) specify that leadership is not about personality but rather about behavior. They explain that behavior consists of skills and abilities that others can observe. Kouzes and Posner (2017) identified five practices of exemplary leadership:

1. *Modeling the way* starts with clarifying personal values and asserting shared ideals and values. Once values and ideals are affirmed, exemplary leaders role model by living out the values and ideals.
2. *Inspiring a shared vision* involves envisioning the future, imagining all possible exciting and ennobling future states, and enlisting others to refine and subscribe to the shared visions.

3. *Challenging processes* means assessing the current ways of doing things for opportunities for improvement, looking externally for innovative ways for improvement, and taking risks to try new ways.
4. *Enabling others to act* necessitates building trust among others, facilitating relationships, fostering collaboration to strengthen others to promote self-determination, and developing increased competence.
5. *Encouraging the heart* emphasizes the importance of recognizing the contributions of others and expressing appreciation for individual excellence through meaningful celebrations that foster creation of a spirit of community.

Take Note!
Exemplary leaders are credible because they display consistency between words and actions they do what they say they will do.

■ QUESTIONS FOR REFLECTION

1. What steps have you taken to develop leadership in yourself or others?
2. Have you encountered any obstacles toward developing leadership? If yes, what were they and how did you handle them?
3. What areas do you need to develop to improve your leadership abilities? Why are these areas important to develop?

KEY LEADERSHIP AND MANAGEMENT SKILLS FOR NURSES

The nature of professional practice dictates that all nurses need to develop leadership skills. Nurses use many **leadership and management skills** when engaged in multiple professional nursing roles (Table 17.3).

The professional nursing roles of critical thinker, caregiver, client advocate, change agent, counselor–teacher, coordinator, and colleague require the use of many leadership and management skills. Nurses must believe they have personal power to execute each role effectively. Hagberg (1994) proposed that the first step in establishing personal power is to perceive oneself as being powerless. Feelings of powerlessness sometimes occur when people encounter new situations. However, as time progresses, all people (including nurses) will develop some sense of power as they succeed in a particular arena.

TABLE 17.3   Key Leadership and Management Skills for Nurses

Leadership Skills	Management Skills	Skills for Leadership and Management
Maintain a focused and intense approach to work.	Clarify organizational goals and expectations.	Expand one's self-awareness.
Challenge others to expand thinking and actions.	Use established relationships to influence others in the organization.	Maintain composure and a high energy level when encountering multiple competing demands (stress management).
Deliver compelling messages.	Create a strong organizational culture.	Learn from experience.
Take risks.	Use all incentives available to motivate others.	Seek feedback from a variety of sources.
Set personal goals.	See that day-to-day operations are executed effectively.	Find common ground with others.
Have a deep, connected, and emotional involvement with subordinates/followers.	Set organizational goals.	Demonstrate sincere empathy toward others.
Keep a strong concern and investment with ideas.	Remain fair by keeping a low level of emotional involvement with employees.	Make self available to others.
See the gestalt of situations.	Be concerned with results.	Listen effectively.
Inspire others.	Make a strong investment in the organization.	Express appreciation for the contributions of others toward goals.
Tolerate ambiguity.	Staff inpatient and outpatient departments.	Abide consistently and constantly by ethics and principles.
Welcome diverse perspectives.	Enhance productivity. Budget to meet operations. Market the organization. Reduce risks in the organization. Write and deliver employee performance appraisals. Follow organizational guidelines and procedures.	Establish trust with all people. Establish and agree on goals using collaboration. Use facts or evidence to clarify expectations rather than assumptions or rumors. Identify rumors, clarify their truth, and dispel them if false. Display optimism in all situations. Analyze situations from multiple perspectives to identify issues and concerns. Network with others to identify issues and concerns that need to be addressed. Monitor the impact of change. Learn new things quickly. Set effective priorities. Generate multiple courses of action. Take decisive action but know when to change to a different course of action. Commit self to effective action plans. Attract others to assume leadership or management positions. Share power with subordinates/followers. Form alliances with key players in any given situation. Communicate precisely and consistently and in ways that are acceptable and clear to others. Manage resistance. Clarify roles of others and encourage them to assume a leadership role. Resolve conflicts. Motivate others to be their best. Manage the vast sea of information.

Leadership Skills	Management Skills	Skills for Leadership and Management
		Master computers and high-tech equipment.
		Meet standards of professional nursing practice.
		Work to attain optimal client outcomes.
		Delegate tasks to others.
		Deconstruct 20th-century barriers and structures.
		Recognize future trends that will point to a need to change to meet the needs of the future.
		Celebrate all progress toward change to meet 21st-century health care demands.

Adapted from Blank, W. (2001). *The 108 skills of natural born leaders*. AMACOM; Donnelly, G. (2003). How leaders work: Myths and theories. In T. Steltzer (Ed.), *Five keys to successful nursing management* (pp. 31–60). Lippincott; Porter-O'Grady, T., & Malloch, K. (2018). *Quantum leadership: Creating sustainable value in health care* (5th ed.). Jones & Bartlett Learning; Van Velsor, E., McCauley, C. D., & Ruderman, M. N. (2010). *The Center for Creative Leadership handbook of leadership development* (3rd ed.). John Wiley & Sons.

Box 17.2, Learning, Knowing, and Growing, "Strategies for Professional Nurses to Develop a Personal Power Base," provides ideas for accomplishing this.

Take Note!

When nurses have personal power, the likelihood of professional power increases.

Like Kouzes and Posner (2017), Marquis and Huston (2021), and Robinson-Walker (2021), Hagberg (1994) stressed the importance of self-awareness and the value of teamwork when establishing personal power. However, Hagberg proposed that true empowerment does not occur until people no longer use power by association (hoping the power of strong people or superiors will be transferred to them) or power by symbols (displaying signs of success such as having an extravagant lifestyle or the newest gadget). True empowerment occurs when people have the freedom to be their true authentic selves (power by reflection), live out their life purposes (power by purpose), or have power by gestalt (turning to higher powers without the need for social prominence). Truly empowered people give power to others by fostering in them their ability to

17.2 Learning, Knowing, and Growing

Strategies for Professional Nurses to Develop a Personal Power Base

- Develop, nurture, and maintain high personal energy.
- Interact with others with authenticity and honesty.
- Display a powerful image to others.
- Listen and speak with care.
- Work hard and diligently to become a valued member of the nursing, interprofessional health care, and administrative teams.
- Identify the powerful people within the organization, remembering that those with informal power are sometimes more influential than those with formal power.
- Study, learn, and master the language, symbols, and entire organizational culture.
- Use the organization's priorities to meet professional and personal goals.
- Increase expertise by expanding professional skills and knowledge.

- Envision broadly by looking upward and outward to expand organizational influence.
- Seek and use counsel from experts and professional role models.
- Be flexible and open to others and change.
- Become a visible person and respected voice within the organization.
- Inform others of personal talents and professional accomplishments without bragging, and compliment others on their talents and accomplishments.
- Accept compliments graciously.
- Use humor carefully to diffuse tense situations.
- Laugh at yourself, and do not take yourself too seriously.
- Empower others by sharing knowledge and experience while building a cohesive team.
- Support others whenever possible.

Adapted from Marquis, B., & Huston, C. (2021). *Leadership roles and management functions in nursing, theory and application* (10th ed., pp. 338-345). Wolters Kluwer; Robinson-Walker, C. (2021). *Leading with mastery and heart, the coaching companion for thriving nurse leaders*. Elsevier.

share special gifts and make meaningful contributions to the world (Bass & Riggio, 2005; Hagberg, 1994).

Leadership in the Role of Critical Thinker

Most nurses engage in critical thinking as they perform all aspects of clinical practice. Critical thinking prevents nurses from blindly following physician orders and jumping to conclusions about client care situations. Nurses use critical thinking to analyze situations, identify problems, set priorities, develop multiple possible approaches to a specific situation, and consider the consequences of a strategy before taking action. Nurse leaders also use critical thinking when clarifying personal values, envisioning missions, challenging processes, and enabling others to act independently.

Leadership in the Role of Caregiver

When driven to do what is in the client's best interest, nurses use power to ensure client care needs are met. Empowered nurses share power with others, thereby empowering clients to manage their own health. When nurses understand levels of power, they use power more effectively. With **empowered caring**, nurses share their knowledge and skills freely with others while valuing the contributions all persons bring to nursing care situations. Changes arising from empowering situations tend to become realistic, genuine, long-lasting habits.

Nurses use a range of power sources while engaging with clients and others in a variety of clinical practice settings. Expert power is used when nurses bring their specialized knowledge and skills to any practice. Nurses use power based on legitimate right and authority (position power) in daily practice situations. Nurses use referent power (based on identification with the personal qualities of the nurse) to mobilize others to facilitate desired outcomes.

Leadership in the Role of Client Advocate

The concept of client advocacy has many meanings. An advocate "supports or defends someone or something and recommends or pleads on another's behalf ... [and] works to change the power structure so that a situation will be improved" (Douglass, 1988, p. 259). Box 17.3, Professional Building Blocks, "What Is Advocacy?" outlines beliefs of the nurse advocate.

17.3 Professional Building Blocks

What Is Advocacy?

Nurses who believe in advocacy share the following beliefs:

- Clients have the right to a nurse–client relationship based on mutuality, shared respect, consideration of information and feelings, and full participation when solving problems regarding their health and health care needs.
- Nurses have the responsibility to ensure clients have access to appropriate services to meet their health care needs.
- Clients are responsible for their own health.
- Nurses are responsible for mobilizing and facilitating client strengths in achieving the highest possible levels of health.

Nurses cannot be effective advocates unless they believe fully in their strengths. Power is shared among nurses and the people they serve. Frequently, nurses serve as resources for clients, subordinates, or colleagues. Because advocacy requires conviction, it is important for the nurse to overcome personal feelings and beliefs about nurses' "powerlessness" to take the first step in the process of empowerment (Richardson, 1992, p. 38).

Client advocacy has been associated with an assumption that nurses have a responsibility to protect their clients. Since the time of Florence Nightingale, nurses have been called on to protect clients from harm. Bandman and Bandman (1995) reported that nurses are often caught in ethical dilemmas especially working with persons during end of life situations.

Perhaps the greatest need for nurses to act as protectors occurs when nurses identify threats to client safety such as situations in which care is inadequate or environmental hazards surface. As client advocates, nurses assume leadership roles in promoting access to health care for all, preserving the rights of people to make health care decisions, keeping clients safe, monitoring care quality, and intervening in a nonadversarial manner when harmful (or potentially harmful) situations arise. Nurses may have to take risks to protect clients. They may need to confront persons who have more organizational power and status. When nurses defend client rights, they act as client advocates even if they must engage in an adversarial struggle against the forces of institutional oppression, including those arising from cost containment or discrimination.

To restructure their working conditions, nurses must be advocates for professional colleagues and for themselves. Chapter 8, "Professional Nursing Processes," and Chapter 10, "Professional Practice Based on Nursing Research and Best Evidence" suggest that an effective method for gaining control over practice is to develop and use evidence as a basis for recommending changes. Evidence, rather than opinion, strengthens the need for change. Advocacy for any client is more effective if the advocate is working from a position of strength, is armed with solid evidence, and holds the steadfast belief that what one proposes will improve the safety and quality of client care.

Leadership in the Role of Counselor–Teacher

Professional nurses provide emotional support and education to clients (see Chapter 4, "Establishing Helping and Healing Relationships," and Chapter 16, "The Professional Nurse's Role in Teaching and Learning"). Nurse leaders also teach and counsel colleagues.

Most nurse practice acts contain clauses that state that RNs teach others in any nursing care activities. Most institutions set basic standards for educating UAP in collaboration with nurses. As direct supervisors, professional nurses assess the educational needs of staff and design educational programs. When nurses keep the client and family at the center of health care, they serve as role models for all health team members regarding the provision of client- and family-centered care. Nurses teach UAP daily when different approaches are required to meet individual client care needs and preferences. Many times, nurses teach other professional team members about new work processes (e.g., electronic documentation changes), potential client safety issues (e.g., reminding physicians to comply with hand hygiene or posted isolation procedures), and specific client home care needs (e.g., imparting information from client stories about home life).

Professional nurses frequently find other members of the health care team experiencing distress. Nurses who spend time listening to the concerns of team members can offer support and guidance. Through this informal counsel, nurses may refer coworkers to community health resources as indicated (see Concepts in Practice, "The Colleague–Counselor Role in Action"). When nurses counsel team members and each other, they acknowledge the humanness of all colleagues, care enough to listen to personal stories

and issues, provide needed emotional support, and display an ability to lead from the heart. Helping colleagues through difficult times and issues builds trust and fosters the development of meaningful team relationships.

Concepts in Practice $\boxed{\text{IDEA}} \longrightarrow \boxed{\text{PLAN}} \longrightarrow \boxed{\text{ACTION}}$

The Colleague–Counselor Role in Action

The following scenario demonstrates how a nurse leader might teach and counsel a colleague.

Luisa, an RN, finds Sara, a UAP, crying in the nurse's lounge instead of performing delegated tasks. Luisa takes time to listen as Sara shares that she discovered a breast lump during her morning shower and believes it must be cancer. Luisa shares her knowledge about various breast tumors and available treatment centers and helps Sara make an appointment for diagnosis. Later that week, Luisa accompanies Sara to a breast care center, where a needle biopsy is performed and the tumor is found to be benign.

Leadership in the Role of Coordinator

Nurses often find themselves in the role of coordinator. Nurses assume responsibility for delivering basic client care, carrying out physician orders, and promoting optimal client outcomes. When competing demands are placed on the nurse's time, they must frequently prioritize activities.

The role of coordinator becomes more apparent when professional nurses assume administrative positions. Managers assume responsibility for utilizing people, supplies, money, and systems effectively to provide high-quality, cost-effective care. They coordinate the efforts of others so that the job is performed efficiently. To meet the challenges of management, nurse managers use a variety of skills, including interpersonal ("people") skills, budgeting and finance skills, information technology skills (see Chapter 14, "Informatics and Technology in Nursing Practice"), and quality management skills (see Chapter 18, "Quality Improvement: Enhancing Patient Safety and Health Care Quality").

Interpersonal Skills for Nursing Management and Supervision

Effective managers strive to bring out the best in their employees while providing them with required resources and support to provide effective client care. Nurse managers need to set and effectively communicate expectations for their departments. Nurse managers must also interact with administrators, other department managers, physicians, and other interprofessional team members. Strategies for developing helpful and healing relationships (outlined in Chapter 4, "Establishing Helping and Healing Relationships") serve as the basis for developing effective communication with staff and all members of the interdisciplinary health care team.

Meetings provide an avenue for employees and managers to process information together. Reasons for meetings include sharing complex information (e.g., major policies, organizational or accreditation changes), generating ideas, solving problems, making decisions, and planning actions. Nurse leaders, managers, and staff nurses (especially those involved in shared governance activities) frequently lead meetings. With careful planning, meetings can be effectively run, provide consistency in communications, and save time because participants receive the same information simultaneously. The cost of running a group meeting is each person's hourly rate of pay multiplied by the length of the meeting.

It is important to consider who should attend the meeting. All key stakeholders (those affected by the decisions) involved in the topics covered in the meeting along with anyone with specialized knowledge or skills in the topic areas should be present. Meetings consisting of more than 12 people can be difficult to manage because of increased likelihood of side conversations. For a working meeting to generate a new policy, three to five people seems ideal (Lofland & Lofland, 1995). Once attendees have been identified, the meeting leader decides when and where the meeting should occur. Many health care organizations have access to computer calendar applications. For larger staff meetings, sometimes an hour prior to a shift change works for many employees.

As the meeting is being planned, the leader must find a meeting location. Some nursing units have a staff break room large enough to suffice. However, if the meeting involves brainstorming or developing new work processes or solutions to current problems, a private location free from interruptions may be preferred. Space may be difficult to find in some facilities. However, other facilities may have classrooms devoted to staff education, private meeting rooms, or small consultation rooms that might provide privacy when sensitive issues are planned for discussion. Most organizations have a scheduling process to follow to reserve rooms.

Once the meeting attendees, time, and location have been established, a meeting agenda serves as a communication tool in advance of the meeting to inform participants of topics to be discussed to facilitate any special preparation that needs to be done prior to the meeting. The agenda also serves as the meeting schedule. A well-developed agenda includes key topics, discussion about each topic, if a topic requires action, and a time frame devoted to each topic. The agenda should have a professional appearance and include the meeting, date, starting time, and location presented using a table or an outline. If a table is used, two additional columns can be added for the note taker to include columns for discussion, actions, and follow-up. Because the meeting leader will need to attend to the deliberations and group dynamics, a designated note taker should be identified prior to the meeting if possible. Some leaders may have administrative assistants who can fill this role or one of the meeting participants volunteers or is appointed.

When leading a meeting, the leader may find it useful to arrive at the room early to verify room setup and that the room has working climate controls, necessary technology, and other materials. A circle or horseshoe chair arrangement will enable attendees to see each other and facilitate discussion.

Because meetings can quickly become time-wasters, the leader should start the meeting on time and begin by welcoming and thanking participants for their time. If a note taker has not been determined earlier, a call for a volunteer should occur before deliberations on topics begin. The role of the note taker must be clearly delineated because sometimes the note taker just takes minutes and the leader may or may not type up and distribute the minutes. Many organizations have standardized templates for minutes. The leader should explain meeting guidelines, such as the process for discussions, voting procedures, technology use, confidentiality, and respect.

As the meeting is conducted, the agenda serves as the itinerary. The leader times discussions or another participant can monitor the time spent on each topic. If too much time is spent on one topic, the leader has to limit discussion, or if the topic is one of prime importance, set a time limit for discussion to end, ask the group if they want to proceed to the next topic, or schedule another meeting to continue revisit the topic. By watching participants' nonverbal behavior, the leader can monitor how the meeting is progressing. Engaged participants make eye contact, nod their heads, lean forward, and smile. Crossed arms, scowls, and frowns may suggest disagreement. Restlessness, looking at watches, cell phones, and yawning may signify boredom or eagerness for the meeting to end.

Meetings rarely follow the agenda exactly. Attendees can drift off topic, express negativity, and talk simultaneously. When the participants drift off topic, the leader should redirect the conversation. Negativity can be addressed by asking direct questions of the persons expressing negative ideas or thoughts about the topic. Sometimes, the negative comment can generate a novel idea that may need to be considered. When multiple people talk at once, no one can hear the discussion. Sometimes, having attendees raise hands, passing an object for the speaker to hold, or requesting one person to speak at a time may alleviate this problem. When a participant repeatedly brings up the same topic, the leader needs to remind the participants to focus on generating new ideas. When participants get weary, conversations may start to ramble. By summarizing the conversation, the leader helps focus participants on key elements of the discussion. Some leaders opt for a quick summary of the discussion prior to a vote or before moving to a new topic on the agenda. Some participants may dominate the conversation, and the leader can handle this by acknowledging a good point and moving on to pose a question to the group. There will always be attendees who fail to contribute to the conversation. When this occurs, the leader can invite these participants by addressing them by name and asking for their opinions.

Productive meetings result in decisions. Multiple decision-making approaches are commonly used during staff meetings. Managerial decisions occur when the person with organizational leadership makes the decisions. This approach may limit buy-in from others for the decision. Majority vote is another way some decisions are made. This requires more than 50% of participants agreeing with the decision. Some organizations may adopt a super majority vote, which requires a two-thirds majority vote in favor of a decision. The group and leader can delegate the decision when the goal is to have the people closest to an issue make the decision or there is a reason to leverage someone's higher level of knowledge and expertise on the subject. Sometimes, delegation can also be used to enhance the skills of a particular participant or small group of participants. Consensus is another form of decision making and works best when strong group commitment is present (discussed in detail in the next section).

Some leaders include time for meeting conclusion on the meeting agenda. During the meeting conclusion, the leader provides a summary of meeting proceedings, reviews decisions made, reviews the next steps, and outlines action plans (i.e., who will perform agreed-upon actions and the time frame for completion). If another meeting is to be scheduled, the end of the meeting is an opportune time to choose a time because all stakeholders are present and can offer input based on their availability. Because participants may have other obligations, the leader should end on time. An effective meeting leader expresses gratitude for participant attendance and toward the group for making decisions and achieving goals.

Empowering Team Members: Decisions by Consensus

Decisions related to problems or changes in practice tend to work better when made by consensus rather than by an individual. A major tenet of transformational leadership is to inspire and empower others to achieve the best possible future state (Burns, 1978, 2003). In any given clinical situation, everyone involved has a unique perspective and a specific skill set that must be used to facilitate optimal outcomes. Sharing power and responsibility for outcomes is facilitated when all stakeholders participate in the process.

Consensus provides an avenue for participatory decision making because it relies on all parties sharing key information, generating alternatives, listening with respect to the views of others, and taking time to explore all options and their consequences. In most situations, generating several options for action may be more effective than generating an exhaustive list. Singular solutions are rare in human health concerns or in work situations. Although reaching consensus takes more time than other decision-making processes, the people making the decision will have a commitment to execute it (Burns, 1978; Porter-O'Grady & Malloch, 2018; Van Velsor et al., 2010).

Connectedness underlies the process of consensus. When a team works together toward a common goal (e.g., optimal client outcomes), team cohesion is enhanced when decisions are made by consensus. Consensus means that everyone will try to implement the decision even though each person may not agree fully with it. All people participating in the process feel they played a significant role in decision making, especially if participants engaged in meaningful dialogue (Wesorick & Shiparski, 1997). See Concepts in Practice, "Nursing in Action: Making Decisions by Consensus," for an example of consensus decision making.

Concepts in Practice   IDEA ⟶ PLAN ⟶ ACTION

Nursing in Action: Making Decisions by Consensus

The following scenario demonstrates how nurses can work together to attain a common goal that benefits all parties.

Because of low client census on a hospital unit, nurses have been sent home on a rotating basis as a cost-saving measure. Nurses who have accrued vacation time may use it. The policy states that each nurse must take a turn being sent home. A group of older nurses with more seniority (and more vacation time) collaborate with younger nurses who have recently been hired. The nurses reach a consensus that those with more vacation time will go home twice for every one time that a new nurse is sent home. With their revised plan fully designed, all the nurses meet with the nurse manager, who agrees to its implementation. In the process of working together, these nurses developed more meaningful working relationships and feel more connected to each other.

All people in consensus share equal accountability and responsibility for the quality of the decisions made. However, when hierarchical relationships are established in the health care setting, health care providers (including some nurses) tend to use command styles rather than participatory styles when coordinating efforts of the health team (Porter-O'Grady & Malloch, 2018) or attempting to influence client decision making (Taylor et al., 1989). Participatory decision making is a hallmark of transformational leadership (Burns, 2003; Porter-O'Grady & Malloch, 2018).

Team-Building Skills

Positive work environments are enhanced when all workers display commitment to the work and work together as a cohesive team (Porter-O'Grady & Malloch, 2018; Wesorick & Shiparski, 1997). Effective teamwork enables all team members to use their skills. Effective teams have members who collaborate to set visions and goals while identifying how they will work together to attain them.

Effective teamwork balances unity with diversity. If a group is too unified, new ideas and divergent thinking may become stifled, resulting in groupthink. Groupthink occurs when group members' drive for unanimity supersedes their motivation to consider alternative actions. Antecedents to groupthink include decision-maker cohesiveness, group insulation, leadership responsibilities assigned to a select few members, deeply shared norms, homogeneity of members, high levels of external stress, low member self-esteem, reduced acceptance for individualism, and time constraints. Symptoms of groupthink are closed-mindedness, overestimation of group abilities, and peer pressure toward uniformity. Groupthink results in defective decision making stemming from incomplete information (failure to consider things external to the group) and poor outcomes (Shirey, 2012).

Divergent opinions allow the team to remain open to alternative processes and new possibilities (Van Velsor et al., 2010). When teams express openness to new ideas, they are better equipped to adapt to the continual change that is so prevalent in today's health care organizations (Kouzes & Posner, 2017). If a group has too much diversity, however, conflicts may impede progress toward attaining mutually agreed goals.

Strategic Planning

A **strategic plan** provides a long-term roadmap for ensuring the future and sustainability of an organization. Organizations must continually adapt to keep pace with the ever-changing world. Strategic plan development requires a detailed analysis of internal and external factors affecting offered services. Strategic plan time frames typically range from 3 to 10 years (Harrison, 2021; Marquis & Huston, 2021).

The strategic planning process typically begins with a thorough analysis of the current situation, followed by identification of an ideal future state. Organizational vision, mission, and philosophy are reviewed and revised as needed. Next, the organization identifies goals to fulfill its vision and mission. To ensure organizational sustainability, strategic planning should include goals for the organization's environmental impact (carbon footprint and pollution from health care services waste), sociocultural relevance (how well services meet the demographics and cultural idiosyncrasies of the targeted service areas), financial stability (feasibility of acquiring monetary and other requisite resources), political commitment (internal governance and external legal and governmental issues), and organizational development capacity (new operational systems, current and new facilities, human resources plan, assessment of current and new technology, creation of a strong organizational culture, continuous quality improvement and safety programs, and effective management of knowledge and information) (Harrison, 2021; Ramirez et al., 2011).

Some organizations identify current strengths, weaknesses, opportunities, and threats ("SWOT") during the organizational analysis phase (Harrison, 2021; Marquis & Huston, 2021). After the strategic goals have been finalized, the organization outlines a deployment plan, which includes providing a culture, structures, and resources for plan implementation. Some organizations manage the plan using a strategic planning matrix that includes departmental goals (broadly written statement depicting a desired state), objectives (things to complete within a specific time frame), measurements or benchmarks (targeted dates and data collection to verify objective attainment), target date (deadline), and people responsible for achievement of each goal (Harrison, 2021). Table 17.4 outlines considerations for strategic plan development and deployment.

Strategic plans work best when organizations hold individuals accountable for successful implementation. To track progress toward meeting objectives outlined in a strategic plan, a means to evaluate progress must be devised. Some organizations opt for the use of balanced scorecards to ensure strategic objectives are accomplished by all departments. Balanced scorecards collect and analyze data regarding four aspects of organizational performance: (1) financial, (2) customers,

(3) processes, and (4) learning and growth. Balanced scorecards may be completed at the organizational, departmental, and individual employee levels. Balanced scorecards typically contain the measurement methods and action steps outlined by the strategic plan. When the annual action steps do not happen as outlined by the strategic plan, a detailed analysis takes place to determine why. If results indicate that step failure was a result of unpredictable events (such as a major economic downturn), the organization reviews and revises the strategic plan appropriately. However, if the analysis reveals that the action steps were not executed because of managerial inaction, the organization may demote or terminate the manager (Harrison, 2021; Marquis & Huston, 2021).

Budgeting Skills

To implement a personal or organizational mission, resources must be acquired, mobilized, and used. Human and material resources are required to provide health care services. Viability of a health care organization (from a large medical center to the smallest office or clinic) relies on effective use of human and material resources.

Budgeting is a process to plan for attaining the required material and human resources to accomplish an organizational (or personal) mission. Budgets outline the costs of organizational operations. For example,

TABLE 17.4 Key Elements of a Strategic Plan

Direction Statement	Strategic Objectives	Strategic Priority Issues
Mission statement: purpose and why	Measures performance on the direction statements	Broad issues that should be addressed to meet a desired future state
Vision statement: desired future state	Measures success in meeting intentions	Internal changes to continue to hold a competitive advantage over competitors
Business definition: clear and concise presentation of products, offered services, target consumers, technology, distribution of products and services, and geographic area served	Frequently addresses performance on profitability, shareholder value (if a for-profit), market position, services, quality, and innovations	Target areas in which to develop measurable action plans
Competitive advantage: what makes you better than other organizations offering the same or similar services		
Core competencies: key systems, assets, intellectual prowess, programs, and special skills to enhance the competitive advantage		
Values/beliefs: philosophy and values that guide organizational behavior and processes		

Adapted from Fogg, C. D. (1999). *Implementing your strategic plan.* AMACOM; Harrison, J. P. (2021). *Essentials of strategic planning in healthcare* (3rd ed.). Health Administration Press; Marquis, B., & Huston, C. (2021). *Leadership roles and management functions in nursing: Theory and application* (10th ed.). Wolters Kluwer.

acquiring the resources needed to go to school requires planning, determining the amount of money needed to finance educational costs, and developing a plan to verify that all personal responsibilities can be met. Likewise, an organization must be certain that it has the capital, equipment, and people to meet its mission effectively. The planning phase of the budgeting process is not an exact science but rather a process in which nurse managers look at the current direction of health care, anticipate what future services may be needed, and make decisions based on sound business principles and education. For example, the staffing budget projects the amount of money and the number of nursing personnel needed to provide safe, effective client care.

Nurse managers use critical thinking skills when developing departmental budgets. Budgets are typically determined for a 12-month time frame and include costs for staff (i.e., staff salaries and fringe benefits), client care (i.e., supplies and equipment), and environmental maintenance. Some nurse managers also submit budgets for capital expenditures along with expected revenue (Rundio, 2016). Capital expenditures include material resources that are expensive and have a projected lifespan (e.g., cardiac monitors, computers). In contrast, the supply budget consists of inexpensive or disposable items that are used for a short time (e.g., syringes, dressings, office supplies).

Once the budget is approved by a governing body (e.g., board of directors), nurse managers compare actual spending with the projected amounts outlined in budget reports. Periodic review of reports enables nurse managers to monitor resource utilization and control excessive spending. Nurse managers must account for budgeting variances. A budget variance occurs when there is a difference between estimated and actual costs, revenue, or activity. For example, if more money was spent on nurses' salaries than projected on a cardiac unit, the nurse manager must discover why this occurred and justify the reason for the variance. Sometimes, reasons may be beyond the manager's control (Rundio, 2016). For example, a nurse manager discovered that unit census was above projections because of increased numbers of invasive cardiac procedures resulting from the addition of a new staff cardiologist. However, if the overtime was the result of ineffective delegation of tasks to UAP, then the manager must submit an action plan to remedy the situation.

Staffing

Ensuring that enough nurses are available to deliver client care can be one of the most challenging tasks for nurse managers. The **staffing** process estimates how many people are needed to provide quality nursing care and then finding qualified people to those fill positions. Many staffing plans use the fulltime equivalent (FTE) model to develop staffing plans. An FTE is defined as a person who would work 2080 hours annually if no vacations, holidays, or sick days were taken (Rundio, 2016). The formula used to calculate the number of FTEs to staff a nursing department in a hospital is a number of hours worked per shift multiplied by number of shifts worked per week and then divided by 40 hours.

When nurses work fewer than 40 hours per week, the nurse manager must hire additional nurses to fill the gap in settings that provide services 24 hours a day, 7 days a week. Along with productive employee hours (hours actually spent working), managers must budget for nonproductive hours such as paid time off (e.g., vacation, sick leave), jury duty, holidays, education time, and other benefits (Rundio, 2016).

To determine daily staffing requirements, the nurse manager must consider client census, client acuity, and the number of nursing care hours needed for each client. To accomplish staffing projections, nurses calculate the nursing hours per client day. The number of nursing hours per client day varies across nursing units, with intensive care units requiring more hours of nursing care than short-stay surgical units. To determine daily staffing needs, the unit manager multiplies the average daily census times the nursing hours per client day. With daily census fluctuations, some nurse managers prefer to use a staffing matrix, which is a staffing plan based on the number of clients who need nursing care. The matrix also presents a ratio of RNs, licensed practical/vocational nurses, UAP, and unit secretaries/clerks for each shift (Marquis & Huston, 2021; Rundio, 2016).

Of the workload on a nursing unit, 80% can be predicted (Porter-O'Grady & Malloch, 2018). Prudent nurse managers realize that in health care settings, staff workloads and the timing of essential nursing tasks cannot always be predicted accurately. Therefore, they build overtime expenses into the staffing budget. For example, in acute care nursing, the following situations might result in unplanned overtime: (1) a client may have a medical emergency as nurses are changing shifts, (2) a nursing unit could receive unexpected multiple admissions within a short time, (3) a family emergency may require a staff member to leave work, or (4) a staff member may experience exposure to a health hazard or sustain a work-related injury.

When staff nurses have input into staffing plans, they are more apt to understand the process, feel capable of making decisions about unit staffing, and have increased job satisfaction. Dent (2015) suggests that the following dimensions should be considered when formulating staffing plans for nursing units: using evidence-based staffing guidelines determined by the National Nursing Database of Quality Indicators, include planning for staff turnover (increasing staffing during the orientation of newly hired nurses), using acuity-based client classification systems for making staff assignments, accommodating for travel nurse use, and considering nurse fatigue management. Nurses should not be permitted to work more than 12.5 hours in a given day, 36 hours in any 3-day period, and 602 hours within a 7-day time frame because working more than these amounts produces fatigue and increases the chance or care errors (Dent, 2015).

Marketing Skills

When nurse leaders engage in promotional activities to bring someone to something, they are using **marketing** skills. Many nurses find themselves marketing the facility (engaging in promotional activities to bring clients or employees to a facility in which they work) and/or marketing the nursing profession. Marketing goals might include increasing volume, maximizing client and staff satisfaction, and improving quality of life for the community. The steps of the marketing process mirror the steps of nursing process, starting with

assessing the current situation. Considerations for a marketing assessment include listing services offered and assessing the community served by the facility. The next step is selecting strategies to inform potential clients about the organization and its services. Sometimes, health care organizations have marketing budgets that nurses can use. Marketing strategies used in nursing are outlined in Table 17.5. Of all the strategies outlined, personal recommendation tends to be the most effective (Hunt, 2003).

Leadership in the Role of Change Agent

One constant throughout the world is **change**. When people are actively involved in designing and implementing change, the change is usually sustained. Henriksen et al. (2006) defined transformational change as the process of reinventing an organization or a single work unit to improve performance, thereby enabling it to respond more effectively to external environmental changes and forces. As health care organizations look for ways to continually improve the quality and safety of health care, they seek ways to streamline work processes and use resources more efficiently. Some people find moving from a current, comfortable state (or process) distressing, whereas others find it exciting. The professional nurse confronts change on a daily basis. As **change agents**, nurses steer change while helping themselves and others cope with it.

TABLE 17.5	**Marketing Strategies for Nurses**	
Strategy	**Description**	**Expense**
Personal recommendation	Word-of-mouth compliment	None
Newspaper advertisement	Print ad	Rates depend on circulation of the newspaper
Radio or television advertisement	Broadcast message	Free for a public service announcement; charge rates vary
Printed materials	Brochures, fact sheets, catalogs	Printing costs Free distribution if volunteer time Mailing costs Fee for distribution racks housed in hotels, restaurants, or businesses
Community outreach	Speaking engagements, health screenings at health fairs, or contacting agencies where potential customers may be	Free if services volunteered Work release time for employees Cost for health screening supplies, props, and printed materials
Introductory offers	Health promotion classes on a trial basis Reduced cost for a new service	Costs of running program and delivering services
Traditional sales call	Sell health-related services to other companies	Salesperson salary, supplies, and fringe benefits

Adapted from Hunt, P. (2003). Marketing your facility. In T. Stelzer (Ed.), *Five keys to successful nursing management* (pp. 276–286). Lippincott Williams & Wilkins.

Organizational change requires resources and energy (Perlman & Takacs, 1990). Change often has an emotional meaning for people and is often associated with feelings of loss or pain (Bridges & Bridges, 2019). Based on the Kübler-Ross model of death and dying, Perlman and Takacs (1990) proposed a 10-stage model to explain the psychological issues associated with change, the signs and symptoms of each stage, and nursing interventions to help others grow during the change process (Table 17.6).

In another model, Carnall (1990, pp. 141–146) proposed five stages in coping with change:

- Stage 1: Denial of the validity of new ideas
- Stage 2: Defense (experiencing depression and frustration)
- Stage 3: Discarding (acknowledging change as inevitable or necessary)
- Stage 4: Adaptation (feeling anger)
- Stage 5: Internalization

TABLE 17.6 Growing With Change: The Emotional Voyage of the Change Process

Stage	Characteristics	Interventions for Successful Change
1. Equilibrium	High energy level, state of emotional and intellectual balance, sense of inner peace with personal and professional goals in sync.	Make employees aware of changes in the environment that will impact the status quo.
2. Denial	Energy is drained by the defense mechanism of rationalizing a denial of the reality of the change. Employees experience negative changes in physical health, emotional balance, logical thinking patterns, and normal behavior patterns.	Employ active listening skills (e.g., being empathic, nonjudgmental, using reflective listening techniques). Nurturing behavior, avoiding isolation, and offering stress management workshops also will help.
3. Anger	Energy is used to ward off and actively resist the change by blaming others. Frustration, anger, rage, envy, and resentment become visible.	Recognize the symptoms; legitimize employees' feelings and verbal expressions of anger, rage, envy, and resentment. Active listening, assertiveness, and problem-solving skills are needed by managers. Employees need to probe within for the source of their anger.
4. Bargaining	Energy is used in an attempt to eliminate the change. Talk is about "if only." Others try to solve the problem. "Bargains" are unrealistic and designed to compromise the change out of existence.	Search for real needs/problems and bring them into the open. Explore ways to achieve desired changes through conflict management skills and win–win negotiation skills.
5. Chaos	Diffused energy, feeling of powerlessness, insecurity, sense of disorientation, loss of identity and direction, no sense of grounding or meaning, breakdown of value system and belief, and defense mechanisms begin to lose usefulness and meaning	Quiet time for reflection, listening skills, inner search for both employee and organization identity and meaning, approval for being in state of flux.
6. Depression	No energy left to produce results; former defense mechanisms no longer operable; self-pity, remembering past, expressions of sorrow, feeling nothingness, and emptiness.	Provide necessary information in a timely manner. Allow sorrow and pain to be expressed openly. Exhibit long-term patience, take one step at a time as employees learn to let go.
7. Resignation	Energy expended in passively accepting change; lack of enthusiasm	Expect employees to be accountable for reactions to behavior. Allow them to move at their own pace.
8. Openness	Availability to renewed energy, willingness to expend energy on what has been assigned to individual	Patiently explain again in detail the desired change.
9. Readiness	Willingness to expend energy in exploring new events, and reunification of intellect and emotions begins.	Assume a direct management style, assign tasks, and monitor tasks and results so as to provide direction and guidelines.
10. Reemergence	Rechanneled energy produces feelings of empowerment, and employees become more proactive. Growth and commitment are reborn. Employee initiates projects and ideas. Career questions are answered.	Mutual answering of questions; redefinition of career, mission, and culture; mutual understanding of role and identity; employee's action based on own decisions

Adapted from Perlman, D., & Takacs, G. J. (1990). The ten stages of change. *Nursing Management, 21,* 33–38. Used with permission of the publisher.

Bridges and Bridges (2019) approached change from the perspective of psychological adaptation that expands on the initial work of William Bridges in 2003. Unlike other approaches to change, William Bridges proposed that transitions start with endings and end with beginnings. He acknowledged that during any change, people enter a period of uncertainty (the neutral zone) when they fail to fully understand the meaning of and their role in implementing the change. Too much time in the neutral zone causes extreme psychological distress for people involved in change, contributing to dissatisfaction or even depression. People affected by change need to be encouraged and supported throughout the process. Bridges and Bridges (2019) also warn about dangers associated when multiple changes occur too quickly as people need time to recover from being in the neutral zone.

Table 17.7 compares the Perlman and Takacs model, Carnall model, and Bridges model of change. These models address various psychological responses people experience when confronted with change. Before change can be internalized, people tend to progress through various stages of acceptance. Pritchett and Pound (1995) outlined pitfalls that frequently arise when coping with organizational change (see Box 17.4, Learning, Knowing, and Growing, "Common Mistakes when Coping with Organizational Change").

 17.4 Learning, Knowing, and Growing

Common Mistakes When Coping With Organizational Change

- Assuming that the role of management is to keep you comfortable
- Expecting another or others to reduce your stress
- Aiming for a low-stress work setting
- Attempting to control uncontrollable factors
- Refusing to abandon the expendable
- Facing the future with fear
- Choosing the wrong battles to fight
- Disconnecting psychologically from your job
- Avoiding acceptance of new assignments

Team Roles in the Change Process

Roles of the Professional Nurse Change Agent

Based on a comparative analysis of the literature, Wooten and White (1989) identified five basic change roles: (1) educator/trainer, (2) model, (3) researcher/theoretician, (4) technical expert, and (5) resource linker. The change agent (the person who brings about a change) must model appropriate behaviors in an atmosphere of trust and openness, accept responsibility for getting data in an appropriate manner, provide skills and expertise, and link necessary resources in ways that make the intervention effective. The selection and timing of particular roles depend on the specific needs of the situation.

Roles of the Client System

Effective change depends on the client system assuming various roles. Wooten and White (1989) also described four basic roles of the client system: (1) resource provider, (2) supporter/advocate, (3) information supplier, and (4) participant. The client system provides effort, time, and money resources; advocates the change; provides information involving the self and others; and participates in the change process. It is crucial that the change agent and the client collaborate to promote effective change.

Mutual Roles

Wooten and White (1989, p. 657) indicated that "mutual role enactment is at the heart of the change process." The mutual roles include (1) problem solver, (2) diagnostician, (3) learner, and (4) monitor. Instead of relegating full responsibility for the entire change

TABLE 17.7	**Comparison of Theoretical Stages in Coping With Change**	
Perlman and Takacs (1990)	**Carnall (1990)**	**Bridges and Bridges (2019)**
Equilibrium		*Endings* Disengagement Disidentification Disenchantment
Denial	Denial	*The Neutral Zone* Disequilibrium
Anger	Defense	Disidentification
Bargaining		
Chaos		
Depression		
Resignation	Discarding	
Openness	Adaptation	*New Beginnings* Reengagement
Readiness		Realignment
Reemergence	Internalization	Reidentification

process to the change agents, this model focuses on joint responsibility and action.

Problem solving involves identifying a problem, generating alternatives, and testing assumptions. Diagnosis necessitates sensitivity to issues in the relationship. Learning includes knowledge, skills, and new attitudes, and monitoring involves "remain[ing] aware of alternatives, ascertain[ing] the consequences of action, [and] gaug[ing] the effectiveness of the change effort and relationship at each stage of the intervention" (Wooten & White, 1989, p. 657). Each role can be adopted independently or simultaneously.

Selecting a Change Strategy

As change agents, professional nurses select specific change strategies to use in practice situations. The strategy selected depends on the type of change involved. Change strategies are classified into the following six categories: empirical–rational, normative–reeducative, power–coercive, facilitative, reeducative, and persuasive and power. The following discussion defines each major category and provides examples of how they are used in professional nursing practice.

Empirical–Rational Strategies

The empirical–rational category assumes people will act in a way that is rational and in their own self-interest. These strategies focus on educating a person about the available options and assuming the individual will change behavior because they know the new behavior will be beneficial and desirable.

For example, in-service education may include a demonstration of the latest techniques available for a particular task with the expectation that nurses will apply that knowledge to improve care of clients. Another example is nurses who do not take breaks during work hours and have an increased chance of making an error in client care. Nurses who attend a staff in service on the need to take breaks during their shifts may incorporate this idea into practice. However, if the nurses have the deep personal value that clients come first, they may not take breaks. Thus, sometimes the empirical–rational strategy may be ineffective in establishing and maintaining a desired change, especially if the change involves shifting personal values and beliefs.

Normative–Reeducative Strategies

The normative–reeducative category assumes sociocultural norms are fundamental to a person's behavior. In addition to rationality and intelligence, change must involve modification of attitudes, values, skills, and significant relationships. Thus, when working with clients and colleagues, the change process must be based on mutuality and collaboration. This allows for the problem solving and personal growth necessary to promote effective change.

For example, a young client who needs to have surgery for ovarian cancer refuses to have it because of her belief that the purpose of her life is to bear children. When listening to the client, the RN discovers that the client had an aunt who did not have children, received undivided attention of her partner, had a lavish lifestyle, and was considered by the rest of the family to be spoiled and selfish. Once widowed, the aunt made demands of the other family members, and the client internalized the family's negative response. She expresses fear that she will become like her aunt. The nurse acknowledges the fear, and the two of them engage in meaningful dialogue about the purpose of life. The client's attitude changes, and she consents to having the surgery.

Power–Coercive Strategies

Power–coercive strategies are based on the use of power. The belief is that despite the need for knowledge and modification of attitudes and values, change will occur only when it is supported by power based on potential punishment and rewards. This rationale is the basis for much political action, and it may imply the use of legitimate channels of authority or violent, non-sanctioned methods (Chin, 1976). This strategy effects change more quickly than do other strategies, but the change that results is not usually lasting (Haffer, 1986).

For example, a professional nurse working with a particular UAP notices that every time they work together, the UAP fails to complete delegated tasks in a timely manner. Because the nurse supervises the UAP, the nurse initiates the first step of a progressive discipline process, which is documenting the conversation held with the UAP about not fulfilling job responsibilities. For a month, the UAP completes delegated tasks quickly but returns to previous habits thereafter.

Facilitative Strategies

Facilitative strategies are used to make clients and others aware of the availability of help in sufficient detail and clarity so that they know exactly how to access and use assistance. Facilitative strategies are appropriate when there is openness to change. This type of strategy can include (1) simplifying data, providing feedback, and providing other necessary tools to help others recognize a problem; (2) providing multiple potential solutions to a problem; and (3) involving others in the decision-making process. These strategies produce greater commitment to change, but the change agent must be sure that there are sufficient resources, commitment, and capability to maintain the change after leaving the situation.

For example, a nursing research consultant is hired to help staff nurses develop and implement evidence-based practice or nursing research on hospital nursing units. The consultant meets with interested nurses every other month, helps them develop research projects, and coaches them on project implementation. When the consulting contract ends, the nurse researcher contacts doctoral-prepared nursing faculty from a local nursing program to continue helping the nurses execute and publish their research projects. The unit nurses select the faculty with whom they will work to finish their projects.

Reeducative Strategies

Reeducative strategies are based on empirical–rational theory but are different because the person needs to acquire new skills and knowledge. They also facilitate change when resistance is prevalent, when people have inaccurate information, when the change involved is a radical departure from past practices, and when the person lacks confidence about the ability to implement the new practices. However, reeducative strategies work to bring about change only when there is a strongly felt need and a strong motivation to change.

Reeducative strategies work slowly, so they are feasible only when time is not a pressing factor. Examples of reeducative strategies include creating awareness that a problem exists by indicating how much better things could be when symptoms can be connected with causes, and outlining the benefits of new practices. Reeducative strategies work well when people receive a new diagnosis of a chronic illness, such as diabetes or renal disease that requires special self-monitoring and compliance with strict regimens for optimal outcomes. Reeducative strategies heighten awareness of a problem and possible solutions, but they fail to increase the motivation to change.

Persuasive and Power Strategies

Persuasive and power strategies involve active participation of all people involved and consume much time. Research findings and other forms of evidence serve as useful tools when presenting a case to move from one way of doing things to another (see Chapter 10, "Professional Practice Based on Nursing Research and Best Evidence").

Persuasive and power strategies involve active discussion and debate. Process participants each bring an idea of what should be done and how the change should be implemented. They also outline the consequences if change does not occur.

For example, persuasive and power strategies permeate the federal and state legislative process (see Chapter 19, "The Professional Nurses Role in Public Policy"). As a result of shifting legislation (see Chapter 9, "Health Care Delivery Systems"), many health care organizations are preparing for reductions in federal and state reimbursement for services rendered to older adults and impoverished clients. Hospital administrators (including nursing administrators) possess a global perspective of the implications of reduced income to provide safe, effective health services. Nurses and other care providers have undertaken the challenge to look for ways to reduce costs for client care services. If costs cannot be contained, then many health care organizations may have to close, resulting in reduced access to care and increased unemployment of health care providers. Motivation for change is driven by aversion to potentially undesired consequences rather than the need for improved processes or relationships.

Benefits of Change Strategies

Professional nurses who understand the basic types of change strategies may select the best ways to proceed when confronted with situations where change is indicated. People vary in their responses to the many change strategies. For example, sometimes the power–coercive strategy may be met with much resistance, whereas at other times, it may be successful.

The professional nurse also must assess the ability of individuals to cope with change and how many changes are occurring simultaneously. When one strategy fails, the nurse can try another one to bring about the desired change. At times, the professional nurse must prioritize changes for clients, health care team members, or organizations to avoid extreme psychological distress arising from too much change in too little time.

Cultivating an Environment Supportive of Change and Innovation

Nursing leaders can cultivate environments that are supportive of change and innovation. Innovation begins with divergent thinking, a spontaneous, fluid thought process resulting in creative and nonconforming ideas. Divergent thinking is not a linear thought process and results in multiple, frequently innovative approaches to address an issue or problem. Nursing leaders and managers can promote divergent thinking among members of their professional nursing staff by providing them with education on how to engage in divergent thinking, listening to different views and solutions of their staff, and trying out solutions generated by divergent thinkers (Cianelli et al., 2016).

Sometimes, ideas generated by divergent thinking may seem risky for implementation. Because of the emphasis on safety in health care delivery, taking risks may be discouraged and avoided (Cianelli et al., 2016). Before implementing any solutions generated by divergent thinking, a benefit-to-risk ratio should be considered. If the idea has the potential to place a client or staff member in harm's way or if it is questionable from a legal or ethical perspective, it should not be implemented. However, some divergent ideas may not directly affect safety and may be a way to effectiveness of work processes or improve staff satisfaction. Low-risk divergent ideas should be implemented because they can be a source of innovative ways to improve clinical practice and the work environment.

Risk-taking behaviors by employees can be supported in several ways. The key for safely promoting risk-taking behaviors is to establish a firm policy of openness about risk taking, educating employees about the organization's view and policies related to risk taking, addressing risk taking routinely in staff meetings, refraining from blaming employees for failed attempts at innovation, and rewarding employees who act proactively to solve problems and address risks (Cianelli et al., 2016).

Nurse leaders who tolerate failure during innovation attempts create a climate that enhances innovation. Instead of blaming or punishing people for failed attempts, nurse leaders can provide emotional support and emphasize that the most important aspect of failure is that it provides an opportunity for learning (Cianelli et al., 2016). Staff members frequently observe how leaders handle aversive situations (like failure), and if leaders do not forgive themselves for shortcomings, staff are likely to infer that leaders will not tolerate staff failures when they occur.

The constant, fast-paced changes that occur in health care demand that health care organizations and workers possess agility and flexibility (Cianelli et al., 2016). Adverse man-made or natural disasters can occur with or without warning. Agility is the ability to move quickly with ease and grace (Mish, 2020) and requires the ability to be resourceful and adaptable. Flexibility is the "ready capability to adapt to new, different, or changing requirements" (Mish, 2020, p. 479). Ways to cultivate agility and flexibility within a health care organization include:

- Creating organizations that include agility and flexibility within mission statements, structures, and processes
- Hiring new staff that display the knowledge, attitudes, and skills needed for quick adaptation to change
- Developing employee policies and procedures that promote, support, and reward flexibility and agility
- Anticipating future changes by analyzing trends, staying abreast of world events, and developing ways to meet future challenges within the work environment
- Forming employee and management teams to provide input and steer anticipated changes
- Fostering the development of shared governance systems, sharing of stories related to similar situations, and using lessons learned from past experiences
- Avoiding developing overconfidence or inertia (Cianelli et al., 2016).

The COVID-19 pandemic challenged hospitals to demonstrate agility and flexibility, as discussed in the Concepts in Practice, "Acute Care Hospitals Demonstrate Agility and Flexibility during the COVID-19 Pandemic."

Concepts in Practice

Acute Care Hospitals Demonstrate Agility and Flexibility During the COVID-19 Pandemic

Acute care hospitals were required to demonstrate agility and flexibility during the COVID-19 pandemic starting in 2020. In the early days of the COVID-19 pandemic, little was known about how quickly the disease would spread across the United States. To free up personal protective equipment and ventilators, many acute care hospitals and outpatient facilities canceled nonemergency surgeries and procedures. In some states, governors signed executive orders providing waivers for health care providers from out of state to practice telehealth and provide medical services during the pandemic.

Concepts in Practice (*Continued*)

Some of the waivers also included relaxing practice restrictions for nurse practitioners. Hospitals in these states had to revise policies for staff privileges and limitations on nurse practitioners to ensure adequate numbers of providers. Some hospitals furloughed nurses without compensation, and some nurses were required to use accrued paid time off to make up the shortfall between hours worked and fulltime compensation. Some areas experienced high numbers of cases resulting in nurses volunteering to leave their homes, risk their lives, and work in high-risk situations. Some hospitals found themselves dependent on travel nurses for meeting staffing needs.

Based on the trajectory of the 1918 to 1919 influenza epidemic, history indicated that the second wave of the illness was worse in terms of numbers of people infected and deaths (Brook, 2020). An American second surge in COVID-19 cases reflected this trend, starting in November 2020 before leveling off in January 2021. The concept of a medical surge is not new; it occurs when there is a marked increase in the volume of clients that challenges or exceeds the capacity of a hospital. Owing to the nature of the COVID-19 pandemic, the medical surge was expected to overwhelm entire health care infrastructures of both rural and urban communities.

Proactive surge preparations included the development of COVID-19 surge teams consisting of multidisciplinary team members.

Planning committees bore the responsibility for maximizing available operational resources and determining locations within the facility for supplies, equipment, and personnel. Additional planning included rapid education for frontline providers for ensuring that infected individuals were accurately identified, evaluated, and treated. In addition, RNs received specialized training so they could work with clients with COVID-19 in the intensive care unit or specialized acute care COVID-19 unit. COVID-19 response teams formed for organizing and delivering care to large numbers of inpatients with COVID-19 (DiSilvio et al., 2020; Shaffer, 2020).

Response teams were led by physicians with specialization in critical care medicine who coordinated multidisciplinary teams. Nursing personnel were taught how to consolidate care by clustering all client care assessments, medication administration, other treatments, and basic care into single trips to the client's bedside (DiSilvio et al., 2020). Surge planning ensures that all material and human resources are ready for rapid deployment when needed, illustrating agility and flexibility.

For some nurses and nurse leaders, agility seems to occur naturally. However, other nurses and leaders may seem stuck in their ways and rigid. Many nurses and nurse leaders learn from clinical practice or experiences that help them become expert nurses who are able to be flexible and agile. Others continue to practice using methods that produced successful outcomes. Sometimes, stellar clinical nurses are promoted to managerial or leadership experiences without being fully prepared. In an ideal world, nurses in leadership positions engage in succession planning, which involves identifying staff nurses with leadership potential, sponsoring them for leadership positions, and mentoring them as they experience their first leadership role (Robinson-Walker, 2021). Eichinger and Lombardo (2004) investigated individuals with high leadership potential and discovered they tended to be active learners who learn quickly and possess the ability to craft novel responses to address constantly fluctuating situations. These individuals also possess learning agility, defined as "willingness and ability to learn new competencies in order to perform under first-time, tough, or different conditions" (Eichinger & Lombardo, 2004, p. 323).

Some nurses working during the COVID-19 pandemic willingly learned new skills to work in critical care units, and some had to develop novel work practices so that hospitals could adapt and provide care for large numbers of critically ill clients. Some nurses developed creative team approaches for caring for COVID-19 by having certified critical care nurses familiar with medication drips commonly used in intensive care units set and titrate intravenous medication drips with the infusion pump outside the client's room, whereas other nurses with strong procedural skills provided bedside client care.

Eichinger and Lombardo's (2004) five domains of leaning agility include four types of agility and self-awareness. *People agility* is found in individuals who know themselves well, learn from experience, critique others constructively, and remain cool and resilient under the pressure of change. *Results agility* is the ability to get favorable results under tough conditions, inspire others to go beyond their comfort zones, and build confidence in others. *Mental agility* is the ability to think through problems from a fresh viewpoint, feel comfortable with complexity and ambiguity, and be able to explain their thinking to others. *Change agility* is displayed by a curious nature, passion for ideas, affinity for experimenting, and enjoyment in skill building. *Self-awareness* is possessing deep personal insight, understanding one's own strengths and weaknesses, freedom from blind spots, and using

awareness for effective performance (Eichinger & Lombardo, 2004). Robinson-Walker (2021) identifies many of the same or similar concepts as characteristics of effective leadership and uses them while coaching nursing leaders.

Nurses with high levels of learning agility display high potential for successful careers in nursing administration. The following "Focus on Research" box outlines how learning agility can be used by nurse managers and leaders to identify areas for leadership development, use it for performance improvement, and predict success in nursing leadership roles.

FOCUS ON RESEARCH
Learning Agility in Nurse Managers

The investigator conducted a pilot study to explore the concept of learning agility in a group of nurse leaders employed in a single academic medical center, focusing on its effects on the nurse manager in the areas of adaptation to change, attainment of leadership competencies, and development of staff. Another purpose (if the results were positive) was to lay the foundation for identifying leadership talent to develop future nursing leaders within the organization.

Using an exploratory descriptive study design, data were collected using the learning agility scale (LAS) that measures the five domains of learning agility using a subscale for each type or agility (people agility, results agility, mental agility, change agility, and self-awareness). The LAS contains 53 items and took 30 minutes to complete. The mean score on each of the subscales were summated to determine the overall learning agility score. To assess current manager ability, the investigator used an internal institutional performance management matrix (PPM). The PPM is a nine-celled rubric that plots contributions and potential for careers in the following paths: specialized clinical, nursing management, or chief nursing officer. All 48 nurse managers were invited for study participation, but only 17 managers completed all the study requirements.

The nursing directors supervising the nurse managers completed the PPM for each participating nurse manager as a group. Each nursing director submitted a completed performance evaluation on each participating nurse manager using a 1-to-5 scoring

system, with the highest score on a single item indicating "significantly exceeding expectations." The six scores on the LAS were recorded, and the total learning agility score was calculated by summating the score on the six subscales.

The investigator analyzed data using factor analysis to confirm construct validity, even though the sample size was too small to support this conclusion. Cronbach's alpha for internal consistency was calculated to be 0.7, which is acceptable. Nonparametric correlations were run to compare nurse learning agility scores of each subscale and total learning agility scores to the PPM results. Results revealed a moderate correlation among performance ratings and total learning agility and people agility scores. The investigator plotted out scores using different colored stars to represent LAS score results with PPM results, and it was revealed that high performers tended to have total learning ability scores and higher subscale scores. None of the nurse managers scored high enough to demonstrate leadership potential at the nurse executive level, and all but two nurse managers had scores consistent with the nurse manager role.

The investigator concluded that learning agility can be used to identify areas for development and performance improvement and to predict success in a nursing leadership role. The investigator also acknowledged that more research needs to be done exploring the use of learning agility for identifying future nurse leaders and for other areas of clinical practice.

FOCUS ON RESEARCH (*CONTINUED*)

The findings and conclusions presented by the investigator need to be viewed with caution because of the small sample size and the setting of a single academic medical center. This hampers the ability to generalize the findings to other groups of nurses and other settings. The clinical significance of this study is that it is one of few nursing research studies to address the need for nursing leadership succession and offers a possible way to identify talented nurses who might be candidates. The concept of learning agility has not been studied in professional nurses. Ideas for future research include exploring the effects of learning agility on compassion satisfaction, compassion fatigue, burnout, and nurse turnover. If there appears to be a positive effect of leaning agility in nurses, then intervention studies to develop it should be conducted.

Glassman, K. S. (2018). Nurse manager learning agility and observed leadership ability: A case study. *Nursing Economics, 36*(2), 74–82.

For optimal organizational agility and flexibility, nurses and other employees with specialized expertise need the autonomy and freedom to act independently on ideas generated by divergent thinking. Nurse leaders can promote autonomy and freedom in staff by allowing them to think for themselves and act without consulting leaders. Nurses who work in shared governance systems have the responsibility, freedom, and autonomy to make decisions related to the scope of professional nursing practice within the organization. Nurse leaders can provide opportunities and support for nurses to engage in political processes at the local, state, and national levels as well (Cianelli et al., 2016). Along with the aforementioned ideas, nurse leaders can role model freedom and autonomy when working with upper-level organizational management and community leaders.

Nurse leaders have the ability to develop innovative organizations that contain necessary and multiple components for success. Employee feedback sometimes provides information needed to create environments capable of innovation, such as in areas for organizational changes and opportunities for improvement. Human resources are a critical component for successful innovation and include staff selection for innovative potential, education on innovation theory and processes, and active participation in innovation, increasing the likelihood of success. When job descriptions outline the expectation for innovation, staff members know they will be evaluated on this dimension during performance reviews. Nurse leaders with expertise in innovation can become role models, mentors, teachers, and coaches for staff members when they engage in organizational innovations (Cianelli et al., 2016).

Frequently, time is a barrier to success in the innovation process. Budgetary constraints prevent staff members from having the resources and time needed to develop, implement, and evaluate innovations in clinical practice. Some required resources include access to current nursing research findings and other evidence-based clinical practices. Therefore, having computers and online subscriptions to literature databases and professional organizations would assist staff in discovering what is known in potential areas of innovation. When an organization values innovation in clinical practice, managers reward nurses for their efforts (Cianelli et al., 2016). Rewards can be in the form of professional recognition or something tangible (e.g., gift cards, printed certificates).

In some cases, the organization reaps benefits from nurse engagement in innovation. Innovations to work processes may result in the reduction of time and supplies, resulting in a return on investment for the organization (Cianelli et al., 2016). Sometimes, staff nurses publish their innovations in nursing journals. Typically, author credentials specify the organization for which the nurses work. The health care organization receives state or national exposure that can sometimes be used for marketing or staff recruitment processes.

Leadership in the Role of Colleague

Whether working with individual clients, client groups, other health care team members, or an entire organization, nurses must establish collegial partnerships with others. Collegial partnerships enable equality among all people involved in an interaction. Over time, health care team members develop collegial partnerships with each other in which each person acknowledges the contributions and skills that the other members bring to client service.

A collegial partnership is a relationship in which all people view each other as providing equal contributions to a mutually defined outcome. Collaboration begins when individuals realize they need others to attain an envisioned goal (Porter-O'Grady & Malloch, 2018; Wesorick & Shiparski, 1997). Collegial partnerships may occur between nurses and clients, nurses and UAP, nurses and other nurses, nurses and physicians, nurses and other health team members, and even nurses and a community group. Partnerships may be short-lived or last for an extended time. When working in partnership with others, various partners assume leadership when an issue arises that falls within the realm of their expertise. The development of clinical paths or client care maps within health care organizations represents one outcome of interdisciplinary collegial partnerships.

Various barriers can undermine the development of effective collaboration among health care partners (Wilson & Porter-O'Grady, 1999):

- Old animosities, such as perceived physician superiority, sometimes prevent the nurse from trusting and relating effectively to physicians.
- Incongruence of philosophy related to the partnership may create tension. However, when these philosophical differences are acknowledged and a new common ground is found, professional partnerships may flourish.
- Competitive behavior may limit the ability to form effective collegial partnerships.
- Social status and inequality in educational levels may interfere with the development of partnerships. Information sharing is critical, and systems must be designed so all partners have access to the same information and so responsible decisions and behaviors can occur.
- Partners sometimes equate collaboration with total agreement on every issue, and processes must be in place for negotiating differences between and among partners when disagreements arise.

Take Note!
Collaboration serves as the foundation for professional partnerships in health care.

LEADERSHIP EFFECTIVENESS

Professional nurses serve as experts on health issues, care coordinators, client advocates, counselors, educators, and change agents. Box 17.5, Professional Building Blocks, "Forms of Influence within the Nurse–Client Relationship," outlines different forms of nurse influence in the nurse–client relationship. These forms of influence may also apply when the nurse works with UAP. For example, nurses make legitimate requests to UAP when delegating tasks to them. At times, nurses may use coercion or rational

17.5 Professional Building Blocks

Forms of Influence Within the Nurse–Client Relationship

1. **Legitimate request:** Responding to legitimate power, the client complies with the nurse's request because the client recognizes the nurse's right to make such a request. The client's compliance represents internalized values of obedience, cooperation, courtesy, respect for tradition, and loyalty to the organization.
2. **Instrumental compliance:** Responding to reward power, the client complies because the nurse has made an explicit or implicit promise to ensure some tangible outcome that the client desires.
3. **Coercion:** Responding to the threat of adverse outcomes, such as economic loss, embarrassment, or expulsion. Because the influence is motivated by fear, it is most effective when it is credible.
4. **Rational persuasion:** Responding to a logical argument, the client is convinced that the nurse's suggested behavior is the best way to satisfy needs or attain objectives.
5. **Rational faith:** Acting out of faith in the nurse's expertise and credibility. Such a response is based on expert power.
6. **Inspirational appeal:** Responding to expressions of values and ideals without any tangible reward, the client acts from obedience to authority figures, reverence for tradition, self-sacrifice, and so forth.
7. **Situational engineering:** Responding to manipulation of relevant aspects of the physical and social situation. The nurse must have control, and the client must accept the situation.
8. **Personal identification:** Responding to referent power. The client imitates the behavior of an admired nurse.
9. **Decision identification:** Responding to involvement in decision making.

persuasion to get them to perform the delegated tasks. With time, UAP may recognize nurses as experts, internalize some of the values of nurses they respect, relinquish control of independence to comply with nurse requests, participate actively in client care decisions, and begin to emulate nurses whom they admire. Likewise, some professional nurses acknowledge the valuable and unique contributions UAP make to client care.

In transformational leadership, rational persuasion and shared decision making serve as the most valid forms of influence because they promote empowerment. Research findings suggest transformational leadership promotes staff empowerment, increased job satisfaction for staff and managers, improved client satisfaction with care, supportive work environments, the development of mutual team goals, and an optimal mix of nursing skill and expertise (Marquis & Huston, 2021; Porter-O'Grady & Malloch, 2018). When a seasoned nurse leaves a nursing position, the organization loses the nurse's intellectual capital and professional expertise. They also lose money in terms of productivity and time replacing the nurse who left. Increased staff nurse retention saves money because recruitment and replacement costs for new professional nurse employees range from $28,400 to $51,700, with an average cost of $40,038. Based on the mean cost, a hospital would spend over $400,380 to replace 10 nurses who left the facility in a given year (Nursing Solutions Inc., 2021). The areas of high turnover in hospitals occur in specialty practice areas of behavior health units (22.7%), step-down units (24.4%), and emergency departments (20.0%). Lower rates of turnover occur in critical care nursing (18.7%), medical-surgical units (17.1%), women's health (14%), and pediatrics (14.9%). Over 27% of hired nurses left new positions within a year, and 49.1% of all new RNs left their first professional nursing position within 2 years (Nursing Solutions Inc., 2021). Thus, effective development of transformational leadership competencies in nurse managers can reduce the costs for acute care health care delivery from increased nurse retention rates.

> **Take Note!**
> The sharing of power—rather than the wielding of power—characterizes the transformational relationship of the nurse with all members of the health care team, including the client.

Transformational Leadership Competencies

Gurka (1995, p. 170) identified certain qualities of transformational leaders:

- Individual consideration: Promoting others' growth, recognizing and supporting others' needs and feelings, and giving positive feedback and recognition
- Charisma: Inspiring and motivating, demonstrating enthusiasm, and communicating in a positive manner
- Intellectual stimulation: Creating a questioning environment, acting as a mentor, and challenging others to grow and learn
- Vulnerability: Communicating authentically and openly, expressing emotions as well as ideas, and sharing the self with others
- Knowledge, concern, and courage: Seeking knowledge through study and experience, showing concern and caring for others, and being willing to take risks
- "Feminine" attributes: Maintaining accessibility, paying attention to process as well as outcomes, and practicing balance in lifestyle

Based on these and other transformational leadership concepts (Bennis & Nanus, 1985), Box 17.6, Learning, Knowing, and Growing, "Leadership Competencies," suggests way to foster your own personal and professional growth. When these actions become part of the nurse's character, they are called habits. Leadership habits of the nurse also determine the nurse's effectiveness in practice.

Covey's Habits of the Effective Leader

Covey (1989, p. 47) defined a habit as "the intersection of knowledge, skill, and desire that has great power in a person's life." Covey has described knowledge as the "what to do and why," skills as the "how to do," and desire as the motivation or the "want to do" (p. 47). He emphasized that without desire or motivation, essential, effective leadership skills such as sharing knowledge confidently and listening intently to others will never become ingrained habits. Covey outlined seven habits of highly effective people in 1989 and an eighth habit was published in 2004. Although they have been around for over 30 years, they remain relevant for today's nursing leaders.

Habits of effective leaders are the internalized principles and patterns of behavior that reflect the three interrelated factors of knowledge, skills, and

17.6 Learning, Knowing, and Growing

Leadership Competencies

- Acknowledging and using the inner wisdom of self and others
- Setting goals and working to achieve them
- Working with others to achieve a common vision and mission
- Recognizing the interconnection of everyone on everything
- Abandoning the hierarchical approach to leadership
- Recognizing that people performing the work are specialists
- Engaging in systems thinking
- Recognizing patterns
- Synthesizing new ideas and processes
- Knowing and following the laws and regulations associated with the leadership role
- Ensuring ethical principles are followed
- Committing to lifelong continuous learning
- Adapting to and accepting chaos
- Facilitating each team member's involvement and accountability
- Sharing knowledge freely with others
- Empowering others
- Being receptive to new ideas and the ideas of others
- Facilitating group meetings and participation of everyone in organizational processes (especially decision making)
- Coaching
- Acting with immediacy and equality
- Displaying technical expertise (organizational culture and design, financial management, economics, business ethics, evaluation methods, health care jurisprudence, information technology, and strategic planning for the long term)
- Practicing knowledge of relationship dynamics
- Sharing administrative functions
- Learning from mistakes
- Favoring collaboration over competition
- Mentoring others for leadership

desire. Seven habits that Covey (1989) designated for effective leadership are based on the theoretical premise of sequential growth—moving people from dependence to independence and finally to interdependence, the phase in which true mutuality can occur.

Covey's eighth habit is hearing one's own voice and inspiring others to find theirs. Finding one's own voice means periodic analysis of values and beliefs and finding quiet time to listen to oneself. Once found, the voice must be expressed by developing a personal vision, practicing discipline, showing passion in action, and not doing anything against one's conscience. Inspiring others means being a "trim-tab" (a small rudder that turns the large rudder of a ship), modeling character and competence, instilling trust, and blending voices to develop shared vision. Once others have discovered their voices, the great leader aligns goals and systems to achieve desired results (the shared vision) while empowering others to use their talents and live out passions.

Covey identified the four roles of leadership as modeling (inspiring trust), path finding (creating order), aligning (nourishing vision and empowerment), and empowering (getting others to internally unleash their human potential). Great leaders use their influence to serve others. Box 17.7, Learning, Knowing, and Growing, "Covey's Eight Habits, Adapted for the Nurse," outlines the eight habits identified by Covey (1989, 2004; Covey, 2020) in terms of nursing leadership and enhanced personal and professional growth. Habits represent the integrated principles of the professional nurse while providing consistency in action.

Take Note!
When leaders use effective habits, they earn the trust of their followers.

EVALUATING LEADERSHIP EFFECTIVENESS

As professionals, nurses engage in the process of self-evaluation and look for ways to improve their leadership performance. Unfortunately, not all leaders are effective. Competing demands force leaders (especially managers) to make difficult decisions, which may result in win–lose situations. Ineffective leadership takes many forms, including in the person who assumes a leadership position without proper qualification, the person who bides their time until retirement, and the person who received a leadership appointment because of success in a previous appointment. Frequently, personal insecurities of people in charge result in dysfunctional leadership (Robinson-Walker, 2021). Poor nursing leadership may also occur when the well-respected, competent, professional nurse is forced into accepting a leadership position. The quality of

17.7 Learning, Knowing, and Growing

Covey's Eight Habits, Adapted for the Nurse

1. Be proactive: Nurses need to set a goal and work to achieve it. They commit themselves to the client's perceptions and serve as a model for health, not a critic of those with expressed concerns. They accept their own ability to be "response-able" in dealing with clients' whole human responses to their health concerns. They believe that it is the response to what happens that results in harm and hurt.

2. Begin with the end in mind: The nurse should identify what is really important and try to do what really matters the most every day. The nurse also must differentiate management from leadership. Management, representing the bottom line, focuses on how the nurse can best accomplish certain things with the client, whereas leadership, representing the top line, focuses on what the nurse wants to accomplish. Leadership determines the vision, goals, and direction, and management focuses on the most efficient way to achieve the goals.

3. Put first things first: The formula for the nurse who wants to stay focused on the important business of nursing and expend less energy on the unimportant is to set priorities, organize, and perform. The challenge for the nurse is to manage time in such a way that most of the time is used for urgent activities, such as crises, pressing problems, and deadline-driven projects, as well as the not urgent but important projects, such as health promotion/illness prevention, relationship building, recognizing new opportunities, planning, and recreation.

4. Think win–win or no deal: Interdependence is the most mature goal for any relationship; thus, in professional relationships, interdependence would emphasize mutual benefits. Activities would reflect a commitment to both parties' growth, development, and satisfaction. For example, a client benefits from being empowered by the professional nurse providing informational support, and the nurse benefits by having the interventions validated and the sense of presence with the client valued. When such mutuality is experienced, neither person in the relationship loses or feels powerless.

5. Seek first to understand, then to be understood: Empathy is the habit reflected in this principle. The ability to focus on the client's reality as they experience it is vital to positive communication. (Empathy is discussed in detail in Chapter 18, "Quality Improvement: Enhancing Patient Safety and Health Care Quality"). Credibility problems, such as the client's feeling that "you just don't understand," are prevented to the extent that the nurse empathizes with the client.

6. Value differences and bring all perspectives together: Respect is the characteristic that enables the nurse to develop this habit. (Respect is discussed further in Chapter 15, "Nursing Approaches to Client Systems"). To the extent that the nurse facilitates respect for differing perspectives, the client is likely to feel freer to seek the best possible alternative. If the nurse also experiences respect for their perspectives, synergistic relationships are enhanced. Using the principle of synergy, the nurse and client multiply their individual talents and abilities, and the outcome of their efforts is greater than the sum of the parts.

7. Have a balanced, systematic program for self-renewal: Consistency in having a regularly planned and balanced program for self-renewal prevents weakening of the body, mechanization of the mind, exposure of raw emotions, and desensitization of the spirit. Clearly, nurses' leadership ability is enhanced if they consistently participate in activities that renew four aspects of the self: physical, mental, emotional–social, and moral. Renewal energizes capabilities that are necessary for productive helping relationships in nursing.

8. Find your own voice and inspire others to find theirs: Being truly authentic toward one's personal life mission and helping others find themselves foster the development of new leaders and promote deep satisfaction with life and work. Others quickly detect lack of authenticity in a relationship, especially when nurses establish helping and healing relationships with clients and health team members.

Adapted from Covey, S. R. (2020). *The 7 habits of highly effective people* (30th Anniversary ed.). Simon & Schuster; Covey, S. R. (2004). *The 8th habit.* Free Press.

leadership suffers when the person assuming the leadership position would rather be doing something different. Nurses who know themselves and have a clear idea of their life passions can thwart the influences of others before assuming a leadership position that they do not really want.

Unfortunately, dysfunctional leadership behaviors can be displayed in a variety of ways. Vertical violence occurs when someone in an authority position repeatedly acts aggressively or rudely toward a team or individual. Such behavior may result in inability to complete work, annoyance, emotional trauma, and demoralization. Overt behaviors are openly hostile and easy to observe, whereas covert behaviors occur discreetly and may be difficult to see. Some overt behaviors used by dysfunctional nurse managers include displaying openly disrespectful attitudes, blaming staff or individual nurses for shortcomings, ridiculing others, emphasizing staff weaknesses, and isolating themselves and others. Dysfunctional managers frequently create hostile workplaces characterized by "an aggressive, unproductive, or otherwise oppressive atmosphere that interferes with a person's ability to function at work" (Bond & Birkholz, 2020, p. 50).

When these behaviors occur among peers, horizontal or lateral violence has occurred. Horizontal and lateral violence are forms of bullying defined as "covert or overt acts, actions, or behaviors that are intentionally abusive, demeaning and intimidating, and repeated over a period of at least 6 months which interferes with other staff members' ability to complete their work" (Bond & Birkholz, 2020, p. 50). If a nurse perceives they have been a target of bullying, they need to directly confront the offender using assertive communication. Sometimes, an offender may be unaware of the impact of their behavior. If the offending behavior persists, staff nurses can report repeated instances to the offender's supervisor or human resources department (Bond & Birkholtz, 2020).

Micromanagement is another form of dysfunctional leadership. Leaders who have little trust in their followers may attempt to control every detail of the work being done so they do not allow workers to make decisions. Micromanagers tend to not delegate tasks to others because they feel they are the only people who can perform the work correctly. They also insist on receiving frequent reports and updates. Their failure to delegate and trust others creates an inordinate amount of work for them, so they will frequently complain about how hard they have to work and not having enough time to complete their jobs. They set unrealistically high standards for themselves and others. Instead of looking at the global nature of the work being done, they often find flaws with some insignificant work detail and angrily confront workers about it. Because they perceive knowledge and their expertise as the value they offer, micromanagers may be reluctant to share it with others, perhaps using lack of time as an excuse. Finally, micromanagers typically display no interest in receiving feedback from others; they would rather look for weaknesses in the performance of others (Robinson-Walker, 2021).

Van Velsor et al. (2010) and Robinson-Walker (2021) proposed that people who assume leadership positions should conduct periodic self-evaluations of their performance. They suggest self-reflection and eliciting information from followers to provide a complete, accurate picture of one's leadership. Box 17.8 , Professional Prototypes, "Nursing Leadership Self-Evaluation Criteria," provides pertinent questions to use for nurse leaders to consider in their own **nursing leadership self-evaluation criteria**.

Take Note!
Periodic evaluation of one's leadership provides information for future learning and professional development.

17.8 Professional Prototypes

Nursing Leadership Self-Evaluation Criteria

1. Can I be trusted?
2. Do I use effective verbal and nonverbal communication skills?
3. Am I accessible to the people I serve as a leader?
4. Am I aware of all the issues encountered by nurses engaged in client care activities?
5. Do I provide support to staff when problems arise?
6. Can I initiate, maintain, and terminate effective professional relationships?
7. Do I understand my own impact on others, leading to effective use of myself?
8. Can I effectively modify my behavior and that of others?
9. Do I effectively delegate tasks to others, or do I try to micromanage everything?
10. Do I provide the necessary resources to provide quality nursing services?
11. Do I set high standards and hold others and accountable for them?
12. Do I welcome feedback from others and use this information for professional growth?
13. Am I willing to help others grow as professional nurses?

Data from Van Velsor, E., McCauley, C. D., & Ruderman, M. N. (2014). *The Center for Creative Leadership handbook of leadership development* (3rd ed.). John Wiley & Sons.

Summary and Significance to Practice

Effective nursing leadership is critical in today's complex, chaotic health care environment. Because all professional nurses are leaders, they need to use cognitive and communication skills to empower others to make decisions, facilitate access to care services, share knowledge, coordinate care delivery, plan for the future, use resources judiciously, and facilitate adaptation to change. Effective leaders in nursing display caring, compassion, commitment, confidence, and competence in their roles and periodically conduct self-evaluations to discover additional areas for lifelong learning.

REAL-LIFE REFLECTIONS

Recall Elena from earlier in the chapter. Which of the leadership theories would be most useful to Elena as she leads the group of parent volunteers to determine how to get an RN in every school? Why do you think your selected theory would work best? What are the potential outcomes of having an RN in every school for students, faculty, school administration, the local school board, and school district taxpayers? What obstacles do you think Elena and the task force might encounter in achieving the goal of a nurse in every school?

From Theory to Practice

1. How do you rate your effectiveness as a nurse leader? What are your strengths? Your weaknesses?
2. What are your opportunities for future growth as a leader? Outline an action plan to facilitate your growth as a nursing leader.

Nurse as Author

Think about the best leader/manager/teacher/coach you have encountered in your working career or as a student. Think about the worst leader/manager/teacher/coach you have encountered in your working career or as a student. Write a two- to three-page essay comparing the traits and practices of these two people. In one paragraph, include each person's strengths and weaknesses.

In another paragraph, specify what you learned from each. Do not identify either person by name. In your concluding paragraph, specify what you plan to do in a future leadership role based on your experiences with both people.

Your Digital Classroom

Online Exploration

American Academy of Nursing: **www.aannet.org**

American Organization for Nursing Leadership: **https://www.aonl.org/**

American Nurses Association: **https://www.nursingworld.org/ana/**

Changing Minds—Transformational Leadership: **http://changingminds.org/disciplines/leadership/styles/transformational_leadership.htm**

Center for Servant Leadership: **https://www.greenleaf.org/**

Sigma Theta Tau International: **https://www.sigmanursing.org/**

The Centre for Innovative Leadership: **http://cil.net/**

Expanding Your Understanding

Visit the Sigma Theta Tau International website and view the following microlearning presentations located in the "Find Your Forward: Resources for Advocacy and Resilience" section.

1. Watch "Leadership Resilience" at **https://nursingcentered.sigmanursing.org/find-your-forward/view/leading-through-crisis**. After watching the video, download Dr. Love's "Resilience Plan." For each of the 10 suggestions, generate a list of two to three action items.
2. Watch "The Fragility of Our Trust in Our Workplace: Easily Broken Necessary to Repair" at **https://nursingcentered.sigmanursing.org/find-your-forward/view/re-establishing-trust**. Download and read Ann Bandar's "How to Establish Trust." What are your initial thoughts on this presentation? Do you agree or disagree with her perceptions of trust? Why or why not?

Beyond the Book

Visit the Point® at **www.thePoint.lww.com** for activities and information to reinforce the concepts and content covered in this chapter.

REFERENCES

Anderson, T. (1998). *Transforming leadership* (2nd ed.). St. Lucie Press.

Bandman, E. L., & Bandman, B. (1995). *Nursing ethics through the life span* (3rd ed.). Appleton & Lange.

Barrett, R. (1998). *Liberating the corporate soul: Building a visionary organization.* Butterworth-Heinemann.

Bass, B., & Riggio, R. (2005). *Transformational leadership* (2nd ed.). Erlbaum.

Bennis, W. (1989). *Why leaders can't lead: The unconscious conspiracy continues.* Jossey-Bass.

Bennis, W., & Nanus, B. (1985). *Leaders: The strategies for taking charge.* Harper & Row.

Blake, R., & Morton, J. (1964). *The managerial grid: Key orientations for achieving production through people.* Gulf Publishing.

Blanchard, K., Carlos, J. P., & Randolph, A. (1996). *Empowerment takes more than a minute.* Berrett-Koehler.

Bond, M. F., & Birkholz, L. J. (2020). What if the bully is the manager? *Nursing, 5*(3), 48–52. https://doi.org/10.1097/01.NURSE.0000654048.73369.b8

Bondas, T. (2006). Paths to nursing leadership. *Journal of Nursing Management, 14*(5), 332–339. https://doi.org/10.1111/j.1365-2934.2006.00620.x

Bridges, W. (2003). *Managing transitions* (2nd ed.). Perseus.

Bridges, W., & Bridges, S. (2019). *Transitions: Making sense of life changes* (40th Anniversary Ed.). *Lifelong Books* and Perseus.

Brook, D. P. (2020). *The Spanish Influenza, the deadliest pandemic. A lesson from history 102 years after 1918. The FLU epidemic in the world and critical moments. Origin, symptoms, outbreak, spread and contagion.* Damina P. Brook.

Burns, J. (1978). *Leadership.* Harper & Row.

Burns, J. (2003). *Transformational leadership.* Grove/Atlantic.

Carnall, C. A. (1990). *Managing change in organizations.* Prentice Hall.

Chin, R. (1976). The utility of systems models and developmental models for practitioners. In W. G. Bennis, K. D. Benne, & R. Chin (Eds.), *The planning of change* (3rd ed., pp. 90-122). Holt, Rinehart & Winston.

Cianelli, R., Clipper, B., Freeman, R., Goldstein, J., & Wyatt, T. (2016). *The innovation roadmap: A guide for nurse leaders.* Retrieved November 24, 2020, from www.nursing world.org/globalassets/innovations-roadmap-english.pdf.

Covey, S. R. (1989). *The 7 habits of highly effective people.* Simon & Schuster.

Covey, S. R. (1996). *Three roles of the leader in the new paradigm.* In F. Hesselbein, M. Goldsmith, & R. Beckhard (Eds.), *The leader of the future: New visions, strategies, and practices for the next era* (pp. 149–160). Jossey-Bass.

Covey, S. R. (2004). *The 8th habit.* Free Press.

Covey, S. R. (2020). *The 7 habits of highly effective people, (30*th Anniversary ed.). Simon & Schuster.

Dent, B. (2015). Nine principles for improved nurse staffing. *Nursing Economics, 35*(1), 44–44, 66. Retrieved April 23, 2021, from https://pubmed.ncbi.nlm.nih.gov/26214937/

DiSilvio, B., Virani, A., Patel, S., Finoli, L., Singh, A., DuMont, T., & Cheema, T. (2020). Institutional COVID-19 protocols: Focused on preparation, safety, and care consolidation. *Critical Care Nursing Quarterly, 43,* 413–427. https://doi.org/10.1097/CNQ.0000000000000327.

Donnelly, G. (2003). *Why leadership is important to nursing.* In T. Stelzer (Ed.), *Five keys to successful nursing management* (pp. 31–60). Lippincott Williams & Wilkins.

Dotlich, D., Noel, J., & Walker, N. (2004). *Leadership passages.* Jossey-Bass.

Douglass, L. M. (1988). *The effective nurse: Leader and manager* (3rd ed.). Mosby.

Eichinger, R. W., & Lombardo, M. M. (2004). *The leadership machine: Architecture to develop leaders for any future.* Lominger Ltd., Inc.

Fiedler, F. (1967). *A theory of leadership effectiveness.* McGraw-Hill.

George, B. (2003). *Authentic leadership.* Jossey-Bass.

Greenleaf, R. (1977). *Servant leadership: A journey into the nature of legitimate power and greatness.* Paulist Press.

Gurka, A. M. (1995). Transformational leadership: Qualities and strategies for the CNS. *Clinical Nurse Specialist, 9,* 169–174. Retrieved April 23, 2021, from https://journals.lww.com/cns-journal/Abstract/1995/05000/Transformational_Leadership__Qualities_and.15.aspx

Haffer, A. (1986). Facilitating change: Choosing the appropriate strategy. *Journal of Nursing Administration, 16,* 17–22. Retrieved April 23, 2021, from https://journals.lww.com/jonajournal/Abstract/1986/04000/Facilitating_Change__Choosing_the_Appropriate.5.aspx

Hagberg, J. (1994). *Real power: Stages of personal power in organizations* (2nd ed.). Sheffield.

Hames, C. C., & Joseph, D. H. (1980). *Basic concepts of helping: A holistic approach.* Appleton-Century-Crofts.

Harrison, J. P. (2021). *Essentials of strategic planning in healthcare* (3rd ed.). Health Administration Press.

Henriksen, K., Keyes, M., Steens, D., & Clancy, C. (2006). Initiating transformational change to enhance patient safety. *Journal of Patient Safety, 2*(19), 20–24. Retrieved April 23, 2021, from https://journals.lww.com/journalpatientsafety/Abstract/2006/03000/Initiating_Transformational_Change_to_Enhance.4.aspx

Hershey, P., & Blanchard, K. (1977). *Management of organizational behavior: Leading human resources* (3rd ed.). Prentice Hall.

House, R., & Mitchell, T. (1974). Path–goal theory of leadership. *Journal of Contemporary Business, 3,* 81–97. Retrieved April 23, 2021, from https://www.scirp.org/(S(czeh2tfqyw2orz553k1w0r45))/reference/ReferencesPapers.aspx?ReferenceID=2233851

Hunt, P. (2003). *Marketing your facility.* In T. Stelzer (Ed.), *Five keys to successful nursing management* (pp. 276–286). Lippincott Williams & Wilkins.

King, E. C. (1984). *Affective education in nursing.* Aspen Systems.

Kouzes, J., & Posner, B. (2011). *The five practices of exemplary leadership.* Pfeiffer.

Kouzes, J., & Posner, B. (2017). *The leadership challenge* (6th ed.). Jossey-Bass.

Lofland, J., & Lofland, L. H. (1995). *Analyzing social setting a guide to qualitative observation and analysis* (3rd ed.). Wadsworth Publishing.

Marquis, B., & Huston, C. (2021). *Leadership roles and management functions in nursing: Theory and application* (10th ed.). Wolters Kluwer.

McGregor, D. (1960). *The human side of enterprise.* McGraw-Hill.

Mish, F. C. (Ed.). (2020). *Merriam-Webster's collegiate dictionary* (11th ed.). Merriam-Webster, Inc.

Noddings, N. (1984). *Caring: A feminine approach to ethics and moral education.* University of California Press.

Nursing Solutions Inc. (2021). *2021 NSI National Health Care Retention & RN Staffing Report.* Retrieved May 29, 2021, from https://www.nsinursingsolutions.com/Documents/Library/NSI_National_Health_Care_Retention_Report.pdf

Ouchi, W. (1981). *Theory Z: How American business can meet the Japanese challenge.* Addison-Wesley-Longman.

Perlman, D., & Takacs, G. J. (1990). The 10 stages of change. *Nursing Management, 21,* 33–38. Retrieved April 23, 2021, from https://journals.lww.com/nursingmanagement/Citation/1990/04000/The_10_Stages_of_Change__To_cope_with_change.10.aspx

Porter-O'Grady, T., & Malloch, K. (2018). *Quantum leadership: Building better partnerships for sustainable health* (5th ed.). Jones/Bartlett Learning.

Pritchett, R., & Pound, R. (1995). *A survival guide to the stress of organizational change.* Pritchett & Associates.

Ramirez, B., Oetjen, R., & Malvey, D. (2011). Sustainability and the health care manager. *The Health Care Manager, 30*(2), 13–138. https://doi.org/10.1097.HCM.0b013e317216f4e5

Richardson, P. (1992). Hospital practices that erode nursing power by promoting job dissatisfaction. *Revolution: The Journal of Nurse Empowerment, 2,* 34–39. Retrieved April 23, 2021, from https://greatnurses.com/wp-content/uploads/2020/03/spring-1992-5.pdf

Robinson-Walker, C. (2021). *Leading with mastery and heart, the coaching companion for thriving nurses leaders.* Elsevier.

Rundio, A. (2016). *The nurse manager's guide to budgeting and finance* (2nd ed.). Sigma Theta Tau International.

Shaffer, J. (2020). From surge plans to a culture of readiness. *American Nurse Today, 15*(11), 6–13. Retrieved April 23, 2021, from https://www.myamericannurse.com/from-surge-plans-to-a-culture-of-readiness/

Shirey, M. (2012). Group think, organizational strategy and change. *Journal of Nursing Administration, 42*(2), 67–71. https://doi.org/10.1097/NNA.0b013e3172433510

Snowball, J. (1996). Asking nurses about advocating for patients: "Reactive" and "proactive" accounts. *Journal of Advanced Nursing, 24,* 67–75. https://doi.org/10.1046/j.1365-2648.1996.01719.x

Taylor, S. G., Pickens, J. M., & Geden, E. A. (1989). Interactional styles of nurse practitioners and physicians regarding patient decision making. *Nursing Research, 38,* 50–55. doi: 10.1097/00006199-198901000-00011

U.S. Army. (2004). *Be-know-do: Leadership the Army way.* Jossey-Bass.

Van Velsor, E., McCauley, C. D., & Ruderman, M. N. (2010). *The Center for Creative Leadership handbook of leadership development* (3rd ed.). John Wiley & Sons.

Videbeck, S. (2008). *Psychiatric-mental health nursing* (4th ed.). Wolters Kluwer Health/Lippincott Williams & Wilkins.

Vroom, V., & Yetton, P. (1973). *Leadership and decision making.* University of Pittsburgh Press.

Wesorick, B., & Shiparski, L. (1997). *Can the human being thrive in the workplace? Dialogue as a strategy of hope.* Practice Field Publishing.

White, R., & Lippitt, R. (1960). *Autocracy and democracy: An experimental inquiry.* Harper & Row.

Wilson, C. K., & Porter-O'Grady, T. (1999). *Leading the revolution in health care* (2nd ed.). Aspen.

Wooten, K. C., & White, L. P. (1989). Toward a theory of change role efficacy. *Human Relations, 42,* 651–669. https://doi.org/10.1177/001872678904200801

Quality Improvement: Enhancing Patient Safety and Health Care Quality

LEARNING OUTCOMES

By the end of this chapter, the learner will be able to:

1. Define the term "quality."
2. Outline the history and evolution of quality improvement in health care.
3. Compare and contrast the four different types of medical care errors that may occur during health care delivery.
4. Compare and contrast quality assurance, quality control, total quality management, and continuous quality improvement.
5. Explain the plan, do, check, act (PDCA) cycle used in quality improvement programs.
6. Identify internal and external customers in health care settings.
7. Explain Six Sigma and how it could be used to improve health care quality.
8. Describe the process of benchmarking.
9. Specify core measures and nursing-sensitive outcomes for client care delivery.
10. Outline the professional nurse's roles in quality improvement.
11. Explain how recent quality and safety initiatives improve the quality of health care services.

REAL-LIFE REFLECTIONS

Laura is a nurse working on a busy cardiac care unit. During a half-hour time frame this evening, she has admitted two people with chest pain and transferred another of her assigned clients to the intensive care unit. Upon returning to the unit, Laura notices that one of her other clients did not receive ordered medications per the scheduled time. Laura missed giving an ordered antibiotic on time by 2 hours. She notifies the attending physician who yells at her. Laura completes an incident report. Because she is new to the unit, Laura wonders how the nurse manager and her colleagues will react to her mistake.

■ QUESTIONS FOR REFLECTION

1. How does the organization in which you practice nursing handle medication errors? How does your nursing program handle medication and other care errors made by students?

2. What steps could you take to prevent the medication error Laura made?

3. Are you afraid to complete incident reports? Why or why not?

4. Who is at fault when a nurse makes an error?

Swanwick and Vaux (2020, p. 1) define **quality** generally as "the degree of excellence of something"—basically how good or bad something is. Quality in health care can mean different things depending on individual perspectives:

■ The Institute of Medicine (IOM) considers **quality health care** to be safe, timely, efficient, equitable, effective, and client-centered (IOM, 2001, 2011).

■ Consumers look for caring providers, timely services, technical competence, error-free care, accurate bills, and improved health status as indicators of quality.

■ Nurses consider nurse–client ratios, adequate time spent with clients, availability of supplies, quality of ancillary staff, easy access to resources for procedures, and educational information and assistance to be quality indicators (IOM, 2011).

Take Note!
The hallmarks of quality health care are safety, timeliness, efficiency, equitability, effectiveness, and client-centeredness.

Most health care consumers assume health care providers and organizations will keep them safe. However, according to a 2016 study from Johns Hopkins University, safety experts have estimated that more than 250,000 Americans died as a result of medical care errors in 2013. Thus, medical care errors across care settings have become the third highest cause of death in the United States (Makary & Daniel, 2016). A literature review conducted by James (2013) suggested that the number of Americans dying as a result of medical care errors could be as high as 440,000. Currently, the reporting of care errors is voluntary, and there is no centralized system for tracking them in the United States (Duffour, 2019). Deaths from medical errors, however, are extremely

hard to track as they do not appear on death certificates as the cause of death. Manufacturing companies and the travel industry would likely be out of business if they had as many errors as those that occur in the health care arena.

Medical care errors are unintentional. Outcomes of medical care errors may be no adversity, reversible problems, temporary or permanent disability, and even death. When care interventions are either overlooked or not performed, an **error of omission** has occurred. For example, the prescribing provider forgot to order a medication from the standardized guidelines for disease management or a nurse overlooked delivering a treatment. **Errors of commission** happen when the provider performs the right action but does so improperly (James, 2013; Makary & Daniels, 2016). For example, a surgeon may nick the colon when removing an ovary, causing the client to develop an infection or a nurse breaks aseptic technique when inserting an indwelling catheter causing a urinary tract infection leading to urosepsis. Equipment failures fall into this classification of medical care errors. **Errors of communication** occur when there is miscommunication between and among health care team members or between the client and health team members. **Diagnostic errors** happen when there is a misdiagnosis or a delayed diagnosis resulting in a prolonged problem (James, 2013; Makary & Daniels, 2016). For example, because a person with severe respiratory symptoms tests negative for COVID-19, the health care provider may treat the client for pneumonia. However, if the test provided a false negative, the person could spread COVID-19 throughout the community. **Contextual errors** occur when members of the health care team fail to identify unique situations in the life of a client that might hamper proper follow-up care and treatment (James, 2013). For example, an older adult is discharged from the hospital into the care of a partner, but both have impaired cognitive skills.

Hospital nurses today care for more acutely ill clients than in the past, requiring nurses to be able to change their thinking rapidly, keep a mental list of multiple tasks to accomplish, document all care activities, and supervise unlicensed care providers. According to McMullen and colleagues (2017), nurses tend to make more errors of omission than other forms of errors. The following "Focus on Research" box, "Examining Nurse Errors of Omission," identifies the most commonly made errors by nurses working in acute care settings.

FOCUS ON RESEARCH

Examining Nurse Errors of Omission

The investigators replicated a study conducted in 2009 that examined the types and reasons for errors of omission that occurred in acute care practice. The purpose of this study was to answer the following questions:

1. What are the types and amounts of missed nursing care?
2. What are the reasons for missed care?
3. Do the type and amount of missed care vary by the demographic characteristics of the nurse?
4. Do the reasons for missed care vary by the demographic characteristics of the nurse? (p. 9)

Using a cross-sectional, descriptive research design and convenience sampling of full-time registered nurses (RNs), licensed practical nurses (LPNs), and unlicensed assistive personnel (UAP), data were collected using an email survey that consisted of demographic information and the administration of the MISCARE survey. Data were collected from three hospitals, and nurses at two of the hospitals had the option of completing the survey anonymously in paper format returned to a locked drop box. The MISCARE survey contains 22 items about specific nursing care tasks and 16 items regarding reasons for missed care tasks.

Participants included 537 nursing staff members who completed the survey (65% RNs), They worked on a variety of units (medical–surgical, critical care, emergency department, and obstetrics). Most of the respondents identified as females (92%), ages were primarily 25 to 52 years (71%), and 28% of the respondents had more than 10 years of experience in their current units. Of the respondents, 450 reported working more than 30 hours per week with 137 working 12-hour shifts and 89 working 8.5-hour rotating shifts.

A factor analysis of the MISCARE revealed three main areas of missed care: assessment, interventions, and planning. Three main areas for missed care were also identified—communication, material resources, and labor resources. The most frequently missed care items identified were bedside glucose monitoring, client assessment, and handwashing. Of the nurses, 93% reported missing one intervention. However, setting up clients for meals who were able to feed themselves was the most frequently missed intervention (54%). Of the respondents, 82% reported missing at least one planning activity, and the most frequently missed one was discharge planning and teaching (74%).

Lack of labor resources was the top reason identified for missed care, followed by lack of material resources and communication tied for second place. The only demographics identified as resulting in increased incidences of missed care were education and job title. Missed care was in the area of planning, and nurses with higher levels of education and positions with more responsibility reported missed care more frequently. No statistically significant differences were found among the demographic variables and reasons for missed care.

The investigators identified inclusion of UAP who do not have responsibility for developing care plans and educating clients as limitations. The self-report nature of the survey with no opportunity to clarify was also identified as an issue. A number of nurses not included in the sample only completed the demographic information section of the emailed survey, which may mean they might have felt uncomfortable reporting missed care.

The investigators concluded that adequate staffing, good communication, effective teamwork, and strong leadership with accountability are ways to reduce missed care. The findings of this study are in line with studies conducted over a decade ago. They proposed that additional studies should be completed by administering different surveys to RNs, LPNs, and UAPs, examining the relationship of short staffing, teamwork, and leadership quality on missed care as well as exploring possible interventions for preventing missed care.

The clinical significance of this study reveals that working short-staffed, ineffective communication, and lack of material resources for care completion have been associated with missed care for decades. Frequently, nurses have to deliver safe, effective nursing care without the necessary equipment and personnel needed to avoid care errors. More research should be conducted about the role of computer-generated care reminders and quality of the work environment on the number of errors of omission.

From McMullen, S. L., Kozik, C. A., Meyers, G., Keenan, K., Wheelock, M., & Kalman, M. (2017). CNE SERIES. Improving nursing care: Examining errors of omission. *MEDSURG Nursing*, *26*(1), 9–19. Retrieved May 1, 2021, from https://www.thefreelibrary.com/Improving+nursing+care%3a+examining+errors+of+omission.-a0482392057/

There are multiple reasons why nurses commit errors. When recent research findings are compared with findings from many years ago, inadequate staffing, miscommunication, lack of necessary equipment and supplies, ineffective teamwork, and complex work processes remain key precipitating factors (American Nurses Association [ANA], 2013; Kalisch & Lee, 2010; Kalisch & Williams, 2009; McMullen et al., 2017; Porter-O'Grady & Malloch, 2018; Schroers, 2021). Other nurse factors associated with errors include fatigue and rotating shift work (Gander et al., 2020; Scott et al., 2010).

Take Note!

Because nurses work in environments where errors may frequently and quickly occur, they must be totally engaged when providing care to health care consumers.

▌ QUESTIONS FOR REFLECTION

1. As a consumer, what do you consider elements of quality care when you receive health care services? Why are these important?

2. As a professional nurse, what do you consider the elements of quality care? Why are they important?

3. How well do your lists of quality care match?

HISTORY OF CONTINUOUS QUALITY IMPROVEMENT IN HEALTH CARE

Quality management became popular in business and industry after American manufacturers lost market share to Japanese competitors in the late 1970s (Ouchi, 1981). As American businesses began incorporating quality management principles in the 1980s, they noticed improved sales. American workers also became involved in shaping work processes and a new sense of pride emerged. In 1980s, the American automobile industry lost market share as American consumers noted better quality in Japanese-made vehicles. American car companies adopted quality management techniques to improve the quality of American-built vehicles. The Japanese management techniques involve direct participation of workers doing the work. In health care, adoption of these techniques resulted in the direct participation of nurses in the development of and decisions about direct client care work processes. At the same time, the Rand Corporation conducted a health insurance experiment with the aim of identifying plausible ways to improve health delivery processes

and care outcomes. The results of the experiment proposed that if health care organizations would adopt a total quality improvement approach, the quality of American health care would improve (Sollecito & Johnson, 2020). However, efforts at improving health care had been occurring since the 19th century.

Florence Nightingale can be considered the first nurse who engaged in **continuous quality improvement** (QI) activities. During the Crimean War, Nightingale's work at the Barrack Hospital demonstrated the effects of quality nursing care on wounded and frail soldiers. The mortality rate at the Barrack Hospital was 60% when Nightingale arrived. By the time she departed, it had fallen to just a fraction over 1%. Nightingale kept detailed records that included statistics about the effects of cleanliness, good nutrition, and fresh air on the survival of the soldiers (Kalisch & Kalisch, 2004). Her diligent attention to detailed records and continuous analysis of the data provided evidence that nursing care could reduce mortality. In 1855, Nightingale's interventions resulted in a reduction of mortality from 33% in January through March to just 2% by July through September of the same year (Gill & Gill, 2005).

In 1913, a group of surgeons concerned about the quality of care in American hospitals formed the American College of Surgeons. By 1918, their work led to the implementation of the Hospital Standardization Program (HSP), which evolved into an accreditation process for hospitals. The HSP developed minimum standards for physician credentialing, hospital privileges, and methods to evaluate physician care and medical equipment. To create a standardized system for record keeping, the HSP established the first known standards for health care recipient medical records. Along with developing standards, hospitals engaging in HSP conducted mortality and morbidity conferences to see what hospital-associated factors contributed to death and permanent disability. By the 1920s, tumor registries became a standard of practice so that more data regarding cancer could be collected and recorded (Sollecito & Johnson, 2020).

The Evolution of The Joint Commission and Hospital Accreditation

In 1951, the HSP evolved into The Joint Commission on Accreditation of Hospitals (JCAH), a private, nonprofit, voluntary agency that ascertained that a hospital met American College of Surgeons standards. Concerned about the quality of care received by subscribers during hospitalizations, the insurer Blue Cross required that participating hospitals be accredited by the JCAH by the early 1970s. Eventually, JCAH accreditation became a way for hospitals to prove they met quality care requirements to receive Medicare program payments. By the mid-1970s, JCAH accreditation automatically guaranteed Medicare reimbursement (the other option for hospitals was to design their own system for meeting all Medicare program quality of care requirements) (Sultz & Young, 2004; The Joint Commission [TJC], 2013c).

Hospitals began to develop health care systems that also included primary care services for consumers in the mid-1980s. Accreditation by JCAH meant that each health care–providing organization demonstrated effective, high-quality services. JCAH accreditation became a requirement for many health care organizations to qualify for insurance company reimbursement (Sultz & Young, 2004). In addition to ensuring health care quality, Joint Commission on Accreditation of Healthcare Organizations (JCAHO) accreditation standards addressed efficacy of health care interventions and appropriateness of services delivered. Aspects for quality services include (Sultz & Young, 2004; TJC, 2013c):

- Availability of the necessary health care intervention
- Timeliness of services
- Effectiveness of health care interventions
- Continuity of health care services across various health care settings
- Safety of clients and others
- Efficiencies of provided care and services
- Respect given to consumers and caring with which services are rendered

In 2003, JCAHO recognized the impact of nursing care on client quality outcomes and established a Nursing Advisory Council to address evolving nursing and client care issues (TJC, 2013d). Today, the Nursing Advisory Council has nursing organization, chief nursing officer, staff nurse, magnet hospital, research, academic, and nurse leader representation (TJC, 2016). The Joint Commission collaborates with the American Nurses Association and has posted ANA materials related to workplace violence on its website.

JCAHO, known as **The Joint Commission** (TJC) since 2007, accredits approximately 21,000 health care organizations that include general, pediatric, long-term, acute, rehabilitation, and specialty hospitals, home health agencies, laboratories, and extended-care and outpatient facilities. TJC uses standards, performance outcomes, and consumer perceptions of rendered services as criteria for accreditation. When an organization has earned accreditation from TJC, it means it has met all standards and requirements for delivering high-quality care. By meeting these requirements, health care organizations are eligible to be reimbursed for rendered services under federal, state, and private insurance plans (TJC, 2020f). In 2006, the World Health Organization (WHO) acknowledged TJC's contributions to ensuring quality health services, and today, Joint Commission International (JCI) accredits health care organizations in more than 100 countries. JCI works internationally with health care organizations to "promote rigorous standards of care and provide solutions for achieving peak performance" (2020a, para. 2). In honor of World Patient Safety Day, JCI published a digital book entitled *Health Care Safety Worker Checklists: Protecting Those Who Serve*. The book covers all potential hazards encountered by health care workers and provides governmental standards–based checklists for demonstrating effective staff education and competencies (JCI, 2020b).

In 1997, TJC launched an initiative called ORYX to provide comparative outcomes and other performance measures into the accreditation process. The system was named ORYX®. TJC works with the Centers for Medicaid and Medicare Services (CMS) to align measures as closely as possible to CMS requirements. ORYX reports data charts that are submitted to them by accredited facilities. Facility reporting requirements depend on the size and type of health care organization as well as the number of client encounters. Organizations can submit required data electronically and directly to TJC using TJC's direct data submission platform, a requirement starting in 2021. Electronic clinical quality measures must be submitted on an annual basis (TJC, 2020c). Along with these measures, accredited agencies must submit data related to sentinel events (care errors resulting in either death, permanent disability, or temporary harm requiring immediate monitoring or intervention to save a life or preserve function); actual errors; near-miss events (errors that could have occurred, but someone intervened and prevented them); hospital readmission rates; and nosocomial infection rates. The data are compiled and compared with other TJC-accredited facilities and then presented on TJC's quality check website (TJC, 2020d). TJC awards a gold star seal to health care organizations that display outstanding services and quality improvement efforts. The Gold Star Seal of Approval designation means the organization has a deep commitment to and emphasis on quality of care. Consumers can visit the website and type in their location or zip code to help determine where they want to receive hospital care in nonemergent situations (e.g., scheduled procedure or surgery). The website lists facility accreditation status, TJC certification of specialties, and TJC certification of advanced certifications (TJC, 2020d).

TJC and the CMS set annual National Patient Safety Goals aimed at preventing errors that compromise client safety in hospitals, home care agencies, outpatient facilities, and laboratories (see Box 18.1, Professional Prototypes, "The Joint Commission's 2021 Critical Access Hospital National Patient Safety Goals"). TJC's 2021 National Patient Safety Goals for hospital programs included improving accuracy of client identification, effective communication among caregivers, safety of medication usage, identification of safety risks with specific client populations (e.g., risk for suicide and surgical errors); reducing client harm from clinical alarm systems; and reducing the risk of health care–associated infections (TJC, 2020b). The annual safety goals are broadly written. For most of the goals, TJC outlines elements of performance that typically include client and health provider education along with a series of critical steps to follow. For example, 13 performance elements are identified before an invasive procedure is performed. TJC accreditation process requires that health care organizations compile data on the safety goals, communicate findings to staff, and develop plans to address each of the safety goals (TJC, 2020b).

Along with the development of National Patient Safety Goals, TJC has collaborated with CMS since 2003 to align specific core measures for the management of disease processes. CMS and TJC work in collaboration with physician specialty organizations to develop the core measures for performance. In 2020, core measures for performance were available for cardiac care, emergency department care, health care staffing services, inpatient psychiatric care, immunization, palliative care, perinatal care, stroke, substance use, tobacco treatment, total knee and hip replacement, and venous thromboembolism (TJC, 2020a). For professional nurses, this typically means that there will be a checklist outlining a series of required actions that must be documented so that the data from the client electronic health record can be uploaded to TJC's direct data submission platform.

CMS reimburses health care organizations on how well each performance core measure has been met, thereby creating accountable care organizations (ACOs). ACOs are voluntary-provider partnerships that integrate and align providers to provide coordinated care services to a specifically defined group of clients (e.g., older adults with congestive heart failure). CMS pays organizations with higher levels of performance more and has established a competitive reimbursement structure in which the best performers attain the highest reimbursement. ACOs deliver the right care at the right time, avoid duplication of services, and focus on error prevention while constantly looking for ways to improve the quality of health care delivered to the defined client group. In the future, measurement related to client engagement in the health care delivery process is expected to become part of the core performance measures for ACOs (Joyner & Kreitzer, 2021). TJC (2020a) identifies accountability measures as quality measures that meet the following four criteria:

1. Research: Performance of evidence-based care processes that have been supported by research to influence desired client outcomes
2. Proximity: Performance of direct care process most closely linked to a desired outcome
3. Accuracy: Correctly measuring the care process associated with a positive outcome
4. Adverse effects: Implementation of a measure is unlikely to produce undesired, negative outcomes

TJC uses these measures for evaluating organizations for accreditation, reporting comparative results of organizations, and determining pay-for-performance (TJC, 2020a). Accountability measures form the basis for continuous quality improvement processes for many hospitals.

Quality Assurance Programs

Quality assurance programs became part of the hospital accreditation process in the 1970s. **Quality assurance** (QA) is defined as a "planned, systematic process of gathering evidence to provide confidence that a system is meeting internal or external standards" (Swanwick & Vaux, 2020, p. 2). The process involves evidence collection retrospectively or after health care is delivered. In contrast, **quality control** is an internal process that compares performance levels of a system against internal standards or benchmarks (predetermined performance goals). People who are closest to and responsible for work implementation should continuously assess the quality of work processes and outcomes (Swanwick & Vaux, 2020).

TJC standards require that health care organizations (especially hospitals) regularly review the

18.1 Professional Prototypes

The Joint Commission's 2021 Critical Access Hospital National Patient Safety Goals

2021 Critical Access Hospital National Patient Safety Goals

The purpose of the National Patient Safety Goals is to improve patient safety. The goals focus on problems in health care safety and how to solve them.

Identify patients correctly

NPSG.01.01.01 — Use at least two ways to identify patients. For example, use the patient's name *and* date of birth. This is done to make sure that each patient gets the correct medicine and treatment.

Improve staff communication

NPSG.02.03.01 — Get important test results to the right staff person on time.

Use medicines safely

NPSG.03.04.01 — Before a procedure, label medicines that are not labeled. For example, medicines in syringes, cups and basins. Do this in the area where medicines and supplies are set up.

NPSG.03.05.01 — Take extra care with patients who take medicines to thin their blood.

NPSG.03.06.01 — Record and pass along correct information about a patient's medicines. Find out what medicines the patient is taking. Compare those medicines to new medicines given to the patient. Give the patient written information about the medicines they need to take. Tell the patient it is important to bring their up-to-date list of medicines every time they visit a doctor.

Use alarms safely

NPSG.06.01.01 — Make improvements to ensure that alarms on medical equipment are heard and responded to on time.

Prevent infection

NPSG.07.01.01 — Use the hand cleaning guidelines from the Centers for Disease Control and Prevention or the World Health Organization. Set goals for improving hand cleaning. Use the goals to improve hand cleaning.

Identify patient safety risks

NPSG.15.01.01 — Reduce the risk for suicide.

Prevent mistakes in surgery

UP.01.01.01 — Make sure that the correct surgery is done on the correct patient and at the correct place on the patient's body.

UP.01.02.01 — Mark the correct place on the patient's body where the surgery is to be done.

UP.01.03.01 — Pause before the surgery to make sure that a mistake is not being made.

This is an easy-to-read document. It has been created for the public. The exact language of the goals can be found at www.jointcommission.org.

From The Joint Commission. (2021). *Critical access hospital national patient safety goals.* https://www.jointcommission.org/-/media/tjc/documents/standards/national-patient-safety-goals/2021/simplified-2021-cah-npsg-goals-final-11420.pdf. Reprinted with permission.

following data as part of their QA programs: mortality rates by department or service; hospital-acquired infections; client falls; adverse drug reactions; unplanned returns to surgery; and hospital-incurred trauma (TJC, 2020a). QA programs examine client outcomes retrospectively. QA also includes planning operational and strategic plans for an organization to compare past performance with current performance including communication of standards, identifying key indicators for mentoring compliance to standards as well, and assessing compliance to standards. Because of its punitive nature toward individual health care providers and reactive approach to errors, QA has been losing popularity (Joshi et al., 2014).

Total Quality Management and Continuous Quality Improvement

The terms "total quality management" and "continuous quality improvement" (CQI) are sometimes used synonymously in the business and health care–related literature. Both outline structures and processes for improving health care delivery. However, **total quality management** (TQM) uses fundamentals based on scientific management emphasizing fact-based management and management becoming the master of facts by collecting information. After seeking employee input into work processes, methods, and decisions for improvements, management assumes responsibility for making the final decision for determining which work processes and methods to implement. Management also consistently implements work processes and methods so that variance is reduced. Variance in work processes and methods are linked to inferior quality of products and service delivery (Sollecito & Johnson, 2020). Unlike QA programs, the evidence for improvements is collected prospectively, and an improvement cycle is followed after a change has been instituted. For example, a plan is developed, the change is executed, the effects of the change are measured, and if the change is successful, it becomes a standard practice. If the change is not successful, the cycle repeats itself. In TQM, the organization constantly strives to improve work processes, outcomes, and products.

CQI evolved from TQM when managers embraced the human relations approach to management. The human relations management perspective recognizes the importance of people and the abilities they bring to the organization. An early but relevant and accurate definition of CQI in health care is "the combined efforts of everyone—health care professionals, patients and their families, and researchers. Planners and educators make changes that will lead to better patient outcomes (health), better system performance (care), and professional development (learning)" (Batalden & Davidoff, 2007, p. 2).

Sollecito and Johnson (2020) identify the eight characteristics of CQI. Because CQI has a visionary and strategic focus, there is a link to the organization's strategic plan. To promote the involvement of all engaged in a process for organizational improvement, the facility creates a quality council consisting of members of the organization's top management team. The quality council creates structures and processes that include formal training for personnel, mechanisms for selecting which improvement opportunities will be addressed, formation of specific process improvement teams, and personnel policies to support and motivate employees' active participation in process improvement efforts. CQI also uses the most current and rigorous methods for evaluating evidence and substantiating results. This includes advanced statistical techniques and complex statistical process controls.

CQI tackles four types of institutional improvements, which may be discrete or may blend with each other. The first is localized improvement efforts in which an ad hoc team is created to examine a specific process problem or opportunity (e.g., the need to revise approaches to client pain control because of low rankings on a follow-up survey). Second, organizational learning occurs when the QI process is finalized and policies and procedures are developed and implemented (e.g., development of evidence-based and new clinical pathways resulting from new research findings). Process reengineering, the third type, occurs when the organization makes a major investment, blending internal and external resources (e.g., urgent care visits conducted via telehealth) that result in radically different organizational processes. Finally, evidence-based practice and management involve integration of best health and management practices determined by comprehensive professional literature analyses, evidence generated by internal organizational experiences, and accreditation requirements (Sollecito & Johnson, 2020; Swanwick & Vaux, 2020).

Organizations participate in CQI for many reasons, including meeting accreditation requirements, facilitating cost control, competing for customers, and responding to pressures from third-party payers (i.e., insurance providers). CQI is a management method that promotes effective leadership and management. Sollecito and Johnson (2020) identify the following CQI leadership and management characteristics and functions:

- Knowing about, understanding, and adapting to the external environment
- Empowering clinicians and managers engaged in practice to identify, analyze, and improve work processes in their areas of clinical practice
- Adopting a view that customers include both clients (external customers) and providers (internal customers) and that their preferences are key determinants in the quality of health care delivery processes
- Developing a multidisciplinary approach that crosses departmental and professional boundaries in which all perspectives and ideas are given equal importance
- Adopting a well-planned and articulated organizational philosophy that specifies the value and importance of ongoing change and adaptation
- Developing and implementing well-defined processes to promote and ensure execution of best practices via planned organizational learning
- Motivating internal customers for using "a rational, data-based, cooperative approach to process analysis and change" (Sollecito & Johnson, 2020, p. 5)
- Creating an organizational culture that promotes all the aforementioned characteristics

CQI can also be a philosophy that underpins health care delivery and practices. CQI possesses a strategic focus that means organizational vision, mission, values, and objectives include valuing, designing, prioritizing, and supporting process improvement. The organization emphasizes the importance of placing customers first (i.e., clients, providers, and third-party payers) so satisfaction and health outcomes become key performance measures. A systems view is adopted so the organization engages in analyzing the whole system that provides a service or influences an outcome. This requires systems thinking that entertains both internal and external situations and occurrences. CQI also focuses on involving all stakeholders of all system components who work together to seek a common understanding of service delivery processes. Instead of focusing on a single cause, CQI philosophy asserts there are multiple root causes of occurrences within and outside of the organization. Processes, not people, are sources of errors. Solutions for organizational improvement sometimes involve a series of simultaneous changes in several normally independent functions in order to enhance organizational performance (e.g., billing processes may require considering how orders are entered into a computer, how the software informs

the department, ways to decrease time for implementation, and how the supplies used for procedures are tracked and recorded). Systems optimization involves how to enhance meeting customers' needs and preferences, which may mean disregarding previous and current practices along with crossing departmental boundaries and ignoring fiefdoms. Improvement is continuous, meaning even when a successful solution is found, the work process analysis continues. Organizational learning is critical so that the capacity of the organization to generate improvements in processes and outcomes is enhanced, and personal and professional growth of internal customers is fostered and supported (Sollecito & Johnson, 2020; Swanwick & Vaux, 2020).

Most CQI initiatives require that certain structural elements facilitate organization and support for improvement processes. The process improvement (PI) team is a group of employees and providers (internal customers) who meet to develop current solutions for problems and opportunities for improvement. A variety of CQI instruments provide the PI team and others affected by the proposed improvement implementation to analyze and track multiple causes and progress toward process improvements (e.g., fishbone diagrams, flow charts, checklists, cause-and-effect diagrams, Pareto charts, frequency distributions, run charts, control charts). Typically, a parallel organization separate from organizational management is formed to determine organizational priority improvements and monitor the CQI strategy and implementation efforts (commonly called a quality council). In order to ensure the material and human resources are available for CQI, organizational leadership bears the responsibility to make the improvement processes effective, motivate participants, provide support to PI team members, and integrate CQI "into the institutional fabric of the organization" (Sollecito & Johnson, 2020, p. 9). Resources for statistical thinking and analysis must be in place to identify common and special causes of variation in practices and processes and also to develop the visual displays outlining root causes of events and track progress toward attainment of incremental and final goals and objectives of the improved process. An established customer satisfaction measure that is used over time to detect trends in satisfaction or dissatisfaction is essential for determining areas of opportunity for improvement (the tabulation and statistical analysis of the survey used can be done by the publisher of the instrument or could be done by an internal statistical department). Benchmarking sets realistic goals to identify best practices within and across organizational settings to simulate processes or for use as performance targets. Redesign of processes may need to be done from scratch. However, the redesigning process should start with customer requirements and preferences so these are included in the redesign efforts before deployment occurs (Sollecito & Johnson, 2020; Swanwick & Vaux, 2020).

Health care organizations have a variety of additional resources to generate evidence for CQI. Evidence-based practice can be enhanced by using epidemiologic studies, clinical trials, research studies, insurance payment records, and data from electronic health records. QA and risk management data can facilitate the identification of problems to address. Risk-adjusted outcomes can facilitate the development of evidence-based individualized clinical tools such as clinical pathways. Cost-effectiveness data can be analyzed, and results can be used to create value-based policies and procedures. Involvement of the medical staff is key to success in CQI, as physicians frequently participate in self-governance activities including membership in pharmacy and therapeutics, QA, and organ and tissue donation committees (Sollecito & Johnson, 2020; Swanwick & Vaux, 2020). Medical staff members also frequently attend medical educational conferences in order to stay abreast of new developments in their areas of practice, thereby having access to the newest information that can be used for CQI.

TJC standards for accreditation emphasize the importance of QA and QI. Success in QI is based on the premise that if staff members who are closest to the point of service delivery are empowered and educated on the process of incremental change, the quality and efficiency of client care will improve. TQM and CQI differ from QA in that QA programs tend to be reactive in nature and focus on the correction of specific identified causes of problems. In contrast, TQM and CQI are proactive processes aimed at anticipating and correcting common system problems; CQI holds everyone involved in a process responsible for continually improving it. In contrast, TQM designates managers who actively lead and guide improvement efforts from identifying opportunities for improvement to evaluating implemented improvements. Table 18.1 outlines the differences between QA, TQM, and CQI.

Take Note!
CQI and TQM use consistent processes with the goal of improving all aspects of goods and services offered to consumers.

TABLE 18.1	Comparison of Quality Assurance, Total Quality Management, and Continuous Quality Improvement	
Quality Assurance	**Total Quality Management**	**Continuous Quality Improvement**
Conformance-focused	Improvement focus based on facts with management driving the improvement processes including identification of necessary innovations and driving an improvement cycle used for implementation	Innovation and change are the keys for value-driven growth, and each individual in the organization is responsible for engagement in improvement processes.
Reactive in nature	Proactive in nature	Proactive in nature and more future-focused
Looks for special sources of variation within a system	Focuses on internal variations within a system and looks for ways to reduce variation, thereby improving the system	Strategically and customer focused using the systems view for data-driven analysis to identify multiple causations to generate solutions for process optimization Improvement is continual and emphasizes organizational learning, and all stakeholders are actively involved in the process.
Variation results from actions of specific people or work groups.	Variation results from increased complexity of work processes or may be random in nature.	Variation is reduced by forming process improvement teams, using tools such as checklists, control charts, cause-and-effect diagrams, statistical analysis and thinking, and setting performance benchmarks.

Adapted from Sollecito, W. A., & Johnson, J. K. (2020). The global evolution of continuous quality improvement: From Japanese manufacturing to global health services. In J. K. Johnson & W. A. Sollecito (Eds.), *McLaughlin & Kaluzny's Continuous quality improvement in health care* (5th ed., pp. 1–31). Jones & Bartlett Learning.

THE NEED FOR IMPROVED CLIENT SAFETY AND CARE QUALITY

The Institute of Medicine's Quality Chasm Series

In light of concerns for client safety and health care quality, the IOM conducted a series of quality studies known as the **Institute of Medicine Quality Chasm Series.** The findings of the first study, *To Err Is Human: Building a Safer Health System* (2000), shocked many health care consumers and providers. This landmark study, with findings derived from the analysis of aggregate data, estimated that between 44,000 and 98,000 people die annually as a result of preventable medical errors. The report also concluded that medical errors in health care settings were the leading cause of unexpected deaths in the United States, more than any other form of sudden, unexpected death (including motor vehicle accidents). The report identified ineffective communication as the root cause of 65% of errors that resulted in death or permanent disability. As a result of the report, the U.S. Congress appropriated funds starting in fiscal year 2001 to 2002 to establish the Patient Safety Network within the Agency for Healthcare Research and Quality (AHRQ) that would also establish national safety goals, track progress in safety improvement, and fund research on preventing health care–related errors.

The second IOM study (2001), *Crossing the Quality Chasm: A New Health System for the 21st Century*, proposed radical reforms for the American health care system. The report determined a set of performance expectations to ensure that client care is safe, timely, effective, efficient, equitable, and client-centered. The goal of the reforms was to align payment and accountability with QI initiatives. The report identified the complexity of current health care organizations that resulted in increased risk for errors and higher care delivery costs. Complicated work processes and ineffective communication were cited as two key factors interfering with health care safety and quality.

Results from the 2001 IOM study led to additional recommendations for education of the health care professions outlined in *Health Professions Education: A Bridge to Quality* (IOM, 2003). The report called for education based on five competencies: (1) client-centered care, (2) teamwork and collaboration, (3) evidence-based practice, (4) QI (and safety), and (5) informatics. Key recommendations included the development of a common language for interdisciplinary team members; educational experiences including all members of the interprofessional health care team; creating evidence-based health professions curricula; providing evidence-based teaching and learning methods; initiating faculty development programs for effective role modeling of desired competencies; and developing and implementing plans for monitoring student, graduate, and faculty proficiency in the five competencies.

The 2004 IOM report, *Keeping Patients Safe: Transforming the Work Environment of Nurses,* linked the work environment of nurses with the quality and safety of client care. The report acknowledged high-stress, complex work processes; inadequate resources (human and material); and environmental barriers nurses face in providing safe, effective client care. Key recommendations included the creation and maintenance of a satisfying and rewarding work environment for nurses, adequate nurse staffing levels, increased focus on client safety at the bedside *and* by governing boards, use of evidence-based nursing management strategies, determination of ways to build and maintain trust between nurses and facility administration, participative decision making, development of ways to support and promote learning for all nurses, establishment of interdisciplinary collaboration, work environment redesign for improving client care processes, and creation of a culture of client safety.

Aspen et al. (2007) conducted a study aimed at discovering the prevalence and reasons for medication errors by nurses. This final study in the IOM Quality Chasm series, *Identifying and Preventing Medication Errors*, found that over 7000 clients died as a result of medication errors each year and that most inpatients are subjected to at least one medication error per day on average. The authors projected that 1.5 million preventable adverse drug events occur annually; adverse drug events account for 2% of hospital admissions; and the annual cost for these events is $2 billion in national health care expenditures.

The federal government examined societal trends and noted increasing diversity of citizenship, numbers of older adults, and demands for high-quality health care services. Analysis of data and literature revealed the important roles that nurses fill. To plan for the future of health care delivery, the IOM formed an ad hoc committee to explore how to maximize the use of professional nurses in reshaping the American health care delivery system. In 2011, the IOM published the findings of the committee in the report, *The Future of Nursing: Leading Change, Advancing Health.*

To meet the future health care needs of American society (increased diversity of the population and numbers of older adults), the National Health Workforce Commission and the Health Resources and Services Administration must improve the way nursing workforce data are collected. Current predictions are made from the National Registered Nurses Sample Survey (NRNSS) conducted every 4 years and from state licensing boards reports. Suggested ways to improve data include conduction of the NRNSS biannually and developing state nursing workforce centers to determine regional health care workforce needs, set regional health care workforce targets, and plan appropriately to expand the supply of health professionals to meet future needs (IOM, 2011). Once these programs are in place, efforts to improve their quality will be needed.

In response to the IOM *Future of Nursing Report*, the Robert Wood Johnson Foundation and the American Association of Retired Persons collaborated with the nursing profession to develop a Nursing Campaign for Action to design and implement programs to achieve the four key messages in the report. In the action campaign, each state formed a State Nursing Coalition in order to prevent duplicative efforts for each key message. The Future of Nursing Campaign for Action (2021) reported the following progress on the four key messages 10 years after the report was published:

1. Message 1: "Nurses should practice to the full extent of their education and training" (IOM, p. 4).: In 2010, only five states permitted independent practice for APRNs. In 2020, nine states now permit full scope of independent practice for RNs. During the COVID-19 pandemic, seven states granted temporary full scope of independent practice for APRNs. In 2010, 16 states allowed APRNs to have full prescriptive authority, whereas in 2018, APRNs enjoyed full prescriptive authority in 23 states and the District of Columbia.

2. Message 2: "Nurses should achieve higher levels of education and training through an improved educational system that promotes seamless academic progression" (IOM, 2011, p ,4). The number of practicing RNs with a bachelor of science in nursing (BSN) rose 59% from 2010 to 2019, and the number of RNs with earned doctorates increased from 11,589 to 37,852 from 2010 to 2019.

3. Message 3: "Nurses should be full partners with physicians and other health professionals, in redesigning health care in the United States" (IOM, 2011, p. 4). At the top-ranked nursing schools by *U.S. News and World Report*, the number of graduate clinical nursing courses that required collaboration

with other graduate student health team members rose from 6 to 15 from 2010 to 2019. The Center for Workforce Analysis reported that 98% of graduate nursing programs provided opportunities for interprofessional education during 2018 to 2019 academic year (Health Resources and Services Administration, 2019).

4. Message 4: "Effective workforce planning and policy making require better data collection and an improved information infrastructure" (IOM, 2011, p. 4). Thirty-one states collected data related to nursing education program enrollment, current nurse supply, and projected demand for nurses in 2010. With the exception of Delaware, all other states have data related to the supply of nurses within their state; 41 have enrollment and graduation data on all nursing programs within their states.

The National Academy of Medicine (formerly the IOM) has a task force working on a 2020 to 2030 *Future of Nursing Report*. The timeline for completion was disrupted because of the need to include information on the future of the profession related to the impacts of the COVID-19 pandemic.

Improving the Quality and Safety of Health Care Delivery

Progress toward meeting the recommendations of the IOM Quality Chasm reports has been slow. Brady (2015) reported that from 2010 to 2013 with the implementation of Comprehensive Unit-Based Safety Programs and TEAMSTEPPS, there were 1.3 million fewer hospital-associated complications (a 17% decline), 50,000 lives saved, and $12 billion in health care expenditures avoided. Client safety has also improved because of tougher accreditation standards and mandatory error reporting requirements. National and international campaigns aimed at improving client safety and care quality include the "5 Million Lives Campaign" by the Institute for Healthcare Improvement (IHI), evidence-based care protocols from the AHRQ, TJC's National Patient Safety Goals, and the Millennium Development Goals of the WHO.

The National Quality Forum (NQF) is "a nonprofit, private, nonpartisan, membership-based organization that works to catalyze improvements in health care" (NQF, 2020a, para. 1). NQF is interested in improving the quality (effectiveness and efficiency) of health care delivery in the United States. Its mission is to "be the trusted voice driving measurable health care improvements" (NQF, 2020d, para. 2). The NQF was formed following the 1999 Presidential Advisory Commission on Consumer Protection and Quality in the Health Care Industry. The NQF sets performance standards for health care and establishes routine measures of quality outcomes that have been determined by consensus of all individuals involved in health care delivery represented by specialty councils (consumers, health care plans, health professionals, public/community health providers, suppliers, and industries). Federal, state, and private organizations use NQF-endorsed measures to evaluate performance of health care facilities and share this information with consumers (NQF, 2020c). Participating members have access to a dashboard that displays collected data on key performance indicators of delivery of high-quality health care (NQF, 2020b). The NQF also engages in CQI/TQM and constantly updates data reports using the best possible evidence to set quality performance standards. Nursing-sensitive outcome measures are included in NQF performance standards. Currently, nearly 300 NQF-endorsed measures are used by federal and state pay-for-performance reimbursement systems (National Quality Forum, 2020e).

Many health care organizations have adopted a "just culture" for managing errors when they occur; such a culture emphasizes that work processes rather than people are usually the cause of mistakes in health care delivery. According to the just culture approach, there are four main categories of failures, and the levels have differing remedies. The first failure level is that of unintentional harm when an unintended result occurs typically as a result of ambiguous work processes or systems. In this case, focus is placed on the system and how it might be improved. The second failure level is provider carelessness or at-risk behavior such as inattentiveness to details that resulted in an error. When this happens, the provider receives counseling and education about how to avoid repeating the same mistake. The next two levels require some form of punishment because of the severity of their nature. A level-three situation involves recklessness with complete disregard for established work processes or norms resulting in a care error (such as a health care provider coming to work under the influence of alcohol). The fourth level arises when providers simply refuse to follow standards and procedures or show flagrant disregard for organizational authorities. The last two levels typically result in either a suspension from duty or cessation of employment (Joshi et al., 2014). Just culture promotes accountability for error management. However, effective implementation requires effective communication, comprehensive information surrounding a situation, strong and fair management, and healthy workplace environment (Foster, 2020).

The CMS has moved to value-based purchasing (VBP). Once the industry began looking for ways to provide the best possible health insurance coverage for employees, VBP represents a shift from reimbursement based on fee-for-service and high volume to reimbursement for the quality of care received in inpatient hospitals. Hospitals receive incentive payments for achieving optimal client outcomes. Hospital participants work to achieve error reduction or elimination, adoption of best-practice standards that are based on sound evidence, development or processes to enhance client experiences, improved transparency of care equality for consumers and providers, and increased efficiency to reduce the cost of care delivery (CMS, 2020). Hospitals receive a score of achievement of a score of needing improvement in the following areas: "(a) mortality and complications, (b) hospital-acquired infections, (c) client safety, (d) client experience, (e) process, and (f) efficiency and cost reduction" (CMS, 2020, para. 5). Hospitals receive payments based on how well they performed compared to each other and improved performance compared to a baseline measurement (CMS, 2020).

Using data from national quality organizations, companies could compare outcomes for disease processes for hospitals, individual health care providers, and how services were organized and delivered across the continuum of care. In response to the rising costs of health care and prevalence of potentially avoidable complications, the United States initiated the Provider Payment Reform for Outcomes, Margins, Evidence, Transparency, Hassle-Reduction, Excellence, Understandability, and Sustainability (PROMETHEUS) model (CMS, 2020; Joshi et al., 2014, p. 533). By instituting the PROMETHEUS model, the NQF was able to collect detailed data and compare outcomes for health care providers and settings. The NQF discovered that 27% of health care costs were the result of potentially avoidable complications arising from health care interventions. Therefore, CMS has evidence for using a payment-for-performance reimbursement structure (CMS, 2020; Joshi et al., 2014).

In 2005, the NQF endorsed the Hospital Consumer Assessment of Healthcare Providers and Systems (HCAHPS) survey to collect data regarding the quality of health care received by consumers in hospitals. The HCAHPS survey was developed by the CMS in 2005 to collect information about the hospital experiences of program recipients. The survey includes 27 items, 18 of which request client perspectives of care in the following eight areas: communication with physicians, communication with nurses, hospital staff responsiveness, pain management, communication about prescribed medications, discharge information, environmental cleanliness, and hospital environmental quietness. The survey also collects four screener questions and five client demographic items (CMS, 2020). Under the implementation of the Patient Protection and Affordable Care Act (PPACA), Medicare and Medicaid reimbursement rates to hospitals are adjusted based on HCAHPS survey scores. Higher scores mean higher rates of reimbursement. Hospital administrators and nurse managers have begun directing staff to use key phrases when communicating with clients, families, and visitors so that they will be able to answer HCAHPS items correctly. For example, when a nurse provides dismissal instructions to a client or family member, the nurse may use the term "side effect" when discussing prescribed medication administration at home.

▌ QUESTIONS FOR REFLECTION

1. How does VBP change care delivery using a fee-for-service approach?
2. What problems do you see for different health care organizations when receiving reimbursement for client outcome attainment?
3. How do nurses contribute to optimal client outcomes across the continuum of care?

Along with TJC's National Patient Safety Goals, TJC has developed the SPEAK UP initiative to educate clients and their families to do the following when receiving health care services:

- *S*peak up if you have questions or concerns.
- *P*ay attention to the care you get.
- *E*ducate yourself about your illness.
- *A*sk a trusted family member or friend to be your advocate, advisor, and supporter.
- *K*now what medicines you take and why you take them.
- *U*se a health care organization that has been carefully vetted.
- *P*articipate in all decisions about your treatment.

The SPEAK UP initiative emphasizes the importance of all individuals to actively participate and be knowledgeable about personal health and health issues. Currently, TJC offers online videos and brochures that can be downloaded without charge on topics covering the use of SPEAK UP, anesthesia and sedation, physician office situations, avoiding hospital readmission, depression, dialysis, diabetes, safe surgery, client rights, infant and child health, medical imaging, memory problems and dementia, organ donation, preventing medical errors, research studies, serious illness and palliative care, fall prevention, stroke, and infection prevention (TJC, 2020d).

Quality and Safety Education for Nurses

Starting in 1995, several annual invitational Dartmouth Summer Symposia were led by Paul Batalden, a pediatrician who was concerned about the quality of health care in the United States. Meeting participants included physicians, nurses, hospital administrators, and educators who referred to themselves as "an interprofessional community of educators devoted to building knowledge for leading improvement in health care" (Cronenwett, 2012, p. 6). Using basic principles of QI (i.e., identification of ways to improve, developing an action plan, implementing the plan, measuring plan results, comparing results with baseline data, and determining the effectiveness of the plan), the participants designed a program to improve the safety and quality education for the health professions, especially nursing. The Robert Wood Johnson Foundation agreed to fund the project, which would start by educating faculty on the quality and safety goals outlined in *Transforming Care at the Bedside*; this became known as **Quality and Safety Education for Nurses (QSEN)**.

Starting in 2005 and ending in 2015, the project participants identified key knowledge, skills, and attitudes (competencies) for nurses to use in order to continuously improve and enhance the quality and safety of health care delivery. The following areas were identified for the competencies: "patient-centered care, teamwork and collaboration, evidence-based practice, quality improvement, safety, and informatics" (Cronenwett, 2012, p. 52). The program was developed and implemented across four phases. With each phase, more nurses and faculty became involved, the competencies were empirically tested, teaching methods were developed, learning outcomes were assessed, and interprofessional education strategies were developed. They also established a website for sharing teaching strategies for QSEN competencies.

QSEN continues its work and publishes a monthly newsletter that highlights current projects. The QSEN website offers resources to professional nursing programs for integrating the competencies into courses and curricula. Resources can also be used for interprofessional and nursing continuing education programs. QSEN sometimes offers contests for nurses to submit educational materials addressing key topics. For example, in fall 2020, QSEN announced a contest for nurses and nurse educators to submit entries for COVID-19 teaching and practice strategies (QSEN, 2020).

QUALITY IMPROVEMENT APPROACHES

QI education appears as a QSEN competency for nursing undergraduate and graduate programs. The American Association of Colleges of Nursing (AACN) also lists QI education as an essential element of undergraduate and graduate nursing education (AACN, 2021). The expectation is that nurses will be capable of using data to monitor care process outcomes and utilizing methods outlined in the QI process to identify targeted areas for improvement, design ways to change current work systems and processes, test new ways of care delivery, and determine whether tested innovations enhance the quality and safety of health care. If the innovations are shown to improve health care systems, they will become the new standard practices. The AACN 2021 Essentials document clusters client safety and quality improvement into one domain. Expected outcomes for this domain are that the BSN graduate will be able to "apply quality improvement principles in care delivery." This broadly written outcome means graduates will need to have a knowledge of QI theory and principle processes and tools. They must have the skill to use the processes for TQI in practice, act with the attitude that things can always be improved, and be open to constant change. Because knowledge of the process is critical to meeting QI outcomes, key QI models are presented in the order of their historical development.

W. Edwards Deming

W. Edwards Deming, a physicist, mathematician, and engineer, was responsible for postwar construction in Japan. In 1950, he presented a quality management workshop that emphasized the importance of statistical control for managers. To maintain a competitive edge, Deming proposed that dedication to quality and productivity was essential. He suggested errors increased and productivity declined as a result of flawed work processes rather than individual actions. He also

FIGURE 18.1 Deming's plan, do, check, and act cycle, the first quality improvement method.

believed that productivity and quality would improve when workers became empowered to make decisions about work processes (Walton, 1986).

Deming developed a cycle, today known as the Deming cycle, to improve quality (Fig. 18.1). The cycle is a continuous loop consisting of four steps: **plan, do, check, and act (PDCA)**. Using the Deming cycle, organizations *plan* what improvements need to be made, *do* by implementing the plan, *check* results of plan implementation using statistical data, and *act* by correcting work processes to improve the quality of services or products. The IHI uses a variation of the PDCA cycle (Sollecito & Johnson, 2020; Walton, 1986).

Deming also emphasized that a successful QI program requires total commitment and accountability from all workers, including management. He created 14 points that must be applied for successful QI processes (see Box 18.2, Professional Prototypes, "Deming's 14 Points for Successful Quality Improvement Processes").

Along with proposals for successful QI programs, Deming warned of seven "deadly diseases" and obstacles that could derail the process:

1. Lack of constancy of purpose (everyone working toward different goals without a single strategic plan to ensure organizational survival)
2. Emphasis on short-term profits (quality and productivity may decline if quarterly goals are met or exceeded, which may result in workers or managers scaling back efforts)

18.2 Professional Prototypes

Deming's 14 Points for Successful Quality Improvement Processes

1. Create a constancy of purpose for improvement of products and services.
2. Adopt the philosophy that poor workmanship and services must not be tolerated.
3. Cease dependence on mass inspection by trusting and expecting workers to develop ways to improve production processes and have them make decisions during the production process whether to discard or rework a product.
4. End the practice of awarding business based solely on the lowest cost.
5. Work constantly and endlessly to improve the systems of production and service.
6. Institute training for all workers.
7. Reconfigure leadership so that supervisors help workers perform better.
8. Drive out fear in the workplace because fear prevents people from asking questions or expressing ideas and perpetuates errors in performance.
9. Remove all barriers between staff areas by bringing various departments together to work toward the common purpose and find more opportunities for improvement.
10. Replace slogans, exhortations, and targets for the workforce by having the workers write their own slogans and specify production targets.
11. Eliminate numerical quotas as they create the perception that employment status is based only on meeting quotas rather than on producing high-quality goods and services.
12. Remove barriers to the pride of workmanship by providing workers with the best equipment and materials so products and services can be improved continually.
13. Institute a vigorous program of education and retraining so that all managers and workers understand the statistical techniques and teamwork skills needed for an effective QI program.
14. Take action to accomplish the transformation by defining the action plan required to lead the quality mission with dedication (Walton, 1986).

and quality, which means managers must be on the job long enough to accomplish these tasks)
5. Running a company solely on visible figures (the effects of a satisfied or dissatisfied customer remain unknown)
6. Excessive medical costs (reveal potential problems within the work environment or no time for employees to engage in health promotion activities)
7. Excessive costs of warranty, fueled by lawyers working for contingency fees (high losses reveal that inferior goods or services are being provided to customers) (Walton, 1986)

Deming provided businesses with an innovative approach. He outlined strategies for success that empowered workers. In addition, his obstacles warned about potentially catastrophic effects arising from failure to develop strategic plans, relying on technology rather than people to solve problems, and generating excuses for suboptimal performance (Walton, 1986). CQI scholars frequently refer to Deming as the father of QI (Sollecito & Johnson, 2020; Swanwick & Vaux, 2020).

If Deming's principles are applied to clinical nursing practice, QI efforts would be made to streamline work processes related to direct client care. For example, nurses would not be blamed if errors occurred while taking care of clients. Each error that occurred would be analyzed fully to determine all contributing factors. Work processes would be changed to prevent the error's recurrence. Nurses would be empowered to make changes in clinical policies and procedures as well as assume control over their clinical practice environments.

Joseph Juran

Like Deming, management consultant and engineer Joseph Juran stressed the importance of careful planning to generate product quality. In 1945, Juran took his concepts to Japan, where he used statistical quality control as a management tool. He created the Juran Trilogy, consisting of quality planning, quality control, and QI:

- Quality planning consists of identifying specific customers and their needs, developing products to meet customer needs, developing processes to produce product features, and transferring production plans and product features to operating forces.
- Quality control consists of evaluating actual performance, comparing it with product goals, and acting on the difference.

3. Evaluation by performance, merit rating, or annual performance reviews (sets up a competitive environment with the potential for destroying teamwork, instilling rivalry, creating despondency, and encouraging management upward mobility)
4. Mobility of management away from production or service (management must understand the work and complete changes for improved productivity

- QI consists of establishing an infrastructure; identifying specific improvement projects; establishing project teams; and providing improvement teams with resources, training, education, and motivation. The QI team works to diagnose causes of inferior quality, propose and simulate remedies to identified causes, and establish control systems to maintain the gains (Juran, 1989).

Juran (1989) also differentiated quality circles from QI project teams. Quality circles serve primarily to improve human relationships and secondarily to improve quality. They usually occur within a single department where members volunteer to tackle many QI projects. Managers and workers hold equal status in quality circles. In contrast, QI project team membership crosses departmental boundaries, has a primary mission of improving quality, is run by a manager (or professional), and disbands once the project ends.

Juran (1989) outlined eight factors to distinguish institutions that have improved quality and reduced quality-related costs:

1. Upper managers lead the quality process and serve on quality councils (QI teams) as guides.
2. **Internal customers** (people working within the organization) and **external customers** (people outside the organization receiving products or services) needs are considered as QI processes are applied to businesses and usual operating processes.
3. Senior managers are given clear responsibility to adopt mandated annual QI with a defined infrastructure that identifies opportunities for improvement, and they are held accountable for making the improvements.

4. Managers involve everyone who affects the plan in the QI process.
5. Managers use modern quality methodology rather than empirical methods in quality planning.
6. Senior managers train all management team members in quality planning, quality control, and QI.
7. Managers train all workers in how to participate actively in QI.
8. QI becomes a major feature in the strategic planning process.

Juran's major contributions to QI include the Juran Trilogy that distinguishes the concepts of quality planning, quality control, and QI. He also adopted the Pareto principle, named after Vilfredo Pareto, a 17th-century Italian economist. The Pareto principle asserts that about 80% of consequences result from 20% of causes, the "vital few." By addressing the "vital few," Juran noted larger impacts could be made when identifying areas for quality planning, control, and improvement. Juran incorporated the Pareto chart into the QI process (Fig. 18.2). It displays information about a process using a bar graph with a line indicating numbers of outcomes. Reasons for an observed outcome are plotted along a horizontal axis with the most common reasoning appearing first on the left, closest to the vertical axis. The vertical axis represents the number of observed incidences of an event until 100% of the observations are plotted. The line is plotted along the tops of the bars. Thus, the least common reason for an outcome appears on the far right of the graph (Sollecito & Hardison, 2020; Swanwick & Vaux, 2020). This format can provide a quick and easy visualization of reasons for near-miss events or health care errors.

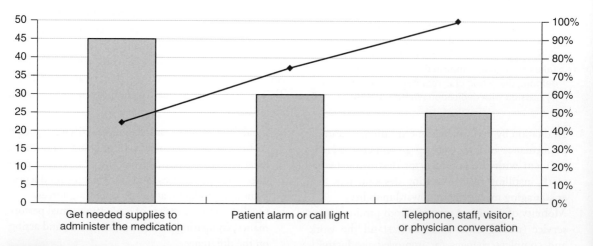

FIGURE 18.2 A Pareto chart analyzing nurse interruptions during medication administration.

Philip Crosby

Businessman Philip Crosby (1979) asserted that quality is free, but time, manpower, and resources cost money. Crosby advocated for doing things right the first time, stating that quality saves money, thereby increasing profits. He defined quality as "conformance to requirements" (Crosby, 1979, p. 8). Crosby's emphasis on doing things right the first time particularly resonates in health care delivery because health care professionals usually only get one chance to deliver effective, safe client care (e.g., the nurse has only one chance to administer the right medication to a client). He proposed that organizations needed to create climates in which attitudes and controls make error prevention possible.

Like Deming, Crosby saw the need for all within an organization to be committed to the QI process. However, Crosby believed that "management needs to understand their personal roles in implanting quality and engaging employees in the vision of the company" (Crosby, 1979, p. 78). Crosby identified 14 essential elements of a quality management program:

1. Management commitment to the QI process
2. QI teams to oversee actions
3. Measurement tools appropriate to specific activities going through the QI process
4. Consideration of the costs of quality evaluation (using estimates as needed)
5. Quality awareness promotion from all involved
6. Corrective action as needed to correct measurement tools and reduce costs associated with the QI process
7. Planning for zero defects
8. Supervisory education and training for management at all levels
9. Holding a zero defects day to celebrate the new standard of performance
10. Goal determination for individual workers and work teams
11. Worker rather than management removal of causes of error after notification
12. Recognition of all involved once performance goals are attained
13. Quality circle sharing of ideas, experiences, and problems
14. Constant repetition of all steps (QI is a continuous, never-ending process)

Crosby's thesis of the importance of doing things right the first time has been recently expanded by Toyota's lean operations and Six Sigma design approach to quality management.

Genichi Taguchi and Kaoru Ishikawa

Deming's QI concepts introduced in Japan continued to evolve. Genichi Taguchi and Kaoru Ishikawa contributed significant advances to the CQI process. Taguchi used statistical techniques to design experiments to rapidly identify problematic variations in services and products. He proposed the idea of evaluation quality from a process and end-user approach. He developed a forgiving design that removed blaming individuals for variances that resulted in defects (Sollecito & Johnson, 2020).

Ishikawa's work focused on identifying multiple steps in processes. He developed a cause-and-effect diagram known as the fishbone diagram (Fig. 18.3) (Sollecito & Johnson, 2020). The fishbone diagram is a starting point to identify common causes of variance in stabilized documented processes. Once completed, the diagram resembles a fish skeleton. The process of creating a fishbone diagram is multilayered and begins with an identified gap in performance. A horizontal line or arrow points to the gap. Lines or arrows pointing to the initial shaft of the arrow (or intersecting with the horizontal line) are drawn at a 45-degree angle to indicate major causes. For example, in health care, they might be people, procedures, policies, equipment, or plans. Each main cause contains specific causes that point to each main cause. The fishbone diagram can provide a detailed view of factors contributing to near-miss events or care errors. Work processes can also be mapped out using fishbone diagrams. QI teams find this tool useful because it provides a quick and easy format for sorting ideas into useful categories as well as for brainstorming (Sollecito & Hardison, 2020; Swanwick & Vaux, 2020).

Because of its unlimited capacity for detail, the fishbone diagram is useful for conducting a root cause analysis for sentinel events. Some sentinel events identified by TJC include client suicide, abduction, assault, or elopement (client leaving the hospital without permission or dismissal); unanticipated death of a full-term infant; sending a newborn home with the wrong family; hemolytic blood transfusion reactions in response to administering the wrong blood type; medication error resulting in death; invasive procedure or surgery performed on the wrong client, the wrong site, or the wrong procedure; any injury caused by fire, smoke, heat, or flashes; radiation therapy delivered to the wrong body part; high radiation doses from prolonged fluoroscopy procedures; and any intrapartum maternal death or severe unanticipated maternal morbidity. Because of the serious outcomes of sentinel events, the goal is to try to understand why they occurred and

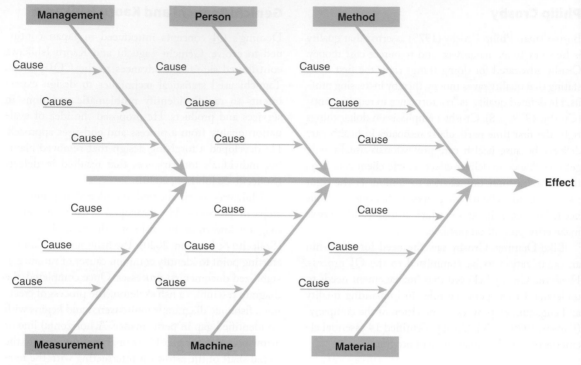

FIGURE 18.3 A fishbone diagram.

to keep them from happening again. The root cause analysis is a detailed review of the situation from beginning to end and maps out all potential sources that contributed to the event. The fishbone diagram has no limits to the number of main and specific causes that can be added. Sometimes factors contributing to specific causes are added. When the diagram is completed, the review committee identifies all contributing factors leading to the event. For each identified contributing factor, the committee generates ways to prevent each factor from happening. The facility generates an action plan for preventing the sentinel event from recurring, and the report is submitted to TJC or other required entities and is stored in confidential organization files.

Walter A. Shewhart

In the early 1960s, physicist Walter A. Shewhart modified the PDCA cycle, substituting the word "study" for "change." The study phase encompasses examining the results of changes, especially looking at what went right, what went wrong, and what was learned. Deming agreed with the changes and attributes this improvement to Shewhart (Sollecito & Johnson, 2020). The IHI adopted this cycle to guide its

QI processes to focus on its triple aim of health care improvement—improved experience of care, improved population health outcomes, and reduced per capita costs of health care (Institute of Healthcare Improvement, 2020c). By studying the change effects, health care organizations redesign work processes based on multiple form of evidence, including information regarding safety, efficiency, improved customer experience, and impact on costs.

Lean

Since the 1980s, Toyota automobiles have had a reputation for their quality construction and performance. The company emphasized elimination of waste, focusing on the terms "muda" (wasting resources), "muri" (overburdening staff and equipment), and "mura" (uneven process workflow). The uneven workflow was identified when there was an abundance of supplies in storerooms. Instead of spending resources on storage and excess inventory of parts needed for vehicle production, Toyota developed the "just-in-time" production system. In health care organization, this translated to the development of consolidating services and delegating them to specific departments or individuals to process (Popovich et al., 2020). An example of batching would be sending multiple requests for mammography to an outpatient radiology department for scheduling followed by sending the films once a day to the radiologist to view and establish findings.

The Toyota production system also created a learning environment that uses four key practices:

1. How people work: Workers follow strict production specifications, are encouraged to identify changes in work processes, and then perform controlled trials of new work processes.
2. How workers connect: Workers across all levels of the organization interact directly following standardized methods. These practices reduce ambiguity, prevent key issues from losing attention, encourage requests for help (to which assistance is provided immediately), set deadlines for problem resolution, and foster trust among everyone in the organization.
3. How work is constructed: Work processes are designed to attain maximum reliability, eliminate repetition, and follow principles to promote worker health and well-being.
4. How work is improved and errors are reduced: All workers are trained in how to effect change, assume responsibility for making errors, and use the scientific method to identify and propose changes to improve productivity and product quality and reduce errors (Joshi et al., 2014).

Toyota also uses **lean** operation techniques that advocate the use of desired, value-added activities while eliminating undesirable activities and waste in all work processes. Lean techniques eliminate waste by using visual controls, streamlined physical plant layouts, standardized work processes (eliminating variation), and point-of-use storage. If a health care organization operates using lean principles, operations flowcharts outlining steps for delivering various services would be posted in departments (Joshi et al., 2014). Nursing units and other ancillary departments would be designed to promote the flow of activities required for client care. Routine work processes would be standardized (many institutions already use standardized clinical care pathways for commonly encountered diseases, surgeries, and invasive diagnostic and intervention procedures). Finally, supplies, equipment, information, and procedures would be housed in convenient locations where client services are delivered (IOM, 2004).

Lean management systems (LMSs) operate using five principles:

1. Customers define value.
2. The value stream of every process should be identified, and any wasted steps should be eliminated because they do not add value to the process.
3. Organization should subject their products continuously through the steps of the value-added process (in health care, the product is client flow through care processes).
4. Organizations should pull products from previous steps of processes rather than causing them to back up waiting for the next step.
5. Organizations should work to continuously improve processes to reduce steps, time, costs, and information needed to provide services or products (Popovich et al., 2020).

Because client flow through health care processes remains one of the keys to high-quality care, each step in the process requires special attention. When possible, variations need to be eliminated. However, health care consumers enter the system with a variety of conditions, and many consumers have multiple health problems, creating complexity. Client flow can be calculated by using the "VUT" equation (Popovich et al., 2020, p. 152):

$$\text{Average client flow care time} = \text{Variation (V)} \times \text{Utilization (U)} \times \text{Process time (T)}$$

Reductions in variation, utilization, and process time reduce the time each consumer spends in a care delivery process. Reduced time spent in receiving health care provides consumers with more time for engagement in the things they would prefer to be doing. Besides reducing time for care delivery, the VUT equation can also predict when a system is operating close to saturation and/or capacity (Popovich et al., 2020).

The lean system outlines seven categories of waste: (1) poor utilization of resources, (2) excess motion, (3) unnecessary waiting, (4) transportation, (5) process inefficiency, (6) excess inventory, and (7) defects/quality control. Another approach to root cause analysis is asking a series of why questions, which is an effective way for identifying reasons for waste or lost productivity. The following "Concepts in Practice" provides an example of using this method to determine why nurses on a unit cannot find supplies, resulting in reduced productivity (see Concepts in Practice, "Using Root Cause Analysis and Learning to Discover Quality Defects Leading to Reduced Nursing Productivity").

When nurses need to search for equipment for client care, hospitals are practicing poor utilization

Concepts in Practice [IDEA] → [PLAN] → [ACTION]

Using Root Cause Analysis and Learning to Discover Quality Defects Leading to Reduced Nursing Productivity

Location: A medical–surgical nursing unit

Problem: The nurses cannot find basic client care equipment such as a bedpan, toothbrushes, and soap. This results in wasted time searching for client care supplies.

- *Why do the nurses have difficulty finding a bedpan?* Because a new bedpan is not available in the supply room

- *Why is the equipment not in the supply room?* Because the bedpan was not specified on the list of supplies that should be restocked

- *Why are the supplies not on the list?* Because the nursing staff did not scan the computer-based barcode and charge the client for the bedpan when one was taken from the supply room

- *Why did the nursing staff not scan the bedpan?* Because the nurse was in a hurry to get the client a bedpan

- *Why was the nurse in such a hurry?* Because the nurse did not want the client to eliminate in the bed because the client was ordered on complete bed rest

Possible Resolutions

- Stock a bedpan in each client room (excess inventory possible).

- Position the computer-based barcoding device in a strategic location to make scanning quick and easy (may be a process inefficiency or excessive motion by staff).

- Educate the nursing staff about how the scanning device is used for supply inventory control (correct a quality defect).

- Install cameras to record staff as supplies are removed from the supply room, and then generate reports for specific staff members who fail to comply with scanning supplies when removing them from a supply room (correct a process inefficiency; however, this process is incongruent with QI philosophy).

of resources, excess motion, unnecessary waiting, and process inefficiency. Many times, clients wait for long periods after undergoing diagnostic tests because of the unavailability of personnel to return them to their rooms (waste from transportation, unnecessary waiting, and process inefficiency). Nurses may make

medication errors because they engage in multitasking to meet client care needs (waste in terms of process inefficiency). Hospitals frequently buy supplies in bulk to reduce cost per unit, resulting in a higher inventory of supplies than actually needed; some supplies may become outdated and have to be discarded (excess inventory) (IOM, 2004).

However, health care organizations constantly look for ways to reduce delivery costs. Some health care organizations have identified that by removing waste and improving workflow processes (e.g., the use of interprofessional team–developed client care paths), better client outcomes occur.

Six Sigma

In the late 1980s, Motorola developed the Six Sigma strategy as a means to sharpen its focus on QI and help accelerate the pace of change in a highly competitive technologic and telecommunications market (Pande et al., 2000). The concept was expanded by other companies, including General Electric, Allied Signal, and Honeywell (Pande et al., 2000). Six Sigma has its basis in the quality principles outlined by Deming, Juran, and Crosby and in the lean model, but takes quality to a new level. "In a nutshell, **Six Sigma** is a management philosophy focused on eliminating mistakes, waste, and rework" (Chowdhury, 2002, p. 4).

Sigma (the Greek letter for deviation) measures variation within a process. The standard deviation of a process quantifies how far a process functions from its ideal. Instead of using percentages (based on a system of 100 performances), Six Sigma looks at "defects per million opportunities" (Chowdhury, 2002; Pande et al., 2000). Table 18.2 summarizes the levels of Six Sigma, translates them in terms of performance accuracy, and presents health care–based scenarios using Six Sigma.

Six Sigma methodology strives to improve products and work processes during the design rather than the quality control stage. Its processes emphasize providing the highest possible quality of goods and services to consumers. The methodology focuses on understanding variation and then reduces variation within processes to improve results. Six Sigma can be combined with lean because lean focuses on flow improvement and waste reduction, whereas Six Sigma focuses on reductions in errors and variations in process (Evans, 2020). Six Sigma provides statistical control that lean lacks. Six Sigma lacks the ability to improve process speeds dramatically while reducing capital investments (Popovich et al., 2020). Pande and colleagues (2000, p. 68) outlined a Six Sigma roadmap consisting of the

Sigma Level	Performance Accuracy/Million	Defective Performance/Million	Implication for Nursing Practice
	TABLE 18.2	**Six Sigma Levels, Performance Accuracy, and Implications for Nursing Practice**	
1	310,000 (30.9% accuracy)	690,000	309 of 1,000 client interactions make clients feel that the nurse truly understood their concerns.
2	692,000 (69.2% accuracy)	308,000	692 of 1,000 IVs are inserted successfully on the first attempt.
3	933,200 (93.3% accuracy)	66,800	933 of 1,000 postoperative complications are detected and treated effectively.
4	993,790 (99.4% accuracy)	6,210	994 of 1,000 medications are administered accurately.
5	999,680 (99.98% accuracy)	320	4,999 of 5,000 physician orders are transcribed accurately.
6	999,996.6 (99.9997% accuracy)	3.4	Between three and four errors are made per million client care documentation entries in medical records.

Data from Pande, P., Neuman, R., & Cavanagh, R. (2000). *The Six Sigma way*. McGraw-Hill.

following five sequential steps: (1) identify core processes and key customers; (2) define customer requirements; (3) measure current performance; (4) prioritize, analyze, and implement improvements; and (5) expand and integrate the Six Sigma system.

The steps apply to situations related to business transformation, strategic improvement, and problem solving. When transforming business, Pande and colleagues (2000) suggested limiting the scope of change to one or two core processes. However, in health care, Six Sigma may best be used for strategic improvement (finding out what clients and families need and want, followed by implementation of initiatives to fulfill client and family expectations) and for problem solving (looking for ways to improve effective health care delivery while reducing costs).

Six Sigma uses a cyclical process similar to the PDCA cycle (Fig. 18.4):

1. Define: Identify the problem, determine requirements, and set goals.
2. Measure: Validate the problem or flawed process, refine problems or goals, and measure key steps and inputs.
3. Analyze: Develop causal hypotheses, identify the "vital few" root causes, and validate a causal hypothesis.
4. Improve: Develop ideas to eliminate root causes, test solutions, standardize to a single solution, and measure results.
5. Control: Establish standard measurements to maintain performance and correct problems as needed (Evans, 2020; Sollecito & Johnson, 2020).

Six Sigma sets a no-nonsense but ambitious goal of 3.4 defective parts per million opportunities (Chowdhury, 2002; Pande et al., 2000) rather than using benchmarking (comparing outcomes or results with those of other

FIGURE 18.4 The Six Sigma process incorporates customer focus and wise use of facts to improve and manage work processes.

similar organizations) systems as indicators for improvement. Six Sigma has the ability to detect incremental and exponential change. TQM/CQI initiatives focus on product quality, whereas Six Sigma solutions attend to all business processes. Six Sigma may hold the key to satisfying both clients and nurses in health care environments as Morgan and Cooper (2004) used the process, for example, to change the methods for making staff assignments and to increase the availability of client care supplies. Results of improved work processes included higher consumer satisfaction score, less overtime, and increased job satisfaction (Morgan & Cooper, 2004).

However, the professional nurse's job in the hospital environment remains highly complex. Complex work processes increase the likelihood of errors, especially when nurses experience multiple interruptions when performing essential client care tasks (Cooper, Tupper & Holm, 2016).

Experience-Based Co-design

The Point of Care Foundation in Great Britain developed the **experience-based co-design (EBCD) model** to develop simple solutions to enhance client experiences with health care services. The EBCD method uses qualitative storytelling approaches to develop a deep understanding of how consumers and providers experience a service. Information is generated using in-depth interviewing, direct observation of the experience, and group discussions. Key touch points (emotionally significant points within the experience) are identified, and a group of providers and consumers rate them as positive or negative. Short films consisting of client interviews about their experiences are produced and then shown to small groups of consumers and providers. The small group identifies areas for improvement, creates ways to change the experience, and implements activities to improve the service or established clinical pathway (Evans, 2020).

The EBCD method embraces the partnership of health care consumers and providers. CQI efforts using this framework consider the values and preferences of providers and consumers. Improvements are co-designed using the experiences and expertise of all involved in health care delivery. The EBCD approach also creates person-centered care strategies within the confines of what is feasible from provider and organizational perspectives.

▉ QUESTIONS FOR REFLECTION

1. Which of the QI approaches seems best to you? Why do you think it is superior to the others presented in the chapter?
2. What is the QI approach used in your current clinical practice setting? What QI approaches are used in your nursing program?
3. How have you participated in the QI process in your current clinical practice setting or nursing program?
4. Is it important for nurses or students to participate in the QI process? Why or why not?

IMPLEMENTING CONTINUOUS QUALITY IMPROVEMENT

Standardizing Continuous Quality Improvement

CQI may be viewed as an organizational value and process to deliver the best possible goods and services to consumers. CQI works to improve constancy in actions while meeting and exceeding product and service standards; this requires standardization.

All CQI programs focus efforts on four areas: (1) customer service (both internal and external customers); (2)

ways to improve the quality of key work processes; (3) development and use of quality tools and statistics; and (4) involvement of all people and organizational departments that provide service to the consumer.

Benchmarking

Effectiveness of QI initiatives relies on institutional **benchmarking**, a process that compares performance with a predetermined standard. Some organizations have set benchmarks (a certain score for goal attainment) that apply to all departments for performance in customer service and delivery. Organizational benchmarks are included in company policies. Standardized performance evaluation tools rate and compare results within the institution to track gains in quality or with similar institutions to determine how well the organization is performing against others. Comparative benchmarks are frequently determined by external agencies in the health care industry such as CMS or TJC. When performance fails to reach the benchmark, everyone in the organization works together to fix processes rather than blaming specific individuals.

Balanced Score Card

A balanced scorecard is a tool that provides useful information about an organization in four areas: financial, customers, internal processes, and organizational learning and growth. The balanced scorecard is useful in strategic planning and developing quality improvement strategies (Sherr et al., 2017). Besides having the ability to translate strategy into actions, it facilitates translation of a strategic vision into clear and realistic goals and objectives. The balanced scorecard collects data on metrics for performance measurement standards and indicators to track organizational performance in attaining its goals (Hall et al., 2008; Sultz & Young, 2004). Some organizations post periodic charts containing recently collected data regarding specific initiatives, including those for QI to increase staff awareness of progress.

International Organization for Standardization 9000

The International Organization for Standardization (ISO) is a nongovernmental organization composed of a network of national standards institutes from 146 countries. Its goal is to set international standards for all businesses and for the broader needs of the global human society. ISO standards benefit society by promoting fair trade; compatibility of technology; conformity of consumer products in terms of safety, quality, and reliability; and scientific knowledge and technology for health. They also provide guidelines to prevent global environmental contamination (ISO, 2017). The ISO outlines eight key principles for TQM known as ISO 9000, which ensures consistency among all international efforts aimed at TQM and CQI (Table 18.3).

Celebrating Successes

One of Deming's 14 principles for QI is to recognize participants when performance goals are attained (Walton, 1986). Responding to the perception in the 1980s that the American manufacturing industry was trailing the Japanese manufacturing industry, Congress enacted the "Malcolm Baldrige National Quality Improvement Act" (Public Law 100–107) with the "objective of encouraging American business and other organizations to practice effective quality control in the provision of their goods and services." The law was named after the Secretary of Commerce who had been killed in a rodeo accident that year and provided funding for recognizing organizations that excel in QI implementation. Only three **Malcolm Baldrige National Quality Awards** per category (manufacturing, small business, service, education health care, and nonprofit) are given in any year (National Institute of Standards and Technology [NIST], 2020b).

TABLE 18.3   Key Principles and Health Care Examples of TQM Based on ISO 9000

TQM/ISO Principle	Goal/Purpose	Examples
Customer focus	Satisfy external and internal customers.	▪ Provide external customers (recipients of health care services) with "the little extras" that make big differences, such as customized menus, backrubs, and aesthetically appealing rooms. ▪ Create an open, trusting work environment for internal customers (physicians, interdisciplinary health care professionals, nursing staff members, and other supportive client services staff) that encourages collaboration and suggestions to improve work-related processes that are studied and, if feasible, implemented.
Leadership	Provide vision, direction, and understanding of the constancy of purpose among all members of the organization.	▪ Empower all workers by inviting them to participate in departmental strategic planning. ▪ Provide education about the mission, values, goals, and objectives of the organization to all workers.
Involvement of people	All people within the organization should feel ownership in the TQM values and processes.	▪ Form a nursing unit and other department-based quality circles. ▪ Form interdepartmental and interdisciplinary QI teams to improve work processes that involve more than one department or discipline. ▪ Institute interdisciplinary shared governance systems for nursing and other professional disciplines.
Process approach	Desired results are more effectively accomplished when related resources and activities are defined and managed as a process.	▪ Constantly monitor organizational performance, comparing results with similar organizations (benchmarking), and share results on a regular basis with all organization members. ▪ Consistently use client care pathways.
Systems approach to management	Leaders and people in the organization must look outside the organization to plan how best to use physical, monetary, and human resources.	▪ Analyze local, regional, and global trends to plan future services. ▪ Review and analyze current work processes to determine how to improve health care and health education services. ▪ Stay abreast of the latest scientific advancements in disease management, illness prevention, health promotion, and health care delivery.
Continual improvement	Constant improvement becomes a permanent organizational objective.	▪ Always look for ways to improve delivery of health care services. ▪ Continually reinforce with staff the importance of improving quality via education, informing staff of performance results. ▪ Share data with all organizational members who deliver specific services.
Factual approach to decision making	Actual data, current trends, and other forms of objective information serve as the basis for decision making within the organization.	▪ Stay informed of current trends and advances in health care. ▪ Use data generated by QI processes to guide actions, changes, and plans. ▪ Pilot new equipment before making purchases.
Mutually beneficial supplier relationships	The organization forms partnerships with external contractors based on the quality of goods and services they can provide.	▪ Identify vendors that provide high-quality products. ▪ Secure exclusive purchasing contracts with identified vendors.

Adapted from Institute of Medicine. (2004). *Keeping patients safe: Transforming the work environment of nurses.* National Academies Press; *St. Luke's Hospital of Kansas City Organizational Manual.* (2018). Saint Luke's Health System.

The NIST (2019a) revised the criteria for the awards and presents them annually. Criteria are built on 11 core values:

1. Systems perspective
2. Visionary leadership
3. Customer (client, student)-focused excellence
4. Valuing people
5. Organizational learning and agility
6. Focus on success
7. Managing for innovation
8. Management by fact
9. Societal contributions
10. Ethics and transparency
11. Delivering value and results

The 11 values are embedded in the systematic processes of strategy, leadership, operations, workforce, customers, measurement analysis, and knowledge management. The systematic processes are then evaluated for results in the areas of leadership and governance, product and process, workforce sustainability, customer -focused excellence, and financial management, market share, and organizational strategy (NIST, 2020a). Several integrated health care systems and hospitals have won this prestigious award but only one health care organization, the Southcentral Foundation, a nonprofit organization that provides health services to Alaskan Natives and Native Americans, has won the award more than once (NIST, 2017).

In addition to these awards, health care systems in most states are eligible for state-sponsored Balridge-based quality award programs. Many national award recipients start their journey to the national award by entering and winning a state quality award. Winning a state or a national quality award serves as a valuable marketing strategy in a health care system increasingly driven by competition and the need to reduce costs (NIST, 2019b).

To showcase the accomplishment of QI goals, some institutions prominently post baseline and improvement data for health care team members and consumers to see. Materials highlighting goal attainment frequently recognize members of PI teams. Sometimes, intra-agency publications express appreciation to workers for gains in quality. Ceremonies for nurses and other team members who achieve performance improvement goals provide recognition of those achievements. To inform staff of progress and necessary improvements, some units limit their posting of QI data exclusively to staff areas.

Using CQI Processes in Health Care

Key principles of CQI consider people who receive services and attend to people providing services. Therefore, CQI enhances the health care delivery experience for everyone.

CQI places consumers first. People providing services seek to find ways to streamline work processes. Deming asserted that more complex work processes have a greater chance for error. Consistency of action reduces error rates (Sultz & Young, 2004; Walton, 1986). CQI programs use a variety of instruments to identify variations in work processes (Table 18.4). With the exception

TABLE 18.4 Instruments Used in TQM/CQI Programs

Instrument	Description	Advantages
Check sheet	Generic instrument to collect data over time to identify "patterns, trends, defects, or causes of defects" (Joshi et al., 2014, p. 94).	Excellent for tracking progress over time, and captured data is easily converted to visual tool such as a histogram or Pareto chart.
Five whys	Asking repetitive why questions helps drill down to identify the flaws in a process or design failure to identify the root cause. Caution is needed to avoid ceasing prematurely, which may result in failure or misidentification of a root cause.	Provides a structured process to identify a root cause
Flowchart	Graphic representation of a sequence of events required to attain a specific outcome. Specific symbols depict steps of a process (e.g., rectangle, activity; diamond, decision; triangle, wait; large circle, file; small circle, go to another point); arrows indicate the direction of the overall process. Symbols may vary according to organizational practices.	Easily identifies sources of variation and easily updated to remain current
Fishbone diagram	A horizontal line depicts the work process with the desired outcome appearing at the far left side of the diagram. Inputs into the work process are represented as lines (or spines) that intersect the horizontal line drawn obliquely from the baseline in upward or downward directions. The diagram looks like a fish skeleton.	Depicts work processes during brainstorming sessions, readily stratified to show details, and identifies causes and effects in a work process
Run chart	Displays the frequency of events or a particular observation over time; frequency counts are connected by a line.	Depicts alterations arising from changes and key for determining whether improvements have resulted from changes

Instrument	Description	Advantages
Pareto chart	Displays data using a rank order; factors with the most frequent observation appear first followed by less frequent observations.	Offers the ability to stratify causes and identify the top causes, helpful for prioritizing changes, and useful for showing results of changes
Histogram	Bar graph that displays the frequency of an occurrence.	Offers the ability to detect the frequency of root causes in a process and useful for tracking results of changes
Control chart	Depicted as a run chart but with statistically determined upper and lower limits of variation above and below the average performance	Essential to see if the process remains under control
Scatter diagram	Points are placed across a vertical and horizontal axis to demonstrate the relationship between two variables.	Useful to see if any relationships between two variables are occurring to detect causes and monitor the effects of changes
Regression analysis	Statistical testing of correlational models	Tests hypothesis used by organizations for decision making

Adapted from Joshi, M. S., Ransom, E. R., Nash, D. B., & Ransom, S. B. (2014). *The healthcare quality book, vision strategy and tools* (3rd ed.). Health Administration Press & Association of University Programs in Health Administration; Koch, M., & Fairly, T. (1993). *Integrated quality management, the key to improving nursing care quality*. Mosby; Sollecito, W. A., & Hardison, D. (2020). Understanding variation, tools, and data sources for CQI in health care. In J. K. Johnson & W. A. Sollecito (Eds.), *McLaughlin & Kaluzny's continuous quality improvement in health care* (5th ed., pp. 107–142). Jones & Bartlett Learning.

of regression analysis, most of the instruments diagram the steps of a given process, thereby providing CQI team members with a picture and facilitating identification of variations along with potential sources for error.

Once the work process has been fully described, participants in the CQI process can proceed to implement Deming's PDCA cycle or Shewhart's plan–do–study–act (PDSA) cycle. Note that the process starts with planning, requires implementation of plans, and concludes with the final step that restarts the cycle by looking for ways to improve the process. The "Concepts in Practice" box, "Use of the TQM/CQI Process to Reduce Medication Errors," provides an example of the CQI process in action.

Concepts in Practice

Use of the TQM/CQI Process to Reduce Medication Errors

The following example shows how Laura, the nurse presented at the beginning of the chapter, and the nursing department where she works could use TQM/CQI to avoid the problem of medication errors.

1. Step 1: Identify a work process to be improved—Accuracy of antibiotic administration
2. Step 2: Organize a CQI team—Select health team members to serve on the CQI/TQM team who are involved in this work process. In this case, members would include a physician who writes antibiotic orders; a unit secretary who transcribes the physician order; a pharmacist who checks the order against the client electronic health record (EHR), validates its safety for client administration, and enters the medication into the client EHR; a pharmacist who fills the order; a courier who delivers daily doses to the nursing units; and a nurse who verifies the

physician order and administers the antibiotics to clients.

3. Step 3: Clarify the current work process—The team meets and diagrams the current process from the time the order is written until the client receives the ordered medication.
4. Step 4: Identify and understand all variation sources—The team notices that six people are involved in the process of antibiotic administration (physician; unit secretary; pharmacist who reviews the client data, validates that it is safe for the client to receive the medication, and enters it into the client electronic medication administration record; another pharmacist who mixes and prepares the intravenous (IV) antibiotics and places it in the box for delivery to the nursing unit; the pharmacy courier; and the nurse who administers the antibiotic dose to the client). The team also notes that antibiotic orders may be written at any time during the day,

(continued)

Concepts in Practice (*Continued*)

leading to scheduling issues. The team analyzes all the medication incident reports filed related to antibiotic administration to confirm the information generated from the brainstorming session. In addition, the team creates a checklist for collecting data regarding administration of intravenous antibiotics in the 2 weeks before the next meeting.

5. Step 5: Select the improvement—The team discovers after its data collection that delay in administration was a prevalent quality problem. Therefore, the team decides that commonly administered dosages could be placed in the computerized medication-dispensing station so that the nurse can access it more readily and not have to wait for unit delivery. Another suggestion is that nurses on the unit should notify at least two nursing colleagues when they leave the unit for more than 5 minutes and inform their colleagues of any client care needs, especially antibiotic administration.

6. Step 6: Implement the improvement—The nurses obtain ordered antibiotic doses from the computerized medication-dispensing system and comply with the recommended notification of other nurses when leaving the unit for longer than 5 minutes.

7. Step 7: Check and compare results with the desired outcome—Within a month of implementing step 6, the number of incident reports filed related to antibiotic administration decreases by 80%.

8. Step 8: Take steps to maintain improved performance and suggest ways to further improve the process—Proposals are made for hospital-wide implementation. The first proposal is that all nurses will contact a minimum of two other nurses on the unit when leaving the unit for more than 5 minutes and provide them with the status of medication administration and other client care needs. The second proposal is that commonly ordered antibiotics will be placed in all hospital-computerized medication-dispensing systems.

Using a CQI approach, Laura does not receive a reprimand for missing the ordered dose of antibiotics; rather, work processes are found that contributed to her error. In health care, the professional nurse plays a pivotal role in CQI because they are instrumental in providing direct consumer service and possess evidence-based knowledge to improve work processes, clinical procedures, and standardized care pathways.

To recognize their success in implementing the TQM/CQI project, the hospital acknowledges contributions of the QI team in the organizational newsletter. The team also posts graphs to promote reduction in warfarin administration errors in the staff lounge of the cardiac unit.

▮ QUESTIONS FOR REFLECTION

1. What do you like about using a CQI/TQM process when quality issues arise in health care delivery?
2. What are the benefits of the process?
3. What barriers might interfere with the process?
4. Would you be willing to participate as a CQI/TQM team member? Why or why not?

COLLABORATIVE AND EVIDENCE-BASED EFFORTS TO IMPROVE THE QUALITY OF HEALTH CARE

The Institute for Healthcare Improvement

In 1986, a group of health care providers saw the gap between ideal and actual health care safety and quality. Their efforts to improve health care for all people worldwide led to the formation of the IHI in 1991, a nonprofit organization that works collaboratively with professional health care teams to establish a scientific foundation for improving the quality and safety of health care delivery (IHI, 2018). The mission of the IHI is "to improve health and health care worldwide" to achieve a vision of "everyone [having] the best care and health possible" (IHI, 2020a). IHI works with all members of the health care team, academics, executives, and systems (IHI, 2020a). Using the goals outlined by the IOM, the IHI developed an "always events" list that captures what is vitally essential to clients and families when they receive health care as well as a "never events" list. A "never events" list results in a client death, permanent disability, or severe, intense suffering of any nature (Balik, 2016). The IHI also addresses helplessness in health care consumers and providers, undesirable waiting for services, wasteful expenditure of health care resources, and denial of access to care. The IHI strives to reinstill the passion that health care professionals have toward their work and started facilitating interprofessional education for health care professionals in 1994 (IHI, 2018). Some of the key IHI contributions to health care that have become practice standards include the ventilator bundle (specific care protocols for people on respirators); applying operations research to health care; transitions home program (a program that reduces hospital readmission rates and improves client outcomes); rapid response teams; and a medication reconciliation process (IHI, 2018). The IHI offers free information and education for health care professionals and students about how to improve quality and safety in health care and coordinates interprofessional QI teams.

Current initiatives of the IHI include evidence-based current resources on COVID-19, practices for improving clinician well-being, ways to improve nursing home care, workforce keys to client safety, a client safety executive development program, and ways to increase teamwork while reducing costs. IHI offers over 35 interprofessional continuing education courses as well as a basic certificate in quality and safety in its open school (IHI, 2020b).

The Leapfrog Group

The Leapfrog Group was established in 2000 when 60 businesses came together over concerns about the quality, safety, and affordability of health care in the United States (The Leapfrog Group, n.d.-c, 2020a). The Leapfrog Group is a not-for-profit watchdog organization that drives movement by proposing big leaps toward improving the American health care system (The Leapfrog Group, n.d.-a). Starting in 2001, they developed and deployed a hospital performance survey and reported the findings publicly in 2002. The survey is completed by over 2,000 hospitals each year. The Leapfrog Group uses survey results for transparent reporting of hospitals meeting specific standards of care to assign letter grades to hospitals for their safety results and VBP programs. In 2020, they initiated a survey for ambulatory surgical centers and hospital outpatient departments (The Leapfrog Group, 2020b).

The Leapfrog Group website enables anyone to view how any hospital meets its standards for safe care, view the letter grade assigned for hospital safety, and describes its VBP program. Health care consumers can view and use this information to make decisions about where to receive hospital and ambulatory surgical services when possible. The Leapfrog Group makes data available from surveys administered to researchers (The Leapfrog Group, n.d.-a).

The Leapfrog Group also surveys employers who purchase health insurance plans to cover the health care needs of employees. They work with health insurance plans to assist them in the selection of preferred providers when plans use a network approach to reduce delivery costs.

The Leapfrog Group convenes expert panels representing various members of the interprofessional health care team to confirm currently used measures are valid, relevant, meaningful, and actionable for clients, their families, and health care providers. Current expert panels are addressing outpatient surgery, culture of safety, hand hygiene, the nursing workforce, intensive care unit physician staffing, computerized physician order entry, barcode medication administration, inpatient surgery, pediatric care, maternity care, and client and family caregiver standards. The addition of client and family caregiver standards is aimed at increasing consumer involvement in the process (The Leapfrog Group, n.d.-b).

PROFESSIONAL NURSING ROLES IN QUALITY IMPROVEMENT

TQM/CQI provides professional nurses with an opportunity to showcase the unique contributions they make to interdisciplinary health care delivery. Because nurses have always been concerned with client safety and quality of care, they can assume leadership roles in TQM/CQI processes. Data collection by nurses as part of routine care delivery sometimes identifies a quality initiative (an area for improvement). In addition, the professional nurse serves as a key player in developing work processes and strategies to improve care quality. The following discussion outlines how nurses might use professional nursing roles to promote QI.

Role of Caregiver

Professional nursing continues to study the effects of nursing care on client outcomes. Client outcomes that arise directly from nursing assessment and intervention are known as **nursing-sensitive outcomes**. Box 18.3, Professional Building Blocks, "Client-Related Nursing-Sensitive Outcomes," displays nursing-sensitive outcomes that have been identified to date. Most of these outcomes have been identified through nursing research or comprehensive literature reviews of nursing research studies examining the impact of professional nursing care on client outcomes (Doran, 2003; Dunton, 2008; Dunton et al., 2011; Press Ganey, 2020). Research suggests that the increased presence of RNs and RNs with specialty certifications improves client outcomes, reduces hospital-acquired complications, and decreases health care costs (Boltz et al., 2012; Gigli et al., 2020; Park et al., 2012; Roche et al., 2012; Twigg et al., 2012).

The ANA (2021) incorporates nurse participation in QI programs as a required professional practice standard (Standard 15, Quality of Practice). Required

18.3 Professional Building Blocks

Client-Related Nursing-Sensitive Outcomes

- Safety from medication and other treatment-related errors
- Functional status
- Self-care
- Effective symptom management
- Effective pain management
- Satisfaction with received health care services
- Effective management of fatigue
- Effective management of nausea and vomiting
- Effective management of dyspnea
- Early detection and effective management of postoperative complications
- Reduced incidence of urinary tract infections
- Reduced incidence of pneumonia
- Increased incidence of successful rescue following cardiac or respiratory arrest
- Reduced rate of injury from falling
- Reduced rates of institutionally acquired pressure injuries
- Reduced use of physical or chemical restraints
- Reduced incidence of bloodstream infections from central line use
- Failure to rescue

National Quality Forum Nursing-Sensitive Measures

- Hospital-acquired pressure injuries
- Nursing staff skill mix
- Nursing hours per client day
- RN Survey: Practice Environment Scale
- Restraint use prevalence
- Nurse turnover
- Ventilator-associated pneumonia
- Central line–associated bloodstream infection
- Catheter-associated urinary tract infections

Adapted from Doran, D. (Ed.). (2003). *Nursing-sensitive outcomes: The state of the science*. Jones & Bartlett; Dunton, N. (2008). Take a cue from the NDNQI. *Nursing Management, 39*(4), 20, 22, 23; Institute of Medicine. (2004). *Keeping patients safe*. National Academies Press; Dunton, J., Montalvo, I., & Dunton, N. (2011). *NDNQI case studies in nursing quality improvement*. American Nurses Association; National Quality Forum. (2016). *Reports*. Retrieved June 26, 2016, from http://www.qualityforum.org/Publications.aspx; Press Ganey. (2020). *Capture nursing-specific measure: Assess performance across domains that drive nursing excellence*. Retrieved December 3, 2020, from https://www.pressganey.com/solutions/clinical-excellence/capture-nursing-specific-measures

QI competencies include identifying areas of practice for quality monitoring; using indicators to monitor the quality, safety, and effectiveness of practice; collecting, analyzing, and interpreting data to improve practice; developing, implementing, and evaluating policies,

procedures, and guidelines to improve quality of practice; and analyzing factors, systems, and processes to remove barriers to safety and quality. To practice ethically, nurses must assert themselves when needed to question practices that may endanger client safety, jeopardize the best interests of consumers, or affect QI (Standard 7, Ethics).

To facilitate attainment of Standard 15 (Quality of Practice), the ANA has compiled the National Database of Nursing Quality Indicators (NDNQI), which addresses the structures, processes, and outcomes of nursing care. The database collects information and reports some findings to the NQF. Specific data collected by the NDNQI include information on client falls; fall injuries; pressure injuries; physical/sexual assault; all aspects of pain assessment and management; peripheral IV infiltration; use of physical restraints; health care–associated infections (e.g., central line, ventilator-associated pneumonia, catheter-associated urinary tract infections); nursing staff mix; nursing care hours provided per client day; nurse turnover; RN education/certification; and RN practice environment scales and job satisfaction (ANA, 2010; Press Ganey, 2020). In 2014, Press Ganey acquired the NDNQI from the ANA (Press Ganey, 2015).

In daily practice, nurses collect data that substantiate adherence to Centers for Disease Control and Prevention (CDC) and institutional standards for care when they document routine care processes. Some institutions have a quality council that determines what work processes need evaluation to determine QI opportunities. For example, for hospitals to receive third-party reimbursement for IV tubing and supplies, the information must be documented in client medical records. If a hospital is interested in determining how well nurses are following CDC and institutional standards for IV therapy, the nurse working at the bedside is the best-qualified person to perform EHR audits (a review of records) to identify when nurses are changing IV sites and tubing. After audit data are tabulated, nurses receive the results. If results reveal that standards are not being followed, a QI team analyzes the work processes for changing IV sites and tubing. Depending on the outcome of the analysis, the team then determines how to change work processes and provides staff education to ensure that all nurses follow outlined processes rather than taking shortcuts. However, if the chart audits reveal that the performance meets or exceeds the desired performance, some form of recognition is given to the staff responsible for effective IV management.

Because cost-effectiveness has been identified as an indicator of quality health care, nurses in clinical practice look for ways to use human and material resources judiciously. Professional nurses use cost-effective strategies when they take time to attend to the little details associated with care delivery that, if ignored, could result in poor client outcomes.

Role of Critical Thinker

Critical thinking is an essential cognitive skill used by nurses in clinical decision making. To ensure safe and quality nursing care delivery, professional nurses engage in multiple activities requiring critical thinking, from determining what assessments are appropriate for a clinical situation to evaluating how well clients have met desired care outcomes.

Nurses use critical thinking to develop theoretical approaches to evaluate and improve the quality of nursing care (Sidani et al., 2004). Five key characteristics produce direct effects on client outcomes, thereby accounting for individual and variable responses to nursing and health care interventions.

1. Client characteristics: Personal, factors and social determinants of health
2. Professional characteristics: Personal factors (dedication, commitment, and finding meaning in work), educational preparation, keeping current with new practice advances, and sociocultural factors
3. Health care setting: Physical layout, availability of supplies, and organizational culture
4. Health care interventions for client: Invasiveness, risks, type, and if individualized to specific client
5. Nature and timing or attainment of expected outcomes for health care interventions

---

Concepts in Practice [IDEA] → [PLAN] → [ACTION]

Mediating Variables in a Client Case

Mr. Jones is a client with a preexisting condition of diabetes and knows that recovering from an infection is a complex process. He notices that his right leg has become warm, red, and swollen after his beloved cat scratched him 3 days ago. He opts to seek care for the infection in a large teaching hospital where there will be multiple specialty physicians available to attend to his complex needs, especially an endocrinologist who will manage his blood sugar.

Mr. Jones knows that in clients with limited access to veins for starting an IV for antibiotics, the hospital uses an IV team to initiate IV lines. He anticipates being on antibiotics for a long time and will request the insertion of a peripherally inserted central catheter (PICC) so that the number of sticks to maintain an IV line will be limited.

Mr. Jones is admitted to the hospital, and his antibiotics are not started until 6 hours after admission because of the need for the IV team to insert a PICC. Knowing the risks of bloodstream infections with central catheter use, Eugenia, the nurse recognizes that Mr. Jones will be at higher risk for a bloodstream infection because of his diabetes. She also realizes that the delay in starting the antibiotic means that Mr. Jones also has an increased risk of systemic complication from his right leg cellulitis.

Sidani and team (2004) also identified two forms of indirect effects: "moderating and mediating" (p. 61). Moderating effects address the effectiveness of care to produce desired outcomes according to different levels of the five factors. An example of this would be how soon a client admitted to the hospital for a severe infection receives the first dose of an antibiotic. Mediating effects explain variance based on all factor effects on the intervention provided to the client (see Concepts in Practice, "Mediating Variables in a Client Case").

A nursing-specific theoretical approach to evaluate nursing care is more valuable to nurses than relying on approaches used by medicine or business. As critical thinkers, nurses who use a theoretical approach can generate questions to gather data for a holistic approach to nursing care concerns and choose instruments to consistently measure the effects of nursing care. A theoretical approach also fosters an understanding of the unique contributions nurses make in the health care setting. A consistent approach to evaluating nursing care fosters QI initiatives because comparisons can be tracked over time.

Role of Client Advocate

Nurses work hard to consider the client's best interests. When participating in QI activities, nurses advocate for all clients. Improvements in work processes reduce care errors.

For example, nurses who acknowledge the effects of physical and mental fatigue advocate for clients when they refuse to work overtime. Nurses who provide direct client care services for 12.5 hours or longer triple the chance of making errors (Rogers et al., 2004). Working extra shifts also increases the chance of committing nursing care errors (IOM, 2004; Rogers et al., 2004). However, despite the research evidence linking long shifts and overtime to nursing errors, some nurses volunteer for overtime shifts to fill staffing shortages. Some institutions require nurses to work overtime. Many nurses consider long hours and overtime acceptable and agree to work them despite the effects of fatigue on judgment. Nurses who refuse extra shifts may be perceived as not being good members of the nursing care team. Nevertheless, refusing to work long hours and overtime may be the best way to prevent nursing care errors, increasing the quality of health care services while ultimately looking out for the client's best interests.

Role of Change Agent

Professional nurses act as change agents when they identify necessary changes in work processes to improve the quality of nursing care. Change occurs rapidly in the health care arena. As new health care devices, medications, and treatment advances become available, nurses need to change practice procedures. Because they are stakeholders in the delivery of health care services, nurses must continuously determine which rituals and routines remain applicable and which should be discarded (Porter-O'Grady & Malloch, 2018).

As leaders of a nursing care team, professional nurses must clearly communicate changes in practice procedures to all team members. Some staff members (especially those who have worked in nursing for a long time) need to learn new approaches, new skills, and new equipment procedures. Replacing traditional practice may create distress for some older nurses. Successful integration of change requires that the innovation fits well with the practice setting, has congruence with staff roles, improves client outcomes, and complements values and beliefs. Empowering staff to make work-related decisions and empowering clients to assume responsibility for their own health increases the chance of successful change (Porter-O'Grady & Malloch, 2018). Because change requires unlearning old ways and learning new ones, the role of counselor/teacher becomes critical.

Role of Counselor/Teacher

Before adopting an innovation, the staff must be educated about the reasons for the innovation, changes in practice policies, and how to operate new equipment, if applicable. Staff educational programs may be planned using the teaching/learning principles outlined in Chapter 17, "Leadership and Management in Professional Nursing." Interdepartmental educational programs provide staff with the opportunity to network, share successes with change, and support each other.

Along with education, nurses and other care providers need emotional support during times of change. Psychological effects of change are discussed in Chapter 17, "Leadership and Management in Professional Nursing." Staff need time to grieve for the way things have been done traditionally before they can fully embrace innovations. When the innovation process becomes tough or stagnant, staff relationships may be the only glue holding the nursing care team together. Taking time to listen to peers and team members fosters capturing the messages and the meanings that surround continual change processes associated with TQM/CQI programs (Porter-O'Grady & Malloch, 2018).

Role of Coordinator

As coordinators of care, professional nurses must seek ways to provide quality care while using resources effectively. Nursing unit characteristics directly affect client outcomes. Increased nurse perception of autonomy and collaboration has been instrumental in reducing incidences of urinary tract infections and failure-to-rescue events. When specialized nurses provide care with continuity, lower rates of pneumonia and cardiac arrests are reported along with shorter length of hospital stays. Likewise, high levels of nurse manager support have been associated with reduced levels of pressure injury prevalence in clients and client mortality (Aiken et al., 1994, 2000; Boyle, 2004; Haven & Aiken, 1999; Porter-O'Grady & Malloch, 2018; Twigg et al., 2012).

Role of Colleague

American culture traditionally values independence and self-sufficiency. Nurses frequently have a strong sense of responsibility for individual vigilance that emphasizes independence and self-sufficiency. Some nurses believe that asking for help with client assignments might be viewed as a sign of incompetence, whereas others are afraid of being perceived as weak if they need to ask for assistance with a problem. The CQI process discourages this line of thinking, instead giving all health team members the responsibility to point out work process flaws.

As a colleague on an interdisciplinary health care team, nurses have an equal responsibility to engage in collaboration with team members to promote safe, effective health care delivery. Nurses have the responsibility to share concerns about clients when they arise with other members of the health care team.

Establishment of a culture of safety in health care organizations requires trust among nurses, physicians, hospital administration, and all health team members. A culture of safety uses errors as an opportunity for learning rather than blaming. Team training for client emergencies using simulated experiences helps team members identify each other's roles, learn how to best execute their roles confidently, create a venue to dispel stereotypes associated with each team member, and provide an opportunity for collegial networking (Barnsteiner et al., 2007; Finkelman, 2017; Grey & Connolly, 2008; Weaver, 2008).

When flaws are identified with work processes, multidisciplinary CQI teams are formed. Participation in the QI project team provides opportunities for nurses to network with other members of the health care team, thereby strengthening working relationships with them. During team deliberations, members of the CQI team have opportunities to see and value the unique skills and approaches they bring to client health care delivery.

Take Note!
Effective teamwork facilitates safety and quality in health care.

▮ QUESTIONS FOR REFLECTION

1. Can you think of other roles held by nurses that might affect QI efforts?
2. Which of the nursing roles discussed do you believe is most critical to QI? Why?

AN INTEGRATED APPROACH TO QUALITY IMPROVEMENT AND SAFETY IN HEALTH CARE

Since the inception of nursing, nurses have assumed the obligation of keeping clients safe. Improving the quality and safety of health care requires a fully integrated approach from all stakeholders. CQI initiatives from various stakeholders tend to overlap. Nurse educators establish desired knowledge, skills, and attitudes associated with each QSEN competency to provide guidance for basic and continuing nursing education.

The competencies, standards, and safety goals of these organizations cross the entire health care continuum; although they differ slightly, improving the quality and safety of health care delivery is the ultimate goal of each group.

Effectiveness and safety are two hallmarks of quality health care (Sollecito & Johnson, 2020; Swanwick & Vaux, 2020). To ensure fiscally responsible tax expenditures, the federal government no longer covers expenses incurred from hospital-acquired injuries and illnesses. The government also bestows awards (e.g., the Baldrige National Quality Award) and recognizes health care organizations by publishing lists for consumer use to facilitate decision making about where to access quality health care. TJC publishes and posts online lists of fully accredited providers along with deficiencies found in others. For-profit health care insurance companies sometimes follow the lead of the federal government in these ways of cutting health care costs.

Consumers play a key role in CQI and safety in health care. When they enter the health care system, consumers must communicate their needs to providers. Consumers also need to freely share all information (such as a complete list of all medications, including those obtained over the counter, herbal supplements, and other home remedies) that could impact the health care provider's decisions for a safe treatment plan. Consumers are more apt to share detailed information when providers develop helping and healing relationships with them (see Chapter 4, "Establishing Helping and Healing Relationships"). Along with freely shared information about themselves, consumers provide valuable input into health care delivery processes when they complete satisfaction questionnaires for rendered services.

The development of a culture of safety and quality may mean that some stakeholders might have to change behaviors and attitudes. When all have access to knowledge and take time to listen to each other, health care safety and quality improve. Everyone involved in health care delivery becomes capable of making evidence-based decisions. Evidence ranges from individual client values and preferences to a meta-analysis of research studies and/or clinical trials to determine best practices.

Take Note!
Many people play key roles in developing and maintaining a culture of safety and quality for health care.

Summary and Significance to Practice

The process of delivering high-quality and safe health care is highly complex. Professional nurses use cognitive, communication, and clinical skills when working as partners with clients and in multidisciplinary teams. CQI programs look for opportunities to change the processes of health care delivery in order to improve safety, effectiveness, client focus, and efficiency. When nurses and health team members subscribe to a CQI approach, they constantly look for ways to improve care delivery. Professional nurses bring a unique perspective and offer valuable skills to enhance health care quality. All health team members must be invested in developing and maintaining a culture of safety and CQI to maximize the quality of health care services.

REAL-LIFE REFLECTIONS

Recall Laura from the beginning of the chapter, who was unable to administer the client antibiotic as ordered. What advice would you give her based on the information presented in this chapter? Do you feel that writing a care variance report is a sign of professional weakness? Why or why not? What suggestions would you make to improve unit practices to prevent a similar error from occurring again?

From Theory to Practice

1. Do you think the health care industry should be held to the same quality standards as those in business and industry? Why or why not?
2. How would you have to change your practice and practice environment to attain the same level of quality that is required of the business and manufacturing industries?
3. How does your clinical practice setting view incident reports? What are the advantages of having staff complete incident reports for quality monitoring purposes? Are you afraid to complete incident reports? Why or why not?
4. How would you change your nursing program to improve its quality? What steps would you take to present these ideas to nursing program administration? Would you be afraid to share your ideas with program administration? Why or why not?

Nurse as Author

In four to six paragraphs, report on how you have seen CQI used in a clinical setting among an interprofessional health care team. How did this collaboration enhance the quality of client care? In what ways did the collaboration fall short? Using one of the QI processes outlined in this chapter, briefly describe a way to improve such interprofessional collaboration in a clinical practice setting.

Your Digital Classroom

Online Exploration

Baldrige Performance Excellence Program: **https://www.nist.gov/baldrige**
   Institute for Healthcare Improvement: **www.ihi.org**
   Juran Institute: **https://www.juran.com**
   National Quality Forum: **www.qualityforum.org**
   The Joint Commission: **www.jointcommission.org**
   The W. Edwards Deming Institute: **deming.org**

Expanding Your Understanding

1. Visit the NQF and TJC websites, and compare the information you find. Which site do you think offers the best information for nurses? Why? Which site offers the best health-related information for consumers? Why?
2. Visit the Juran Institute, and read the case study on "Improving Patient Satisfaction Via Lean Six Sigma" at **https://www.juran.com/results/case-studies/patient-satisfaction-improve-patient-experience/**. What are your initial reactions to the process used by this health care organization? Do you think it would be viable in your practice work setting if you are an RN or in your assigned clinical unit if you are a nursing student? Why or why not?
3. Visit "Quality Check" at **http://www.qualitycheck.org**. Type in your zip code, and click "Locate" to see if there are any facilities close to you that have the TJC Gold Seal of Approval. Make a list of things you would want to have in place if you were to go to a hospital. Is the hospital where you would likely seek care on the list? Would this information change your mind about where to seek care? Why or why not?

Beyond the Book

Visit thePoint® at **www.thePoint.lww.com** for activities and information to reinforce the concepts and content covered in this chapter.

REFERENCES

Aiken, L., Clarke, P., & Sloane, D. (2000). Hospital restructuring: Does it adversely affect care and outcomes? *Journal of Nursing Administration*, *30*, 457–465. Retrieved May 1, 2021, from https://journals.lww.com/jonajournal/Abstract/2000/10000/Hospital_Restructuring__Does_It_Adversely_Affect.3.aspx

Aiken, L., Smith, H., & Lake, E. (1994). Lower Medicare mortality among a set of hospitals known for good nursing care. *Medical Care*, *32*, 771–787. Retrieved May 1, 2021, from https://www.jstor.org/stable/3766652?seq=1m

American Association of Colleges of Nursing. (2021). The Essentials: Core competencies for professional nursing education. Retrieved June 15, 2021, from https://www.aacnnursing.org/Portals/42/AcademicNursing/pdf/Essentials-2021.pdf

American Nurses Association. (2010). *NDNQI: Transforming data into quality care.* Retrieved March 10, 2013, from https://www.nursingquality.org/discover.aspx

American Nurses Association. (2013). *Safe staffing saves lives: Safe nursing staffing poll results.* Retrieved February 6, 2013, from http://www.safestaffingsaveslives.org/WhatisANADoing/PollResults.aspx

American Nurses Association. (2015). *Nursing: Scope and standards of practice* (3rd ed.). Author.

Aspen, P., Walcott, J., Bootman, L., & Cronenwett, L.; the Committee on Identifying and Preventing Medication Errors (Eds.). (2007). *Identifying and preventing medication errors.* National Academies Press.

Balik, B. (2016). *What is an 'Always event'?* Retrieved July 1, 2016, from http://www.ihi.org/education/IHIOpenSchool/resources/Pages/Activities/Balik-WhatIsAnAlwaysEvent.aspx

Barnsteiner, J., Disch, J., Hall, L., Mayer, D., & Moore, S. (2007). Promoting interprofessional education. *Nursing Outlook*, *55*(3), 144–150. https://doi.org/10.1016/j.outlook.2007.03.003

Batalden, P., & Davidoff, F. (2007). What is "quality improvement" and how can it transform health care? *Quality and Safety in Health Care*, *16*, 2–3. https://doi.org/10.1136/qshc.2006.022046

Boltz, M., Capezuti, E., Fulmer, T., & Zwicker, D. (2012). *Evidence-based geriatric nursing protocols for best practice* (4th ed.). Springer Publishing.

Boyle, S. (2004). Nursing unit characteristics and patient outcomes. *Nursing Economic$*, *22*, 111–123. Retrieved May 1, 2021, from https://www.researchgate.net/publication/8496149_Nursing_Unit_Characteristics_and_Patient_Outcomes

Brady, J. (2015). *Health care safety: Progress & opportunities.* Retrieved June 6, 2021 from https://www.genome.gov/Pages/Research/ResearchFunding/DGM/HealthCare_Safety_052115.pdf

Centers for Medicare and Medicaid Services. (2020). *The hospital value-based purchasing system.* Retrieved December 2, 2020, from https://www.cms.gov/Medicare/Quality-Initiatives-Patient-Assessment-Instruments/Value-Based-Programs/HVBP/Hospital-Value-Based-Purchasing

Chowdhury, S. (2002). *The power of six sigma.* Dearborn Trade.

Cooper, C. H., Tupper, R., & Holm L. (2016). Interruptions during medication administration: A descriptive study. *MEDSURG Nursing*, *25*(3), 186–191. Retrieved May 1, 2021, from https://www.thefreelibrary.com/Interruptions+during+medication+administration%3a+a+descriptive+study.-a0456907463

Cronenwett, L. (2012). *A national initiative: Quality and safety education for nurses (QSEN).* In G. Sherwood & J. Barnsteiner (Eds.), *Quality and safety in nursing, a competency approach to improving outcomes* (pp. 49–64). John Wiley & Sons, Inc.

Crosby, P. (1979). *Quality is free: The art of making quality certain.* Mentor.

Doran, D. (Ed.). (2003). *Nursing-sensitive outcomes: State of the science.* Jones & Bartlett.

Duffour, M. N. (2019). Filling voice promotion gaps in healthcare through a comparative analysis of error reporting and learning systems and open communication and disclosure policies in the United States and Germany. *American Journal of Law & Medicine*, *44*(4), 579–605. https://doi.org/10.1177/0098858818821137

Dunton, J., Montalvo, I., & Dunton, N. (2011). *NDNQI case studies in nursing quality improvement.* American Nurses Association.

Dunton, N. (2008). Take a cue from the NDNQI. *Nursing Management*, *39*(4), 20, 22, 23. https://doi.org/10.1097/01.NUMA.0000316054.35317.bf

Evans, K. (2020). *Models of improvement.* In T. Swanwick & E. Vaux (Eds.), *ABC of quality improvement in healthcare* (pp. 14–20). John Wiley & Sons, Inc.

Finkelman A., & Kenner, C. (2007). Teaching IOM/HMD: Implications of the Institute of Medicine & Health and Medicine Division reports for nursing education, (4th ed.). American Nurses Association.

Foster, S. (2020). Just culture and staff wellbeing. *British Journal of Nursing*, *29*(6), 381. https://doi.org/10.12968/bjon.2020.29.6.381

Future of Nursing Campaign for Action. (2021). *Welcome to the future of nursing: Campaign for action dashboard.* Retrieved April 2021 from https://campaignforaction.org/wp-content/uploads/2020/09/dashboard-indicator-updates-Winter2021.pdf

Gander, P., O'Keeffe, K., Santos-Fernandez, E., Huntington, A., Walker, L., & Willis, J. (2020). Development and evaluation of a matrix for assessing fatigue-related risk, derived from a national survey of nurses' work patterns. *International Journal of Nursing Studies*, *112*, 103573. https://doi.org/10.1016/j.ijnurstu.2020.103573

Gigli, K. H., Davis, B. S., Ervin, J., & Kahn, J. M. (2020). Factors associated with nurses' knowledge of and perceived value in evidence-based practices. *American Journal of Critical Care*, *29*(1), e1–e8. https://doi.org/10.4037/ajcc2020866

Gill, C. J., & Gill, G. C. (2005). Nightingale in Scutari: Her legacy reexamined. *Clinical Infectious Diseases*, *40*(12), 1799–1905. https://doi.org/10.1086/430380

Grey, M., & Connolly, C. (2008). "Coming together, keeping together, working together": Interdisciplinary to transdisciplinary research and nursing. *Nursing Outlook*, *56*(5), 102–107. https://doi.org/10.1016/j.outlook.2008.02.007

Hall, L., Peterson, J., Baker, G. R., Brown, A. D., Pink, G. H., McKillop, I., Daniel, I., & Pedersen, C. (2008). Nursing staffing and system integration and change indicators in acute care hospitals: Evidence from a balanced scorecard. *Journal of Nursing Care Quality*, *23*(3), 24–52. https://doi.org/10.1097/01.NCQ.0000324589.91837.cd

Haven, D., & Aiken, L. (1999). Shaping systems to promote desired outcomes. *Journal of Nursing Administration*, *29*, 14–20. Retrieved May 1, 2021, from https://www.nursingcenter.com/journalarticle?Article_ID=102058

Health Resources and Services Administration, *National Center for Workforce Analysis.* (2019). *Nursing education and practice programs, academic Year 2018–2019.* Retrieved June 6,

2020, from https://bhw.hrsa.gov/sites/default/files/bureau-health-workforce/funding/nursing-education-practice-programs-2019.pdf

Institute for Healthcare Improvement. (2018). *More than 25 years of driving improvement*. Retrieved December 4, 2020, from http://www.ihi.org/about/pages/history.aspx

Institute for Healthcare Improvement. (2020a). *About us. Vision, mission and values*. Retrieved December 4, 2020, from http://www.ihi.org/about/Pages/IHIVisionandValues.aspx

Institute for Healthcare Improvement. (2020b). *Ready to start improving?* Retrieved December 4, 2020, from http://www.ihi.org/education/ihiopenschool/Pages/default.aspx

Institute for Healthcare Improvement. (2020c). *IHI triple aim measures*. Retrieved December 3, 2020, from http://www.ihi.org/Engage/Initiatives/TripleAim/Pages/MeasuresResults.aspx

Institute of Medicine. (2000). *To err is human: Building a safer health system*. National Academies Press.

Institute of Medicine. (2001). *Crossing the quality chasm: A new health system for the 21st century*. National Academies Press.

Institute of Medicine. (2003). *Health professions education: A bridge to quality*. National Academies Press.

Institute of Medicine. (2004). *Keeping patients safe: Transforming the work environment of nurses*. National Academies Press.

Institute of Medicine. (2011). *The future of nursing, leading change, advancing health*. National Academies Press.

International Organizations for Standardization. (2017). *About ISO*. Retrieved April 14, 2017, from https://www.iso.org/about-us.html

James, J. T. (2013). A new, evidence-based estimate of patient harms associated with hospital care. *Journal of Patient Safety*, *9*(3), 122–128. https://doi.org/10.1097/PTS.0b013e3182948a69

Joint Commission International. (2020a). *Our purpose*. Retrieved November 30, 2020, from https://www.jointcommissioninternational.org/about-jci/

Joint Commission International. (2020b). *World Patient Safety Day. Health care safety worker checklists: Protecting those who serve*. Retrieved November 30, 2020, from https://www.jointcommissioninternational.org/products-and-services/publications/books-and-e-books/world-patient-safety-day-2020/

Joshi, M. S., Ransom, E. R., Nash, D. B., & Ransom, S. B. (2014). *The healthcare quality book, vision strategy and tools* (3rd ed.). Health Administration Press & Association of University Programs in Health Administration.

Joyner, J. C., & Kreitzer, M. J. (2021). *Patient engagement and public policy*. In D. J. Mason, E. Dickson, M. R. McLemore, & G. A. Perez (Eds.), *Policy & politics in nursing and health care* (8th ed., pp. 171–179). Elsevier.

Juran, J. (1989). *Juran on leadership for quality*. Free Press.

Kalisch, B. J., & Lee, K. H. (2010). The impact of teamwork on missed nursing care. *Nursing Outlook*, *58*(5), 233–241. https://doi.org/10.1016/j.outlook.2010.06.004

Kalisch, B. J., & Williams, R. A. (2009). Development and psychometric testing of a tool to measure missed nursing care. *Journal of Nursing Administration*, *39*(5), 211–219. https://doi.org/10.1097/NNA.0b013e3181a23cf5

Kalisch, P. A., & Kalisch, B. J. (2004). *The advance of American nursing* (4th ed.). Lippincott Williams & Wilkins.

Makary, M. A., & Daniel, M. (2016). Medical error: The third leading cause of death in the U.S. *British Medical Journal*, *353*, i2139. https://doi.org/10.1136/bmj.i2139

McMullen, S. L., Kozik, C. A., Meyers, G., Keenan, K., Wheelock, M., & Kalman, M. (2017). CNE SERIES. Improving nursing care: Examining errors of omission. *MEDSURG Nursing*, *26*(1), 9–19. Retrieved May 1, 2021, from https://www.thefreelibrary.com/Improving+nursing+care%3a+examining+errors+of+omission.-a0482392057

Morgan, S., & Cooper, C. (2004). Shoulder work intensity with six sigma. *Nursing Management*, *35*, 28–32. Retrieved May 1, 2021, from https://journals.lww.com/nursingmanagement/Fulltext/2004/03000/Shoulder_work_intensity_with_Six_Sigma.12.aspx

National Institute of Standards and Technology. (2017). *Southcentral foundation*. Retrieved December 3, 2020, from https://www.nist.gov/baldrige/southcentral-foundation-2017

National Institute of Standards and Technology. (2019a). *Core values and concepts*. Retrieved December 3, 2020, from https://www.nist.gov/baldrige/core-values-and-concepts

National Institute of Standards and Technology. (2019b). *State, local and regional Baldrige-based award programs*. Retrieved December 3, 2020, from https://www.nist.gov/baldrige/how-baldrige-works/baldrige-community/state-local-baldrige-based-programs

National Institute of Standards and Technology. (2020a). *Baldrige excellence framework*. Retrieved December 3, 2020, from https://www.nist.gov/baldrige/publications/baldrige-excellence-framework

National Institute of Standards and Technology. (2020b). *Malcolm Baldrige quality award*. Retrieved December 3, 2020, from https://www.nist.gov/baldrige/baldrige-award#:~:text=The%20Malcolm%20Baldrige%20National%20Quality%20Award%20is%20the,receive%20the%20award%20for%20specific%20products%20or%20servicesNational Quality Forum. (2020a). *About us*. Retrieved December 2, 2020, from https://www.qualityforum.org/About_NQF/

National Quality Forum. (2020b). *NQF's history*. Retrieved December 2, 2020, from https://www.qualityforum.org/about_nqf/history/

National Quality Forum. (2020c). *NQF members: Leading the quality community*. Retrieved December 2, 2020, from https://www.qualityforum.org/membership/

National Quality Forum. (2020d). *NQF's mission, vision and values*. Retrieved December 2, 2020, from https://www.qualityforum.org/about_nqf/mission_and_vision/

National Quality Forum. (2020e). *NQF's work in quality measurement*. Retrieved December 2, 2020, from https://www.qualityforum.org/what_we_do.aspx

Ouchi, W. (1981). *Theory Z: How American business can meet the Japanese challenge*. Addison Wesley.

Pande, P., Neuman, R., & Cavanagh, R. (2000). *The six sigma way: How GE, Motorola and other top companies are honing their performance*. McGraw-Hill.

Park, S., Blegen, M., Spetz, J., Chapman, S, & De Groot, H. (2012). Patient turnover and the relationship between nurse staffing and patient outcomes. *Research in Nursing & Health*, *35*, 277–288. https://doi.org/10.1002/nur.21474

Popovich, E., Wiggin, H., & Barach, P. (2020). *Lean and six sigma management: Building a foundation for optimal patient care using patient flow physics*. In J. K. Johnson & W. A. Sollecito (Eds.), *McLaughlin & Kaluzny's continuous quality improvement in health care* (5th ed., pp. 143–174). Jones & Bartlett Learning.

Porter-O'Grady, T., & Malloch, K. (2018). *Quantum leadership: Creating sustainable value in health care* (5th ed.). Jones & Bartlett Learning.

Press Ganey. (2015). *Press Ganey acquires national database of nursing quality indicators NDNQI®*. Retrieved May 1, 2021, from https://www.pressganey.com/resources/reports/press-ganey-acquires-national-database-of-nursing-quality-indicators-(ndnqi-)

Press Ganey. (2020). *Capture nursing-specific measure: Assess performance across domains that drive nursing excellence*. Retrieved May 1, 2021, from https://www.pressganey.com/solutions/clinical-excellence/capture-nursing-specific-measures

QSEN. (2020). *The QSEN news November 2020*. Retrieved December 2, 2020, from http://hosted.verticalresponse.com/1428573/182fb5b4e6/578281903/ba324c8ec8/

Roche, M., Duffield, C., Aisbett, C., Diers, D., & Stasa, H. (2012). Nursing work directions in Australia: Does evidence drive the policy? *Collegian, 18*(4), 231–238. https://doi.org/10.1016/j.colegn.2012.03.006

Rogers, A., Hwang, W., Scott, L., Aiken, L., & Dinges, D. (2004). The working hours of hospital staff nurses and patient safety. *Health Affairs, 23*, 202–212. https://doi.org/10.1377/hlthaff.23.4.202

Schroers, G., Ross, J. G., & Moriarty, H. (2021). Nurses' perceived causes of medication administration errors: A qualitative systematic review. *Joint Commission Journal on Quality & Patient Safety, 47*(1), 38–53. https://doi.org/10.1016/j.jcjq.2020.09.010

Scott, L. D., Hofmeister, N., Rogness, N., & Rogers, A. E. (2010). An interventional approach for patient and nurse safety: A fatigue countermeasures feasibility study. *Nursing Research, 59*(4), 250–258. https://doi.org/10.1097/NNR.0b013e3181de9116

Sherr, K., Fernandes, Q., Kanté, A. M., Bawah, A., Condo, J., Mutale, W., & AHI PHIT Partnership Collaborative. (2017). Measuring health systems strength and its impact: Experiences from the African Health Initiative. *BMC Health Services Research, 17*, 29–38. https://doi.org/10.1186/s12913-017-2658-5

Sidani, S., Doran, D., & Mitchell, P. (2004). A theory-driven approach to evaluating quality of nursing care. *Journal of Nursing Scholarship, 36*, 60–65. https://doi.org/10.1111/j.1547-5069.2004.04014.x

Sollecito, W. A., & Hardison, D. (2020). *Understanding variation, tools, and data sources for CQI in health care*. In J. K. Johnson & W. A. Sollecito (Eds.), *McLaughlin & Kaluzny's continuous quality improvement in health care* (5th ed., pp. 107–142). Jones & Bartlett Learning.

Sollecito, W. A., & Johnson, J. K. (2020). *The global evolution of continuous quality improvement: From Japanese manufacturing to global health services*. In J. K. Johnson & W. A. Sollecito (Eds.), *McLaughlin & Kaluzny's continuous quality improvement in health care* (5th ed., pp. 1–31). Jones & Bartlett Learning.

Sultz, H., & Young, K. (2004). *Healthcare USA: Understanding its organization and delivery* (4th ed.). Jones & Bartlett.

Swanwick, T., & Vaux, E. (2020). *What is quality:?* In T. Swanwick & E. Vaux (Eds.), *ABC of quality improvement in healthcare* (pp. 1–4). John Wiley & Sons, Inc.

The Joint Commission. (2013a). *Nursing advisory council fact sheet*. Retrieved March 10, 2013, from http://www.jointcommission.org/assets/q1/18/Nursing_Advisory_Council2.pdf

The Joint Commission. (2013b). *Core measure sets*. Retrieved March 10, 2013, from http://www.jointcommission.org/core_measure_sets.aspx

The Joint Commission. (2013c). *Facts about the joint commission*. Retrieved February 6, 2013, from http://www.jointcommission.org/about_us/fact_sheets.aspx

The Joint Commission. (2013d). *Fact about ORYX® for hospitals*. Retrieved March 10, 2013, from http://www.jointcommission.org/facts_about_oryx_for_hospitals

The Joint Commission. (2016). *Facts about the nursing advisory council*. Retrieved April 11, 2016, from https://www.jointcommission.org/facts_about_the_nursing_advisory_council/

The Joint Commission. (2020a). *Measures*. Retrieved November 30, 2020, from https://www.jointcommission.org/measurement/measures/#592065b7f1d44a5691c528709db19784_bbebaad4025e4900b8f28a00580c26c9

The Joint Commission. (2020b). *National patient safety goals effective January 2021 for the hospital program*. Retrieved November 30, 2020, from https://www.jointcommission.org/standards/national-patient-safety-goals/hospital-national-patient-safety-goals/

The Joint Commission. (2020c). *ORYX® performance measurement reporting*. Retrieved November 30, 2020, from https://www.jointcommission.org/measurement/reporting/accreditation-oryx/

The Joint Commission. (2020d). *Quality check*. Retrieved December 2, 2020, from https://www.qualitycheck.org/

The Joint Commission. (2020e). *Speak up campaigns*. Retrieved December 2, 2020, from https://www.jointcommission.org/resources/for-consumers/speak-up-campaigns/#first=10

The Joint Commission. (2020f). *The value of Joint Commission accreditation and certification*. Retrieved November 30, 2020, from https://www.qualitycheck.org/the-value-of-accreditation-certification/The Leapfrog Group. (n.d.-a). *About us*. Retrieved December 4, 2020, from https://www.leapfroggroup.org/about

The Leapfrog Group. (n.d.-b). *Expert panelists*. Retrieved December 4, 2020, from https://www.leapfroggroup.org/about/expert-panelists

The Leapfrog Group. (n.d.-c). *Mission and vision*. Retrieved December 4, 2020, from https://www.leapfroggroup.org/about/mission-and-vision

The Leapfrog Group. (2020a). *Employers rank CIGNA highest, UnitedHealthcare lowest for driving health care quality in a new survey of employee benefits executives*. Retrieved December 4, 2020 from https://www.leapfroggroup.org/news-events/employers-rank-cigna-highest-unitedhealthcare-lowest-driving-health-care-quality-new

The Leapfrog Group. (2020b). *History*. Retrieved December 4, 2020, from https://www.leapfroggroup.org/about/history

Twigg, D., Duffield, C., Bremner, A., Rapley, P., & Finn, J. (2012). Impact of skill mix variations on patient outcomes following implementation of nursing hours per patient day staffing: A retrospective study. *Journal of Advanced Nursing, 68*(12), 2710–2718. http://dx.doi.org/10.1111/j.1365-2648.2012.05971.x

Walton, M. (1986). *The Deming management method*. Putman.

Weaver, T. (2008). Enhancing multiple disciplinary teamwork. *Nursing Outlook, 56*(3), 108–114. https://doi.org/10.1016/j.outlook.2008.03.013

The Professional Nurse's Role in Public Policy

LEARNING OUTCOMES

By the end of this chapter, the learner will be able to:

1. Define the terms politics, public policy, political competence, lobbyist, and political action committee.
2. Explain the key concepts and relationships of the Kingdon model for agenda development and policy formation.
3. List the strategies used to lobby elected officials.
4. Outline a plan for a personal visit with an elected official.
5. Discuss the key elements of effectively written letters to elected officials.
6. Differentiate between the roles of lobbyists and political action committees.
7. Specify strategies to stay abreast of current legislative and public policy issues.

REAL-LIFE REFLECTIONS

As a result of budget cuts and loss of grant funding, school districts in Florida no longer have the resources to provide registered nurses (RNs) for student health services. Some counties in the state have a licensed practical nurse (LPN) in every school who keeps records of specific health encounters with students. In other schools, students, health issues, and concerns are managed by health aides, teachers, or school staff members, resulting in many children automatically being sent home for complaints of physical illness. Without RNs to manage complex chronic student illnesses, provide preventive health care services, and develop and implement health promotion education, there has been an increase in adolescent health problems, including alcohol abuse, drug abuse, sexually transmitted infections, teenage pregnancy, obesity, and immunization noncompliance.

Several nurses with school-aged children band together to work to overturn state policy. Assuming the roles of client advocate and change agent, these nurses approach the members of the state legislature and the governor to see if they would propose legislation mandating "an RN in every school." They cite the example of Delaware, which requires an RN in every school (Roth, 2011).

Assisting to draft legislation to make violence against health care workers illegal, petitioning the city to install stoplights at a busy intersection, visiting an elected official to discuss supporting nurse-friendly legislation, and volunteering for a candidate's campaign are some examples of how professional nurses can influence public policy. Governmental and institutional policies greatly affect nursing practice and health care delivery.

This chapter provides an overview of public policies, including the various levels of governmental influence on the development and implementation of public policies and how nurses influence public policies. It offers strategies for nurses to use when working with people in charge of public policy development and implementation. Finally, it highlights nurses who have influenced public policy development and outlines strategies to help other nurses learn the art and science of political action.

Politics plays a key role in policy development. *Merriam-Webster's Collegiate Dictionary* (11th edition) defines politics as "1. the art or science of governmental policy; 2. The art or science of guiding or influencing governmental policy" (Mish, 2020, p. 960). Being "political" means being engaged in the process of policy development. Frequently, political action means "taking sides or prudently crafting a plan." People use political activities to influence policy development, revision, and implementation. Most laws are public policies, but not all public policies are laws. Some policies may evolve into law. Laws are a set of established rules that create a system of privileges and a process for people to solve problems with minimal force. **Laws** outline and govern the relationships between citizens, between citizens and organizations, and between citizens and their government. In democratic societies, citizens use political action to influence the legislative process required for law enactment.

Once laws become established, policies must be developed to ensure their uniform enforcement. **Policies** are consciously selected courses of action such as an administrative action, law, regulation, rule, procedure, incentive, or voluntary practice of government and other institutions (Milstead & Short, 2019). Formal expressions of policy occur in position statements, resolutions, goals, objectives, programs, procedures, laws, and regulations (Mason et al., 2021; Milstead & Short, 2019). Public policy is developed and enforced by the government. Allocative policies denote decisions and actions that benefit a group of people or organizations at the expense of others. Regulator policies are decisions aimed at influencing the actions, behaviors, and decisions of people or groups to fulfill public policy objectives. The policy-making process in a nonlinear, nonsequential (and sometimes illogical) process that involves problem or issue identification; agenda setting; outlining alternative solutions; debating the alternative approaches (e.g., economic, financial, societal costs); selection of policy (usually through legislation or regulation); implementation; and evaluation of policy outcomes (Mason et al., 2021; Milstead & Short, 2019). Rules specify how things are to be done. In contrast, regulations are rules that outline the details and specifics of how laws are to be implemented. Rules and regulations may be part of legislation that is approved or they may be developed after legislation is signed into law (Loversidge, 2019).

THE KINGDON MODEL FOR POLITICAL PROCESSES

The processes of law passage and policy development are highly complex. Political action that results in policy changes requires the cooperation of legislators, special interest groups, and administrative agencies (Furlong, 2019; O'Grady, 2021). To bolster their policy-making efforts, nursing experts in political processes identify and use models from political science. The research-based **Kingdon model for political processes** attempts to make sense of the complex American political process by offering a conceptual approach that can be used by nurses to aid in the development of legislative agendas and public policies.

Kingdon's model addresses how issues become part of the political agenda and how alternative approaches for resolving them are developed. Kingdon (1995) specified that people within and outside the government play key roles in the processes of agenda development and policy formation. These processes are dynamic and fluid rather than linear and sequential and include three key streams: (1) problem streams, (2) policy streams, and (3) political streams. A window of opportunity affects each of the three streams, thereby influencing the development of an agenda.

The problem stream starts with the recognition of conditions (issues that ought to be solved). Conditions become problems when people believe that something ought to be done about them. Triggers for conditions to transform into problems might be a key study report, an unexpected crisis, media attention to an issue, or a thoughtful, well-executed plan from a special interest group (Kingdon, 1995). For example, if the unemployment rates were to rise sharply, many Americans would lose health care insurance benefits. Conditions affecting disenfranchised members of society or those without resources to grant political favors, however, are sometimes ignored (Kingdon, 1995). Sometimes, a group of people interested in publicizing an issue can develop a media campaign to illuminate the issue for the public.

The policy stream involves determining viable approaches to solving an identified problem. Stakeholders (people who have an interest in how the issue is addressed) present their views on how to best resolve it. During this phase, multiple approaches are generated and studied. Experts from the governmental, private, and academic arenas provide testimony about the issues. Before addressing the problem in the formal agenda, ideas must be "softened up," which is the process of getting people accustomed to new approaches, building support for new ideas, and gaining acceptance for new proposals (Kingdon, 1995). For example, if too many people lose health care coverage, health care providers, insurance companies, public health officials, and special interest groups might collaborate to generate alternative solutions.

The political stream aims at creating a political culture in elected bodies that supports tackling the problem. This stream involves changing the public mood, using pressure group campaigns, influencing election results, and changing the partisan composition of the legislature and administration. During this phase, coalitions are built based on negotiation and persuasion. Political parties reach consensus on campaign platforms. Frequently, trading favors becomes a key way to build coalitions (Kingdon, 1995). For example, if there were to be a spike in gun violence in schools, the political climate might indicate the need for more restrictive gun control laws and regulations. Public pressure and media advertisements might change the attitude of many citizens who believe that the right to bear arms is a basic fundamental right for all Americans and there may be real benefits toward tighter restrictions of gun ownership. Thus, the outcomes of the next election might put into office, officials who espouse to work diligently to pass strict gun control laws.

Agenda formation occurs when streams couple together during a window of opportunity. A formal agenda is developed when a group of people who share similar interests (such as a professional nursing organization) band together and decide on what issues they would like to see resolved. Members of the group agree to work toward achieving desired action on agenda issues. In the United States during general elections,

each major political party develops a platform. A party's platform is a formal agenda that outlines key positions on issues confronting American society that may be solved by changing laws or regulations (Kingdon, 1995).

According to Kingdon (1995), windows of opportunity rapidly open and close. Kingdon specified that the problem and political streams drive agenda formation, whereas alternative solutions tend to be driven by the policy stream.

Kingdon (1995) acknowledged the contributions that elected officials bring to the processes of agenda development and policy formation. Elected officials bring issues to legislative bodies that are merged to become the formal agenda. The ability of the elected official to influence formal agenda development depends on their position as a member of the body. A legislative committee chairperson determines which issues are brought before a committee, a ranking member of the minority party on a committee has the power to influence committee proceedings, and a committee member with long tenure as an elected official may be viewed as being more powerful than their colleagues. Each elected official wants to serve constituent interests to ensure reelection, enhance their reputation, and pass sound public policy legislation.

Take Note!
A political model such as Kingdon's provides a framework to understand the complex art and science of influencing public policy and guide nurses as they engage in that process.

THE NURSE'S ROLE IN INFLUENCING PUBLIC POLICY

Nurses have a great deal of knowledge about health and the delivery of health care. Practicing nurses frequently identify flaws in the health care delivery system. Although nurses represent the largest health care professional group in the United States, they have historically failed to play a proportionate role in shaping health policies for Americans at all levels of government (Mason et al., 2021; Milstead & Short, 2019). According to Wakefield (2004), nursing lacks the financial resources prevalent in more highly influential groups such as organized medicine, insurance corporations, and pharmaceutical firms. In the United States (and elsewhere), money determines how much political power and influence a group possesses.

The Nurse's Role as a Responsible Citizen

The U.S. Constitution ensures the right of American citizens to have a voice in the government. Americans have the freedom to ask questions, offer suggestions, and debate the effects of public policies.

Nurses have a history of political activism. During the women's suffrage movement of the early 1900s, the American Federation of Nursing (now the American Nurses Association [ANA]) joined forces with other women's groups to enfranchise women. Nurses quickly discovered that they could affect public policy by working independently and with other likeminded organizations to exert pressure on elected officials to develop policies that also support health promotion and disease prevention (Feldman & Lewenson, 2000).

The degree of political action varies among nurses. Cohen and colleagues (1996) outlined four stages of political activism in nursing that still apply:

1. Buying in: Nurses become aware of the importance of political activism to attain professional goals, and use the political system to provide input into public policy development.
2. Self-interest: Nurses use the political system exclusively to advance their own agenda.
3. Political sophistication: Nurses engage in complex political activity such as building coalitions and running for political office.
4. Leading the way: Nurses influence other people by holding key governmental positions and in the process select the course for public policy changes.

Nurses participate in public policy formation in a variety of ways; most nurses, however, tend to be in the first stage of political activism. Casting an informed vote during an election is the first level of responsible citizenship in a democracy. **Responsible citizenship** consists of being an active participant in the governing process. The second level of responsible citizenship is engaging in the process of affecting governmental policies. Once they are successful in affecting public policy by providing input, some nurses progress to higher levels of political activism.

Political activism in nursing started with Florence Nightingale's efforts during the Crimean War, fitting with professional nursing goals of enhancing health and improving the quality of life for all. The public perceives nurses as being trustworthy and credible. Nurses advocate for large groups of clients when they use their specialized knowledge to influence policy makers to create and fund public health programs. Nurses also have well-refined communication and assessment skills that enhance their ability to determine what types of health programs are needed (and wanted). Because they understand nursing and health-related research, nurses can present strong cases based on solid evidence to document the need for new programs and to continue existing ones. Politically active nurses frequently use the nursing process to guide their thinking for public policy development and evaluation (Mason et al., 2021; Milstead & Short, 2019).

Nurses who have **political competence** possess knowledge of the political process, a perception that they can be effective in working with the process to achieve desired results, effective communication with all involved in the political process (elected officials, their aides, persons with similar interests, other health care team members and special interest groups), and engagement in the political process (Han & Kim, 2020). When nurses have knowledge of the political process and current issues, they can systematically analyze them to present solid evidence to influence elected officials to take specific action on an issue. Political competence enables nurses to steer the direction of the profession and the delivery of health care services. In a few cases, some nurses decide to embark on a political career.

Feldman and Lewenson (2000) noted that some nurses begin political careers because of grassroots efforts to accomplish a particular public policy goal. **Grassroots efforts** start at the basic unit of society (local community or special interest group) and expand to reach more centralized areas of influence. These efforts frequently start as an action to improve a local community that snowballs into a larger action. Grassroots activities involve building coalitions, contacting and visiting elected officials, and testifying before governmental committees. When nurses successfully attain political action goals, they directly affect public policy (Mason et al., 2021; Milstead & Short, 2019). Successful grassroots efforts can be personally rewarding and can lead to the development of personal relationships with legislators and their staff members. Strong relationships with legislators and their staff members facilitate nurses getting appointments to visit with lawmakers, being sought out for providing a nursing and health care perspective to pending legislative issues, providing volunteer or civil service (e.g., membership on a governor-appointed state board of nursing, government task force, or committee), and enhancing the power of professional nurses. Participating in grassroots efforts builds the self-confidence of nurses. By following through with requests from legislators and staff who want nurse input in political processes, nurses earn the reputation that they can be trusted to get the job done.

The second stage of political activism is that of self-interest. An analysis of the current American government reveals that many times, small groups of people expend great resources and much energy to have their agendas approved (especially when competing for a piece of the federal budget). During the third stage of political activism, individuals and groups collaborate and reach consensus about how to best use available resources to better society. Running for office or receiving a political appointment to a governmental agency are the key elements of the fourth stage of political involvement (Feldman & Lewenson, 2000). Examples of nurses serving in legislative bodies and governmental posts are presented later in this chapter. There is little research that has been done to address political activity of nurses, and none has been published in the last decade in peer-reviewed journals. The Focus on Research box, "Empowerment Skills and Values among Nurses and Social Workers," describes and compares the political activity levels of nurses and social workers.

Governments and institutions create policies to achieve their missions. However, policy development and implementation are not limited to governments and institutions. Any health care–providing agency, professional organization, nonprofit organization, or family may make policies for its members to follow. Professional nurses bring special expertise to the process of developing and revising health care policies.

Take Note!

Being part of a successful grassroots effort builds the nurse's confidence and enhances the nurse's reputation.

■ QUESTIONS FOR REFLECTION

1. In which stage of political activism do you fit?
2. What are the current barriers to your participation in the political process?
3. Do you want to be more politically active? Why or why not?
4. What current behaviors do you need to change to become more politically active?

FOCUS ON RESEARCH

Empowerment Skills and Values Among Nurses and Social Workers

The investigators sought to discover the differences between nurses' and social workers' perceptions and reported actions using the skills and values of the concept of empowerment. Participants in this cross-sectional survey study included 213 social workers and 152 RNs in Israel. Participants completed Frans's Social Worker Empowerment Scale, Alperin and Richie's Social Service Skills Scale, and Schwartz's Human Values Survey.

Using multiple analysis of variance techniques, the investigators identified the following differences:

1. The nurses scored higher than social workers in knowledge, self-concept, critical awareness, and propensity to act; social workers scored higher on the scale measuring collective identity.
2. Nurses scored higher than social workers in therapeutic communication skills.
3. Social workers ranked higher than nurses in social action skills (including finding government resources, lobbying, and contacting elected officials).

4. Nurses reported having more emphasis on spiritual and material values than social workers did.
5. Social workers had higher levels of political activity than nurses.

These findings reveal that nurses and social workers, though both employed in helping professions, have distinct differences. The investigators suggested that the differences could have arisen because nurses use therapeutic communication daily. Results also reveal that nurses tended to think of themselves as individuals rather than as a collective group. Results of this study must be interpreted with caution because the study was conducted in Israel. However, the study points to the need to increase nurses' awareness of the political process and how they could influence public policy. More research is needed to see how all members of the interdisciplinary health team perceive empowerment and how they use their influence in helping shape public policy and health care delivery.

Itzhaky, H., Gerber, P., & Dekel, R. (2004). Empowerment skills and values: A comparative study of nurses and social workers. *International Journal of Nursing Studies, 41,* 447–456.

The Role of Government in Public Policy Development

The federal government and most state governments are organized into three branches: legislative, executive, and judicial. The legislative branch develops and approves legislation for executive branch consideration. The executive branch approves legislative acts and administers and regulates governmental policies. Once laws are passed, the administrative and executive branches of government develop policies to enact them. The judicial branch interprets laws and their applications as well as the meaning of approved policies.

Legal bases for legislative action in health care are found in Article I, Section 8 of the U.S. Constitution, which states that the government bears the responsibility to provide for the general welfare of its citizens, regulate interstate commerce, fund the military, and provide funds for governmental operations. Each state bears the responsibility to enforce national policies while protecting the safety, health, and welfare of its citizens. Local governments implement national programs and develop laws, regulations, and policies to ensure public health.

The Role of Nurses in Public Policy Development

Nurses have a dual stake in public policy legislation and enforcement; laws not only govern professional nursing practice, but they also impact research, professional education, and the scope of and access to health care by citizens. Nurses shape legislative proposals by contacting their elected officials to influence actions during the legislative process. Some nurses engage in proactive political action by proposing legislation, persuading an elected official in the legislature to introduce a bill, devising public relations campaigns around their proposals, **lobbying** (attempting to sway an elected official to take a desired action) to get the bill passed by legislative bodies, and influencing the head of the executive branch to sign it. A national or statewide effort to pass legislation requires the participation of many for success. Once legislation becomes law, some nurses continue to work with the state or federal agencies responsible for devising the regulations and/or policies to implement the law.

Nursing's Legislative Agenda and Priorities

Nurses need to stay abreast of current legislative and public policy issues because professional practice is governed by laws and regulations. Federal and state governments also provide funding for health care services and nursing education. Nurses can become aware of current legislative and public policy issues by reading, listening to, or watching national and local news reports. Other avenues for increasing awareness of public policy issues include engagement in community service activities and networking. Some nurses with higher levels of political involvement track legislation by accessing federal Congressional records and state Congressional websites where legislative calendars are posted, drafts of legislation are available for reading, and local elected officials' actions can be reviewed. FastDemocracy.com is an online legislative platform that enables users to stay informed and track legislative action at the federal and state levels. Free membership enables users to stay abreast of legislation and contact elected officials for desired action on introduced legislation. Users can select to track and receive email alerts about legislative initiatives in their areas of interest (FastDemocracy, n.d.). Because of the multitude of legislative initiatives introduced within a Congressional session at the national and state levels, nurses must set priorities for legislative action.

Every 2 years, the ANA develops and publishes a list of legislative and regulatory priorities for each session of the U.S. Congress. The identified priorities help shape the goals of an organization and the actions it will take to influence the passage of legislative proposals and the development of governmental policies. ANA's legislative goals are developed by the ANA's Department of Governmental Affairs, approved by its Board of Directors, and accepted by the House of Delegates at the ANA Annual Convention (ANA, n.d.). Once finalized, the ANA publicizes its **legislative and regulatory agendas**. Its membership bears the responsibility for supporting the agenda, while the ANA staff advances it. State nursing associations (SNAs) follow a similar process.

The ANA and SNAs also hire professional lobbyists to help draft and promote legislation that favorably affects professional nursing practice (Inouye, 2021; Milstead & Short, 2019). The ANA's legislative priorities are developed collaboratively by the ANA Membership Assembly and the ANA Board of Directors. Frequently, priorities are carried over from one Congressional session to another. The 117th Congressional session started January 3, 2021, and will end January 2, 2023. Each Congressional session lasts 2 years, and they are sequentially numbered. At the start of the 117th session, the ANA (2021f) identified legislative issues that apply to nursing, health care delivery, and the health and well-being of American citizens. The following list highlights some of the key issues that appear on the ANA legislative agenda:

1. COVID-19-specific safety issues: These concerns focus on protecting nurses and other health care providers during the COVID-19 pandemic, including improving the medical supply chain so that high-quality personal protective equipment is available for all health care providers working in any health care setting; improving mental health services for nurses and other providers; and mandating hazard pay for nurses and other care providers who work directly with clients with COVID-19. This topic also looks at providing an ample supply of personal protective equipment for any future pandemics or public health threats (ANA, 2021a).

2. Workplace violence: In 2021, The Workplace Violence Prevention for Healthcare and Social Worker Act was introduced in the House and Senate. This bill would require the Occupational Safety and Health Administration to develop enforceable standards mandating that employers develop and implement workplace violence prevention plans (ANA, 2021g). At the time of printing, no similar bill had been introduced into the Senate.

3. Opioid epidemic: The ANA advocates for legislation targeted to develop guidelines for pain management and substance use disorder therapies, including medication-assisted treatment. In 2021, the Mainstreaming Addiction Treatment Act of 2021 was introduced into the House of Representatives by Democratic Congressman Paul Tonko from New York and the Senate by Democratic Senator Maggie Hassan from New Hampshire. This bill would permit eliminating separate registration for dispensing schedule III, IV, and V medications, including buprenorphine, a medication frequently used for detoxification, for addiction treatment. Current law permits a waiver after a health care provider completes an educational course on safe use and prescribing of buprenorphine for treating opioid withdrawal and maintenance therapy to prevent a relapse (ANA, 2021d). At the time of printing, the ANA was continuing to monitor these introduced bills (ANA, 2021d).

4. Improving public health infrastructure and processes: The ANA advocates for legislation aimed at improving infrastructure and increasing personnel for public health services in order to fight the COVID-19 pandemic as well as to improve structures, processes, and personnel available to confront future pandemics or other public health threats (ANA, 2021b).

5. Advanced practice full practice: The ANA supports ensuring the full use of RN and advanced practice nurse (APRN) leadership abilities, knowledge, and skills to optimize nursing practice and quality of health care. Legislative efforts include continued support and reauthorization of Title VIII Nursing Workforce Development programs and removing barriers to APRN full scope of practice. Some states require continuous physician-nurse collaborative agreements; limit the medications that APRNs can prescribe; require that a physician be within a certain physical distance from the location where the APRN offers services; require that a physician chart reviews of APRN care; and require an APRN to meet a certain number of hours working alongside a physician annually (ANA, 2021b).

6. Safe staffing: The ANA supports legislation focused on protecting clients from receiving care in an unsafe environment and protecting nurses from working in these situations. This legislation that would ensure that RNs with no experiences or education in practice areas receive orientation before working; that assignments consider the intensity, complexity, and stability of clients; provide whistleblower protections for nurses who report unsafe staffing situations; eliminate mandatory overtime; establish procedures for receiving and investigating violations; require public reporting regarding staffing information; and allow the Secretary of Health and Human Services to issue and impose monetary fines on institutions for each violation (ANA, 2021e).

7. Nursing workforce development: Even though annual Title VIII funding has been approved through 2024, legislative initiatives are needed to increase the supply of RNs and to provide currently practicing nurses with incentives to remain in professional practice (ANA, 2021c).

8. Gun violence legislation: The ANA supports requiring mandatory background checks on all individuals who purchase firearms; current law includes a loophole that does not mandate background checks when people buy guns from unlicensed gun dealers. At the time of printing, the ANA had not listed gun violence as a legislative priority even though it has been on their list of priorities for several legislative sessions (ANA, 2018b).

The first step in publicizing action toward achieving legislative priorities is to develop position papers for each of the identified legislative goals. A position paper is a brief (usually one page) paper that specifies a goal, and clearly and concisely communicates the rationale behind the agenda based on solid facts and persuasive arguments. Supportive evidence such as research findings, statistics, and published articles are used to solidify the position. Typically, nursing organizations print the paper using their official logo, thereby adding credibility to the publication. The position papers also provide data that are useful for developing printed educational materials to legislators when nurses engage in lobbying.

The Art of Lobbying

The world of politics can move quickly—sometimes a piece of legislation changes in less than an hour. To stay abreast of the proposed legislation and its changes, nursing organizations hire lobbyists. The ANA has lobbyists for federal legislation. Most SNAs hire a lobbyist for state legislation. Lobbyists visit with elected officials in the hopes of influencing action on a piece of pending legislation. In addition, lobbyists are responsible for keeping their organizational membership informed of the proposed changes to a piece of legislation. At the local level, nurses directly engage in lobbying activities by attending city council and other community organizational meetings.

In addition to hiring lobbyists, the ANA and SNAs offer the Nurses Strategic Action Team (N-STAT), a grassroots lobbying group organized to ensure that nurses' voices are heard at the federal and state governmental levels.

When presenting information on a legislative or local issue, nurses and lobbyists must do their homework to develop expertise on the impending issue. Before briefing an elected official on an issue, it is mandatory to develop expertise on it. Having the facts and statistics related to an issue provides a solid foundation for the art of persuasion. Effective use of statistics involves (1) putting the numbers in human terms; (2) reporting the statistics in simple terms while avoiding the use of percentages; (3) including practical and statistical significance when reporting numbers; (4) using national, state, and local statistics (elected representatives are most concerned with the local impact of an issue on the constituents whose votes will affect their electability); and (5) citing the source of information (Hebda, 2019; Price et al., 2021).

Along with statistics, the use of personal stories may be effective in influencing elected officials. Effective use of personal stories involves (1) telling a personal story about a citizen who resides in the elected official's district; (2) telling the story in clear, concise, declarative, strong, and simple terms; (3) requesting a specific action by the legislator; and (4) emphasizing the importance of the issue (Short & Milstead, 2019).

Take Note!

Because elected officials deal with multiple issues every day, they appreciate a clear, concise, precise, and persuasive presentation of the individual's or the organization's goal.

Before effective lobbying can occur, nurses must be aware of current changes in any proposed legislation. To stay aware of current and proposed legislation and policies, nurses must have access to information. Information on legislative issues may be found in newspapers and news magazines (print and online), television and radio, nursing and professional publications, and websites. Along with these sources, legislative bodies offer their own websites to inform constituents of pending legislation and the legislator's position on that legislation. The U.S. Library of Congress has a website that links to federal legislative information. This site posts the status of pending legislation and committee hearing transcripts, which may be studied, downloaded, and printed. In addition, legislative body websites have features for citizens to find the legislators representing them.

Professional nursing associations post legislative issue information on their websites. The ANA and the Canadian Nurses Association websites also contain information about pending national legislation affecting health care and professional nursing practice. The ANA offers an online *Capitol Update* newsletter as well as opportunities for its membership to participate in RN Action. RN Action is the ANA's initiative to publicize key political issues affecting the professional nursing practice, access to care, and client care quality and safety.

Availability of information regarding state issues depends on the state or provincial nursing association. Several SNAs reserve access to information on current state legislative issues for their members while others post key information on the public pages of their website. Some SNAs also have social media accounts.

Elected legislators frequently provide their constituents with periodic reports during the legislative session, such as weekly electronic updates and annual reports from state representatives and state senators. Reports may be delivered to constituents via email or the postal service. Reports sent to constituents before the end of the legislative session usually ask for voter opinions on pending legislative issues. When nurses return questionnaires addressing pending legislation, they are participating in the legislative process.

Because of the complex process set forth in the Constitution, the path of legislation provides ample opportunity for citizen input. The **federal legislative path** specifies the required steps for an idea to become law in the United States. Nurses and other citizens can offer suggestions and express support or rejection for proposed legislation at any of the steps in the process. Box 19.1, Learning, Knowing, and Growing, "The Federal Legislative Path," outlines the complicated process by which an idea becomes law and how nurses can influence that process.

Lobbying Strategies

Lobbying strategies are techniques that are used by citizens to influence others to take a desired action. Lobbying strategies are classified into two types: direct and indirect (Table 19.1). Direct lobbying involves personal contact with elected officials. Indirect lobbying involves influencing public opinion on a particular issue.

Before implementing lobbying strategies, nurses should outline a plan that contains a timeline for

recording lobbying activities and their results. By keeping records of reactions and responses from elected officials, nurses may use this information in future interactions. Appointment of a spokesperson can help maintain a consistent lobbying approach and enhance public recognition of a particular issue viewpoint.

Constituent pressure is perhaps the most effective weapon for the lobbyist, and mobilization of a group of individuals for collective action provides numbers that influence action. Letter writing and email campaigns are effective when a bill is pending in Congress or in a state legislative body. Communicating by form letter or form email is superior to sending nothing. If a specific piece of legislation is supported by a nursing organization, the organization may have a sample letter or email message drafted for membership use. The ANA's RN Action initiative provides form email messages for members to personalize prior to sending. Communications are most effective when the constituents share a

---

19.1 Learning, Knowing, and Growing

The Federal Legislative Path

When you step into the voting booth on election day, you set in motion the legislative process. Your elected representatives are charged with taking your ideas and beliefs and carrying them forward to their ultimate enactment into law.

A member of the U.S. House of Representatives or the Senate must introduce a bill before it can be considered. They may do so based on their perception of a public need, in support of their elected colleagues, or at the urging of their constituents or of professional associations such as the ANA. Once a bill is introduced, it goes to a committee where it may be referred (passed to another committee), become the topic of a hearing, be marked up (rewritten and amended), or be reported out (sent to the House or Senate for floor action).

The chair of the committee considering the bill decides on its action. This person possesses much power because they may delay the presentation of the bill to the committee. During this phase of the legislative process, interested individuals and groups, including nurses, may brief the committee chair to attempt to influence the scheduling of the bill for committee discussion or action on the floor.

Bills that make it out of committee go to the legislative chamber for debate. Once either chamber passes a bill, it goes to the other chamber and is subjected to the entire legislative process again. After the second chamber approves the bill, it is submitted to a conference committee that consists of members from both chambers. The conference committee negotiates differences between the two versions of the bill, adopts the bill, and submits

(reports) it to both chambers for adoption or rejection. If both chambers adopt the conference bill, it becomes an Act of Congress (or of the state legislature). At each of the stages through which a bill moves, constituent input, including that of nurses, can be critical to the outcome.

Each adopted act (also known as an enrolled bill at the federal level) is referred to the president (or governor in state legislatures), who signs or vetoes it. The influence of the public is key at this stage as well—likely, you have seen stories in the news of individuals and groups demonstrating to have the president sign or veto a bill. If the bill is signed, it becomes law. If the bill is vetoed, the House and Senate may override the veto by a two thirds majority vote, and the bill becomes public law. If the veto is sustained, the bill dies. The U.S. Constitution gives the president 10 days (excluding Sundays) to act on an enrolled bill. The president has four possible options. The bill may be approved by signature, approved by inaction (i.e., the president takes no action within 10 days, an option used when it is considered unnecessary or politically unwise to sign a bill, or if there are questions regarding its constitutionality), pocket vetoed (used at the end of a legislative session when the Congress adjourns before the 10-day expiration date), or vetoed (the president refuses to sign the bill and presents both bodies of the Congress with a message stating their objections to it) (Bowers-Lanier, 2019; Schumann, 2021). When the enrolled bill is submitted for executive approval, nurses should contact the president or governor via phone, fax, or email to voice the desired action.

TABLE 19.1 Lobbying Strategies

Direct Lobbying Through a Legislative Body	Indirect Lobbying Through Public Opinion
Participate in party platform development.	Publicize nursing organizational agendas.
Contribute time and money to political campaigns.	Use traditional media (especially television) and social media (such as Facebook, Twitter, TikTok) to further the agenda.
Influence the legislative committee members by personally visiting, messaging, emailing them, preferably using forms on their websites. Calling them will usually result in a conversation with one of their aides.	Write editorial pieces for print and electronic media, such as newspapers or news magazines, email newsletters, and blogs, and/or establish a website or social media page that promotes the cause.
Influence the agency regulators by personally visiting, writing, or emailing them, preferably using the form on the agency's website.	Seek public opinion by polling the public and publishing the results.
Engage in direct lobbying by visiting and emailing elected officials or hiring a professional lobbyist.	Use paid media advertisements (e.g., television, radio, print, online).
Attend social events at which elected officials appear.	Print and distribute books or pamphlets, or set up a website or social media page.
Develop an understanding of elected officials' key positions on issues.	Develop and execute educational campaigns.

From American Nurses Association. (2018a). *ANA advocacy toolkit*. Retrieved April 11, 2021, from https://ana.aristotle.com/SitePages/toolkit.aspx; de Vries, C., & Vanderbilt, M. (1992). *The grassroots lobbying handbook: Empowering nurses through legislative and political action*. American Nurses Association; Glassman, M. E., Straus, J. R., & Shogan, C. J. (2010). *Social networking and constituent communications: Member use of Twitter during a two-month period in the 111th Congress. Congressional Research Service 7-5700*. Retrieved April 19, 2013, from https://fas.org/sgp/crs/misc/R43018.pdf; Short, N. M., & Milstead, J. A. (2019). An insider's guide to engaging in policy activities. In J. A. Milstead & N. M. Short (Eds.), *Health policy and politics: A nurse's guide* (6th ed., pp. 215–232). Jones & Bartlett Learning.

personal story related to the issue or bill, specific reasons to support or oppose a particular bill or issue, and key information about the impact pending legislation would have on the legislator's district or state.

Since 2009, email has made it possible for elected officials to receive a flood of messages from people beyond their constituents. An elected official may receive thousands of messages in one day and only a fraction of them may have been sent by their constituents. Most elected officials now post a contact form for constituent use that requires detailed identification about who is sending the message, thereby facilitating the separation of messages sent to an official from a constituent (Congress.org, 2021).

Electronic media and technology have become essential vehicles for elected officials to communicate with constituents. Along with traditional face-to-face town hall meetings, personal visits, telephone calls, and mailed letters, elected officials use email updates, web sites, teleconference town hall meetings, online videos, social networking sites, and other forms of technology to connect with the constituents. Between 1995 and 2008, postal mailings to Congressional members declined 50%. In 2008, members of the U.S. House of Representatives received close to 190 million email messages. Twitter has become a relatively inexpensive way for members of the Congress and other federal bodies to inform interested individuals of events, views, and new products or services (Glassman et al., 2010).

Because elected officials rely on voter support for re-election, each letter, email, tweet, and personal contact counts. Follow-up messages of appreciation for action on an issue enhance relationships among elected officials and their constituents. Box 19.2, Learning, Knowing, and Growing, "Characteristics of Effective Written Communication to an Official," provides strategies to enhance the impact of your communication with your elected officials.

Using email to lobby an elected official has advantages and disadvantages. It is economical and quick and enables users to send messages at any time. The message is not dependent on postal delivery, and delivery is instantaneous, which can be particularly crucial when a critical vote is only minutes or hours away. In light of security issues with chemically and infectious-agent tainted letters, some elected officials prefer email messages over handwritten letters for personal safety (Roll Call CQ, 2013; Roll Call CQ Staff, 2009). Many members of the Congress also use software to tabulate constituent views and positions on pieces of pending legislation (Roll Call CQ Staff, 2009).

However, email also has some disadvantages. The ease of email also means that its impact may be watered down by sheer numbers especially when form email messages are sent. Some special interest groups bombard legislators with emails, many of which may be identical, as group members simply forward the

19.2 Learning, Knowing, and Growing

Characteristics of Effective Written Communication to an Official

1. Limit letters or emails to one page (approximately 250 words) if possible, and not longer than two pages. Focus on one issue for each email or letter.
2. Identify the issue in the subject heading if using email.
3. Correctly address the person to whom you are writing, referring to an elected official as The Honorable (first name followed by surname; verify that you have the correct spelling of legislator's name).
4. Greet the official according to the title (e.g., Dear Senator _____, Dear Representative _____, Dear Congressperson _____, Dear Mr. Chairman or Madam Chairwoman _____, or Dear Mr./Madam Speaker _____), using a colon for punctuation after the greeting.
5. Identify yourself as a constituent, a health care expert, a member of a large organization, and a credible source on the issue within the first paragraph.
6. Refer to the specific piece of legislation by title (H.R. [number] for a House bill; S. [number] for a Senate bill) in the first paragraph if the letter pertains to a specific legislative proposal.
7. Emphasize the local importance of the proposed issue.
8. Be brief and specific when presenting key information.
9. Add personal experiences and views, thus eliminating the tone of a form letter.
10. If you are sending a letter or document, use professional but personalized letterhead.
11. Verify that the email or letter is free of spelling, grammatical, or typographical errors.
12. Be specific about the desired action on the part of the elected official.
13. Offer personal assistance or the organization's assistance in the closing.
14. Thank the official for their anticipated action.
15. Provide your contact information.

From American Nurses Association. (2018). *ANA advocacy toolkit*. Retrieved December 6, 2020, from aristotle.com; Short, N. M., & Milstead, J. A. (2019). An insider's guide to engaging in policy activities. In J. A. Milstead & N. M. Short (Eds.), *Health policy and politics: A nurse's guide* (6th ed., pp. 215–232). Jones & Bartlett Learning.

messages without bothering to personalize them. If an individual tries to send multiple messages on a subject to one representative, the messages may get trapped as spam or flagged as such by staffers. Messages from individuals who fail to identify themselves clearly as a constituent may not be given as much attention (with mailed letters, postmarks help identify the writer's location). As is the case with traditional letters, many elected officials receive large volumes of email and must rely on staff to read it, sort it, and to relay crucial information (Roll Call CQ, 2013). Because legislators tend to hear exclusively from dissatisfied constituents, they may be led to believe falsely that large numbers of their constituents disagree with a pending issue when a large volume of email is received.

A bill may be introduced years before it is passed, and in multiple sessions of the Congress or state legislatures. "Persistence and patience are two key factors in lobbying" (de Vries & Vanderbilt, 1992, p. 59). When nurses stay in regular contact with elected officials, the officials are more likely to remember them and work to help support nursing's agenda.

A telephone call offers a way to deliver a brief and quick message to an elected official. A legislator's staff members frequently keep a tally of how many calls support and how many calls disapprove of pending

legislation. Many nurses find it beneficial to have the desired message scripted for reading to an elected official. A phone call, like an email, is superior to traditional written and mailed media because it best communicates the urgency of an issue.

All national elected officials have offices in Washington, D.C., as well as in the locality they represent. When legislators return home during breaks, nurses can arrange to meet with them to share their views, eliminating time and travel barriers to this personal communication. Email messages are effective tools to send quick messages requesting prompt action. Petitions containing large numbers of signatures are usually effective only for public relations because it is difficult for the staff to verify whether all signatures on the document represent constituents.

In addition to written communication, a personal visit is an effective method of lobbying. Constituents are often invited to meet with elected officials in the local or governmental office. A personal visit lays the foundation for future contacts. A scheduled appointment usually ensures a personal meeting with an elected official. Frequently, visits are limited to 15 to 30 minutes. Because of legislative emergencies, appointments may be canceled, especially if a floor vote is scheduled during the planned meeting. Box 19.3,

19.3 Learning, Knowledge, and Growing

Steps for Facilitating a Personal Visit With an Elected Official

1. Confirm the appointment and arrive several minutes early, using this time to establish relationships with the official's staff members.
2. Wear professional attire. Avoid dressing casually, such as in jeans, shirts with logos, or exercise clothes.
3. Bring a prepared speech and a fact sheet summarizing the issue, your position on it, and any requested action.
4. Be patient and flexible if the meeting does not occur exactly as scheduled.
5. Provide the official with a business card after greeting them with a firm handshake and confident personal introduction. State that you are a registered nurse and provide information about your current role and setting as well as a brief description of the types of clients to whom you provide care.
6. Start the meeting by establishing a tie between you and the legislator (such as where you live) so that the official knows you are a constituent who may be responsible for their reelection.
7. Inform the official of your mission and clearly identify the issue. If there is pending legislation, refer to it

by the bill number and the title. Limit the number of issues for a single visit to no more than three.
8. Present statistics and personal stories when appropriate, while emphasizing the issue's importance to the local community.
9. Request the name of the staff member who handles the issue, and request follow-up.
10. Be concise and focus solely on the issue of the meeting.
11. Leave a one- or two-page fact sheet summarizing the issue and your position on it.
12. Conclude the meeting by thanking the official for spending time with you.
13. Send a thank you note or email shortly after the meeting.
14. If the legislator requests more information about the bill and issue, provide all requested information promptly the visit.
15. Stay in contact with the legislator's relevant staff who address and manage information about the bill or issue that was discussed during the visit.

From American Nurses Association. (2018). *ANA advocacy toolkit*. Retrieved December 6, 2020, from aristotle.com; de Vries, C., & Vanderbilt, M. (1992). *The grassroots lobbying handbook: Empowering nurses through legislative and political action*. American Nurses Association; Mason, D. J., Gardner, D. S., Hopkins Outlaw, F., & O'Grady, E. T. (Eds.). (2016). *Policy and politics in nursing and health care* (7th ed.). Elsevier; and Short, N. M., & Milstead, J. A. (2019). An insider's guide to engaging in policy activities. In J. A. Milstead & N. M. Short (Eds.), *Health policy and politics: A nurse's guide* (6th ed., pp. 215–232). Jones & Bartlett Learning.

Learning, Knowing, and Growing, "Steps for Facilitating a Personal Visit with an Elected Official," provides suggestions for how you can effectively visit with your elected official. Box 19.4, Learning, Knowing, and Growing "Creating a Legislative Fact Sheet" offers guidance for preparing a fact sheet for requested actions that you can leave at the legislators' offices so they can readily refer to information when making decisions about pending legislation.

When lobbying for specific action on an issue, inviting an elected official for a personal tour of a local hospital or to participate in a local community service event may assist in advancing the cause. These activities increase the official's visibility and provide an opportunity for interaction with constituents. Because this may be viewed as an opportunity for press coverage, special attention to the press secretary at this time may increase the likelihood of future access to the elected official (de Vries & Vanderbilt, 1992; Short & Mason, 2019).

Once reliable relationships are established with elected officials, nurses may be invited to testify at legislative committee hearings. When this happens,

careful preparation is required, and a technical expert or attorney may accompany a witness. ANA's president frequently testifies at committee hearings when issues regarding professional nursing practice are debated. Karen Daley, PhD, MPH, RN, FAAN, a former ANA president, provided testimony regarding the 2013 fiscal year appropriations for the Title VIII Nursing Workforce Development Programs and in support of nurse-managed health clinics. In 2020, ANA President Ernest Grant, PhD, RN, FAAN, testified before Congress about the disparate impact of COVID-19 on communities of color and the shortage of personal protective equipment for nurses during the pandemic (Grant, 2020a, 2020b). Rich sources of evidence for testimony include the Agency for Health Care Research and Quality (AHRQ; formerly the Agency for Health Care Policy and Research), the Center for Telehealth and e-Health Law, the National Council of State Boards of Nursing (NCSBN), and the U.S. Department of Health and Human Services.

Sending emails or letters and visiting the legislators are the most effective lobbying techniques. Traditionally, people lobby the officials they have elected

19.4 Learning, Knowing, and Growing

Creating a Legislative Fact Sheet

General Guidelines

- Limit the length of the document to one page (front and back).
- Use an easily read font with no type smaller than 12 points.
- Use larger font and boldface type for major headings.
- Keep typeface and font consistent for major headings.
- If any boxes or figures are used, make certain that they are easily read.
- Use boldface type for important facts.
- Make sure you have no spelling or typographical errors.
- No references are needed as this is not an academic assignment.

Specific Information

- Title of issue: Use a major heading format with the largest font point that will appear in the document.
- State the desired action using a major heading format.

- Bulleted list format is acceptable.
- Boldface type key terms in the request for impact.
- Fast facts
  - Include statistics when possible.
  - If known, list the financial and human costs of the current state of the issue.
  - Include any personal stories or how the current state of the issue is affecting constituents.
- Your contact information: Include your name, credentials, email, and telephone number at the bottom of front of the page if preferred with all information in a major heading format.
- Projected costs
  - List the financial impact of the proposed legislation if known.
  - If this is not known, omit this section.
- Summary: List three summary points.
- Supporting organizations
  - List any supporting organizations if known.
  - If none are known, omit this section.

From American Nurses Association. (2018a). *ANA advocacy toolkit*. Retrieved April 11, 2021, from https://ana.aristotle.com/SitePages/toolkit.aspx; Short, N. M., & Milstead, J. A. (2019). An insider's guide to engaging in policy activities. In J. A. Milstead & N. M. Short (Eds.), *Health policy and politics: A nurse's guide* (6th ed., pp. 215–232). Jones & Bartlett Learning.

into office while ignoring powerful legislators, such as party leaders and committee chairs. Different lobbying strategies work more effectively during different phases of the legislative process. Table 19.2 outlines specific lobbying strategies recommended for use during each phase of the legislative and regulatory process.

Obstacles to Effective Lobbying

Major obstacles encountered by nurses include not knowing whom to lobby, where to contact officials, or the best time for contact. Some do not know the names of their elected officials. Before contacting an elected official, nurses should find out about the official's personal biography, political party affiliation, committee memberships, voting record, and introduced or cosponsored legislative activity. Knowledge of the official's personal causes or pet projects may also be useful.

The Importance of Legislative Staff Members

Because of their enormous responsibilities, all elected officials have staff (elected officials may work with thousands of pieces of legislation during one legislative session). Staff members routinely handle much of the elected official's work. Good relationships with

legislative staff at the national and local offices provide invaluable contacts and advantages when engaging in lobbying activities.

An elected official's personal staff may include an administrative assistant, a legislative director, legislative assistants, legislative correspondents, a press secretary, caseworkers, a secretary, an office manager, and a receptionist. Staff members are responsible for scheduling appointments and activities. More importantly, officials fill staff posts with highly qualified people who assist them in making decisions, including members of the nursing profession. For example, Sheila Burke, RN, MPA, FAAN, served as chief of staff for Senator Robert Dole when he was the Senate Majority Leader (Goldwater & Zusy, 1990). Mary Wakefield, PhD, RN, was a member of Senator Tom Daschle's staff as well as a legislative assistant and chief of staff to North Dakota Senators Ken Conrad and Quentin Burdick. Both of these nurses advised their respective senators on issues related to health care delivery and workforce development.

Dr. Wakefield served as the Administrator for the U.S. Health Resources and Services Administration from 2009 to 2015. In March 2015, she was appointed Deputy Secretary of the U.S. Department of Health

TABLE 19.2   The Legislative Process: Steps and Suggested Lobbying Strategies

Steps in the Legislative Process	Suggested Lobbying Strategy
Legislation introduction	Hold a technical expert meeting to map out a strategy. Form a coalition of people and organizations with the same goal. Identify a legislator in each legislative chamber (House and Senate) who would be likely to introduce the proposal. Schedule a meeting with the legislator's staff members. Initiate emailing or letter writing campaigns to other legislative members who may wish to cosponsor the bill.
Immediately following introduction of legislation before committee assignment	Meet with interest groups to map out additional lobbying strategies. Create a one-page fact sheet to distribute to interested parties. Initiate email or letter writing campaigns to elected officials to urge bill cosponsorship. Draft proposed amendments to bill.
Committee consideration	Send emails or write letters to all committee members to emphasize the need for a public hearing. Enlist members of other interested organizations in emailing and letter writing. Submit written information about oral or written testimony if a hearing is to occur. Have someone monitor the mark-up session and share information with letter writers. Conduct an emailing or letter writing campaign to committee members either supporting or disagreeing with the bill amendments added in the committee. Conduct an emailing or letter writing campaign to elected officials from the local district outlining support or disapproval of the revised bill or to enlist their support by contacting committee members or testifying at a committee meeting. Call a meeting of interested people to verify whether new amendments are tolerable. Work with committee staff in drafting the final draft of the bill. Notify the press about the bill.
Rules Committee action	Work with Rules Committee members to determine whether amendments can be made while the bill is debated on the floor of either chamber.
Legislation on the floor of a chamber	Send short messages to all members of the chamber in great quantities (e.g., emails, telephone calls, postcards). Develop a swing list of officials. Initiate personal visits to officials on undecided, leaning no, and leaning yes lists.
Conference Committee action	Meet with other interested people to verify which version (House or Senate) is to be supported. Email, write, visit, or call district officials and members of the Conference Committee
Return to both chambers for approval	No lobbying strategies are needed if work has been consistent. Email, write, or call elected officials from district.
Presidential or gubernatorial signature	Call the White House or governor's staff, leaving a message for veto or signature.
Veto override	Email, write, or call locally elected official. Intensify lobbying efforts at those who appeared on the leaning yes list.

From American Nurses Association. (2018a). *ANA advocacy toolkit.* Retrieved April 11, 2021, from https://ana.aristotle.com/SitePages/toolkit.aspx; de Vries, C., & Vanderbilt, M. (1992). *The grassroots lobbying handbook: Empowering nurses through legislative and political action.* American Nurses Association.

and Human Services, a post she held until January 20, 2017 (Josiah Macy Jr. Foundation, n.d.). In November 2020, Dr. Wakefield was appointed to President Joe Biden's transition team following the 2020 presidential election (Shirley, 2020).

Nurses who serve as staff members bring their expertise on health and safety issues to the team. To become a staff member, nurses should get to know political candidates, join political parties, donate time to work for election campaigns, contribute funds to campaigns, and market their nursing expertise on issues related to health care and health promotion.

Maintaining a Working Relationship

Expressing appreciation is a frequently overlooked step in the lobbying process. Elected officials should be acknowledged for introducing and supporting legislation that enhances professional nursing practice. Some SNAs bestow honors on elected officials who have developed records for supporting "nursing-friendly" legislation. A thank you note that includes a statement about informing other nurses living in the district about an official's action in supporting legislation increases the support for an official running for reelection.

Honesty is perhaps the most important factor contributing to effective lobbying. When lobbying, nurses must be willing to spend the time to explore the issues and collect valid and reliable data surrounding them. When encountering questions that cannot be answered accurately with complete certainty, nurses should refer the question to another expert or offer to find the desired information and present it to the official at a later date. Attempts to "wing it" or inadvertently sharing untrue information could sabotage the personal relationships established with officials (de Vries & Vanderbilt, 1992; Short & Mason, 2019).

There are multiple ways to cultivate a working relationship with an elected official. Wakefield (2004) suggested that working for an election (or reelection) campaign and becoming a member of a political party foster networking with elected officials. Attendance at events where legislators are scheduled to speak or fundraise serves as an additional opportunity for access. Some SNAs offer programs to meet political candidates at district meetings or during special programs held in state capitols. During the programs, the SNAs typically provide participants with a list of legislative initiatives along with fact sheets to present to legislators when visiting with them. A political campaign contribution offers a token of appreciation (Wakefield, 2004). Taking time to listen to candidates running for office when they canvass neighborhoods enables nurses to meet the candidates.

In the United States, public policy development and implementation are affected by money, power, and societal position. To maintain their position and power, elected officials must work for reelection. Because officials acknowledge the importance of satisfying their constituents, their actions are aimed at protecting and serving their voters. Politically astute people acknowledge the importance of building coalitions (forming a larger group from smaller groups of people with similar goals and interests) and contributing resources to a political campaign to get their candidate elected to office.

Take Note!
Without nurses' active participation in the legislative and election processes, public policy may not remain friendly to the nursing profession or health care consumers.

■ QUESTIONS FOR REFLECTION

1. Do you know the number of the congressional district in which you reside?
2. Who are the senators serving your state in Congress?
3. Who is your congressional district's House of Representatives member?
4. Who are your representatives in the state legislature?
5. Which of the lobbying strategies is most appealing to you? Why?

Coalition Building

Although difficult to establish and maintain, **coalitions** unite diverse groups, organizations, and people for a common specific purpose. Coalitions operate under the assumption that "there is strength in numbers." Many coalitions begin with an informal structure that formalizes as the coalition evolves and becomes more active. Before extending an invitation for membership, a background check verifies any strengths or weaknesses individuals or organizations bring to the coalition. The goal of building a coalition is to capitalize on all members' strengths (Bowers-Lanier, 2021). Usually, the organization that started the coalition becomes its leader. When the ANA, American Hospital Association, and American Medical Association (AMA) work together to support a piece of legislation, they build a coalition of health care providers. Once a formal structure has been established, a coalition may need to hire employees to accomplish its goals.

The ANA (2016b) has built coalitions with a variety of groups in order to advance efforts for improving health care funding, protecting the environment, enhancing public safety, seeking funding to advance health care delivery, and protecting client rights. Current coalitions in place include 50 States United for Healthy Air, Alliance of Nurses for Healthy Environments, Coalition for Health Funding, Coalition for Patient Rights, NDD United (a group aimed at securing funding for nondefense discretionary spending at all government levels), Get Covered America, Friends of the National Institute of Occupational Health and Safety, Nursing Community, the Public Affairs Council, Smart Disposal and Safe Chemicals, and Healthy Families.

Political Action Committees

Political action committees (PACs) are created by existing organizations for the purpose of financing campaigns for political office. Federal election guidelines prohibit nonprofit groups from contributing to political campaigns. Funding for a PAC is independent of the founding organization's funding.

Federal election guidelines mandate that PAC donations may be solicited from an organization's membership only for candidates of public office. However, general organizational funds may finance a political education program for members of the PAC's founding organization. Sometimes candidates for office receive political contributions from the PAC. However, some candidates may request only a public endorsement of their campaigns.

The ANA-PAC, founded in 1972, supports political candidates with "nursing-friendly" agendas (Flanagan, 1976). "The ANA-PAC is an unincorporated committee of the ANA Board of Directors" (Conant & Jackson, 2007, p. 24). Conant and Jackson reported that the ANA-PAC has a separate fund dedicated for the sole use of supporting candidates running for federal office. The ANA broke its tradition and decided not to endorse a 2020 presidential candidate. In 2020, the ANA-PAC dispersed $231,500 to candidates running for the U.S. House of Representatives and $31,500 to U.S. Senate candidates; 66% of the funds went to candidates from the Democratic National Party. Of the candidates the ANA-PAC endorsed, 100% of Republican candidates and 83% of Democrat candidates won their elections (Hatmaker, 2020).

Before supporting candidates, the ANA offers them the opportunity to complete a questionnaire about their positions on issues important to nurses. The ANA-PAC Board sets concrete endorsement criteria and then forwards information to the ANA-PAC Board of Trustees to review relevant information addressing the criteria. The ANA-PAC Board votes to endorse candidates for federal office. However, each constituent SNA may agree or disagree with endorsements for federal political offices. Once a candidate is endorsed, ANA staff members notify the candidate. Once the candidate agrees to the endorsement, the ANA-PAC contributes funds to their campaigns and receives ANA candidate endorsement (ANA, 2016a). The ANA-PAC often supports a political candidate for president and frequently the candidate wins the election as Barack Obama did in the 2008 and 2012 presidential elections. Many SNAs also have PACs, and each designates specific criteria for endorsing a candidate running for office and contributing to state candidate political campaigns.

According to the Federal Election Commission (FEC), the American Hospital Association PAC is one of the largest PACs, having dispersed over $3.11 million from 2019 to 2020 (FEC, 2020b). The American Medical Association PAC (AMPAC) reported dispersing over $1.58 million (FEC, 2020d). The American Association of Nurse Anesthetists PAC dispersed over $1.85 billion (more than the AMPAC) (FEC, 2020a). The ANA-PAC dispersed more than $499,000 (FEC, 2020d).

Even though the nursing profession has many more members than the other groups, they have fewer donors to the ANA-PAC. There are likely multiple reasons for the lack of ANA-PAC political support. First, professional nurses generally earn less than physicians, and some nurses refuse to join the ANA because of the perception that it primarily supports the Democratic National Party. Some nurses with strong pro-life beliefs fail to join ANA because of its support for a pregnant person's right to choose.

CURRENT POLITICAL AND LEGISLATIVE ISSUES AFFECTING PROFESSIONAL NURSING PRACTICE AND HEALTH CARE

Laws regulate nursing practice and health care delivery. Each state regulates nursing practice through its nurse practice act. Federal and state governments regulate health care access and health care service reimbursement. Many issues confronting legislators affect citizen safety, health care policy, and the control of nursing practice.

Many bills addressing health care are introduced into the Congress and state legislatures annually. If a bill is not passed during the session of Congress in which it is introduced, it dies. However, the bill may be reintroduced during each successive session of Congress until it passes. Issues that are current today may become irrelevant tomorrow.

In the recent past, nurses have been successful in influencing the passage of legislation related to client safety, nursing and health care research funding, human immunodeficiency virus (HIV) programs, family leave, tobacco settlements, abuse programs, direct Medicare reimbursement to APRNs, Medicare prescription coverage, expanded scope of practice for APRNs, and nursing education funding. Often, a particular issue surfaces over several legislative sessions before legislative action occurs. For example, health care reform has remained on the legislative table for decades. The following section discusses pending legislative issues that may be of interest to professional nurses.

Annually, the federal government develops a budget for all expenditures, including a number of long-standing programs related to public health, nursing education, and nursing research. Nurses need to be aware of the funding proposals made for such programs (Wakefield, 2004). Nurses can become aware of proposed program cuts or increases through efforts of the ANA and other specialty nurse organizations.

The American Nurses Association's 117th Congress Federal Legislative Priorities

When the Institute of Medicine (IOM) released the report *To Err Is Human: Building a Safer Health System* in 1999, health care consumers and providers began questioning the general safety of health care delivery. An IOM follow-up report issued in 2011, *The Future of Nursing: Leading Change, Advancing Health*, offered suggestions to improve the quality of health care by increasing the educational level and optimizing the use of professional

nurses (RNs and APRNs) to create a more efficient, patient-centered health care system (see Chapter 9, "Health Care Delivery Systems," and Chapter 18, "Quality Improvement: Enhancing Patient Safety and Health Care Quality"). Nurses seized the opportunity to validate their contributions to quality health care by conducting studies and sharing results that demonstrated improvements in hospitalized client outcomes with increased RN hours per patient day (Agency for Healthcare Research and Quality [AHRQ], 2007; Institute of Medicine [IOM], 2011). The ANA's *114th Congress Federal Legislative Priorities* outlined ways to implement recommendations from the 2011 Institute of Medicine's study and to promote the overall health for all Americans. The ANA develops a new list of legislative priorities for each new session of Congress, and SNAs also create legislative agendas for each state legislative session (see Box 19.5, Professional

---

 19.5 Professional Prototypes

Items from the ANA 117th Congress Federal Legislative Priorities

Health System Transformation (ANA, 2021f)

- Universal access to a standard essential package of health care services for all American citizens including Medicaid expansion in all states.
- Prohibit practice of limiting insurance coverage for preexisting conditions.
- Health insurance coverage for persons under age 26 on parents' policies.
- Community-based and preventive health care services that include sustainable and equal payment for services.
- Health care services across the care continuum that are client-centered and involve engaged partnership among providers and consumers.
- Removal of all barriers and restrictions that prevent RNs and APRNs from practicing within their full scope of practice.
- Payment systems rewarding evidence-based protocols, quality outcomes, and effective resource use.
- Affordable health insurance without lifetime caps or annual limits.
- Develop programs to ensure equity in health care services, disease burden, and costs (ANA, 2021b).

Nursing Workforce Development (ANA, 2021f)

- Increase funding (e.g., scholarships, grants, loans with realistic repayment plans) for educating an adequate supply of RNs to meet the needs of the American population, increasing the primary care workforce (i.e., APRNs).

- Facilitate longer nursing careers by requiring national safe staffing guidelines, providing improved mental health services for nurses, protecting whistleblowers, and promoting healthy work environments.
- Continue annual federal funding for Title VIII Nursing Workforce Development programs that provide grants for advanced nursing education, workforce diversity grants, National Nurse Service Corps, nurse faculty loan programs, and other grants funding geriatric specialization, nursing centers, and nursing education. (ANA, 2021c).

Workplace Violence (ANA, 2021f)

- Require all health care employers to develop suitable workplace violence prevention plans.
- Provide a mechanism for mandatory reporting of incidences of workplace violence.
- Develop a process for receiving and investigating reports of workplace violence incidences.
- Provide whistleblower protection for nurses reporting incidences of workplace violence and abusive situations (ANA, 2021g).

Opioid Epidemic (ANA, 2021f)

- Develop guidelines for pain management and substance use disorder treatments that include medication-assisted treatment.
- In 2021, the Mainstreaming Addiction Treatment Act of 2021 was to permit eliminating separate

19.5 Professional Prototypes

Items from the ANA 117th Congress Federal Legislative Priorities

registration for dispensing schedule III, IV, and V medications for detoxification, addiction treatment (ANA, 2021d).

Safe Staffing (ANA, 2021f)

- Assurance that nurses are not required to work on units on which they have not received education and training or when lacking experience without orientation.
- Establishment of procedures for receiving and investigating nurse complaints about unsafe staffing situations.
- Determination of specific civil monetary fines for violation of safe staffing policies.
- Provision of whistle-blower protection for nurses who report incidences of unsafe staffing.
- Reporting of staffing information to the general public (ANA, 2021e).

COVID-19 (ANA, 2021a)

- Require health care providers to report shortages of personal protective equipment so that they can be alleviated and that an adequate supply will be placed in stockpiles for future health care disasters.
- Improve public health infrastructure to support enhanced community-based care, emergency preparedness and response, eliminate disparities to access for care.
- Provide funding for mental health services for nurses and hazard pay for nurses caring for COVID-19 clients and future disasters.
- Prioritize nurses and other health care providers for additional vaccinations if needed and improve mass distribution and administration of vaccines including funding education for vaccination compliance (ANA, 2021a).

Prototypes, "Items from the ANA 117th Congress Federal Legislative Priorities").

The federal government spends billions of dollars to monitor and improve the quality of health care services. It funds the AHRQ, the National Institutes of Health, the Centers for Disease Control and Prevention, the Food and Drug Administration, the Health Care Financing Administration, and the Health Resources and Services Administration. Federal funding is directly related to the quality of health and health care in the United States.

Safe Nursing and Client Legislation and Nursing's Legislative Efforts

Legislative initiatives on safe nursing and client care have been introduced with each session of Congress since 2003. All of the legislative proposals on this issue have had provisions that would prohibit mandatory overtime for RNs and other licensed members of the interdisciplinary care team, but would not set limits on voluntary overtime (IOM, 2004; McKeon, 2008). Despite IOM (1999) evidence-based findings denoting increased errors made by nurses when they work for more than 96 hours per week or longer than 12 hours at a time, no federal legislation has been enacted to reduce the number of hours that RNs can work within a week's time frame. Passage of any law limiting the

amount of overtime or hours nurses work might create a financial hardship for some nurses.

At time of printing, the 117th session of Congress had not addressed the issue of mandatory nurse overtime. However, several states have enacted laws prohibiting health care organizations from requiring nurses to work mandatory overtime, though some states have provisions requiring nurses to work overtime in the event of a natural or man-made disaster.

Nursing Workforce

The U.S. Bureau of Labor Statistics [BLS] (2020) projects an RN demand of approximately 221,900 by 2029. To keep RNs active in the workforce, the federal and state governments have introduced health care workforce legislation. Each year, Congress approves funding for Title VIII Nursing Workforce Development programs. However, funding for nursing education was incorporated into the Coronavirus Aid Relief and Securities (CARES) Act of 2020. The 2020 fiscal year final budget was $259.72 million annually through fiscal year 2024. The amount was a $28 million increase over allocations in the 2019 fiscal year budget (American Association of Colleges of Nursing [AACN], 2020). The funding is for all levels of nursing education (i.e., nursing students, advanced practice nursing students, and nursing faculty pursuing doctoral studies) (AACN, 2020). With multiyear funding appropriated, nurses should expect to see this issue as a legislative priority starting in 2023. At the time of printing, there were no legislative initiatives aimed at keeping currently employed nurses in the workforce.

State Legislative Initiatives

States frequently address similar health care issues in their legislative bodies. Some SNAs hire lobbyists to work on their behalf. The lobbyists work with members of the state legislatures to draft nurse-friendly legislation, seek cosponsors for legislative actions, attend legislator fundraising events, network with members of established coalitions, meet regularly with legislatures to request specific actions on legislative initiatives, track the status of pending legislation, and establish meaningful relationships with legislators and their staff members. To track state legislative initiatives, SNAs monitor pending legislation that affects health care and professional practice. Some of the issues that are active in various state legislatures include the prohibition of mandatory overtime, safe client handling, minimum nurse–client ratios, malpractice tort reform, whistleblower protection for nurses, mandatory development of valid nursing staffing systems for acute and long-term care, state funding for nursing education, and passage of mutual state compacts for nursing licensure.

Mutual Recognition State Compact Legislation

The NCSBN developed a system in which professional nurses wishing to practice across state lines would not have to secure individual state licenses; this system is known as the **Nurse Licensure Compact (NLC)**. Under this provision, the RN holds a professional nursing license in the state of primary residence but would not have to hold another professional nursing license in states abiding by the NLC in order to practice. However, the RN is held accountable to the nurse practice act of the state in which nursing practice occurs. The compact is beneficial to nurses who live close to state lines and to those employed by traveling nurse agencies (Interstates Commission of Nurse Licensure Compact Administrators [ICNLCA], 2018).

Each state regulates professional nursing practice within its borders. For a state to participate in the mutual recognition program, the state legislature must adopt the NLC. Currently, 34 states have approved NLC and five states have introduced legislation for its approval. When the previous compact was dissolved in 2018, Rhode Island became the first and only state to remove itself from participating in the NLC (National Council of State Boards of Nursing [NCSBN], 2020).

∎ QUESTIONS FOR REFLECTION

1. What are your views on some of the current nursing legislative issues at the federal level? Which of these do you feel is the most important to you as a student or a practicing nurse?
2. Do your political views match those of the professional nursing organizations to which you belong?
3. Do the legislative goals of the professional nursing organizations make you more or less likely to join those organizations? Why?

EXAMPLES OF NURSES INFLUENCING PUBLIC POLICY

Although politics is frequently equated with corruption and abuse of power, the combination of political activity and professional nursing does not create cognitive dissonance. Nurses bring a caring perspective to the political process. Health care delivery and access are greatly affected by the political process. Nurses can fulfill the roles of client advocates and change agents by becoming politically active.

In addition to influencing legislation, as noted earlier in this chapter, nurses may assume responsibility in the legislative process by becoming members of legislative bodies. In 2016, 60 nurses held seats in state legislatures. Minnesota had the highest number of RNs serving in their state legislature (three RNs as state senators and three state representatives). Sixteen states do not have an RN in their legislative bodies (ANA, 2015). At the time of printing, there was no updated information regarding the number of nurses serving in political offices at the state level. Currently, only two nurses serve in the U.S. Congress (see Box 19.6, Professional Prototypes, "Nurses in Congress"). The number of RNs serving in the U.S. Congress fell from a high of five in 2014 to two following the 2018 election. Both nurses won reelection in 2020.

19.6 Professional Prototypes

Nurses in Congress

Membership of the 117th Congressional session in the U.S. House of Representatives includes the following nurses (ANA, n.d.-a):

- Eddie Bernice Johnson, RN (D-TX), was the first nurse elected to the Congress in 1992 and won her most recent election with more than 77.49% of the popular vote. Representative Johnson currently serves as the Democratic deputy whip of the House, a ranking member of the Transportation and Infrastructure Committee, and the chair of the Science, Space, and Technology Committee. She also serves as the secretary of the Congressional Black Caucus and was inducted as a fellow in the American Academy of Nursing in 2020 (Johnson, 2020).
- Lauren Underwood, RN (D-IL), was the first African American millennial elected to Congress in 2018. She won her most recent election with 50.67% of the popular vote. Prior to her run for Congress, she worked in the Department of Health and Human Services and facilitated implementation of the Affordable Care Act as well as assisting communities in prevention and preparation for responding to disasters, bioterrorism, and public health emergencies. She graduated from the University of Michigan and Johns Hopkins University. Before assuming her congressional seat, she taught nurse practitioner students online at Georgetown University. She founded and cochairs the Black Maternal Health Caucus; serves on the Education, Labor, Veterans Administration committees; is vice chair of the House committee on Homeland Security; and is a member of the Gun Violence Prevention Task Force (Underwood, n.d.).

Take Note!
Nurses fulfill the roles of client advocate and change agent when they become politically active.

Many nurses, officers of nursing organizations (ANA, SNAs, specialty nursing organizations), and nursing education program deans and directors testify before congressional committees when issues regarding health care and nursing arise. Elected officials and executive directors of SNAs frequently provide testimony before state legislative bodies. At the federal level, the president of the ANA frequently shares nursing expertise before the Congress. Since starting his term as ANA president in 2020, Grant has provided testimony twice to Congress. Mary Wakefield frequently provided Congressional Testimony as the Administrator of the Health Services Resource Administration regarding the current and future health care workforce needs.

Individuals are asked to provide testimony because of their position of special expertise. They will receive a letter requesting participation in the hearing from the committee chair conducting the hearing (LaForge, 2010; Spafford, n.d.). If called upon to provide testimony related to a committee or governmental agency, it is best to prepare a written document according to the guidelines presented in Box 19.7, Learning, Knowing, and Growing, "Guidelines for Preparing and Providing Testimony to a Committee or Governmental Agency."

OPPORTUNITIES TO LEARN THE ART OF INFLUENCING PUBLIC POLICY

There are many ways nurses can learn the art of influencing public policy development and legislative activity. ANA membership and involvement provide an avenue to learn how to participate in politics. The ANA employs political action specialists who educate nurses about the political process, communicate directly with elected officials about pending legislation, collect information about elected officials' voting records, identify politicians who are friends of nursing, and advise the ANA-PAC Board on potential candidates for ANA endorsement. In addition to active involvement in national politics, some SNAs offer daylong or weeklong internships on influencing public policies.

Fellowships and internships also offer the nurses an opportunity to learn the process of public policy development through actual experience. Fellowships and internships inform participants about the complexities of health care policy and legislative priorities and provide knowledge and skills to function in the public policy arena. Nurses may participate in formal fellowships and internships or create their own internship in the nation's capital. Some colleges and university graduate programs offer college credit to students who complete a Congressional practicum. Internships offer nurses the ability to network professionally with members of Congress and their staff. An internship may start a long-term relationship with a legislator or an influential staff

19.7 Learning, Knowing, and Growing

Guidelines for Preparing and Providing Testimony to a Committee or Governmental Agency

- Study and review material related to the issue for which the testimony is to be given.
- Learn about the congressional committee members (chair, ranking members) and committee staff.
- Prepare three versions of your testimony—an official written statement, a shorter version consisting of opening remarks and verbal statements, and abbreviated opening remarks.
- Make sure all versions are consistent and free of grammatical and spelling errors as the official statement will be entered into the record; the other versions are provided to expedite committee proceedings.
- Anticipate possible questions and prepare answers to them.
- Know the location of the hearing room and arrive 10 to 15 minutes before the hearing is scheduled to begin.
- While waiting, rehearse all three versions of your testimony.
- Upon arrival, sign the witness list (witnesses are called to testify starting at the top of the witness list).
- The typical time allotted for a single witness to testify is 3 to 5 minutes.
- Memorize the shorter version and have all materials printed with large font and on the top half of the sheet (this prevents head bobbing).
- Limit the opening remarks to three key points.
- Write each version using concise sentences.
- In the document, provide the following:
  - Your name, the issue being addressed, and the group receiving the testimony (provide this in the heading)

- Salutation of persons receiving the testimony and group name
- Identification of yourself, your professional credentials, and any people you represent
- Background information of the group if you are representing one
- Evidence for desired action (cite relevant research findings, societal trends)
- Personal request for desired action
- Describe the specifics of the program to resolve or help the issue being presented including potential negative results if the program is not developed, funded, or continued.
- State the desired action again.
- Be open and willing to discuss alternative views and actions politely and calmly if any comments or questions are presented.
- Express appreciation for the committee's
- time and attention and then offer to answer questions.
- If any follow-up information is requested following the hearing, provide clear, concise written information as soon as possible.
- If there are minutes from the hearing, they should be received within 4 to 8 weeks. Carefully review them for accuracy and submit changes within a week's time.
- Prepare statements for the press that include your key presented points. If you have access to a media department in your organization, reach out to them for assistance.
- Thank the person who invited you to testify (usually a staff member) and if you have any additional information of future ideas, share these with them.

From Short, N. M., & Milstead, J. A. (2019). An insider's guide to engaging in policy activities. In J. A. Milstead & N. M. Short (Eds.), *Health policy and politics: A nurse's guide* (6th ed., pp. 215–232). Jones & Bartlett Learning; Spafford, E. H. (n.d.). *Advice on government testimony.* Retrieved December 6, 2020, from purdue.edu

member and increase political passion within the nurse.

Internships can be applied for sending a brief cover letter and résumé (by email or post office) to an elected official. The information should be sent to the member's administrative assistant or chief of staff. A number of groups offer formal public policy fellowships (see Box 19.8, Professional Building Blocks, "Groups Offering Formal Public Policy Fellowships").

Summary and Significance to Practice

In fast-paced times, change is needed to provide safe, effective, client-centered, timely, and efficient health care. By virtue of their training, nurses possess the cognitive and communication skills necessary to successfully navigate the complex political processes required to influence public policy. To change the health care system, nurses can use critical thinking to analyze issues and communication skills to illuminate elected officials, policy makers, and the public about pressing health care issues. A model for political processes such as Kingdon's provides nurses with an evidence-based framework to guide political action efforts. Developing expertise in influencing public policy requires dedication, time, practice, and a willingness to work with others. When nurses succeed with political action, they become confident in their ability to influence public policy, resulting in improved health care for all.

Issues affecting personal and public health are too important to be left to politicians alone. They and their constituents need nurses to ensure that future public health care policies are based on solid evidence and improve access to health care.

19.8 Professional Building Blocks

Groups Offering Formal Public Policy Fellowships

- The Robert Wood Johnson Foundation
- David A. Winston
- The W.K. Kellogg Foundation
- The Congressional Black Caucus Foundation
- The White House Commission
- The Women's Research and Education Institute
- The Coro Foundation
- The American Association of University Women Educational Foundation
- The Business and Professional Women's Foundation
- The Everett McKinley Dirksen Congressional Leadership Research Center
- The U.S. Supreme Court
- The Woodrow Wilson National Fellowship Foundation
- The Employee Benefit Research Institute
- The Margaret Mahoney Fellowship in Health Policy
- The Office of Technology Assessment of the United States Congress
- The U.S. Department of Health and Human Services Office of the General Counsel
- IOM
- AHRQ
- The American Public Health Association
- The Centers for Disease Control and Prevention's Health and Aging Policy Fellows Program
- SNAs

From Mason, D. J., Gardner, D. S., Hopkins Outlaw, F., & O'Grady, E. T. (Eds.). (2016). *Policy and politics in nursing and health care* (7th ed.). Elsevier; Sharp, N., Biggs, S., & Wakefield, M. (1999). Public policy: New opportunities for nurses. *Nursing & Health Care, 12*(1), 16–22; Johnson, V. (2018). *10 fellowships for early and mid-career nurses*. Retrieved December 8, 2020, from https://www.profellow.com/fellowships/10-fellowships-for-early-and-mid-career-nurses/

Take Note!
Through advocacy and lobbying efforts and by serving as elected officials, nurses influence the future of health care delivery, public safety, and nursing practice.

Recall the scenario presented at the beginning of the chapter in which state school districts no longer have the resources to provide RNs for student health services. Do you think that all schools within a state should have an RN on the premises at all times during school hours? Why or why not? What impact would having an RN on school premises during school hours have on students, faculty, school staff, school administration, parents, and taxpayers? Does your state provide resources for RNs in its schools? What actions might you take to change your state's policies?

From Theory to Practice

1. Identify a currently introduced national or state bill. Using information from the ANA or your SNA, create a legislative fact sheet using the guidelines outlined in Box 19.4, Learning, Knowing, and Growing "Creating a Legislative Fact Sheet." Find position papers and white papers on the topic to provide information related to the issue that should be included in your fact sheet. Write an email message or letter to a legislator considering the initiative. After your message and fact sheet are approved by your instructor, send them to your legislator. Most legislators have websites with forms for sending email messages.

2. Write a personal story related to one of the ANA's legislative priorities found in Professional Prototypes Box 19.5.

Nurse as Author

Identify a legislative proposal at either the federal or state level that you think may affect your future as a nurse, your current nursing practice, or client care delivery. Write a one- to two-page position paper on the pending legislation using research and other evidence to support your position. Give the paper to a colleague to critique in terms of clarity, conciseness, and strength of your argument. Revise the paper based on your colleague's critique.

Your Digital Classroom

Online Exploration

Agency for Healthcare Research and Quality: **ahrq .gov**

American Academy of Nursing Health Policy Issues: **aannet.org**

American Hospital Association (Advocacy Issues): **https://www.aha.org/advocacy/2020-01-30-2020-aha-advocacy-agenda**

American Nurses Association Political Advocacy efforts: **nursingworld.org**

Canadian Nurses Association: **https://www.cna-aiic.ca/en/**

Find your legislator: **https://fiscalnote.com/find-your-legislator**

Centers for Medicare and Medicaid Services: **https://www.cms.gov**

Department of Health and Human Services: **www.hhs.gov**

Government Made Easy (database of more than 1.5 million U.S. government web pages): **www.usa.gov**

Institute of Medicine: **https://www .nationalacademies.org/hmd/health-and-medicine-division**

Library of Congress: **https://www.loc.gov/**

National Council of State Boards of Nursing: **www.ncsbn.org**

Occupational Safety and Health Administration: **www.osha.gov**

RN Action: **http://www.rnaction.org**

U.S. House of Representatives: **www.house.gov**

U.S. Senate: **www.senate.gov**

Expanding Your Understanding

1. Visit the websites of the U.S. Senate and House of Representatives and complete the following exercises:
   a. Visit the home pages of your state Senators and Representative. If you do not know their names, you can find them by entering your home zip code, clicking your home location on a map, or typing in the number of your legislative district found on your voter registration card in the information request section.
   b. Search for the current legislation. In the search bar, type in the words "nursing," "health care," or "nursing practice" to see current legislative initiatives affecting nursing and health care delivery.
   c. Find a relevant bill and click to read the summary and the text.
   d. Send an email to your Senators and Representative using the strategies for composing letters and messages found in this chapter.
   e. Find your state legislature by conducting a search for "(your state's name) legislature." On your state's legislative site, search for "nursing" and "health care delivery" as key words to find information about the current legislative efforts affecting professional nursing in your state.
2. Visit RN Action at www.rnaction.org.
   a. Click on the tab "Nurses Vote" and choose "Nursing Priorities" to find a list of the ANA's legislative priorities. Select an issue that interests you and click "Learn More" to find current information on the issue. If any legislation is active in either the House of Representatives or Senate, the bill number will be listed and you can find out more about it by clicking on the bill numbers within the information text block. You will also be invited to contact your elected official regarding the legislation. You will find a link to directly share ANA's views on the introduced legislation with your Senator or House Representative.
   b. On the home page, click on "Action Centers" and select one of the issues for action. You will be able to take the requested action on it by contacting one of your elected officials.
   c. When you come to class or participate in a course online discussion board, report on the action you took. Include the reasons why you selected to act on one alert over another, the action that you took, and if you received any follow-up communication from your legislator(s). How did it feel to take political action? Would you take action on another issue? Why or why not?
3. Visit the NCSBN website at www.ncsbn.org, and complete the following exercises:
   a. At the top of the page, click on "Licensure Compacts." On the next page, click on "NLC Model Legislation and Rules," and read the rules and

regulations that must be followed by states and nurses practicing in NLC states. On this page, scroll down until you see a map of the United States that identifies current states that have enacted the NLC. You will see a map of the United States, with certain states highlighted in blue. These are the states that participate in the compact. What states participate in it? Does your state participate in the interstate nursing licensure compact?

b. Scroll down and continue reading information that appears below the map of the United States that specify NLC compact states. On a piece of paper, write down information to explain the NLC to a nurse who does not live in a participating state and to a nurse who lives in a participating state but is considering a move to a nonparticipating state.

c. Once you have read all the information posted to answer questions for part b, scroll to the top of the page. On the left side of the screen, click on "NLC FAQs," and read answers to frequently asked questions about the NLC. In addition, download the NLC Toolkit that contains NLC Fact Sheets and Flow Charts. Click on the flow charts for "Licensure by Examination" and "Licensure by Endorsement." Compare and contrast this information. Consult with a nursing faculty member from your program if you have any questions. Click on the following Fact Sheets: "What Nurses Need to Know" and "Fact Sheet for New Graduates." What did you find important and interesting? Why did you find this information important and interesting?

Beyond the Book

Visit the Point at **www.thePoint.lww.com** for activities and information to reinforce the concepts and content covered in this chapter.

REFERENCES

Agency for Healthcare Research and Quality. (2007). *Nursing staffing and quality of patient care* (AHRQ Publication No. 07-E005). Author. Retrieved July 2008, from www.ahrq.gov/clinic/tp/nursesttp.htm

American Association of Colleges of Nursing. (2020). *AACN applauds increased federal investment in nursing education and research*. Retrieved December 8, 2020, from https://www.aacnnursing.org/News-Information/Press-Releases/View/ArticleId/24546/Federal-Investments-FY20

American Nurses Association. (2015). *Nurse state legislators and administrative leaders directory*. Retrieved June 5, 2016, from http://nursingworld.org/NurseLegislatorDirectory.aspx#mo

American Nurses Association. (2016a). *ANA-PAC endorsement process*. Retrieved June 16, 2016, from http://www.rnaction.org/site/PageNavigator/nstat_pac_endorsement_process.htmll

American Nurses Association. (2016b). *Coalitions*. Retrieved June 11, 2016, from http://www.rnaction.org/site/PageNavigator/nstat_ana_coalitions.html

American Nurses Association. (2018a). *ANA advocacy toolkit*. Retrieved April 11, 2021, from https://ana.aristotle.com/SitePages/toolkit.aspx

American Nurses Association. (2018b). Gun violence. *RN Action*. Retrieved April 11, 2021, from https://ana.aristotle.com/SitePages/gunviolence.aspx

American Nurses Association. (2021a). COVID-19. *RN Action*. Retrieved April 9, 2021, from https://ana.aristotle.com/SitePages/Personal_Protective_Equipment.aspx

American Nurses Association. (2021b). Health system transformation. *RN Action*. Retrieved April 9, 2021, from https://ana.aristotle.com/SitePages/health_system_transformation.aspx

American Nurses Association. (2021c). Nursing workforce development. *RN Action*. Retrieved April 9, 2021, from https://ana.aristotle.com/SitePages/nursingworkforcedevelopment.aspx

American Nurses Association. (2021d). Opioid epidemic. *RN Action*. Retrieved April 9, 2021, from https://ana.aristotle.com/SitePages/Opioid.Epidemic.aspx

American Nurses Association. (2021e). Safe staffing. *RN Action*. Retrieved April 9, 2021, from https://ana.aristotle.com/SitePages/safestaffing.aspx

American Nurses Association. (2021f). Top federal legislative priorities. *RN Action*. Retrieved April 9, 2021, from https://rnaction.org/SitePages/Homepage.aspx/issues.aspx

American Nurses Association. (2021g). Workplace violence. *RN Action*. Retrieved April 9, 2021, from https://ana.aristotle.com/SitePages/WorkplaceViolence.aspx

American Nurses Association. (n.d.-a). *Nurses currently serving in ongress*. Retrieved April 11, 2021, from https://www.nursingworld.org/practice-policy/advocacy/federal/nurses-serving-in-congress/

American Nurses Association (n.d.-b). Practice and Advocacy. State. Retrieved May 17, from https://www.nursingworld.org/practice-policy/advocacy/state/

Bowers-Lanier, R. R. (2021). *Coalitions: A powerful political strategy*. In D. J. Mason, E. Dickson, M. R. McLemore, & G. A. Perez (Eds.), *Policy and politics in nursing and health care* (8th ed., pp. 543–549). Elsevier.

Bureau of Labor Statistics. (2020). Occupational outlook handbook. *Registered Nurses*. Retrieved December 8, 2020, from https://www.bls.gov/ooh/healthcare/registered-nurses.htm

Cohen, S. S., Mason, D. J., Kovner, C., Leavitt, J. K., Pulcini, J., & Sochalski, J. (1996). Stages of nursing's political development: Where we've been and where we ought to go. *Nursing Outlook, 44*, 259–266. https://doi.org/10.1016/s0029-6554(96)80081-9

Conant, R., & Jackson, C. (2007). Brief overview of ANA political action committee. *American Nurse Today, 2*(3), 24. Retrieved April 11, 2021, from https://www.myamericannurse.com/brief-overview-of-ana-political-action-committee/

Congress.org. (2021). *Advocacy 101 A new age of online advocacy*. Retrieved May 17, 2021, from https://www.congress.org/advocacy-101/

de Vries, C., & Vanderbilt, M. (1992). *The grassroots lobbying handbook: Empowering nurses through legislative and political action*. American Nurses Association.

FastDemocracy. (n.d.). *Which version of FastDemocracy is right for you.* Retrieved April 11, 2021, from https://fastdemocracy.com/

Federal Election Commission. (2020a). *American Association of Nurse Anesthetists PAC*. Retrieved December 6, 2020, from https://www.fec.gov/data/committee/C00173153/

Federal Election Commission. (2020b). *American Hospital Association political action committee*. Retrieved December 6, 2020, from https://www.fec.gov/data/committee/C00106146/

Federal Election Commission. (2020c). *American Medical Association political action committee*. Retrieved December 6, 2020, from https://www.fec.gov/data/committee/C00000422/

Federal Election Commission. (2020d). *American Nurses Association political action committee*. Retrieved December 6, 2020, from https://www.fec.gov/data/committee/C00017525/

Feldman, J. R., & Lewenson, S. B. (Eds.). (2000). *Nurses in the political arena*. Springer.

Flanagan, L. (1976). *One strong voice: The story of the American Nurses Association*. ANA.

Furlong, E. A. (2019). Agenda setting: What rises to a policy-maker's attention? In J. A. Milstead & N. M. Short (eds.), *Health policy and politics a nurse's guide* (6th, ed. pp. 17–56). Jones & Bartlett Learning.

Glassman, M. E., Straus, J. R., & Shogan, C. J. (2010). *Social networking and constituent communications: Member use of Twitter during a two-month period in the 111th Congress* (Research Report No. 7-5700). Retrieved April 11, 2021, from https://fas.org/sgp/crs/misc/R43018.pdf

Goldwater, M., & Zusy, M. (1990). *Prescription for nurses: Effective political action*. Mosby.

Grant, E. (2020a). *May 27, 2020 testimony from ANA President Ernest Grant to the House Ways and Means Committee regarding COVID-19 disparities in communities of color*. Retrieved April 11, 2021, from https://www.nursingworld.org/practice-policy/work-environment/health-safety/disaster-preparedness/coronavirus/may-27-2020-testimony-from-ana-president-ernest-grant-regarding-covid-health-disparities/

Grant, E. (2020b). *July 30, 2020 testimony form ANA President Ernest Grant to the Senate Finance Committee regarding personal protective equipment*. Retrieved December 6, 2020, from https://www.nursingworld.org/practice-policy/work-environment/health-safety/disaster-preparedness/coronavirus/covid-19-interview-with-debbie-hatmaker-on-cnn/senfin-grant/

Han, N. K., & Kim, G. S. (2020). Concept development of political competence for nurses. *Journal of Korean Academy of Nursing, 50*(1), 81–100. https://doi.org/10.4040/jkan.2020.50.1.81

Hatmaker, D. D. (2020). *Fourth edition of the 2020 ANA PAC Quarterly Newsletter*. Retrieved December 6, 2020, from https://contentsharing.net/actions/email_web_version.cfm?ep=7tWQbl9aHr4va6V3BNw5-_AOycRE7b-jpV85i4td13GtTBchlhYkfIVhpak-BJTDftSHBMCIhDex-zdT6qn5HO7D-Ly7tAxJoJLcdYNru_PwlxDlxdtc7FSlUx-nh5hsXv9

Hebda, T. (2019). The impact of EHRs, big data and evidence-informed practice. In J. A. Milstead & N. M. Short (Eds.), *Health policy and politics: A nurse's guide* (6th ed., pp. 133–150). Jones & Bartlett Learning.

Inouye, L. M. (2021). Lobbying policymakers: Individual and collective strategies. In Mason, D. J., Dickson, E., McLemore,

M. R. & Perez, G. A. (Eds.), *Policy & politics in nursing and health care* (8th ed., pp. 343–348). Elsevier.

Institute of Medicine. (1999). *To err is human: Building a safer health system*. National Academies Press.

Institute of Medicine. (2004). *Keeping patients safe: Transforming the work environment of nurses*. National Academies Press.

Institute of Medicine. (2011). *The future of nursing: Leading change, advancing health*. National Academies Press.

Itzhaky, H., Gerber, P., & Dekel, R. (2004). Empowerment skills and values: A comparative study of nurses and social workers. *International Journal of Nursing Studies, 41*, 447–456. https://doi.org/10.1016/j.ijnurstu.2003.10.012

Johnson, E. (2020). *About Eddie Bernice Johnson*. Retrieved April 11, 2011, from https://ebjohnson.house.gov/

Johnson, V. (2018). *10 fellowships for early and mid-career nurses*. Retrieved December 8, 2020, from https://www.profellow.com/fellowships/10-fellowships-for-early-and-mid-career-nurses/

Josiah Macy Jr. Foundation. (n.d.). *About the foundation. Leadership and staff. Mary K. Wakefield, PhD, RN, FAAN*. Retrieved December 5, 2020, from https://macyfoundation.org/about/our-leadership-and-staff/mary-k-wakefield

Kingdon, J. (1995). *Agendas, alternatives and public policy*. Harper Collins College.

LaForge, W. N. (2010). *Testifying before Congress*. The Capital-Net.Net Inc.

Loversidge, J. M. (2019). *Government response: Regulation*. In J. A. Milstead & N. M. Short (Eds.), *Health policy and politics: A nurse's guide* (6th ed., pp. 57–86). Jones & Bartlett Learning.

Mason, D. J., Dickson, E., McLemore, M. R., & Perez, G. A. (2021). Frameworks for action in policy and politics. In D. J. Mason, E. Dickson, M. R. McLemore, & G. A. Perez (Eds.), *Policy and politics in nursing and health care* (8th ed., pp. 1–15). Elsevier.

McKeon, E. (2008). Legislative updates: 110th Congress wrap-up. *Capitol Update, 6*(9). Retrieved January 3, 2009, from www.capitolupdate.org/Newsletter/index.asp?nlid=199&nlid=1054

Milstead, J. A., & Short, N. M. (2019). Informing public policy: An important role for registered nurses. In J. A. Milstead & N. M. Short (Eds.), *Health policy and politics: A nurse's guide* (6th ed., pp. 1–16). Jones & Bartlett Learning.

Mish, F. C. (2020). *Merriam-Webster's Collegiate Dictionary* (11th ed.). Merriam-Webster.

National Council of State Boards of Nursing. (2020). *NLC member jurisdictions*. Retrieved May 17, 2021, from https://www.ncsbn.org/nlcmemberstates.pdf

O'Grady, E. T. (2021). The policy process. In J. A. Milstead & N. M. Short (Eds.), *Health policy and politics a nurse's guide* (6th ed., pp. 52–64). Jones & Bartlett Learning.

Price, L., Lessard, K., & Mumm, E. (2021). Research as a political and policy tool. In D. J. Mason, E. Dickson, M. R. McLemore, & G. A. Perez (Eds.), *Policy and politics in nursing and health care* (8th ed., pp. 81–88). Elsevier.

Roll Call CQ. (2013). *Communicating with congress*. Retrieved April 19, 2013, from www.congress.org/ Roll Call news/communicating-with-congress/

Roll Call CQ Staff. (2009). *Why congress prefers email*. Retrieved April 19, 2013, from www.congress.org/news/why-congress-prefers-e-mail/

Roth, L. (2011). A nurse in every school? Not in Florida—Not even close. *The Orlando Sentinel*. Retrieved April 19, 2012, from http://articles.orlandosentinel.com/2011-09-26/business/os-fewer-school-nurses-florida-20110925_1_school-nurses-practical-nurses-students-with-chronic-illnesses

Schumann, M. J. (2021). An overview of legislative and regulatory processes. In D. J. Mason, E. Dickson, M. R. McLemore, & G. A. Perez (Eds.), *Policy and politics in nursing and health care* (8th ed., pp. 333–342). Elsevier.

Sharp, N., Biggs, S., & Wakefield, M. (1999). Public policy: New opportunities for nurses. *Nursing & Health Care, 12*(1), 16–22. Retrieved April 11, 2021, from https://eric.ed.gov/?id=EJ420867

Shirley, H. (2020). *Former UND nursing instructor selected for Biden-Harris transition team*. Retrieved November 16, 2020, from https://www.grandforksherald.com/news/government-and-politics/6764665-Former-UND-nursing-instructor-selected-for-Biden-Harris-transition-team

Short, N. M., & Milstead, J. A. (2019). An insider's guide to engaging in policy activities. In J. A. Milstead & N. M. Short (Eds.), *Health policy and politics: A nurse's guide* (6th ed., pp. 215–232). Jones & Bartlett Learning.

Spafford, E. H. (n.d.). *Advice on government testimony*. Retrieved April 11, 2021, from https://spaf.cerias.purdue.edu/usgov/testimony.html

The Interstate Commission of Nurse Licensure Compact Administrators. (2018). *The Interstate Commission of Nurse Licensure Compact Administrators final rules*. Retrieved December 8, 2020, from https://www.ncsbn.org/FinalRulesadopted81120clean_ed.pdf

Underwood, L. (n.d.). *Lauren Underwood, 14th District of Illinois, About, Biography*. Retrieved April 11, 2021, from https://underwood.house.gov/about/biography

Wakefield, M. (2004). Health policy and politics: A call to political arms. *Nursing Economic$, 33*, 166–167. Retrieved April 11, 2021, from https://www.researchgate.net/publication/8496161_A_call_to_political_arms

Envisioning and Creating the Future of Professional Nursing

As a profession, nursing can count on change. Nurses have many career options. A rewarding and satisfying career depends on the interests and passions of each individual nurse. Once nurses discover what they want to do, they can use specific career development strategies to ensure success. Many nurses move from one area of professional practice to another throughout their professional nursing career. To meet the future needs for professional nursing and to secure a future for the profession, nurses need to examine current trends, develop future scenarios, and envision a preferred future. Once a preferred future is envisioned, professional nurses can develop plans to create a future that optimizes the contributions that nurses make in enhancing the health and well-being of all people.

4

ENVISIONING AND CREATING THE FUTURE OF PROFESSIONAL NURSING

Career Options for Professional Nurses

LEARNING OUTCOMES

By the end of this chapter, the learner will be able to:

1. Outline universal job skills.
2. Specify which universal job skills nurses possess.
3. Identify career options for nurses educated at the generalist level.
4. Explain the differences between general and advanced nursing practice.
5. Distinguish certification from advanced nursing practice.
6. Describe advanced nursing practice roles and responsibilities.

REAL-LIFE REFLECTIONS

Laura is thinking about entering the nursing profession. As she explores professional nursing, Laura interviews four nurses and finds that there are many career options within the profession. One nurse Laura interviewed remained employed for over 20 years as a staff nurse at the same clinical site where she had her capstone nursing experience as an undergraduate student. Another nurse shared her experiences in a nursing career that began as a nursing assistant, followed by several years each of hospital staff nursing, school nursing, and outpatient clinic nursing that resulted in more education to work as a **nurse practitioner** *(NP) in a small rural clinic. The third nurse told Laura she had been a nurse for 15 years and started her career in the Army Nurse Corps. She shared stories about multiple areas of clinical practice including medical–surgical nursing, critical care nursing, and now the neonatal intensive care unit. The nurse explained she likes to constantly challenge herself to learn new things and thrives on different experiences. The fourth nurse Laura interviewed was a nurse faculty member who held a nursing doctorate and enjoyed researching and teaching. After learning about the diverse career options in nursing, Laura realizes she does not have to decide on a specialized area of practice and will keep her options open until she finds her preferred niche.*

TABLE 20.1   Universal Job Skills and How Professional Nurses Use Them

Occupational Outlook Handbook (BLS, 1992)	Yee-Litzenberg (2011) (University of Michigan)	Professional Nurse Example
Leadership/persuasion	Management	Supervising unlicensed assistive personnel
Problem solving/creativity	Analytical/problem-solving skills	Utilizing nursing process
Working as part of a team	Multidisciplinary team experience/interpersonal skills	Working in partnership with clients, families, and other health care providers
Manual dexterity	Technical skills	Executing complex clinical nursing and computer skills (e.g., starting intravenous lines and accessing from and entering information in computers)
Helping or instructing others	Interpersonal skills	Establishing and maintaining therapeutic relationships Teaching
Initiative	Leadership/initiative	Performing surveillance activities to detect complications before they arise
		Providing optimal, high-quality client care services
Frequent contact with the public	Interpersonal skills	Working with clients, families, visitors, and communities
Physical stamina		Meeting physical demands of client care activities Working long hours
	Communication/media	Developing client, family, and community education materials Giving public presentations

Setting career goals begins with self-assessment. Ideally, career goals should match personal values and acquired skills. This chapter explores many of the possible career options in professional nursing.

UNIVERSAL JOB SKILLS

In 1992, the *Occupational Outlook Handbook* published by the U.S. Bureau of Labor Statistics delineated the following **universal job skills** for all types of work: (1) leadership/persuasion, (2) problem solving/creativity, (3) working as part of a team, (4) manual dexterity, (5) helping or instructing others, (6) initiative, (7) frequent contact with the public, and (8) physical stamina. These skills remain relevant today. Yee-Litzenberg (2011) identified similar universal job skills but expanded the skill set to include media use and technical skills (including computer software abilities); physical stamina does not appear on her list. Table 20.1 compares these two sets of universal job skills and provides examples of how professional nurses use them. The comprehensive skill set required by professional nurses may be one reason for the diversity of nursing career opportunities.

Individuals rank the importance of job skills differently, thereby providing clues to how nurses perceive what is important to them. For example, a nursing position that limits direct communication with clients and families would be a suboptimal choice for a nurse who values establishing and maintaining therapeutic relationships with others. By taking time to rank each job skill, nurses discover what type of a nursing career fits in with their personal values.

Take Note!
The job skills mastered by nurses readily transfer to multiple fields within and outside the nursing profession.

QUESTIONS FOR REFLECTION

1. How might you use each of the eight universal job skills in your daily professional nursing practice?
2. How do people with non-nursing jobs use the skills differently than nurses?
3. Why does nursing require mastery of all eight universal job skills?

LEVELS OF NURSING PRACTICE

In the United States, state legislatures and state boards of nursing regulate practice. In most of Canada (except Ontario and Quebec), provincial/territorial professional nursing associations regulate practice. In Ontario, diploma nursing programs are approved and monitored by the Ministry of Training Colleges and the Council of Ontario University Programs in Nursing (COUPN). All university nursing programs in Ontario are also approved by each university senate or governing council. In 2008, COUPN delegated its authorship for approving university-based nursing programs to the Canadian Association of Schools of Nursing (CASN). CASN accreditation constitutes nursing program approval. In Quebec, diploma nursing programs are approved and monitored in the Collège d'enseignement général et professionnel, and university programs are monitored by the particular university in which they reside (Ross-Kerr, 2011). In both countries, regulation of practice involves determining educational qualifications, setting standards of professional practice, limiting the use of the title "registered nurse (RN)," approving nursing education programs, determining the extent of continuing education and competency, disciplining professional members who endanger the public, and specifying the scope of nursing practice (National Council of State Boards of Nursing [NCSBN], 2012; Ross-Kerr, 2011).

When nurses complete a preparatory nursing education program (associate degree, diploma, or baccalaureate degree), successfully pass the NCSBN Licensure Examination for Registered Nurses (NCLEX-RN), and pay nursing licensure fees, they begin professional practice as RNs. **Licensure** is a process of legal authorization for nursing practice. **Registration** encompasses a listing of qualified, licensed nurses in good standing that is available to the public. Newly licensed nurses initially practice as generalists. However, with increased experience in a particular area of practice, many nurses become specialized.

Professional nurse associations recognize competence in a particular nursing field through certification. **Certification** means that an individual meets specified requirements, which usually include specialized knowledge and skills in a particular area of nursing practice. Most certifications in professional nursing practice require a specified number of years of experience within a specialty along with successful completion of a competency examination. Each nursing organization sets criteria for nurses to maintain specialty certification. Most organizations require a combination of clinical practice hours along with a determined number of continuing education contact hours. Some nursing regulatory agencies recognize certification from professional nursing associations as credentials for an advanced nursing practice licensure.

Advanced nursing practice extends the scope and responsibilities beyond what is typically expected of an RN. According to the American Nurses Association's *Nursing: Scope and Standards of Practice, 4th ed.* (American Nurses Association, [ANA]), advanced practice registered nurses (APRNs) are defined as "a subset of graduate-level prepared registered nurses who have completed an accredited graduate-level education program preparing the nurse for special licensure recognition and practice for one of the four recognized APRN roles: certified reigisterd nurse anesthestist (CRNA), certified nurse-midwife, clinical nurse specialst (CNS) or certified nurse practiioner (CNP)" (ANA, 2021, p. 3). Along with earning a graduate nursing degree, APRNs pass a national certification exam measuring specific APRN roles and population-based competencies. APRNs are also licensed for advanced practice by the state in which they practice and must undergo periodic recertification, which typically includes a minimum number of clinical practice hours in their area of practice. Hallmarks of advanced nursing practice include **graduate nursing education** (master's degree or doctorate in nursing), national certification for the role, and a focused population for whom they will be providing services.

Early in the profession's history, a graduate nursing education was not required for entry into advanced nursing practice. Nursing practice laws, rules, and regulations for APRNs vary from state to state and depend upon the practice role. Some states require additional nursing licensure for advanced practice. Depending on the state, APRN practice may fall under the auspices of the state board of healing arts (BHA), the state board of nursing (SBN), or both. For example, a clinical nurse specialist may attain licensure with the SBN and a certified nurse-midwife must be licensed through the BHA. According to the American Association of Nurse Practitioners (2020b), 28 states require that NPs, who deliver primary, secondary, or tertiary health care services to clients, sometimes in collaboration with a physician, enter into collaborative practice agreements with physicians licensed in the state of practice. However, 22 states and the District of Columbia offer APRNs full practice authority, which means that a collaborative practice agreement is not required (AANP, 2020b). During the COVID-19 epidemic, some states issued waivers reducing restrictions on advanced nursing practice. Some of these states passed legislation (and governors signed resolutions) making these changes permanent.

GENERAL NURSING CAREER OPPORTUNITIES

The nursing profession offers a wide array of opportunities. Nurses have the flexibility to focus on one area of practice or work in several practice areas. In addition, nurses may work for an organization or for themselves. **General nursing practice** encompasses areas of practice in which no additional or specialized formal education is required. **Specialized nursing practice** occurs when nurses work in a specific clinical area (e.g., obstetrics, oncology, intensive care) in which additional education and training are needed to meet specific client concerns or to master unique clinical nursing skills. In many specialty areas of nursing practice, nurses become certified in the area of practice, which means they have mastered specific skills and possess a unique knowledge to deliver client care.

When a nurse identifies a problem in practice, a potential opportunity arises for a new area of nursing practice. An identified problem sometimes leads to the development of a personal business or an entirely new health service to be offered by a large medical center.

This section briefly summarizes the more common areas of nursing practice. Detailed information about specific nursing careers can be found in this and other chapters, including advanced practice nursing (later in this chapter), nursing informatics (Chapter 14, "Informatics and Technology in Nursing Practice"), lobbying as a nurse (Chapter 19, "The Professional Nurses Role in Public Policy"), and nursing careers in community health nursing (Chapter 15, "Nursing Approaches to Client Systems").

Acute Care or Hospital Nursing Options

When asked about professional nursing, people not involved in health care tend to describe a nurse as someone who provides direct care to clients in inpatient settings. According to the U.S. Bureau of Labor Statistics (BLS) (2020f), about 1.86 million (60%) of employed RNs worked in hospitals in 2020, with most of them being engaged in direct client care. Recent changes in the health care delivery system have resulted in a variety of career options for nurses working in acute care.

Staff Nursing

Nurses engaging in direct client care find themselves in a fast-paced and challenging position. Within the past decade, the acuity of hospitalized clients has increased dramatically. Nurses today often care for clients who once would have been admitted only to intensive care units. As complex specialized skills become requirements for various types of staff nursing (such as oncology and cardiac specialties), many nurses become certified in specialty practice areas. Experience and certification in specialty areas of practice result in highly trained experts delivering client care. As nurses develop more technical expertise in specific areas, they cannot be expected to provide expert nursing care to clients outside those areas of clinical specialties. However, because basic nursing education effectively prepares nurses to assume safe care responsibilities as nurse generalists, hospitals sometimes assign nurses to work outside their clinical specialty areas.

In all practice settings, professional nurses must become experts at juggling multiple tasks simultaneously as they fulfill numerous obligations. Nurses confront competing client care priorities such as balancing the quality of care with cost containment. They use leadership skills for effective delegation and supervision of unlicensed assistive personnel (UAP) and licensed practical/vocational nurses (LPNs/LVNs) rather than performing direct care activities themselves. They serve as the primary coordinators of client care when consumers receive care in health care organizations. In order to remain in control of and have a voice in daily practice, some nurses assume shared governance responsibilities. When getting clients the services they need, nurses coordinate care activities. They also use therapeutic communication skills to effectively soothe disgruntled clients, families, and physicians. Sometimes they judiciously use humor for optimal management of emotionally charged situations (especially when work colleagues are involved). Above all, professional nurses keep health care consumers safe and look for ways to enhance environmental safety for all parties involved in health care delivery.

Keeping nurse experts at the client bedside poses challenges for acute care organizations. Some hospitals have designed nursing clinical ladders as a means to keep highly qualified and experienced nurses at the bedside. **Clinical ladders** recognize and reward staff nurses for years of bedside nursing experience, engagement in shared governance activities, and participation in ongoing professional development activities. Rewards typically include increased income and job titles that denote professional accomplishments and experience; these can be viewed as promotions without nurses having to leave direct client care. Each acute care facility has criteria for climbing the clinical ladder. Many employers use educational status, specialty professional nurse certification, integration of nursing research in clinical practice, and participation in shared governance activities as criteria for promotion. Frequently, nurses who climb clinical ladders have the opportunity to serve as mentors or preceptors to novice nurses.

Take Note!

Due to changes in the health care delivery system, a variety of career options have recently arisen for all professional nurses.

QUESTIONS FOR REFLECTION

1. What are the benefits for nurses of having nursing clinical ladders? For hospitals?

2. Would a clinical nursing ladder keep you at the bedside? Why or why not?

Forensic Nursing

Forensic nurses provide care to victims of violent crimes. Many hospital emergency departments (EDs) have a nurse who has special education in working with victims of violent crimes. Nursing care provided by forensic nurses includes caring for the victim's injuries; identifying and documenting injuries (including taking photographs); determining wound patterns; collecting evidence (samples of hair, tissue, and body fluids) for future investigations and potential trials; and testifying in court to present and explain evidence and examination findings (Commission for Forensic Nursing Certification [CFNC], 2020; International Association of Forensic Nurses [IAFN], 2020; Lehmann, 2020).

Victims of violent crimes benefit from having forensic nurses because these nurses have special training in how to approach and counsel survivors while collecting evidence. Some EDs have special rape crisis or abuse crisis programs where victims receive care in specially designated rooms from RNs educated as sexual assault nurse examiners (SANEs).The education for SANEs includes 40 hours of classroom didactic instruction followed by 40 hours of clinical training supervised by a nurse with SANE certification. The International Association of Forensic Nurses offers two certifications for SANEs, SANE-A (for adolescent and adult victims) and SANE-P (for pediatric victims). SANEs preform physical, psychological, developmental, and safety client assessments; collect and document evidence; manage the care of sexually assaulted clients from a holistic perspective; respond to subpoenas and court orders; and provide factual or expert witness testimony during trials. Initial management of victims of sexual assault following evidence collection involves referrals to social workers (CFNC, 2020; IAFN, 2020; Lehmann, 2020).

Professional Nursing Development Educators

Concerns related to staff competency and improving the quality of care have spurred hospitals to maintain nursing staff education and training departments (sometimes called *staff or professional nursing development*). The roles of the professional nurse development educator (PNDE) vary from organization to organization. Typically, the PNDE plans, executes, and evaluates nursing staff orientation and continuing education programs. Planning programs frequently involve meeting with nurse learners so that the programs are relevant to their needs. The PNDE plans educational offerings with staff input, and submits the offerings for continuing educational credit approval to a SBN or another nursing organization. Frequently, the PNDE has the responsibility for maintaining American Nursing Credentialing Center (ANCC) certification for the department in order to provide continuing education credit for all offered continuing education programs (an essential part of the job in states that have continuing education requirements for nursing license renewals). The PNDE may also be required to submit an organizational continuing education report to the SBN.

Professional nursing development departments sometimes manage professional nurse competencies that must be verified on a regular basis (e.g., annual reviews for infection control and safety or biannual cardiopulmonary resuscitation [CPR]). Professional nursing development departments also become involved in offering education for professional nurses on new equipment and new nursing protocols that may arise from new care regulations, quality improvement, and new evidence-based initiatives. Verification of professional nurse competence to perform specific clinical skills may be centralized through this department or may occur within individual nursing units. Because client safety is a primary concern for the PNDE, frequent rounds to clinical units may be made to ask staff about their learning needs as well as observing staff as care is delivered to note any performance gaps in adhering to established policies and procedures. PNDEs also develop, plan and execute transition programs for new graduate nurses as they assume their first professional nurse positions (Association for Nursing Professional Development [ANPD], 2016).

When a facility trains its own UAP, the professional development department offers and coordinates training efforts to ensure consistency in UAP preparation. The staff development educator may also manage UAP competencies and provide additional education and training for new equipment, policies, and procedures. Some hospitals require graduate degrees in nursing or education for PNDE positions. However, most long-term care facilities do not have this requirement. ANCC offers certification for nursing staff development educators (ANPD, 2016). Titles for nurses working in this field include staff educator, clinical education specialist, in-service educator, and educational specialist. Some institutions (usually smaller ones) also use staff development personnel to plan community education programs. When a hospital is used as a clinical site for multiple nursing programs, staff educators frequently coordinate clinical day availability, set up programs to verify clinical faculty competence, ensure students have met all clinical requirements, develop student clinical orientation programs, and keep records related to nursing program satisfaction with the agency as a clinical site.

Utilization Review and Hospital Case Management

In response to Medicare regulations, many hospitals have utilization review programs. To verify the effective use of hospital services, hospitals and insurance companies use nurses to streamline inpatient care. Because they have the education and experience to understand effective use of resources, some nurses obtain employment as utilization reviewers. Some managed care organizations employ nurses as preadmission coordinators who prepare clients for hospital admission by coordinating preadmission testing and providing clients with education related to the usual hospital course, especially for surgical procedures. In addition, some managed care organizations use nurses as case managers who act as client care advocates to make care-related decisions, recommend medical treatments, certify insurance coverage, and listen to customer expectations and problems.

Nurses working in utilization usually work behind the scenes. They engage in chart reviews and audits to verify that clients receive required services, as efficiently as possible. The goal of utilization is to eliminate any ineffective treatments or unnecessary procedures. Utilization nurses advocate for care that maximizes client quality of care and life and prevents complications associated with hospital care. Because inpatient acute care is so expensive, the utilization review nurse questions any prolonged hospital stays. They work closely with social workers on dismissal planning. Along with promoting optimal effectiveness in care delivery, utilization nurses also conduct chart audits to verify that government regulations are followed. Working as a utilization reviewer requires a strong clinical background, refined communication skills, good research skills, and well-developed analytical skills. Nurses in these positions often serve as liaisons among the provider, physician, and consumer.

Risk/Quality Management

Most hospitals have departments to monitor care quality, track unusual reported incidents, identify potential liability areas, provide staff education on the documentation and reporting of incidents, and assist the staff when legal actions or malpractice suits arise. Risk management focuses on reducing institutional financial losses because of care errors and accidents. Nurses employed in risk management departments sometimes hold law degrees.

Although all nurses play a role in managing the quality of health care provided within their institutions, some larger organizations may have centralized quality management departments to evaluate the quality of services provided. Some quality management departments employ nurses who have earned graduate degrees or doctorates in quality management. Because a large portion of the services offered by hospitals is nursing care, nurses may be members of the quality department. However, some organizations opt for a decentralized approach to quality management. In these cases, staff nurses assume a larger role in monitoring the quality of nursing care and may be required to perform periodic review of client care documentation to verify that quality indicators have been met. With increased emphasis on pay-for-performance and accountable care organizations, nurses have been employed for managing quality in the arena of client care delivery. Because of their knowledge of health care delivery systems, many organizations look for a nursing background when they are looking for individuals who can assume leadership positions in quality management departments.

Travel Nursing

With regional and seasonal RN shortages, some nurses (especially those who like variety, taking risks, and traveling) elect to travel to different inpatient institutions to practice bedside client care. Travel nurses accept staff nurse assignments in all areas of the hospital. Travel nurses may contract with a travel nurse agency or work as independent contractors. Most traveling agencies require that a nurse has 1 to 2 years of acute care experience before a contract is offered.

Travel nurse agencies may contract with hospitals to fill vacant staff nurse positions. The agency offers nurses positions from which to choose as well as assistance with housing, moving, and professional licensure expenses; some agencies may offer benefits (health insurance, life insurance, and retirement plans). Salary for travel nursing may be substantially higher than that of nurses working within facilities, but some travel nurses do not receive fulltime benefits (e.g., employer contribution to Social Security, pension, health insurance contributions, vacation time, retirement pension). Employment benefits account for approximately 35.2% of a nurse's salary for nurses working as employees (not as agency-contracted nurses in private hospitals) (Faller et al., 2018). For most travel nurses, they must submit estimated taxes and make full tax contributions to Social Security. During the COVID-19 pandemic, some travel nurse agencies offered RNs a salary between $6,200 and $10,000 per week (i.e., hazard pay) to accept positions working with clients with COVID-19. Some agencies may offer some fringe benefits as well (Hawryluk & Bichell, 2020).

Terms of contracts with travel nurse agencies vary greatly. Most temporary agencies require nurses to fulfill their current contract and then wait for a period of time before accepting a position once held as a travel nurse (Morrison, 2014). For example, conditions of a contract may specify that the nurse may not accept employment at a hospital where the agency sent the nurse for 2 years after severing ties with the nursing agency.

Extended Care Facility Nursing

The BLS (2020f) estimated that close to 21,000 (7%) RNs worked in extended care facilities in 2020. Most of these nurses were educated in diploma or associate degree programs.

Older Adult Long-Term Care

For nurses who wish to escape the fast pace of acute care nursing and establish long-term relationships with clients, long-term care (LTC) nursing provides these opportunities. In most LTC facilities, professional nurses assume supervisory roles and delegate tasks to LPN/LVNs, certified medication technicians, and other UAP. With the push for earlier hospital dismissals, complex care needs (e.g., mechanical ventilation, tracheotomy, hyperalimentation, tube feeding) have become common among clients in LTC facilities. Some LTC clients are residents only long enough to complete rehabilitative therapy or to regain strength after a hospital stay. Thus, the professional nurse can maintain some acute care clinical skills when working in LTC.

Some LTC facilities offer assisted living services. Professional nurses conduct initial periodic client assessments, screen clients for health problems, see clients when health-related problems arise, develop the client care plan, manage client medications, supervise licensed and unlicensed personnel as they provide client care, and determine staff in-service educational needs (Mitty, 2003). Instead of providing an institutional approach to client care, most LTC facilities view themselves as the client's home.

Some nurses find great rewards in working with older adults. Some older adult clients have no families or support systems, and members of the LTC staff become their primary social interactions. Many clients develop strong personal relationships with LTC staff. Because death is viewed as a normal part of life in LTC facilities, residents may receive palliative care. Most LTC facilities permit visits to hospice when death is imminent.

Rehabilitation Nursing

Advances in trauma care and increases in chemical dependency have resulted in an increase in the number of rehabilitation facilities. Insurance companies have identified that transferring clients to rehabilitation facilities after bouts of acute illness or surgery saves money. Rehabilitation units have opened as part of acute care and LTC facilities as well as freestanding rehabilitation centers. Some centers specialize in specific rehabilitation needs for particular health problems, such as stroke, head injury, spinal cord trauma, chemical dependency, amputation, or blindness.

In contrast to nurses working in acute care, rehabilitation nurses participate as equal partners of an interdisciplinary health team. Rehabilitation nurses need to be cooperative team players and have excellent organizational and communication skills. In rehabilitation, there is a strong focus on client education because the goal of rehabilitation is to get the clients to care for themselves or coach someone on how to care for them. Rehabilitation nurses may become very involved with clients and families and experience great satisfaction from being part of the client's journey toward mastering an independent lifestyle. The Association of Rehabilitation Nurses offers special certification in rehabilitation nursing.

Outpatient Nursing Opportunities

Many nursing opportunities occur in outpatient settings. Some outpatient nursing opportunities demand specialized education and training.

Ambulatory Care Centers, Outpatient Clinics, and Physician Offices

Nurses working in ambulatory care centers, outpatient clinics, and physician offices usually work with clients who have less acute conditions. In 2020, ambulatory care centers employed close to 558,000 (18%) RNs (BLS, 2020f). Many nurses choose these settings because of better hours (usually daytime hours with no weekend shifts) and less stressful working conditions. Depending on the clinic or office, the professional nurse may be a specialist or a generalist. Some nurses work in clinic settings, where a specialized clinic may be held on a specific day of the week. Clinics and offices may be located close to a hospital, in professional office buildings, shopping malls, pharmaceutical retail establishments, or even department stores. Some urgent care clinics offer services 24 hours a day, 7 days a week for illnesses and injuries not requiring emergency services.

Ambulatory Surgery Centers

Many surgical procedures do not require a postoperative hospital stay. Although outpatient centers do not have all the resources available in an acute care setting, they do have emergency equipment available and policies to guide staff should life-threatening emergencies arise. Many nurses working in outpatient surgery centers have operating room experience. In this setting, some nurses admit clients, assist with surgical procedures, provide care after anesthesia administration, give clients discharge instructions, and accompany them to vehicles for the ride home. Some outpatient surgery centers have nurses call to check on client progress the day after a procedure.

Take Note!
There are myriad nursing opportunities in outpatient settings, some of which require specialized education and training.

Special Care Centers

In addition to outpatient clinics and surgery centers, disease-focused centers provide expert care to people with health problems such as diabetes, heart disease, renal failure, and cancer. Some large urban medical centers have opened breast care centers that provide a comprehensive approach to breast health. Services include screening mammography, breast self-examination education, a comprehensive library related to breast cancer, ultrasound testing, and breast biopsy. In these settings, nurses work as interdisciplinary team members to provide holistic, comprehensive client care. Some oncology centers assign nurse navigators to clients to provide education and support throughout the cancer experience, starting with diagnosis and ending when the client has been cancer-free for 5 years. If a recurrence occurs after 5 years, the same nurse navigator is assigned if possible.

Community Nursing Centers/Clinics

Community nursing centers/clinics offer primary health care services to middle- and low-income clients at lower costs than traditional clinics and physician offices. Community nursing centers or nurse-run clinics may be freestanding or may be part of a rescue center, school, or place of worship. Some nurses run mobile clinics in converted buses or recreational vehicles. Nurse-run centers usually have an NP and nurses with specialized skills in health education, stress reduction, weight-related concerns, lifestyle management, and other wellness-focused health topics to deliver services. Many community nursing centers have affiliations with collegiate nursing programs. According to a literature review by Coddington and Sands (2008), nurse-managed clinics provide an important safety net for delivering health care services to the underinsured and uninsured. Along with removing barriers to care, nurse-managed centers encourage meaningful, therapeutic relationships between clients and NPs; reduce the incidence of emergency use for primary care and minor illnesses; reduce hospitalizations; promote health; improve client compliance with treatment plans; and have the same level of consumer satisfaction compared to the care received from a physician's office. The University of California Los Angeles Health Center at the Union Rescue Mission started serving those living in poverty and those without homes in 1983. In 2019, the center provided 8,000 visits, many for pediatric clients with chronic illnesses who were without homes or experiencing unstable home lives. NPs from the University of California San Francisco had 13,000 client encounters in 2019 at Glide Health Services, a facility providing care for those living in poverty and those without homes.

If the required care is not available at the community nursing center, nurses make referrals and sometimes arrange for services. Depending on funding, the nursing center may pay for services arranged within a provider network or government grants (The Regents of the University of California, 2020).

Cardiac Rehabilitation

Clients with cardiovascular disease frequently participate in cardiac rehabilitation programs after undergoing cardiac catheterization, pacemaker implantation, or open heart surgery. People recovering from myocardial infarctions also qualify for cardiac rehabilitation. Cardiac rehabilitation centers can be found in hospital settings, physician offices, or fitness centers. These programs rely on the expertise of professional nurses and exercise physiologists to develop and supervise physical workouts for clients with cardiac disease.

Most cardiac rehabilitation nurses have backgrounds in critical care nursing and have advanced cardiac life support (ACLS) certification. Many also have certification in critical care and/or cardiovascular nursing. Cardiac rehabilitation nursing responsibilities include observing cardiac monitors as clients exercise, performing periodic pulse and blood pressure measurements, assessing for signs of overexertion, and teaching relaxation and stress reduction techniques. Some cardiac rehabilitation programs use nurses for nutritional lifestyle counseling and mental health counseling when nutritionists or dietitians and psychologists are not part of the program.

Travel Health Nursing

Travel health nursing is a service offered for people planning international trips for medical tourism, volunteer service, disaster relief, and pleasure. In 2020, more than 25,000 nurses were working as travel health nurses (ANA, 2020). Travel health nurses typically work in travel health clinics, ideally staffed with physicians, RNs, laboratory technicians, and social workers.

However, some smaller travel health clinics may be staffed with only a nurse and physician with laboratory tests provided by a different laboratory. In collaboration with the American Travel Nurses Association, the ANA developed a set of scope and standards for travel nursing practice (ANA, 2020). Travel health nurses conduct pretravel consultations (e.g., assessment, review of the itinerary for the upcoming trip, needed immunizations, destination disease prophylaxis, any specific health care needs during the trip) review travel precautions, and provide posttrip consultations. The travel health nurse assists clients in creating a travel health kit that contains first aid supplies and medications to manage common and travel-related conditions (e.g., jet lag, altitude sickness, diarrhea, minor pain). The travel kit also contains a signed physician attestation for the need for the medication as some countries do not allow tourists to bring medications into their nation. Posttrip follow-up includes the management of trip-related illnesses such as persistent fever, diarrhea, or new onset of jaundice, skin lesions, or genitourinary conditions. Some clients may also need laboratory testing follow-up if they have taken medications to prevent malaria (Priyadharishini, 2017).

Qualifications for becoming a travel health nurse often include general nursing experience with travel experience. For nurses without international travel experience, the travel health clinic provides training during employment orientation. Key skills include computer literacy, ability to understand various governmental laws and regulations, venipuncture, immunization administration (intramuscular, subcutaneous, and intradermal), teamwork skills, effective communication, and knowledge of home country regulations and laws regarding health care delivery in an outpatient clinic setting. Nurses who manage a travel health clinic must ensure the clinic has ample room to provide privacy; enough personnel to meet needs of clients; equipment for drawing blood and administering vaccines; safe storage of medications and vaccines; a small laboratory to confirm and manage travel-related diseases; proper storage for equipment; safe waste disposal units; and financial support. Some travel health clinics are owned and operated by RNs (Priyadharishini, 2017).

Hospice and Palliative Care Nursing: Outpatient and Inpatient Settings

As the older adult population increases, so does the incidence of life-limiting diseases. Palliative care occurs across a continuum in which nurses provide care and support to clients and families who experience serious or potentially life-limiting progressive illnesses. The goal of hospice and palliative care nursing is to help clients and families live full and comfortable lives as much as possible when managing serious, life-altering illnesses. In recent years, palliative care has become an option for people undergoing medical treatments that have profound adverse effects (e.g., cancer chemotherapy). When an illness is diagnosed as terminal, hospice care is initiated. Hospice care recognizes death as a natural process and attempts to cure the illness are terminated. Palliative care aims to maximize comfort and acknowledges that keeping clients comfortable helps them live fully during the time they have remaining. Palliative care measures do not hasten or postpone death (Hospice & Palliative Nurses Association [HPNA] & ANA, 2014).

Hospice and palliative care nursing occurs in homes, residential hospices, extended care facilities, and hospitals. This special area of practice offers employment opportunities for nurse generalists, clinical nurse specialists (CNSs), and NPs. RNs can take the certification examination in adult and pediatric hospice nursing offered by the Hospice and Palliative Credentialing Center. Certification exams are also available for LPNs/LVNs and nursing assistants who work in hospice and palliatives care. Currently 15,500 health professionals hold this certification (Hospice and Palliative Credentialing Center, n.d.). Some university nursing education programs offer graduate degrees whereas others offer postgraduate certificates in palliative care. Nursing roles in hospice and palliative care also include case managers, first-line and middle nurse administrative opportunities, and executive positions (HPNA & ANA, 2014).

Business Opportunities

Nurses can also find employment opportunities in the business sector. Business career opportunities enable nurses to make an impact on client care by bringing the care ethic to corporations that supply products and reimbursement for health care.

Insurance and Managed Care Companies

Insurance and managed care companies use nurses to evaluate care delivered to customers. Third-party payers frequently use nurses as gatekeepers to verify that company resources have been used effectively to provide services. Responsibilities of nurses employed by these companies include reviewing medical records and activities to evaluate the need for care, ensuring that the appropriate level of care was received, and determining whether quality care was delivered in a timely fashion.

Along with quality management, third-party payers use nurses to staff telephones to certify insurance coverage before service delivery. Nurses who fill certification positions need strong clinical backgrounds and the ability to grasp the global picture of the issues surrounding care delivery. However, nurses employed in these positions frequently encounter many ethical dilemmas when working with complex clinical issues and deciding when to certify care. If a wrong decision is made, the nurse may be solely accountable for it, especially if the nurse is a company manager.

Telephone Triage and Health Care Advice Lines

Managed care companies, physician offices, clinics, and hospitals frequently use professional nurses to staff call centers devoted to determining the urgency of care needed, providing health information, referring clients to appropriate health care providers, scheduling appointments with health care providers, and offering health advice. Although triage and health care advice lines started out as a marketing strategy, they quickly demonstrated the ability to streamline the use of health care services, thereby reducing health care costs. Some managed care companies require that subscribers call the triage nurse to certify trips to EDs.

Nurses use assessment and therapeutic communication skills to determine the extent of the health problems of callers. Because some clients become frequent callers, telephone triage nurses may develop long-term relationships with them. Some nurses report that they schedule the time to call clients to follow up on the decisions they made.

Marketing and Sales

Companies that sell products such as pharmaceuticals, equipment, and monitors often hire professional nurses as sales representatives. Nurses provide credibility for product promotion, especially when they have used the product in clinical practice. Nurses also provide insight into product improvements and future products that may be useful in client care delivery. When complex equipment is purchased, the company often provides staff education in the use of the equipment.

Nurses can be effective sales representatives because they know how to approach other nurses and anticipate questions and problems that nurses may experience. Sales representatives must be energetic and self-motivated. Because most sales representatives work from their homes and travel a lot, they work flexible hours. Much time is spent meeting with prospective customers. Nurses entering the corporate sales world require knowledge related to the business world and principles of operating a home office. Some companies provide a base salary that does not meet the salary earned in clinical practice. However, significant bonuses can be earned on commissions from successful sales.

Take Note!
With a career in the business sector, nurses can influence client care by bringing the care ethic to pharmaceutical and medical device companies and to organizations that provide reimbursement for health care.

Occupational Health Nursing

Many businesses have occupational health departments or contract with businesses that offer occupational health services to offer employee health services. Occupational health nurses (OHNs) engage in case management, employee counseling, crisis intervention, workplace hazard detection, worker hazard reduction, and verification of compliance with legal and regulatory standards in work settings. As case managers, they manage and coordinate care of injured or ill employees for work-related and non–work-related situations. This includes all aspects related to employee health coverage, worker's compensation, short- and long-term disability, and provisions of the Family Medical Leave Act (American Association of Occupational Health Nurses [AAOHN], 2020c). Most importantly, OHNs are often the first to respond to work-related injuries or medical emergencies that occur.

OHNs frequently counsel employees about work-related conditions, health promotion, psychosocial needs, and other health-related issues. They also screen employees for signs of mental illness and substance abuse. When workers are a danger to themselves or others, OHNs intervene to manage the crisis. This may involve calling for law enforcement, an ambulance, or referring an employee to employee assistance programs or community mental health resources. When this occurs, OHNs provide follow-up care in the work setting (AAOHN, 2020c).

To keep workers healthy and productive, OHNs create programs aimed at supporting the development of healthy lifestyles among employees. These programs address preventing workplace injuries (e.g., safe use of equipment and chemicals, effective body mechanics) and illness (e.g., immunizations, smoking cessation, exercise/fitness, nutrition, stress management) (AAOHN, 2020c).

Concepts in Practice   IDEA → PLAN → ACTION

Occupational Health Nursing During the COVID-19 Pandemic

During the COVID-19 pandemic beginning in 2020, OHNs played a key role in promoting employee health and well-being. Their services facilitated keeping the supply chain for goods and services open during the pandemic. OHNs screened employees for COVID-19 before they started working using a variety of strategies including reviewing employee symptom surveys, completing worker daily symptom checklists, taking temperatures, and determining if employees were well enough to engage in work. Some OHNs had the ability to conduct virtual visits with employees who thought they had the virus and offer guidance to manage their situations. OHNs provided education on proper hand hygiene, surface cleaning protocols, social distancing, and mask use. In some cases, they supervised cleaning processes and assisted with them. OHNs also role-modeled effective cleaning of frequently touched surfaces, social distancing, mask use, and hand hygiene. In some businesses, they made rounds on hand sanitizing stations to verify they were operable. If an employee became ill with the virus, the OHN sent the person home, conducted contract tracing, and determined who should be placed in quarantine. In many companies, the OHN also monitored and enforced employee compliance for hand hygiene, barrier controls, cleaning protocols, social distancing, and mask wearing. OHNs kept records on employee cases and determined when workers in quarantine could return to work. Along with managing the complexities of worker physical health during the pandemic, OHNs also screened and monitored employees for signs of deteriorating mental health (AAOHN, 2020b).

Because of regulations surrounding workplace safety, OHNs need to know all Occupational Safety and Health Administration (OSHA), state, and local laws and regulations and monitor for compliance with them. These nurses work with employers, managers, and sometimes owners to ensure all resources are available for meeting legal and regulatory mandates (AAOHN, 2020c).

Most workplaces have some health hazards. OHNs assess the work environment for hazards that may result in employee illness or injury. Using knowledge of the research process, OHNs identify the frequency of occurrence, develop and implement control measures, and determine the effectiveness of implementations to prevent recurrence of worker injury or illness. Some examples of situations addressed by OHNs include toxic chemical exposures, work-related accidents, patterns of illnesses, and changes in trends among individuals and groups of employees (AAOHN, 2020c).

Due to the complexity of OHN practice, most OHNs enter this specialty with a baccalaureate degree and experience in ambulatory care, community health critical care, and/or emergency room nursing. Some OHNs have graduate degrees in public health, business, or advanced practice nursing (AAOHN, 2020c). The American Board of Occupational Health Nurses offers certification for this specialized area of nursing practice (AAOHN, 2020a).

Nurse Entrepreneurs and Private Consulting

Entrepreneurs are individuals "who organize, manage and assume the risk of a business or enterprise" (Mish, 2020, p. 417). Nurses who create, open, and run businesses are **nurse entrepreneurs**. Florence Nightingale was the first nurse entrepreneur when she created, opened, and managed the Nursing School at St. Thomas Hospital in London. There are three categories of entrepreneurs. The first category, the startup entrepreneur, is someone who creates and runs new businesses. Some startup entrepreneurs earn livings by starting successful businesses and later selling them for a profit. The second category, the corporate entrepreneur, is someone within an organization who creates, steers, and manages change within the organization. The final category, the social entrepreneur, is a person who creates enterprises with a specific social mission (Ribeiro Lima et al., 2019).

Starting and running an independent business is a complex undertaking. Some nurses who have specialized education in complementary health care practices, such as massage, therapeutic touch, aromatherapy, or magnet therapy, may assume the role of nurse consultant when they use these practices or help others to incorporate them into client care. The possibilities for nurses to engage in entrepreneurship are nearly endless.

However, becoming an entrepreneur can be a complex and risky undertaking.

Many nurse entrepreneurs experience some life-defining event that serves as the reason for a career change. Life-defining events may be a singular event, such as reaching a personally significant age, changing marital status, or having a child or children, or they may be a compilation of factors, such as job boredom, frustration with administration, an unfulfilled need, or a general feeling that life is being wasted. Setting out to become an entrepreneur can be a challenging yet fulfilling move (Box 20.1, Learning, Knowing, and Growing, "The Road to Entrepreneurship").

Not all nurses have the necessary personality to embark on an entrepreneurial career path. Key personality characteristics shared by successful entrepreneurs include a willingness to take risks, self-confidence, internal locus of control, determination, perseverance, interpersonal communication skills, willingness to delay gratification, business awareness, desire for total control, ability to direct others, physical stamina, mental resilience, and a strong need for achievement. Running a personal business requires detailed knowledge of the corporate world and governmental policies that guide small businesses (McKinnon, 2019; Norton, 2020).

McKinnon (2019) and Norton (2020) identify the advantages and disadvantages of being a nurse entrepreneur. Advantages include a high level of autonomy, flexible working hours, constant change, meeting new people, using previously untapped skills (creativity and interpersonal), and being paid high hourly rates. Disadvantages include loss of employee-based fringe benefits, having to secure accounts payable, taking risks, loss of daily contact with other nurses, no paid time off, and loss of job structure. However, many nurses, especially those who enjoy working independently, find being an entrepreneur satisfying and rewarding.

As companies outsource employee services, demands for consultants increase. Some nurse entrepreneurs form consulting firms based upon their area of expertise. Health care organizations use consulting firms to prepare for accreditation visits, apply for quality awards, meet employee educational needs, engage in work redesign, and look for ways to reduce operating costs. Some consultants have insider status, with which they provide special services within a system that employs them. Other consultants have outsider status; they work either as an independent contractor or for a company that provides services to organizations (Norwood, 1998). For example, a hospital may employ an enterostomal therapist

20.1 Learning, Knowing, and Growing

The Road to Entrepreneurship

Making the move from nursing practice to entrepreneurship generally follows these steps (Bennis, 2016; McKinnon, 2019; Norton, 2020; Vogel & Doleysh, 1997):

The nurse entrepreneur discovers an idea for a viable business. Frequently, the idea for a business appears while practicing professional nursing in a traditional institution.

1. The nurse entrepreneur gathers more information about the idea to provide a solid foundation for the new business concept.
2. The nurse entrepreneur develops the business concept by verifying the idea through the gathering of more information.
3. The nurse entrepreneur develops a detailed business plan for testing the business concept that includes a clear definition of the business concept; list of targeted customers; developing policies and procedures; budget (e.g., income, expenses for human and material resources); marketing plan; contingencies for managing cash flow issues; and schedule for

obtaining and renewing a business license, securing and renewing contracts, paying estimated taxes, and filing taxes.

4. The nurse entrepreneur performs an initial test of the business concept for success.
5. The nurse entrepreneur consults someone to navigate the complex legal aspects of developing and running a business. Possible resources include the Small Business Administration, Service Corps of Retired Executives, and legal counsel.
6. The nurse entrepreneur revises the business plan based on the advice of consultants and the issues encountered during pilot tests of the business.
7. If needed, the nurse entrepreneur seeks out a business loan or financial partner for the business.
8. The nurse entrepreneur expands the number and types of offered products or services.
9. The nurse entrepreneur expands the business as needed to include organizational structures, employees, policies, and procedures.

Vogel, G., & Doleysh, N. (1997). *Entrepreneuring: A nurses' guide to starting a business* (NLN Publication No. 41–2201). National League for Nursing; Bennis, P. A. (2016). *Self-employed RN: Earn respect, independence & a higher income*. P.A. Bennis; McKinnon, A. (2019). Lessons learned in year one of business. *Journal of Legal Nurse Consulting, 30*(4), 26–28; Norton, L. W. (2020). The business of consulting psychology: Lessons from the field. *Consulting Psychology Journal: Practice and Research, 72*(1), 68–76.

specifically to provide ostomy care and education for clients and families. However, when the need arises for staff education related to ostomy care, the hospital uses the same enterostomal therapist to provide a staff program. Extended care facilities may use external nurse consultants for monthly client assessments or to provide client services such as foot care.

Legal Nurse Consultants

Legal nurse consultants (LNCs) have practiced for many years. As our society grows more litigious, the demand for LNCs continues to rise. Because of the nature of the work, the skills required for an LNC include an ability to quickly find relevant nursing and medical literature pertaining to a case, effective computer skills (e.g., internet search proficiency), well-developed critical thinking skills, and detailed knowledge of legal issues surrounding nursing and health care delivery. LNCs assume the following roles and responsibilities:

- Obtain and analyze health records, medical literature, and practice guidelines and standards.
- Review and study health records to identify any omissions, contradictions, tampering, or inconsistencies with standards of care or customary practice.

- Prepare a detailed summary of the case, chronologically based on the content of health records.
- Identify and retrieve applicable standards of care relevant to cases.
- Interview and support clients and witnesses associated with a specific medical case.
- Evaluate the health records for evidence of duty, breach of duty, damages, and causation (the four elements that constitute medical-related tort claims).
- Outline and evaluate the defensibility or merit of any claim or merits of cases in filed medical tort claims.
- Educate attorneys, clients, and others about the aspects of health care and clinical practice, especially those related to the case or claims (e.g., explaining usual and customary care compared to what occurred).
- Determine the validity and credibility of expert witnesses to determine the value they bring to the case.
- Confer with expert witnesses (e.g., sharing case strategy and practice testimony).
- Assume the role of liaison to clients, parties involved in suits, and fact and expert witnesses.
- Draft medical and health-related sections of legal documents.
- Collaborate with members of the legal team regarding case strategy.

- Identify client injuries.
- Determine cost estimates for covering short- and long-term care associated with injuries, pain, and suffering that occurred directly from accidents, crimes, or the action or inaction of health care providers.
- Attend all independently conducted medical examinations.
- Assist with arbitration of the final judicial decision of a medical case or claim.
- Provide testimony as a fact or nurse expert witness. (American Association of Legal Nurse Consultants [AALNC], 2018; Magnusson et al., 2020).

LNCs may be entrepreneurs, independent contractors, or employees of law firms, health care facility insurance companies, government agencies, LNC consulting firms, health maintenance organizations, or business and industry legal departments. When working for an organization, the LNC enjoys the benefits of working within an organization and does not need to assume the responsibility of running their own business (AALNC, 2018). To become an LNC, an RN may enroll and complete a 17-module online course offered by the American Association of Legal Nurse Consultants. Propriety schools, businesses, community colleges, 4-year universities, and law schools also offer educational programs for nurses interested in becoming LNCs. Some universities offer graduate nursing programs leading to master's degrees in legal nurse consulting (Huff et al., 2019). The American Association of Legal Nurse Consultants offers certification examinations that assess the key knowledge and skills required for legal nurse consulting as well as demonstrating a commitment to this specialized area of professional nursing through their certification board. Eligibility criteria for the certification examination include a current, unrestricted registered license in a state or U.S. territory, 5 years of practice as an RN, and 2,000 hours of legal nurse consulting within the last 5 years. Examples of LNC requirements include activities performed at the request of a client (law firm, insurance company, hospital or other firm engaged in legal processes); involvement of claims or cases for which the nurse has the necessary education, skills, and expertise; and billable services (American Legal Nurse Consultant Certification Board, 2020; Huff et al., 2020).

ADVANCED NURSING PRACTICE

Most APRN careers require some education beyond the baccalaureate degree. Currently, APRN practice is recognized in the roles of NP, certified nurse-midwife (CNM), certified registered nurse anesthetist (CRNA), and CNS.

In the United States, the practice of nursing is determined at the state level. Some states recognize professional certification as a nurse-midwife or practitioner as the credential to obtain an advanced practice nursing license. However, because of the multiple entry paths into professional nursing, the NCSBN and professional nurses have pushed for APRNs to obtain a second nursing license to provide assurance that a minimum set of professional competencies is met. In addition, licensure as an APRN enables some nurses to prescribe medications and receive direct insurance (private and/or government policies) reimbursement for rendered services in most states. In most states, APRN licensure and statutes for advanced practice fall under the jurisdiction of the SBN. However, some states may have legal statutes and regulations for APRN practice with the BHA. There are some states (especially those who do not require collaborative practice agreements) where statutes and regulations for APRN practice are determined by both the SBN and BHA.

As APRNs move across state and national borders, credentialing becomes increasingly important. Credentialing provides documentation that an individual is recognized by a regulatory body and has met the standards to use a particular title. In health care, credentialing serves as a vehicle to protect the public against people who fail to meet the set standards and preparation to execute certain duties. Because of the variance among state nurse practice acts, some states require credentialing prior to attainment of the second advanced nursing practice license. Along with providing initial documentation of qualifications for advanced practice, most states require that the APRN fulfill continuing education and specific practice requirements (a certain number of clinical practice hours) to maintain certification (Blair, 2019). In 2020, the NCSBN adopted an APRN Compact that will be activated once seven states approve it. The APRN Compact will allow an APRN to hold one multistate license that will permit APRN practice privileges in all other participating states. At the time of manuscript preparation, North Dakota passed legislation to become a participant in the APRN Compact and Delaware has introduced legislation to become an APRN Compact member state (NCSBN 2021).

Doctor of Nursing Practice

The American Association of Colleges of Nursing (AACN, 2006) passed a resolution recommending that all APRNs be educated in a new program called the *Doctor of Nursing Practice (DNP)*. In 2010, the NCSBN and the AACN adopted the licensure, accreditation, certification, and education (LACE) model to regulate advanced practice nursing in the United States. Although recommended, the DNP is not an educational requirement for nurses to take advanced practice nurse certification examinations, thereby making nurses with master's degrees eligible to take APRN certification exams.

Under the LACE model, the nurse would be licensed according to role and population focus after passing a national certification examination. Licensure in an advanced practice role is a legal requirement before engaging in advanced nursing practice. The APRN would pass an examination in one of six population foci: family (across the lifespan), adult gerontology, neonatal, pediatric, women's health/gender-related, and psychiatric/mental health. Certifying bodies include the ANCC; American Academy of Nurse Practitioners; American Association of Critical Care Nurses; American Psychiatric Nurses Association; Association for Women's Health, Obstetrics, and Neonatal Nursing; National Board of Pediatric Nurse Practitioners and Associates; and the Oncology Nursing Society. The Council for the Advancement of Comprehensive Care has developed a certification examination for DNP graduates who have undertaken comprehensive care programs (Blair, 2019).

The DNP remains controversial for several reasons. Some states do not recognize the DNP for APRN practice, and others have statutory restrictions regarding the use of the title "Doctor," limiting its use in health care settings to medical or osteopathic physicians and surgeons, podiatrists, and dentists. Rhodes (2011) outlined facilitating factors and barriers to the DNP as entry level for APRNs. Adoption of the DNP by the NCSBN and individual states would provide APRNs with advanced competencies for the ever-increasing complexity of clinical, faculty, and leadership roles; enhance knowledge to improve nursing practice and client outcomes; improve the match between program requirements and earned degree; provide parity with other professional health team members; attract people to nursing from non-nursing backgrounds; increase the supply of clinical nursing faculty; and improve the image of the nursing profession. Currently, there are 357 DNP programs (up by 93 in 2015) and 104 new programs. Of these new programs, 60 are postbaccalaureate programs (BSN to DNP) and 46 are post master's degree programs (AACN, 2015a; AACN, 2020). In 2018, the National Organization of Nurse

Practitioner Faculties released a statement specifying that all entry-level NP education should occur at the DNP level by 2025 (Higher Number of NP Graduates, 2018). Movement toward BSN to DNP education facilitates a seamless education progression for nurses to become NPs.

With the shortage of primary care physicians, the increased time required to prepare APRNs for preventive and primary care services to consumers could mean reduced access for the public to health care services, increased health care costs, and the rise of physician assistants (who have poorer outcomes than APRNs) as the cost-effective primary care provider (Newhouse et al., 2011). In addition, faculty with nursing doctorates would need to complete postgraduate education in DNP programs, resulting in fewer qualified faculty to teach in undergraduate nursing programs and exacerbating the current and projected professional nursing shortage. However, in 2018, 27,967 new NPs and 8,788 physician assistants entered clinical practice and exceeded the influx of new physicians (approximately 33,000) into the health care delivery system (Higher Number of NP Graduates, 2018).

The DNP as entry level for APRN practice has been rejected by the ANA, American College of Nurse Midwives, American Organization of Nurse Executives, and the National Association of Nurse Practitioners in Women's Health. The American Association of Nurse Anesthetists (2019) has accepted DNP as the entry degree into practice and have enrollment in a doctoral program for students starting approved programs in January 2022.

Take Note!

The DNP, which may become the entry level for APRN practice, remains controversial.

Additional Advanced Practice Opportunities

In addition to opportunities as an NP, CNS, CRNA, or CNM, other emerging advanced practice opportunities include parish nurses, case managers, clinical transplant coordinators, childbirth educators, advanced diabetes managers, genetic advanced practice nurses, and wound, ostomy, and continence nurses (Hamric & Tracy, 2019). However, many of these practice areas may not require graduate collegiate education. Instead, nurses who enter these specialized practice areas typically take specific continuing education courses and practice a specified number of hours within a given specialty to qualify to take certification exams (offered by a specialty nurse organization or the ANCC). Once they pass the certification exam, they become recognized nurse specialists.

Global APRN Practices

The APRN movement is not confined to the United States. Progress toward education, regulation, and utilization has occurred globally, especially in Australia, Africa, the Americas, and Europe. The United States remains the only nation with specified regulations for APRN practice in the NP, CNM, CNS, and CRNA roles. Canada has regulations for the CNS and NP roles. Less defined roles and regulations for NPs are present in Latin America, South Africa, and Botswana. In Mexico, Honduras, and Bolivia, there is no requirement for advanced nursing education. Japan and China have embraced the role of CNS, but there is no formalized regulation. South Korea started developing APRN practice roles in the 1950s starting with CNMs. In South Korea, 10 types of APRNs are recognized across multiple specialty areas, each of which requires an advanced nursing degree and is regulated by the Ministry of Health. In Thailand, thousands of NPs provide care across a variety of specialties. Australian APRNs practice as CNSs and NPs and abide by regulations similar to those in the United States. Advanced practice is common in Europe, with the CNS and NP roles dominating, and in all European countries with the exception of Nordic countries, which have formal regulations for APRN practice (Bryant-Lukosius & Wong, 2019).

Effectiveness of APRNs

Multiple research studies indicate NPs provide safe, efficient, cost-effective care to consumers (Sheer & Wong, 2008). Newhouse et al. (2011) conducted a comprehensive systematic review of studies comparing physician

and APRN outcomes, looking at various APRN roles. NP and physician outcomes were the same and there was no significant differences in physician and APRN outcomes. While comparing outcomes between physicians and NPs, there were equivalent outcomes of satisfaction with received care, perceived health status, functional abilities, glucose levels, blood pressure, use of inpatient care, emergency room visits, and mortality rates. There was a high level of evidence that NPs managed client serum lipid levels more effectively than physicians. For CNM and physician comparisons, there were equivalent outcomes for physicians and CNMs for Apgar scores, levels of labor augmentation, and low-birth weight infants. Evidence showed CNMs had lower rates of epidural use, labor induction, vaginal operative deliveries, labor analgesia, third- and fourth-degree lacerations, and lower rates of infant admissions to neonatal intensive care units. CNMs were found to facilitate higher rates of breastfeeding compared to physicians. When CNS outcomes were compared to physician outcomes, evidence showed CNS outcomes resulted in shorter hospital stays, lower care costs, and fewer complications. Studies of CRNAs were focused on clinical interventions, and few outcome studies could be found. Only single observational studies were found that suggested equivalent mortality and complications from anesthesia when comparing CRNA care and anesthesiologist care.

In 2017, Woo, Lee, and Tam published an integrative review comparing NP and physician outcomes in the areas of ED, critical care, stroke center (SC), and trauma center (TC) care. The results are presented in the Focus on Research box, "The Impacts of APRNs." Studies that generate evidence that APRN services result in similar outcomes from those generated by physicians provides a solid foundation for governmental agencies and health insurance companies to approve APRN care services.

 FOCUS ON RESEARCH
The Impacts of the APRNs

Woo, Lee, and Tam sought to identify the impact of APRNs on the quality of care, clinical outcomes, client satisfaction, and costs in the ED and critical care health settings. They conducted a systematic literature review that examined published articles that compared APRN outcomes to physician outcomes.

Using nine electronic databases and a manual search of two journals, the two investigators searched for published studies dating from 2006 to 2016. They found a total of 12,061 studies of varying quality. They read the studies to determine which studies met review criteria according to desired content, using the population–intervention–comparison–outcome framework. They determined that the following outcomes would be included for comparisons: client length of stay in the critical care unit (CCU) or ED; client mortality; time to consultation or treatment; client satisfaction; and cost of care delivery. This narrowed the number of articles to 68. The remaining 68 studies were then analyzed according to client ages, and 20 studies were identified that included clients aged 16 and older.

Data extracted from the remaining 20 studies were subjected to review by using the Joanna Briggs Institute (JBI) Data Extraction Form for Experimental/Observational Studies. The extraction was cross-checked for accuracy. The form was adjusted to tabulate characteristics and findings for the study. Any incidences of disputed data were resolved.

Two of the investigators then performed independent assessments of the quality of the studies using the JBI Critical Appraisal Checklist for Randomized Clinical Trials and the JBI Critical Appraisal Checklist for Cohort Studies. They determined that studies attaining a score of at least 40% (indicating medium quality) or higher would be included in the systematic review. This resulted in a total of 15 studies that were carefully reviewed and analyzed.

Six of the studies were conducted in the EDs, six in CCUs, two in TCs, and one in an SC. There were a total of 23,681 clients across the 15 studies. Nine of the studies addressed independent nurse practitioner (INP) practice compared to physician practice, and six of the studies compared NP and physician collaborative practice (NPPCP) to physician-only practice.

Results of the data analysis conducted by the investigators revealed no differences in client mortality across all 15 studies. Statistically significant care reductions were noted in two of the NPPCP practice studies (one in a CCU and one in a TC). A statistically significant increase in the length of stay in CCU was found in a study looking at NPPCP, but there was no increase in the length of total hospital stay. Statistically significant decreases were noted in INP in ED setting studies regarding decreased length of stay (two studies), reduced time to treatment (two studies), and reduced time to consultation (one study). Client satisfaction scores were statistically higher among NPs who engaged in INP in the ED in one study.

The investigators concluded that NPs add value to delivery of care in ED and CCU settings. NPs achieve comparable outcomes with physicians in these settings. Use of NPs will improve access to care while reducing care costs. They proposed that the use of NPs for less complex cases in the ED would free physicians to manage the more complex, critical ones. The researchers acknowledged the lack of high-quality studies in numbers to perform a true meta-analysis of the data as a study weakness. In addition, they only examined literature published in English.

The significance of this study is that it indicates APRNs, primarily NPs, positively affect health care delivery in the ED and CCU settings. There needs to be more research comparing physician and NP outcomes related to care delivered across the health care continuum as well as across specialty areas of medical and nursing practice. The evidence suggesting NP care is as safe as a physician's care and that they can deliver similar clinical outcomes but at a reduced cost will further expand the use of NPs as providers of care, either in independent or collaborative practice.

Woo, B. F. Y., Lee, J. X. Y., & Tam, W. W. S. (2017). The impact of the advanced practice nursing role on quality of care, clinical outcomes, patient satisfaction, and cost in the emergency and critical care settings: a systematic review. *Human Resources for Health 15*, 63. https://doi.org/10.1186/s12960-017-0237-9

Opportunities for APRNs

The following discussion presents information on the most common forms of advanced nursing practice. NPs, CNSs, and CNMs sometimes practice case management as a way to coordinate health care services across the continuum of care. According to the U.S. BLS (2020e), there were 263,400 NPs, CNMs, and CRNAs earning a median salary of $115,800 in 2019. In acute care settings, NPs and CNSs assist clients and their significant others as they negotiate the complex maze of health care delivery, set realistic health outcomes, determine health care needs following facility dismissal, and develop strategies to improve health (education or supportive services). Home health agencies and community health centers use APRNs as case managers to coordinate needed health care services to keep people at home. Providing home care is more cost-effective than providing inpatient or residential care.

Nurse Practitioners

NPs provide primary health care services to consumers, including assessing client health using a holistic framework; identifying medical and nursing diagnoses; planning and prescribing treatments; managing health care regimens for individuals, families, and communities; promoting wellness; preventing illness and injury; and managing acute and chronic health conditions. The NP role surfaced during a physician shortage in the 1960s. The first NPs attended certification programs that lasted from a few weeks to as long as 2 years. NPs carved out a distinct difference in practice from the medical model by using a holistic approach to care based on nursing theory.

As the recognition of NPs grew (mostly related to the reduced cost of primary care and positive health outcomes for clients), NP programs in higher education settings proliferated. Education at the master's level dominates education of NPs. Specialty practice areas for NPs include family care, adult care, pediatrics, geriatrics, acute care, and women's health. Primary care NPs typically practice in outpatient settings; provide health care services aimed at health promotion, disease prevention, and management of simple, acute, and chronic health conditions; and establish partnerships with their clients.

Acute care NPs provide health care services to clients who may be hospital inpatients or clients seeking care in emergency room, urgent care, or clinic settings. They work in a variety of clinical specialties, including diabetes management, orthopedics, oncology, neurology, neurosurgery, and cardiovascular services. Acute care NPs frequently perform procedures that residents perform in teaching hospitals, such as lumbar punctures (neurologic acute NP); bone marrow aspirations (oncology acute NP); harvesting saphenous vein grafts during coronary bypass surgery (cardiovascular surgery acute NP); or serving as first assistants during surgery. They may work with physicians or they may have independent practice privileges at hospitals (Blair, 2019). NPs also provide health care services to the underprivileged and people living in underserved areas. According to the AANP (2020a), more than 290,000 NPs were licensed in the United States with a median base income of $110,000 in 2019. Psychiatric-mental health NPs earned the highest median salary ($125,000), and ED NPs earned the highest hourly wage at $70 an

hour. To qualify for direct third-party reimbursement, NPs must obtain certification. Most NPs are required to renew their certification every 5 years. This process requires documented practice and evidence of continuing education (Blair, 2019). NPs have earned the respect of clients and other health team members.

Certified Nurse-Midwives

CNMs independently manage women's health care with a special emphasis on pregnancy, childbirth, postpartum care, newborn care, family planning, and well-woman care. Well-woman care focuses on family planning, screening for reproductive system cancer, and management of perimenopause and postmenopause. CNM care supports the natural processes of birth, growth, development, and aging; CNMs intervene only when absolutely indicated (Avery & Saftner, 2019).

Of all the advanced practice roles, midwifery is the oldest. Records of midwifery practice are documented in the Bible. As the profession of medicine arose, midwifery declined. Mary Breckenridge, who received midwifery education in Scotland, became the first practicing nurse-midwife in the United States when she established the Frontier Nursing Service in 1925. In 1932, the first American nurse-midwifery education program opened in the Maternity Center of the Lobenstein Clinic in New York City. Nurse-midwifery experienced slow growth, and it was not until 1955 that the American College of Nurse-Midwives was established. By the 1970s, nurse-midwifery was in demand by consumers seeking a more natural approach to childbirth. In 1971, a national certification examination became the standard for entry into practice by the American College of Nurse-Midwives. However, CNM practice is regulated by individual states, thereby creating variances in prescriptive authority, educational preparation, employment contracts, and practice arrangements. In 2019, the U.S. BLS (2020b) reported that there were 6,930 CNMs employed in the United States earning a mean income of $108,810.

Although they started as certificate programs, nurse-midwifery programs progressed to graduate nursing education. By the 1990s, many CNMs were graduating from university-based programs (Avery & Saftner, 2019). Forty-seven nurse-midwifery programs are housed in American universities, all but seven of which are incorporated into master of nursing programs.

Research indicates CNMs contribute substantially to the quality of maternal–child health care. The Bureau of Health Professions (BHPR) (2003) reported reduced cesarean section rates and fewer medical interventions for clients at low risk cared for by CNMs when compared with clients at low risk cared for by physicians. Studies report significantly lower neonatal mortality and infant mortality, as well as higher birthweights of infants when clients were attended by CNMs. Along with improved outcomes, CNMs provide clients with health care at reduced costs (Avery & Saftner, 2019; Rosseter, 2013).

Clinical Nurse Specialists

CNSs are highly skilled clinical experts in a specialized area of nursing practice and use all the steps of the nursing process to promote health, prevent complications, and manage health problems. CNSs work in many settings, including hospitals, schools, extended care facilities, homes, and community agencies. In 2020, close to 72,000 CNSs were in practice, earning an average annual salary of 87,500 (ExploreHealthCareers .org, 2020).

In 1954, Hildegard Peplau established the first graduate-level CNS program at New Jersey's Rutgers University to prepare psychiatric CNSs. CNSs provide expert client care, serve as professional role models, and act as client advocates. They also provide indirect care services when they act as consultants or resources to other health team members, supervise care delivery, act as liaisons between the client system and the care providers, initiate and direct change for client care, and engage in research and evidence-based nursing projects through clinical research. Some CNSs have prescriptive privileges. Second licensure as an APRN is not required for CNS practice in some states.

Tracy and Sendelbach (2019) noted that changing population demographics, health care cost containment issues, accessibility and affordability of care delivery, the ever-expanding knowledge base for specialty nursing practice arenas, and shortages of physicians and nurses have resulted in the role blending of CNSs and NPs. When CNSs have prescriptive privileges, most states typically require a second advanced practice nursing license. Nurses who have merged the roles of NP and CNS usually have had graduate educational preparation in both roles. The blended role offers nurses an opportunity to cross health care settings, provide comprehensive health care services to a narrowly defined clinical population, and serve as team members in primary, secondary, and tertiary care settings.

Early CNSs worked primarily in hospitals to provide support for clients and nursing staff. However, with the advent of managed care, many hospitals enlisted CNSs to serve as case managers. CNSs coordinate care of highly acute clients within the hospital and have been used as discharge planners. They practice in many subspecialty fields, including pulmonology, oncology, neuroscience, geriatrics, rehabilitation, diabetes, hospice, and palliative care. In the 1990s, CNSs assumed case management positions within their specialty area of practice. Case management by APRNs is expected to evolve and perhaps become more commonplace as the population ages and more older adults with chronic illnesses have complex health care needs (Tracy & Sendelbach, 2019). In 2006, the AACN proposed a new academic degree, the clinical nurse leader (CNL), which is a master's degree aimed at facilitating seamless health care delivery across the health care continuum. The role of the CNL outlined by the AACN includes the following: "care coordination, outcome measurement, care transitions, interprofessional team communication and leadership, risk assessment, implementation of evidence-based best practices, and quality improvement" (AACN, 2021, para. 2).

Certified Registered Nurse Anesthetists

CRNAs provide anesthesia and anesthetic-related services to health care consumers. Along with completing the 24-month program consisting of advanced study in anatomy, physiology, chemistry, and pathophysiology, and 90 hours emphasizing the principles of anesthesia, an RN must administer at least 450 anesthetics before taking the certification examination (Callahan & Kremer, 2019).

All 50 states recognize CRNA practice. According to the American Association of Nurse Anesthetists (2013), CRNA practice includes preanesthetic assessment; anesthetic plan development and implementation; anesthesia induction; selection, application, and insertion of noninvasive and invasive monitoring devices; anesthetic selection, acquisition, and administration; fluid and ventilatory support; administration of medications and fluids to facilitate the emergence and recovery from anesthesia; client discharge and follow-up care after anesthesia administration; airway support and management in medical emergencies; and implementation of various acute and chronic pain treatment modalities. Despite rigorous, standardized education requirements, approximately 80% of CRNAs practice anesthesia with a group of physician anesthesiologists. The other 20% practice independently to provide anesthesia services in outpatient clinics and rural hospitals (more than 70% of rural hospitals rely on CRNAs for anesthesia services). CRNAs receive payment for services directly from third-party payers and assume full legal responsibility for their own actions (Callahan & Kremer, 2019). During the COVID-19 pandemic, CRNAs intubated many infected clients experiencing respiratory failure. Because this procedure results in spraying of respiratory secretions, CRNAs were at a higher risk of contracting COVID-19 than many of the other health care team members. The U.S. BLS (2020a) reported that in 2019, there were 43,570 employed CRNAs who earned a mean income of $181,040.

Registered Nurse First Assistants

Registered nurse first assistants (RNFAs) may be employed by hospitals and physicians or may work as independent contractors. Practice settings for RNFAs include hospitals, ambulatory surgical centers, and physician offices. RNFAs work collaboratively with surgeons during surgery; they may prepare the skin for incisions, hold retractors, assist with clamping vessels, perform suction, perform cautery, irrigate surgical wound beds, and close incisions. Along with working in the operating room, RNFAs collect client histories, perform preoperative assessments, make client preoperative visits, educate clients about procedures, and conduct postoperative visits (Association of periOperative Registered Nurses [AORN, 2018]). They assist surgeons during surgery but not as surgical scrub nurses (AORN, 2020). RNFAs are widely used in rural hospitals.

The scope of responsibility of RNFAs varies according to the employment setting. RNFAs working in surgeons' offices tend to have more autonomy and responsibilities than those employed by hospitals. AORN published the first official statement on RNFAs in 1984 and created an educational and certificate program for RNFAs in 1985. Qualifications for certification as an RNFA include current licensure as an RN, certification from AORN as a certified operating room nurse, a bachelor's degree in nursing or a master's degree in nursing with a bachelor's degree in another field of study, and successful completion of an approved RNFA course. Approved courses range from private courses with the equivalent of 6 credit hours (90 clock hours) with collegiate programs that provide intensive 1-year programs taught by surgeon–nurse teaching teams consisting of didactic classroom instruction and surgeon-supervised clinical practice in surgery. All approved programs must meet criteria specified by the AORN Standards for RN First Assistant Education Programs (AORN, 2018, 2020). Starting in January 2020, all new RNFAs must have baccalaureate nursing

degrees but current RNFAs without this educational credential are grandfathered in and may continue to practice in this role. AORN posts a list of approved RNFA programs on its website (AORN, 2018).

RNFAs are reimbursed for their services at lower rates than are assisting surgeons. Medicare does not reimburse RNFAs for their services. Many RNFAs receive payment from the surgeons or hospitals for which they work. Some states require insurance companies to pay RNFAs directly for their services. RNFA salaries vary according to the number of cases, types of cases, and location of practice (National Institute of First Assisting, n.d.).

INDIRECT CLIENT CARE ADVANCED NURSING CAREER OPTIONS

Nursing Administration

Most health care organizations and systems employ nurses as administrators or managers. Positions in **nursing administration** range from departmental heads (head nurse or nurse manager) to hospital chief nursing officers to system chief nursing executives (heads of nursing for multiple hospitals that are part of comprehensive health systems). In some hospitals, nurse managers may be responsible for one unit and other hospitals require nurse managers to run several units. Long-term care facilities or small rural hospitals may have only one nurse administrator with the title *director of nursing*. Many hospitals require advanced degrees for management or administrative positions. Many colleges and universities offer graduate nursing education in nursing administration. However, some nurse administrators have opted to pursue graduate degrees in business or health administration to enhance role performance.

According to the U.S. BLS (2020a), health and medical manager (including nurse manager and executive) positions numbered 432,000. The mean salary for managers was $109,980. The U.S. Bureau of Labor Statistics does not separate nursing administration from other health and managerial positions.

The practice of nursing administration is complex. Most of the roles and responsibilities of nurse administrators are discussed in Chapter 18, "Nursing Leadership and Management." Nurse executives and managers must engage in proactive risk management; display proficiency using technology; possess the ability to navigate and draw conclusions from large databases; bridge gaps between organizational departments and health professions; provide human and material resources for client care; engage in effective collaboration (especially with chief medical officers, business executives, and nursing staff); track facility census (inpatient facilities) and visits (outpatient facilities); derive value from data; build effective teams; facilitate value-base care; and remain visible while engaging in work. To create sustainable organizations, they must influence innovation by engaging in and encouraging divergent thinking, tolerate failures, display flexibility and agility, and give freedom and autonomy to individuals providing client care (Larson, 2017; Porter-O'Grady & Malloch, 2018).

Nursing Academia

Teaching a generation of nurses is rewarding for nursing faculty members. A career in **nursing academia** (nursing education) enables experienced nurses to share their knowledge and expertise with future professional nurses. As a faculty member, the nurse has opportunities to polish clinical skills, expand the knowledge of clinical nursing, engage in nursing research, and participate in community service. Although most nursing programs require a master's degree in nursing and recent clinical experience for faculty appointment, some associate degree and vocational nursing programs may hire baccalaureate-prepared nurses. Most programs preparing certified nursing assistants use baccalaureate-prepared nurses as faculty. Nursing programs offering baccalaureate degrees prefer to hire faculty with nursing or educational doctorates. The AACN (2015a) recognized both the doctor of philosophy degree in nursing and DNP as terminal degrees in nursing. Both degrees enable nurses with these advanced degrees to teach in collegiate and university settings. However, the AACN recommends that additional optional coursework in education should be added to DNP programs that would prepare nurse educators (AACN, 2015b). However, many institutions of higher learning require a PhD as a qualification for tenure (Rees et al., 2019).

Nursing faculty have a variety of settings to teach the art and science of nursing. State- and privately sponsored research universities require faculty to develop a program of nursing research. In these settings, faculty members develop research proposals, write grants to fund projects, engage in research, disseminate research findings, and fulfill teaching responsibilities. Some small liberal arts colleges and universities have teaching as their main missions. Nursing faculty members in these settings teach as their major responsibility but also frequently apply for grants to improve

instructional efforts. Nursing programs in the community college setting emphasize the technical aspects of nursing and faculty members concentrate on teaching students clinical skills. Many faculty members practice nursing outside the academic setting to maintain their clinical competence.

Distance learning programs pose different challenges for faculty. In addition to being content and practice experts, nurse faculty in these programs must have the knowledge and expertise to run computer hardware, use software to engage learners, design online instructional activities, work with technology support staff, and establish online student relationships. Faculty teaching online have more flexibility than in the classroom setting, but they still need to be available for assisting students with course questions and assignments. When teaching in institutions of higher learning, faculty members are expected to engage in institutional and departmental governance. This means serving on committees at the college level along with serving on committees for the nursing program. According to the U.S. BLS (2020c), there were 59,680 fulltime employed nursing faculty in postsecondary settings. In 2019, nurses employed in academia earned a mean $83,160, and entry-level educators earned salaries as low as $41,130. For the academic year 2020 to 2021, 52.1% of nursing programs responding to an AACN special survey on faculty vacancies reported having fulltime faculty positions that needed to be filled. Because of the low pay for entry-level nursing faculty members, noncompetitive wages were reported to be the biggest obstacle for nursing programs to fill their vacant faculty positions (Fang et al., 2020).

Nurse Researcher

As health care facilities strive to deliver the best quality care, many have hired nurse researchers to fill director of nursing research positions. Director of nursing research roles vary across institutions. The Institute of Medicine's (2011) recommendation to include the use of best practices to provide safe, effective, and efficient health care has created a climate that values the input of evidence-based practices and protocols. In many facilities, the director of nursing research educates staff about the research process and how to critique research studies effectively. The director of nursing research also guides, supports, and assists staff as they engage in evidence-based quality improvement and nursing research. The preferred preparation for nurse researchers is a PhD in nursing (Rees et al., 2019).

■ QUESTIONS FOR REFLECTION

1. What career options sound like they might appeal to you in the short term? In 10 years?
2. What further information about the career options presented in this chapter would you like?
3. What additional education or skills would you need to obtain to pursue a specific career option in nursing?

Summary and Significance to Practice

Professional nursing offers many career options for committed, caring nurses. Nurses have opportunities not afforded to the other health professions to change their specialty and practice areas. Many expanded and most advanced nursing practice roles require additional education beyond undergraduate education. Most APRN roles require certification and additional licensure in some states. In the future, the educational preparation for these roles might be a nursing doctorate. Some nurses find that discovering one's personal niche in the profession can be a challenging and complex process. Exploring all nursing career options takes time. Nurses proceed with confidence after making a career choice when they find a nursing career that matches their personal and professional goals and one that instills great passion in their hearts.

REAL-LIFE REFLECTIONS

Recall Laura from the beginning of the chapter. How would you respond to Laura if she asked you about your current nursing practice or your career plans? Why would you respond this way?

From Theory to Practice

1. Whom would you contact if you wanted to explore one of the nursing career options presented in this chapter? Why would you select this person? What other resources might you use?

Nurse as Author

Based on the information you learned in this chapter, write an essay about what career in professional nursing most interests you. In the opening paragraph, identify the career and explain why it appeals to you. In the next two to four paragraphs, outline the steps you will need to take to become a practicing nurse in this area. What current barriers do you face and what resources will you need to overcome them? In the final paragraph, share your plans for an ideal career in this nursing practice area.

Your Digital Classroom

Online Explorations

All Nursing Schools: **www.allnursingschools.com**
American Association of Nurse Anesthetists: **https://www.aana.com/**
American Association of Nurse Practitioners: **https://www.aanp.org**
American Nurses Association: **https://www.nursingworld.org/ana**
Health Resources and Services Administration: **https://www.hrsa.gov**
International Association of Forensic Nurses: **https://www.forensicnurses.org**
The Johnson & Johnson Commitment to Nursing: **https://nursing.jnj.com**
Sigma Theta Tau International Honor Society of Nursing: **www.sigmanursing.org**
TravelNursing.com: **www.travelnursing.com**
U.S. Department of Labor, Bureau of Labor Statistics Occupational Outlook Handbook: **https://www.bls.gov/ooh/**

Expanding Your Understanding

1. Visit the Nursing Careers and Specialties for RNs website at https://www.registerednursing.org/nursing-careers/. Scroll down the page and select an area of specialized nursing practice that you find appealing. Click on the specialty and note what you need to do to prepare for and pursue a career in your desired nursing specialty. After reading about this specialty, would you still like to continue pursing it? Why or why not? Share this information with your classmates in a discussion forum or in class.
2. Visit the ANCC website and look for information about specialty practice certification and advanced practice nursing. Was this information useful? Why or why not? Do you see yourself becoming an advanced practice nurse? Why or why not?

Beyond the Book

Visit thePoint® at **www.thePoint.lww.com** for activities and information to reinforce the concepts and content covered in this chapter.

REFERENCES

American Association of Colleges of Nursing. (2006). *DNP roadmap task force report*. Retrieved February 26, 2013, from www.aacn.nche.edu/DNP/roadmapreport.pdf

American Association of Colleges of Nursing. (2015a). *DNP fact sheet*. Retrieved June 18, 2016, from http://www.aacn.nche.edu/media-relations/fact-sheets/dnp

American Association of Colleges of Nursing. (2015b). *The doctor of nursing practice: Current issues and clarifying recommendations report from the task force on the implementation of the DNP*. Retrieved June 18, 2016, from http://www.aacn.nche.edu/aacn-publications/white-papers/DNP-Implementation-TF-Report-8–15.pdf

American Association of Colleges of Nursing. (2020). *Current DNP facts*. Retrieved December 13, 2020, from https://www.aacn-nursing.org/News-Information/Fact-Sheets/DNP-Fact-Sheet

American Association of Colleges of Nursing. (2021). *Clinical nurse leader (CNL)*. Retrieved April 3, 2021, from https://www.aacnnursing.org/cnl

American Association of Legal Nurse Consultants. (2018). *What is an LNC?* Retrieved December 12, 2020, from https://www.aanlc.org/page/what-is-an-nlc

American Association of Nurse Anesthetists. (2013). *Certified registered nurse anesthetists at a glance*. Retrieved February 26, 2013, from https://www.aana.com/ceandeducation/becomeacrna/Pages/Nurse-Anesthetists-at-a-Glance.aspx

American Association of Nurse Anesthetists. (2019). *Certified registered nurse anesthetist fact sheet*. Retrieved December 13, 2020, from https://www.aana.com/membership/become-acrna/crna-fact-sheet

American Association of Nurse Practitioners. (2020a). *More than 290,000 nurse practitioners licensed in the U.S. AANP News*. Retrieved December 13, 2020, from aanp.org

American Association of Nurse Practitioners. (2020b). *State practice environment*. Retrieved December 9, 2020, from https://www.aanp.org/advocacy/state/state-practice-environment

American Association of Occupational Health Nurses. (2020a). *Careers, becoming certified*. Retrieved December 11, 2020, from https://www.aohn.org/page/certification

American Association of Occupational Health Nurses. (2020b). *Covid-19 FAQs*. Retrieved April 3, 2021, from wwww.aaohn.org/page/covid-19-resources-for-ohns

American Association of Occupational Health Nurses. (2020c). *Occupational health nursing as a career*. Retrieved April 3, 2021, from www.aohn.or/page-become-an-ohn

American Legal Nurse Consultant Certification Board. (2020). *About certification*. Retrieved April 3, 2021, from www.lncc.aalnc.org/about-certification

American Nurses Association. (2015). *Scope and standards of nursing practice* (3rd ed.). Author.

American Nurses Association. (2020). American Nurses Association Recognizes Travel Health Nursing as New Specialty Nursing Practice. Retrieved May 18, 2021, from https://www.nursingworld.org/news/news-releases/2020/american-nurses-association-recognizes-travel-health-nursing-as-a-new-specialty-nursing-practice/

Association for Nursing Professional Development. (2016). *About ANPD*. Retrieved June 12, 2016, from http://www.anpd.org/?page=about

Association of periOperative Nurses. (2018). *AORN's position statement on RN first assisting*. Retrieved April 3, 2021, from https://www.aorn.org/guidelines/clinical-resources/rn-first-assistant-resources

Association of periOperative Nurses. (2020). *Registered nurse first assistants*. Retrieved December 14, 2020, from https://www.aorn.org/-/media/aornguidelines/rnfa/RNFA-Standards-of-Practice%20.pdf

Avery, M. D., & Saftner, M. A. (2019). The certified nurse midwife. In M. F. Tracy & E. T. O'Grady (Eds.), *Hamric and Hanson's advanced nursing practice: an integrative approach* (6th ed., Chapter 17, pp. 436–459). Elsevier.

Blair, K. (2019). Practice issues: Regulations, including prescriptive authority, title protection, certification, clinical privileges/credentialing and liability. In K. Blair (Ed.), *Advanced practice nursing core concepts for professional development* (6th ed., Chapter 10, pp. 1870210). Springer Publishing Co. LLC.

Bryant-Lukosius, D., & Wong, F. K. (2019). International development of advanced nursing practice. In M. F. Tracy & E. T. O'Grady (Eds.), *Hamric and Hanson's advanced nursing practice: an integrative approach* (6th ed., Chapter 6, pp. 129–141). Elsevier.

Bureau of Health Professions. (2003). *A comparison of changes in the professional practice of nurse practitioners, physician assistants, and certified nurse midwives: 1992–2000*. Retrieved July 1, 2005, from http://bhpr.hrsa.gov/healthworkface/reports/scope/scope1–2./htm

Bureau of Labor Statistics. (1992). *Occupational outlook handbook: Universal job skills*. Author.

Bureau of Labor Statistics. (2020a). *Occupational employment statistics. Occupational employment and wages 2019. 29–1151. Nurse Anesthetists*. Retrieved December 13, 2020, from bls.gov

Bureau of Labor Statistics. (2020b). *Occupational employment statistics, Occupational employment and wages, 2019. 29–1161. Nurse Midwives*. Retrieved December 13, 2020, from bls.gov

Bureau of Labor Statistics. (2020c). *Occupational employment statistics. Occupational employment and wages 2019. 25–1072. Nursing Instructors*. Retrieved December 14, 2020, from bls.gov

Bureau of Labor Statistics. (2020d). *Occupational outlook handbook. Medical and health services managers*. Retrieved December 14, 2020, from bls.gov

Bureau of Labor Statistics. (2020e). *Occupational outlook handbook. Nurse anesthetists, nurse midwives, and nurse practitioners*. Retrieved December 13, 2020, from https://www.bls.gov/ooh/healthcare/nurse-anesthetists-nurse-midwives-and-nurse-practitioners.htm

Bureau of Labor Statistics. (2020f). *Occupational outlook handbook. Registered nurses*. Retrieved December 12, 2020, from bls.gov

Callahan, M. F., & Kremer, M. J. (2019). The certified registered nurse anesthetist. In M. F. Tracy & E. T. O'Grady (Eds.), *Hamric and Hanson's advanced nursing practice: an integrative approach* (6th ed., Chapter 18, pp. 460–485). Elsevier.

Coddington, J. A., & Sands, L. P. (2008). Cost of health care and quality outcomes of patients at nurse-managed clinics. *Nursing Economic, 26*(2), 75–83. https://www.researchgate.net/publication/51400682_Cost_of_health_care_and_quality_of_patients_at_nurse-managed_clinics

Commission for Forensic Nursing Certification. (2020). *Sexual assault nurse examiner (SANE-A® and SANE-P® 2021 certification examination handbook*. Retrieved December 10, 2020, from https://cdn.ymaws.com/www.forensicnurses.org/resource/resmgr/certification/2021_cert_exam_hb_and_links_.pdf

ExploreHealthCareers.org. (2020). *Clinical nurse specialist*. Retrieved December 13, 2020, from https://explorehealth-careers.org/career/nursing/clinical-nurse-specialist/#:~:text=There%20are%20approximately%2072%2C000%20clinical%20nurse%20specialists%20 in,private%20practice%2C%20schools%2C%20nursing%20homes%2C%20corporations%20and%20prisons

Faller, M., Dent, B., & Gogek, J. (2018). The ROI of travel nursing: A full-cost comparison of core staff pay rates to travel nurse bill rates. *Nursing Economic*, *36*(4), 177–181. Retrieved May 19, 2021, from https://search-ebscohost-com.lib.rockhurst.edu/login.aspx?direct=true&AuthType=cookie,ip,url&db=c8h&AN=131366442&site=ehost-live

Fang, D., Keyt, J., & McFadden, T. (2020). *Special survey on vacant faculty positions for academic year 2020-2021*. Retrieved December 14, 2020, from http://aacnursing.org/Portals/42/Neews/Surveys-Data/2020-Faculty-Vacancy-Report.pdf

Hamric, A. B., & Tracy, M. F. (2019). A definition of advanced nursing practice. In M. F. Tracy & E. T. O'Grady (Eds.), *Hamric and Hanson's advanced nursing practice: an integrative approach* (6th ed., Chapter 3, pp. 61–79). Elsevier.

Hawryluk, M., & Bichell, R. E. (2020). *Need a COVID-19 nurse? That'll be $8,000 a week*. Retrieved April 3, 2020, from https://khn.org/news/highly-paid-traveling-nurses-fill-staffing-shortages-during-covid-pandemic/

Higher Number of NP Graduates. (2018). *AACN Bold Voices*, *10*(10), 8. Retrieved May 18, 2021, from https://www.aacn.org/journalassets/Bold%20Voices/10/10/BV%2010_18.pdf

Hospice and Palliative Credentialing Center. (n.d.). *Certification*. Retrieved from December 11, 2020, from https://www.advancingexpertcare.org/HPNA/HPNA/certification

Hospice and Palliative Nurses Association & American Nurses Association. (2014). *Palliative nursing: Scope and standards of practice*. Nursesbooks.org

Huff, K. J., West, T., & King, I. (2020). History, entry into practice and certification. In J. Dickinson & A. Meyer (Eds.), *Legal nurse consulting principles and practice* (4th ed., Chapter 1, pp. 1–38). Routledge.

Institute of Medicine. (2011). *The future of nursing, leading change, advancing health*. The National Academies Press.

International Association of Forensic Nurses. (2020). *What is forensic nursing?* Retrieved December 10, 2020, from https://www.forensicnurses.org/page/WhatisFN

Larson, L. (2017). The rapidly evolving role of NURSE EXECS. *Hospitals & Health Networks*, *91*(3), 28–31. www.hhmag.com/articles/8029-the-rapidly-evolving-role-of-nurse-executives

Lehmann, D. (2020). Specialty spotlight: Forensic nursing. *Maryland Nurse*, *21*(2), 18. https://d3ms3kxrsap.50t.cloudfront.net/uplads/publication/pdf/2012/Maryland_Nurse_2_20_updated.pdf

Magnusson, J., Zorn, E. K., & Dickinson, J. (2020). Professionalism, ethics, scope and standards of practice. In J. Dickinson & A. Meyer (Eds.), *Legal nurse consulting principles and practice* (4th ed., Chapter 2, pp. 39–56). Routledge.

McKinnon, A. (2019). Lessons learned in year one of business. *Journal of Legal Nurse Consulting*, *30*(4), 26–28. http://viewflipdocs.com/?ID=10004296_332282

Mish, F. C. (Ed.). (2020). *Meriam-Webster's Collegiate Dictionary*, (11th ed.). Merriam-Webster, Inc.

Mitty, E. (2003). Assisted living and the role of the nurse. *American Journal of Nursing*, *103*, 32–44. https://journals.lww.com/ajnonline/Citation/2003/0800/Policy_Perspectives_Assisted_Living_and_the_Role.14.aspx

Morrison, D. (2014). Travel nursing anyone? *American Nurse Today*, *9*(11), 41–42. https://www.myamericannurse.com/travel-nursing-anyone/

National Council of State Boards of Nursing. (2012). *Mutual recognition: Frequently asked questions*. Retrieved September 2, 2012, from www.ncsbn.org/2002.htm

National Council of State Boards of Nursing. (2021). *APRN compact*. Retrieved April 3, 2021, from https://www.ncsbn.org/aprn-compact.html

National Institute of First Assisting. (n.d.). *Reimbursement*. Retrieved from December 14, 2020, from https://www.rnfa.org/rnfa-billing/reimbursement

Newhouse, R., Stanik-Hutt, J., White, K. M., Johantgen, M., Bass, E. B., Zangaro, G., Wilson, R. F., Fountain, L., Steinwachs, D. M., Heindel, L., & Weiner, J. P. (2011). Advanced practice nursing outcomes 1990–2008: A systematic review. *Nursing Economic*, *29*(5), 230–251. https://www.researchgate.net/publication/22186828_Advanced_Nurse_Practice_Outcomes_1990-2008_A_Systematic_Review

Norton, L. W. (2020). The business of consulting psychology: Lessons from the field. *Consulting Psychology Journal: Practice and Research*, *72*(1), 68–76. https://doi.org/10.1037/cpb0000159

Norwood, S. L. (1998). *Nurses as consultants: Essential concepts and processes*. Addison-Wesley.

Porter-O'Grady, T., & Malloch, K. (2018). *Quantum leadership: creating sustainable value in health care* (5th ed.). Jones & Bartlett Learning.

Priyadharishini, J. (2017). Travel health nursing. *International Journal of Nursing Education*, *9*(2), 167–171. https://doi.org/10.5958/0974-9357.2017.00057.5

Rees, S., Ousey, K., Koo, K., Ahmad, N., & Bowling, F. L. (2019). Higher degrees in nursing: traditional research PhD or professional doctorate? *British Journal of Nursing*, *28*(14), 940–945. https://doi.org/10.12968/bjon.2019.28.14.940

Rhodes, M. K. (2011). Using effect-based reasoning to examine the DNP as the single entry degree for advanced practice nursing. *The Online Journal of Issues in Nursing*, *16*(3), 8. https://doi.org/10.3912/OJIN.Vol16No03PPT01

Ribeiro Lima, K. F., Pinheiro, A. S., da Silva, P. L., Maltezi Cavalini, A. F., dos Santos Bispo, A., de Carvalho Andrade, A., & de Medeiros, J. S. (2019). Nurse entrepreneur profile: Contribution of academic training. *Journal of Nursing UFPE/Revista de Enfermagem UFPE*, *13*(4), 904–914. https://doi.org/10.5205/1981-8963-v13i04a238347p904-914-2019

Rosseter, R. (2013). *Nurse practitioners: The growing solution in health care delivery*. Retrieved February 25, 2013, from www.aacn.nche.edu/media-relations/fact-sheets/nurse-practitioners

Ross-Kerr, J. (2011). *Credentialing in nursing*. In J. Ross-Kerr & M. Wood (Eds.), *Canadian nursing issues & perspectives*. Elsevier Canada.

Sheer, B., & Wong, F. (2008). The development of advanced nursing practice globally. *Journal of Nursing Scholarship*, *40*(3), 204–211. https://doi.org/10.1111/j.157-5069.2008.00242.x

The Regents of the University of California. (2020). *Community impact: Nurse-run clinics*. Retrieved December 11, 2020, from https://nursing.ucsf.edu/news/commnity-impact-nurse-run-clinics

Tracy, M. F., & Sendelbach, S. (2019). The clinical nurse specialist. In M. F. Tracy & E. T. O'Grady (Eds.), *Hamric and Hanson's advanced nursing practice: an integrative approach* (6th ed., Chapter 14, pp. 343–373). Elsevier.

Woo, B. F. Y., Lee, J. X. Y., & Tam, W. W. S. (2017). The impact of the advanced practice nursing role on quality of care, clinical outcomes, patient satisfaction, and cost in the emergency and critical care settings: A systematic review. *Human Resources for Health*, 15, 63. https://doi.org/10.1186/s12960-017-0237-9

Yee-Litzenberg, L. (2011). *Universal job skills: Skills to highlight in your resume/cover letter/job interview*. Retrieved April 27, 2013, from www.rackham.umich.edu/downloads/examples/snre_universal_job_skills.pdf

Development of a Professional Nursing Career

LEARNING OUTCOMES

By the end of this chapter, the learner will be able to:

1. Discuss the relationship between values and career goals.
2. Use a process to discover a passion for a specific area of professional practice.
3. Compose personal vision and mission statements for professional nursing practice.
4. Specify strategies to develop a professional nursing network.
5. Explain how networking and mentoring enhance career opportunities.
6. Design a career map for their future professional career.
7. Prepare a professional cover letter and résumé.
8. Compile a professional nursing portfolio.

REAL-LIFE REFLECTIONS

Glen and Patricia work together on an inpatient oncology unit. They both started as new graduates a year ago. During a shift report, Glen mentions he is thinking about changing jobs because he no longer enjoys his work. Patricia responds, "Oh, I'm sorry to hear that you don't love this work the way I do. I feel so satisfied if I can get patients to smile, even for a minute, or have them share how they are coping with cancer. I think that I want to spend my entire career specializing in oncology nursing. But if you no longer enjoy the work, it might be best for you to consider something else."

- *What steps do these nurses need to take to establish careers tailored to best meet their personal needs and desires?*
- *How can other nurses support these two novice nurses as they pursue their career goals?*

As the health care delivery system changes, new opportunities for professional nursing practice arise. Nurses live in an exciting time in which their specialized and complex skills can dramatically affect client care and outcomes. Developing required competence for effective professional nursing practice, especially in specialty areas, takes many years. As a profession, nursing offers a wide array of career opportunities. Nurses decide what type of nursing they wish to pursue and where they want to practice. How a nursing career develops depends on the individual nurse. Some nurses create detailed written career plans with established timelines for implementation. Other nurses rely on seizing opportunities as they arise. This chapter outlines how to match career goals with personal values, discover ways to instill personal passion into practice, consider factors to envision a future career, develop strategies to create and implement a career map, and successfully apply and interview for a new nursing position.

Take Note!

The responsibility for professional nursing career development lies within each nurse.

▊ QUESTIONS FOR REFLECTION

1. Do you have a particular nursing career goal in mind? If so, what is it? Are you flexible enough to consider other available nursing career options? Why, or why not?

2. Why is it important for nurses to support each other as they pursue their career goals?

VALUES AND CAREER GOALS

Values are what a person perceives as being important in life, and they provide guidance as people interact with each other and the environment. Examples of values include truth, integrity, justice, peace, health, education, conservation, possessions, money, security, safety, career, and family. Life has many important values, and selecting which ones are the most important can be a difficult task. A clue to defining a personal set of values may reside in what people enjoy doing. In early life, values are formed in families, but a person's values may change over time. Self-betrayal occurs when personal behaviors fail to match a personal set of values.

When people share values, communities are formed (Barrett, 1998). However, even within the profession of nursing (a community), no two nurses share an identical set of values.

Nurses learn professional values as part of socialization into the profession. Certain areas of nursing cater to different value sets. Nurses who value technologically complex skills tend to pursue critical care, emergency, or perioperative nursing, for example. Nurses who value long-term relationships and the wisdom of older adults find great rewards in working with geriatric populations in long-term care facilities. Hospice nursing is rewarding

21.1 Learning, Knowing, and Growing

Values Clarification Exercises

- **Step 1**: Find a quiet, peaceful place where you can spend some time alone and free from interruption.
- **Step 2**: Close your eyes and ask yourself: What things in life are important to me as a person? Record the list.
- **Step 3**: Close your eyes and ask yourself: What things in life are important to me as a professional nurse? Record the list.
- **Step 4**: Identify the entries that are common to both of your lists to identify similarities between your personal and professional values. Create a list for these results.
- **Step 5**: Generate a list of activities in which you engaged during the past week and include the approximate amount of time spent in each activity. Place each activity in a list according to how much time you spent on it, with the activity in which you spent the most time at the top of the list.
- **Step 6**: Compare this list with the lists generated in Steps 2 to 4. This represents the congruence between how you spend your time and your sets of personal and professional values.
- **Step 7**: Answer the following questions:
    1. Am I living in accordance with my personal values?
    2. Am I living in accordance with my professional values?
    3. Are there any things that I could do differently to live out my personal and professional values?

to nurses who value providing comfort and peace in the dying process above preserving life at all costs. Nurses for whom the generation of knowledge is a cherished value may become nurse researchers or theorists. Unlike some other professions, nursing offers many career paths that mesh with one's personal values. Most nurses use personal values when determining their **career goals** (specific professional nursing aspirations). Box 21.1, Learning, Knowing, and Growing, "Values Clarification Exercises," can help you determine your values.

DISCOVERING YOUR PASSION IN NURSING

Chang (2000) defined passion as a "personal intensity, an underlying force that fuels our strongest emotions," and distinguished this from **passions**, which are described as "activities, ideas, and topics that elicit these emotions" (p. 19). When people perform with passion, they perceive the world as being full of opportunities, rather than obstacles, and they focus on personal abilities, rather than limitations. People who live out their life's passions follow their hearts. Passions change as life evolves. A life without passion becomes a life of regrets (Chang, 2000). Nursing is a content-based and context-based passion (the personal, intense desire to help others) with multiple passions (activities and specialized knowledge to care for others). Client care involves activities that require specialized knowledge and skills (passions) centered on a theme of helping others (passion).

Take Note!
All people have the capacity to live passionate lives.

Chang (2000) outlined a seven-step process to develop a passion plan for living that requires feeling, thinking, and acting. These steps are outlined in Box 21.2,

21.2 Learning, Knowing, and Growing

Developing a Passion Plan for Living

1. **Start from the heart:** Acknowledge all your emotions and desires and recognize their power. Engage in a gradual process that requires identifying things that inspire or elicit deep, strong emotions. (This may mean rediscovering things from childhood.)
2. **Discover all your passions:** Make a list of everything in life that is meaningful to you and all that you wish to accomplish during your life.
3. **Clarify the purpose of your passions:** Identify the results of living out your life's passions. The purpose of each passion helps determine how it will be followed.
4. **Define the actions to achieve each passion:** Develop an action plan for each passion.
5. **Perform with passion:** Implement the action plan developed in Step 4, which may require some form of risk taking.
6. **Spread the passion:** Share the passion and how it excites you with others, and let it permeate all your interactions with others.
7. **Persist in the passion:** Stay the course, despite any unexpected circumstances or obstacles that may arise.

Data from Chang, R. (2000). *The passion plan.* Jossey-Bass.

Learning, Knowing, and Growing, "Developing a Passion Plan for Living."

Passionate nurses provide client care from the depths of their hearts and souls. They hold to high ideals and have no fear in confronting situations that compromise client care. Their nursing colleagues and other members of the health care team "catch" their enthusiasm. Passionate nurses demonstrate authentic caring, making clients and their significant others and families feel safe and important. Nurses and clients deeply connect with each other, and the fond memories of the nursing situation last a lifetime.

QUESTIONS FOR REFLECTION

1. What deep emotions surface when you engage in nursing practice or think about your future nursing career?
2. What activities in clinical practice result in extremely high levels of personal satisfaction for you?
3. What passions, other than nursing, do you currently have in life?
4. Why is it important to have passions or interests other than nursing?

ENVISIONING YOUR NURSING CAREER

Envisioning means picturing oneself (Mish, 2020, p. 418). A **personal vision** specifies a future desired state for oneself. Developing a **career vision** statement assumes that change in one's career will occur. The ideal professional nursing career vision would include nursing-related passions.

Like all people, nurses progress through life transitions, so personal career vision statements may be revised to address changes in physical, mental, and spiritual health status. For example, a nurse may leave a position to stay home with their children. A nurse may reenter clinical practice because of a change in marital status, spousal unemployment, or reduced child care responsibilities. Because physical stamina declines with age, a nurse may decide to pursue a nursing position that requires less physical exertion.

Reviewing personal values and strengths facilitates the development of a career vision. Values and beliefs affect attitudes. Attitudes shape behaviors. When nurses give themselves permission to dream, they are ready for developing career visions. All visions start with dreams. When developing a personal vision, let ideas flow freely. Visions may be articulated in the

21.3 Professional Prototypes

Sample Vision and Mission Statements

Sample Vision Statement

I envision myself to be a professional nurse who demonstrates authentic caring toward and appreciation of all living people and things.

Sample Mission Statement

As an authentic professional nurse, my personal mission is to take time to genuinely listen to clients, families, nursing colleagues, and other members of the interdisciplinary health team to provide them with the highest quality of service that is humanly possible.

present or future tense. A **vision statement** is a written declaration of a desired future state and may incorporate ideas for future improvement (Barrett, 1998; Covey, 2004).

Vision statements relate closely to mission statements. A **mission statement** specifies how a vision may be actualized (Barrett, 1998) or the meaning and purpose behind work (Covey 2004). Florence Nightingale (1929) viewed nursing as a spiritual calling. Barrett (1998) presented the concept of "soul work" as activities to be performed by the energy field occupying a living human body. For some, professional nursing may be one way to fulfill one's life purpose.

Mission statements clearly and concisely outline specific services using action verbs with meaning that comes from the heart (Meadows & Buckley, 2014). Mission statements related to a professional nursing career usually focus on client care. Box 21.3, Professional Prototypes, "Sample Vision and Mission Statements," provides a look at some commonly addressed areas.

When nurses create a career vision based on passions, they commit to living out a meaningful life as they engage in activities of the soul, rather than of the mind. Passionate nursing practice enables nurses to live out their life purpose of caring for others. Once personal visions and mission statements have been developed, nurses need to find a nursing position to fulfill them. Nurses use a variety of strategies to find and obtain a desired position.

NETWORKING

Networking consists of exchanging ideas and information among individuals, groups, or institutions (Mish, 2020). Professional networks are interconnected groups of people who share similar work roles. Professional networks may be interprofessional in nature or consist of people within a single profession. Networking consists of building and maintaining beneficial relationships for all involved parties. When nurses network, they become cognizant of commonly encountered practice issues, learn about variances in care practices across settings, collaborate to address common issues, provide support to each other, and discover career opportunities. Strategies for developing effective professional networks include having the courage and willingness to reach out and connect with others as well as a genuine desire to help others, freely sharing information with others, distributing professional business cards, and actively participating in collaborative projects. Networking can occur face-to-face or electronically (Goolsby & Knestrick, 2017).

Opportunities for networking occur at work, schools, professional organizational meetings, professional development conferences, and community service activities. Networking beyond the boundaries of the nursing community enables nurses to expand their knowledge outside of the profession, share information about professional nursing with people who are not nurses, and explore other career options. Many nurse consultants and entrepreneurs rely on professional and community networking to generate business (Norton, 2020). Nurses who network effectively may have a goal when interacting in professional or community groups. However, once the non-nursing professional or community group learns they have a nurse member, the nurse may be called upon to address issues within the realm of nursing expertise.

Take Note!

When nurses interact with each other, their professional networks expand.

QUESTIONS FOR REFLECTION

1. Why is it important to have strong collegial relationships?
2. What have you done during the past week to strengthen your relationships with your fellow students or nursing colleagues?

3. What networking opportunities are available to you as a nursing student?

4. Why is networking important in nursing education and practice?

NURSING CAREER PHASES

Nursing career phases consist of various time frames that denote expected nurse value in the workforce, specify developmental milestones within a nurse's career trajectory, and outline some of the key decisions that nurses make within their careers. Career phases may be interrupted when nurses decide to quit practicing. Some nurses may quit the profession entirely. However, other nurses may decide to reenter practice after new career phases have been designated, resulting in an experienced nurse who left practice returning to an earlier career phase. For example, nurses who are on hiatus from practice may return to a vastly different practice environment. When they return, these nurses may lack confidence in their abilities, needing to relearn and refine nursing skills. However, once they get accustomed to any changes that occurred, they can move more quickly into their next career phase.

In 2009, Shirey proposed that nurses experience three different phases in a professional nursing career. She provided the following labels for the phases: promise (early career, years 1 to 10), momentum (middle career, years 11 to 29), and harvest (late career, years 30 and beyond). The promise phase of a nursing career encompasses the first 10 years of professional practice during which nurses progress through the stages of Benner's novice-to-expert model (see Chapter 1, "The Professional Nurse"). According to Shirey (2009), nurses in the promise phase are viewed as having high potential value but lacking clinical experience. The developmental milestones for nurses in this phase include socialization into the professional nursing role; acquisition of knowledge, skills, abilities, formal education, and credentials; exposure to multiple clinical situations; identification of professional strengths; attainment of confidence; and procurement of positioning for a professional future. Nurses in the promise phase usually start with an idealistic view of nursing but then find themselves in the thralls of reality shock. During the promise phase, career decisions will typically impact future career trajectories. Sometimes, nurses in this phase overlook the importance of making wise career choices (Shirey, 2009). For example, a nurse with a career goal of becoming a certified registered nurse

anesthetist may work in critical care nursing during this career phase.

During the second phase, momentum, nurses are perceived as having high experiential value but mixed potential value. Continuing education and professional growth opportunities are needed for career sustainability. The developmental milestones for nurses in this phase include continued building of professional competence and confidence, development of mastery in practice, experience in managing more clinical situations, and establishment of a professional track record. Nurses in the momentum phase typically make decisions regarding career progression (e.g., administrative, advanced practice, or academic careers) or continued practice in the same area, resulting in renewed significance or stagnation in one's work (Shirey, 2009). For example, students seek out a particular nurse in the momentum phase during their clinical learning experiences because this nurse displays great patience and has a way of linking knowledge the students have learned in the classroom to clinical practice situations. After discussions with the nurse manager, the nurse decides to start preparations for a career as a nursing faculty member.

For the final phase, the harvest phase, Shirey (2009) outlined two stages: prime harvest (years 30 to 40) and legacy (more than 40 years). In the harvest phase, nurses are perceived as having mixed potential value. They sometimes must reinvent themselves to remain relevant. However, they bring high experiential value because they are likely to have seen and experienced a wide variety of situations in their long careers. Unfortunately, nurses with prolonged career longevity can sometimes be viewed by others as obsolete and in the way. Some nurses during the harvest phase reach a career peak and then start to decline. However, these well-seasoned nurses can bring a stabilizing perspective to practice and remain valued team members when they share their expertise with others and continue lifelong learning. The developmental milestones for the harvest phase include the elevation of professional practice to a level of sage practice. Professional nurse sages use their wisdom to advance the profession, position themselves as valued scholars or practitioners, and leave a valuable legacy for future nurses (Shirey, 2009). Key decisions for nurses in the harvest phase include preparing for retirement, deciding if and when to retire, and planning for position or leadership succession. For example, the department chair of undergraduate nursing programs may notice a reduction in physical stamina and occasional difficulty remembering student names. Instead of continuing to work because of the feeling of losing capabilities, the chair hires someone who is capable of filling the position and offers mentorship in preparation for a pending retirement.

MENTORING

For centuries, novices in various professions have sought the advice of experienced professionals. The term "mentor" has its roots in Greek mythology, when Odysseus entrusted the education of his son to his friend named Mentor (Mish, 2020). Today, the word **mentoring** has come to mean the process of enlisting an experienced guide or trusted adviser who assumes responsibility for the professional growth and advancement of a less experienced person, called the protégé. Mentors open doors, create opportunities, and provide career role modeling for protégés while inspiring them. Mentors provide directions for nurses just entering the profession as well as those entering a specialized area or new role of nursing practice. They also provide wisdom and help protégés develop professional networks. Mentors often actively sponsor protégés when career opportunities in the selected field arise. In addition, protégés help mentors by serving as trusted assistants who help clarify ideas (Malone, 1999).

Mentoring does not need to be reserved for nurses who are just beginning their professional careers. Professional nurses can seek out mentors for advice and guidance for making decisions; actively pursuing professional nurse specialty certifications; continuing formal education; career ladder advancement; opportunities for publishing, public speaking, or professional presentation events; engagement in political advocacy; precepting nursing students and new nurses; improving interprofessional communication; learning organizational politics; and resolving issues related to adversity, conflict, and work–life balance (Jakubik et al., 2017).

Mentoring Models and the Mentoring Process

Allen et al. (2004) identified four distinct models for approaching mentorship. The first one is based on apprenticeship; it involves the pairing of an inexperienced person with the most experienced person within a work or educational setting. This form works best for instructing novices to build and develop skills. The second model consists of cloning; the mentor role models for the protégé in hopes of the protégé succeeding the mentor in the same role. This method works effectively

for leadership succession. The third model involves nurturing, a process designed to create a conductive environment and relationship between the mentor and protégé so that the protégé feels willing and comfortable to share strengths, weaknesses, and fears with the mentor. The nurturing model of mentoring works best when new professionals are assuming their professional roles and duties for the first time. The final model of mentoring is based on friendship, meaning the mentor and protégé have equal status. This model works effectively when experienced nurses change jobs and receive orientation to the new work setting and/or practice area.

Olaolorunpo (2019) conducted a concept analysis on mentoring and noted that the antecedents to mentoring are time for regular meetings, effective match of protégés with mentors, solid knowledge and understanding of the mentoring process, and willingness of the protégé to accept any struggling that may be encountered during interactions with the mentor. She identified defining attributes of mentoring as role modeling by the experienced person, nurturing environment and relationship, friendship, regular meetings, and endurance on the part of the protégé. Consequences of mentoring identified in the concept analysis included recognition and gratitude.

Strategies for Successful Mentoring

Successful mentoring relationships require personal chemistry between the people involved. A novice nurse may not want to impose on a potential mentor's time, fear relationship failure, or have difficulty identifying the right person. Some mentoring relationships unfold naturally over the course of a career. People become mentors for various reasons, including the desire to help another, admiration for the novice's personal and professional goals and vision, recollection of a former younger self, and past experience as a protégé in a successful mentoring experience. Successful mentoring requires mutual respect, complementary personalities, open attitudes, proper timing, confidential conversations, appropriate quality and quantity of guidance, and regular meetings (Grossman, 2013; O'Neill Hewlett et al., 2020).

Effective mentoring requires regular meetings between the protégé and mentor. Because mentors and protégés may not work at the same place, finding the time to connect may be difficult. Traditionally, mentors and protégés meet in person. However, not all locations have enough mentors available to provide mentoring to new or nurses looking to change careers (e.g., a staff nurse moving to nursing academia). Virtual or online mentoring may fill this gap and eliminate the need for scheduling sessions because the mentor and protégé interactions can occur asynchronously. Online meeting software programs enable the mentor and protégé to meet synchronously with video capability as long as both parties have a computer or smart phone. Email and online discussions offer ways for asynchronous mentoring to occur. Social media and other web-based platforms have the ability to provide meeting space for synchronous or asynchronous sessions (O'Neill Hewlett et al., 2020).

To ease the burden of professional transition to clinical practice for new graduate nurses, some health care institutions offer mentoring, coaching, preceptor, or residency programs. Preceptors differ from mentors because they work alongside the nurse in the orientation phase of employment (O'Neill Hewlett et al., 2020). Many nursing programs use the preceptor model in the final clinical course of the program. Some of the strategies for successful mentoring apply to an effective preceptorship experience for the preceptor and the novice nurse.

Sometimes, these programs result in effective mentoring relationships. However, mentoring requires reciprocal investment in the relationship. Because most mentors have years of experience within a given field, they have much knowledge to impart to protégés (Grossman, 2013). Mentoring provides mentors with the opportunity to fulfill developmental tasks such as nurturing the new generation of nurses commonly encountered by older professional nurses. Sometimes, the mentor finds a protégé willing to continue the mentor's professional contributions as the mentor retires or loses interest in them as part of a natural career trajectory.

Residency programs differ from mentorship and other nursing orientation programs. Residency programs provide new graduate nurses entering the profession with expanded opportunities to understand and experience the transition arising from graduation from a nursing program to learning how to be a professional nurse in the clinical arena. In a nursing residency program, new graduate nurses receive detailed information of issues encountered during the first year (or two) of clinical practice. Along with understanding the transition process, new nurses are provided opportunities to refine their clinical skills, develop time management strategies, sharpen priority setting skills, and improve interprofessional and consumer communication skills. They also discuss transitions with each other. Residency programs assign each new nurse a seasoned

nurse preceptor who guides them through agency (and unit) orientation and the professional transition processes (Bong, 2019; Institute of Medicine, 2011).

Nurses often experience a wide array of issues resulting in psychological distress during their first year of practice (Box 21.4, Professional Building Blocks,

---

 ### 21.4 Professional Building Blocks

Issues Encountered by New Nurses That Lead to Psychological Distress

- Lack of self-confidence
- Unrealistic expectations from clinical staff, supervisors, and other health team members
- Role ambiguity
- Lack of social support from nursing colleagues, unlicensed care providers, and/or supervisors
- Inadequate staffing
- High demands of the work of nursing
- Inability to use all capacities and qualifications to choose how to do one's work
- Job strain
- Imbalance between individual efforts and rewards from the work
- Unanticipated physical demands of the work of nursing
- Perceptions of being unprepared to work long hours
- Horizontal violence (bullying) by other nurses and health team members
- Feelings of being unprepared to manage clients or other staff members
- Perceptions of being unprepared to assume independent leadership roles
- Being unable to communicate effectively with physicians, residents, and/or interns
- Inability to organize all the tasks needed for effective delivery of nursing care
- Lack of confidence and ability to perform the complex skills required in practice
- Increasingly complex client care requirements
- Difficulty in assertive communication resulting in the inability to advocate for oneself
- Lack of confidence in decision-making abilities
- Discomfort when working with dying clients and their significant others

From Bong, H. E. (2019). Understanding moral distress: How to decrease turnover rates of new graduate pediatric nurses. *Pediatric Nursing*, *45*(3), 109–114. Institute of Medicine. (2011). *The future of nursing: Leading change, advancing health.* The National Academies Press; Lavoie-Tremblay, M., Wright, D., Desforges, N., Gélinas, C., Marchionni, C., & Drevniok, U. (2008). Creating a healthy workplace for new generation nurses. *Journal of Nursing Scholarship, 40*(3), 200–297; Zimmerman, C., & Ward-Smith, P. (2012). Attrition of new graduate RN: Why nurses are leaving the profession. *The Missouri Nurse–Missouri Nurse*, Spring, 15–17.

"Issues Encountered by New Nurses That Lead to Psychological Distress") (Lavoie-Tremblay et al., 2008; Zimmerman & Ward-Smith, 2012). New graduate turnover has been reported to be 27.3% within the first year of licensure, and 49.9% of nurses leave their first nursing position by the second year (Nursing Solutions, 2021). Residency programs typically last 1 year and have been shown to facilitate transition to independent practice and reduce turnover rates. The following Focus on Research brief "Transition to Practice Study in Hospital Settings" conducted by Spector et al. (2015) compares 6-, 9-, and 12-month outcomes of new nurses who were employed in acute care facilities with new transition-into-practice programs, established onboarding or nurse residency programs, and no program other than new employee orientation.

FOCUS ON RESEARCH

Transition to Practice Study in Hospital Settings

The National Council of State Boards of Nursing (NCBSN) developed a transition-in-to-practice model program (TIPP) using the core competencies identified by the Quality and Safety Education in Nursing (QSEN) Institute. They wanted to know if the TIPP program provided a better transition for new graduate nurses in hospital settings. The TIPP program contains basic facility orientation combined with five online modules addressing patient-centered care, teamwork and collaboration, evidence-based practice (EBP), quality improvement, and informatics. They wanted to examine the effects of TIPP on client safety, overall nurse competence, specific QSEN competencies, job stress, job satisfaction, and retention of new graduate nurses.

Using a longitudinal, randomized comparative design, they looked at the study outcomes in 105 hospitals in the states of Illinois, Ohio, and North Carolina. Hospitals ranged in size of less than 100 to over 400 beds and were evenly distributed across urban, suburban, and rural locations. The hospitals were randomly assigned to TIPP and established programs for onboarding new nurses ranging from basic facility orientation to well-established new graduate programs with preceptorships.

Data were collected on safety and negative safe practices, overall competence, work stress, and job satisfaction at 6-, 9-, and 12-month intervals. Participants included 544 new nurses and 691 preceptors who completed data collection at the 6-month interval, 518 new nurses and 675 preceptors who provided data at the 9-month interval, and 281 new nurses and 336 preceptors who completed data collection at the 12-month interval. The following tools were used to collect data: the *NCSBN Practice Issues Index Revised* (self-report data on errors and positive and negative safety practices), *Overall Competency Tool* (perception of overall competence as a professional nurse), *Specific Competency Tool* (perception of competence in each of the QSEN competencies), *NCSBN 4 Questions on Job Stress* (self-reported levels of job stress), *Brayfield and Roth Index of Job Satisfaction*, and retention rates reported at 12 months. The investigators reported elements of validity and reported reliabilities of 0.77 or higher for all tools used for data collection. They also reported minimum sample size required to achieve a power of 0.98 for the study.

Data were analyzed using χ^2 for categorical data, analysis of variance for continuous data, and paired *t*-tests to compare measurements on tools used in the study. Initial data analysis comparing TIPP with control hospitals revealed control group hospitals had fewer errors, reported negative safety practice, and reduced levels of job stress ($p < 0.05$). There were no statistical significant differences in overall competence and job satisfaction. TIPP participants reported statistically significant higher scores on patient-centered care, use of technology, and teamwork and collaboration ($p < 0.05$), and there were no statistically significant differences in quality improvement and EBP. Post hoc data analysis was done separating control groups with established preceptor orientation programs and those with only facility orientation. Established programs with preceptorships were found to have statistically significant lower job stress levels at the 6-month time frame. The only statistically significant difference reported was that TIPP had higher scores on the use of technology compared to all other programs. The study revealed no statistical significant differences in new graduate nurse retention.

This study provides solid support for preceptor use when onboarding new graduate nurses to acute care settings. Job stress peaked at 6 months into the role of professional nurse for all groups and then starts to decline. Job satisfaction showed steady declines until 9 months on the job and then it stabilized or increased. Therefore, new graduate nurses need someone to help them during this difficult professional transition. More research is needed to address the effectiveness of the NCSBN TIP model and how it might be used in hospitals that provide only basic facility orientation for new graduate nurses and other interventions that might ease the stress of the transition to professional practice.

Spector, N., Blegen, M. A., Silvestre, J., Barnsteiner, J., Lynn, M. R., Ulrich, B., Fogg, L., & Alexander, M. (2015). Transition to practice study in hospital settings. *Journal of Nursing Regulation, 5*(4), 24–38. https://doi.org/10.1016/S2155-8256(15)30031-4

■ QUESTIONS FOR REFLECTION

1. What are the characteristics of an ideal mentor?
2. Why are these characteristics important?
3. If you were to select a professional nursing mentor today, whom would you choose?

CAREER DEVELOPMENT STRATEGIES

Once a nurse identifies a career direction on which to focus, they can use a variety of strategies to make their ideal career happen. Most authors addressing career development suggest beginning the process with a self-assessment of personal values followed by a period of dreaming about what a future career may look like (ANA Career Center Staff, 2015; Chang, 2000; Donner & Wheeler, 2009; Malone, 1999; McGillis Hall et al., 2004). A career in nursing equips nurses with many life skills that can transfer to other professions, while basic nursing knowledge transfers to a variety of professional nursing specialty areas.

Career Paths

No one career-planning process has proven to be superior to others. The process may be linear or nonlinear, and nurses select which path to follow based on their ability to tolerate uncertainty and ambiguity (Bongard, 1997a).

Linear career paths require nurses to follow a sequential series of steps. For example, staff nurses who enjoy working with students may decide they will pursue a career in nursing academia. They usually earn a master's degree in nursing before assuming nursing faculty positions. Once employed by nursing programs, they closely follow a tenure track system with specific criteria for advancement from instructor to full professor. Nurses who like structure and meeting designated deadlines prefer this approach to career development (Bongard, 1997b).

Nonlinear career paths rely on life circumstances and critical incidents that result in career changes. Nurses who follow nonlinear career paths frequently create careers by using their interests, outside experiences, and nursing skills. They seize opportunities as they arise. Nurses using a nonlinear approach to career development frequently create new nursing positions within a health care organization or become entrepreneurs. Today, nurses and other health care professionals following nonlinear career paths have a better chance of professional survival, especially during times when health care organizations engage in restructuring and sometimes eliminating nursing positions (Chin, 2020).

Take Note!
No two nurses follow identical paths for career development.

Career Development Model

Donner and Wheeler (2009, p. 2) viewed career development as "an iterative and continuous" process and combine linear and nonlinear approaches to career development. They developed a five-phase career planning and development model, which starts with scanning the environment to understand current realities and future trends in society that have implications for nursing and create possibilities for new areas of clinical practice. Their model emphasizes the importance of periodic self-assessments and reality checks related to self-identity and how others view the individual nurse. If nurses find that their current employment situations do not fit with attributes discovered from their self-appraisals, Donner and Wheeler suggest it may be time to pursue an alternative career path. They also advocate for the creation of a career vision to link current status with future possibilities. Nurses may then use the career vision as a motivating source for remaining in a current practice setting or making a change. Donner and Wheeler suggest that designing a strategic career plan around the career vision facilitates attainment of career goals. Finally, once a career plan has been established, efforts should be channeled into marketing professional skills by forming an expansive professional network, developing a mentoring relationship, and further refining verbal and written communication skills.

Career Mapping

Malone (1999) used the term **career mapping** to denote a continuous process of nursing career development in which career moves unfold as a person engages in professional practice and lifelong learning. This process starts with identifying values, determining the importance of each value, and envisioning a future. The following questions can facilitate the career-mapping process:

- Why did I select a nursing career?
- Why do I have a specific job?
- What can I do now to impact my career?
- What strengths have I brought to clinical practice settings while serving the clients under my care?
- What is my 5-year career goal? (ANA Career Center Staff, 2015)

The future vision creates a blueprint for personal action to make that envisioned future become a reality.

To facilitate the preferred career vision, nurses can use a variety of resources that outline career trends. Resources for learning about current and future needs for professional nursing include the U.S. Department of Labor, the Bureau of Health Professions, the Bureau of Labor Statistics, the American Association of Colleges of Nursing, the National League for Nursing, and the American Nurses Association.

Once nurses determine their preferred career, specialty certification serves as an important step in the career-mapping process. Professional certification provides public acknowledgment of professional competence, enhances career opportunities, demonstrates the ability of the profession for self-regulation, and increases personal power (Malone, 1999). The American Nurses Credentialing Center offers 19 certification examinations across a variety of nursing practice areas (5 in advanced practice nursing, one in disaster certification interprofessional team members, and 13 in nurse specialty practice areas). Nurses can also earn certification from a variety of nurse specialty organizations. Nurse specialty certifications are a contributing factor to better client outcomes (Kendall-Gallagher et al., 2011).

For developing successful career maps, Malone (1999) identified networking and finding a mentor as key strategies. Nurses frequently overlook the importance of networking with professionals from other disciplines. Networking with other members of the health care team and with other professionals within the community enables nurses to gain a more global perspective on the meaning of health and the needs for future health care delivery. Malone specified that personal and professional mentors serve vital roles in the career-mapping process because mentors help shape professional values and instill confidence in young professionals to pursue their dreams.

MAKING A NURSING CAREER CHANGE

Nurses make career changes for a variety of reasons. Some pursue part-time employment to spend more time with families or pursue outside interests. Some nurses experience intense value conflicts with employers that result in a desire for an employment change. Some nurses follow partners to new locations when their employment situations change. Others lose their jobs during periods of economic downturns. During the COVID-19 pandemic, some hospitals and ambulatory surgery and diagnostic centers placed nurses on hiatus while all nonemergent procedures were canceled. Nurses who earn advanced degrees may frequently change jobs. Finally, when nurses get bored or burned out with their current position, they embark on a journey to either change jobs or pursue a different area of nursing practice.

Several strategies prove useful for nurses who wish to remain hirable in today's employment market:

- Maintaining an updated résumé enables immediate action when an opportunity for employment surfaces.
- Refining personal interview skills facilitates confidence when interacting with future employers.
- Networking with other nurses at professional organizational meetings, career fairs, conventions, on online platforms, and during community service activities enables acquisition of key information about employment opportunities.
- Making lists of personal assets, strengths, and preferred professional activities helps identify the type of position best suited to the individual nurse.
- Exposing oneself to motivational information (print, audio, video, or online) arms the nurse considering change with a "can do" attitude.
- After accepting a new position, easing out of the old one gracefully makes it easier to return if the new job fails to meet expectations.

Questions for Reflection

1. What is your ideal picture of your future nursing career?
2. How can you make this picture a reality?
3. What are the consequences of not envisioning an ideal future nursing career?

Finding Available Nursing Opportunities

Nurses can use a variety of resources to locate employment opportunities. Most hospitals and integrated health systems post internal job openings in areas accessible to employees and in human resources departments. Many organizations also list employment opportunities on their company websites. The internet also offers many commercial online job search sites. Nursing journals and periodicals contain classified advertisements with available nursing opportunities. Nursing staffing agencies post openings, and sometimes when their sites are visited, they automatically contact site visitors about available openings. Many professional nursing organizations have career centers within their websites and nurses can find jobs related to their nursing specialties. Nurses who subscribe to electronic list services may also find job opportunities posted or be automatically notified by email when new positions become available. Nurses can learn about career opportunities from networking with colleagues during professional nursing organizational events as well. In times of nursing shortages, some health care agencies turn to radio and television advertising to recruit nurses. Local newspapers publish classified advertisements related to employment opportunities in nursing. Social networking websites (e.g., Facebook, LinkedIn) and other online applications also serve as useful tools for nurses to find employment and market themselves.

Marketing Your Skills

Employers need to verify that applicants have the necessary skills to meet the demands of the position. Tailoring cover letters and résumés to address specific skills outlined for a particular position may prove to be more successful in securing a new job than using generic cover letters and résumés. Documents showcasing professional skills should be saved as computer files and edited to fit the requested skills and previous professional experience delineated by the posted job. Special care must be taken to verify that all information sent to prospective employers and clients has no spelling or punctuation errors, and if being shared in person, is visually appealing. Poorly constructed documents readily find their way into the trash (Bongard, 1997b; Enelow & Kursmark, 2010; Hawkes, 2017; VGM Career Horizons, 2008).

Writing a Cover Letter

Cover letters provide a general introduction to prospective employers and offer an opportunity for the applicant to showcase their personality. If the organization specifies a person to contact in its advertisement for the position, the cover letter should be addressed to this designated person.

Two forms of cover letters provide information to prospective employers. The traditional cover letter gives reasons for contact, expands on the rationale for applying for the position, and details how to contact the applicant to set up an interview. The second form, a skill-matched cover letter, not only provides the same information as the traditional cover letter but also outlines how the applicant's acquired credentials and skills match the job requirements. The skill-matched cover letter format saves time for people who screen applicants for interview invitations because they can easily read specific applicant qualifications. For an example of each type, see Box 21.5, Professional Prototypes, "Sample Cover Letters."

The general rules for cover letters apply regardless of how applicants communicate with prospective employers. Nurses who use the cover letter as a method to market themselves and showcase their experiences and accomplishments frequently get noticed by human resources representatives. When human resources personnel become interested in a job candidate, they invite the candidate for an employment interview.

Preparing a Résumé

The résumé originated as a solution for employers who wanted to interview only qualified job applicants. Human resources personnel find most résumés dull and boring. A good **professional nursing résumé** presents individual strengths while showcasing special skills and professional accomplishments (Enelow & Kursmark, 2010; Hawkes, 2017; Poulin, 2015; VGM Career Horizons, 2008). A good résumé will get the candidate an interview, and preparation of the résumé assists in interview preparation, especially for the common request during interviews for applicants to "tell me about yourself." Résumé preparation also provides time for reflection about one's career. All résumés should showcase professional achievements, attributes, and experience

21.5 Professional Prototypes

Sample Cover Letters

Jane Doe, RN, BSN, OCN
111 E. Lilac Avenue
Springfield, MO 65106

October 3, 2020

Ms. Mary Ashcraft, RN
Nurse Recruiter
Human Resources Department
Springfield Medical Center
803 North Maple Street
Springfield, MO 65107

Dear Ms. Ashcraft:

As I was reading the latest edition of the <u>Missouri Nursing News</u>, I spotted your advertisement for a nursing position on your oncology unit. I have recently moved to Springfield, Missouri, and would like to work for Springfield Medical Center, the premier hospital in the area. My professional nursing background includes previous oncology nursing experience and certification.

I am enclosing a copy of my resume so that you may review my credentials. I would appreciate the opportunity to discuss my qualifications in person. Please call me at my home, 417-888-6464 at any time to schedule an interview. If I am not available to take your call, please leave a message and telephone number so I can contact you. My email address is jdoe82@gmail.com if you prefer to use email to contact me.

Thank you for reviewing my credentials. I look forward to meeting you soon.

Sincerely,

Jane Doe, RN, BSN, OCN

Jane Doe, RN, BSN, ONC

FIGURE 21.1 Traditional cover letter.

Jane Doe, RN, BSN, OCN
111 E. Lilac Avenue
Springfield, MO 65106

October 3, 2020

Ms. Mary Ashcraft, RN
Nurse Recruiter, Human Resources Department
Springfield Medical Center
803 North Maple Street
Springfield, MO 65107

Dear Ms. Ashcraft:

As I was reading the latest issue of the <u>Missouri Nursing News</u>, I spotted your advertisement for a nursing position on your oncology unit. I have recently moved to Springfield, Missouri, and would like to work for Springfield Medical Center, the premier hospital in the area. I have also read about the exciting news about the current expansion of the oncology services at Springfield Medical Center.

My professional nursing background includes previous oncology nursing experience and the following summary outlines how my qualifications fit your nursing position requirements:

<u>Your requirements</u>	<u>My qualifications</u>
* Current MO Professional Nursing License	* Current, unencumbered Missouri Professional Nursing License
* One year's experience in oncology nursing	* Five years' experience in oncology nursing at St. Luke's Hospital, Omaha, NE
* OCN certification	* Current OCN certification

I am enclosing a copy of my resume so that you may review my credentials. I would appreciate the opportunity to discuss my qualifications in person. Please call me at my home, 417-888-6464 or email me at jdoe82@gmail.com (if you prefer to use email) to schedule an interview. If I am not available to take your call, please leave a message and telephone number so I can contact you. Thank you for reviewing my credentials. I look forward to meeting you soon.

Sincerely,

Jane Doe, RN, BSN, OCN

Jane Doe, RN, BSN, OCN

FIGURE 21.2 Skill-matched cover letter.

TABLE 21.1 Comparison of the Chronologic and Functional Résumé Formats

	Chronologic Résumé	Functional Résumé
Description	Lists job titles and responsibilities in reverse chronologic order	Highlights professional skills (also called skill-based résumé)
Components	Contact information Job and career objectives Career summary that highlights dates of each position Education Special awards or honors Community service	Contact information Job and career objective List of skills specific for job Dates of previous positions, usually listed at the end or in smaller type Education and skills acquired from employment or community service activities
Situations for best use	Documentation of personal career growth Continued employment in a field without too many job changes	Professional career established Beginning of a career Career change with the goal to focus on relevant skills Stagnant or declining career Returning to the workforce after a prolonged absence
When best not to use	Frequent job changes (every 1–2 years) Just finishing school Seeking a career change	No situations
Advantages	Showcases detailed employment history Outlines specific job responsibilities and previous employers	Highlights skills, rather than employment history Makes it easier for human resources personnel to determine if skills match posted job description Can include skills gained from outside areas of past employment

Adapted from Enelow, W., & Kursmark, L. (2010). *Expert resumes for health care careers* (2nd ed.). JIST Works; Yate, M. (2012). *Knock 'em dead resumes: How to write a killer resume that gets you job interviews* (10th ed.). Adams Media; VGM Career Horizons. (2008). *Resumes for nursing careers* (2nd ed.). Author.

while minimizing any potential weaknesses and stimulating enough interest in the applicant to ensure an invitation for an interview (Enelow & Kursmark, 2010; Hawkes, 2017; Poulin, 2015). Many companies today use automated programs to screen résumés for key terms, and résumés should be modified as needed to ensure the specific skill terminology mentioned in a job posting is included in the document.

The majority of job applicants use either a chronologic or a functional résumé format. Of the two, the chronologic format is the most common. Some people opt to combine the two formats when developing a résumé (Hawkes, 2017; Poulin, 2015; Yate, 2012). Table 21.1 outlines the chronologic and functional résumé formats and highlights the strengths of each. The selection of format depends on where a person is within their career trajectory, employment experiences, and the type of opportunity being considered. For an example of each type, see Box 21.6, Professional Prototypes, "Sample Résumés." Résumé experts disagree on many aspects of résumé preparation. However, they do agree on several preparation principles.

Human resources personnel spend little time reading individual résumés. Résumés containing more than one to two pages will most likely not be read. Some potential employers use automated programs to screen résumés;

résumés not containing critical key terms will be automatically rejected. Many experts on résumé preparation suggest inclusion of a job/career goal over an objective. When a job/career objective is present, some human resources department employees assume that if the objective fails to match the open position, the applicant will reject an offer if made. Therefore, when using a job/career objective, it is imperative that the objective matches the desired position and editing the résumé to match each job application is advisable. Résumés that incorporate the following suggestions are more likely to be efficiently processed:

1. Organize résumé categories in a logical manner.
2. For paper-based and electronic formats:
   - Use a font size of 11 to 14 pt in an easily readable font (e.g., Arial, Bookman, Times New Roman, Verdana), and keep the font style consistent throughout the résumé (a larger size font and boldface type can be used effectively to present headings).
   - Use 8½ by 11-in. paper (or standard letter size for electronic format) because employers may photocopy the résumé for distribution to department managers and human resources files.
   - Select high-quality, white, cream, or pastel (avoid pink) paper of 16- to 25-lb weight if printing.

21.6 Professional Prototypes

Sample Résumés

Jane Doe, RN, BSN, ONC
111 E. Lilac Avenue
Springfield, MO 65106
(417) 888-6464 jdoe82@gmail.com

Objective   Obtain a professional nursing position on an oncology client care unit.

Experience   St. Luke's Hospital, Omaha NE
                           Oncology Unit
                           Evening Charge Nurse   **July 2015 to present**

                           University of Nebraska Medical Center, Omaha NE
                           Post Anesthesia Care Unit
                           Staff Nurse   **June 2013 to July 2015**

                           University of Nebraska Medical Center, Omaha NE
                           East Seven (Surgical Nursing Unit)
                           Staff Nurse   **June 2011 to May 2013**

                           Longview Extended Care
                           Licensed Practical Nurse   **May 2009 to June 2011**

Education   BSN, University of Nebraska   **May 2011**
                           LPN, Clarkson Technical School,
                           Omaha, NE   **May 2007**

Professional   Missouri Professional Nursing License
Credentials   ACLS Certification
                               Oncology Nursing Society Certification
                               Oncology Nursing Society
                               American Nurses Association

Professional & Personal References Available Upon Request

FIGURE 21.3 Sample chronologic résumé.

(continued on page)

21.6 Professional Prototypes (*continued*)

Sample Résumés

Jane Doe, RN, BSN, OCN
111 E. Lilac Avenue
Springfield, MO 65106
(417) 888-6464 jdoe82@gmail.com

Goal: Full-time position to provide compassionate person-centered nursing care on an adult inpatient oncology unit

Skills
- Certification in Oncology Nursing since June 2017
- 5 years nursing experience in Oncology Nursing
- Experienced in insertion and removal of percutaneous intravenous central catheters
- Taught oncology certification review courses on chemotherapy administration and radiation therapy for oncology staff
- Published newsletter for the local chapter of the Oncology Nursing Society
- Supervised staff of 2 RNs and 3 Patient Care Technicians as evening charge nurse

Education
- BSN, University of Nebraska Medical Center, May 2011
- Oncology Certification Course, Omaha Chapter of the Oncology Nursing Society, May 2016
- 30 hours of continuing education in Oncology Nursing, May 2015 to July 2017
- LPN, Clarkson Technical School, May 2009

Professional Credentials
- Certification in Oncology Nursing by the Oncology Nursing Society
- Missouri Professional Nursing License #556087352
- Nebraska Professional Nursing License #N6670889
- Current certification in ACLS and BCLS

Professional Organizations
- Oncology Nursing Society (past secretary of the Omaha, Nebraska Chapter)
- American Nurses Association

Employment History

St. Luke's Hospital, Omaha NE
Oncology Unit
Evening charge nurse   July 2015 to present

University of Nebraska Medical Center, Omaha NE
Post Anesthesia Care Unit
Staff nurse   June 2013 to July 2015

University of Nebraska Medical Center, Omaha NE
East Seven (Surgical Nursing Unit)
Staff nurse   June 2011 to June 2013

Longview Extended Care, Hastings, NE
Licensed Practical Nurse   May 2009 to June 2011

Professional and Personal References Available on Request

FIGURE 21.4 Sample functional (skill-based) résumé.

- Maintain strict alignment of margins within sections.
- Keep a free-flowing appearance without any noticeable breaks.

3. Limit résumé blocks to five to seven lines (two to three sentences).
4. Use action verbs to describe all job skills and responsibilities. If key job skills are mentioned in an advertisement for a position, make sure those terms are used in your résumé.
5. Have a friend or family member proofread the résumé before sending it.

Take Note!
The typical résumés receive about a 30-second review.

Nurses may develop a résumé independently, seek the advice of career counselors, or have their résumés generated by a résumé specialist. Résumé preparation software can also be useful. The internet is a great source of information for creating a professional résumé and for résumé templates. State employment agencies may also offer online assistance with résumé generation. Today, many organizations prefer electronic submission of job application materials over paper copies, either through portals on their websites or via email.

The résumé should include the applicant's name without any titles, physical mailing address, telephone number, and email address. Applicants should refrain from using their current employer's email address or telephone number unless they have informed the current employer of their search for another job (Bongard, 1997b; Hawkes, 2017; VGM Career Horizons, 2008; Yate, 2012). If the applicant does not have an email address that sounds professional, they should create one. Google, Yahoo, and others offer free email accounts.

Finally, résumés lose power if they contain mistakes or possess certain characteristics. Yate (2012) and Hawkes (2017) offer the following suggestions for what *not* to do on a résumé.

1. Never give the document a title, such as "résumé" or "fact sheet."
2. Never state availability for employment.
3. Never specify reasons for leaving a previous or current job.
4. Never outline references (employers are legally obligated to obtain written consent from prospective employees before they check references).

The résumé provides applicants with a systematic format to showcase their professional skills and written communication abilities to prospective clients and employees. Usually, no verbal interaction occurs between the person screening the résumé and the applicant (and some are screened by computers). Thus, utmost care should be taken when preparing a résumé to create the best impression.

References

As stated earlier, personal and professional references should not be listed on a résumé (Hawkes, 2017; VGM Career Horizons, 2008; Yate, 2012). The type and number of references required vary across organizations (typically three to six are required). Applicants usually find out how many references are required when they complete an employment application. When specifying references, common courtesy suggests that applicants inform the people whose names appear on the reference list. In addition, if people have used more than one surname during their employment, this information should be included somewhere because verifying references can become difficult if previous employers know the person by a different name from the one on application documents (Hawkes, 2017; Moore & Pierce, 2016; Yate, 2012).

Moore and Pierce (2016) offer suggestions for selecting and contacting people to use as professional references. Human resources personnel typically ask professional references about job applicant knowledge, skills, attitudes, and work ethic. Because professional nurses may change positions throughout a career, some nurses keep a record of significant contacts with whom they have worked. Suggested professional references include past and present employers and professional colleagues. If the nurse has not informed anyone in their current work setting that they are applying externally, then they would use past employers and colleagues. For new graduate nurses, Moore and Pierce suggest using professors, clinical instructors, preceptors, and professional mentors. Classroom professors can address applicant's work ethic and knowledge, and clinical instructors can address applicant's clinical skills. When making decision about whom to include in a reference list, the job applicant should determine if the person being considered would share positive information about their abilities to fulfill the desired job responsibilities. Before finalizing a professional reference, nurses should considerer how much time has lapsed since having a working relationship. For example, a favorite professor from a nursing program would be an excellent choice as a reference especially for graduate nurses pursuing their first nursing position. However, if several years have lapsed and the nurse has had no contact with the professor, the professor would not be able to provide recent information about the nurse's professional abilities.

After professional references are identified, applicants should contact them, inform them about the nursing position and its requirements, and request how the identified reference might address job requirements. Professional references appreciate receiving a current résumé, especially if the applicant is applying after some time has lapsed since working together. Because employers and graduate nursing programs use a variety of ways to secure information from professional references, job applicants should inform each reference of the expectations (e.g., phone call, online survey, formal letter) and if there is a specific deadline for completing required materials (Moore & Pierce, 2016).

Professional references appreciate learning about career accomplishments for people for whom they have provided information. Moore and Pierce (2016) suggest sending each reference a brief note expressing thanks to them for providing information to prospective employers and notifying them whether they got the position. Additional ways of contacting references can also be email or through social media.

Professional Portfolios

Some nurses have developed **professional portfolios** to showcase their skills and accomplishments (Fig. 21.5). Some nursing programs have students generate nursing portfolios as part of the curriculum (Peddle et al., 2016). In clinical practice, the professional nursing portfolio is used by some health care organizations as evidence that the employee deserves a promotion. In many Magnet facilities, a career ladder serves as a means for keeping experienced nurses at the bedside while offering them financial rewards for providing requisite nursing care and participating in shared governance activities. Nurses who have professional portfolios may elect to take them to interviews to display evidence of professional accomplishments. Some nurses leave the portfolio with a prospective employer for review after all interviews have been completed along with a specific time for the nurse to retrieve it (Bell, 2001). Box 21.7, Learning, Knowing, and Growing, "Building Your Portfolio," outlines the most common components you should consider including.

 21.7 Learning, Knowing, and Growing

Building Your Portfolio

Whether you are new to nursing or have many years of experience, it is never too soon to start building your portfolio. Your portfolio components may vary according to its intended use and the stage of your career. Williams and Jordon (2007) offered the following suggestions for things that may be included in a professional portfolio:

- Résumé
- Nursing philosophy statement
- Letter(s) of recommendation or appreciation
- Professional license
- Professional certifications
- Diplomas and continuing education certificates
- Special recognition such as honors or awards
- List of professional organizational memberships
- Copies of publications
- Photographs of podium or poster presentations
- Evidence of organizational service (e.g., shared governance committee participation) and community service
- List of inventions
- Written documentation of professional behaviors to facilitate client outcome attainment

From Williams, M., & Jordon, K. (2007). The nursing professional portfolio: A pathway to career development. *Journal for Nurses in Staff Development*, 3, 125–131; Peddle, M., Jokwiro, Y., Carter, M., & Young, T. (2016). A professional portfolio of learning for undergraduate nursing students. *Australian Nursing & Midwifery Journal, 24*(4), 40.

FIGURE 21.5 Presenting oneself as a polished professional is the first step in attaining a desired professional nursing position.

Williams and Jordon (2007) specify that besides being a vehicle to document professional accomplishments, portfolio development gives nurses the opportunity to reflect on practice endeavors and determine future career goals.

Take Note!

Professional portfolios provide documented evidence for meeting criteria for promotion.

Interview Skills

A face-to-face, phone, or remote interview enables potential employers or clients to assess applicants on a personal level and determine how they may fit with the organization. When an interview invitation is extended, applicants are one step closer to getting the desired position. Successful interview performance relies on adequate preparation. Table 21.2 outlines tips for effective performance during an interview. Although some nurses find the interview process stressful, it is

TABLE 21.2 Tips for Effective Interviewing

Tips	Rationale
Learn as much as possible about the organization.	Knowledge of the organization's mission and philosophy enables the applicant to anticipate questions related to their personal fit with the organization.
Be prepared to answer questions related to your personal strengths, problem-solving skills, teamwork experiences, assessment for safe practice, organizational skills, priority setting, your expectations, areas for future professional growth and career.	Employers want to hire someone who has the capability to perform the roles and responsibilities of professional nursing safely and effectively. They also want nurses who have realistic appraisals of themselves.
Dress conservatively in a business suit or well-tailored dress, not a uniform or scrubs.	Present a professional appearance. The employment interview rule is to dress one level above the position being considered.
Avoid wearing fragrances, smoking, or filling your car's gas tank right before the interview.	Fragrances create impressions. Some scents trigger allergies.
Groom any facial hair, have clean neat hair, and wear conservative makeup.	Facial appearance and hair create an initial impression when interacting with others.
Groom the feet and lower legs impeccably with well-polished, clean shoes with no signs of wear and stockings or socks that blend with clothing.	A neat, clean appearance signifies attention to detail.
Rehearse the employment interview with a friend or family member.	This can allay nervousness and anxiety.
Bring nursing license and certification requirements with you.	Prospective employers may want to copy these for your file.
Prepare a set of questions related to the agency and position.	Asking questions may generate information to continue or stop pursuing the position. Questions also reveal interest.
Be prepared with information related to the local market salary, bonus, and job expectations.	Verify that the position is aligned with others in the current market.
Arrive 5–10 minutes before the scheduled interview time.	Extra time allows you to relax immediately before the interview, allays potential anxiety related to tardiness, and demonstrates punctuality. However, arriving too early may make the interviewer feel rushed with any previous appointments.
Stay busy while waiting: read a magazine, look over a list of questions, or review your résumé.	The interviewer may accompany their previous appointment to the waiting area, and making use of waiting time creates a positive first impression.
Do not bring friends or relatives to the interview site.	Concern for them may keep you from focusing on the interview and may give the impression that you lack self-confidence.
Greet the interviewer with direct eye contact and a firm handshake.	Business etiquette dictates use of a firm handshake when first meeting someone, and eye contact denotes assertiveness in Western culture.

(continued)

TABLE 21.2 **Tips for Effective Interviewing (*continued*)**	
Do not chew gum.	Chewing gum disrupts articulation of words and creates an unprofessional appearance.
Always ask a question when asked if you have any questions.	Asking questions implies interest in the organization and shows that you are focused on the interview.
Be honest and forthcoming with all answers.	Dishonesty or perceptions of covert information provide reasons for the interviewer not to continue the job application process.
If asked why you left previous places of employment, describe the situation specifically using positive terms.	Employers will assume that if an applicant speaks negatively about previous employment experiences, this will happen if they leave.
Wait for the interviewer to address salary, hours, and working conditions.	These topics are usually not covered in the first interview. However, they must be discussed before accepting a position.
Limit answers to each question to three statements, and share something about yourself related to the question.	Brief, targeted answers facilitate the interview process.
Come prepared to address professional experiences and include information related to teamwork.	Applicants are expected to share specific examples of how they executed various aspects of professional nursing and evidence of working in teams.
Carry a briefcase or folder to store a portfolio or evidence of accomplishments, extra résumés, reference letters, and reference list.	Briefcases and folders keep materials neat and project an air of professionalism.
Conclude the interview with a question related to the next step of the interview process.	This communicates continued interest in pursuing the position.
Send a thank-you note to the interviewer as soon as possible after the interview.	A follow-up note shows appreciation and highlights courtesy as a personal strength; it also provides one last opportunity to highlight a personal strength.

From Bongard, B. (1997b). Managing your career. In B. Case (Ed.), *Career planning for nurses*. Delmar Publishers; Pagana, K. (2012). Presenting yourself professionally. *American Nurse Today, 7*(7), 16–17; Ulrich, D. L., & Stalter, A. M. (2015). Securing your first clinical nursing position. *Nursing, 45*(8), 60–63. https://doi.org/10.1097/01NURSE.0000466447,19807.6b

important to remember that interview skills improve with practice. Rehearsing with someone who assumes the role of interviewer can be an effective strategy for interview preparation.

Some organizations prefer to conduct online interviews with video technology, especially if the applicant lives far away but is relocating to the area. The same tips for preparing and executing a face-to-face interview apply to online interviews. However, special care needs to be exercised in the environment to minimize interruptions and undesired background noise where the online interview is conducted. Prospective employers have legal limitations regarding the questions they may ask during an employment interview. Some organizations have prospective employees interview with a member of the human resources department, the nursing department manager, and staff members before an employment offer is extended. Nurses who inquire about the hiring process during the initial interview can better prepare themselves for any future interviews.

In times of nursing shortages, some employers offer large sign-on bonuses and other amenities to attract qualified nurses. When applying for positions with attractive bonuses and incentives, nurses should be aware of the risks associated with such enticements. Some incentives require nurses to sign contracts agreeing to a specified time commitment for employment. If nurses do not abide by conditions for the incentives, they usually must reimburse the employer for all or a portion of funds received.

Follow-Up Communication

Applicants should send a thank you note within 24 hours after the interview, either by postal service or by email. Manners mean a lot to organizations that value customer service and teamwork. A thank-you note also gives applicants a chance to summarize interview highlights and make a final positive impression.

Summary and Significance to Practice

Developing a meaningful nursing career requires an open attitude, periodic self-assessment, lifelong learning, creativity, courage, and confidence. Along with personal characteristics, nurses rely on others for effective career development. Networking and mentoring are effective strategies for career development. Both require commitment, caring, and effective communication skills. To live out a preferred career vision, professional nurses must develop a plan and market their personal and professional skills to make the vision become a reality.

REAL-LIFE REFLECTIONS

Recall Glen and Patricia from the beginning of the chapter. What advice would you give to Glen as he looks for ways to change his nursing career? Why is this advice important? Why do you suppose that Patricia is content in her current nursing position?

From Theory to Practice

1. What are the positive and negative consequences of staying in a particular nursing position for a long time?
2. Develop a professional nursing résumé and compile a portfolio. Analyze both projects. Are you on target to meeting your desired career goals? Why, or why not?
3. Determine a nursing career goal. Design a career map to meet your desired career goal. You might find the four-step career-planning process designed by the New Zealand Health Workforce website listed in the "Online Exploration" section useful as it contains a downloadable template. Share your plan with another nurse or your nurse manager (if you are already practicing nursing) or with a clinical nurse preceptor or nursing faculty (if you are a nursing student who has not engaged in professional clinical nursing practice). What are the advantages and disadvantages of having a career map?

Nurse as Author

1. Write a cover letter to accompany your résumé that could also be used as an email message to introduce yourself when applying for a nursing position. It is your choice whether to write a traditional or a skill-matched cover letter.
2. Create your own professional nursing résumé using either a chronologic or functional format.

Your Digital Classroom

Online Exploration

American Nurses Association Career Center (click on the "Nurse Focus Resources" and "blog" tab): **https://www.nursingworld.org/education-events/career-center**

Bureau of Labor Statistics *Occupational Outlook Handbook:* **www.bls.gov/ooh**

Nursing Solutions Inc.: Welcome to NSI Nursing Solutions Inc.: **https://nsinursingsolutions.com/Home.php**

Monster: **www.monster.com**

New Zealand Health Workforce: Nurses: Four-Step Career-Planning Process: **http://www.health.govt.nz/our-work/health-workforce/career-planning**

Nurse.com job listings: **www.nurse.com/jobs**

PONGO: **https://www.pongoresume.com/**

Résumé Writers: **www.resumewriters.com**

Sigma Theta Tau International: **https://www.sigmanursing.org/**

Expanding Your Understanding

1. Develop two brief professional nursing résumés, one using PONGO and the other using a computer software program or website. Print the résumés and compare them. Would you use one of these while applying for a nursing position? Why, or why not?
2. Visit the Résumé Writers website and determine if it would be worth it for you to pay for a professionally generated résumé and cover letter. Why, or why not?
3. Visit Nurse.com and click on "Find a Nursing Job." Read about current job openings, including travel nursing positions and prospective employers. Do any of these positions appeal to you? Why, or why not?

Beyond the Book

Visit the**Point** at **www.thePoint.lww.com** for activities and information to reinforce the concepts and content covered in this chapter.

REFERENCES

Allen, T. D., Eby, L. T., Poteet, M. L., Lentz, E., & Lima L. (2004). Career benefits associated with mentoring for protégés: A meta-analysis. *Journal of Applied Psychology, 89*(1):127–136 https://doi.org/10.1037/0021-9010.89.1.127

ANA Career Center Staff. (2015). *5 Considerations for nurses facing ethical challenges on the job.* Retrieved May 11, 2021, from https://www.nursingworld.org/education-events/career-center/nursing-career-resources/

Barrett, R. (1998). *Liberating the corporate soul, building a visionary organization.* Butterworth-Heinemann.

Bell, S. K. (2001). Professional nurse's portfolio. *Nursing Administration Quarterly, 25*(2), 69–73. https://doi.org/10.1097/00006216-200101000-00012

Bong, H. E. (2019). Understanding moral distress: How to decrease turnover rates of new graduate pediatric nurses. *Pediatric Nursing, 45*(3), 109–114. Retrieved March 31, 2021, from http://www.pediatricnursing.net/ce/2021/posttest4503109114.html

Bongard, B. (1997a). Creating your own job: Using nonlinear strategies to reach your career goals. In B. Case (Ed.), *Career planning for nurses.* Delmar.

Bongard, B. (1997b). Managing your career. In B. Case (Ed.), *Career planning for nurses.* Delmar.

Chang, R. (2000). *The passion plan.* Jossey-Bass.

Chin, J. L. (2020). Successfully navigating career paths. *Women & Therapy, 43*(1/2), 182–196. https://doi.org/10.1080/02703 149.2019.1684677

Covey, S. (2004). *The 8th habit: From effectiveness to greatness.* Free Press.

Donner, G. J., & Wheeler, M. M. (2009). *Taking control of your career: A handbook for health professionals.* Mosby/Elsevier.

Enelow, W., & Kursmark, L. (2010). *Expert resumes for health care career* (2nd ed.). JIST Works.

Goolsby, M. J., & Knestrick, J. M. (2017). Effective professional networking. *Journal of the American Association of Nurse Practitioners, 29*(8), 441–445. https://doi.org/10.1002/2327-6924.12484

Grossman, S. C. (2013). *Mentoring in nursing: A dynamic and collaborative process.* Springer.

Hawkes, B. (2017). *Your last nursing class: How to land your first nursing job: The ultimate guide to landing your first nursing job… and your next.* Beth Hawkes.

Institute of Medicine. (2011). *The future of nursing: Leading change, advancing health.* The National Academies Press.

Jakubik, L. D., Weese, M. M., Aliades, A. B., & Huth, J. J. (2017). Leadership series: "How To" for mentoring. Mentoring in the career continuum of a nurse: Clarifying purpose and timing. *Pediatric Nursing, 43*(3), 149–152. Retrieved May 11, 2021, from https://www.thefreelibrary.com/Mentoring+in+the+career+continuum+of+a+nurse%3a+Clarifying+purpose+and...-a0502001270

Kendall-Gallagher, D., Aiken, L., Sloane, D., & Cimiotti, P. (2011). Nurse specialty certification, inpatient mortality, and failure to rescue. *Journal of Nursing Scholarship, 43*(2), 188–194. https://doi.org/10.1111/j.1547-5069.2011.01391.x

Lavoie-Tremblay, M., Wright, D., Desforges, N., Gélinas, C., Marchionni, C., & Drevniok, U. (2008). Creating a healthy workplace for new-generation nurses. *Journal of Nursing Scholarship, 40*(3), 200–297. https://doi.org/10.1111/j.1547-5069.2008.00240.x

Malone, B. L. (1999). Career mapping: Visioning your future. In C. A. F. Anderson (Ed.), *Nursing student to nursing leader: The critical path to leadership development.* Delmar.

McGillis Hall, L., Waddell, J., Donner, G., & Wheeler, M. (2004). Outcomes of a career planning and development program for registered nurses. *Nursing Economics, 22*(5), 231–238. Retrieved March 31, 2021, from https://www.researchgate.net/publication/8142439_Outcomes_of_career_planning_and_development_program_for_registered_nurses

Meadows, K. L., & Buckley, J. J. (2014). You, Inc. *Journal of Healthcare Management, 59*(3), 173–176. Retrieved March 31, 2021, from https://pubmed.ncbi.nlm.nih.gov/24988671/

Mish, F. C. (Ed.) (2020). *Merriam-Webster's Collegiate Dictionary* (11th ed.). Merriam-Webster.

Moore, G., & Pierce, Y. (2016). Selecting and preparing professional references. *American Nurse Today, 11*(1), 31–32. Retrieved January 13, 2016, from https://www.myamerican-nurse.com/selecting-and-preparing-professional-references/

Nightingale, F. (1929). *Notes on nursing.* D. Appleton.

Norton, L.W. (2020). The business of consulting psychology: Lessons from the field. *Consulting Psychology Journal: Practice and Research, 72*(1), 68–76. https://doi.org/10.1037/cpb0000159

Nursing Solutions. (2021). *2021 NSI National Health Care Retention & RN Staffing Report.* Retrieved May 11, 2021, from https://www.nsinursingsolutions.com/Documents/Library/NSI_National_Health_Care_Retention_Report.pdf

Olaolorunpo, O. (2019). Mentoring in nursing: A concept analysis. *International Journal of Caring Sciences, 12*(1), 142–148. Retrieved March 31, 2021, from http://www.internationaljournalofcaringsciences.org/docs/16_olorufremi_12_1.pdf

O'Neill Hewlett, P., Santolla, J., & Devi Persaud, S. (2020). Investing in nursing's future: Mentoring across the profession. *American Journal of Nursing, 120*(8), 58–63. https://doi.org/10.1097/01.naj.0000694592.98888.10

Peddle, M., Jokwiro, Y., Carter, M., & Young, T. (2016). A professional portfolio of learning for undergraduate nursing students. *Australian Nursing & Midwifery Journal, 24*(4), 40. Retrieved from https://www.researchgate.net/publication/30945426_A_professional_portfolio_of_learning_for_undergraduate_nursing_students

Poulin, R. (2015). *Nurse résumé hacking: Shortcuts to outshining your peers & getting interviews.* Richard Poulin.

Shirey, M. R. (2009). Building an extraordinary career in nursing: Promise, momentum, and harvest. *The Journal of Continuing Education in Nursing, 40*(9), 394–402. https://doi.org/10.3928/00220124-20090824-01

Spector, N., Blegen, M. A., Silvestre, J., Barnsteiner, J., Lynn, M. R., Ulrich, B., Fogg, L., & Alexander, M. (2015). Transition to practice study in hospital settings. *Journal of Nursing Regulation, 5*(4), 24–38. https://doi.org/10.1016/S2155-8256(15)30031-4

VGM Career Horizons. (2008). *Resumes for nursing careers* (2nd ed.). VGM Career Horizons.

Williams, M., & Jordon, K. (2007). The nursing professional portfolio: A pathway to career development. *Journal for Nurses in Staff Development, 23*(3), 125–131. https://doi.org/10.1097/01.NND.0000277181.24959.3b

Yate, M. (2012). *Knock 'em dead resumes: How to write a killer resume that gets you job interviews* (10th ed.). Adams Media.

Zimmerman, C., & Ward-Smith, P. (2012). Attrition of new graduate RN: Why nurses are leaving the profession. *Missouri Nurse, Spring, 2012,* 15–17. Retrieved May 11, 2021, from https://www.thefreelibrary.com/Attrition+of+new+graduate+RN%3a+why+nurses+are+leaving+the+profession.-a03043 20755

Shaping the Future of Nursing

LEARNING OUTCOMES

By the end of this chapter, the learner will be able to:

1. Compare and contrast the terms "possible future," "plausible future," "probable future," and "preferable future."
2. Explain the implications of current trends on the nursing profession for each future scenario presented.
3. Specify ways nurses can create a preferable future.
4. Outline how nursing education might better prepare nurses to meet the challenges of future health care delivery.
5. Discuss the role of nursing scholarship in the future of the nursing profession and health care.
6. Outline strategies nurses can use to plan for the future.

REAL-LIFE REFLECTIONS

Jing is a registered nurse (RN) who learned that the hospital where she has worked for 15 years is closing. Reasons for closing the hospital include the declining local economy, fewer service demands, increased competition for clients among local health care providers, high unemployment, reduced government reimbursement for rendered care, inability to meet financial demands, and difficulty with nursing staff recruitment and retention. Jing is upset and wonders why she did not foresee the hospital closure. Jing has worked for the past 10 years on the day shift in the postpartum unit, and she is concerned her work hours and special area of practice will change in a new hospital.

QUESTIONS FOR REFLECTION

1. How can you prepare yourself so that you maximize your knowledge, skills, and talents as a professional nurse?
2. Where would you like to be in the nursing profession 10 years from now?
3. What steps do you need to take to accomplish your future career vision?
4. What are the consequences for you as a professional nurse if you fail to consider what changes may occur within health care and the nursing profession in the next decade?

Humans have attempted to predict the future for centuries. Egyptian pyramids, for example, contain hieroglyphics that predict the future of the human race. Today, computer software programs and advanced statistical techniques have led to the development of sophisticated forecasting models. The random nature of the universe, however, prevents even the best forecasting methods from definitively predicting the future. Humans have come to realize that the only thing they can reliably predict is change.

Dramatic environmental and societal changes have influenced human health, health care delivery, professional nursing practice, nursing education, and nursing scholarship. Many of the forces influencing change have been detailed in earlier chapters in this text. Because the forces influencing professional nursing are intertwined with these changes in the world, an effort has been made to avoid redundancy. This chapter focuses on the future as a concept and outlines potential future scenarios so that the nursing profession and individual nurses can plan to meet the challenges of the 21st century and beyond. An entire book could be written about the myriad issues that impact the future of the nursing profession. To keep the subject manageable, this chapter provides a conceptual approach to the future and then uses it to address three critical societal issues: an aging American population, disasters, and increased rates of obesity.

A CONCEPTUAL APPROACH TO THE FUTURE

Depending on the context in which it is used, the word **future** means "that is to be … existing or occurring at a later time … a time that is to come … what is going to happen" (Mish, 2020, p. 576). In English (and many other languages), verbs have a future tense to communicate proposed actions. Whatever the definition, unless time ceases, the future will arrive soon.

Futurists use a variety of forecasting methods. Minkin (1995) proposed using a format that identifies and analyzes trends and determines their implications before making predictions. Other futurists use similar approaches to forecasting with varying degrees of success (Canton, 2015; Johnson & White, 2000; Naisbitt, 1996; Sachs, 2008; Toffler & Toffler, 2006). Some futurists, such as Thomas Alva Edison, started with a vision (the concept of electric lighting) and then took steps to make the vision a reality. In terms of the future, the meaning of **vision** expands to include forecasting or prophecy.

There is much scholarly debate about the ability of mankind to shape the future. Minkin (1995) said the future is the only part of life that people can change based on their actions or inactions. Sullivan (1999, p. 5) identified two relevant assumptions about the future: "First, the future is uncertain. … Second, we choose and create major aspects of the future by what we do or fail to do." In contrast, many religions hold the belief that the future unfolds as part of a grand plan by a higher power.

Henchley (1978) specified four ways of looking at the future: possible, plausible, probable, and preferable. Henchley's approach considers the future from standpoints ranging from the wildest possible ideas to probable concepts based on human history and trends. This chapter presents definitions and scenarios for Henchley's four ways to approach the future, followed by select key issues confronting the nursing profession and health care delivery.

The **possible future** considers all potential things that may occur, including the wildest ideas, even if they violate the laws of science (Henchley, 1978). Examples include unpredicted catastrophes, such as the catastrophic earthquake and tsunami that affected the Japanese northwestern coastline in 2011; potential, coordinated, multiple worldwide terrorists attacks; or a large meteor hitting and destroying the planet. Science fiction media and doomsday prediction include examples of the possible future.

The **plausible future** focuses on what may occur based on current trends that may be combined to describe a range of potential futures (Henchley, 1978). Examples include increasing tensions between the United States and other nations, developing clean alternative energy sources, technologic advances, increasing disparity of income between the rich and poor, and increasing global warming and pollution.

The **probable future** presents a picture of what most likely will happen, with the future being primarily a mirror to the present with little or no actual change. Examples include continued financial strain on health care providers and businesses, a complex system of health care delivery, continued scientific and technologic advances, and the multifaceted dimensions of making life decisions.

The **preferable future** proposes the desired state for the future. Development of a preferred vision requires the evolution of common visions, shared values, and strategic plans among many groups of people. The preferable future starts by identifying a vision and taking steps to make that vision a reality. This future results from deliberate actions or inactions. Examples include the effectiveness of the government (federal, state, and local levels), insurance companies, and all health care providers to develop and implement a realistic health care system without resulting in national bankruptcy; the elimination of culturally biased health care service delivery by actively recruiting the best and the brightest of all cultural groups into the health care professions; and the development of strategies to integrate holistic health care practices into traditional scientific-based medical care methods.

Scenarios are a sequence of imagined events including accounts or synopses of possible courses of action. Forecasts can be "prophecies, estimates, or predictions of a future happening or condition" (Mish, 2020, p. 489). Scenario use is compatible with "new thinking about complexity and the uncertainties of prediction" (Staley, 2010, p. 35). Scenarios are worlds built with imagination to describe the large range of possibilities. Constructing scenarios involves using logic and evidence to generate them. Staley proposed that a major event occurs approximately every 80 years (e.g., Civil War in the 1860s, World War II in the 1940s) (Staley, 2010). Although this is one historian's perspective, it should be noted that the United States entered World War I in 1917, 52 years following the end of the Civil War. Since World War II, there appeared to be no major event affecting the entire world until 2019, when the COVID-19 pandemic started. If Staley's predictions are correct, the COVID-19 pandemic serves as a major event that historically will characterize the 2020s. In addition, the next major world event would occur sometime in the last decade of the 21st century. However, a major global event could happen sooner.

Prophecies are based on visions, whereas forecasts, estimates, and predictions are typically based on numbers and trends. Forecasts raise awareness of the wide range of possible implications of external forces, sensitize people to potential threats and opportunities, and allow examination of alternative options for action. Historians propose that because events tend to repeat themselves, people should look backward to see the actions resulting in today's outcomes and to use history as a platform for planning new developments and addressing future issues (Staley, 2010).

The scenarios presented in this chapter barely skim the issues that affect the future of professional nursing. Some of the presented scenarios are controversial. The scenarios without reference citations represent the author's predictions of what could happen.

FUTURE SCENARIOS FOR SOCIETY AND HEALTH CARE

Many of the forces that shape the future are beyond human control. Humans have yet to find ways to control acts of nature, such as weather patterns, earthquakes, some epidemics, and famines. However, people do control governments, laws, and policies. Unfortunately, professional nurses lack the societal status and resources to become highly influential in the determination of laws, policies, and regulations. Thus, nurses must build coalitions with more influential members of society to create a solid united front to create change. The following scenarios contain factors that cannot be controlled by the nursing profession alone. Nevertheless, nurses play a key role in being prepared to either confront these challenges or work collaboratively with others to steer action in a desired direction.

The Aging American Population

In 2014, 46.2 million Americans were over age 65 years (14.5% of the population) Roberts et al., 2018. The number of Americans aged 65 or older increased to 52.8 million (17.5% of the population) in 2019 (U.S. Census Bureau, 2020). In 2030, one in five Americans is projected to be 65 or older; by 2040, 21.7% of the American population is expected to be over the age of 65. The percentage of older Americans is expected to account for 23% of the population by 2060. The old age dependency ratio is expected to rise over the next four decades. In 2020, there were 3.5 working adults for every person eligible to receive social security benefits. Projections indicate that by 2060, there will be 2.5 working adults for each person eligible for social security (Vespa et al., 2020). The increase of the aging American population results in the need for more RNs in order to meet their needs for health care services. The Institute of Medicine (IOM) (2008) proposed a three-step approach to prepare for this increase that includes improving the way health care is delivered, increasing the number of care providers specializing in geriatric care, and enhancing the geriatric competence of the health care workforce.

Demonstration of essential knowledge and competence in the care of older adults has become part of licensure and has been incorporated into some advanced practice nursing certification examinations (e.g., geriatric and family nurse practitioner examinations). More home health care nurses will be needed because increasing numbers of the older adults at home will need help with activities of daily living and management of complex drug regimens. Older adult clients (if they have the cognitive ability to make sound, reasonable decisions) and their informal caregivers (family members and friends) will need to become active members of the health care team. New technologic devices such as computer-chipped bracelets, home alarms (for doors and stoves), and pressure sensor devices enable older adults to stay at home safely under the care of family members, friends, or hired aides. Nurse geriatric consultants will help caregivers cope with the declining health of this population. Older adults living independently or receiving home care services may be issued an electronic, waterproof bracelet to wear. The monitoring device can detect all movements, including activity, sleep, balance, food and fluid intake, and can issue medication reminders and track compliance to prescribed medications (Sharma, 2019). These devices will automatically notify relatives and/or hired caregivers of any significant changes in activity or eating. When the monitor detects activity indicating a life-threatening event, the device automatically contacts local emergency management systems.

When older adults can no longer manage their own personal and health care needs independently and become homebound, a primary or acute care geriatric nurse practitioner can make home visits aimed at keeping the client stable and safe at home. Placement of older adults in long-term residential care facilities can remain an option of last resort. Because of the increased demand for nurses specializing in geriatric care, nursing research can be conducted to see what is needed to attract nurses and advanced practice nurses to work with the older adult population. Home health agencies offer competitive wages for nurses for care for these clients in their homes, and governments may pay for relatives who care for their loved ones at home. In the future, personal care robots may serve as a viable alternative to in-person care services. Health insurance providers and federal, state, and local government programs sometimes cover a portion of costs for hired caregivers.

Take Note!
All health care professionals, especially nurses, need to prepare for the special needs of older adult clients.

An aging nurse workforce adds to the health care issues of an aging population. In 2018, the mean age of employed nurses was 50, and 28.9% of nurses were over age 60. By 2030, 1 million RNs are expected to retire (U.S. Department of Health and Human Services, Health Resources and Services Administration, 2019). Many of the older nurses reported reducing their working hours because of the physical demands

of the job. Experts estimate that the United States will need to replace 900,000 to 2 million retiring nurses by 2030 (American Association of Colleges of Nursing [AACN], 2019; IOM, 2011; U.S. Bureau of Health Professions, Health Resources and Services Administration, 2017). In 2019, the AACN reported a 5.1% increase in enrollment in nursing programs, but programs turned away 80,407 qualified students to member undergraduate and graduate programs. The AACN reported that reasons for turning students away were faculty shortages, insufficient clinical sites, limited classroom space, too few clinical preceptors, and budgetary constraints (AACN, 2020). Aging nurses might have an increased understanding of the needs of older adult clients as they experience caring for older adult relatives and recognize their own age-associated changes in physical abilities. Clinical issues projected to arise from the aging of the population include prevention of infectious diseases (especially human immunodeficiency virus [HIV], as sexually active older adults may refrain from condom use as pregnancy is not a potential outcome of intercourse); health promotion strategies for older adults; supporting older adults with physical and cognitive limitations; and finding ways to support caregivers who care for loved ones in their homes.

Strategies for reversing the aging process may appear. Biotechnology also may provide artificial body parts, tissue transplants, and implanted computer chips for people. Gene therapy, herbal therapies, and more drugs will be used to limit or reverse the aging process (Canton, 2015; Kaku, 2011; Toffler & Toffler, 2006). Kaku (2011) presents cutting-edge information on the use of nanotechnology to detect and treat life-threatening diseases, including breath analysis for health status in private home bathroom mirrors and the use of nanotechnology to detect and treat many forms of cancer, diabetes, and renal, hepatic, and cardiovascular disease.

Healthy lifestyle choices, including proper exercise, diet, and stress management, will continue to be essential because of their positive effects on physical and mental fitness. With reduced costs of DNA testing at birth, everyone born may be genetically tested to obtain a DNA profile that might effectively predict lifespan and provide specific dietary recommendations and exercise prescriptions to enhance health and prolong life (Canton, 2015).

Possible Future

Often, older adults with financial resources must exhaust them to pay for health care services. As people age, they often consume more health care services (IOM, 2008, 2011). By 2030, 20% of the American population will be over the age of 65, and less than 20% will have defined pension plans (U.S. Department of Health and Human Services, Administration on Aging, 2012). Many retired individuals will rely on 401K savings accounts, reverse mortgages, and additional employment to supplement social security income. Fixed-benefit pension plans no longer exist, and employers provide matches to employee contributions to retirement savings accounts. Some fixed pension plans underestimated the amount of future payouts and dissolved. Retirees too young for Medicare benefits find themselves scrambling to secure health care coverage and paying much more for coverage than they did in the past. Because most retirees cannot afford to be without health care coverage to supplement Medicare, many of them purchase additional insurance. Decisions retirees face will affect their health, well-being, and quality of life. For example, some older adults must choose between buying food or prescription medications, move in with children, buy less nutritious food to reduce their grocery bill, or set thermostats to potentially dangerous settings (e.g., not using air conditioners during a heat wave) to stretch the financial resources they need to survive.

Forecasters predict that a possible intergenerational conflict may arise worldwide as Japan and several European nations have a similar problem with increasing older adult populations. Younger workers may resist paying high social security taxes to support older adults (Canton, 2015; Kaku, 2011; Toffler & Toffler, 2006). This resistance may be paired with ageism in public spaces and family conflict between younger and older relatives (Van Den Huevel, 2015).

In the author's version of a worst-case possible scenario, American society perceives the older adult population as valueless people who do nothing but drain limited resources. Because of increased government debt and possible insolvency, federal plans for income security become defunded. When hospitalized, care providers follow specific care paths created by the government that restrict the use of expensive interventions based upon age. Therefore, older adults must die in order to preserve precious commodities for younger, more productive citizens. Governments enact laws to make euthanasia and assisted suicide legal and potentially mandatory (e.g., with diagnosis of a terminal or expensive chronic illness). The older adults who no longer want to burden their families or society willingly end their lives.

Plausible Future

A plausible scenario (especially for nations that have democratic governments and large older adult populations) is that older individuals with healthy cognitive capabilities exert energy in political activism, resulting in massive reformation in available older adult services sponsored by government, businesses, and nonprofit agencies. For the financially solvent older adults, specialized residences and extended care facilities will be built to provide desirable, individualized, and culturally relevant services. Older people without vast resources will find themselves living with children who gladly welcome them, thereby creating multigenerational family units. As working adults serve as primary caregivers for older adults, geriatric day care programs will increase in number and some may even be employer-sponsored. Caregiver programs will be developed to provide social and emotional support for exhausted and depressed family members caring for an aging adult with declining health. Legislation to provide funding for aging services, caregiver programs, medical care, and tax credits for home caregiving will be enacted. In this possible scenario, basic needs of the older adult population are met and younger members of society value these individuals.

Probable Future

The probable scenario regarding the aging American population is that older adults might benefit from improved health from advances in medical science, remain a strong lobbying group, and demand increased governmental support for life and health care needs. Societal and governmental support for the health care of older adults remains similar to what they are today.

Preferable Future

In the preferable scenario, the aging population makes health-promoting lifestyle choices (starting in middle adulthood) and develops strong ties with younger people. People of all ages, governmental agencies, businesses, and nonprofit foundations and organizations work together to develop policies related to health care delivery that provide equal access to services for all. Physically able older adults engage in volunteerism that results in a meaningful societal contribution. Older adults with sufficient financial resources willingly assume financial responsibility for their health care services and residential care requirements. A universal design for senior housing is adopted, and the floor plan consists of all living areas on one level with technology that detects falls or other significant activity changes (such as changes in gait). Older adults also have access to self-driving cars so they can independently get to the store, senior centers for activities, and health care appointments. They also wear small but smart hearing aids that automatically turn up the volume, improve word clarity, and schedule health care appointments with transportation as needed (Institute for Alternative Futures [IAF], 2018). Public funding is reserved exclusively for the older population and other people who cannot pay for basic life needs, including health care.

■ Questions for Reflection

1. How can the nursing profession prepare for increased numbers of older adult clients who will need nursing services?

2. What are the possible consequences for the nursing profession if it fails to address aging population issues?

3. What are the possible consequences for the nursing profession if it fails to address the aging of the nursing workforce?

Man-Made Disasters and Terrorism

Any event resulting in great harm or damage can be considered a disaster. Man-made disasters occur because of human action or error. Human history is rife with instances of people acting in violent ways that result in human and environmental catastrophes (e.g., government corruption, rebellions, wars, terrorism). In addition, accidents arising from business and industry have created disasters. For example, nuclear power plant accidents such as on Three-Mile Island in New York, in Chernobyl in the Soviet Union, and in Fukushima in Japan caused devastating effects on the environment and health issues because of high levels of radiation experienced. Before September 11, 2001, the United States largely considered itself immune to major foreign terrorist attacks or acts of war. However, there were warnings of a coordinated terrorist attack plan (National Institute of Medicine and National Research Council, 1999). Terrorist acts occur across the world, and countless acts have been averted. The ease of securing plans for building bombs (some with nuclear, disease-producing, or noxious chemical capability) increases the likelihood of a large-scale terrorist attack. Technologic advances in nanotechnology, biotechnology, and robotics offer the possibility of destroying the

human race while leaving buildings and infrastructures intact. Sources of energy production become prime targets for terrorists because of human reliance on these power sources for health, safety, and business (Kaku, 2011). Cyberattacks threaten national security, critical infrastructure (e.g., utility companies, public transportation, financial institutions, health care organizations, and protected health information), businesses, and individuals. Balancing societal needs for safety while preserving individual rights challenges those entrusted to provide public safety.

The terrorist attacks in the United States sparked a war on terrorism, with most of the actual combat occurring in Iraq and Afghanistan. Uprisings against oppressive governments trigger civil wars or government attacks against rebels. Terrorist attacks across the globe create fear and uncertainty for people as they live their lives. As in all wars and terrorist attacks, much environmental destruction has occurred and many people have died (including many innocent civilians) or sustained physical and/or psychological injury.

Possible Future

A possible and bleak scenario is that terrorists obtain access to computers controlling essential infrastructure, nuclear and biologic weapons. Within a short time frame (perhaps weeks), terrorists execute a well-coordinated series of attacks on American soil, resulting in many civilian casualties and widespread destruction. The United States launches a unilateral attack against terrorist cells with total disregard for national borders. The American action fuels international opinion that the United States will conquer the world to force democratic and capitalistic values on other countries. In response, other nations support the terrorists in their efforts against the United States and another world war decimates the planet.

Plausible Future

A more plausible scenario results in the strengthening of the coalition of countries engaging in the war on terrorism because of attacks happening in many countries. In this scenario, the United Nations (UN) becomes the place where strategic plans are made to rid the world of terrorist acts initiated by well-organized groups with global networks. The UN also develops a global response plan to chemical and biologic attacks. However, acts of terrorism performed by individuals remain unpredictable, and the people responsible for such acts remain elusive.

Probable Future

Unfortunately, the probable scenario results in a future not much different from today. The United States and certain allies develop stronger ties, and the war on terrorism lasts for many years. In response to identified potential biologic attacks, the United States stockpiles medical supplies, medications, and vaccines for future use if needed. Most Americans refuse to be intimidated by terrorist threats and continue with their usual life practices—working, shopping, and attending sporting and other recreational events. Some anxious citizens stockpile supplies in anticipation of a terrorist attack using nuclear devices. The government tries to stimulate the economy while spending vast amounts of money to preserve homeland security. Less money becomes available to provide services to those with limited resources (e.g., food subsidies, health care) and to repair infrastructure (e.g., roads, sewage systems, power plants). American citizens live with minor inconveniences, such as having to arrive earlier and wait longer in lines when traveling by air. Health care workers voluntarily register to become members of federal, state, or local medical response teams (Veenema, 2019).

Preferable Future

The preferable future is one in which people have no need for violent acts because diverse values and approaches to life are valued. Rich nations foster the economic development of poorer countries. Agreement occurs on defining basic human rights and values across cultures while allowing for diversity. All people are valued. People with more resources than what they can use support those who cannot meet basic human needs (e.g., food, water, shelter, safety). Because all people feel valued and respected, there is no need for violence.

▪ QUESTIONS FOR REFLECTION

1. How can the nursing profession prepare to confront the effects of terrorist acts?
2. Why is it important for nurses to be prepared for possible acts of terrorism?

Natural Disasters

Natural disasters occur as the result of climate or geologic events. Some climate changes are linked to the actions of humans (see Chapter 13, "Environmental and Global Health") (Canton, 2015; Kaku, 2011;

Sachs, 2008; Veenema, 2019). Natural disasters can occur quickly and without warning (e.g., earthquakes, volcanic eruptions, some tornadoes, flash floods), quickly and with warning (e.g., storms, tsunamis), or slowly and with warning (e.g., downstream flooding, environmental contamination, famines from prolonged drought). The COVID-19 pandemic revealed what can happen when a well-coordinated disaster response plan at the federal, state, and local state governmental levels is lacking. However, the pandemic also resulted in beneficial effects of reduced human activity. For example, Milan, Italy, reported a 30% to 70% reduction in greenhouse emissions in various areas of the city from reduced traffic congestion (Institute for the Future [IFTF], 2020). Some local municipalities propose limiting automobile access to areas and promote walking and cycling to reduce air pollution that can lead to later natural disasters (IFTF, 2020).

Predicted effects of global climate change include more intense storms, rising sea levels, and geographic climate shifts (i.e., tropical forests become deserts, temperate zones become tropical, tundra becomes fertile farmland). An increase in infectious diseases follows climate change, and disease becomes prevalent in more temperate climate zones (Canton, 2015; Kaku, 2011; Sachs, 2008).

Possible Future

The possible future is one in which humans show an increasing disregard for the earth. The need for human survival and desire for extravagant lifestyles dominate all human activities. Humans ravage the planet and expand residential areas with total disregard for wildlife and plant life. Environmental impacts consolidate and result in catastrophic climate effects, that results in climate change produces rapidly rising sea levels and a series of massive storms that culminate with rapidly falling temperatures affecting Europe, North America, and the northern half of Asia. Falling temperatures result in deep freezes that cannot support human existence. Not even the most powerful government can intervene to prevent the catastrophe (Emmerich, 2004).

Plausible/Preferable Future

A plausible (and perhaps preferable) scenario includes increased human awareness of our impact on the environment. The UN spearheads a binding global environmental treaty for all nations (even developing countries with fewer resources). The world works cohesively and collaboratively to reduce greenhouse gas emissions and air, soil, and water pollution, and facilitates action by offering incentives. For example, olivine, a naturally occurring volcanic mineral, has been shown to have the ability to capture greenhouse gases. When transferred into the ocean, the greenhouse gases can be absorbed by shells and coral reefs. By making sand from olivine and spreading it on beaches, the sand can transfer greenhouse gases to the oceans and permanently remove more carbon dioxide that humans have produced since the beginning of the Industrial Revolution (IFTF, 2020). Nature flourishes and counteracts the damage done by humans.

Probable Future

The probable future involves the continuation of existing international, national, and local environmental policies. Economic considerations supersede required actions for energy conservation and environmental preservation, with most people abiding by them and other people looking for ways around them because of increased personal expenditures. However, many realize the effects they have on the environment and have taken action to reduce their individual carbon footprints. By implementing required climate change instruction in elementary and secondary schools, children and adolescents can follow environmentally healthy lifestyles, share them with their parents, and reinforce them with their own future children (IFTF, 2020). If and when sea levels begin to rise enough to threaten human life, storms become highly destructive, and plants and wildlife disappear (Canton, 2015; Kaku, 2011), the human race might then develop and implement stronger, environmentally friendly global policies.

FUTURE SCENARIOS FOR HEALTH CARE DELIVERY

Health care delivery has become increasingly complex. Along with providing services for the older adult population who have more complex health care needs, the health care system will need to become more adept with providing linguistic and culturally appropriate care services. In 2030, the main driver for increasing the U.S. population will be immigration (Vespa et al., 2020).

The National Academies of Science, Engineering, and Medicine (NASEM, 2021) identified that social determinants of health play a key role in the health of people. Social determinants of health include economic stability (income, employment, stable housing, and food security), education (early childhood education and development, high school graduation, enrollment in higher education, language [English proficiency] and literacy levels), social and community context (discrimination, engagement in the community, incarceration rates, and social cohesion), access to all forms of health care (including primary care services), health literacy, and quality of the neighborhood and built environment (access to healthy food, environmental conditions, crime rate, incidence of violence, and quality of housing). In the Future of Nursing 2020–2030 Report, they incorporated the Social Determinants of Health and Social Needs Model developed by Castrucci and Auerbach (2019) that outlines upstream, midstream, and downstream strategies use by nurses to improve health of clients they serve.

Upstream strategies involve nurses working to affect local, state, and federal health-related policies. (See Chapter 19, The Professional Nurse's Role in Public Policy). Midstream strategies focus on screening individuals for societal factors that prevent them from attaining optimal health. Nurses who work in outpatient clinics and public health departments engage in client education and initiate referrals for improving living conditions, providing safe environments, access to healthy foods, and mental health services. Downstream strategies occur in the home, urgent care, and acute care settings and consist of nursing interventions (including client education) required for treatment of acute conditions and management of chronic disease (NASEM, 2021).

In recent times, emerging health issues from vaping (use of e-cigarettes), legalization of medical and recreational cannabis, and the emergence of COVID-19 may affect health care delivery. Some of the long-term effects of consistent use of vaping and cannabis are known, and long-term effects of COVID-19 infection are continuing to be studied. Between 10% and 30% of people who became ill with COVID-19 suffered from lingering effects of the disease, "long COVID" (Stone, 2021). All three factors are likely to result in increased cases of chronic illness that may develop earlier in life and may contribute to long-term disability (Leduc-Pessah et al., 2019; Patterson et al., 2020). Table 22.1 outlines some of the health issues encountered with heavy use of medical marijuana and vaping along with long-term effects of COVID-19. The health care delivery system must be prepared to confront these future challenges. These sequelae have special care needs; in fact, some health care systems began opening special care centers for COVID-19 "long-haulers" to address these special needs (Castellucci, 2020). As COVID-19 long-haulers receive COVID vaccines, preliminary research findings in a study conducted by Dr. Griffin at Columbia University in New York City

▪ TABLE 22.1	Possible Negative Health Effects Associated with Long-Term Use of Medical Cannabis, Vaping, and COVID-19		
Facet of Health	**Medical Cannabis**	**Vaping**	**COVID-19**
Mental health	Increased risk of cannabis use disorder if used frequently and use starts at younger ages Increased association with schizophrenia Anxiety disorder Depression Rare cannabis-induced psychosis	Increased risk of nicotine addiction and other substance use disorders Increased risk of aggressive behavior Increased risk of depression and suicidal ideation Poor sleep quality	Depression Difficulty sleeping Anxiety disorder Mood changes
Cognition	Ongoing cognitive impairment with heavy, frequent use	Increased likelihood of problems with memory and attention	Difficulty thinking and concentrating ("brain fog") Reduced memory
Respiratory system	Earlier decline in lung function if smoked or inhaled Chronic bronchitis if smoked or inhaled	Permanent, irreversible lung damage if vaping substances contain tetrahydrocannabinol (THC), vitamin E acetate, or acrolein (a weed-killing substance)	Shortness of breath Persistent cough Chest pain Reduced pulmonary function Pulmonary fibrosis
Cardiac system	No long-term permanent changes Chronic use can cause bradycardia	No known effects	Palpitations Myocarditis
Gastrointestinal system	Cannabinoid hyperemesis syndrome with heavy use	No known effects	Loss of taste and smell resulting in inadequate nutrition in some people
Pregnancy	Subtle neurodevelopmental infant abnormalities and low birth weight	Low infant birth weight	Possible 2% increase in premature birth No evidence of vertical transmission
Cancer development	Possible increase in testicular cancer with heavy use and lung cancer development	Possible increased risk of lung cancer as antifreeze and formaldehyde may be present in the aerosol of higher-voltage e-cigarettes in two popular brands of vaping substances	No known effects
Youth	Possible adverse effects on brain development Early initiation of use increases risks for mental health effects	Adverse effects on the developing brains resulting in learning problems and poor academic performance	Unknown
Injuries	Increased motor vehicular accidents when driving while under the influence	Exploding devices can result in head injuries, loss of teeth, eyes, and tongues, and severe burns	Not applicable
Other known effects	None	None	Chronic fatigue Joint pain Muscle pain Headache Intermittent chilling with or without fever Rash Hair loss Acute kidney failure resulting in decline or loss of kidney function

From Centers for Disease Control and Prevention. (2021) *Post-Covid conditions: Information from health care providers*. Retrieved April 24, 2021, from https://stacks.cdc.gov/view/cdc/105028; Kahan, M., Srivastava, A., Spithoff, S., & Bromley, L. (2014). Prescribing smoked cannabis for chronic noncancer pain: Preliminary recommendations. *Canadian Family Physician, 60*(12), 1083–1090. Retrieved April 24, 2021, from https://www.cfp.ca/content/60/12/1083; Leduc-Pessah, H., Jensen, S. K., & Newell, C. (2019). An overview of the adverse effects of cannabis use for Canadian physicians. *Clinical & Investigative Medicine, 42*(3), E17–E34. https://doi.org/10.25011/cim.v42i3.33089; Ogamba, I., Kliss, A., Rainville, N., Chuang, L., Panarelli, E., Petrini, J., & Zilberman, D. (2021) Initial review of pregnancy and neonatal outcomes of pregnant women with COVID-19 infection. *Journal of Perinatal Medicine, 49*(3), 263–268. https://doi.org/10.1515/jpm-2020-0446; Patterson, M., William-Jones, P., & Lewis, T. (2020). Consequences of the vaping epidemic on adolescents. *Nursing, 50*(7), 30–38. https://doi.org/10.1097/01.NURSE.0000668600.70206.8f; Sturrock, S., Williams, E., Ambulkar, H., Dassios, T., & Greenough, A. (2020) Maternal smoking and cannabis use during pregnancy and infant outcomes. *Journal of Perinatal Medicine, 48*(2), 168–172. https://doi.org/10.1515/jpm-2019-0422

reveal that up to 30% to 40% of them are reporting significant improvement in symptoms (Stone, 2021). However, other studies show only small numbers or no improvements in their clients (Stone, 2021).

When value-based care payment systems are used to constrain costs, health care providers experience more complexity in care delivery because of the attention paid to increased safety and quality initiatives. Staying abreast of new discoveries about the human body (e.g., genetics, genomics, physiology, biochemistry, stem cells), healthy lifestyle strategies, and technology create distress for some health care providers. Constant change seems to be the only thing on which providers and consumers can rely. In 1996, Bezold identified possible health care delivery scenarios for the 21st century—hard times, buyer's market, business-as-usual, and healthy, healing communities—that capture the essence of possible, probable, and preferable futures.

Hard Times Scenario (Possible Future)

This possible future assumes that times are tough for the economy as a whole and for health care. The federal government has amassed massive debt, inflation is uncontrolled, businesses close, and residents cannot afford to purchase health insurance. As unemployment increases and health insurance costs skyrocket, Americans approve an amendment to the Constitution making health and health care a right of citizenship. The federal government overhauls the health care system to assure equity of health and health care access and creates a mandatory universal health care insurance plan. Because of consistent increases in government deficits, the plan offers a frugal benefit package and sets strict reimbursement schedules for providers and specifies wages for all health care providers (including nurses). The government refuses to pay providers for costs incurred from all preventable hospital-acquired conditions. Government health care plans cover only treatments based on comparative research. Care providers must strictly adhere to federally developed care algorithms that contain implicit biases toward older adults and other marginalized citizens (Allen & Dreyer, 2019). Citizens who fail to comply with governmental guidelines for health promotion are denied services for "preventable" conditions. Governmental controls increase the amount of documentation health care providers must complete to justify reimbursement, and cost containment reduces the amount of federal funding for all forms of health care research. As a result, some hospitals close because of incurred debt. Health care innovations slow dramatically. Heroic measures once used to prolong life are limited to clients who are younger, have something to offer society, or can pay for them. A three-tiered health care system emerges, one for people relying exclusively on the government, another for those with resources for private insurance coverage, and another for people who have the ability to pay for health care costs independently. People who pay for their own health care may choose to engage in travel tourism to countries that cater to medical tourists. Medical trips become a means for individuals with nonemergent care needs and the resources to pay for them to receive cheaper, more immediate care. The outcomes for medical care received internationally are the same as care received in the United States. For people unable to afford private health care services, they have to bear long lines to be seen by health care professionals. Some people may be denied services because of age or lack of governmental funding for needed procedures. Eventually, health care costs bankrupt the government and the United States collapses. Anarchy becomes widespread, and violence becomes a means to gain power.

Buyer's Market Scenario (Probable/Preferable Future)

In this probable future scenario, Bezold (1996) and Herzlinger (2004) propose that the responsibility for health and health care expenditures is returned to the consumer. Insurance coverage includes a tax to help pay for the cost of care given to impoverished individuals. Health care providers are certified in their specialized areas of practice through professional organizations. Health care providers, especially nurses, use evidence-based guidelines for practice. Competition for health care consumers becomes fierce, and health care organizations work hard to please consumers. People rely less on health care providers and have better tools with access to online resources for changing their lifestyles and preventing or managing illnesses. They also have the ability for testing for a variety of health conditions at home with results immediately sent to them and their primary care providers (and specialists) if warranted. Consumers, rather than third-party payers, choose from various types of providers and treatments. Because health becomes a highly valued aspect of human life, consumers seek health care for illness prevention rather than disease treatment and utilize community center programs for health promotion (IAF, 2018; NASEM, 2021). To ensure an adequate supply of health care professionals, all health professions' educational programs are offered free in exchange for 2 years of service in an area of designated need (IFTF, 2020).

This scenario offers real potential for nursing to achieve greater power and influence. Nursing practice based on scientific evidence elevates the level of professionalism for nurses. Nurses present solid evidence for optimal staffing patterns for positive client outcomes (Gordon et al., 2008; NASEM, 2021). Because nurses are seen by society as professionals who have altruistic concerns for clients and have reasonable workloads, more people choose to enter the profession. Nurses develop independent practices and demonstrate superiority in primary health care delivery. Nurse practitioners become the major source of primary care and noncomplex disease management. To address the ever-increasing mental health issues encountered by people living in a highly complex, technical world that is constantly changing, all nurse practitioners receive extra education and clinical experience so that they can also manage clients with psychiatric and mental health illnesses (IFTF, 2020; NASEM, 2021). By caring for consumers directly, nurses have a major role in health promotion. Education emphasizes ways of teaching consumers how to promote individual, family, and community health. This scenario might be a preferable future for professional nursing because of its benefits for both nurses and consumers.

Business-as-Usual Scenario (Probable Future)

Another probable future, the business-as-usual scenario, assumes continued technologic ingenuity, proliferation of new pharmaceuticals, sophisticated communication, and high levels of consumption. Although most Americans are better off in this scenario, poverty rates continue to rise. The Affordable Care Act remains in place, and every American has health insurance. However, advances in biomedical knowledge and technology make it possible to forecast, prevent, and manage illnesses earlier and more successfully. High-tech interventions such as performance-enhancing bionic implants and organoids (a new organ or organ part grown outside the body and then implanted) are widely available to those who can pay for them (Hsia et al., 2021; IAF, 2018; Kaku, 2011). Small hospitals continue to close, client acuity levels rise, early hospital dismissals become desired, and health care becomes more efficient. Wealthy for-profit and non-profit hospitals develop integrated health systems and negotiate discounts with health insurance companies to obtain and maintain a stable client base. Administrators rule and fewer hospitalists (but more acute care nurse practitioners) staff hospitals as employees. Insured consumers receive health care using inpatient, outpatient,

and home health care services. Health insurance plans cover emergency department–incurred costs only if the reason for the visit is determined to be a life-threatening or potentially disability-producing event.

Because innovations continue, health care costs outpace inflation and eventually consume 20% of the gross domestic product. Increased efficiency demands require providers to carry higher client loads. Health professions become more devalued by society, and fewer people enter professional nursing, thereby compounding the nursing shortage.

Healthy, Healing Communities Scenario (Preferable Future)

This preferable and plausible scenario involves a focus on "healing the body, mind, and spirit of individuals and communities" (Bezold, 1996, p. 38). Neighbors look out for each other, and people work together to eliminate problems such as substance abuse, teenage pregnancy, and the effects of poverty. However, information and technology advances result in job losses in the manufacturing and retail industries. Displaced workers seek training and gain employment in service industries. Community health centers serve as medical homes within neighborhoods. Health promotion efforts begin in early childhood. Older people find rewarding ways to contribute to the community, reducing disability and the time spent in long-term care facilities. Community centers offer classes in health promotion to prevent unhealthy behaviors and violence (IAF, 2018; NASEM, 2021). Advanced technologies lead to a comfortable life for most people, and bionics, robotics, smarter homes, and more caring neighborhoods allow older adults and individuals with disabilities to remain in their homes.

Consumers become involved in decision making regarding their health as they learn how to access and evaluate health-related information through computer applications that track personal health information using semantic computing (i.e., looking at quantifiable personal health data and making clinical decisions). People become more comfortable sharing personal health data using electronic health records that connect to large databases used for research. Telehealth provides services for people who are homebound (NASEM, 2021), have work schedules incompatible with care provider office hours, or live in remote rural areas (IAF, 2018; Kaku, 2011; NASEM, 2021).

Technology becomes so advanced and inexpensive that consumers can swallow pills that safely collect comprehensive internal body information about their health that is automatically sent to primary health care providers. Health care providers then send consumers advice for enhancing their health or treating any identified health conditions. In addition, individuals can add sensors and cameras in their homes to collect information about health status and lifestyle measures that are automatically added to their health data cards. The health data cards consist of tiny microchips with wireless technology that are embedded into a piece of wearable technology. Finally, physical home environments help people manage disease, enhance health, and facilitate healthy aging. Some of the physical environmental changes involve verbal reminders from devices like computers, tablets, and smart phones that respond to either the aforementioned pill or in response to the home sensors or cameras (IFTF, 2016). All people, not just those who are affluent, have access to and can afford this technology for personal health management (NASEM, 2021).

Nurses are full partners with consumers in this scenario, helping people with self-care and health promotion activities, interpreting the complex information coming from technology, and providing information to support fully informed decision making. Consumers select a "medical home," a private outpatient office or community clinic that provides them with preventive and health promotion services in a coordinated care effort across the care continuum from primary care providers, including nurse practitioners. The medical home offers specialized services based on lifespan and specific health care needs (IAF, 2012; IOM, 2011). Older adults are valued and cared for at home whenever feasible. Nurses are recognized as highly educated professionals who make valuable contributions, such as providing psychosocial support to clients, engaging in surveillance activities to detect subtle changes in client health status, executing complex evidence-based clinical procedures and protocols confidently, and coordinating health care activities across the continuum of care (IOM, 2011; NASEM, 2021).

EVOLVING HEALTH CARE NEEDS AND HEALTH CARE DELIVERY

Along with the aforementioned issues, the IFTF (2020) and the IAF (2018) have identified additional trends that impact consumer health care needs and the delivery of health care services in the United States. Demographic trends reveal an ever-increasing population with increased immigration to meet labor shortages. Immigration creates a diverse workforce and more culturally diverse clients seeking health care services. Issues on the economic and occupational fronts include globalization, high unemployment (especially in the service sector), younger people entering the workforce, a shrinking industrial workforce, and the continued expansion of information-based organizations. Rising education levels, changing attitudes about gendered roles, increased citizen political participation, increasing technologic sophistication and complexity, reliance on power, and knowledge dependency are societal trends that also impact health care needs and delivery.

Increased cultural diversity and immigration will force all health care providers to become more adept at delivering culturally sensitive and linguistically appropriate services. Health care providers must be attuned to signs of diseases never before seen in the United States when working with people who have lived in other countries. Differences in genetic profiles and genomics also must be considered when caring for culturally diverse clients. In an ideal world, health care provider demographics should match the demographics of health care consumers. In 2019, the U.S. Health Resources and Services Administration reported that 90.4% of nurses are biologically female and only 9.6% are biologically male. The ethnicity breakdown is 73.3% White, non-Hispanic; 10.2% African American; 7.9% Hispanic/Latinx; 5.2% Asian; 0.6% Native Hawaiian/Pacific Islander; 0.3% Native American/Alaska Native; and 1.7% other or multiracial. These demographics do not mirror the demographics of American society. Some health care consumers may find it difficult to feel at ease when receiving care from someone from a different background or someone who has not experienced cultural exclusion and oppression (IOM, 2011; NASEM, 2021; Sullivan Commission, 2004).

Internet technology builds algorithms based on the videos people watch, the information searches they conduct, and the way they engage and interact with social media. The algorithms generate personalized ads and suggestions for further online and television viewing. The technology platforms then individualize content that reinforces rigid personal views (Sharma, 2019) or may contain some unintended biases; (Allen & Dreyer, 2019). Instead of creating common views capable of uniting people, uncompromising polarization fuels incivility, obstructs democratic processes, and impairs the exercise of individual freedoms (IFTF, 2020). When people view and read information that is consistent with their personal views, they are not exposed to diverse ideas. Their possibly biased and unsubstantiated opinions become calcified. They carry these ideas with them as they interact with others in the world. When ideas become excessively polarized, people sometimes refuse to listen to alternative viewpoints. Lack of trust can permeate in the community with health care delivery systems. Care recipients and providers sometimes fail to trust each other. For example, COVID-19 vaccine hesitancy in 2020 and 2021 was fueled by misinformation and disinformation online. Some misguided reasons for vaccine hesitancy included the perception that the government was exercising too much control over personal freedom and choice, the vaccine contained a microchip for tracking purposes, the vaccine caused infertility, the rapid development of the vaccines meant they were unsafe, and that the government would be experimenting on marginalized communities with the new vaccine technology (Marshall & Salahi, 2021). Until people with diverse views can effectively communicate with and learn from each other, distrust will prevail and it will be more difficult for individuals with different perceptions to be united for the common good, including to provide equal and effective health care services to all.

Creating a culturally diverse workforce poses challenges to future health care delivery. Currently, the United States attracts internationally educated health care providers because the American health care system offers a higher income, and social status for nurses is typically higher in the United States than in other countries (Kirk, 2007; Ghazal et al., 2020).

Facilitating migration of nurses is a potential solution for the ever-growing nursing shortage. Currently, internationally educated nurses working in the United States come primarily from 10 countries: the Philippines, India, South Korea, Canada, Cuba, China, Nigeria, Taiwan, Russia, and Jamaica (Squires et al., 2016). Clusters of internationally educated nurses work primarily in California, Florida, New York, Texas, and New Jersey. Unfortunately, nurse migration to developed nations like the United States creates or exacerbates nursing shortages in the donor nations. In 2004, the World Health Organization (WHO) issued a code for ethical recruitment of nurses by affluent countries. The WHO Global Code of Practice on the International Recruitment of Health Personnel provided a globally applied regulatory framework for recruiters to follow to prevent affluent countries from creating shortfalls of health personnel in less affluent nations. It specified that nurses should not be recruited from Nigeria, Nepal, Kenya, Haiti, Pakistan, Ethiopia, Sierra Leone, and Zimbabwe. Since the implementation of this code, the number of internationally educated nurses from these countries markedly decreased. However, in 2008, the National Council of State Boards of Nursing (NCSBN) updated the NCLEX-RN to include changes that ultimately resulted in reduced success of nurses educated in other countries. In addition, the exam also changed test format items (Squires et al., 2016).

When working with a culturally diverse health care team, all members must demonstrate authenticity and encourage the full participation of everyone so that each person feels they make a valuable contribution to the team's efforts (see Chapter 11, "Multicultural Issues in Professional Practice"). Little things such as failure to include culturally diverse team members in informal conversations or outside-of-work activities may "have cumulative and profoundly negative effects" (Myers & Dreachslin, 2007, p. 294) on a team member's overall well-being and professional performance.

Take Note!
A large majority of RNs in the United States are White, non-Hispanic cisgender women, a demographic profile that in large part does not match that of the clients they serve.

Technologic advances in health care also pose challenges to health care delivery. All health team members need effective computer skills to access client health data; find current evidence-based best practice protocols; order client medications, interventions, and supplies; and document client plans, interventions, and outcomes (see Chapter 14, "Informatics and Technology in Nursing Practice"). In the future, people may carry computerized identification cards or wear devices that contain microchips or wireless technology for accessing online electronic health records or a summary of their comprehensive health information (Canton, 2015; IAF, 2012; IFTF, 2016; Kaku, 2011; NASEM, 2021). Identification cards, online cell phone applications, and wearable devices will verify client identity and include health insurance coverage information to prevent health insurance fraud and provide a detailed, consistent health history, reducing the time spent conducting the history for each health care service encounter. Summaries for each time the person accesses and uses health care services will be recorded on the card, online application or wearable device, thereby fostering integration of health care services across the care continuum.

Many persons may decide to wear devices that track all movements and their physiologic responses to them. The insurance company that provides the devices may have clients sign waivers allowing the company to access the information sent to the primary health care provider. What is now considered routine laboratory work from a health provider's office may be monitored through the use of special chips on wearable devices or swallowing a pill. The insurance company can then use the data related to health promotion activities as consumer incentives to lower the cost of health insurance premiums.

■ QUESTIONS FOR REFLECTION

1. What do you think the current health care system will look like in 10 years?
2. What knowledge and skills will be needed for effective nursing practice in 10 years?
3. How can nurses best prepare for the future health care delivery system?
4. What can the nursing profession do to help other nurses prepare for the challenges in the future health care delivery system?

THE FUTURE OF PROFESSIONAL NURSING PRACTICE

Many issues confront the nursing profession as it works to maintain sustainable numbers to meet the needs of society. Initiatives (including IOM recommendations to improve the quality and safety of American health care delivery from a series of IOM quality chasm series) (IOM, 2000, 2001, 2003, 2004, 2006) and Quality and Safety Education in Nursing (QSEN) (Sherwood & Barnsteiner, 2012) calling for improved quality and safety provide an opportunity for nurses to present evidence demonstrating the valuable contributions they make to health care. In addition, the profession needs to develop plans to accommodate a mobile society and increased geographical demands for nurses. If nurses fail to seize current opportunities for leadership in health care delivery and fail to recruit new nurses, the profession may cease to exist. Nurses represent the largest percentage of all health team members.

Take Note!
Actions taken by the nursing profession today have profound implications for future clients, health care delivery, nurses, and society.

Evidence-Based Nursing Practice (Preferable/Probable Future)

Nursing research findings, quality improvement data results, and clinical experience provide the foundation for evidence-based nursing practice. **Evidence-based nursing practice** uses the best available sources of information to enable cost-effective and clinically effective client care. Systematic nursing research and detailed evaluations of health care interventions provide strong evidence nurses can use as foundations for practice. Large databases such as those generated by the National Database of Nursing Quality Indicators (Press Ganey, 2020) and the Omaha System (Sezgin & Esin, 2019) facilitate the generation of sound evidence for use in nursing research, quality management, and clinical protocol development. In the past, nurses performed many tasks based on tradition and ritual. Evidence-based practice enables nurses to determine the effects of newly developed technology, alternative and complementary treatments, and the differences professional nurses make in client care outcomes. Nurses are doing a better job of producing and disseminating information about their impact on the delivery of high-quality care (IOM, 2011; NASEM, 2021; Porter-O'Grady & Malloch, 2018). However, more needs to be done to inform the public and policy makers of the substantial contributions professional nurses make to health care.

Evidence-based practice enables nurses to be taken more seriously by other health care providers and society. Scientific justification for nursing actions raises the level of professional practice. In addition, evidence-based practice may serve as the vehicle for the nursing profession to clearly define the term "nursing."

Multistate Compacts for Nursing Licensure in the United States (Probable Future)

Despite the recommendation by the Pew Health Professions Commission (1995) for health care professional regulation to remain controlled by individual states, the NCSBN has initiated an effort for a mutual recognition model for professional nurse registration. The multistate compact started in 2000 and underwent a major revision in 2015, and additional revisions in 2017, 2018, 2019 and 2020 (NCSBN, 2020b, 2021). Under a mutual recognition model, RNs practicing nursing across state lines do not need a separate state nursing license provided that the states in which they practice participate in the enhanced **Nurse Licensure Compact** (eNLC).

The interstate compact helps states with shortages of professional nurses by allowing nurses from bordering states to practice without needing to obtain an additional nursing license. Electronic- and telecommunication-based nursing practice frequently crosses state borders. The nurse would obtain licensure in the state of legal residence. To protect the integrity of individual state nurse practice acts, the nurse abides by the practice act of the state in which the client receives care (NCSBN, 2020b).

A single professional nursing license facilitates interstate practice, improves tracking of nurses with disciplinary problems, increases cost-effectiveness, simplifies the nursing licensure process, eliminates duplicate listing of licensed nurses, and enhances interstate commerce. In addition, interstate licensure simplifies the licensing process for nurses who are employed by traveling nursing agencies (NCSBN, 2020b). Also, multistate compacts enable nurses to practice in diverse geographical locations, potentially increasing health care access for clients in underserved areas.

Although multistate professional licensure may seem appealing, several disadvantages accompany it. State boards of nursing may need to raise licensing fees for professional nurses to replace the revenue generated by nurses who formerly would have held more than one state nursing license. Nurses with disciplinary action records may not be able to obtain a fresh start in professional nursing after recovering from addiction, for example, or after meeting the disciplinary requirements of a state board of nursing. Multistate licensure also would enable nursing agencies to provide replacement nurses for institutions experiencing shortages because their nurses decide to engage in collective bargaining or strikes to improve working conditions.

To maintain state control of professional nursing licensure, individual states must pass legislation to participate in the multistate licensure compact. As of December 2020, efforts to enact legislation for participation in the eNLC have been successful in 33 states with implementation dates pending for New Jersey. One state, Rhode Island, failed to pass legislation for participation in the eNLC (NCSBN, 2020a). Some failures in states attempting to participate in the eNLC have been the result of failure of all nurses to support the idea. For example, some state nurse associations oppose some elements contained in the language of the compact. The national registration with NURSYS seems to be an obstacle in some states because of perceived

nurse privacy issues. **NURSYS** is a secure database of nursing licenses (RN, LPN, and LVN) and disciplinary actions taken on nursing licenses. The information for each nursing license in the system comes from each state board of nursing. However, NURSYS is the only national database used in the United States for validating nursing licensure for licensed practical/vocational nurses, RNs, and advanced practice RNs. Nurses who practice in states participating in the eNLC must register themselves with NURSYS, which provides electronic notifications to nurses when it is time for license renewal, enables immediate verification of license from any compact-participating state board of nursing, and quick confirmation of a nurse's licensure status and any acts of discipline against a licensee (NCSBN, 2021). In some states, participation in a multistate compact is prohibited by the state constitution, thereby creating another obstacle for multistate nursing licensure compact legislation.

The Demise of the Profession (Possible Future/Worst-Case Scenario)

The demise of the nursing profession is a possible future scenario. Instead of focusing on basic academic skills, the public school system focuses upon educating political activists. The prevailing view becomes that everyone is a victim and, therefore, are entitled to special treatment. Society begins to devalue success based upon hard work. Because nursing is physically, emotionally, and spiritually challenging work, no one expresses a desire to enter the profession. The nursing workforce continues to age with a mean age 50 and 25.8% over age 60, and the proportion of practicing nurses holding baccalaureate degrees or graduate degrees was 63.8% (NCSBN, 2019). However, increasing higher education costs and lack of financial aid programs make nursing education in 4-year colleges too expensive for some who want to enter the nursing profession. Instead of focusing on clients, many nurses feel pressured to focus on meeting documentation requirements, reducing care costs, participating in care rationing decisions, and managing complex technology, resulting in increased client mortality, morbidity, and adverse care events. The few Bachelor of Science in Nursing (BSN)-prepared nurses enter the world of advanced practice nursing within a few years of graduation. Some states expand practice of emergency medical technicians to include providing services that currently fall within the scope of professional nursing practice in emergency departments and intensive care units.

Increased pressure for health care organizations to make profits or stay financially viable results in professional nurses assuming a subservient role to health care administrators. Creative ideas have surfaced to measure individual nurse productivity. For example, wireless communication devices enable administration to track every move made by every nurse. Although such devices reduce the time for nurses to meet client care requests, nurses receive negative performance evaluations for spending too much time providing education and emotional support to clients, completing required documentation, reporting to colleagues during shift changes, and taking breaks. The devices also track the time nurses spend attending to their basic physical needs. Frustrated nurses dissuade others from entering the profession and the nursing workforce shrinks even more.

Efforts at private and federal funding for nursing students prove to be unsuccessful in attracting persons to enter the profession. Nursing ceases to be perceived by the public as the most ethical of all the professions because nurses must cater to the whims of employers. In response to the loss of professional power, nurses engage in conflict with each other.

Because nurses fail to produce a united front for resolving practice and educational issues, they continue to lose power and autonomy. The lack of unity confuses policy makers and society. The marginalized status of nurses means they are denied participation in health care reform efforts, and a system is created that encourages increased workloads, lower pay, and requirements to work in multiple facilities if employed by a large health care system. Because employers know nurses represent the largest single group in the health care workforce, they create work environments that divide nurses. The polarization of relevant ethical issues also continues to fuel division within the profession. Instead of looking at systemic problems as the reasons for declining quality, employers blame nurses. Thus, nursing becomes the weakest link in acquiring and maintaining high-quality and safe health care delivery.

Nursing Gains Clout in Health Care (Preferable/Possible Future)

A more optimistic approach to and preferable scenario for the future of professional nursing would be that the profession becomes more cohesive, provides solid evidence for contributions made to health care, and is valued by society and other health professionals. Nurses have debated with each other for generations on issues such as entry-level education for professional practice,

collective bargaining, defining professional nursing practice, and control of professional practice. Professional nurses work to safeguard the public against threats to health, even sometimes to the detriment of their own health. Nurses have assumed the role of client advocate for many decades by protecting consumers from unscrupulous care providers and serious treatment errors. The movement toward a multidisciplinary health team approach to client care provides nurses with an opportunity to showcase their knowledge and expertise.

Research efforts demonstrate that outcomes are improved when clients receive care from professional nurses. Reductions in mortality, failure to rescue, nosocomial infections, client falls, and readmission rates occur when professional nurses provide direct care to clients (Coto et al., 2020; Harrison et al., 2019; NASEM, 2021; O'Brien et al., 2018). However, conducting studies that support the use of BSN-prepared nursing does not mean changes in health care delivery happen automatically. Changes in public health care policy require an integrated and unified approach by the public, government, and nurses (Milstead & Short, 2019; NASEM, 2021). Thus, professional nurses must determine a means to disseminate research findings to the public, inform the government of their needs and desires, and involve elected officials who draft legislation for policy changes (see Chapter 19, "The Professional Nurse's Role in Public Policy").

Take Note!

As nurses provide solid evidence for the contributions they make to health care, society and other health team members will realize their value.

Along with improved societal status, professional nurses also become valued members of the health care team. Shared governance shifts from an exclusively nurse form of governance to an interdisciplinary form of governance (Porter-O'Grady & Malloch, 2018). Because of increased efforts of collaborative interdisciplinary teamwork, the health professions embark on providing interprofessional learning experiences that result in long-lasting effects. All team members understand their roles and gain increased respect for nursing's contributions to the interprofessional team efforts (IOM, 2011; NASEM, 2021).

When nurses demonstrate specialized knowledge and expertise that make differences in client care outcomes, society and other health team members will greatly value the profession. Nurses will enjoy greater autonomy and higher salaries. The profession of nursing will then have no difficulty attracting the best and brightest young people.

▍ QUESTIONS FOR REFLECTION

1. What areas of nursing knowledge need further development?

2. How can nursing research affect the nursing profession and clinical practice?

3. What are the advantages and disadvantages of a multidisciplinary approach to health and health care research?

4. What might be some specific areas where a nursing approach to health and health care research might be beneficial to health care consumers and the delivery of health care services?

THE FUTURE OF NURSING SCHOLARSHIP

Within the past two decades, nursing research has received increased support from professional nurses and policy makers. In 2021, the National Institute of Nursing Research (NINR) celebrated its 35th anniversary as part of the National Institutes of Health. The NINR provides grant funding for nurse researchers, including studies that look at specific clinical care situations, ways to improve client safety, and strategies to increase the professional nurse workforce. Results of funded nursing research are disseminated at annual NINR meetings.

Nursing research–based protocols have been developed for client care in the areas of skin management, cognitive impairment, culturally relevant care, pain control, and postoperative and chemotherapy-induced nausea and vomiting. Nursing research findings frequently cross health care disciplines. As interdisciplinary approaches to health care demonstrate improved client outcomes, nurses will be asked to participate in multidisciplinary research efforts. The National Institutes of Health's Roadmap to the Future offers opportunities for nurses to engage in multidisciplinary research projects.

Rapid development in nursing theory and research during the past few decades leads to a promising outlook for the future. Nursing needs to develop and explicate theories to predict nursing outcomes. Increasingly, nursing research has validated models and theories for nursing care to provide foundations for care. As this trend continues, nursing will develop a unique knowledge base to fulfill the criteria defined for a profession.

The National Academies of Science, Engineering, and Medicine (NASEM) outlines 10 desired outcomes for the nursing profession in The Future of Nursing 2020–2030: Charting a Path to Achieve Health Equity. The following list presents an abbreviated version of each outcome while capturing the essence of its message:

1. Nurses have the preparation "to act individually, through teams and across sectors to meet the challenges associated with current and future factors that contribute to disproportionate disease burden carried by certain segments of the U.S. population (e.g., high maternal mortality and morbidity, increasing numbers of older adults, mental health issues, structural racism, unequal access to primary care)." (p. 356)

2. Nurses address the social determinants of health that underlie poor health "individually and in partnership with other disciples and sectors" and create individual- and community-focused interventions to achieve solutions as well as working to change health care policies. (p. 356)

3. "Nurses reflect the people and communities served throughout the nation, helping to ensure that individuals receive culturally competent, equitable health care services." (p. 356)

4. "Health care systems enable and support nurses to tailor care to meet the specific medical and social needs of diverse patients to optimize their health." (p. 356)

5. Nurses' contributions to health care "are quantified, extended, and strengthened." Institutional and regulatory barriers that prevent nurses from practicing to the full extent of their education are removed. Historically, uncompensated nursing services that are rendered in the school and public health sectors are reimbursed at a comparable rate to the same services rendered in other health care settings. (pp. 356–357)

6. All sectors of health care along with nurses and health care leaders "create organizational structures and processes" to facilitate professional nurses to expeditiously acquire "relevant content expertise to serve flexibly in areas of greatest need in times of public health emergencies and disasters." (p. 357)

7. "Nurses consistently incorporate a health equity lens learned through revamped academic and continuing education." (p. 357)

8. Nurses collaborate across their affiliated organizations to develop and deploy a shared agenda to contribute to substantial, measurable improvement in health equity: All national professional nursing organizations develop and maintain "an orientation of diversity, equity, and inclusion within and across their organizations." (p. 357)

9. While focusing on primary prevention, nurses consistently look for ways to innovate, capitalize on opportunities for professional growth and development, "expand their roles, work in new settings and in new ways, and markedly expand their partnerships connecting health and health care with all individuals and communities." (p.357)

10. "Nurses attend to their own self-care and help to ensure that nurse well-being is addressed in educational and employment settings through the implementation of evidence-based strategies." (p. 357)

Table 22.2 outlines actions that each professional nurse can take to facilitate implementation of the NASEM's recommendations for nurses to lead the challenge to

TABLE 22.2   Individual Professional Nurse Actions to Implement National Academies of Science, Engineering, and Medicine (NASEM) Recommendations

Simplified NASEM Recommendation	Nurse Action
Using a collaborative process involving all national professional nursing organization and regulatory bodies, create a comprehensive shared professional nursing agenda (priorities, goals, actions, and methods for measuring success) "to address social determinants of health and to achieve health equity that can be used in practice, education, leadership, and health policy development" (p. 13). Project to start in 2021.	Join a professional nursing organization and engage in activities to create the shared nursing agenda. Respond to any surveys sent by regulatory agencies or professional organizations seeking nurse input into the agenda. Educate self about the social determinants of health and issues related to disparities of health conditions, health status and well-being (independent study by reading or online activities or attend a professional conference addressing social determinants of health, health equity and/or heath care access equity).
"By 2023, agencies at the federal, state, and local levels, all private and public health care organizations, third-party payers, and foundations should provide support and start real and enduring action to enable" (p.13) each nurse in the workforce to address social determinants of health and health equity in a comprehensive manner in any practice setting.	Verify that all client history and visit computer templates have entries for data related to the social determinants of health, and if not all are present, request that Information Technology update them. If uncomfortable in addressing certain social determinants of health with clients, role play a client care interview with a professional colleague. Assist grant developers with data collection for evidence to help to get fund for projects that help nurses learn and address social determinants of health in all areas of clinical practice. Engage in political activism at the local, state, and federal levels to secure funding for programs and costs associated with enhancing the use of social determinant of health in clinical practice. Document thoroughly any nursing interventions associated with the social determinants of health.
"By 2021, nursing education programs, employers, nursing leaders, licensing boards, and nursing organizations should initiate the implementation of structures, systems, and evidence-based interventions to promote nurses' health and well-being, especially as they take on new roles to advance health equity".	Inform nursing administrators of education programs and in clinical practice settings of ideas to promote health and well-being of professional nurses. Assist in the development of programs to enhance nurse health and well-being in the employment setting, educational setting, or those offered by professional nursing organizations or regulatory bodies. Report any incidences that threaten the health and well-being to human resources (employment setting) or nursing program administration or student services (academic setting). If any incidences are not addressed using proper channels, report them to the proper local, state, or federal governmental agency. Engage in legislative process or lobbying to pass legislation aimed at keeping nurses physically and psychologically safe.
"Remove all legal, regulatory, public or private entity, commercial barriers that prevent nurses from being able "to practice to the full extent of their education and training" and hinder them from "addressing social needs and social determinants of health" of their clients and "improving health care access, quality, and value" (p. 13).	Engage in the legislative process to change laws and regulations related to advanced practice nursing to assure full scope of practice. Keep time logs regarding time spent engaging with clients addressing the social determinants of health, health equity concerns, and access to care issues. Negotiate with nursing administration to change job descriptions to be more inclusive of addressing the social determinants of health, access to health care, improve health care quality and value including TIME and STAFFING required to address these factors when providing client care based upon data generated from time logs. Set limitations on using nurses as social workers in clinical practice settings.

Simplified NASEM Recommendation	Nurse Action
"Federal, tribal, state, local, and private payers and public health agencies should establish sustainable and flexible payment mechanisms to support nurses in both health care and public health, including school nurses, in addressing social needs, social determinants of health, and health equity" (p. 13).	Network with school and public health nurses to learn about their practice and how they address social determinants of health, provide health promotion education and interventions, manage acute and chronic illnesses, and provide emergent care. Encourage school and public health nurses to keep logs of client/student encounters to document their interventions and their effectiveness to share with the public and legislators. Engage in the legislative process to enact legislation for reimbursing public health and school nurses for rendered health care services at a rate comparable to that given in other outpatient settings.
"All public and private health care systems should incorporate nursing expertise in designing, generating, analyzing, and applying data to support initiatives focused on social determinants of health and health equity using diverse digital platforms, artificial intelligence, and other innovative technologies" (p. 13).	Volunteer to service on interprofessional tasks forces to revise computer documentation templates to address social determinants of health and health equity. Analyze current computerized templates, care paths, decision making algorithms for any evidence of explicit or implicit biases and if any found, inform the organization to have them revised. Become aware of any new innovative technology for clinical practice and if there is perceived value, request to pilot study them in the clinical setting. Collect data on any new digital platforms, artificial intelligence, telemedicine, point of care testing, or other innovative technologies for ease of use, value added to the clinical setting and effectiveness. Be one of the first to adopt promising clinical innovations.
"Nursing education programs, including continuing education, and accreditors and the National Council of State Boards of Nursing should ensure that nurses are prepared to address social determinants of health and achieve health equity" (pp. 13-14).	Keep diaries of how addressing social determinants of health with clients has affected you personally & professionally for future sharing with nursing students. Join your alma mater's nursing alumni association and share your experiences of how addressing the social determinants of health and efforts toward achieving health equity are being implemented in professional practice. Recruit culturally diverse persons to enter the nursing profession. Accept invitations to serve on focus-groups when asked by local nursing programs. Participate in developing continuing education programs addressing social determinants of health and health equity. Serve as an item writer for the NCLEX-RN.
"To enable nurses to address inequities within communities, federal agencies and other key stakeholders within and outside the nursing profession should strengthen and protect the nursing workforce during the response to such public health emergencies as the COVID-19 pandemic and natural disasters, including those related to climate change" (p. 14).	Review employer policies related to public health emergencies and natural disasters and propose any revisions. Educate future nurses about the importance of their availability to serve the public in incidences of public health emergencies and natural disasters. Have a personal plan for your family to follow should you be unavailable at home due to fulfilling professional obligations. Report any unsafe working conditions that might arise during a public health emergency or natural disaster to human resources of your employer and if they persist to the appropriate local, state, or national authority.
"The National Institutes of Health, the Centers for Medicare & Medicaid Services, the Centers for Disease Control and Prevention, the Health Resources and Services Administration, the Agency for Healthcare Research and Quality, the Administration for Children and Families, the Administration for Community Living, and private associations and foundations should convene representatives from nursing, public health, and health care to develop and support a research agenda and evidence base describing the impact of nursing interventions, including multisector collaboration, on social determinants of health, environmental health, health equity, and nurses' health and well-being" (p. 14).	As policies and procedures are developed for nurses to address the social determinants of health with each client encounter, generate ideas for future interventions and how to test them along with current procedures. When asked, volunteer to become a participant in a research study. Share ideas for future research on social determinant of health nursing interventions, effect of interprofessional approaches to them, environmental health issues, health equity and how to enhance nurses' health and well-being with graduate and doctoral students, nursing faculty and nurse researchers.

From Institute of Medicine. (2011). *The future of nursing: Leading change, advancing health* (pp. 3–7). National Academies Press with permission of NAP.

promote health and healthcare access equity while preparing the profession to meet the challenges of the future. Because some recommendations were long, comprehensive and prescriptive, selected ones in the table has been simplified to facilitate display without compromising the key concepts.

Summary and Significance to Practice

Although the future cannot be predicted with great certainty, nurses can look to history, current trends, and reports to predict how health care delivery and the profession will change. By visualizing several possible futures and identifying possible future scenarios, nurses can be prepared for the worst, planning for potential problems while working to shape a desired future for their practice and profession. The preferable future is one in which health care consumers, policy makers, and other providers value the contributions nurses make to health care. To create the preferred future, nurses must use their cognitive skills (e.g., to develop research projects demonstrating the value of professional nurses, make effective clinical decisions in practice, and find meaning in their careers); clinical skills (e.g., to effectively execute safe client care and promote client comfort and well-being); and communication skills (e.g., to collaborate with all health team members, including clients and families, promote public awareness of nursing's valuable contributions to society, shape health care policies, and recruit future nurses and sustain them once they enter the profession).

Take Note!
Competent nurses see opportunities to improve health care delivery and have the ability to work in today's increasingly complex health care environment while navigating constant change.

REAL-LIFE REFLECTIONS

Recall Jing from the beginning of the chapter. What assumptions did Jing make regarding her nursing career? How did these assumptions create a future problem for her? What advice would you give Jing to help her deal with her situation? How might Jing react to your advice? Specify reasons for each possible reaction that you identify.

From Theory to Practice

1. Make a list of the scenarios in this chapter that seem implausible. Conduct a literature search to substantiate your viewpoints on the list of identified scenarios. Develop more realistic scenarios.
2. What actions can you take to promote a preferable future for the nursing profession? Why are these actions important?

Nurse as Author

Pretend you are a time traveler visiting the year 2050. Describe the condition of the nursing profession in the United States, taking into account the quality of nursing education and health care delivery. What challenges confront the profession? How might the profession as it exists today prepare to meet the future challenges you describe?

Your Digital Classroom

Online Exploration

American Association of Colleges of Nursing: **www.aacnnursing.org**
    American Nurses Association: **www.nursingworld.org/ana**
    Institute for Alternative Futures: **http://altfutures.com/**
    Institute for the Future: **www.iftf.org/home/**
    National League for Nursing: **www.nln.org**
    Sigma Theta Tau International: **www.sigmanursing.org**
    Stem Cell Information (National Institutes of Health): **https://stemcells.nih.gov**
    The Future of Nursing Campaign for Action: **https://campaignforaction.org**

Expanding Your Understanding

1. Visit the "After the Pandemic" page of the Institute for the Future at **https://www.iftf.org/whathappensnext/**. Click on the video under the heading "What Happens Next?" to see what may occur. Just below the video, there is a heading "Four Scenarios: Explore What Might Be"; click on "download the full map here." Read all the content and critique each of the major ideas for relevance. Identify areas you could personally affect with your actions. Select

one of the areas that you feel is the most important. Why do you feel this area is the most important? Create an action plan for you to address the area selected. Bring this information to class for discussion or post this information in a course discussion forum per faculty instruction.

2. Visit the AACN website at aacnnursing.org and view resources on the nursing shortage. What can we do collectively as a profession to alleviate the nursing shortage? What can you do as an individual? What are the potential consequences of inaction in this future crisis for health care and the nursing profession?

Beyond the Book

Visit thePoint® at **www.thePoint.lww.com** for activities and information to reinforce the concepts and content covered in this chapter.

REFERENCES

Allen, B., & Dreyer, K. (2019). The role of the ACR Data Science Institute in advancing health equity in radiology. *Journal of the American College of Radiology, 16,* 644–648. doi: 10.1016/j.jacr.2018.12.038

American Association of Colleges of Nursing. (2013). *Competencies and curricular expectations for clinical nurse leader education and practice. October 2013.* Retrieved June 1, 2021, from https://www.aacnnursing.org/Portals/42/News/White-Papers/CNL-Competencies-October-2013.pdf

American Association of Colleges of Nursing. (2019). *Nursing fact sheet.* Retrieved December 19, 2020, from https://www.aacnnursing.org/Portals/42/News/Factsheets/Nursing-Shortage-Factsheet.pdf

American Association of Colleges of Nursing. (2020). *Fact sheet: Nursing shortage.* Retrieved December 19, 2020, from https://www.aacnnursing.org/Portals/42/News/Factsheets/Nursing-Shortage-Factsheet.pdf

Bezold, C. (1996). Your health in 2010: Four scenarios. *The Futurist, 30,* 35–39. Retrieved April 25, 2021, from https://www.researchgate.net/publication/279905284_Aspirational_futures/link/5ec2dcfaa6fdcc90d67fdadb/download

Canton, J. (2015). *Future smart: Managing the game-changing trends that will transform your world.* Da Capo Press.

Castellucci, M. (2020). Health systems launching care centers for COVID "long-haulers." *Modern Healthcare, 50*(39), 10. Retrieved April 24, 2021, from https://web-a-ebscohost-com.lib.rockhurst.edu/ehost/detail/detail?vid=3&sid=03f288ab-daba-4361-848f-0d3b918e1810%40sessionmgr4007&bdata=JkF1dGhUeXBlPWNvb2tpZSZzcxpcCx1cmwm-c2l0ZT11aG9zdC1saXZl#AN=146707775&db=a9h

Castrucci, B., & Auerbach, J . (2019). Meeting individual social needs falls short of addressing social determinants of health. *Health Affairs Blog.* doi: 10.1377/hblog20190115.234942

Cazzell, M., & Anderson, M. (2016). The impact of critical thinking on clinical judgment during simulation with senior nursing students. *Nursing Education Perspectives, 37*(2), 83–90. https://doi.org/2109/10.5480/15–1553

Coto, J. A., Wilder, C. R., Wynn, L., Ballard, M. C., Webel, D., & Petkunas, H. (2020). Exploring the relationship between patient falls and levels of nursing education and certification. *Journal of Nursing Administration, 50*(1), 45–51. https://doi.org/10.1097/NNA.0000000000000838

Curl, D., Smith, S., Chisholm, L. A., McGee, L. A., & Das, K. (2016). Effectiveness of integrated simulation and clinical experiences compared to traditional clinical experiences for nursing students. *Nursing Education Perspectives, 37*(2), 72–77. https://doi.org/2109/10.5480/15–1647

Emmerich, R. (2004). *The day after tomorrow [motion picture].* 20th Century Fox.

Fang, D., & Kesten, K. (2017). Retirements and succession of nursing faculty in 2016–2025. *Nursing Outlook, 65*(5), 633–642. doi: 10.1016/j.outlook.2017.03.003

Forneris, S. G., Neal, D. O., Jones, T., Keihn, M. B., Meyer, H. M., Blazovich, L. M., Holland, A. E., & Smerillo, M. (2015). Enhancing clinical reasoning through simulation debriefing: A multisite study. *Nursing Education Perspectives, 36*(5), 304–310. https://doi.org/10.5480/15–1672

Ghazal, L. V., Ma, C., Djukic, M., & Squires, A. (2020). Transition-to-U.S. practice experiences of internationally educated nurses: An integrative review. *Western Journal of Nursing Research, 42*(5), 373–392. https://doi.org/10.1177/0193945919860855

Gordon, S., Buchanan, J., & Bretherton, T. (2008). *Safety in numbers: Nurse-to-patient ratios and the future of health care.* Cornell University Press.

Harrison, J. M., Aiken, L. H., Sloane, D. M., Brooks Carthon, J. M., Merchant, R. M., Berg, R. A., & McHugh, M. D. (2019). In hospitals with more nurses who have baccalaureate degrees, better outcomes for patients after cardiac arrest. *Health Affairs, 38*(7), 1087–1094. https://doi.org/10.1377/hlthaff.2018.05064

Haverkamp, J., Chovan, J. D., Justice, S., Ball, K., Ballard, K. C., Batross, D., Becker, J. D., Butz, S., Chavez, R., Garrett, B., Hummer, K., Johnson, V., Prusinski, R., Shoemaker, J., Smith, A. L., & Zamaripa, C. (2020). Transforming nursing education through interprofessional collaborative innovation: A project story. *Computers, Informatics, Nursing, 38*(4), 176–182. https://doi.org/10.1097/CIN.0000000000000587

Henchley, N. (1978). Making sense of the future. *Alternatives, 7,* 24–26. Retrieved April 25, 2021, from https://www.jstor.org/stable/45030200?seq=1

Herzlinger, R. (2004). *Consumer-driven health care.* Jossey-Bass.

Hsia, G. S. P., Esposito, J., da Rocha, L. A., Ramos, S. L. G., & Okamoto, O. K. (2021). Clinical application of human induced pluripotent stem cell-derived organoids as an alternative to organ transplantation. *Stem Cells International,* 1–16. https://doi-org.lib.rockhurst.edu/10.1155/2021/6632160

Institute for Alternative Futures. (2012). *Primary care 2025: A scenario exploration.* Author. Retrieved June 1, 2021, from http://kresge.org/sites/default/files/IAF-PrimaryCare2025Scenarios.pdf

Institute for Alternative Futures. (September 2018). *Human progress and human services 2035: A scenario exploration.* Retrieved December 21, 2020, from http://altfutures.org/projects/human-progress-and-humanservices-2035/

Institute for the Future. (2016). *Health aware world map.* Retrieved July 3, 2016, from http://www.iftf.org/our-work/health-self/health-horizons/healthaware/

Institute for the Future. (2020). *Deck 2. Innovations for the future. After the pandemic.* Retrieved December 21, 2020, from https://www.iftf.org/fileadmin/user_upload/downloads/ourwork/IFTF_After_the_Pandemic_2_Innovationsforthe Future_PandemicToolkt_ReaderPDF.pdf

Institute of Medicine. (2000). *To err is human: Building a safer health system.* National Academies Press.

Institute of Medicine. (2001). *Crossing the quality chasm: A new health system for the 21st century.* National Academies Press.

Institute of Medicine. (2003). *Health professions education: A bridge to quality.* National Academies Press.

Institute of Medicine. (2004). *Keeping patients safe: Transforming the work environment of nurses.* National Academies Press.

Institute of Medicine. (2006). *Identifying and preventing medication errors.* National Academies Press.

Institute of Medicine. (2008). *Retooling for an aging America.* National Academies Press.

Institute of Medicine. (2011). *The future of nursing: Leading change, advancing health.* The National Academies Press.

Ironside, P., & Valiga, T. (2006). Creating a vision for the future of nursing education: Moving toward excellence through innovation. *Nursing Education Perspectives, 27*(3), 120–121. Retrieved April 25, 2021, from https://web-b-ebscohost-com.lib.rockhurst.edu/ehost/pdfviewer/pdfviewer?vid=6&sid=c451519b-8c60-46a3-9ebf-fe4af165dd73%40sessionmgr102

Johnson, T., & White, A. (2000). Six business principles for the 21st century. *Civilization, 61*(2), 57.

Kaku, M. (2011). *The physics of the future.* First Anchor Books.

Kirk, H. (2007). Towards a global nursing workforce: The "brain circulation." *Nursing Management, 12*(10), 26–30. https://doi.org/10.7748/nm2007.03.13.10.26.c4338

Koplow, S., Morris, M., Rone-Adams, S., Hettrick, H., Litwin, B., Soontupe, L. B., & Vatwani, A. (2020). Student experiences with engagement in a nursing and physical therapy interprofessional education simulation. *Internet Journal of Allied Health Sciences & Practice, 18*(1), 1–9. Retrieved April 25, 2021, from https://nsuworks.nova.edu/cgi/viewcontent.cgi?article=1842&context=ijahsp

Leduc-Pessah, H., Jensen, S. K., & Newell, C. (2019). An overview of the adverse effects of cannabis use for Canadian physicians. *Clinical & Investigative Medicine, 42*(3), E17–E34. https://doi.org/10.25011/cim.v42i3.33089

Marshall, S., & Salahi, L. (2021). *Vaccine hesitancy.* Retrieved April 25, 2021, from https://www.everydayhealth.com/coronavirus/track-the-vax-understanding-the-reasons-for-covid-vaccine-hesitancy/

Milstead, J. A., & Short, N. M. (2019). *Health policy and politics: A nurse's guide (6th ed.).* Jones & Bartlett Learning.

Minkin, B. H. (1995). *Future in sight.* Macmillan.

Mish, F. C. (Ed.). (2020). *Merriam-Webster's collegiate dictionary* (11th ed.). Merriam-Webster, Inc.

Myers, V., & Dreachslin, J. (2007). Recruitment and retention of a diverse workforce: Challenges and opportunities. *Journal of Healthcare Management, 52*(5), 290–298. https://doi.org/10.1097/00115514-200709000-00004

Naisbitt, J. (1996). *Megatrends Asia.* Simon & Schuster.

National Academies of Sciences, Engineering, and Medicine. (2021). The Future of Nursing 2020-2030: *Charting a Path to Achieve Health Equity.* The National Academies Press. https://doi.org/10.17226/25982.

National Council of State Boards of Nursing. (2019). *2017 National nursing workforce study.* Retrieved December 19, 2020, from https://www.ncsbn.org/workforce.htm

National Council of State Boards of Nursing. (2020a). *NLC member states.* Retrieved December 18, 2020, from https://www.ncsbn.org/nurse-licensure-compact.htm

National Council of State Board of Nursing. (2020b). The Interstae Commission of Nurse Licensure Comapct Administrators Final rules - Effective January 2021.

National Council of State Boards of Nursing. (2021). *NURSYS® overview.* Retrieved April 25, 2021, from https://ncsbn.org/nursys.htm

National Institute of Medicine and the National Research Council. (1999). *Chemical and biological terrorism.* National Academies Press.

O'Brien, D., Knowlton, M., & Whichello, R. (2018). Attention health care leaders: Literature review deems baccalaureate nurses improve patient outcomes. *Nursing Education Perspectives), 39*(4), E2–E6. https://doi.org/10.1097/01.NEP.000000000000030

Ogunyemi, D., Haltigin, C., Vallie, S., & Ferrari, T. M. (2020). Evolution of an obstetrics and gynecology interprofessional simulation-based education session for medical and nursing students. *Medicine, 99*(43), 1–7. https://doi.org/10.1097/MD.0000000000022562

Okun, S., & Wicks, P. (2018). DigitalMe: a journey towards personalized health and thriving. *BioMedical Engineering OnLine, 17*(1). https://doi-org.lib.rockhurst.edu/10.1186/s12938-018-0553-x

Olesen, D. E. (1996). Technology with a human touch: The top 10 innovative products for 2006. *Executive Speeches, 11*(1), 13. Retrieved June 2, 2021, from https://search-ebscohost-com.lib.rockhurst.edu/login.aspx?direct=true&AuthType=cookie,ip,url&db=a9h&AN=9609202090&site=ehost-live

Orique, S. B., & Phillips, L. J. (2018). The effectiveness of simulation on recognizing and managing clinical deterioration: Meta-analyses. *Western Journal of Nursing Research, 40*(4), 582–609. https://doi.org/10.1177/0193945917697224

Patterson, M., William-Jones, P., & Lewis, T. (2020). Consequences of the vaping epidemic on adolescents. *Nursing, 50*(7), 30–38. https://doi.org/10.1097/01.NURSE.0000668600.70206.8f

Pew Health Professions Commission. (1995). *Critical challenges: Revitalizing the health professions for the twenty-first century.* University of California, San Francisco Center for the Health Professions.

Porter-O'Grady, T., & Malloch, K. (2018). *Quantum leadership: Creating sustainable value in health care* (6th ed.). Jones & Bartlett Learning.

Press Ganey. (2020). *Capture nursing-specific measures, assess performance across domains that drive nursing excellence. Retrieved* December 22, 2020, *from* https://pressganey.com/solutions/clinical-excellence/capture-nursing-specific-measures

Rice, S. (2015). *IOM to rebrand as the National Academy of Medicine.* Retrieved June 2, 2021, from https://www.modernhealthcare.com/article/20150428/NEWS/150429895/iom-to-rebrand-as-national-academy-of-medicine

Roberts, A. W., Ogunwole, S. U., Blakeslee, L., et. al. The population 65 years and older in the United States. Retrieved June 1, 2021, from https://www.census.gov/library/publications/2018/acs/acs-38.html

Sachs, J. (2008). *Common wealth: Economics for a crowded planet.* Penguin.

Sezgin, D., & Esin, M. N. (2019). Use of the Omaha System to identify musculoskeletal problems in intensive care unit nurses: A case study. *British Journal of Nursing, 28*(5), 300–306. https://doi.org/10.12968/bjon.2019.28.5.300

Sharma, S. (2019). *AI and the death of exploration.* Retrieved April 25, 2021, from https://www.forbes.com/sites/forbestechcouncil/2019/12/12/ai-and-the-death-of-exploration/?sh=469f73d0ef39

Sherwood, G., & Barnsteiner, J. (2012). *Quality and safety in nursing.* John Wiley & Sons.

Squires, A., Ojemeni, M. T., & Jones, S. (2016). Exploring longitudinal shifts in international nurse migration to the United States between 2003 and 2013 through a random effects panel data analysis. *Human Resources for Health, 14,* 11–21. https://doi.org/10.1186/s12960-016-0118-7

Staley, D. J. (2010). *History and future: Using historical thinking to imagine the future.* Lexington Books.

Stone, W. (2021). *Mysterious ailment, mysterious relief: Vaccines help some COVID long-haulers.* Retrieved April 25, 2021, from https://www.npr.org/sections/health-shots/2021/03/31/982799452/mysterious-ailment-mysterious-relief-vaccines-help-some-covid-long-haulers

Sullivan, E. J. (Ed.). (1999). *Creating nursing's future.* Mosby.

Sullivan, E. J., & Clinton, J. F. (1999). *Achieving a multicultural nursing profession.* In E. J. Sullivan (Ed.), *Creating nursing's future: Issues, opportunities, and challenges* (pp. 317–333). Mosby.

Sullivan Commission. (2004). *Missing persons: Minorities in the health professions: A report of the Sullivan Commission on diversity in the healthcare workforce.* Retrieved April 25, 2021, from https://campaignforaction.org/resource/sullivan-report-diversity/

Toffler, A., & Toffler, H. (2006). *Revolutionary wealth: How it will be created and how it will change our lives.* Currency Doubleday.

Turrise, S. L., Thompson, C. E., & Hepler, M. (2020). Virtual simulation: Comparing .critical thinking and satisfaction in RN-BSN students. *Clinical Simulation in Nursing, 46,* 57–61. https://doi.org/10.1016/j.ecns.2020.03.004

U.S. Bureau of Health Professions, Health Resources and Services Administration. (2017). *The U.S. Nursing Workforce: Nursing workforce projections by ethnicity and race 2014–2030.* Retrieved April 25, 2020, from https://bhw.hrsa.gov/sites/default/files/bureau-health-workforce/data-research/hrsa-bhw-rn-lpn-factsheet-12-17.pdf

U.S. Census Bureau. (2020). *Age and sex composition in the United States: 2019. Detailed tables by age and sex. Table 1. Population by age and sex 2019.* Retrieved June 1, 2021, from https://www.census.gov/data/tables/2019/demo/age-and-sex/2019-age-sex-composition.html

U.S. Department of Health and Human Services, Administration on Aging. (2012). *Older Americans 2012 key indicators or well-being.* Retrieved April 25, 2021, from https://agingstats.gov/docs/PastReports/2012/OA2012.pdf

U.S. Department of Health and Human Services, Health Resources and Services Administration, National Center for Health Workforce Analysis. (2019). *Brief summary results from the 2018 National sample survey of registered nurses.* Retrieved April 25, 2021, from https://data.hrsa.gov/DataDownload/NSSRN/GeneralPUF18/2018_NSSRN_Summary_Report-508.pdf

Van Den Huevel, W. J. A. (2015). Value reorientation and intergenerational conflicts in ageing societies. *Journal of Medicine & Philosophy, 40*(2), 201–220. https://doi.org/10.1093/jmp/jhu079

Veenema, T. G. (Ed.). (2019). *Disaster nursing and emergency preparedness for chemical, biological and radiological terrorism and other hazards* (4th ed.). Springer.

Vespa, J., Medina, L., & Armstrong, D. M. (2020). *Demographic turning points for the United States: Population projections 2020 to 2060.* Retrieved April 25, 2021, from https://www.census.gov/content/dam/Census/library/publications/2020/demo/p25-1144.pdf

American Nurses Association Standards of Professional Nursing Practice*

STANDARDS OF PRACTICE

Standard 1. Assessment
The registered nurse collects pertinent data and information relative to the healthcare consumer's health or the situation.

Standard 2. Diagnosis
The registered nurse analyzes the assessment data to determine actual or potential diagnoses, problems, and issues.

Standard 3. Outcomes Identification
The registered nurse identifies expected outcomes for a plan individualized to the healthcare consumer or the situation.

Standard 4. Planning
The registered nurse develops a collaborative plan encompassing strategies to achieve expected outcomes.

Standard 5. Implementation
The registered nurse implements the identified plan.

Standard 5A. Coordination of Care
The registered nurse coordinates care delivery.

Standard 5B. Health Teaching and Health Promotion
The registered nurse employs strategies to teach and promote health and wellness.

Standard 6. Evaluation
The registered nurse evaluates progress toward attainment of goals and outcomes.

STANDARDS OF PROFESSIONAL PERFORMANCE

Standard 7. Ethics
The registered nurse integrates ethics in all aspects of practice.

Standard 8. Advocacy
The registered nurse demonstrates advocacy in all roles and settings.

Standard 9. Respectful and Equitable Practice
The registered nurse practices with cultural humility and inclusiveness.

Standard 10. Communication
The registered nurse communicates effectively in all areas of professional practice.

Standard 11. Collaboration
The registered nurse collaborates with the healthcare consumer and other key stakeholders.

Standard 12. Leadership
The registered nurse leads within the profession and practice setting.

Standard 13. Education
The registered nurse seeks knowledge and competence that reflects current nursing practice and promotes futuristic thinking.

Standard 14. Scholarly Inquiry
The registered nurse integrates scholarship, evidence, and research findings into practice.

Standard 15. Quality of Practice
The registered nurse contributes to quality nursing practice.

Standard 16. Professional Practice Evaluation
The registered nurse evaluates one's own and others' nursing practice.

Standard 17. Resource Stewardship
The registered nurse utilizes appropriate resources to plan, provide, and sustain evidence-based nursing services that are safe, effective, financially responsible, and used judiciously.

Standard 18. Environmental Health
The registered nurse practices in a manner that advances environmental safety and health.

Note: Page number followed by b, f, and t indicates text in box, figure, and table, respectively.